KU-821-444

# NUTRITION IN SPORT

## IOC MEDICAL COMMISSION

## SUB-COMMISSION ON PUBLICATIONS IN THE SPORT SCIENCES

Howard G. Knuttgen PhD (Co-ordinator)
*Boston, Massachusetts, USA*

Francesco Conconi MD
*Ferrara, Italy*

Harm Kuipers MD, PhD
*Maastricht, The Netherlands*

Per A.F.H. Renström MD, PhD
*Stockholm, Sweden*

Richard H. Strauss MD
*Los Angeles, California, USA*

# NUTRITION IN SPORT

VOLUME VII OF THE ENCYCLOPAEDIA OF SPORTS MEDICINE

AN IOC MEDICAL COMMISSION PUBLICATION

IN COLLABORATION WITH THE

INTERNATIONAL FEDERATION OF SPORTS MEDICINE

EDITED BY

## RONALD J. MAUGHAN

b

**Blackwell
Science**

LIVERPOOL
JOHN MOORES UNIVERSITY
AVRIL ROBARTS LRC
TITHEBARN STREET
LIVERFOO⸱    ⸱ R
TEL. 0151

© 2000 by
Blackwell Science Ltd
Editorial Offices:
Osney Mead, Oxford OX2 0EL
25 John Street, London, WC1N 2BL
23 Ainslie Place, Edinburgh EH3 6AJ
350 Main Street, Malden
  MA 02148 5018, USA
54 University Street, Carlton
  Victoria 3053, Australia
10, rue Casimir Delavigne
  75006 Paris, France

Other Editorial Offices:
Blackwell Wissenschafts-Verlag GmbH
Kurfürstendamm 57
10707 Berlin, Germany

Blackwell Science KK
MG Kodenmacho Building
7–10 Kodenmacho Nihombashi
Chuo-ku, Tokyo 104, Japan

The right of the Author to be
identified as the Author of this Work
has been asserted in accordance
with the Copyright, Designs and
Patents Act 1988.

All rights reserved. No part of
this publication may be reproduced,
stored in a retrieval system, or
transmitted, in any form or by any
means, electronic, mechanical,
photocopying, recording or otherwise,
except as permitted by the UK
Copyright, Designs and Patents Act
1988, without the prior permission
of the copyright owner.

First published 2000
Reprinted 2000

Set by Excel Typesetters Co., Hong Kong
Printed and bound in the United Kingdom
at the University Press, Cambridge

The Blackwell Science logo is a
trade mark of Blackwell Science Ltd,
registered at the United Kingdom
Trade Marks Registry

Part title illustrations by Grahame Baker

DISTRIBUTORS

Marston Book Services Ltd
  PO Box 269
  Abingdon, Oxon OX14 4YN
  (*Orders*: Tel: 01235 465500
      Fax: 01235 465555)

USA
  Blackwell Science, Inc.
  Commerce Place
  350 Main Street
  Malden, MA 02148 5018
  (*Orders*: Tel: 800 759 6102
          781 388 8250
    Fax: 781 388 8255)

Canada
  Login Brothers Book Company
  324 Saulteaux Crescent
  Winnipeg, Manitoba R3J 3T2
  (*Orders*: Tel: 204 837-2987)

Australia
  Blackwell Science Pty Ltd
  54 University Street
  Carlton, Victoria 3053
  (*Orders*: Tel: 3 9347 0300
      Fax: 3 9347 5001)

A catalogue record for this title
is available from the British Library

ISBN 0-632-05094-2

Library of Congress
Cataloging-in-publication Data

Nutrition in sport/edited by Ronald J. Maughan.
    p.    cm.–(Encyclopedia of sports medicine; ISSN
    v.7)
  'An IOC Medical Commission publication in collabora-
tion with the International Federation of Sports Medicine.'
  ISBN 0-632-05094-2
  1. Nutrition. 2. Energy metabolism. 3. Exercise–
Physiological aspects. 4. Athletes–Nutrition.
I. Maughan, Ronald J. II. IOC Medical Commission.
III. International Federation of Sports Medicine.
IV. Series.
QP141.N793    1999
616.3'9'0088796–dc21
                                99-12066
                                CIP

For further information on
Blackwell Science, visit our website:
www.blackwell-science.com

# Contents

## Part 2: Special Considerations

## Part 3: Practical Issues

## Part 4: Sport-specific Nutrition

# List of Contributors

K.P. AULIN MD, PhD, *Department of Medical Sciences, University of Uppsala; Institute of Sport Sciences, Dalarna University, S-79188 Falun, Sweden*

J. BANGSBO PhD, *Department of Human Physiology, August Krogh Institute, University of Copenhagen, 13 Universitetsparken, DK-2100 Copenhagen, Denmark*

A.D.G. BAXTER-JONES PhD, *Department of Child Health, University of Aberdeen, Foresterhill, Aberdeen AB25 2ZD, UK*

D. BENARDOT PhD, *Center for Sports Medicine Science and Technology, Georgia State University, Atlanta, Georgia 30303, USA*

U. BERGH PhD, *Defence Research Establishment, 17290 Stockholm, Sweden*

J.R. BERNING PhD, *Department of Biology, University of Colorado at Colorado Springs, 1420 Austin Bluffs Parkway, Colorado Springs, Colorado 80933, USA*

F. BROUNS PhD, *Department of Human Biology, Maastricht University, 6200 MD Maastricht, The Netherlands*

L.M. BURKE PhD, *Australian Institute of Sport, PO Box 176, Belconnen, Australian Capital Territory 2616, Australia*

L.M. CASTELL MSc, *University Department of Biochemistry, South Parks Road, Oxford OX1 3QU, UK*

J. CHEN MD, *Institute of Sports Medicine, Beijing Medical University, Beijing 100083, China*

P.M. CLARKSON PhD, *Department of Exercise Science, University of Massachusetts, Amherst, Massachusetts 01003, USA*

J.M. DAVIS PhD, *Department of Exercise Science, University of South Carolina, Columbia, South Carolina 29209, USA*

E.R. EICHNER MD, *Section of Hematology (EB-271), University of Oklahoma, Health Sciences Center, Oklahoma City, Oklahoma 73190, USA*

B. EKBLOM MD, *Department of Physiology and Pharmacology, Karolinska Institute, Stockholm, Sweden*

M.A. FEBBRAIO PhD, *Exercise Physiology and Metabolism Laboratory, Department of Physiology, University of Melbourne, Parkville 3052, Australia*

M. FOGELHOLM ScD, *University of Helsinki, Lahti Research and Training Centre, Saimaankatu 11, 15140 Lahti, Finland*

C. FOSTER PhD, *Department of Exercise and Sport Science, University of Wisconsin-La Crosse, La Crosse, Wisconsin 54601, USA*

K.A. GABEL PhD, RD, *School of Family and Consumer Sciences, College of Agriculture, University of Idaho, Moscow, Idaho 8344-3183, USA*

D.F. GERRARD MB, ChB, *Dunedin School of Medicine, PO Box 913, University of Otago, Dunedin, New Zealand*

M. GLEESON PhD, *School of Sport and Exercise*

Sciences, University of Birmingham, Birmingham B15 2TT, UK

A.C. GRANDJEAN Ed.D, International Center for Sports Nutrition, Center for Human Nutrition, 502 South 44th Street, Omaha, Nebraska 68105-1065, USA

P.L. GREENHAFF PhD, School of Biomedical Sciences, Queens Medical Centre, Nottingham NG7 2UH, UK

A.E. HARDMAN PhD, Department of Physical Education, Sports Science and Recreation Management, Loughborough University, Loughborough LE11 3TU, UK

M. HARGREAVES PhD, School of Health Sciences, Deakin University, Burwood 3125, Australia

J.A. HAWLEY PhD, Department of Human Biology and Movement Science, Faculty of Biomedical and Health Science, RMIT University, PO Box 71, Bundoora, Victoria 3083, Australia

J.W. HELGE PhD, Copenhagen Muscle Research Centre, August Krogh Institute, University of Copenhagen, 13 Universitetsparken, DK-2100 Copenhagen, Denmark

R.A. HOWLETT PhD, Department of Medicine, University of California-San Diego, La Jolla, California 92093-0623, USA

E. HULTMAN MD, Department of Medical Laboratory, Science and Technology, Division of Clinical Chemistry, Hiddinge University Hospital, Karolinska Institute, S-14186 Huddinge, Sweden

J.L. IVY PhD, Exercise Physiology and Metabolism Laboratory, University of Texas at Austin, Belmont Hall, Austin, Texas 78712, USA

J. JENSEN PhD, Department of Physiology, National Institute of Occupational Health, PO Box 8149 Dep, N-0033 Oslo, Norway

A.E. JEUKENDRUP PhD, School of Sport and Exercise Sciences, University of Birmingham, Birmingham B15 2TT, UK

B. KIENS PhD, Copenhagen Muscle Research Centre, August Krogh Institute, University of Copenhagen, 13 Universitetsparken, DK-2100 Copenhagen, Denmark

H.G. KNUTTGEN PhD, Department of Physical Medicine and Rehabilitation, Harvard University and Spaulding Rehabilitation Hospital, 125 Nashua Street, Boston, Massachusetts 02114-1198, USA

H. KUIPERS MD, Department of Movement Sciences, Maastricht University, PO Box 616, Maastricht 6200 MD, The Netherlands

W.A. LATZKA ScD, US Army Research Institute of Environmental Medicine, Kansas Street, Natick, Massachusetts 01760, USA

B. LEIGHTON PhD, Zeneca Pharmaceuticals, Alderley Park, Macclesfield SK10 4TG, UK

P.W.R. LEMON PhD, 3M Centre, University of Western Ontario, London, Ontario N6A 3K7, Canada

B.C. LEUTHOLTZ PhD, Department of Exercise Science, Physical Education and Recreation, Old Dominion University, Norfolk, Virginia 23529-0196, USA

L.R. McNAUGHTON PhD, Department of Life Science, Kingston University, Penrhyn Road, Kingston-upon-Thames, Surrey KT1 2EE, UK

M.M. MANORE PhD, Food and Nutrition Laboratory, Department of Family Resources, Arizona State University, Tempe, Arizona 85287-2502, USA

R.J. MAUGHAN PhD, Department of Biochemical Sciences, University Medical School, Foresterhill, Aberdeen AB25 2ZD, UK

S.J. MONTAIN PhD, US Army Research Institute of Environmental Medicine, Kansas Street, Natick, Massachusetts 01760, USA

H.J. MONTOYE PhD, Department of Kinesiology, College of Education, Michigan State University, East Lansig, Michigan 48824-1049, USA

R. MURRAY PhD, Exercise Physiology Laboratory,

*Quaker Oats Company, 617 West Main Street, Barrington, Illinois 60010, USA*

E.R. NADEL PhD, *John B. Pierce Foundation Laboratory, Yale University School of Medicine, 290 Congress Avenue, New Haven, Connecticut 06519, USA (Dr E.R. Nadel unfortunately passed away during publication of this volume)*

E.A. NEWSHOLME MA, PhD, DSc, *University Department of Biochemistry, South Parks Road, Oxford OX1 3QU, UK*

C.W. NICHOLAS PhD, *Department of Physical Education and Sports Science, University of Loughborough, Loughborough, Leicestershire LE11 3TU, UK*

T.D. NOAKES MB, ChB, *Sports Science Institute of South Africa, Newlands, 7800 South Africa*

L. PACKER PhD, *Department of Molecular and Cell Biology, University of California at Berkeley, 251 Life Science Addition, Berkeley, California 94720-3200, USA*

N.J. REHRER PhD, *School of Physical Education, PO Box 56, Otago University, Dunedin, New Zealand*

V.A. ROGOZKIN PhD, *Research Institute of Physical Culture, Pr Dinamo 2, St Petersburg 197110, Russia*

S. ROY PhD, *Department of Molecular and Cell Biology, University of California at Berkeley, 251 Life Science Addition, Berkeley, California 94720-3200, USA*

J.S. RUUD MS, RD, *Center for Human Nutrition, 502 South 44th Street, Omaha, Nebraska 68105-1065, USA*

M.N. SAWKA PhD, *US Army Research Institute of Environmental Medicine, Kansas Street, Natick, Massachusetts 10760, USA*

E.-J. SCHABORT MSc, *Sports Science Institute of South Africa, Newlands, 7800 South Africa*

C.K. SEN PhD, *Department of Molecular and Cell Biology, University of California at Berkeley, 251 Life Science Addition, Berkeley, California 94720-3200, USA*

R.L. SHARP PhD, *Department of Health and Human Performance, Iowa State University, Ames, Iowa 50011-1160, USA*

S.M. SHIRREFFS PhD, *Department of Biomedical Sciences, University Medical School, Foresterhill, Aberdeen AB25 2ZD, UK*

A.C. SNYDER PhD, *Department of Human Kinetics, University of Wisconsin-Milwaukee, PO Box 413, Milwaukee, Wisconsin 53201, USA*

L.L. SPRIET PhD, *Department of Human Biology and Nutritional Sciences, University of Guelph, Guelph, Ontario N1G 2W1, Canada*

J. SUNDGOT-BORGEN PhD, *Department of Biology and Sports Medicine, Norwegian University of Sport and Physical Education, Oslo, Norway*

V.B. UNNITHAN PhD, *Department of Exercise and Sport Science, University of San Francisco, 2130 Fulton Street, San Francisco, California 94117-1080, USA*

A.J.M. WAGENMAKERS PhD, *Department of Human Biology, Maastricht University, PO Box 616, 6200 MD Maastricht, The Netherlands*

M.H. WILLIAMS PhD, *Human Performance Laboratory, Old Dominion University, Norfolk, Virginia 23529-0196, USA*

J.H. WILMORE PhD, *Department of Health and Kinesiology, Texas A&M University, 158 Read Building, College Station, Texas 77843-2443, USA*

# Forewords

On behalf of the International Olympic Committee, I should like to welcome Volume VII of the Encyclopaedia of Sports Medicine series. This new volume addresses nutrition in sport. Emphasis is given to the role of proper nutrition in enhancing good health, well being and the performance capacity of men and women athletes.

I should like to thank all those involved in the preparation of this volume whose work is highly respected and appreciated by the whole Olympic Family.

JUAN ANTONIO SAMARANCH
Marqués de Samaranch


In planning the year-round conditioning programme and making the final preparations for competition, each athlete must carefully consider food intake in order to ensure that all tissues and body systems have available the essential elements for the provision of energy and proper function. Proper nutrition is also essential for maintenance of a body mass and composition appropriate to each sport event.

The new volume, *Nutrition in Sport*, provides a wealth of information on the relationship of the metabolism of carbohydrates, fats and proteins as well as the important involvement of vitamins and minerals to success in sports performance. Special consideration is given to optimal performance in specific sports events. Emphasis is given to the role of proper nutrition in enhancing good health, well being and the performance capacity of men and women athletes. The editor, Professor Ronald J. Maughan, has recruited over 60 of the world's leading nutritionists and physiologists to participate in this project. On behalf of the International Olympic Committee and its Medical Commission I should like to extend our sincere appreciation to the members of our Subcommission on Publications in the Sport Sciences and to Blackwell Science, who have made the publication of this book possible.

PRINCE ALEXANDRE DE MERODE
Chairman, IOC Medical Commission

# Preface

At an international Consensus Conference held in 1991 at the offices of the International Olympic Committee in Lausanne, a small group of experts conducted a comprehensive review of the available information and concluded that 'Diet significantly influences athletic performance'. This statement is unequivocal: what we eat and drink, how much we consume and when it is consumed can all have positive or negative effects on performance in training and in competition. For the athlete striving to succeed at the highest level and training to the limits of what can be tolerated, this offers an avenue that cannot be ignored. Choosing the right foods will not make the mediocre performer into a world beater, but a poor choice of diet will certainly prevent all athletes from realizing their full potential. This may not be a major concern for the recreational athlete or for the 'weekend warrior' who train and compete for enjoyment and for the health benefits that exercise participation confers. For the committed athlete, however, there seems little point in taking other aspects of performance seriously and neglecting diet.

In spite of the importance of diet for health as well as for athletic performance, there are many popular misconceptions, and this reflects in part the limited availability of reliable information. Until recently, there were few books on sports nutrition available to the coach and athlete or to the scientist with an interest in this area, but several have been published in the last decade. Few of these, however, have encompassed the whole breadth of the subject from the basic science to the practical issues that affect training and competition. In keeping with the format of the previous volumes in this series and with the concept that is implied by the term encyclopaedia, this volume has attempted to do that. It brings together sports nutrition—the underlying science that allows identification of nutritional goals—and sports dietetics—the practical application of that science on an individual basis to define the eating strategies that will allow athletes to achieve those goals. This aim has been made possible by the enthusiastic participation in the preparation of this book by leading experts, including both scientists and practitioners, from around the world who have contributed to the 51 chapters of this book. In many cases, individual chapters are the result of a collaborative effort involving authors from more than one country, bringing a true international perspective. This reflects the international dimension of science and the sense of shared purpose among those who work in this field. Although there is an element of competition in science, it is not parochial and the knowledge it generates is available to all. The depth and breadth of the expertise of these authors makes that knowledge available and serves to emphasize those areas where there is a broad consensus of opinion, and to pinpoint areas of uncertainty where more information is required.

The contents of this book are divided into four sections, each emphasizing different aspects of the art and science of sports nutrition. The first, and largest, section covers the basic science that underpins the practice of sports nutrition; these chapters provide definitive information in the form of comprehensive reviews of specific topics. In the second section, a variety of special situations are considered: this begins the move from the underlying science to practical application by bringing together information from different sources to focus on specific issues that affect performance. The second section of the book deals with the nutritional needs of special populations and the strategies that must be developed to meet those needs. The third section focuses on some of the practical issues encountered in working with élite-level athletes. The final section of the book provides a detailed coverage of the specific issues relating to preparing for, and competing in, a wide range of different sports: this section highlights the diversity of sport and reminds the reader that the generalizations that are inevitably made in the pre-ceding sections must be applied with caution when dealing with individuals competing in sports that place very different demands on participants.

The sheer size of this book reflects the breadth and depth of the field of sports nutrition. It is a testimony to the expertise of the authors that the information this volume contains is presented in a way that will be useful to those engaged in research and teaching as well as being accessible to those who can benefit most from its practical application. These include exercise scientists and sports physicians, nutritionists and dietitians. Some background knowledge is necessary for a full appreciation of the contents, but the informed and educated coach and athlete should find much of interest.

Ron Maughan
1999

# PART 1

## NUTRITION AND EXERCISE

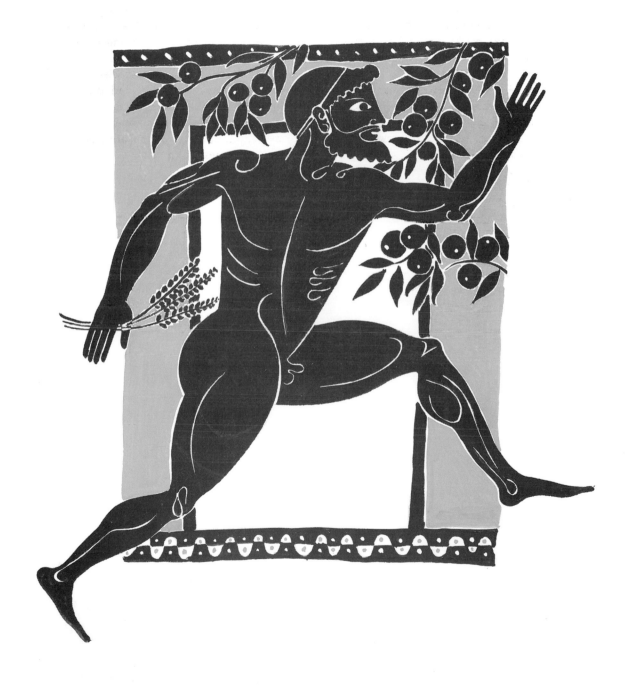

# Chapter 1

# Basic Exercise Physiology

HOWARD G. KNUTTGEN

## Introduction

The performance of sport, as with all physical exercise, is dependent upon the coordinated activation of the athlete's skeletal muscles. The muscles constitute the sources of the forces and power required for skilled movement. Unfortunately, the description and quantification of exercise is frequently made awkward, if not difficult, by a variety of terms, some of which are confusing or inaccurate. Through the years, terms have been regularly misused and units of measurement inappropriately applied.

## Exercise

The term *exercise*, itself, has been defined in different ways by different sources in the literature. For the *Encyclopaedia of Sports Medicine* series of publications, the definition has been accepted as 'any and all activity involving generation of force by activated skeletal muscle' (Komi 1992). This would include activities of daily living, activities of labour, activities for physical conditioning and physical recreation, as well as participation in sport competition. In the *Encyclopaedia of Sports Medicine* series, a sport will be considered as any organized activity that involves exercise, rules governing the event and the element of competition.

To bring about movement of the body parts and coordinate the skills of a sport, the central nervous system activates the striated, voluntary muscle cells which are the principal constituents of the various structures called skeletal muscles. The response of muscle cells to neural stimulation is to produce force.

In order to develop force, skeletal muscle cells are activated by electrochemical impulses arriving via efferent neurones, the cell bodies of which are located in the anterior horn of the gray matter of the spinal cord. When the threshold of excitation of the muscle cells of a motor unit has been attained, electrochemical events within each muscle cell (fibre) result in the cylindrical fibre generating force along its longitudinal axis in order to draw the ends of the cylinder towards its midsection. In this way, the activated fibres develop force between the attachments of the muscle in which they are contained. It has been proposed that this process be referred to as a muscle 'action' (Cavanagh 1988) rather than 'contraction' due to the fact that any activated individual fibre and, indeed, an entire muscle may: (i) shorten the distance along its longitudinal axis, (ii) be held at the same length by an opposing force, or (iii) be forcibly stretched in length by an opposing force. The term *action* has the advantage of being independent of a change in length or of direction. By definition, *contraction* means shortening only.

The terminology employed to identify the three actions thus deserves discussion and explanation. The interaction of muscle force development and the external forces will result in actions that produce static exercise (no movement about the related joints) or in dynamic exercise (resulting in a change in joint angles). Static exercise of

**Table 1.1** Classification of exercise and muscle action types.

| Exercise | Muscle action | Muscle length |
|----------|---------------|---------------|
| Dynamic | Concentric | Decreases |
| Dynamic | Eccentric | Increases |
| Static | Isometric | No change |

activated muscle is traditionally referred to as *isometric*. Force is developed but, as there is no movement, no work is performed. All other muscle actions involve movement and are termed *dynamic*. The term *concentric* is traditionally used to identify a shortening action and the term *eccentric* is used to identify a lengthening action, although the origin of these terms is obscure (Table 1.1) (Knuttgen & Kraemer 1987).

## The International System

Some years ago, the world of science adopted an International System of Measurement (Bureau International des Poids et Mésures 1977; *Le Système International*, abbreviated as SI) to quantify all physical entities and processes. The unit of force in the SI is the newton (N). One newton is quantified as the force which imparts to a mass of 1 kilogram an acceleration of 1 metre per second per second. To develop force, a muscle cell requires energy, and the SI unit for energy is the joule (J).

When force is expressed through a displacement (i.e. movement of body parts is occurring), work is measured as force (N) multiplied by the distance (m) of the displacement, and work can be calculated as force×distance: $1\,N \times 1\,m = 1\,J$. During movement, the performance of work involves conversion of one form of energy (J) to another. The SI unit for energy is the same unit used to quantify work. One joule is the energy of 1 newton acting through a distance of 1 metre.

Any energy used by the muscle for force development that does not result in work becomes heat, the SI unit for heat also being the joule. Obviously, direct relationships exist among energy, work and heat and they are quantified

with the same unit, the joule. Throughout this publication, the term *energy* will most often refer to metabolic energy.

When *time* [SI unit, the second (s)] becomes a factor in quantifying energy release, the performance of work or the generation of heat, then the rate of energy release, work performance or heat generation is presented as power, the SI unit for which is the watt (W) ($1\,J \times 1\,s^{-1} = 1\,W$). In exercise in which 150 W of external power is produced at a metabolic cost of 750 W, then the rate of heat production is 600 W.

Attention should be called at this point to the fact that, when describing exercise and sport, physiologists and nutritionists can be interested in the available energy content that can be metabolized from the food ingested (J), the total stored energy available for the muscle cells (J), the total energy utilized during a conditioning session or sports performance (J), or the rate at which muscle cells are called upon to produce power (W).

### The joule and the calorie

As described above, the joule is the SI unit used to quantify energy, work and heat. This provides a simple and efficient basis for describing the relationship among nutrition, exercise performance, body heat generation and heat dissipation, both in terms of total amounts (in joules) or as power (in watts). Unfortunately, the calorie and its multiple, the kilocalorie (kcal), have been utilized for so long in nutritional circles that a change to the description of the energy content of foods in joules is being implemented very slowly. Instead of utilizing the convenient relationships among newtons, joules, seconds and watts, conversion factors need to be employed. For example, $1\,cal = 4.186\,J$ and $1\,kcal = 4.186\,kJ$.

When a mechanically braked cycle ergometer is used for an exercise bout, one method of obtaining the desired power production would be to have the subject cycle at a pace that would produce a 'velocity' of the flywheel rim of $5\,m \cdot s^{-1}$ and provide an opposing force (sometimes termed 'resistance') of 60 N. The simplest way of quantifying exercise is with SI units. The bout of exercise can be described as follows:

Power developed on the ergometer: 300 W

Duration of exercise: 600 s (10 min)

Metabolic power (derived from oxygen uptake): 1500 W

Total metabolic energy utilized
= 1500 W × 600 s = 900 000 J = 900 kJ

Mechanical efficiency
= 300 W / 1500 W × 100 = 20%

If work is calculated by using a 'kilogram of force' (an improper unit of measurement!), a kilogram-metre can be utilized as an unsanctioned unit to quantify work. Conversion factors would be utilized to convert kilogram-metres per unit of time into the correct unit for power, the watt. If the calorie is used to quantify metabolic energy, conversion factors must be utilized to obtain a measurement of metabolic power that can be compared to the power transferred to the cycle ergometer. It is far easier to utilize SI units throughout all research activity and scientific writing: the newton, the metre, the second, the joule and the watt. (It is important to call attention to the fact that a kilogram-metre [kg-m] in the SI is actually the correct unit of measurement for *torque*.)

There are an infinite number of configurations of force and velocity (determined by cadence on the ergometer) that can produce the desired external power produced and therefore metabolic power desired.

In this volume, the editorial decision was made to acknowledge the continued and extensive use of the kilocalorie (kcal) in much of the scientific literature for the quantification of the energy content of foods and therefore to permit the use of this unit of measurement in the various chapters where considered expedient.

## Energy for muscle activity

The mechanical and biochemical events associated with muscle cell force development are described in detail in Chapter 2. However, it is worth making the following general comments and observations as related to nutrition for sport.

The immediate source of energy for muscle force and power production is adenosine triphosphate (ATP). ATP is the final biochemical carrier of energy to the myofilaments for the generation of force. The breakdown of phosphocreatine (PCr) serves to reconstitute ATP when other sources contribute little or no energy. Each muscle cell then becomes dependent on fat (fatty acids), carbohydrate (glucose and glycogen) and, to a very limited extent, protein (amino acids) as the sources of energy to resynthesize ATP and PCr during exercise. All persons concerned with the nutrition of the athlete must consider the nutritional demands of the long-term conditioning programme, the preparation for competition and the competitive event itself, when planning individual meals as well as the weekly and monthly dietary programmes.

It is generally accepted that the muscle cells obtain all the energy needed for short-term sport performance of a few seconds (as in the throwing and jumping events of track and field, weight-lifting and springboard and platform diving) from ATP and PCr (Fig. 1.1). These compounds are then resynthesized during recovery. When a sport performance lasts approximately 10 s (e.g. the 100-m run), other energy sources, including especially anaerobic glycolysis (resulting in lactic acid formation in the muscle), must also contribute to the resynthesis of ATP. The lower the intensity and the longer the event, the better able is aerobic glycolysis to contribute energy. It is also assumed that, during events that are still considered 'sprints' but that last longer than a few seconds, aerobic metabolism begins to make a contribution to ATP resynthesis.

As the duration of the exercise period increases still further, the energy from the oxidation of a combination of fat and carbohydrate becomes a significant source of energy. If exercise lasts 15 min or longer, such intensities demand a steady-state of aerobic metabolism (i.e. lower than maximum aerobic metabolism) except for any final effort that calls forth all the power the

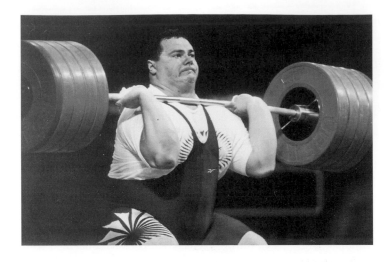

**Fig. 1.1** Olympic weightlifting is an example of a sport in which the competitive performance is so short that all of the energy for the lift is provided by the high-energy phosphates, ATP and PCr. Photo © Allsport.

athlete can generate. The final burst of power (or 'kick') results from a combination of high utilization of both anaerobic glycolysis and aerobic power. In the range of events that last between 30 s and 12 min, a combination of anaerobic glycolysis and oxidative metabolism provides most of the energy necessary to resynthesize ATP and permit the athlete to continue. The lower the demand for power, the better the oxidative metabolism can provide the energy for ATP resynthesis. Anaerobic glycolysis involves only carbohydrate and, at these high intensities, even aerobic metabolism draws upon carbohydrate in preference to fat.

An athlete who performs to exhaustion in approximately 3–12 min challenges the cardiorespiratory and metabolic mechanisms so that aerobic metabolism eventually attains its highest level. When this occurs, the oxygen uptake is identified as either 'maximum oxygen uptake' ($\dot{V}o_{2max}$) or 'maximum aerobic power'.

It is not uncommon to read and hear the term 'maximum exercise' used to refer to intensities that result in maximum oxygen uptake. The term is completely misleading, given the fact that the athlete can produce power anaerobically for short periods of time that is four to five times as great as that which can be developed utilizing maximum aerobic power.

Fat is stored to a limited extent inside the muscle cells but can be mobilized during exercise from depots around the body for transport by the circulatory system to active muscle cells. Carbohydrate is stored inside the muscle cells as glycogen but can also be mobilized as glucose from glycogen stored in the liver.

## Power, energy and endurance

The information presented in the three panels of Fig. 1.2 provides vivid examples of the relationships among human metabolic power production, the sources of energy and the ability to endure at specific exercise intensities. In panel A, the relationship between endurance (or time to exhaustion) is plotted vs. metabolic power. For the sample athlete, power production of about 5000 W can be assumed to come solely from energy stored in skeletal muscle ATP and PCr.

In the range of 2000–4000 W, anaerobic glycolysis assumes major responsibility for the provision of energy. This results in the production of large amounts of lactic acid and lowered pH in the sarcoplasm, which are believed to eventually hinder force and power development by the muscle fibres. Lactic acid values in the blood rise commensurate with muscle concentrations.

For the athlete in the example, oxidative metabolism begins to make a major contribution of energy for ATP and PCr resynthesis once the

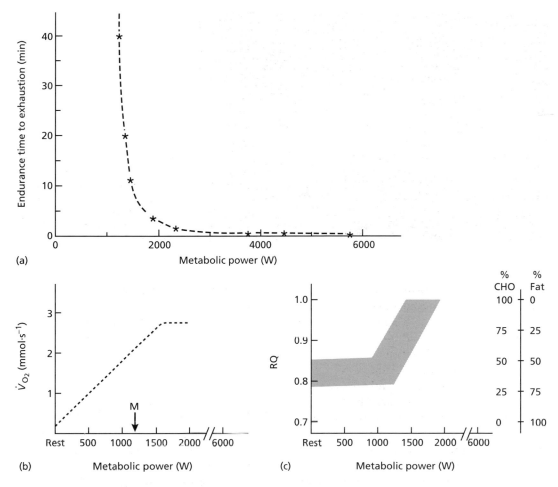

**Fig. 1.2** The relationships of (a) endurance time, (b) oxygen uptake in steady state, and (c) respiratory quotient (RQ) and percentage substrate utilization to human metabolic power production. Values presented for power are representative for an 80-kg athlete.

power output falls to approximately 2000 W. It is at power productions of 1500–1800 W that the maximum oxygen uptake ($\dot{V}o_{2max.}$ of 2.7 mmol·s$^{-1}$) is elicited for this athlete during the final stage of an exercise bout. At 1500 W, the athlete could sustain exercise for approximately 8 min but at 1800 W, for less than 5 min.

Below 1500 W (Fig. 1.2b), the athlete is able to sustain exercise for extended periods with completely or nearly completely aerobic metabolism, utilizing fat and carbohydrate to resynthesize ATP and PCr. The letter 'M' is placed on the

abscissa to indicate the power production corresponding to about 75–80% $\dot{V}o_{2max.}$ that the athlete could sustain for a marathon (42.2 km). At any higher level, the athlete would enlist anaerobic glycolysis, accumulate lactate and lower pH values in the skeletal muscle cells, and be forced, eventually, to reduce power or stop.

Note the relatively narrow range of power production that can be produced completely aerobically by comparing Fig. 1.2b with Fig. 1.2a. Marathon pace in this example would constitute approximately 24% of maximum power produc-

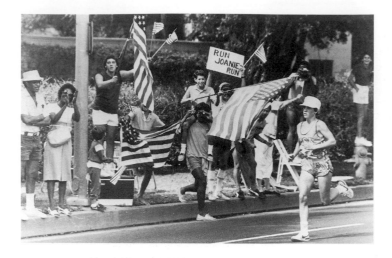

**Fig. 1.3** Marathon pace for a runner requires approximately 75–80% of maximal aerobic power and approximately 24% of the anaerobic power the same muscles could produce for a strength exercise. Photo © NOPP / Larry Bessel.

tion and the range for maximum aerobic power would constitute approximately 30% of maximum power production (Fig. 1.3).

In Fig. 1.2c, the relationship of respiratory quotient (RQ) as determined from steady-state respiratory exchange ratio (RER) to metabolic power is presented. RER, which compares oxygen uptake to carbon dioxide removal in the lungs, attains steady state at lower levels of power production (in this example, less than 1500 W). The values for RQ vs. power production are modified from Åstrand and Rodahl (1986). A range is presented to accommodate different values that might be obtained during different days as a result of variations in the athlete's diet. Utilizing both the left-side and the right-side ordinates, the observed RQs indicate a high utilization of carbohydrate from approximately 75% of maximum aerobic power and upwards. The higher the intensity, the greater is the contribution of carbohydrate.

An athlete maintaining a diet high in carbohydrate will maintain a higher RQ at all levels of aerobic exercise, whereas the RQ of an athlete with a low intake of carbohydrate will remain remarkably lower. During long-lasting events and training bouts, the RQ will become lower at any chosen intensity the longer the exercise lasts, as it is related to increasing free fatty acid availability and falling levels of glycogen in the active muscles. RQ can also be affected by the ingestion of a substance such as caffeine which results in an enhanced utilization of fatty acids for the energy demands of exercise.

**Skeletal muscle**

A skeletal muscle is made up predominantly of extrafusal skeletal muscle fibres, long cylindrical cells which run the length of the muscle, be it short or long (e.g. 1–300 mm). Intrafusal fibres are the small skeletal muscle cells found in the muscle spindles which assist in controlling the body's coordinated movement. The muscle also includes connective tissue which provides some organization to the muscle's internal structure (white connective tissue) and elasticity (yellow connective tissue). Arteries, veins and capillaries made up of smooth muscle, connective tissue and epithelial cells are found throughout each muscle, serving as the combination delivery/removal system. Afferent and efferent neurones connect each muscle to the central nervous system to provide the muscle with motor control and send sensory information to the central nervous system. Fat is found within and between muscle cells in quantities that become reflected in the person's total body composition and percentage body fat. Therefore, each muscle is made up of cells representing the four basic tissue groups: muscle, connective, nervous and epithelial.

Extrafusal fibres can be further divided among groups based upon the interrelated twitch characteristics and metabolic capabilities. Fibres of a particular motor unit (defined as a motor neurone together with the extrafusal fibres it innervates) that attain peak force development relatively slowly are routinely termed 'slow twitch' or type I fibres. Fibres that attain peak force relatively more rapidly are termed 'fast twitch' or type II fibres and further subdivided into type IIa, type IIab and type IIb groups, as based on myosin ATPase staining (Fig. 1.4).

Type I fibres are characterized by high mitochondrial density, high myoglobin content, high aerobic metabolism and modest glycolytic capacity. Early anatomists described muscles with what we now identify as high type I fibre population as 'red muscle' because of the darker colour caused by the high myoglobin content. Type II fibres have high glycolytic capability, low mitochondrial density and low capacity for aerobic metabolism. Types IIa, IIab and IIb fibres are low in myoglobin content, the reason for their being identified many decades ago as white muscle fibres.

The total number of muscle fibres in a particular muscle and the proportion identified as type I and type II appear to be genetically dominated, with small changes occurring through conditioning, injury, ageing, etc. It should also be mentioned that, while type II motor units are termed fast twitch and type I motor units are termed slow twitch, the comparison is on relative terms and all extrafusal muscle fibres attain peak force and shorten extremely fast. The differences among them are great, however, and the shortening velocity is generally considered to be 4–10 times faster for the type II fibres than for type I fibres.

The maximum force that can be developed by an activated muscle is directly related to the physiological cross-section of the muscle, a term that describes the collective cross-sectional area of the muscle cells, excluding the connective tissue (including fat), nervous tissue and blood vessels. The larger the physiological cross-section of muscle, the greater is the muscle's ability to generate peak force (strength). Considerable evidence exists to confirm the importance of the type II fibre population of a muscle to its ability to develop high force and power.

A high type I fibre population and the accompanying increased capillarization to supply oxygen has been shown to be important for sustained, rhythmic exercise which depends on

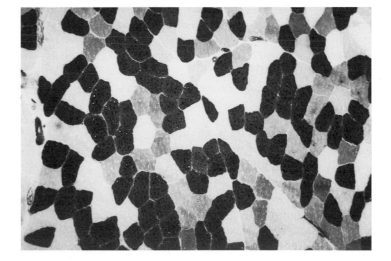

**Fig. 1.4** Cross-section of human muscle showing the mosaic pattern of fibres: darkest stain = type I; lightest stain = type IIa; medium light stain = type IIab; medium dark stain = type IIb. Photo courtesy of William J. Kraemer.

aerobic metabolism. For example, a marathon runner can utilize over 12 000 repeated muscle actions of each leg in completing the 42.2-km course.

The characteristics and capabilities of the muscle fibres can be substantially modified by specific training programmes. Athletes engaging in sports which involve wide ranges of power and continuously varying amounts of aerobic and anaerobic metabolism must utilize a programme of conditioning that raises both the anaerobic and aerobic capabilities of the three fibre types. Examples of such sports are soccer, basketball and tennis.

## Physiological support systems

While muscle cells may obtain energy for force and power production from both anaerobic sources (the breakdown of ATP and PCr; anaerobic glycolysis) and aerobic sources (aerobic glycolysis and β-oxidation of fatty acids, both leading to the provision of electrons to the electron transport system in the mitochondria), the entire human organism and all of its component cells are fundamentally aerobic. Exercise performed at low enough intensities can be performed entirely with energy from aerobic metabolism. The provision of significant amounts of energy for muscular activity by the anaerobic mechanisms, however, is limited in amount and therefore in time. Most importantly, the return to the pre-exercise or resting state following any amount of anaerobic energy release is accomplished exclusively by aerobic metabolism.

Therefore, the essential features in the provision of oxygen for metabolism during aerobic exercise and recovery following anaerobic exercise become pulmonary ventilation (air movement into and out of the lungs), external respiration (exchange of $O_2$ and $CO_2$ between alveoli and pulmonary capillary blood), blood circulation and internal respiration (exchange of $O_2$ and $CO_2$ between systemic capillary blood and interstitial fluid). The essential elements as regards these processes are cardiac output, blood volume, blood composition and skeletal muscle capillarization.

### Pulmonary ventilation and external respiration

Movement of air into and out of the lungs is accomplished by the diaphragm and various muscles of the neck and trunk. Pulmonary ventilation is usually accomplished as a subconscious activity under the influence of chemical stimuli provided by the systemic arterial blood to a nervous centre in the brain stem. While this centre serves the sole function of controlling the minute volume of pulmonary ventilation (by interaction of frequency of ventilation and magnitude of tidal volume), it is interesting to note that it is identified anatomically and physiologically as the 'respiratory centre.'

For continuous aerobic activity that would involve attainment of a 'steady state' of oxygen uptake (and carbon dioxide elimination) via the lungs, pulmonary ventilation corresponds directly to oxygen uptake by an approximate 20:1 ratio (litres per minute are used in the presentation of both variables). Starting at rest, an 80-kg athlete would expect the values presented in Table 1.2 for oxygen uptake and pulmonary ventilation.

The increase in the ratio for the highest level of activity reflects the increased acidity of the blood due to the production in the muscle and appear-

**Table 1.2** Representative data for steady-state oxygen uptake and ventilatory minute volume at rest and during various intensities of constant-intensity exercise (for an 80-kg athlete). The maximum aerobic power is $4.5 \, l \cdot min^{-1}$.

|  | $\dot{V}_{O_2}$ ($l \cdot min^{-1}$) | $\dot{V}_E$ ($l \cdot min^{-1}$) |
|---|---|---|
| Rest | 0.25 | 5 |
| -- | 1.00 | 20 |
| -- | 2.00 | 40 |
| -- | 3.00 | 60 |
| Intense aerobic exercise | 3.50 | 70 |
| Intense aerobic exercise with anaerobic contribution | 4.00 | 100 |

ance in the blood of lactic acid, as related to the anaerobic metabolism.

For the athlete performing aerobic exercise under most conditions, it is considered that the individual's capacity for ventilation is adequate to provide $O_2$ from the atmosphere to the alveoli and to carry $CO_2$ from the alveoli to the atmosphere. In elite endurance athletes who are highly conditioned for aerobic metabolism and are performing near their capacities for aerobic power production, it can be frequently observed that blood leaving the lungs via the pulmonary veins is not as saturated with oxygen as it is under the conditions of rest and submaximal aerobic exercise. It can thus be concluded that, under the very special conditions where a very highly conditioned athlete is performing high-intensity aerobic exercise, pulmonary ventilation serves as a limiting factor for external respiration and therefore oxygen uptake.

**Circulation**

For the delivery of oxygen, the removal of carbon dioxide and the transport of anabolites and catabolites to and from the body cells, the organism is dependent upon the circulation of the blood. With regard to the aerobic metabolism related to exercise and recovery, the most important factors are: the oxygen-carrying capacity of the blood, the blood volume available, the ability of the heart to pump blood (cardiac output) and the capillarization of the skeletal muscles.

The term *cardiac output* can actually refer to the amount of blood ejected through the aorta or the pulmonary arteries per minute ('minute volume' or $\dot{Q}$) or the amount of blood ejected per systole ('stroke volume' or SV). The relationship between minute volume and stroke volume includes the contraction frequency of the heart $(f_H)$ as follows: $\dot{Q} = f_H \cdot SV$.

The relationship of these variables with oxygen uptake includes the unloading factor of oxygen in the tissues as determined from the content of oxygen in systemic arterial blood $(C_aO_2)$ and the content in systemic mixed venous blood $(C_vO_2)$. It is:

$$\dot{V}O_2 = f_H \cdot SV \cdot a\text{-}vO_2\text{diff.}$$

Representative values for an 80-kg athlete are presented in Table 1.3. It can be observed that the relationship between aerobic power (oxygen uptake) and heart rate is essentially rectilinear. Stroke volume increases from a resting value of 104 ml to near maximum values even during low-intensity aerobic exercise. The increase in cardiac minute volume as higher levels of oxygen uptake are attained is accounted for by the increase in heart rate.

Meanwhile, the arteriovenous oxygen difference continues to increase due solely to the lowered concentration of oxygen in systemic mixed venous blood leaving the active tissues. The arterial concentration remains constant at a value of approximately $20\,ml \cdot l^{-1}$ blood, indicating that pulmonary capillary blood becomes

**Table 1.3** Representative data for steady-state oxygen uptake and circulatory variables at rest and during various intensities of constant-intensity exercise (for an 80-kg athlete). The maximum aerobic power for the athlete is $4.5\,l \cdot min^{-1}$ and maximum $f_H$ is 195.

| | $\dot{V}O_2$ (l·min⁻¹) | $\dot{Q}$ (l·min⁻¹) | $f_H$ (beats·min⁻¹) | SV (ml) | $a\text{-}vO_2$diff. (ml $O_2$·l⁻¹) |
|---|---|---|---|---|---|
| Rest | 0.25 | 6.4 | 60 | 104 | 40 |
| -- | 1.00 | 12.3 | 100 | 123 | 81 |
| -- | 2.00 | 14.8 | 120 | 123 | 136 |
| -- | 3.00 | 17.2 | 140 | 123 | 174 |
| Intense aerobic exercise | 3.50 | 19.7 | 160 | 123 | 178 |
| Intense aerobic exercise with anaerobic contribution | 4.00 | 22.1 | 180 | 123 | 180 |

completely saturated with $O_2$ obtained from the alveoli. It should be noted that, at the highest levels of oxygen uptake, highly trained endurance athletes (e.g. distance runners and cross-country skiers) show a lowered oxygen saturation in arterial blood. This is taken to indicate that the blood flow through the lungs during such intense aerobic exercise for these athletes exceeds the capacity of the ventilatory system to provide oxygen to the lungs.

As will be discussed, maximum aerobic power ($\dot{V}o_{2max.}$) can be increased mainly by increasing the stroke volume capability of the heart, which increases the minute volume capability. Maximum heart rate does not increase with aerobic conditioning but, actually, it either remains the same or decreases.

The $\dot{V}o_{2max.}$ of $4.5 \, l \cdot min^{-1}$ corresponds to a metabolic power production of 1500 W. As the athlete in the example is capable of power production for short periods (e.g. 1–20 s) in the range of 3000–6000 W, the question could be raised as to what values for the circulatory variables would be expected during such exercise performance. The answer is that these values, if measured, would be irrelevant. The athlete would be performing in the range of power production where oxidative (aerobic) metabolism contributes little or no energy and the muscles will rely on ATP, PCr and anaerobic glycolysis.

## Adaptations to conditioning

The adaptations of the human organism to programmes of exercise conditioning are highly specific to the exercise programme (i.e. the stimulus) provided. Adaptations to resistance training for strength, to anaerobic training (as in sprinting) and to endurance (aerobic) training are very different and, if used inappropriately, can actually serve to be counterproductive.

### Aerobic conditioning

For athletes engaged in events lasting approximately 3 min or longer, aerobic conditioning is a crucial factor in preparing for competition (Fig. 1.5). For events lasting between 1 and 3 min, aerobic conditioning is important but anaerobic sources of energy for the power demands become more important the higher the exercise intensity and the shorter the accompanying performance time. It also makes a great difference whether or not the athlete performs to exhaustion (such as in the 10-km run) or is involved in one half of a soccer match (45 min) which involves a wide range of aerobic/anaerobic intensities and intermittent activity. Also, skill may be more important than any other performance consideration.

If an increase in aerobic power is required, the athlete must follow a programme designed to increase the cardiac output capability (SV and

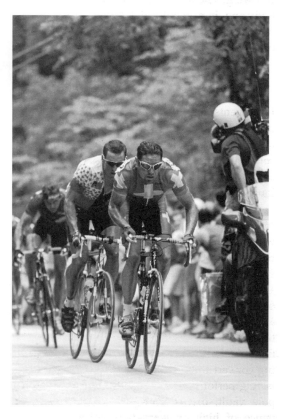

**Fig. 1.5** A sport such as road cycling depends predominantly upon aerobic metabolism. Photo © Allsport / M. Powell.

$\dot{Q}$), the total circulating haemoglobin and the capillarization of the skeletal muscles that are involved. Such conditioning also serves to enhance the aerobic metabolic capacities of the skeletal muscle cells including both type I and type II fibres.

The programme would consist of a combination of interval training and some extended bouts of exercise (e.g. 10–60 min) consistent with the particular competitive event. Depending upon the individual athlete and the point in time relative to the competitive season, the athlete will train vigorously three to seven times per week.

It is important to note that such aerobic conditioning can adversely affect the particular skeletal muscles involved as regards the ability for the generation of high power and the explosive effort involved in activities such as jumping and throwing. The adaptation of the systems of the body and, in particular, the skeletal muscles will be specific to the conditioning stimulus or, in other words, the conditioning programme.

### Anaerobic conditioning

For events lasting less than 10 min, energy obtained from anaerobic glycolysis is an important factor; the shorter the event the greater is the contribution of this source. There is an obvious overlapping with oxidative metabolism the longer the duration of the activity.

With a programme of conditioning that combines a considerable amount of strength training with very high but continuous exercise intensity that mimics the event (e.g. the 100-m run, the 100-m swim, wrestling), the emphasis is on an appropriate increase in the size of type II muscle cells, enhancing the capability of the cells for anaerobic glycolysis, and increasing the concentrations of ATP and PCr. Most, if not all, type IIb fibres that exist at the initiation of such conditioning convert to type IIa. Except for the shortest lasting performances (weightlifting, high jump, pole vault, discus, shot-put, javelin), maintenance of high concentrations of glycogen in the muscle cells through proper nutrition is important.

### Strength conditioning

Increases in maximum force production (strength) and maximal power of the muscles are brought about through exercise programmes of very high opposing force (routinely termed 'resistance') that limits repetitions to approximately 20 or fewer and therefore a duration of less than 30 s. Exercise programmes based on higher repetitions (e.g. 30–50 repetitions leading to exhaustion) develop local muscular endurance but are not conducive to strength development. Exercise involving many repetitions in a bout (e.g. 400–1000 repetitions) brings about physiological adaptations that result in enhanced aerobic performance that can be especially counterproductive to power development and, to a lesser extent, on the performance of strength tests.

'Resistance training' is performed with a variety of exercise machines, free weights or even the use of gravity acting upon the athlete's body mass. Most resistance training (strength) programmes are based on a system of exercise to a *repetition maximum* (RM) as presented in the mid-1940s by DeLorme (1945). Every time the athlete performs a particular exercise, the bout is performed for the maximum number of repetitions, or RM, possible and this number is recorded along with the mass lifted or opposing force imposed by an exercise machine. Repeated testing at increasingly higher opposing force will eventually lead to the determination of a 1RM, in which the athlete can perform the movement but once and not repeat it. In this system, the mass lifted or opposing force is described as the athlete's strength at that particular point in time and for the particular movement.

Bouts of strength exercise and the daily programme can be based on percentages of a 1 RM, preferably, within heavy (3–5), medium (9–10) and light (15–18) RM zones (Fleck & Kraemer 1997). The number of bouts performed in a set, the number of sets performed per day and the number of daily workouts per week are then prescribed for each movement or muscle group as based on the point in time in the competitive season, the physical condition of the athlete, programme variation for both physiological and psychological considerations and programme objectives.

The principal adaptation of the athlete's body is the increase in size (commonly termed hypertrophy) of type II muscle cells. It is generally held that no interchange takes place between type I and type II fibres as the result of specific conditioning programmes.

As the force development capability of a muscle is directly related to its physiological cross-section, the increase in size of the muscle cells is the principal reason for increased force development. The energy requirement for performance of a 1 RM is quite small, as is the performance of any bout of exercise from the 1 RM to a 20 RM. However, the total energy requirement of performing multiple bouts of exercise for each of a number of movements or exercises (e.g. 10) in a daily workout is large. This deserves careful consideration from the standpoint of the athlete's nutrition, both in terms of quantity and content. In addition to the total energy balance and accompanying maintenance of appropriate body mass, consideration must be given to suitable protein intake.

### Adaptations of skeletal muscle

Muscle cells and the structure of an individual muscle, in general, respond in very different ways to the unique exercise stimulus that is provided. The muscles respond to the acute stimulus by providing the forces and power demanded by such widely diverse performances as weightlifting, high jumping, 100-m sprinting and running at marathon pace. Following a single bout of exercise or a single day's conditioning session, however, the individual muscle fibres and the total muscle recover to a physiological state with little or no measurable change.

Repeated workouts over weeks and months elicit adaptations, and these structural and functional changes are highly specific to the conditioning programme (i.e. the stimulus) as appropriate to the competitive event for which the athlete is preparing (Fig. 1.6). A high-resistance (strength) programme which results in significant muscle hypertrophy could be detrimental to distance running performance. A conditioning programme for distance running would definitely be detrimental to weightlifting, high jumping and sprint performance.

Strength training results in an increase in size (girth and therefore cross-sectional area) of type II muscle fibres and the muscles themselves. Capillarization can evidence either no change or a 'dilution effect', where the hypertrophy of muscle cells spreads out the existing capillaries, with the result that an individual capillary serves a larger cross-sectional area of muscle.

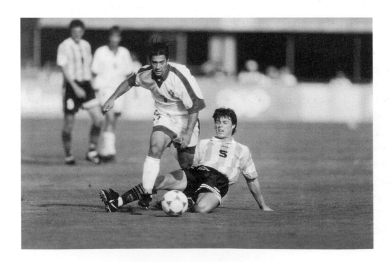

**Fig. 1.6** Many team sports such as international football (soccer) require combinations of aerobic power, anaerobic power and strength, as well as a wide variety of skills. Photo © Allsport / S. Bruty.

A combination of strength and anaerobic conditioning, as appropriate to sprinters, results in some hypertrophy and an increase in the anaerobic metabolic capabilities of type II fibres. The resting concentrations of ATP and PCr increase as well as the capability of the cells to produce force and power with energy from anaerobic glycolysis.

In both strength conditioning and combination strength/anaerobic conditioning, there is little or no adaptation of the cardiovascular system in terms of stroke volume, minute volume or blood composition.

Highly aerobic training involving a large number of movement repetitions (e.g. 500–2000) results in adaptations to both muscle cells and to the cardiovascular system. The aerobic metabolic capacities of type I fibres is greatly enhanced, as is, to a lesser extent, the aerobic capacity of type II fibres. This includes increases in mitochondrial count, myoglobin content and glycogen storage. An increase in capillarization provides enhanced capability for oxygen and substrate delivery and for carbon dioxide and catabolite removal. The abilities of the muscle for high force and power development diminish.

## Nutrition of an athlete

All of the factors involving muscle, ventilation/respiration and circulation are important in determining the success of a particular individual in competing in a particular sport. Additional factors involve coordination (skilled movement), body size and motivation. However, energy is needed for the performance of short-term explosive events, long-term endurance events and the many sport activities that involve the development of varying amounts of power during the course of a contest. Therefore, proper nutrition must be considered to be a key element to success in a wide variety of competitive sports.

Frequently overlooked by athletes when considering the nutrition of sport is the tremendous time and energy involved in the conditioning programme between competitions and/or leading up to a competitive season. Performance of a throwing event in track and field or of Olympic weightlifting events takes but a few seconds of time, but preparation involves many hours of skill practice and conditioning.

The nutrition of an athlete is a 12-months-of-the-year consideration. Too often, the focus of attention is placed on the days or even hours leading up to a competitive event. While pre-event food ingestion is of great importance, optimal health and optimal performance are dependent on year-around planning. Under certain circumstances, nutrition during an event and/or immediately following an event also carry great importance.

Each athlete must perform at an appropriate body weight. In addition to the total mass involved, the relative contribution to total mass by muscle, fat and bone is of importance. Optimal values for the various constituents are best developed through a combination of proper diet and appropriate conditioning that is continuous.

The moment a competitive event begins, the athlete should be at appropriate body mass, sufficiently hydrated, possess proper amounts of vitamins and minerals, and be nourished with sufficient carbohydrate that an appropriate balance of carbohydrate and fat metabolism will provide the energy for the ensuing muscular activity.

## Nutritional and energetic limits to performance

It can be generally accepted that each athlete enters his/her event with fat stores in excess of what will be utilized during the course of a competition. It is well known, however, that the higher the intensity of the muscular activity, the greater the proportion of energy that the muscles will obtain from carbohydrate (glucose and glycogen) compared with that obtained from fat (fatty acids).

Herein lies a major challenge to athletes competing in a wide range of sports involving moderate intensity and long duration, that of ensuring that the carbohydrate stores in the skeletal muscles and liver are optimal as the event starts. Skeletal muscle cells will depend both on endogenous glycogen stores as well as carbohydrate delivered by the blood as glucose. The nervous system depends totally on glucose obtained from the blood for its completely aerobic metabolism. Insufficient glucose for the nervous system results in loss of control and coordination of the muscles and the movements. There is a small amount of glucose circulating in the blood as an event starts, but the blood glucose level must be maintained from glycogen stored in the liver. Low glycogen concentrations in the skeletal muscle cells reduce an athlete's capacity for power production. Low blood glucose can therefore adversely affect both nervous system function and muscle function.

The athlete's conditioning programme must be planned with great care and appreciation for the specific demands of each event or sport activity. The force, power, metabolic and associated nutritional demands of both competition and the conditioning programmes involve great differences among such varied activities as Olympic weightlifting, high jumping, 100-m running, 400-m swimming, tennis, field hockey, basketball, road cycling, cross-country skiing and marathon running.

## References

Åstrand, P.-O. & Rodahl, K. (1986) *Textbook of Work Physiology.* McGraw-Hill, New York.

Bureau International des Poids et Mésures (1977) *Le Système International d'Unités (SI)*, 3rd edn. Sèvres, France.

Cavanagh, P.R. (1988) On 'muscle action' vs. 'muscle contraction.' *Journal of Biomechanics* **22**, 69.

DeLorme, T.L. (1945) Restoration of muscle power by heavy resistance exercises. *Journal of Bone and Joint Surgery* **27**, 645–667.

Fleck, S.J. & Kraemer, W.J. (1997) *Designing Resistance Training Programs.* Human Kinetics, Champaign, IL.

Knuttgen, H.G. & Kraemer, W.J. (1987) Terminology and measurement in exercise performance. *Journal of Applied Sports Science Research* **1**, 1–10.

Komi, P.V. (ed.) (1992) *Strength and Power in Sport.* Blackwell Scientific Publications, Oxford.

## Further reading

Dirix, A., Knuttgen, H.G. & Tittel, K. (eds) (1992) *The Olympic Book of Sports Medicine.* Blackwell Scientific Publications, Oxford.

Komi, P.V. & Knuttgen, H.G. (1996) Sport science and modern training. In *Sports Science Studies*, Vol. 8, pp. 44–62. Verlag Karl Hofmann, Schorndorf.

Shephard, R.J. & Åstrand, P.-O. (eds) (1992) *Endurance in Sport.* Blackwell Scientific Publications, Oxford.

# Chapter 2

# Biochemistry of Exercise

MICHAEL GLEESON

## Introduction

Answers to questions in exercise physiology and sports nutrition, including the most fundamental ones such as the causes of fatigue, can only be obtained by an understanding of cellular, subcellular and molecular mechanisms to explain how the body responds to acute and chronic exercise. Biochemistry usually refers to the study of events at the subcellular and molecular level, and this is where the emphasis is placed in this chapter. In particular, this brief review describes the sources of energy available for muscle force generation and explains how acute exercise modifies energy metabolism. For further details, see Maughan *et al.* (1997) and Hargreaves (1995). Training also modifies the metabolic response to exercise and training-induced adaptations encompass both biochemical responses (e.g. changes in enzyme activities in trained muscles) and physiological responses (e.g. changes in maximal cardiac output and maximal oxygen uptake, $\dot{V}o_{2max.}$) (Saltin 1985).

## Skeletal muscle

Individual muscles are made up of many parallel muscle fibres that may (or may not) extend the entire length of the muscle. The interior of the muscle fibre is filled with sarcoplasm (muscle cell cytoplasm), a red viscous fluid containing nuclei, mitochondria, myoglobin and about 500 thread-like myofibrils, 1–3 mm thick, continuous from end to end in the muscle fibre. The red colour is due to the presence of myoglobin, an intracellular respiratory pigment. Surrounding the myofibrils is an elaborate form of smooth endoplasmic reticulum called the sarcoplasmic reticulum. Its interconnecting membranous tubules lie in the narrow spaces between the myofibrils, surrounding and running parallel to them. Fat (as triacylglycerol droplets), glycogen, phosphocreatine (PCr) and adenosine triphosphate (ATP) are found in the sarcoplasm as energy stores. The myofibrils are composed of overlapping thin and thick filaments and it is the arrangement of these filaments that gives skeletal muscle its striated appearance. The thin filaments are comprised of the protein actin; located on the actin are two other types of protein, tropomyosin and troponin. The thick filaments contain the protein myosin.

When calcium and ATP are present in sufficient quantities, the filaments interact to form actomyosin and shorten by sliding over each other. Sliding of the filaments begins when the myosin heads form cross bridges attached to active sites on the actin subunits of the thin filaments. Each cross bridge attaches and detaches several times during a contraction, in a ratchet-like action, pulling the thin filaments towards the centre of the sarcomere. When a muscle fibre contracts, its sarcomeres shorten. As this event occurs in sarcomeres throughout the cell, the whole muscle fibre shortens in length.

The attachment of the myosin cross bridges requires the presence of calcium ions. In the relaxed state, calcium is sequestered in the sarcoplasmic reticulum, and in the absence of calcium, the myosin-binding sites on actin are physically blocked by the tropomyosin rods (Fig. 2.1). Electrical excitation passing as an action potential along the sarcolemma and down the T-tubules leads to calcium release from the sarcoplasmic reticulum into the sarcoplasm and subsequent activation and contraction of the fila-ment array (Frank 1982). The calcium ions bind to troponin, causing a change in its conformation that physically moves tropomyosin away from the myosin binding sites on the underlying actin chain. Excitation is initiated by the arrival of a nerve impulse at the muscle membrane via the motor end plate. Activated or 'cocked' myosin heads now bind to the actin, and as this happens

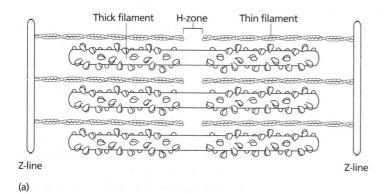

(a)

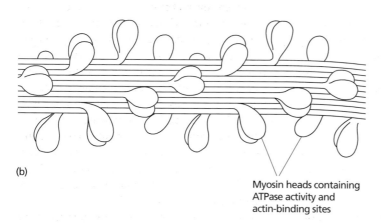

(b)

Myosin heads containing ATPase activity and actin-binding sites

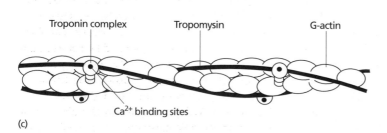

(c)

Troponin complex    Tropomyosin    G-actin

Ca²⁺ binding sites

**Fig. 2.1** (a) Molecular components of the myofilaments and the arrangement of the thick and thin filaments in longitudinal cross section within one sarcomere (the region between two successive Z-lines in a myofibril). (b) The thick filaments are composed of myosin molecules; each of these comprises a rod-like tail and a globular head. The latter contains ATPase activity and actin-binding sites. (c) The thin filaments are composed of actin molecules and several regulatory proteins. Globular (G)-actin monomers are polymerized into long strands called fibrous (F)-actin. Two F-actin strands twisted together form the backbone of each thin filament. Rod-shaped tropomyosin molecules spiral about the F-actin chains. The other main protein present in the thin filaments is troponin, which contains three subunits. One of these, troponin I, binds to actin; another, troponin T, binds to tropomyosin; and the other, troponin C, can bind calcium ions.

the myosin head changes from its activated configuration to its bent shape, which causes the head to pull on the thin filament, sliding it towards the centre of the sarcomere. This action represents the power stroke of the cross bridge cycle, and simultaneously adenosine diphosphate (ADP) and inorganic phosphate ($P_i$) are released from the myosin head. As a new ATP molecule binds to the myosin head at the ATPase active site, the myosin cross bridge detaches from the actin. Hydrolysis of the ATP to ADP and $P_i$ by the ATPase provides the energy required to return the myosin to its activated 'cocked' state, empowering it with the potential energy needed for the next cross bridge attachment–power stroke sequence. While the myosin is in the activated state, the ADP and $P_i$ remain attached to the myosin head. Now the myosin head can attach to another actin unit farther along the thin filament, and the cycle of attachment, power stroke, detachment and activation of myosin is repeated. Sliding of the filaments in this manner continues as long as calcium is present (at a concentration in excess of $10\,\mu mol \cdot l^{-1}$) in the sarcoplasm. Removal and sequestration of the calcium by the ATP-dependent calcium pump (ATPase) of the sarcoplasmic reticulum restores the tropomyosin inhibition of cross bridge formation and the muscle fibre relaxes.

## Fibre types

The existence of different fibre types in skeletal muscle is readily apparent and has long been recognized; the detailed physiological and biochemical bases for these differences and their functional significance have, however, only more recently been established. Much of the impetus for these investigations has come from the realization that success in athletic events which require either the ability to generate a high power output or great endurance is dependent in large part on the proportions of the different fibre types which are present in the muscles. The muscle fibres are, however, extremely plastic, and although the fibre type distribution is genetically determined, and not easily altered, an

appropriate training programme will have a major effect on the metabolic potential of the muscle, irrespective of the fibre types present.

Fibre type classification is usually based on histochemical staining of serial cross-sections. On this basis, human muscle fibres are commonly divided into three major kinds: types I, IIa and IIb. These are analogous to the muscle fibres from animals that have been classified on the basis of their directly determined functional properties as (i) slow twitch fibres, (ii) fast twitch, fatigue resistant fibres, and (iii) fast twitch, fatiguable fibres, respectively. The myosin of the different fibre types exists in different molecular forms (isoforms), and the myofibrillar ATPase activity of the different fibre types displays differential pH sensitivity; this provides the basis for the differential histochemical staining of the fibre types (Åstrand & Rodahl 1986). The biochemical characteristics of the three major fibre types are summarized in Table 2.1.

Type I fibres are small-diameter red cells that contain relatively slow acting myosin ATPases and hence contract slowly. The red colour is due to the presence of myoglobin, an intracellular respiratory pigment, capable of binding oxygen and only releasing it at very low partial pressures (as are found in the proximity of the mitochondria). Type I fibres have numerous mitochondria, mostly located close to the periphery of the fibre, near to the blood capillaries which provide a rich supply of oxygen and nutrients. These fibres possess a high capacity for oxidative metabolism, are extremely fatigue resistant, and are specialized for the performance of repeated contractions over prolonged periods.

Type IIb fibres are much paler, because they contain little myoglobin. They possess rapidly acting myosin ATPases and so their contraction (and relaxation) time is relatively fast. They have fewer mitochondria and a poorer capillary supply, but greater glycogen and PCr stores than the type I fibres. A high activity of glycogenolytic and glycolytic enzymes endows type IIb fibres with a high capacity for rapid (but relatively short-lived) ATP production in the absence of oxygen (anaerobic capacity). As a result, lactic

**Table 2.1** Biochemical characteristics of human muscle fibre types. Values of metabolic characteristics of type II fibres are shown relative to those found in type I fibres.

| Characteristic | Type I | Type IIa | Type IIb |
|---|---|---|---|
| Nomenclature | Slow, red | Fast, red | Fast, white |
|  | Fatigue resistant | Fatigue resistant | Fatiguable |
|  | Oxidative | Oxidative/glycolytic | Glycolytic |
| Capillary density | 1.0 | 0.8 | 0.6 |
| Mitochondrial density | 1.0 | 0.7 | 0.4 |
| Myoglobin content | 1.0 | 0.6 | 0.3 |
| Phosphorylase activity | 1.0 | 2.1 | 3.1 |
| PFK activity | 1.0 | 1.8 | 2.3 |
| Citrate synthase activity | 1.0 | 0.8 | 0.6 |
| SDH activity | 1.0 | 0.7 | 0.4 |
| Glycogen content | 1.0 | 1.3 | 1.5 |
| Triacylglycerol content | 1.0 | 0.4 | 0.2 |
| Phosphocreatine content | 1.0 | 1.2 | 1.2 |
| Myosin ATPase activity | 1.0 | >2 | >2 |

ATP, adenosine triphosphate; PFK, phosphofructokinase; SDH, succinate dehydrogenase.

acid accumulates quickly in these fibres and they fatigue rapidly. Hence, these fibres are best suited for delivering rapid, powerful contractions for brief periods. The metabolic characteristics of type IIa fibres lie between the extreme properties of the other two fibre types. They contain fast-acting myosin ATPases like the type IIb fibres, but have an oxidative capacity more akin to that of the type I fibres.

The differences in activation threshold of the motor neurones supplying the different fibre types determine the order in which fibres are recruited during exercise, and this in turn influences the metabolic response to exercise. During most forms of movement, there appears to be an orderly hierarchy of motor unit recruitment, which roughly corresponds with a progression from type I to type IIa to type IIb. It follows that during light exercise, mostly type I fibres will be recruited; during moderate exercise, both type I and type IIa will be recruited; and during more severe exercise, all fibre types will contribute to force production.

Whole muscles in the body contain a mixture of these three different fibre types, though the proportions in which they are found differ substantially between different muscles and can also differ between different individuals. For example, muscles involved in maintaining posture (e.g. soleus in the leg) have a high proportion (usually more than 70%) of type I fibres, which is in keeping with their function in maintaining prolonged, chronic, but relatively weak contractions. Fast type II fibres, however, predominate in muscles where rapid movements are required (e.g. in the muscles of the hand and the eye). Other muscles, such as the quadriceps group in the leg, contain a variable mixture of fibre types. The fibre type composition in such muscles is a genetically determined attribute, which does not appear to be pliable to a significant degree by training. Hence, athletic capabilities are inborn to a large extent (assuming the genetic potential of the individual is realized through appropriate nutrition and training). The vastus lateralis muscle of successful marathon runners has been shown to have a high percentage (about 80%) of type I fibres, while that of elite sprinters contains a higher percentage (about 60%) of the type II fast twitch fibres (see Komi & Karlsson 1978).

## Sources of energy for muscle force generation

Energy can be defined as the potential for performing work or producing force. Development of force by skeletal muscles requires a source of chemical energy in the form of ATP; in fact, energy from the hydrolysis of ATP is harnessed to power all forms of biological work. In muscle, energy from the hydrolysis of ATP by myosin ATPase activates specific sites on the contractile elements, as described previously, causing the muscle fibre to shorten. The hydrolysis of ATP yields approximately 31 kJ of free energy per mole of ATP degraded to ADP and inorganic phosphate ($P_i$):

$$ATP + H_2O \Rightarrow ADP + H^+ + P_i - 31 \, kJ \cdot mol^{-1} \, ATP$$

Active reuptake of calcium ions by the sarcoplasmic reticulum also requires ATP, as does the restoration of the sarcolemmal membrane potential via the action of the $Na^+$–$K^+$-ATPase. There are three different mechanisms involved in the resynthesis of ATP for muscle force generation:

1 Phosphocreatine (PCr) hydrolysis.

2 Glycolysis, which involves metabolism of glucose-6-phosphate (G6P), derived from muscle glycogen or blood-borne glucose, and produces ATP by substrate-level phosphorylation reactions.

3 The products of carbohydrate, fat, protein and alcohol metabolism can enter the tricarboxylic acid (TCA) cycle in the mitochondria and be oxidized to carbon dioxide and water. This process is known as oxidative phosphorylation and yields energy for the synthesis of ATP.

The purpose of these mechanisms is to regenerate ATP at sufficient rates to prevent a significant fall in the intramuscular ATP concentration. The resting concentration of ATP in skeletal muscle is quite low at about 20–25 mmol $\cdot$ kg$^{-1}$ dry matter (dm) of muscle, which in itself could only provide enough energy to sustain a few seconds of intense exercise. PCr breakdown and glycolysis are anaerobic mechanisms (that is, they do not use oxygen) and occur in the sarcoplasm. Both use only one specific substrate for energy production (i.e. PCr and G6P). The aerobic (oxygen-requiring) processes in the mitochondria can utilize a variety of different substrates. The sarcoplasm contains a variety of enzymes which can convert carbohydrates, fats and proteins into usable substrate, primarily a 2-carbon acetyl group linked to coenzyme A

(acetyl-CoA) which can be completely oxidized in the mitochondria with the resultant production of ATP. A general summary of the main energy sources and pathways of energy metabolism is presented in Fig. 2.2.

## Anaerobic metabolism

### Phosphocreatine

Some of the energy for ATP resynthesis is supplied rapidly and without the need for oxygen by PCr. Within the muscle fibre, the concentration of PCr is about 3–4 times greater than that of ATP. When PCr is broken down to creatine and inorganic phosphate by the action of the enzyme creatine kinase, a large amount of free energy is released (43 kJ $\cdot$ mol$^{-1}$ PCr) and, because PCr has a higher free energy of hydrolysis than ATP, its phosphate is donated directly to the ADP molecule to reform ATP. The PCr can be regarded as a back-up energy store: when the ATP content begins to fall during exercise, the PCr is broken down, releasing energy for restoration of ATP. During very intense exercise the PCr store can be almost completely depleted. There is a close relationship between the intensity of exercise and the rate at which PCr is broken down. The reactions of ATP and PCr hydrolysis are reversible, and when energy is readily available from other sources (oxidative phosphorylation), creatine and phosphate can be rejoined to form PCr:

$$ADP + PCr + H^+ \Leftrightarrow ATP + Cr - 43 \, kJ \cdot mol^{-1} \, PCr$$

Note that the resynthesis of ATP via breakdown of PCr buffers some of the hydrogen ions formed as a result of ATP hydrolysis. The PCr in muscle is immediately available at the onset of exercise and can be used to resynthesize ATP at a very high rate. This high rate of energy transfer corresponds to the ability to produce a high power output. The major disadvantage of this system is its limited capacity (Table 2.2); the total amount of energy available is small. If no other energy source is available to the muscle, fatigue will occur rapidly. An additional pathway to regenerate ATP when ATP and PCr stores are depleted is through a kinase reaction that utilizes two mole-

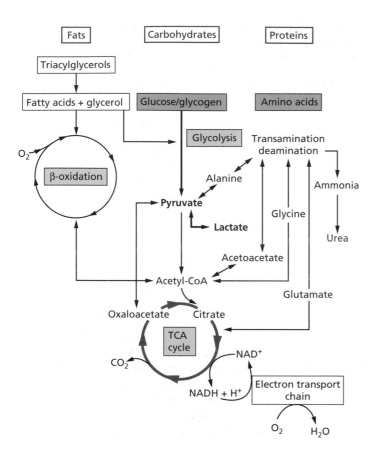

**Fig. 2.2** Summary of the main pathways of energy metabolism using carbohydrate, fats and protein as energy sources. Carbohydrate may participate in both anaerobic and aerobic pathways. In glycolysis, glucose or glycogen are broken down to lactate under anaerobic conditions and pyruvate under aerobic conditions. The pyruvate is converted to acetyl-coenzyme A (CoA) and is completely oxidized in the tricarboxylic (TCA) cycle. Fats in the form of triacylglycerols are hydrolysed to fatty acids and glycerol, the latter entering the glycolytic pathway (in liver but not in muscle) and the fatty acids being converted via the β-oxidation pathway to acetyl-CoA and subsequently oxidized in the TCA cycle. Protein catabolism can provide amino acids that can be converted by removal of the amino group into either TCA cycle intermediates or into pyruvate or acetoacetate and subsequent transformation to acetyl-CoA.

**Table 2.2a** Capacity and power of anaerobic systems for the production of adenosine triphosphate (ATP).

|  | Capacity (mmol ATP $\cdot$ kg$^{-1}$ dm) | Power (mmol ATP $\cdot$ kg$^{-1}$ dm $\cdot$ s$^{-1}$) |
| --- | --- | --- |
| Phosphagen system | 55–95 | 9.0 |
| Glycolytic system | 190–300 | 4.5 |
| Combined | 250–370 | 11.0 |

Values are expressed per kilogram dry matter (dm) of muscle and are based on estimates of ATP provision during high-intensity exercise of human vastus lateralis muscle.

cules of ADP to generate one molecule of ATP (and one molecule of adenosine monophosphate, AMP). This reaction is catalysed by the enzyme called myokinase:

$$ADP + ADP \Rightarrow ATP + AMP - 31\,kJ \cdot mol^{-1}\,ADP$$

This reaction only becomes important during exercise of high intensity. Even then, the amount of energy it makes available in the form of ATP is extremely limited and the real importance of the reaction may be in the formation of AMP which is a potent allosteric activator of a number of enzymes involved in energy metabolism.

It is known that the total adenylate pool can decline rapidly if the AMP concentration of the cell begins to rise during muscle force genera-

**Table 2.2b** Maximal rates of adenosine triphosphate (ATP) resynthesis from anaerobic and aerobic metabolism and approximate delay time before maximal rates are attained following onset of exercise.

| | Max rate of ATP resynthesis (mmol ATP $\cdot$ kg$^{-1}$ dm $\cdot$ s$^{-1}$) | Delay time |
|---|---|---|
| Fat oxidation | 1.0 | >2 h |
| Glucose (from blood) oxidation | 1.0 | Approx. 90 min |
| Glycogen oxidation | 2.8 | Several minutes |
| Glycolysis | 4.5 | 5–10 s |
| PCr breakdown | 9.0 | Instantaneous |

PCr, phosphocreatine.

tion. This decline occurs principally via deamination of AMP to inosine monophosphate (IMP) but also by the dephosphorylation of AMP to adenosine. The loss of AMP may initially appear counterproductive because of the reduction in the total adenylate pool. However, it should be noted that the deamination of AMP to IMP only occurs under low ATP/ADP ratio conditions and, by preventing excessive accumulation of ADP and AMP, enables the adenylate kinase reactions to continue, resulting in an increase in the ATP/ADP ratio and continuing muscle force generation. Furthermore, it has been proposed that the free energy of ATP hydrolysis will decrease when ADP and $P_i$ accumulate, which could further impair muscle force generation. For these reasons, adenine nucleotide loss has been suggested to be of importance to muscle function during conditions of metabolic crisis; for example, during maximal exercise and in the later stages of prolonged submaximal exercise when glycogen stores become depleted (Sahlin & Broberg 1990).

## Glycolysis

Under normal conditions, muscle clearly does not fatigue after only a few seconds of effort, so a source of energy other than ATP and PCr must be available. This is derived from glycolysis, which is the name given to the pathway involving the breakdown of glucose (or glycogen), the end product of this series of chemical reactions being pyruvate. This process does not require oxygen, but does result in energy in the form of ATP being available to the muscle from reactions involving substrate-level phosphorylation. In order for the reactions to proceed, however, the pyruvate must be removed; in low-intensity exercise, when adequate oxygen is available to the muscle, pyruvate is converted to carbon dioxide and water by oxidative metabolism in the mitochondria. In some situations the majority of the pyruvate is removed by conversion to lactate, a reaction that does not involve oxygen.

A specific transporter protein (GLUT-4) is involved in the passage of glucose molecules across the cell membrane. Once the glucose molecule is inside the cell, the first step of glycolysis is an irreversible phosphorylation catalysed by hexokinase to prevent loss of this valuable nutrient from the cell: glucose is converted to G6P. This step is effectively irreversible, at least as far as muscle is concerned. Liver has a phosphatase enzyme which catalyses the reverse reaction, allowing free glucose to leave the cell and enter the circulation, but this enzyme is absent from muscle. The hexokinase reaction is an energy-consuming reaction, requiring the investment of one molecule of ATP per molecule of glucose. This also ensures a concentration gradient for glucose across the cell membrane down which transport can occur. Hexokinase is inhibited by an accumulation of the reaction product G6P, and during high-intensity exercise, the increasing concentration of G6P limits the contribution that the blood glucose can make to carbohydrate metabolism in the active muscles.

If glycogen, rather than blood glucose, is the substrate for glycolysis, the first step is to split off a single glucose molecule. This is achieved by the enzyme glycogen phosphorylase, and the products are glucose-1-phosphate and a glycogen molecule that is one glucose residue shorter than the original. The substrates are glycogen and inorganic phosphate, so, unlike the hexokinase reaction, there is no breakdown of ATP in this first reaction. Phosphorylase acts on the α-1,4 carbon bonds at the free ends of the glycogen molecule, but cannot break the α-1,6 bonds forming the branch points. These are hydrolysed by the combined actions of a debranching enzyme and amylo-1,6-glucosidase, releasing free glucose which is quickly phosphorylated to G6P by the action of hexokinase. There is an accumulation of free glucose within the muscle cell only in very high-intensity exercise where glycogenolysis is proceeding rapidly: because there are relatively few α-1,6 bonds, no more than about 10% of the glucose residues appear as free glucose. The enzyme phosphoglucomutase ensures that glucose-1-phosphate formed by the action of phosphorylase on glycogen is rapidly converted to G6P, which then proceeds down the glycolytic pathway.

The sequence of reactions that convert G6P to pyruvate is shown in Fig. 2.3. Briefly, following a further phosphorylation, the glucose molecule is cleaved to form two molecules of the three-carbon sugar glyceraldehyde-3-phosphate. The second stage of glycolysis involves the conversion of this into pyruvate, accompanied by the formation of ATP and reduction of nicotinamide adenine dinucleotide (NAD+) to NADH.

The net effect of glycolysis can thus be seen to be the conversion of one molecule of glucose to two molecules of pyruvate, with the net formation of two molecules of ATP and the conversion of two molecules of NAD+ to NADH. If glycogen rather than glucose is the starting point, three molecules of ATP are produced, as there is no initial investment of ATP when the first phosphorylation step occurs. Although this net energy yield appears to be small, the relatively large carbohydrate store available and the rapid rate at which glycolysis can proceed mean that the energy that can be supplied in this way is crucial for the performance of intense exercise. The 800-m runner, for example, obtains about 60% of the total energy requirement from anaerobic metabolism, and may convert about 100 g of carbohydrate (mostly glycogen, and equivalent to about 550 mmol of glucose) to lactate in less than 2 min. The amount of ATP released in this way (three ATP molecules per glucose molecule degraded, about 1667 mmol of ATP in total) far exceeds that available from PCr hydrolysis. This high rate of anaerobic metabolism allows not only a faster 'steady state' speed than would be possible if aerobic metabolism alone had to be relied upon, but also allows a faster pace in the early stages before the cardiovascular system has adjusted to the demands and the delivery and utilization of oxygen have increased in response to the exercise stimulus.

The reactions of glycolysis occur in the cytoplasm of the cell and some pyruvate will escape from tissues such as active muscle when the rate of glycolysis is high, but most is further metabolized. The fate of the pyruvate produced by glycolysis during exercise will depend not only on factors such as exercise intensity, but also on the metabolic capacity of the tissue. When glycolysis proceeds rapidly, the problem for the cell is that the availability of NAD+, which is necessary as a cofactor in the glyceraldehyde-3-phosphate dehydrogenase reaction, becomes limiting. The amount of NAD+ in the cell is very small (only about 0.8 mmol·kg$^{-1}$ dm) relative to the rate at which glycolysis can proceed. In high-intensity exercise, the rate of turnover of ATP can be about 8 mmol·kg$^{-1}$ dm·s$^{-1}$. If the NADH formed by glycolysis is not reoxidized to NAD+ at an equal rate, glycolysis will be unable to proceed and to contribute to energy supply.

There are two main processes available for regeneration of NAD+ in muscle. Reduction of pyruvate to lactate will achieve this, and this reaction has the advantage that it can proceed in the absence of oxygen. Lactate can accumulate within the muscle fibres, reaching much higher concentrations than those reached by any of the

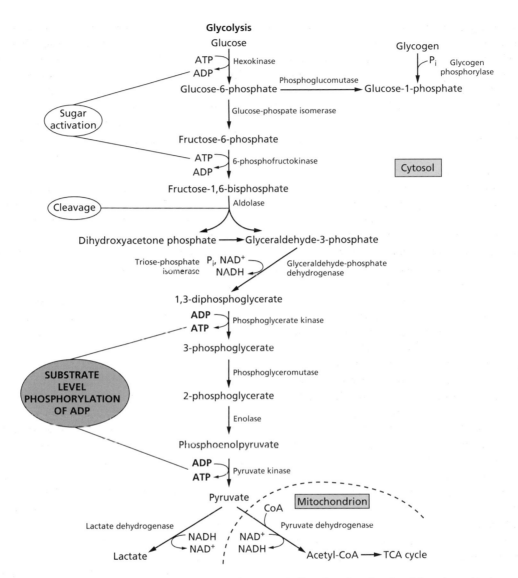

**Fig. 2.3** The reactions of glycolysis. Glucose, a six-carbon sugar, is first phosphorylated and then cleaved to form two molecules of the three-carbon sugar glyceraldehyde-3-phosphate, which is subsequently converted into pyruvate, accompanied by the formation of ATP and reduction of $NAD^+$ to NADH. Glycolysis makes two molecules of ATP available for each molecule of glucose that passes through the pathway. If muscle glycogen is the starting substrate, three ATP molecules are generated for each glucose unit passing down the pathway. Pyruvate may enter the mitochondria and be converted into acetyl-CoA, or be reduced to form lactate in the cytosol. Enzymes are set in small type; $P_i$, inorganic phosphate; TCA, tricarboxylic acid.

glycolytic intermediates, but when this happens, the associated hydrogen ions cause intracellular pH to fall. Some lactate will diffuse into the extracellular space and will eventually begin to accumulate in the blood. The lactate that leaves the

muscle fibres is accompanied by hydrogen ions, and this has the effect of making the buffer capacity of the extracellular space available to handle some of the hydrogen ions that would otherwise cause the intracellular pH to fall to a point where it would interfere with cell function. The normal pH of the muscle cell at rest is about 7.1, but this can fall to as low as 6.4 in high-intensity exercise, when large amounts of lactate are formed. At this pH, the contractile mechanism begins to fail, and some inhibition of key enzymes, such as phosphorylase and phosphofructokinase, may occur. A low pH also stimulates free nerve endings in the muscle, resulting in the perception of pain. Although the negative effects of the acidosis resulting from lactate accumulation are often stressed, it must be remembered that the energy made available by anaerobic glycolysis allows the performance of high-intensity exercise that would otherwise not be possible.

## Aerobic metabolism

As an alternative to conversion to lactate, pyruvate may undergo oxidative metabolism to $CO_2$ and water. This process occurs within the mitochondrion, and pyruvate which is produced in the sarcoplasm is transported across the mitochondrial membrane by a specific carrier protein. The first step to occur within the mitochondrion is the conversion, by oxidative decarboxylation, of the three-carbon pyruvate to a two-carbon acetate group which is linked by a thio-ester bond to coenzyme A (CoA) to form acetyl-CoA. This reaction, in which $NAD^+$ is converted to NADH, is catalysed by the pyruvate dehydrogenase enzyme complex. Acetyl-CoA is also formed from the metabolism of fatty acids within the mitochondria, in a metabolic pathway called β-oxidation which, as its name implies, is an oxygen-requiring process.

Acetyl-CoA is oxidized to $CO_2$ in the TCA cycle: this series of reactions is also known as the Krebs cycle, after Hans Krebs, who first described the reactions involved, or the citric acid cycle, as citrate is one of the key intermediates in the process. The reactions involve combination of acetyl-CoA with oxaloacetate to form citrate, a six-carbon TCA. A series of reactions leads to the sequential loss of hydrogen atoms and $CO_2$, resulting in the regeneration of oxaloacetate:

$$\text{acetyl-CoA} + \text{ADP} + P_i + 3NAD^+ + FAD + 3H_2O \Rightarrow$$
$$2CO_2 + CoA + ATP + 3NADH + 3H^+ + FADH_2$$

Since acetyl-CoA is also a product of fatty acid oxidation, the final steps of oxidative degradation are therefore common to both fat and carbohydrate. The hydrogen atoms are carried by the reduced coenzymes NADH and flavin adenine dinucleotide ($FADH_2$). These act as carriers and donate pairs of electrons to the electron transport chain allowing oxidative phosphorylation with the subsequent regeneration of ATP from ADP.

A summary of the reactions involved in the TCA cycle is shown in Fig. 2.4. Note that molecular $O_2$ does not participate directly in the reactions of the TCA cycle. In essence, the most important function of the TCA cycle is to generate hydrogen atoms for their subsequent passage to the electron transport chain by means of NADH and $FADH_2$ (Fig. 2.5). The aerobic process of electron transport-oxidative phosphorylation regenerates ATP from ADP, thus conserving some of the chemical potential energy contained within the original substrates in the form of high-energy phosphates. As long as there is an adequate supply of $O_2$, and substrate is available, $NAD^+$ and FAD are continuously regenerated and TCA metabolism proceeds. This system cannot function without the use of oxygen. For each molecule of NADH that enters the electron transport chain, three molecules of ATP are generated, and for each molecule of $FADH_2$, two molecules of ATP are formed. Thus, for each molecule of acetyl-CoA undergoing complete oxidation in the TCA cycle, a total of 12 ATP molecules are formed.

The transfer of electrons through the electron transport chain located on the inner mitochondrial membrane causes hydrogen ions or protons ($H^+$) from the inner mitochondrial matrix to be pumped across the inner mitochondrial membrane into the space between the inner and outer mitochondrial membranes. The high concentration of positively charged hydrogen ions in this outer chamber cause the $H^+$ ions to flow back into the mitochondrial matrix through an ATP synthase protein complex embedded in the inner

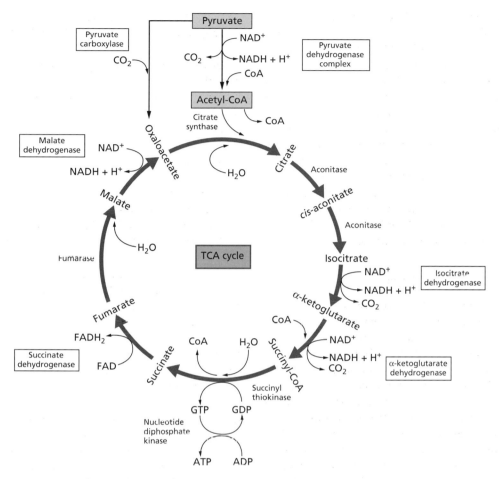

**Fig. 2.4** Summary of reactions of the tricarboxylic acid (TCA) cycle showing sites of substrate level phosphorylation, $CO_2$ production and $NAD^+$ and flavin adenine dinucleotide (FAD) reduction. The two-carbon (2C) acetate units of acetyl-CoA are combined with 4C oxaloacetate to form 6C citrate. The latter undergoes two successive decarboxylation reactions to yield 4C succinate which in subsequent reactions is converted into 4C oxaloacetate, completing the TCA cycle. Enzymes are set in small type; GDP, guanosine diphosphate; GTP, guanosine triphosphate.

mitochondrial membrane. The flow of $H^+$ ions (protons) through this complex constitutes a proton-motive force that is used to drive ATP synthesis. In terms of the energy conservation of aerobic glucose metabolism, the overall reaction starting with glucose as the fuel can be summarized as follows:

$$glucose + 6O_2 + 38ADP + 38P_i \Rightarrow$$
$$6CO_2 + 6H_2O + 38ATP$$

The total ATP synthesis of 38 mol per mole of glucose oxidized are accounted for primarily by oxidation of reduced coenzymes in the terminal respiratory system as follows:

| ATP synthesized | Source |
| --- | --- |
| 2 | Glycolysis |
| 6 | NADH by glycolysis |
| 24 | NADH |
| 4 | FADH$_2$ |
| 2 | GTP |

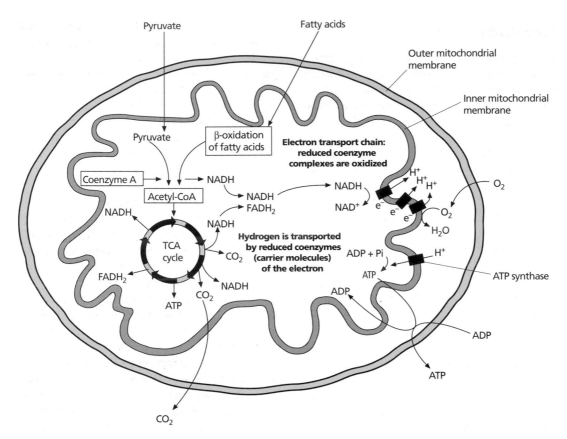

**Fig. 2.5** Schematic diagram showing the relationship of the tricarboxylic (TCA) cycle to the electron transport chain. The main function of the TCA cycle is to reduce the coenzymes $NAD^+$ and flavin adenine dinucleotide (FAD) to NADH and $FADH_2$ which act as carriers of $H^+$ ions and electrons which are donated to the electron transport chain. Molecular oxygen acts as the terminal electron acceptor and the hydrogen ion gradient generated across the inner mitochondrial membrane is used to drive the synthesis of ATP from ADP and $P_i$.

One potential problem with the oxidative regeneration of $NAD^+$ is that the reactions of oxidative phosphorylation occur within the mitochondria, whereas glycolysis is a cytosolic process, and the inner mitochondrial membrane is impermeable to NADH and to $NAD^+$. Without regeneration of the $NAD^+$ in the cytoplasm, glycolysis will stop so there must be a mechanism for the effective oxidation of the NADH formed during glycolysis. This separation is overcome by a number of substrate shuttles which transfer reducing equivalents into the mitochondrion.

Some of the pyruvate formed may be converted to the amino acid alanine. Some may also be converted to the four-carbon compound oxaloacetate by the incorporation of $CO_2$ in a reaction catalysed by pyruvate carboxylase. This conversion to oxaloacetate can be the first step in the resynthesis of glucose by the process of gluconeogenesis. Alternatively, this may be important as an anapleurotic reaction: these are reactions which maintain the intracellular concentration of crucial intermediates (e.g. of the TCA cycle) which might otherwise become depleted.

## Carbohydrate and fat stores

Carbohydrates (CHO) are stored in the body as the glucose polymer called glycogen. Normally, about 300–400 g of glycogen is stored in the muscles of an adult human. Skeletal muscle contains a significant store of glycogen in the sarcoplasm. The glycogen content of skeletal muscle at rest is approximately $54–72\,g \cdot kg^{-1}$ dm (300–400 mmol glucosyl units $\cdot kg^{-1}$ dm). The liver also contains glycogen; about 90–110 g are stored in the liver of an adult human in the postabsorptive state, which can be released into the circulation in order to maintain the blood glucose concentration at about $5\,mmol \cdot l^{-1}$ ($0.9\,g \cdot l^{-1}$). Fats are stored as triacylglycerol mainly in white adipose tissue. This must first be broken down by a lipase enzyme to release free fatty acids (FFA) into the circulation for uptake by working muscle. Skeletal muscle also contains some triacylglycerol (about $50\,mmol \cdot kg^{-1}$ dm) which can be used as energy source during exercise following lipolysis, and this source of fuel may become relatively more important after exercise training. Fat stores in the body are far larger than those of CHO (Table 2.3) and fat is a more efficient storage form of energy, releasing $37\,kJ \cdot g^{-1}$, whereas CHO releases $16\,kJ \cdot g^{-1}$. Each gram of CHO stored also retains about 3 g of water, further decreasing the efficiency of CHO as an energy source. The energy cost of running a marathon is about 12 000 kJ; if this could be achieved by the oxidation of

fat alone, the total amount of fat required would be about 320 g, whereas 750 g of CHO and an additional 2.3 kg of associated water would be required if CHO oxidation were the sole source of energy. Apart from considerations of the weight to be carried, this amount of CHO exceeds the total amount normally stored in the liver, muscles and blood combined. The total storage capacity for fat is extremely large, and for most practical purposes the amount of energy stored in the form of fat is far in excess of that required for any exercise task (Table 2.3).

Protein is not stored, other than as functionally important molecules (e.g. structural proteins, enzymes, ion channels, receptors, contractile proteins, etc.), and the concentration of free amino acids in most extracellular and intracellular body fluids is quite low (e.g. total free amino acid concentration in muscle sarcoplasm is about $50\,mmol \cdot l^{-1}$). It is not surprising, then, that in most situations, CHO and fats supply most of the energy required to regenerate ATP to fuel muscular work. In most situations, protein catabolism contributes less than 5% of the energy provision for muscle contraction during physical activity. Protein catabolism can provide both ketogenic and glucogenic amino acids which may eventually be oxidized either by deamination and conversion into one of the intermediate substrates in the TCA cycle, or conversion to pyruvate or acetoacetate and eventual transformation to acetyl-CoA. During starvation and when glycogen

Table 2.3 Energy stores in the average man.

|  | Mass (kg) | Energy (kJ) | Exercise time (min) |
|---|---|---|---|
| Liver glycogen | 0.08 | 1 280 | 16 |
| Muscle glycogen | 0.40 | 6 400 | 80 |
| Blood glucose | 0.01 | 160 | 2 |
| Fat | 10.5 | 388 500 | 4856 |
| Protein | 12.0 | 204 000 | 2550 |

Values assume a body mass of 70 kg and a fat content of 15% of body mass. The value for blood glucose includes the glucose content of extracellular fluid. Not all of this, and not more than a very small part of the total protein, is available for use during exercise. Also shown are the approximate times these stores would last for if they were the only source of energy available during exercise at marathon running pace (equivalent to an energy expenditure of about $80\,kJ \cdot min^{-1}$).

stores become depleted, protein catabolism may become an increasingly important source of energy for muscular work.

## Regulation of energy metabolism

### Intracellular factors

Experiments in which muscle biopsies were taken before and immediately after exercise indicate that the intramuscular ATP concentration remains fairly constant. Thus, ATP is constantly being regenerated by other energy-liberating reactions, at a rate equal to which it is being used. This situation provides a sensitive mechanism for the control of energy metabolism within the cell. The sum of cellular ATP, ADP and AMP concentrations is termed the total adenine nucleotide pool. The extent to which the total adenine nucleotide pool is phosphorylated is known as the energy charge of the cell, and it is a good indicator of the energy status of the cell. The rate at which ATP is resynthesized during exercise is known to be regulated by the energy charge of the muscle cell. For example, the decline in cellular concentration of ATP at the onset of muscle force generation and parallel increases in ADP and AMP concentrations (i.e. a decline in the energy charge) will directly stimulate anaerobic and oxidative ATP resynthesis. The relatively low concentration of ATP (and ADP) inside the cell means that any increase in the rate of hydrolysis of ATP (e.g. at the onset of exercise) will produce a rapid change in the ratio of ATP to ADP (and will also increase the intracellular concentration of AMP). These changes, in turn, activate enzymes which immediately stimulate the breakdown of intramuscular fuel stores to provide energy for ATP resynthesis. In this way, energy metabolism increases rapidly following the start of exercise.

ATP, ADP and AMP act as allosteric activators or inhibitors of the enzymatic reactions involved in PCr, CHO and fat degradation and utilization (Fig. 2.6). For example, as already mentioned, creatine kinase, the enzyme responsible for the rapid rephosphorylation of ATP at the initiation of muscle force generation, is rapidly activated by an increase in cytoplasmic ADP concentration and is inhibited by an increase in cellular ATP concentration. Similarly, glycogen phosphorylase, the enzyme which catalyses the conversion of glycogen to glucose-1-phosphate, is activated by increases in AMP and $P_i$ (and calcium ion) concentration and is inhibited by an increase in ATP concentration.

The rate limiting step in the glycolytic pathway is the conversion of fructose-6-phosphate to fructose-1,6-diphosphate and is catalysed by phosphofructokinase (PFK). The activity of this complex enzyme is affected by many intracellular factors, and it plays an important role in controlling flux through the pathway. The PFK reaction is the first opportunity for regulation at a point which will affect the metabolism of both glucose and glycogen. The activity of PFK is stimulated by increased concentrations of ADP, AMP, $P_i$, ammonia and fructose-6-phosphate and is inhibited by ATP, $H^+$, citrate, phosphoglycerate and phosphoenolpyruvate. Thus, the rate of glycolysis will be stimulated when ATP and glycogen breakdown are increased at the onset of exercise. Accumulation of citrate and thus inhibition of PFK may occur when the rate of the TCA cycle is high and provides a means whereby the limited stores of CHO can be spared when the availability of fatty acids is high. Inhibition of PFK will also cause accumulation of G6P, which will inhibit the activity of hexokinase and reduce the entry into the muscle of glucose which is not needed.

Conversion of pyruvate to acetyl-CoA by the pyruvate dehydrogenase complex is the rate-limiting step in CHO oxidation and is stimulated by an increased intracellular concentration of calcium, and decreased ratios of ATP/ADP, acetyl-CoA/free CoA and NADH/NAD$^+$ ratio and thus offers another site of regulation of the relative rates of fat and CHO catabolism. If the rate of formation of acetyl-CoA from the β-oxidation of fatty acids is high, as after 1–2 h of submaximal exercise, then this could reduce the amount of acetyl-CoA derived from pyruvate, cause accumulation of phosphoenol pyruvate

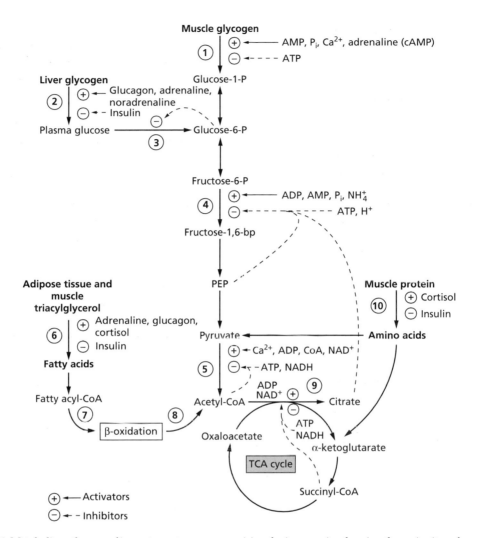

**Fig. 2.6** Metabolic pathways of importance to energy provision during exercise showing the main sites of regulation and the principal hormonal and allosteric activators and inhibitors. Enzymes: **1**, glycogen phosphorylase (muscle); **2**, glycogen phosphorylase (liver); **3**, hexokinase; **4**, phosphofructokinase; **5**, pyruvate dehydrogenase; **6**, hormone-sensitive lipase; **7**, carnitine acyl-transferase; **8**, 3-hydroxyacyl dehydrogenase; **9**, citrate synthase; **10**, proteases. AMP, adenosine monophosphate; cAMP, cyclic AMP; PEP, phosphoenolpyruvate; $P_i$, inorganic phosphate; TCA, tricarboxylic acid.

and inhibition of PFK, thus slowing the rate of glycolysis and glycogenolysis. This forms the basis of the 'glucose–fatty acid cycle' proposed by Randle *et al.* (1963), which has for many years been accepted to be the key regulatory mechanism in the control of CHO and fat utilization by skeletal muscle. However, recent work has challenged this hypothesis and it seems likely that the regulation of the integration of fat and CHO catabolism in exercising skeletal muscle must reside elsewhere, e.g. at the level of glucose uptake into muscle, glycogen breakdown by phosphorylase or the entry of fatty acids into the mitochondria. A detailed discussion is beyond the scope of this review; for further details, see Hargreaves (1995) and Maughan *et al.* (1997).

A key regulatory point in the TCA cycle is the reaction catalysed by citrate synthase. The activity of this enzyme is inhibited by ATP, NADH, succinyl-CoA and fatty acyl-CoA; the activity of the enzyme is also affected by citrate availability. Hence, when cellular energy levels are high, flux through the TCA cycle is relatively low, but can be greatly increased when ATP and NADH utilization is increased, as during exercise.

### Hormones

Many hormones influence energy metabolism in the body (for a detailed review, see Galbo 1983). During exercise, the interaction between insulin, glucagon and the catecholamines (adrenaline and noradrenaline) is mostly responsible for fuel substrate availability and utilization; cortisol and growth hormone also have some significant effects.

Insulin is secreted by the β-cells of the islets of Langerhans in the pancreas. Its basic biological effects are to inhibit lipolysis and increase the uptake of glucose from the blood by the tissues, especially skeletal muscle, liver and adipose tissue; the cellular uptake of amino acids is also stimulated by insulin. These effects reduce the plasma glucose concentration, inhibit the release of glucose from the liver, promote the synthesis of glycogen (in liver and muscle), promote synthesis of lipid and inhibit FFA release (in adipose tissue), increase muscle amino acid uptake and enhance protein synthesis. The primary stimulus for increased insulin secretion is a rise in the blood glucose concentration (e.g. following a meal). Exercise usually results in a fall in insulin secretion.

Glucagon is secreted by the α-cells of the pancreatic islets and basically exerts effects that are opposite to those of insulin. It raises the blood glucose level by increasing the rate of glycogen breakdown (glycogenolysis) in the liver. It also promotes the formation of glucose from non-carbohydrate precursors (gluconeogenesis) in the liver. The primary stimulus for increased secretion of glucagon is a fall in the concentration of glucose in blood. During most types of exercise, the blood glucose concentration does not fall, but during prolonged exercise, when liver glycogen stores become depleted, a drop in the blood glucose concentration (hypoglycaemia) may occur.

The catecholamines adrenaline and noradrenaline are released from the adrenal medulla. Noradrenaline is also released from sympathetic nerve endings and leakage from such synapses appears to be the main source of the noradrenaline found in blood plasma. The catecholamines have many systemic effects throughout the body, including stimulation of the heart rate and contractility and alteration of blood vessel diameters. They also influence substrate availability, with the effects of adrenaline being the more important of the two. Adrenaline, like glucagon, promotes glycogenolysis in both liver and muscle (see Fig. 2.6). Adrenaline also promotes lipolysis in adipose tissue, increasing the availability of plasma FFA and inhibits insulin secretion. The primary stimulus for catecholamine secretion is the activation of the sympathetic nervous system by stressors such as exercise, hypotension and hypoglycaemia. Substantial increases in the plasma catecholamine concentration can occur within seconds of the onset of high-intensity exercise. However, the relative exercise intensity has to be above about 50% $\dot{V}o_{2max.}$ in order to significantly elevate the plasma catecholamine concentration.

Growth hormone, secreted from the anterior pituitary gland, also stimulates mobilization of FFA from adipose tissue and increases in plasma growth hormone concentration are related to the intensity of exercise performed. During prolonged strenuous exercise, cortisol secretion from the adrenal cortex is increased. Cortisol is a steroid hormone that increases the effectiveness of the actions of catecholamines in some tissues (e.g. its actions further promote lipolysis in adipose tissue). However, its main effects are to promote protein degradation and amino acid release from muscle and to stimulate gluconeogenesis in the liver. The primary stimulus to cortisol secretion is stress-induced release of adrenocorticotrophic hormone from the anterior pituitary gland.

## Metabolic responses to exercise

Undoubtedly the most important factor influencing the metabolic response to exercise is the exercise intensity. The physical fitness of the subject also modifies the metabolic response to exercise and other factors, including exercise duration, substrate availability, nutritional status, diet, feeding during exercise, mode of exercise, prior exercise, drugs and environmental factors, such as temperature and altitude, are also important. Several of these factors are dealt with in subsequent chapters and here a brief discussion is limited to consideration of the effects of exercise intensity, duration and training on the metabolic responses to exercise and the possible metabolic causes of fatigue.

### High-intensity exercise

ATP is the only fuel that can be used directly for skeletal muscle force generation. There is sufficient ATP available to fuel about 2 s of maximal intensity exercise and therefore for muscle force generation to continue it must be resynthesized very rapidly from ADP. During high-intensity exercise, the relatively low rate of ATP resynthesis from oxidative phosphorylation results in the rapid activation of anaerobic energy production from PCr and glycogen hydrolysis. PCr breakdown is initiated at the immediate onset of contraction to buffer the rapid accumulation of ADP resulting from ATP hydrolysis. However, the rate of PCr hydrolysis begins to decline after only a few seconds of maximal force generation (Fig. 2.7).

If high-intensity exercise is to continue beyond only a few seconds, there must be marked increases in the contribution from glycolysis to

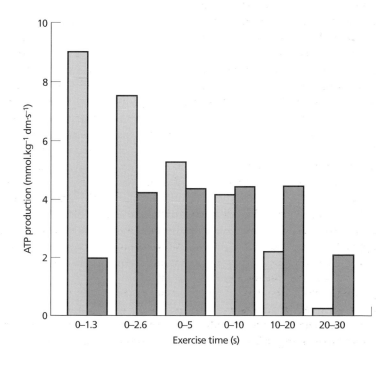

**Fig. 2.7** Rates of anaerobic ATP resynthesis from phosphocreatine (PCr) hydrolysis (▢) and glycolysis (◼) during maximal isometric contraction in human skeletal muscle. Rates were calculated from metabolite changes measured in biopsy samples of muscle obtained during intermittent electrically evoked contractions over a period of 30 s. Note that the rate of ATP resynthesis from PCr hydrolysis is highest in the first few seconds of exercise, but falls to almost zero after 20 s. The rate of ATP resynthesis from glycolysis peaks after about 5 s, is maintained for a further 15 s but falls during the last 10 s of the exercise bout. From Maughan *et al.* (1997).

ATP resynthesis. Anaerobic glycolysis involves several more steps than PCr hydrolysis. However, compared with oxidative phosphorylation, it is still very rapid. It is initiated at the onset of contraction, but, unlike PCr hydrolysis, does not reach a maximal rate until after 5 s of exercise and can be maintained at this level for several seconds during maximal muscle force generation (Fig. 2.7). The mechanism(s) responsible for the eventual decline in glycolysis during maximal exercise have not been resolved. Exercise at an intensity equivalent to 95–100% $\dot{V}_{O_{2max.}}$ can be sustained for durations approaching 5 min before fatigue is evident. Under these conditions, CHO oxidation can make a significant contribution to ATP production, but its relative importance is often underestimated.

Fatigue has been defined as the inability to maintain a given or expected force or power output and is an inevitable feature of maximal exercise. Typically, the loss of power output or force production is likely to be in the region of 40–60% of the maximum observed during 30 s of all-out exercise. Fatigue is not a simple process with a single cause; many factors may contribute to fatigue. However, during maximal short duration exercise, it will be caused primarily by a gradual decline in anaerobic ATP production or increase in ADP accumulation caused by a depletion of PCr and a fall in the rate of glycolysis. In high-intensity exercise lasting 1–5 min, lactic acid accumulation may contribute to the fatigue process. At physiological pH values, lactic acid almost completely dissociates into its constituent lactate and hydrogen ions; studies using animal muscle preparations have demonstrated that direct inhibition of force production can be achieved by increasing hydrogen and lactate ion concentrations. A reduced muscle pH may cause some inhibition of PFK and phosphorylase, reducing the rate of ATP resynthesis from glycolysis, though it is thought that this is unlikely to be important in exercising muscle because the *in vitro* inhibition of PFK by a reduced pH is reversed in the presence of other allosteric activators such as AMP (Spriet 1991). It would also appear that lactate and hydrogen ion accumula-

tion can result in muscle fatigue independent of one another but the latter is the more commonly cited mechanism. However, although likely to be related to the fatigue process it is unlikely that both lactate and hydrogen ion accumulation is wholly responsible for the development of muscle fatigue. For example, studies involving human volunteers have demonstrated that muscle force generation following fatiguing exercise can recover rapidly, despite also having a very low muscle pH value. The general consensus at the moment appears to be that the maintenance of force production during high-intensity exercise is pH dependent, but the initial force generation is more related to PCr availability.

One of the consequences of rapid PCr hydrolysis during high-intensity exercise is the accumulation of $P_i$, which has been shown to inhibit muscle contraction coupling directly. However, the simultaneous depletion of PCr and $P_i$ accumulation makes it difficult to separate the effect of PCr depletion from $P_i$ accumulation *in vivo*. This problem is further confounded by the parallel increases in hydrogen and lactate ions which occur during high-intensity exercise. All of these metabolites have been independently implicated with muscle fatigue.

As described earlier, calcium release by the sarcoplasmic reticulum as a consequence of muscle depolarization is essential for the activation of muscle contraction coupling. It has been demonstrated that during fatiguing contractions there is a slowing of calcium transport and progressively smaller calcium transients which has been attributed to a reduction in calcium reuptake by the sarcoplasmic reticulum and/or increased calcium binding. Strong evidence that a disruption of calcium handling is responsible for fatigue comes from studies showing that the stimulation of sarcoplasmic reticulum calcium release caused by the administration of calcium to isolated muscle can improve muscle force production, even in the presence of a low muscle pH. Alternatively, fatigue during high-intensity exercise may be associated with an excitation-coupling failure and possibly a reduced nervous drive due to reflex inhibition at the spinal level.

In the latter hypothesis, accumulation of interstitial potassium in muscle may play a major role (Sjogaard 1991; Bangsbo 1997).

When repeated bouts of maximal exercise are performed, the rates of muscle PCr hydrolysis and lactate accumulation decline. In the case of PCr, this response is thought to occur because of incomplete PCr resynthesis occurring during recovery between successive exercise bouts. However, the mechanism(s) responsible for the fall in the rate of lactate accumulation is unclear.

It is commonly accepted that nutrition is not of great importance to individuals involved in high-intensity exercise. Muscle glycogen availability *per se* is not usually considered to be responsible for fatigue during high-intensity exercise, providing the pre-exercise glycogen store is not depleted to below $100 \, mmol \cdot kg^{-1} \, dm$. It is even unlikely that glycogen availability will limit performance during repeated bouts of exercise, due to the decline in glycogenolysis and lactate production that occurs under these conditions. However, there is a growing body of evidence to indicate that dietary creatine intake may be a necessary requirement for individuals wishing to optimize performance during high-intensity exercise.

### Prolonged exercise

The term *prolonged exercise* is usually used to describe exercise intensities that can be sustained for between 30 and 180 min. Since the rate of ATP demand is relatively low compared with high-intensity exercise, PCr, CHO and fat can all contribute to energy production. The rates of PCr degradation and lactate production during the first minutes of prolonged exercise are closely related to the intensity of exercise performed, and it is likely that energy production during this period would be compromised without this contribution from anaerobic metabolism. However, once a steady state has been reached, CHO and fat oxidation become the principal means of resynthesizing ATP. Muscle glycogen is the principal fuel during the first 30 min of exercise at 60–80% $\dot{V}O_{2max}$. During the early stages of exercise, fat oxidation is limited by the delay in the mobilization of fatty acids from adipose tissue. At rest following an overnight fast, the plasma FFA concentration is about $0.4 \, mmol \cdot l^{-1}$. This is commonly observed to fall during the first hour of moderate intensity exercise (Fig. 2.8), followed by a progressive increase as lipolysis is stimulated by the actions of catecholamines, glucagon and cortisol. During very prolonged exercise, the plasma FFA concentration can reach 1.5–$2.0 \, mmol \cdot l^{-1}$ and muscle uptake of blood-borne FFA is proportional to the plasma FFA concentration. The glycerol released from adipose tissue cannot be used directly by muscle that lacks the enzyme glycerol kinase. However, glycerol (together with alanine and lactate) is taken up by the liver and used as a gluconeogenic precursor to help maintain liver glucose output as liver

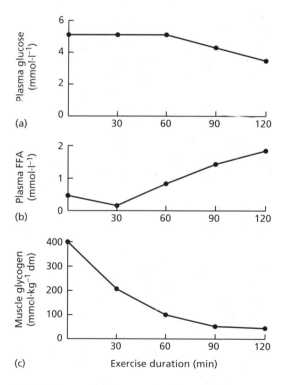

**Fig. 2.8** Changes in the concentrations of (a) plasma glucose, (b) plasma free fatty acids (FFA), and (c) muscle glycogen during continuous exercise at an intensity equivalent to about 70% $\dot{V}O_{2max}$.

glycogen levels decline. The utilization of blood glucose is greater at higher workrates and increases with exercise duration during prolonged submaximal exercise and peaks after about 90 min (Fig. 2.9). The decline in blood glucose uptake after this time is attributable to the increasing availability of plasma FFA as fuel (which appears to directly inhibit muscle glucose uptake) and the depletion of liver glycogen stores.

At marathon-running pace, muscle CHO stores alone could fuel about 80 min of exercise before becoming depleted (Table 2.3). However, the simultaneous utilization of body fat and hepatic CHO stores enables ATP production to be maintained and exercise to continue. Ultimately, though, ATP production becomes compromised due to muscle and hepatic CHO stores becoming depleted and the inability of fat oxidation to increase sufficiently to offset this deficit. The rate of ATP resynthesis from fat oxidation alone cannot meet the ATP requirement for exercise intensities higher than about 50–60% $\dot{V}o_{2max}$. It is currently unknown which factor limits the maximal rate of fat oxidation during exercise (i.e.

why it cannot increase to compensate for CHO depletion), but it must precede acetyl-CoA formation, as from this point fat and CHO share the same fate. The limitation may reside in the rate of uptake of FFA into muscle from blood or the transport of FFA into the mitochondria rather than in the rate of β-oxidation of FFA in the mitochondria.

It is generally accepted that the glucose–fatty acid cycle regulates the integration of CHO and fat oxidation during prolonged exercise. However, whilst this may be true of resting muscle, recent evidence (Dyck *et al.* 1993) suggests that the cycle does not operate in exercising muscle and that the site of regulation must reside elsewhere (e.g. at the level of phosphorylase and/or malonyl-CoA). From the literature, it would appear that the integration of muscle CHO and fat utilization during prolonged exercise is complex and unresolved.

The glycogen store of human muscle is fairly insensitive to change in sedentary individuals. However, the combination of exercise and dietary manipulation can have dramatic effects on muscle glycogen storage. A clear positive relationship has been shown to exist between muscle glycogen content and subsequent endurance performance. Furthermore, the ingestion of CHO during prolonged exercise has been shown to decrease muscle glycogen utilization and fat mobilization and oxidation, and to increase the rate of CHO oxidation and endurance capacity. It is clear therefore that the contribution of orally ingested CHO to total ATP production under these conditions must be greater than that normally derived from fat oxidation. The precise biochemical mechanism by which muscle glycogen depletion results in fatigue is presently unresolved (Green 1991). However, it is plausible that the inability of muscle to maintain the rate of ATP synthesis in the glycogen depleted state results in ADP and $P_i$ accumulation and consequently fatigue development.

Unlike skeletal muscle, starvation will rapidly deplete the liver of CHO. The rate of hepatic glucose release in resting postabsorptive individuals is sufficient to match the CHO demands of

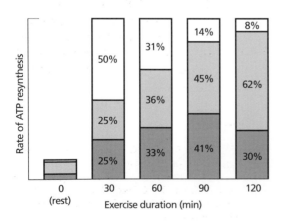

**Fig. 2.9** Changes in the relative contributions of the major fuel sources to ATP resynthesis during prolonged submaximal exercise at an intensity equivalent to about 70% $\dot{V}o_{2max}$ (approximately 10 times the resting metabolic rate). ■, blood glucose; ▨, plasma free fatty acids; □, muscle glycogen and triacylglycerol.

only the central nervous system. Approximately 70% of this release is derived from liver CHO stores and the remainder from liver gluconeogenesis. During exercise, the rate of hepatic glucose release has been shown to be related to exercise intensity. Ninety percent of this release is derived from liver CHO stores, ultimately resulting in liver glycogen depletion.

Thus, CHO ingestion during exercise could also delay fatigue development by slowing the rate of liver glycogen depletion and helping to maintain the blood glucose concentration. Central fatigue is a possibility during prolonged exercise and undoubtedly the development of hypoglycaemia could contribute to this.

## Metabolic adaptation to exercise training

Adaptations to aerobic endurance training include increases in capillary density and mitochondrial size and number in trained muscle. The activity of TCA cycle and other oxidative enzymes are increased with a concomitant increase in the capacity to oxidize both lipid and CHO. Training adaptations in muscle affect substrate utilization. Endurance training also increases the relative cross-sectional area of type I fibres, increases intramuscular content of triacylglycerol, and increases the capacity to use fat as an energy source during submaximal exercise. Trained subjects also appear to demonstrate an increased reliance on intramuscular triacylglycerol as an energy source during exercise. These effects, and other physiological effects of training, including increased maximum cardiac output and $\dot{V}o_{2max}$, improved oxygen delivery to working muscle (Saltin 1985) and attenuated hormonal responses to exercise (Galbo 1983), decrease the rate of utilization of muscle glycogen and blood glucose and decrease the rate of accumulation of lactate during submaximal exercise. These adaptations contribute to the marked improvement in endurance capacity following training.

Alterations in substrate use with endurance training could be due, at least in part, to a lesser degree of disturbance to ATP homeostasis during exercise. With an increased mitochondrial oxidative capacity after training, smaller decreases in ATP and PCr and smaller increases in ADP and $P_i$ are needed during exercise to balance the rate of ATP synthesis with the rate of ATP utilization. In other words, with more mitochondria, the amount of oxygen as well as the ADP and $P_i$ required per mitochondrion will be less after training than before training. The smaller increase in ADP concentration would result in less formation of AMP by the myokinase reaction, and also less IMP and ammonia would be formed as a result of AMP deamination. Smaller increases in the concentrations of ADP, AMP, $P_i$ and ammonia could account for the slower rate of glycolysis and glycogenolysis in trained than in untrained muscle.

Training for strength, power or speed has little if any effect on aerobic capacity. Heavy resistance training or sprinting bring about specific changes in the immediate (ATP and PCr) and short-term (glycolytic) energy delivery systems, increases in muscle buffering capacity and improvements in strength and/or sprint performance. Heavy resistance training for several months causes hypertrophy of the muscle fibres, thus increasing total muscle mass and the maximum power output that can be developed. Stretch, contraction and damage of muscle fibres during exercise provide the stimuli for adaptation, which involves changes in the expression of different myosin isoforms.

## References

Åstrand, P.-O. & Rodahl, K. (1986) *Textbook of Work Physiology*. McGraw-Hill, New York.

Bangsbo, J. (1997) Physiology of muscle fatigue during intense exercise. In *The Clinical Pharmacology of Sport and Exercise* (ed. T. Reilly & M. Orme), pp. 123–133. Elsevier, Amsterdam.

Dyck, D.J., Putman, C.T., Heigenhauser, G.J.F., Hultman, E. & Spriet, L.L. (1993) Regulation of fat–carbohydrate interaction in skeletal muscle during intense aerobic cycling. *American Journal of Physiology* **265**, E852–E859.

Frank, G.B. (1982) Roles of intracellular and trigger calcium ions in excitation–contraction coupling in skeletal muscle. *Canadian Journal of Physiology and Pharmacology* **60**, 427–439.

Galbo, H. (1983) *Hormonal and Metabolic Adaptation to Exercise*. Verlag, New York.

Green, H.J. (1991) How important is endogenous muscle glycogen to fatigue in prolonged exercise? *Canadian Journal of Physiology and Pharmacology* **69**, 290–297.

Hargreaves, M. (1995) *Exercise Metabolism*. Human Kinetics, Champaign, IL.

Komi, P.V. & Karlsson, J. (1978) Skeletal muscle fibre types, enzyme activities and physical performance in young males and females. *Acta Physiologica Scandinavica* **103**, 210–218.

Maughan, R.J., Gleeson, M. & Greenhaff, P.L. (1997) *Biochemistry of Exercise and Training*. Oxford University Press, Oxford.

Randle, P.J., Garland, P.B., Hales, C.N. & Newsholme, E.A. (1963) The glucose fatty acid cycle: its role in insulin sensitivity and the metabolic disturbances of diabetes mellitus. *Lancet* **i**, 786–789.

Sahlin, K. & Broberg, S. (1990) Adenine nucleotide depletion in human muscle during exercise: causality and significance of AMP deamination. *International Journal of Sports Medicine* **11**, S62–S67.

Saltin, B. (1985) Physiological adaptation to physical conditioning. *Acta Medica Scandinavica* **711** (Suppl.), 11–24.

Sjogaard, G. (1991) Role of exercise-induced potassium fluxes underlying muscle fatigue: a brief review. *Canadian Journal of Physiology and Pharmacology* **69**, 238–245.

Spriet, L.L. (1991) Phosphofructokinase activity and acidosis during short-term tetanic contractions. *Canadian Journal of Physiology and Pharmacology* **69**, 298–304.

# Chapter 3

## Exercise, Nutrition and Health

ADRIANNE E. HARDMAN

### Introduction

By virtue of its mass and unique potential to increase metabolic rate, skeletal muscle is man's largest 'metabolic organ'. Energy expenditure is increased profoundly during exercise with the body's large muscles and individuals who engage regularly and frequently in such exercise have enhanced energy requirements. These are met through increased nutrient intake, particularly of carbohydrate, so that the relative contributions of macronutrients to energy intake may be altered. This in itself may constitute a more healthy diet but, in addition, the metabolic handling of dietary fats and carbohydrates is improved, changes which help reduce the risk of developing several chronic diseases, specifically atherosclerotic vascular diseases, non-insulin-dependent diabetes (NIDDM, also known as adult-onset or type II diabetes) and possibly some cancers (Bouchard *et al.* 1994).

An example of an association between disease risk and energy turnover is given in Table 3.1, which shows average daily energy intakes in prospective studies of coronary heart disease (CHD). Men who subsequently had fatal attacks showed lower levels of energy intake than survivors, an apparent paradox in the light of the increase in CHD risk associated with overweight, obesity and the deleterious metabolic sequelae of these. One explanation is that the men with higher energy intakes were more physically active, and that their exercise afforded a level of protection against CHD, compared with more sedentary men who ate less.

Thus, the transition from a sedentary to an active state is associated with a higher energy turnover, with important implications for the transport, storage and utilization of the body's metabolic fuels. All of these are altered in the trained state such that regular exercisers experience a lower risk of what has been called 'metabolic, hypertensive cardiovascular disease'. Higher energy turnover may also be associated with improved weight regulation because food intake appears to be more closely coupled to energy expenditure with more exercise.

Rather than prolonging life, regular exercise protects against premature death, with an estimated increase in longevity in men on average of one or two years (Paffenbarger *et al.* 1986). Moreover, lower all-cause mortality has recently been reported for physically active women (Blair *et al.* 1996), although evidence is much less extensive. People who take exercise also maintain a better quality of life into old age, being less likely than sedentary individuals to develop functional limitations.

This chapter will identify some of the health gains which accrue from the biological interactions between exercise and the body's metabolism of dietary carbohydrate and fats. For discussion of the evidence for a specific role of diet in promoting health, the reader is referred to other sources (WHO 1990).

**Table 3.1** Average daily energy intake (MJ) and future risk of coronary heart disease. Adapted from Wood (1987).

| Cohort | Heart disease victims | Survivors |
| --- | --- | --- |
| English banking and London bus workers | 11.11 | 12.00 |
| Framingham, Massachusetts | 9.91 | 10.97 |
| Puerto Rico | 9.30 | 10.02 |
| Honolulu, Hawaii | 8.99 | 9.70 |

## Atherosclerotic vascular diseases

Pathological changes to the arterial wall give rise to atherosclerotic plaques, complex structures which result from proliferation of the smooth muscle cells and collagen, with deposition of cholesterol-rich lipid. These probably begin as fatty streaks which develop when lipid-laden macrophages accumulate after the integrity of the endothelium is breached and blood components are exposed to collagen in the wall of the artery. The clinical outcome depends on the site(s) and extent of the lesion: in coronary arteries, myocardial blood flow is reduced, leading to chest pain on effort (angina) and a risk of thrombotic occlusion (heart attack) and/or disturbances in the electrical coordination of contraction; blood supply to the limbs is impaired when the arteries supplying the legs are narrowed, imposing severe limits on walking capability; and stroke occurs when there is thrombolytic occlusion of a cerebral artery or a local haemorrhage from a vessel with atherosclerotic damage. Links with nutrition are clear from, for example, the association between levels of saturated fat in the diet and the risk of CHD.

### Coronary heart disease

Epidemiological studies have shown significant associations between indices of both physical activity (a behaviour) and physical fitness (a set of characteristics arising from the regular pursuance of this behaviour) and risk of the commonest manifestation of atherosclerosis, CHD—a disease responsible for one in four male deaths and one in five female deaths in the UK in 1994.

We must be careful in our interpretation of associations, however, because exercisers may be constitutionally different from sedentary people in ways which decrease the likelihood of their developing the disease. Complementary scientific evidence of plausible mechanisms has much to contribute and the role of exercise in this will be discussed later.

More than 50 population studies have compared the risk of CHD in physically active men with that of their sedentary counterparts. Careful scrutiny of their findings shows that sedentary men experience about twice the risk seen in active men (see Whaley & Blair 1995). This relative risk is of the same order of magnitude as that associated with hypertension (systolic blood pressure $>150\,mmHg$ vs. $<120\,mmHg$), smoking ($\geq20$ cigarettes$\cdot$day$^{-1}$ vs. no smoking) and high serum total cholesterol levels ($>6.9\,mmol\cdot l^{-1}$ vs. $\leq5.6\,mmol\cdot l^{-1}$). Estimates of the protective effect of exercise are highest in those studies with the soundest design and methodology and no study has found a *higher* risk in active men. The effect is independent of hypertension, smoking and high total cholesterol levels.

Early studies compared groups of men with different levels of occupational work. For example, postal workers who walked and cycled delivering mail and dock workers with high levels of habitual on-the-job energy expenditure experienced less heart disease than colleagues in less physically demanding jobs. Leisure time physical activity has also been studied and an inverse, graded relationship between leisure time physical activity and CHD was found among graduates (alumni) of Harvard and Pennsylvania universities (Paffenbarger *et al.*

1986); the risk of first attack was one quarter to one third lower in men who expended more than $8.36\,MJ\cdot week^{-1}$ ($2000\,kcal\cdot week^{-1}$) in physical activity (sports, garden work, walking, stair-climbing, etc.) than in classmates whose exercise energy expenditure was lower, i.e. high total energy expenditure in exercise was a determinant of risk.

By contrast, prospective study of English civil servants found no association between total exercise energy expenditure and risk of heart attack (Morris *et al.* 1990); only men reporting 'vigorous' exercise experienced a lower risk than sedentary men. Vigorous was defined as exercise likely to involve peaks of energy expenditure of $31\,kJ\cdot min^{-1}$ ($7.5\,kcal\cdot min^{-1}$) or more. This is about the rate of energy expenditure of a middle-aged man of average weight during fast walking, so it is not surprising that men who reported that their usual speed of walking was 'fast' ($>6.4\,km\cdot h^{-1}$) experienced a particularly low rate of attack. Low rates were also reported for men who did considerable amounts of cycling.

Increasingly, studies have measured physical fitness rather than, or as well as, physical activity. Their findings are broadly similar, i.e. a two- to threefold increase in the risk of cardiovascular death in men when comparing the least fit with the most fit groups (Whaley & Blair 1995). The limited data available suggest an effect of at least this magnitude for women.

Given the diverse methodologies and cohorts studied, the clarity with which the inverse, graded relationship between level of physical activity or fitness and risk of mortality from CHD emerges is noteworthy. Figure 3.1 summarizes the findings of seven studies in which either leisure time activity (questionnaire) or fitness (laboratory exercise test) was assessed prior to a follow-up period of 7–17 years. The precise pattern differs between studies, but it is clear that, whilst men with only moderate levels of activity or fitness experience some degree of pro-tection, higher levels tend to confer greater protection. Some studies, however, suggest that the relationship may be curvilinear—CHD risk decreasing steeply at the lower end of the contin-uum, reaching an asymptote in the mid-range. Thus, for men in the age group most studied (approximately 40–60 years), values for $\dot{V}o_{2max.}$ of around $35\,ml\cdot kg^{-1}\cdot min^{-1}$ have been proposed as being sufficient to confer a worthwhile—not necessarily optimal—decrease in risk; evidence for women is scanty, but a comparable value is probably at least 2 or $3\,ml\cdot kg^{-1}\cdot min^{-1}$ lower.

Two aspects of the evidence strengthen the argument that the relation of activity and fitness with CHD risk may be causal. First, only current

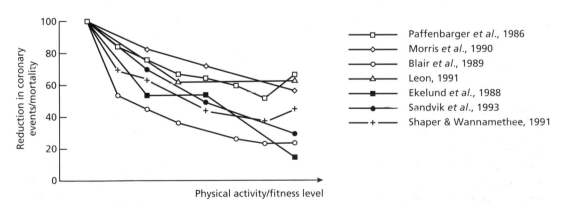

**Fig. 3.1** The relationship between the level of physical activity (Paffenbarger *et al.* 1986; Ekelund *et al.* 1988; Morris *et al.* 1990; Leon 1991; Shaper & Wannamethee 1991) or fitness (Blair *et al.* 1989; Sandvik *et al.* 1993) and risk of coronary heart disease among men in prospective studies. Adapted from Haskell (1994).

and continuing activity protects against heart disease; men who were active in their youth but became sedentary in middle-age experience a risk similar to that of men who had never been active. Second, men who improved either their physical activity level or their fitness level between one observation period and another some years later experienced a lower risk of death than men who remain sedentary. To put these levels of risk reduction into perspective, taking up physical activity was as effective as stopping smoking.

The role of exercise intensity in determining CHD risk is still uncertain. Several key studies have shown substantial reductions in risk with accumulation of physical activity, most of which was at a moderate intensity (see Haskell 1994). However, other evidence argues that more vigorous physical activity may provide unique benefits. These uncertainties should not, however, detract from the wealth of evidence, gathered over a long period and in different populations, that identifies physical inactivity as a major risk factor for CHD.

Mechanisms by which exercise might confer a lower risk of CHD include effects on blood pressure, weight regulation, lipoprotein metabolism and insulin sensitivity—all of which are discussed below. Another suggestion, arising from the evidence referred to above that only current exercise protects against CHD, involves an effect on the acute phase of the disease—the thrombotic component, for example. This possibility is supported by associations between exercise habits and haemostatic factors and is an area justifying more research.

### Stroke

Atherosclerotic damage to cerebral arteries is a prominent feature of stroke, so an effect of habitual exercise on the risk of having a stroke is plausible, but there is little direct evidence. In the British Regional Heart Study (Wannamethee & Shaper 1992), the age-adjusted rate for strokes showed a steep and significant inverse gradient with physical activity category in men with or without heart disease or stroke at baseline; the risk in moderately active subjects was less than half that reported for inactive men. Data from the Honolulu Heart Program (Abbott et al. 1994) show an association between the risk of stroke and a physical activity index in older middle-aged men (55–68 years) but not in younger men (45–54 years); the excess incidence of haemorrhagic stroke in inactive/partially active men was three- to fourfold. For thromboembolic stroke, among non-smokers the risk for inactive men was nearly double that for active men but there was no effect in smokers.

### Hypertension

About 16% of men and 14% of women in England have hypertension (systolic blood pressure >159 mmHg and/or diastolic >94 mmHg). It is a major public health problem; even mild to moderate elevations in blood pressure substantially increase the risk of developing CHD, stroke, congestive heart failure and intermittent claudication in both men and women.

There is some evidence that high levels of physical activity decrease the risk of developing hypertension (see Paffenbarger et al. 1991). For example, of 5500 male Harvard alumni free of hypertension at entry to the study, 14% developed the disease during 14 years' observation. Contemporary vigorous exercise alone was associated with lower incidence, chiefly among men who were overweight-for-height. Similar conclusions arise from study of fitness levels in relation to risk of hypertension: during follow-up of 6000 men and women over 1–12 years (median, 4) the risk of developing hypertension was 1.5 times greater for those with low fitness (the bottom 75% of the sample) than for those deemed to have high fitness (the top 25%).

The rationale for a role for exercise in the prevention of hypertension is that, during exercise, there is marked dilation of blood vessels in active skeletal muscle, decreasing resistance to flow. This persists during the recovery period, possibly contributing to the chronic lowering of (arterial) blood pressure which is often associated with regular aerobic exercise. The proposition that exercise brings blood pressure down has been tested experimentally. Valid conclusions can only be drawn from studies including non-exercising control subjects, because blood pressures tend to fall with repeated measurements when people become accustomed to the procedure. Controlled exercise intervention trials have found an average reduction of 3/3 mmHg (systolic/diastolic) in normotensives, with somewhat greater reductions in borderline hypertensives and hypertensives, i.e. 6/7 mmHg and 10/8 mmHg, respectively (Bouchard *et al.* 1994). These conclusions are based on resting blood pressure measured in clinic or laboratory; reductions in measures made during the normal living conditions tend to be less consistent and smaller but more evidence is needed. Moderate intensity training ($<70\%$ $\dot{V}o_{2max.}$) leads to reductions in systolic blood pressure which are up to 40% greater than those resulting from training at higher intensity, possibly because of the lesser response of the sympathetic nervous system.

The blood-pressure lowering effect of exercise probably occurs very rapidly, possibly after as little as 1 week of exercise training. Repeated short-term effects during recovery from individual exercise sessions may therefore be important. For example, in sedentary hypertensives, blood pressure is reduced for up to 8–12 h after a single exercise session. Longer training programmes produce somewhat larger reductions in blood pressures, however, suggesting that adaptive effects of habitual exercise, i.e. training, may act synergistically to enhance short-term effects.

## Glucose/insulin dynamics

Diabetes mellitus afflicts about 2% of individuals in Western populations. By far the most common type is NIDDM, the incidence of which rises steeply with age. It is characterized by the failure of insulin to act effectively in target tissues such as muscle, liver and adipose tissue. The pancreas responds with enhanced secretion by its β-cells and plasma insulin levels are chronically high. Glucose intolerance (an abnormally high blood glucose response to a standard 75 g oral load) develops gradually, fasting plasma glucose and insulin levels rising in parallel until the former reaches 7–8 mmol·l⁻¹ (compared with normal values of around 4–5 mmol·l⁻¹). At this stage the β-cells of the pancreas fail to maintain adequate insulin secretion and so there is a progressive fall in the fasting concentration. Profound glucose intolerance then develops and the condition worsens to overt NIDDM, the severity of which is determined by the inadequacy of β-cell function.

Resistance to insulin-stimulated glucose uptake is the most important precursor of NIDDM and a common characteristic occurring in approximately 25% of the population. It is a prominent feature of obesity. Normal glucose tolerance is maintained but at the expense of hyperinsulinaemia, which leads to multiple derangements of metabolism—for example, high plasma levels of triacylglyceride (TAG) and low levels of high-density lipoprotein (HDL) cholesterol. In the longer term, these result in damage to blood vessels, with increased risk of developing CHD, hypertension and problems of the microcirculation, including renal disease and retinal damage.

### Risk of NIDDM

Prospective studies show an inverse relationship between energy expenditure in leisure time activity and the risk of subsequently developing NIDDM (Kriska *et al.* 1994). For example, among male ex-students of the University of Pennsylvania the incidence of NIDDM decreased by some 6% for each 2.1 MJ (500 kcal) expended per week in physical activity. US male physicians who exercised 'vigorously' at least once per week experienced only 64% of the risk of developing NIDDM, compared with those who exercised less frequently. Findings have been similar for middle-aged women, those taking part in vigorous exercise experiencing only two thirds of the risk seen in other women. There are indications that the influence of physical activity may be particularly strong in those who are overweight.

## Potential mechanisms

The primary targets for insulin-stimulated glucose disposal are skeletal muscle and adipose tissue and influences on their glucose transport and metabolism dictate whole-body responsiveness to insulin. Muscle, representing some 40% of body mass, is probably the more important tissue.

Insulin-mediated glucose uptake into skeletal muscle proceeds by a series of steps, the first of which is insulin binding to receptors on the outer surface of the cell membrane. Glucose transport is achieved via 'facilitated diffusion', a process which involves a mobile protein carrier (GLUT-4) which facilitates its transport across the membrane and is thought to be rate-limiting. Besides its action on glucose transport, insulin inhibits glycogenolysis, promoting glycogen synthesis. Muscle glycogen is reduced during exercise, creating the need for enhanced uptake and storage and raising the possibility that improved responsiveness of this tissue to insulin might exert an important influence on the body as a whole, explaining the lower incidence of NIDDM in physically active people.

It is more than 25 years since the first report of markedly lower plasma insulin concentrations in endurance-trained middle-aged men—both in the fasted state and after an oral glucose load—than in comparable sedentary men. These findings have generally been interpreted as a sign of increased insulin sensitivity in peripheral tissues, since hepatic glucose output is suppressed after glucose ingestion. Later studies have confirmed this, measuring reduced insulin secretion and a shift in the insulin/glucose disposal response curve, promoting glucose transport and storage. Whole-body non-oxidative glucose disposal during glucose infusion is higher in endurance-trained athletes than in sedentary controls. Total activity of glycogen synthase and insulin-stimulated activation of the enzyme is enhanced as trained muscle adapts to the increased intracellular availability of glucose by developing an enhanced capacity for glucose storage as glycogen.

The mechanisms by which training enhances glucose uptake in skeletal muscle are local rather than systemic and probably involve changes in levels of the muscle glucose transporter GLUT-4. Endurance-trained athletes possess higher levels of GLUT-4 than sedentary controls and levels are markedly higher in trained than in untrained muscle from the same individual, in association with a higher insulin-stimulated glucose uptake. Glucose uptake depends on its rate of delivery to the tissue, however, as well as that tissue's responsiveness to insulin. Insulin stimulates increases in blood flow to muscle in a dose-responsive manner and this effect could, speculatively, be enhanced in athletes because of improved capillarization.

Following each exercise session, glucose uptake into skeletal muscle increases. This is partly an insulin-independent contractile effect which persists for several hours afterwards but, in addition, the response to insulin of the glucose transport system is improved. This usually lasts longer, for at least 48h. As stated above, these may be responses to the need to replenish muscle glycogen; certainly exhaustive, intermittent glycogen-depleting exercise at 85% $\dot{V}o_{2max.}$ results in increased non-oxidative glucose disposal when measured 12h later.

When endurance-trained people refrain from training, their enhanced insulin action is rapidly reversed. The timescale of this reversal is not clear; training effects have been reported to persist for as little as 36h but more typically for about 3 days, so that levels seen in sedentary people are approached within 1 week. Could the good insulin sensitivity which characterizes athletes be attributable to residual effects of their last training session, rather than to any long-term adaptive effects? The answer to this question is 'probably not'. Studies have compared the response of a trained leg to a single session of exercise with that of an untrained (contralateral) leg to identical exercise; insulin action was improved in the trained leg but there was no effect in the untrained leg. The effect of training on insulin-mediated glucose disposal in muscle has therefore been described as a genuine adaptation to training—but short-lived.

Whole-body insulin sensitivity is directly and

positively related to muscle mass and, long-term, there may be additional effects of regular activity if muscle mass increases. By contrast with the effects of endurance training, which leads to predominantly qualitative changes in muscle insulin/glucose dynamics, the main effect of strength, and perhaps sprint, training may be to increase the quantity of muscle. Indeed, increases in lean body mass gained through strength training have been reported to be closely related to reductions in the total insulin response during an oral glucose tolerance test.

## Net effect of training

Laboratory study has shown that exercise increases insulin sensitivity and decreases glucose-stimulated β-cell insulin secretion. It does not follow, however, that training spares insulin secretion and blood glucose levels in real life because training necessitates an increase in food intake. A study from Copenhagen makes the point well (Dela *et al.* 1992). These workers compared trained male athletes with untrained controls during their (different) ordinary living conditions as well as in the laboratory (Table 3.2). The higher daily energy intakes of the athletes — mean of $18.6 \, MJ \cdot day^{-1}$ ($4440 \, kJ \cdot day^{-1}$), compared with $12.5 \, MJ \cdot day^{-1}$ ($2986 \, kcal \cdot day^{-1}$) for the sedentary men — reflected mainly differences in carbohydrate intake ($678$ vs. $294 \, g \cdot day^{-1}$). Following oral glucose loads comprising identical fractions of daily carbohydrate intake, the areas under the plasma glucose and insulin concentration vs. time curves did not differ between athletes and untrained men. The two groups also had identical 24-h glucose responses during a day when they went about their normal activities (including one or two training sessions for the athletes). It seems that training, rather than sparing the pancreas, elicits adaptations in the action of insulin which allow the necessary increases in food intake without potentially harmful hyperglycaemia and overloading of β-cells. During the day of normal activity, arterial insulin concentrations were, however, some 40% lower (NS) in athletes because of enhanced hepatic clearance. As insulin may directly promote both atherosclerosis and hypertension, a lower circulating level of the hormone may in itself be advantageous.

The example just presented is an extreme case, with the athletes (one 800-m runner, one 1500-m runner and five triathletes) consuming some 50% more food energy than the sedentary comparison group. It is not atypical, however, as other researchers have found almost 80% of the increased energy intake associated with high

**Table 3.2** Integrated glucose and insulin responses to the same absolute oral glucose load ($1 \, g \cdot kg^{-1}$ body mass), to the same relative oral glucose load (27.7% of usual daily carbohydrate intake) and to food consumed under ordinary living conditions during a 24-h period. Adapted from Dela *et al.* (1992).

|  | Glucose | Insulin |
|---|---|---|
|  | ($mmol \cdot l^{-1} \cdot 3 \, h^{-1}$) | ($pmol \cdot ml^{-1} \cdot 3 \, h^{-1}$) |
| Same absolute load |  |  |
| Untrained | 1277* | 58* |
| Trained | 1040 | 24 |
| Same % daily carbohydrate intake |  |  |
| Untrained ($1 \, g \cdot kg^{-1}$ body mass) | 1277 | 58 |
| Trained ($2.3 \, g \cdot kg^{-1}$ body mass) | 1173 | 44 |
|  | ($mol \cdot l^{-1} \cdot 24 \, h^{-1}$) | ($pmol \cdot ml^{-1} \cdot 24 \, h^{-1}$) |
| 24-h responses, ordinary living |  |  |
| Untrained | 7.3 | 175 |
| Trained | 7.4 | 124 |

*Significantly different from trained, $P < 0.05$.

volume training was from carbohydrate. Similar, if smaller, effects on carbohydrate intake also tend to occur with more modest, non-athletic, levels of exercise. For example, when a group of middle-aged men took up jogging, their average daily energy intake increased by about $1.25 MJ \cdot day^{-1}$ ($300 kcal \cdot day^{-1}$) after 2 years (12.5%) and this was almost all from carbohydrate (an increase of $70 g \cdot day^{-1}$, about 30%) (Wood *et al.* 1985).

## Lipoprotein metabolism

The body's major energy store is TAG, a hydrophobic molecule which is transported through the watery plasma in particles called lipoproteins. Lipoproteins comprise a core of fatty material (cholesteryl esters as well as TAG) surrounded by a relatively hydrophilic coat comprising phospholipid, free cholesterol and one or more protein molecules known as apolipoproteins. The main categories are (in order of increasing density): chylomicrons, very low density lipoproteins (VLDL), low-density lipoproteins (LDL) and HDL. A brief outline of their metabolism helps understand both the influence of exercise and the potential implications for health.

The function of chylomicrons is to carry TAG and cholesterol derived from the diet. Their main role is to deliver TAG to peripheral tissues and cholesterol to the liver. Secreted by the cells of the intestinal wall, they enter the bloodstream via the lymphatics. As they pass through the capillary beds of adipose tissue and muscle, their TAG is hydrolysed by the enzyme lipoprotein lipase (LPL), the non-esterified fatty acids (NEFA) released mostly being taken up by the tissues. As TAG is lost, the chylomicrons shrink and cholesterol-rich remnant particles are removed by hepatic receptors.

By contrast, VLDL distribute TAG from the liver to other tissues. Like chylomicrons, they are a substrate for LPL and become TAG-depleted as they pass through capillary beds. Their remnants are LDL which carry (in ester form) some 70% of the cholesterol in the circulation, delivering it to

a variety of tissues, according to their needs. Plasma total cholesterol concentration, in epidemiological study shown to be strongly and positively related to the risk of CHD, predominantly reflects LDL cholesterol.

HDL provide a means by which cholesterol is routed from peripheral tissues to the liver where it is disposed of safely, mainly via synthesis into bile acids. HDL receive unesterified cholesterol which is released as excess surface material during the degradation of TAG-rich particles, but also incorporate cholesterol from the body's cells when this is present in excess of needs. This pathway has been termed 'reverse cholesterol transport' and may be the mechanism underlying the inverse relationship between HDL cholesterol and the risk of CHD. In women, for example, an increase of $0.26 mmol \cdot l^{-1}$ (about 20%) in HDL cholesterol is associated with a 42–50% decrease in CHD risk. An alternative explanation is that low HDL-cholesterol may be a marker for some defect in the metabolism of TAG-rich lipoproteins which means that chylomicron remnants and LDL remain in the circulation for longer, becoming correspondingly smaller and more readily taken up into atherosclerotic lesions. There is clear evidence of this for LDL, but also increasing awareness that the chylomicron remnant may also be atherogenic, not least because it may contain 30 times as many cholesterol molecules as a typical LDL particle. The view that atherogenesis is a postprandial phenomenon is gaining support and patients with known coronary artery disease show a more marked and prolonged rise in plasma TAG concentrations following an oral fat load than healthy controls.

Insulin plays an important role in fat metabolism, coordinating events during the postprandial period. LPL activity in adipose tissue is stimulated and mobilization of NEFA is depressed through inhibition of hormone sensitive lipase and plasma NEFA levels fall markedly.

When insulin sensitivity is poor, fat metabolism is disordered: there is failure to stimulate LPL, so TAG-removal rate falls; failure to suppress release of NEFA from adipose tissue, leading to high plasma levels; and inappropriate hepatic VLDL secretion which exacerbates the rise in plasma TAG. Remnant particles of the TAG-rich lipoproteins persist in the circulation for longer, their smaller size increasing their atherogenic potential.

Thus, insulin resistance may lie at the heart of the abnormalities of lipoprotein metabolism which are key features of the 'metabolic syndrome', i.e. low HDL cholesterol, high TAG levels and possibly also a preponderance of small dense LDL. It is not entirely clear, however, which is the 'chicken' and which the 'egg' here because an argument may be advanced for an underlying role of abnormal fat metabolism secondary to the excessive delivery of TAG to adipose tissue and muscle—in the pathogenesis of insulin resistance. Either way, exercise may be beneficial because of its potential to improve fuel homeostasis through its effects on the assimilation, mobilization and oxidation of fat fuels. Alterations to lipoprotein metabolism result.

### Effects of physical activity

Well-trained endurance runners, men and women, possess lipoprotein profiles consistent with a low risk of CHD (Durstine & Haskell 1994). HDL cholesterol is typically 20–30% higher than in comparable sedentary controls. Triglycerides are low, particularly when veteran athletes (>40 years) are studied. Total cholesterol concentrations stand out as low only when the control group is large and representative of the wider population. Athletes trained specifically for strength and power do not differ from sedentary individuals in these ways.

Less athletic, but physically active, people also show lipoprotein profiles which are consistent with a reduced risk of cardiovascular disease. For example, data from the Lipid Clinics Prevalence Study showed that men and women who reported some 'strenuous' physical activity generally had higher HDL cholesterol levels than those who reported none (Haskell et al. 1980). Differences were independent of age, body mass index, alcohol use and cigarette smoking. Even simple exercise like walking has been linked to elevated HDL levels, with relationships between distance walked per day and the concentration of $HDL_2$, the subfraction that accounts for most of the difference in total HDL cholesterol between athletes and controls. In addition, men and women who habitually walk 12–20 km·week$^{-1}$ are only half as likely to possess an unfavourable ratio of total to HDL cholesterol (>5) as a comparable no-exercise group. Thus cross-sectional observations of ordinary men and women, and of everyday activity, provide a basis for proposing that endurance exercise influences lipoprotein metabolism.

Longitudinal studies are less consistent but, for HDL cholesterol, the consensus is that, over months rather than weeks, endurance exercise involving a minimum expenditure of about 15 MJ·week$^{-1}$ (3580 kcal·week$^{-1}$) causes an increase and that the magnitude of this tends to be greater when there is weight loss.

The majority of longitudinal studies have employed rather high intensity exercise, most frequently jogging/running, but evidence is gradually becoming available that more accessible, self-governed exercise regimens may also be effective (Després & Lamarche 1994). For example, in previously sedentary middle-aged women who had rather low levels of HDL cholesterol (mean, 1.2 mmol·l$^{-1}$) at base line, walking briskly for about 20 km·week$^{-1}$ over a year resulted in a 27% increase. Increases in HDL cholesterol do not always mirror changes in fitness, however. Figure 3.2 shows the main findings of one study which examined the effect of the intensity of walking in women over 24 weeks; fast walking at 8 km·h$^{-1}$ produced greater improvements in fitness than walking the same distance at slower speed, but increases in HDL cholesterol did not differ between groups walking at different speeds. Several other studies have confirmed these findings.

Dietary modifications recommended to overweight people invariably combine energy intake restriction with decreases in the intake of saturated fats and cholesterol. Such changes can

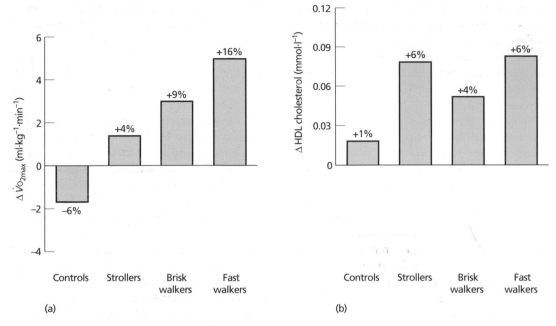

**Fig. 3.2** Changes in (a) maximal oxygen uptake ($\dot{V}O_{2\,max}$) and (b) serum high-density lipoprotein (HDL) cholesterol concentration in control subjects ($n=10/13$) and in three groups of previously sedentary women who walked 4.8 km · day$^{-1}$ for 24 weeks. One group walked at 4.8 km · h$^{-1}$ ($n=17/18$, strollers), one group at 6 km · h$^{-1}$ ($n=12$, brisk walkers) and one group at 8 km · h$^{-1}$ ($n=13$, fast walkers). Adapted from Duncan *et al.* (1991).

reduce HDL levels and, given the inverse association between HDL cholesterol and the risk of CHD, theoretically may diminish the anticipated beneficial effects of decreased low density lipoprotein cholesterol. Exercise may be one way to offset a diet-related fall in HDL cholesterol. Comparison of two different interventions in sedentary overweight men and women, i.e. a low energy, low fat diet alone with the same diet plus exercise (brisk walking and jogging) showed that the addition of exercise to the low fat diet resulted in more favourable changes in HDL cholesterol than diet alone; in men, diet plus exercise provoked in a greater rise in HDL cholesterol than did diet only; and in women only the diet-plus-exercise group showed a favourable change in the ratio of LDL cholesterol to HDL cholesterol.

It was mentioned above that changes in lipoproteins tend to be greater when an exercise regimen is accompanied by weight loss. There is

also an effect which is independent of weight change, which appears to be linked to adaptations in skeletal muscle. During exercise there is a net efflux of HDL$_2$ across a trained leg, but not across the contralateral untrained leg (Kiens & Lithell 1989). The rate of HDL$_2$ synthesis is positively and strongly related to the rate of VLDL degradation. As the rate-limiting step in VLDL degradation is LPL activity, this points to skeletal muscle LPL as an important determinant of the effects of exercise on lipoprotein metabolism.

### Postprandial lipoprotein metabolism

High levels of muscle LPL activity, leading to an enhanced metabolic capacity for TAG may therefore explain the elevated HDL cholesterol levels in physically active people. Endurance trained men and women show high levels of plasma and muscle LPL activity, together with high rates of TAG clearance (compared with sedentary controls). The high LPL levels probably arise from enhanced capillarization in the muscle of athletes because the enzyme is bound to the luminal surface of capillary endothelium.

There are also short-term effects of recent exercise on postprandial TAG clearance. During recovery TAG clearance rates are increased, reducing the postprandial rise in plasma TAG concentration. The effect is greater after moderate intensity exercise (60% $\dot{V}o_{2max.}$) than after low intensity exercise (30% $\dot{V}o_{2max.}$) of the same duration probably because of its greater energy expenditure; if energy expenditure is held constant the effects on lipaemia of low and moderate intensity exercise are strikingly similar (Tsetsonis & Hardman 1996). These short-term benefits may therefore be potentially greater for trained people because their higher $\dot{V}o_{2max.}$ values and greater endurance capability allow them to expend more energy than untrained individuals before becoming fatigued.

People spend the majority of their lives in the postprandial state and exercise-induced decreases in postprandial lipaemia may be clinically important in the long term. When TAG clearance is good, the postprandial rise in TAG is reduced and TAG-rich particles will remain in the circulation for shorter periods, decreasing the atherogenic stimulus. Clinical evidence is consistent with this view because case-control studies have shown that postprandial TAG levels accurately predict the presence or absence of coronary artery disease.

## Energy balance

In the UK, overweight (body mass index 25–30 kg·m⁻²) and obesity (body mass index >30 kg· m⁻²) are a serious problem. More than 50% of men and more than one third of women in the age group 45–54 are overweight, whilst nearly 20% of both sexes are obese. Figures are even worse in the US, where mean body weight increased by 3.6 kg between 1976/80 and 1988/91. The health hazards of carrying excess weight are well documented so its prevalence rightly gives rise to concern. Recent findings have particularly emphasized the importance of the regional distribution on body fat in relation to the risk of atherosclerotic metabolic disease. As with so many aspects of human health, there is substantial genetic control but environmental factors—diet, physical activity—modify these influences profoundly.

The energy stores of the body are, of course, determined by the balance between energy intake and energy expenditure and any exercise contributes to energy expenditure. Although for most people the expenditure in habitual exercise rarely accounts for more than 20% of the total, physical activity is the only way in which energy expenditure can be increased voluntarily. Its importance in helping to control body weight and body fat content—for individuals or for populations—is still a matter of debate, despite the fact that there is a fairly consistent negative relationship between level of activity and body mass index or skinfold thicknesses.

The energy stored in 1 kg of adipose tissue is approximately 32.4 MJ (7740 kcal). Energy expenditure during weight-bearing activities depends on body mass; for example, walking or running 1.6 km expends (net) about 220 kJ (52 kcal) for a 50-kg person, but about 350 kJ (84 kcal) for an 80-kg person, i.e. about 4.2 kJ·kg⁻¹ body weight·km⁻¹ (1 kcal·kg⁻¹ body weight· km⁻¹). Theoretically, therefore (and disregarding the small postexercise elevation of metabolic rate which, in non-athletes, probably never exceeds 10% of exercise expenditure), walking an extra mile every day for a year would expend (net) an estimated total of 80–128 MJ (19100–30580 kJ), i.e. the energy equivalent of 2.5–4 kg of adipose tissue. Resting metabolic rate decreases, however, as body mass falls and energy intake will be stimulated, offsetting this deficit. As planned exercise increases, there may also be a spontaneous decrease in the physical activities of everyday living. The situation is far from simple.

What tends to happen in practice? The consensus in the literature is that relatively small increases in physical activity (for example, walking 3.2 km·day⁻¹, three times per week, adding up to 2.1–2.5 MJ or 500–600 kcal gross) are

LIVERPOOL JOHN MOORES UNIVERSITY
LEARNING SERVICES

not associated with changes in body fatness over 3–6 months (Haskell 1991). Above this amount of exercise, there tends to be a consistent loss of body fat, $0.12\,kg\cdot week^{-1}$ for men (a little less for women), total exercise energy expenditure being the variable most·strongly related to the body mass change. Thus, the natural adjustments to increased exercise levels reduce, but do not eliminate, the theoretical energy deficit. For example, in a study where sedentary men followed a programme of jogging for 2 years with no instructions about dietary intake, energy intake rose over the first 6 months by about $1.3\,MJ\cdot day^{-1}$ ($310\,kcal\cdot day^{-1}$). This compensation, however, did not increase further, remaining less than the energy expenditure of exercise so that a gradual loss of body fat occurred.

Physical activity is increasingly viewed as an important adjunct to restriction of dietary energy. For example, the addition of exercise to a low energy diet has been reported to enhance weight and fat loss and prevent a fall in resting metabolic rate and it may also help with the intractable problem of weight maintenance after weight loss. The most important role for activity is probably that which is least well explored, i.e. prevention of weight gain. Some information on the relationship of activity with longer-term weight change in the general population is available from the NHANES-I Epidemiologic Follow-up Study in the USA; this found that the risk of major weight gain ($>13\,kg$) over a 10-year period was twice as high among inactive men and sevenfold higher among inactive women, compared with men and women of high activity level (Williamson et al. 1993).

Exercise may influence the distribution of body fat as well as the amount. In population studies, individuals practising vigorous activities on a regular basis have lower waist-to-hip ratios than others, even after the effect of subcutaneous fat is adjusted for. Training has sometimes been reported to decrease this ratio even in the absence of a reduction in body weight. One reason may be that the metabolic state of the visceral fat depot is such that it should be readily mobilized during weight loss.

For individuals who are overweight, the health gains from increased physical activity should not be judged solely by the extent of change in body fatness; several prospective studies have shown that overweight men and women who are physically active have lower rates of morbidity and mortality than comparable sedentary people.

### Fat balance

The energy balance equation (change in energy stores = energy intake – energy expenditure) has

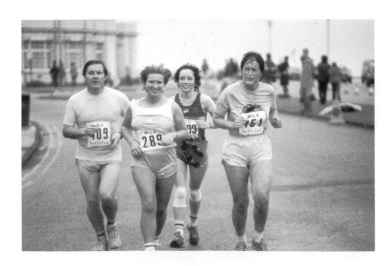

**Fig. 3.3** Sport offers an opportunity to people who wish to take exercise for health reasons rather than as a competitive outlet. Photo courtesy of Ron Maughan.

traditionally provided the theoretical framework for understanding of the nature of energy balance in humans. More recently, alternative approaches have been proposed which take account of how different fuels are partitioned among metabolic pathways. The body responds differently to overfeeding with different nutrients, suggesting that balance equations for separate nutrients might be more informative. Protein balance is achieved on a day-to-day basis, with oxidation of intake in excess of needs; and carbohydrate intake stimulates both glycogen storage and glucose oxidation, with negligible conversion to TAG under dietary conditions of industrialized countries. In marked contrast, fat intake has little influence on fat oxidation so that energy balance is virtually equivalent to fat balance and there is a strong relationship between fat balance and energy balance even over a period as short as 24 h. Chronic imbalance between fat intake and fat oxidation may therefore predispose to increased fat storage.

This line of thinking leads to the conclusion that physical activity has greater potential to influence body energy stores than would be deduced on the basis of the tradtional energy balance equation. Fat oxidation is of course enhanced during submaximal exercise, and more so in people who are well trained. It is also enhanced for some hours afterwards, even when the postexercise elevation of metabolic rate has disappeared (Calles-Escandon et al. 1996). The response to a fatty meal is changed, with greater postprandial fat oxidation (Tsetsonis et al. 1997). There might be synergistic benefits of increased exercise if, as discussed above, there is an increased appetite for high carbohydrate foods.

## Conclusion

Substantial elevations in mortality are seen in sedentary and unfit men and women. With regard to CHD, a biological gradient has been documented convincingly, although its exact pattern remains unclear; high levels of rather vigorous endurance exercise may be necessary for optimal benefit but some studies show that risk decreases steeply at the lower end of the physical activity (or fitness) continuum, reaching an asymptote in the mid-range. Detailed information about the influence of either the amount of exercise or the independent effect of intensity is not available for the relation of physical activity with the development of either hypertension or NIDDM.

Information on the mechanisms by which activity decreases the risk of these diseases is incomplete, but adaptive changes in the metabolism of fat and carbohydrate, giving rise to 'metabolic fitness', are undoubtedly involved. Many of the health gains associated with high levels of physical activity can be explained through the consequences of increased exercise for the intake and metabolism of these macronutrients.

## References

Abbott, R.D., Rodriguez, B.L., Burchfiel, C.M. & Curb, J.D. (1994) Physical activity in older middle-aged men and reduced risk of stroke: the Honolulu Heart Program. *American Journal of Epidemiology* **139**, 881–893.

Blair, S.N., Kohl, H.W., Paffenbarger, R.S. *et al.* (1989) Physical fitness and all-cause mortality: a prospective study of healthy men and women. *Journal of the American Medical Association* **262**, 2395–2401.

Blair, S.N., Kampert, J.B., Kohl, H.W. *et al.* (1996) Influences of cardiorespiratory fitness and other precursors on cardiovascular disease and all-cause mortality in men and women. *Journal of the American Medical Association* **276**, 205–210.

Bouchard, C., Shephard, R.J. & Stephens, T. (eds) (1994) Consensus statement. In *Physical Activity, Fitness and Health*, pp. 9–76. Human Kinetics, Champaign, IL.

Calles-Escandon, J., Goran, M.I., O'Connell, M. *et al.* (1996) Exercise increases fat oxidation at rest unrelated to changes in energy balance or lipolysis. *American Journal of Physiology, Endocrinology and Metabolism* **270**, E1009–E1014.

Dela, F., Mikines, K.J. & von Linstow, M. *et al.* (1992) Does training spare insulin secretion and diminish glucose levels in real life? *Diabetes Care* **15** (Suppl. 4), 1712–1715.

Després, J.-P. & Lamarche, B. (1994) Low-intensity endurance exercise training, plasma lipoproteins and the risk of coronary heart disease. *Journal of Internal Medicine* **236**, 7–22.

Duncan, J.J., Gordon, N.F. & Scott, C.B. (1991) Women

walking for health and fitness: how much is enough? *Journal of the American Medical Association* **266**, 3295–3299.

Durstine, J.L. & Haskell, W.L. (1994) Effects of exercise training on plasma lipids and lipoproteins. *Exercise and Sport Science Reviews* **22**, 477–521.

Ekelund, L.-G., Haskell, W.L., Johnson, M.S. *et al.* (1988) Physical fitness as a predictor of cardiovascular mortality in asymptomatic North American men. *New England Journal of Medicine* **319**, 1379–1384.

Haskell, W.L. (1991) Dose–response relationship between physical activity and disease risk factors. In *Sport for All* (ed. P. Oja & R. Telema), pp. 125–133. Elsevier Science Publications, Amsterdam.

Haskell, W.L. (1994) Health consequences of physical activity: understanding and challenges regarding dose–response. *Medicine and Science in Sports and Exercise* **26**, 649–660.

Haskell, W.L., Taylor, H.L., Wood, P.D., Schrott, H. & Heiss, G. (1980) Strenuous physical activity, treadmill exercise test performance and plasma high-density lipoprotein cholesterol. The Lipid Research Clinics Program Prevalence Study. *Circulation* **62** (Suppl. IV), 53–61.

Kiens, B. & Lithell, H. (1989) Lipoprotein metabolism influenced by training-induced changes in human skeletal muscle. *Journal of Clinical Investigation* **83**, 558–564.

Kriska, A.M., Blair, S.N. & Pereira, M.A. (1994) The potential role of physical activity in the prevention of non-insulin-dependent diabetes mellitus: the epidemiological evidence. *Exercise and Sports Science Reviews* **22**, 121–143.

Leon, A.S. (1991) Physical activity and risk of ischaemic heart disease. In *Sport for All* (ed. P. Oja & R. Telema), pp. 251–264. Elsevier Science Publishers, Amsterdam.

Morris, J.N., Clayton, D.G., Everitt, M.G. *et al.* (1990) Exercise in leisure time: coronary attack and death rates. *British Heart Journal* **63**, 325–334.

Paffenbarger, R.S., Hyde, R.T., Wing, A.L. *et al.* (1986) Physical activity, all-cause mortality, and longevity of college alumni. *New England Journal of Medicine* **314**, 605–613.

Paffenbarger, R.S., Jung, D.L., Leung, R.W. *et al.* (1991) Physical activity and hypertension: an epidemiological view. *Annals of Internal Medicine* **23**, 319–327.

Sandvik, L., Erikssen, J., Thaulow, E. *et al.* (1993) Physical fitness as a predictor of mortality among healthy, middle-aged Norwegian men. *New England Journal of Medicine* **328**, 533–537.

Shaper, A.G. & Wannamethee, G. (1991) Physical activity and ischaemic heart disease in middle-aged British men. *British Heart Journal* **66**, 384–394.

Tsetsonis, N.V. & Hardman, A.E. (1996) Reduction in postprandial lipemia after walking: influence of exercise intensity. *Medicine in Science Sports and Exercise* **28**, 1235–1242.

Tsetsonis, N.V., Hardman, A.E. & Mastana, S.S. (1997) Acute effects of exercise on postprandial lipemia: a comparative study in trained and untrained middle-aged women. *American Journal of Clinical Nutrition* **65**, 525–533.

Wannamethee, G. & Shaper, A.G. (1992) Physical activity and stroke in British middle-aged men. *British Medical Journal* **304**, 597–601.

Whaley, M.H. & Blair, S.N. (1995) Epidemiology of physical activity, physical fitness and coronary heart disease. *Journal of Cardiovascular Risk* **2**, 289–295.

WHO (1990) *Diet, Nutrition, and the Prevention of Chronic Diseases*. World Health Organization, Geneva.

Williamson, D.F., Madans, J., Anda, R.F. *et al.* (1993) Recreational physical activity and ten-year weight change in a US national cohort. *International Journal of Obesity* **17**, 279–286.

Wood, P.D. (1987) Exercise, plasma lipids, weight regulation. In *Exercise, Heart, Health: Conference Report*. Coronary Prevention Group, London.

Wood, P.D., Terry, R.B. & Haskell, W.L. (1985) Metabolism of substrates: diet, lipoprotein metabolism and exercise. *Federation Proceedings* **44**, 358–363.

# Chapter 4

# Energy Costs of Exercise and Sport

HENRY J. MONTOYE

## Introduction

In the middle of the 18th century, Lavoisier conceived the first law of thermodynamics, that energy can be neither created nor destroyed but only changed from one form to another. This principle of the conservation of energy was later formulated by Mayer in 1842 and Helmholtz in 1847, but it remained for Joule, a brewer, to provide experimental data to support the concept (Fenn & Rahn 1964). When Lavoisier and Laplace demonstrated that muscular exercise consumes oxygen and produces carbon dioxide (Chapman & Mitchell 1965), the stage was set for learning how to measure energy expenditure. It was clear then that the energy in the food consumed should equal the energy expended.

Energy is expended in three ways in humans and other warm-blooded animals. A certain amount of energy is required at rest to maintain body temperature and involuntary muscular contraction for functions such as circulation and respiration. This energy level represents the resting metabolic rate. Second, some energy is required to digest and assimilate food. This process, formerly called *specific dynamic action* and now referred to as *dietary induced thermogenesis* or *thermic effect of food*, adds about 10% to the resting metabolic rate. These two represent but a small part of the total energy expenditure and can be altered only very slightly in individuals. By far the most important source of variation between individuals in energy expenditure (when adjusted for body size) is the muscular activity carried out. The sources of this activity are one's daily work, leisure pursuits, and transportation to and from work or other destinations (which some investigators include as part of leisure time activity).

In the International System of Units (SI), the unit of measurement for heat production is the joule (named for James Prescott Joule, who did pioneering work in metabolism).

One observation about energy expenditure is essential to keep in mind. The intake or expenditure of joules is related to body size. A small person who is very active may expend a similar number of kilojoules in 24 h as a large person who is sedentary. So if exercise is to be expressed as energy expenditure in joules or calories, body size must be taken into account. To this end, energy expended or ingested is sometimes given as kilojoules or kilocalories per unit of body weight or, in the case of oxygen ($O_2$) uptake, as millilitres of $O_2$ per kilogram of body weight. The use of METs (an abbreviation for 'metabolic equivalent') is another approach to correcting for body weight. A MET represents the ratio of energy expended in kilojoules divided by resting energy expenditure in kilojoules, either measured or estimated from body size. In estimating resting (not basal) energy expenditure, a value of 4.2 kJ per kilogram of body weight per hour or 3.5 ml $O_2$ utilized per kilogram of body weight per minute gives reasonably satisfactory results in most cases. Although neither method is perfect, the MET approach is more popular and probably more useful. Although he did not use the term MET, LaGrange (1905) almost a century ago expressed the strenuousness of activities as a ratio of exercise metabolism to resting metabolism. The World Health Organization adopted the same principle in its physical activity index. Among exercise physiologists, it is almost universally accepted to use METs to express energy expenditure in relation to body weight. In Appendix 4.1, the energy cost of activities is expressed in METs as well as kilojoules per kilogram of body weight.

## Methods of measurement

The direct measurement of energy expenditure (heat production) by a living animal or human being is possible. Although the engineering problems are formidable, the heat produced while the subject is in a sealed, insulated chamber can be measured.

A room calorimeter measures the heat produced by the subject at rest or during exercise by circulating water through pipes in the insulated chamber and carefully measuring, at frequent intervals, the temperature of the ingoing and outgoing water and the water flow. Sophisticated engineering is required to prevent heat loss from the chamber by other means. The latent heat of the water vaporized must be determined by measuring the vapour in the ventilating air current. Calorimeters have been built in which air flow and temperature are measured by means of thermocouples using the thermal gradient principle (Carlson & Hsieh 1970; Jéquier et al. 1987). Energy exchange during muscular exercise can be measured by installing an exercise device (treadmill, cycle ergometer, etc.) in the chamber.

Webb (Webb 1980; Webb et al. 1980) also describes an insulated, water-cooled suit worn by the subject in which the flow of water through the suit and the temperature of the incoming and outgoing water are measured to determine heat production. The suit has been modified by Hambraeus et al. (1991). When energy is transformed from food to heat and muscular work, oxygen is consumed and thus the oxygen con-

sumed could be measured to ascertain energy expenditure. The term *indirect calorimetry* is applied to the method of estimating energy expenditure from oxygen consumption and carbon dioxide production because heat production is not measured directly.

A room calorimeter can be constructed in which expired air is analysed to estimate heat production. Atwater and Benedict (1905) showed that by measuring the oxygen consumed and carbon dioxide produced, heat production could indeed be estimated with reasonable accuracy. This kind of calorimeter is usually referred to as a respiration chamber.

However, room calorimeters and respiration chambers are confining. Even Webb's water-cooled suit, because of the computer and other necessary equipment, is confined to the laboratory. Hence, although the energy cost of some activities (walking at various grades on a treadmill, riding a stationary cycle at various resistances and speeds, certain calisthenic exercises, for examples) can be measured with calorimeters or respiration chambers, the energy cost of many sports activities or occupational tasks cannot be measured in this way.

There are several simpler techniques for measuring oxygen uptake. One, called the *closed circuit method*, requires the subject to be isolated from outside air. The respirometer originally contains pure oxygen, and as the subject breathes in this closed system the carbon dioxide is continuously removed as it passes through soda lime. The gas volume gradually decreases, and the rate of decrease is a measure of the rate of oxygen consumption. Regnault and Reiset developed this system in 1849, and by measuring the carbon dioxide absorbed they discovered the respiratory quotient (Fenn & Rahn 1964). This method works reasonably well for measuring resting or basal metabolic rate, but absorbing the large volume of carbon dioxide produced during prolonged, strenuous exercise becomes a problem. The *open circuit method* described next is more suited to measuring exercise metabolism.

Two procedures in the open circuit method have been developed. In one, the flow-through

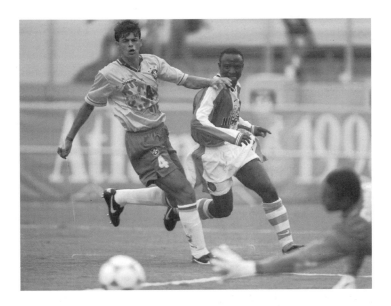

**Fig. 4.1** In most games, the exercise intensity flucuates, and total energy expenditure depends on many factors. In games such as soccer, the most important of these are body mass and total distance covered. Photo © Allsport / A. Bello.

technique (Kinney 1980), a large volume of the equivalent of outside air passes through a hood worn by the subject. The subject inspires and expires into the airstream flowing through the hood. Air flow and percentage of oxygen and carbon dioxide are precisely measured to calculate $\dot{V}o_2$ and RQ. It is necessary to have accurate gas analysers, particularly the one for carbon dioxide, because its concentration may be between 0% and 0.5%. This method is especially useful for long-term measurements with the subject at rest or doing only mild exercise.

The second procedure, the time-honoured Douglas bag method (although a Douglas bag may not necessarily be used), has been found to be accurate and theoretically sound. With this procedure, the subject generally wears a nose clip and mouthpiece or a face mask. Outside air or its equivalent is inhaled through the mouthpiece or mask containing a one-way valve and exhaled into a Douglas bag or Tissot tank. It is important that the mouthpiece and connected tubing provide minimal resistance to airflow, or the cost of breathing will increase the energy expenditure. The volume of air in the bag or tank is measured to calculate ventilation. A sample of exhaled air is obtained to measure the $O_2$ and $CO_2$ concentrations. This is usually done with a Haldane, modified Haldane, or Micro-Scholander apparatus. These techniques use reagents to absorb the carbon dioxide and oxygen, respectively, with the volume of the sample measured before and after the gases are absorbed.

In the laboratory, modern electronic equipment usually replaces the Douglas bag and chemical analysers, whereby ventilation and oxygen and carbon dioxide percentages are determined instantaneously and continuously. Chemical analysers are generally used to analyse standard gas mixes to calibrate the electronic equipment. The electronic equipment confines the procedure to laboratory or clinic. The Douglas bag method is not as restricting because a bag can be carried on the back or by an assistant close by. This method thus can be used in the field.

Nathan Zuntz (1847–1920) recognized the advantage of having the subject carry a self-contained unit if $\dot{V}o_2$ is to be measured during exercise. He developed what was probably the first such unit, which resembled a large rucksack (Zuntz & Leowy 1909). This was a forerunner of the portable calorimeter designed by Kofranyi and Michaelis (1940). Improvements were made during the subsequent 10 years, resulting in the model by Müller and Franz (1952). This also resembles a rucksack but is smaller and lighter than Zuntz's apparatus.

The Müller–Franz calorimeter registers ventilation and siphons off a small percentage of the expired air into a small attached bag for later analysis. This apparatus functions reasonably well during rest or moderate exercise. At airflows of about $80–100 l \cdot min^{-1}$, the meter begins to under-record ventilation (Orsini & Passmore 1951; Insull 1954; Montoye et al. 1958) and hence underestimate energy expenditure. At severe exercise, where instantaneous flows can reach $200 l$ or more per minute, the instrument seriously underestimates energy expenditure. There is also a potential error due to diffusion of the gas through the bag, which becomes more serious the longer the delay in analysing the gas. In addition to these limitations, there may be some interference in particular activities (the calorimeter weighs about 3 kg), although the instrument can be carried in a bicycle basket or by an assistant. Also, the rates of energy expenditure are averaged over the entire collection period.

Wolff (1958) improved the Kofranyi–Michaelis respirometer. His integrating motor pneumotachograph (IMP) is available from J. Langham Thompson Ltd, Bushey Heath, Herts, UK. The IMP has some of the limitations of the Kofranyi–Michaelis respirometer. Ventilation is integrated electrically rather than mechanically lowering the expiratory resistance. Also, samples with smaller percentages are possible. This group (Humphrey & Wolff 1977) later developed a more advanced instrument, the oxylog, available from P.K. Morgan Ltd, Rainham, Kent, UK. This battery-operated, self-contained, portable instrument weighs about the same as the Kofranyi-Michaelis respirometer, but it is engineered for on-line measurement of oxygen consumption. Carbon dioxide is not measured. It has been found to be reasonably accurate in field measurements during rest and up to moderately strenuous exercise (Harrison et al. 1982; McNeill et al. 1987; Collins et al. 1988). The error was reported to be 2–3% at 4 METs, but the error increases at lower and higher workloads

(Patterson & Fisher 1979). Ikegami et al. (1988) added a telemetry capacity to the oxylog so $\dot{V}o_2$ could be recorded remotely at 1-min intervals.

Nutritionists and others have estimated energy expenditure by measuring the energy in food consumed. However, this method estimates an average energy expenditure over days or weeks and hence is not suitable for the measurement of the energy cost of individual activities. Similarly the use of doubly labelled water (Montoye et al. 1996) which some consider the gold standard for estimating habitual energy expenditure, also is not useful for measuring energy expenditure of specific activities because it too only provides an average energy expenditure over a week or two.

Because of the difficulties encountered in measuring $\dot{V}o_2$ in the field, there is interest in the simpler but less direct method—recording physiological data associated with energy expenditure. Advancements in telemetry and other aspects of bioengineering have made such techniques more attractive.

From the beginning of their existence, humans must have observed that pulse rate and ventilation increase during strenuous activity. Systolic blood pressure, electromyographs, and body temperature are also roughly proportional to the intensity of exercise. All of these variables can be telemetered, or entered on portable recorders.

Of the physiological variables, heart rate (HR) is the easiest to measure in the field. The relationship between HR and energy expenditure was shown as early as 1907, when Benedict (1907) reported that changes in pulse rate were correlated with changes in heat production in any one individual. He later suggested that pulse rate may provide a practical and satisfactory method for estimating total metabolism.

Murlin and Greer in 1914 confirmed Benedict's results. They measured respiratory metabolism and HR simultaneously in subjects who were resting and doing moderate work. Their results indicated that HR was a good index of oxygen consumption. Thus, when work can be carefully controlled (as, for example, on a treadmill or bicycle), $\dot{V}o_2$ and HR are closely related and the relationship is linear over much of the range when the measurements are taken on one individual (Montoye 1970). The linear relationship of HR with $\dot{V}o_2$ can be understood from the Fick equation: $\dot{V}o_2 = HR \cdot SV (a - \dot{V}o_{2diff.})$. Over a wide range of exercise, stroke volume and $a - \dot{V}o_{2diff.}$ do not change greatly; consequently, the increase in HR reflects an increase in $\dot{V}o_2$. Some investigators have presented data showing that relationship is not linear over the full range from rest to strenuous activity (Henderson & Prince 1914; Booyens & Hervey 1960; Malhotra et al. 1963; Bradfield et al. 1969; Berg 1971; Viteri et al. 1971; Warnold & Lenner 1977). Most agree that during exercise HR is more consistent and there is a greater tendency toward linearity than when resting values are included.

Under many conditions, considerable error may be expected when energy expenditure is estimated from the heart rate. There is some day-to-day variation in HR at a given energy expenditure. To this must be added other sources of error. High ambient temperature and humidity or emotion may raise the HR with little effect on oxygen requirement of the work. Training lowers the HR at which tasks of a given energy cost are performed. For example, active workers exercise at lower rates than sedentary men when the workload is equal (Taylor & Parlin 1966; Taylor 1967). Females have higher rates during exercise than males (Montoye 1975). Fatigue (Lundgren 1947; Booyens & Hervey 1960) and state of hydration (Lundgren 1947) affect the HR–$\dot{V}o_2$ relationship. Heart rates are higher for a given energy expenditure in anaemic children (Gandra & Bradfield 1971). Furthermore, certain kinds of activities, such as work with the arms only, will elicit higher HR than work done with the legs and arms, even though the oxygen cost is the same (Durin & Namyslowski 1958; Payne et al. 1971; Vokac et al. 1975; Anderson et al. 1981; Collins et al. 1991). Andrews (1971) has shown that HR–$\dot{V}o_2$ slopes were the same for arm and leg exercise but the intercepts were different. Static exercise increases HR above that expected on the basis of oxygen requirement (Hansen & Maggio 1960; Mass et al. 1989).

Saris et al. (1982) showed that over 5 h, changing the strenuousness of activities has an effect on the accuracy of the HR-to-energy expenditure conversion, especially for quiet activities after moderate exercise: the energy expenditure is overestimated. This phenomenon may contribute to the overestimation of total energy expenditure regardless of what $\dot{V}o_2$–HR regression equation is used.

If one wishes to express the energy expenditure in kilojoules from the oxygen utilized (i.e. not measuring heat produced), it must be recognized that the kilojoules of heat produced by the utilization of 1 litre of oxygen varies with the foodstuffs consumed. The combustion of 1 litre of oxygen yields 19.59 kJ (4.68 kcal) from fat alone, 18.75 kJ (4.48 kcal) from protein alone, and 21.18 kJ (5.06 kcal) from carbohydrate starch alone. Even this is not precise because within each of these three main food sources, the kilojoules of heat from 1 litre of oxygen can vary. For example, considering different types of macronutrients, Brody (1974) gives 18.4 kJ (4.4 kcal) for cottonseed oil and corn oil, 19.3 kJ (4.6 kcal) for butterfat, 21.18 kJ (5.06 kcal) for starch, and 21.26 kJ (5.08 kcal) for sucrose. Similarly, the production of heat from 1 litre of carbon dioxide varies with the foodstuffs metabolized. For precise conversion of oxygen utilization to energy expenditure, the proportions of fat, carbohydrates, and protein being utilized can be determined by the nitrogen that appears in the urine during the time of observation. About 1 g of nitrogen is excreted for every 6.25 g of protein metabolized.

The ratio of the volume of carbon dioxide produced to the volume of oxygen consumed, the so-called respiratory quotient (RQ), gives a reasonable approximation of the percentage of carbohydrate and fat being burned, the ratio being 0.7 when pure fat is the source of energy and 1.00 when it is pure carbohydrate. These ratios assume a 'steady state,' which exists when the oxygen uptake equals the oxygen requirement of the tissues and there is no accumulation of lactic acid. Heart rate, ventilation, and cardiac output remain at fairly constant levels during a steady state. RQ is not representative of the foodstuffs being oxidized in a non-steady state, such as at the start of exercise or during the onset of acidosis of alkalosis as may occur during strenuous exercise or some disease states. The term *respiratory exchange ratio* (RER) rather than RQ is used when a steady state does not exist.

Variations in the caloric equivalents of different fat, different carbohydrate, and different protein sources can be ignored because the error produced is very small. This is because in a normal diet the mixture of different types of fat, carbohydrate, and protein balances out the differences in caloric equivalents. Even the error introduced by not measuring the percentage of protein being used can be ignored in most instances because the caloric equivalents of oxygen are similar for carbohydrates and protein. No matter how diverse the actual composition of the food oxidized, the error in estimating energy expenditure is unlikely to be more than 2–4%. An error of 100% in the estimation of urinary excretion of nitrogen leads to only a 1% error in energy expenditure.

## A table of energy costs of exercise and sport

A list of energy costs of various activities is presented in Appendix 4.1. This is a modification of the list shown in appendix C of the publication by Montoye and others (1996) which in turn was a modification of the list by Ainsworth *et al.* (1993). Appreciation is hereby acknowledged for the willingness of these authors to allow the lists to be modified once again and reproduced in this chapter.

Many of the values of this list came from the following sources: Bannister and Brown (1968); the 7-Day Recall Physical Activity Questionnaire (Blair *et al.* 1985); Durnin and Passmore (1967); Howley and Glover (1974); the American Health Foundation's Physical Activity List (Leon 1981); McArdle *et al.* (1988); Passmore and Durnin (1955); Tecumseh Questionnaire (Reiff *et al.* 1967a, 1967b). Some values have been added from the following sources: Collins *et al.*

(1991); Geissler *et al.* (1981); Getchell (1968); Goff *et al.* (1956); Mandli *et al.* (1989); Nelson *et al.* (1988); Seliger (1968); Stray-Gundersen and Galanes (1991); Veicsteinas *et al.* (1984); VonHofen *et al.* (1989); Watts *et al.* (1990); Wigaeus and Kilbom (1980).

Much of the data in this appendix are derived from actual measurement by indirect calorimetry. However, where data are not available, the figures are based on educated guesses. For some activities, the values are not the values obtained exclusively during execution of the activities. For example, folk dancing requires a higher value than that shown. However, in an hour of folk dancing, considerable time is spent standing, receiving directions, and so on, so the value shown represents the estimated average value. On the other hand, walking usually is done continuously, so its values represent the actual energy cost of doing the activity.

Adults (usually young adults) served as subjects in determining most of the metabolic costs of activities that have been reported in the literature. Little data is based on children and the elderly. The energy expended by children in kilojoules per kilogram of body weight in performing even common activities such as walking is significantly higher than when the same activities are done by adults (Montoye 1982). This is probably because of children's greater ratio of surface area to body weight and poorer coordination than adults. Even if the resting energy expenditure is also higher in children, the MET values of activities in the table are probably a little low for children. Data from Torún *et al.* (1983) have shown the same results. This has also been shown to be true for infants (Torún *et al.* 1983). Data on energy cost of activities are needed to create a table for children.

Data on the energy cost of elderly adults are also needed. Although walking at the same rate may elicit an energy expenditure not much different than in young adults, the elderly generally walk slower, play tennis at less intensity, skate less vigorously, and the like, so the estimate of habitual energy expenditure in the elderly requires other energy cost values.

The numerical values in the third column is the MET rating (the energy cost of the activity divided by the resting, not basal, energy expenditure). The last columns contain the approximate energy cost of the activity expressed as kilojoules or kilocalories per hour per kilogram of body mass.

## Acknowledgements

The editorial assistance of Ms Joann Janes is appreciated.

## References

Ainsworth, B.E., Haskell, W.L., Leon, A.S. *et al.* (1993) Compendium of physical activities: classification of energy costs of human physical activities. *Medicine and Science in Sports and Exercise* **25**, 71–80.

Anderson, R.M., Liv, K., Stamler, J., Van Horn, L. & Hoeksema, R. (1981) Assessment of individual physical activity level: intra-individual vs. inter-individual variability (Abstract). *Medicine and Science in Sports and Exercise* **13**, 100.

Andrews, R.B. (1971) Net heart rates substitute for respiratory calorimetry. *American Journal of Clinical Nutrition* **24**, 1139–1147.

Atwater, W.O. & Benedict, F.G. (1905) *A Respiration Calorimeter with Applicances for the Direct Determination of Oxygen.* Publication no. 42. Carnegie Institute of Washington, Washington, DC.

Bannister, E.W. & Brown, S.R. (1968) The relative energy requirements of physical activity. In *Exercise Physiology* (ed. H.B. Falls), pp. 267–322. Academic Press, New York.

Benedict, F.G. (1907) *The Influences of Inanition on Metabolism.* Publication no. 77. Carnegie Institute, Washington, DC.

Berg, K. (1971) Heart rate telemetry for evaluation of the energy expenditure of children with cerebral palsy. *American Journal of Clinical Nutrition* **24**, 1438–1445.

Blair, S.N., Haskell, W.L., Ho, P. *et al.* (1985) Assessment of habitual physical activity by a 7-day recall in a community survey and controlled experiment. *American Journal of Epidemiology* **122**, 794–804.

Booyens, J. & Hervey, G.R. (1960) The pulse rate as a means of measuring metabolic rate in man. *Canadian Journal of Biochemical Physiology* **38**, 1301–1309.

Bradfield, R.B., Huntzicker, P.B. & Fruehan, G.J. (1969) Simultaneous comparison of respirometer and heart rate telemetry techniques as measures of human energy expenditure. *American Journal of Clinical Nutrition* **22**, 696–700.

Brody, S. (1974, original work published 1945) *Bioenergetics and Growth.* Collier Macmillan, New York.

Carlson, L.D. & Hsieh, A.C.L. (1970) *Control of Energy Exchange.* Macmillan, New York.

Chapman, C.B. & Mitchell, J.H. (1965) The physiology of exercise. *Scientific American* **212**, 88–96.

Collins, K.J., Abdel-Rahman, T.A. & Awad El Karim, M.A. (1988) Schistosomiasis: field studies of energy expenditure in agricultural workers in the Sudan. In *Capacity for Work in the Tropics* (ed. K.J. Collins & D.F. Roberts), pp. 235–247. Cambridge University Press, Cambridge.

Collins, M.A., Cureton, K.J., Hill, D.W. & Ray, C.A. (1991) Relationship of heart rate to oxygen uptake during weight lifting exercise. *Medicine and Science in Sports and Exercise* **23**, 636–640.

Durin, N. & Namyslowski, L. (1958) Individual variations in energy expenditure of standardized activities. *Journal of Physiology* **143**, 573–578.

Durnin, J.V.G.A. & Passmore, R. (1967) *Energy Work and Leisure.* Heinemann Educational Books, London.

Fenn, W.O. & Rahn, H. (eds) (1964) *Handbook of Physiology: Section 3. Respiration: Vol. 1.* American Physiological Society, Washington, DC.

Gandra, Y.R. & Bradfield, R.B. (1971) Energy expenditure and oxygen handling efficiency of anemic school children. *American Journal of Clinical Nutrition* **24**, 1451–1456.

Geissler, C.A., Brun, T.A., Mirbagheri, I., Soheli, A., Naghibi, A. & Hedayat, H. (1981) The energy expenditure of female carpet weavers and rural women in Iran. *American Journal of Clinical Nutrition* **34**, 2776–2783.

Getchell, L.H. (1968) Energy cost of playing golf. *Archives of Physical Medical Rehabilitation* **49**, 31–35.

Goff, L.G., Frassetto, R. & Specht, H. (1956) Oxygen requirement in underwater swimming. *Journal of Applied Physiology* **9**, 219–221.

Hambraeus, L., Forslund, A. & Sjödin, A. (1991) The use of a suit calorimeter in combination with indirect respiratory calorimetry for studies on the effect of diet and exercise on energy balance in healthy adults [abstract]. *Federation of American Societies for Experimental Biology Journal* **5**, A1648.

Hansen, O.E. & Maggio, M. (1960) Static work and heart rate. *Internationales Zeitschrift für Angewandte Physiologie Einschleisslich Arbeitsphysiologie* **18**, 242–247.

Harrison, M.H., Brown, G.A. & Belyasin, A.J. (1982) The oxylog: an evaluation. *Ergonomics* **25**(a), 809–820.

Henderson, Y. & Prince, A.L. (1914) The oxygen pulse and the systolic discharge. *American Journal of Physiology* **35**, 106–115.

Howley, E.T. & Glover, M.E. (1974) The caloric costs of

running and walking one mile for men and women. *Medicine and Science in Sports and Exercise* **6**, 235–237.

Humphrey, S.J.E. & Wolff, H.S. (1977) The oxylog (Abstract). *Journal of Physiology* **267**, 120.

Ikegami, Y., Hiruta, S., Ikegami, H. & Miyamura, M. (1988) Development of a telemetry system for measuring oxygen uptake during sports activities. *European Journal of Applied Physiology* **57**, 622–626.

Insull, W. (1954) *Indirect Calorimetry by New Techniques: A Description and Evaluation.* Report no. 146, Medical Nutrition Laboratory. US Army, Fitzsimmons Army Hospital, Denver, CO.

Jéquier, E., Acheson, K. & Schutz, Y. (1987) Assessment of energy expenditure and fuel utilization in man. *Annual Review of Nutrition* **7**, 187–208.

Kinney, J.M. (1980) The application of indirect calorimetry to clinical studies. In *Assessment of Energy Metabolism in Health and Disease*, pp. 42–48. Ross Laboratories, Columbus, OH.

Kofranyi, E. & Michaelis, H.F. (1940) Ein tragbarer Apparat zur Bestimmung des Gasstoffwechsels [A portable apparatus to determine metabolism]. *Arbeitsphysiologie* **11**, 148–150.

LaGrange, F. (1905) *Physiology of Bodily Exercise.* D. Appleton, New York.

Leon, A.S. (1981) Approximate energy expenditures and fitness values of sports and recreational and household activities. In *The Book of Health and Physical Fitness* (ed. E.L. Wynder), pp. 283–341. Watts, New York.

Lundgren, N.P.V. (1947) The physiological effects of time schedule work on lumber workers. *Acta Physiologica Scandinavica* 13 (Suppl. 41), 1–137.

McArdle, W.D., Katch, F.I. & Katch, V.L. (1988) *Exercise Physiology: Energy, Nutrition, and Human Performance*, 2nd edn. Lea & Febiger, Philadelphia.

McNeill, G., Cox, M.D. & Rivers, J.P.W. (1987) The oxylog oxygen consumption meter: a portable device for measurement of energy expenditure. *American Journal of Clinical Nutrition* **45**, 1415–1419.

Malhotra, M.S., Sen Gupta, J. & Rai, R.M. (1963) Pulse count as a measure of energy expenditure. *Journal of Applied Physiology* **18**, 994–996.

Mandli, M., Hoffman, M.D., Jones, G.M., Bota, B. & Clifford, P.S. (1989) Nordic ski training: in-line skates or roller skis? (Abstract) *Medicine and Science in Sports and Exercise* 21, S64.

Mass, S., Kok, M.L., Westra, H.G. & Kemper, H.C.G. (1989) The validity of the use of heart rate in estimating oxygen consumption in static and in combined static/dynamic exercise. *Ergonomics* **32**, 141–148.

Montoye, H.J. (1970) Circulatory-respiratory fitness. In *An Introduction to Measurement in Physical Education*, Vol. 4 (ed. H.J. Montoye), pp. 41–87. Phi Epsilon Kappa Fraternity, Indianapolis, IN.

Montoye, H.J. (1975) *Physical Activity and Health: an Epi-demiologic Study of a Total Community.* Prentice-Hall, Englewood Cliffs, NJ.

Montoye, H.J. (1982) Age and oxygen utilization during submaximal treadmill exercise in males. *Journal of Gerontology* **37**, 396–402.

Montoye, H.J., Kemper, H.C.G., Saris, W.H.M. & Washburn, R.A. (1996) *Measuring Physical Activity and Energy Expenditure.* Human Kinetics, Champaign, IL.

Montoye, H.J., Van Huss, W.D., Reineke, E.P. & Cockrell, J. (1958) An investigation of the Müller–Franz calorimeter. *Arbeitsphysiologie* **17**, 28–33.

Müller, E.A. & Franz, H. (1952) Energieverbraughsmes-sungen bei beruflicher Arbeit mit einer verbeserten Respirationsgasuhr (The measurement of energy consumption during occupational work with an improved respirometer). *Arbeitsphysiologie* **14**, 499–504.

Murlin, J.R. & Greer, J.R. (1914) The relation of heart action to the respiratory metabolism. *American Journal of Physiology* **33**, 253–282.

Nelson, D.J., Pells, A.E. III, Greenen, D.L. & White, T.P. (1988) Cardiac frequency and caloric cost of aerobic dancing in young women. *Research Quarterly for Exercise and Sport* **59**, 229–233.

Orsini, D. & Passmore, R. (1951) The energy expended carrying loads up and down stairs: experiments using the Kofranyi–Michaelis calorimeter. *Journal of Physiology* **115**, 95–100.

Passmore, R. & Durnin, J.V.G.A. (1955) Human energy expenditure. *Physiological Reviews* **35**, 801–840.

Patterson, R.P. & Fisher, S.V. (1979) Energy measurements in ambulation and activities of daily living: development and evaluation of a portable measuring system (Abstract). *Archives of Physical and Medical Rehabilitation* **60**, 534–535.

Payne, P.R., Wheeler, E.F. & Salvosa, C.B. (1971) Prediction of daily energy expenditure from average pulse rate. *American Journal of Clinical Nutrition* **24**, 1164–1170.

Reiff, G.G., Montoye, H.J., Remington, R.D., Napier, J.A., Metzner, H.L. & Epstein, F.H. (1967a) Assessment of physical activity by questionnaire and interview. *Journal of Sports Medicine and Physical Fitness* **7**, 1–32.

Reiff, G.G., Montoye, H.J., Remington, R.D., Napier, J.A., Metzner, H.L. & Epstein, F.H. (1967b) Assessment of physical activity by questionnaire and interview. In *Physical Activity and the Heart* (ed. M.J. Karvonen & A.J. Barry), pp. 336–371. Charles C. Thomas, Springfield, IL.

Saris, W.H.M., Baecke, J. & Binkhorst, R.A. (1982) Validity of the assessment of energy expenditure from heart rate. In *Aerobic Power and Daily Physical Activity in Children* (ed. W.H.M. Saris), pp. 100–117. University of Nymegen, Meppel, Krips-Repro, The Netherlands.

Seliger, V. (1968) Energy metabolism in selected physical exercises. *Internationale Zeitschrift für Angewande Physiologie Einschliesslich Arabeitsphysiologie* **25**, 104–120.

Stray-Gundersen, J. & Galanes, J. (1991) The metabolic demands of roller skating compared to snow skiing [abstract]. *Medicine and Science in Sports and Exercise* **23**, S107.

Taylor, H.L. (1967) Occupational factors in the study of coronary heart disease and physical activity. *Canadian Medical Association Journal* **96**, 825–831.

Taylor, H.L. & Parlin, R.W. (1966) The physical activity of railroad clerks and switchmen: Estimation of the on-the-job caloric expenditure by time and task measurements and classification of recreational activity by a questionnaire. Paper presented at 'Three Days of Cardiology,' Seattle, WA, June.

Torún, B., Chew, F. & Mendoza, R.D. (1983) Energy cost of activities of preschool children. *Nutrition Research* **3**, 401–406.

Veicsteinas, A., Ferretti, G., Margonato, V., Rosa, G. & Tagliabue, D. (1984) Energy cost of and energy sources for alpine skiing in top athletes. *Journal of Applied Physiology* **56**, 1187–1190.

Viteri, F.E., Torún, B., Galicia, J. & Herrera, E. (1971) Determining energy costs of agricultural activities by respirometer and energy balance techniques. *American Journal of Clinical Nutrition* **24**, 1418–1430.

Vokac, Z., Bell, H., Bautz-Holter, E. & Rodahl, J. (1975) Oxygen uptake/heart rate relationship in leg and arm exercise, sitting and standing. *Journal of Applied Physiology* **39**, 54–59.

VonHofen, D., Auble, T.E. & Schwartz, L. (1989) Aerobic requirements for pumping vs. carrying 9 kg hand weights while running (Abstract). *Medicine and Science in Sports and Exercise* **21**, S7.

Warnold, T. & Lenner, A.R. (1977) Evaluation of the heart rate method to determine the daily energy expenditure in disease: a study in juvenile diabetics. *American Journal of Clinical Nutrition* **30**, 304–315.

Watts, P.B., Martin, D.T., Schmeling, M.H., Silta, B.C. & Watts, A.G. (1990) Exertional intensities and energy requirements of technical mountaineering at moderate altitudes. *Journal of Sports Medicine and Physical Fitness* **30**, 365–376.

Webb, P. (1980) The measurement of energy exchange in man: an analysis. *American Journal of Clinical Nutrition* **33**, 1299–1310.

Webb, P., Annis, J.F. & Troutman, S.J. Jr (1980) Energy balance in man measured by direct and indirect calorimetry. *American Journal of Clinical Nutrition* **33**, 1287–1298.

Wigaeus, E. & Kilbom, A. (1980) Physical demands during folk dancing. *European Journal of Applied Physiology* **45**, 117–183.

Wolff, H.S. (1958) The integrating pneumotachograph: a new instrument for the measurement of energy expenditures by indirect calorimetry. *Quarterly Journal of Exercise Physiology* **43**, 270–283.

Zuntz, N. & Leowy, A. (1909) *Lehrbuch der Physiologie bes Menschen* (*Textbook of Human Physiology*). F.C.W. Vogel, Leipzig, Germany.

## Appendix 4.1  A compendium of the energy costs of different physical activities.

| Activity category | Specific activity (kcal h$^{-1}$·kg$^{-1}$) | METs | kJ·h$^{-1}$·kg$^{-1}$ (kcal·h$^{-1}$·kg$^{-1}$) body wt |
|---|---|---|---|
| Bicycling | Mountain biking | 8.5 | 35 (8.3) |
| Bicycling | <16 km·h$^{-1}$, general, leisure, to work or for pleasure | 4.0 | 17 (4.0) |
| Bicycling | 16–19 km·h$^{-1}$, leisure, slow, light effort | 6.0 | 25 (5.9) |
| Bicycling | 19.1–22.4 km·h$^{-1}$, leisure, moderate effort | 8.0 | 33 (7.8) |
| Bicycling | 22.5–25.5 km·h$^{-1}$, racing or leisure, fast, vigorous effort | 10.0 | 42 (10.0) |
| Bicycling | 25.6–30.5 km·h$^{-1}$, racing/not drafting or >30.5 km·h$^{-1}$ drafting, very fast, racing general | 12.0 | 50 (11.9) |
| Bicycling | >30.5 km·h$^{-1}$, racing, not drafting | 16.0 | 67 (15.9) |
| Bicycling | Unicycling | 5.0 | 21 (5.0) |
| Conditioning exercise | Bicycling, stationary, general | 5.0 | 21 (5.0) |
| Conditioning exercise | Bicycling, stationary, 50 W, very light effort | 3.0 | 13 (3.1) |
| Conditioning exercise | Bicycling, stationary, 100 W, light effort | 5.5 | 23 (5.5) |
| Conditioning exercise | Bicycling, stationary, 150 W, moderate effort | 7.0 | 29 (6.9) |
| Conditioning exercise | Bicycling, stationary, 200 W, vigorous effort | 10.5 | 44 (10.5) |
| Conditioning exercise | Bicycling, stationary, 250 W, very vigorous effort | 12.5 | 52 (12.4) |
| Conditioning exercise | Calisthenics (e.g. push-ups, pull-ups, sit-ups), heavy, vigorous effort | 8.0 | 33 (7.8) |

| Activity category | Specific activity | METs | kJ·h⁻¹·kg⁻¹ (kcal·h⁻¹·kg⁻¹) body wt |
|---|---|---|---|
| Conditioning exercise | Calisthenics, home exercise, light or moderate effort, general (e.g. back exercises), going up and down from floor | 4.5 | 19 (4.5) |
| Conditioning exercise | Circuit training, general | 8.0 | 33 (7.8) |
| Conditioning exercise | Weight lifting (free weight, nautilus or universal-type), power lifting or body building, vigorous effort | 6.0 | 25 (5.9) |
| Conditioning exercise | Health club exercise, general | 5.5 | 23 (5.5) |
| Conditioning exercise | Stair-treadmill ergometer, general | 6.0 | 25 (5.9) |
| Conditioning exercise | Rowing, stationary ergometer, general | 9.5 | 40 (9.5) |
| Conditioning exercise | Rowing, stationary, 50 W, light effort | 3.5 | 15 (3.6) |
| Conditioning exercise | Rowing stationary, 100 W, moderate effort | 7.0 | 29 (6.9) |
| Conditioning exercise | Rowing, stationary, 150 W, vigorous effort | 8.5 | 35 (8.3) |
| Conditioning exercise | Rowing, stationary, 200 W, very vigorous effort | 12.0 | 50 (11.9) |
| Conditioning exercise | Ski machine, general | 9.5 | 40 (9.5) |
| Conditioning exercise | Slimnastics | 6.0 | 25 (5.9) |
| Conditioning exercise | Stretching, hatha yoga | 4.0 | 17 (4.0) |
| Conditioning exercise | Teaching aerobics exercise class, assumes participation | 6.0 | 25 (5.9) |
| Conditioning exercise | Water aerobics, water calisthenics | 4.0 | 17 (4.0) |
| Conditioning exercise | Weight lifting (free, nautilus or universal-type), light or moderate effort, light workout, general | 3.0 | 13 (3.1) |
| Conditioning exercise | Whirlpool, sitting | 1.0 | 4 (0.9) |
| Dancing | Aerobic, ballet or modern, twist | 6.0 | 25 (5.9) |
| Dancing | Aerobic, general | 6.0 | 25 (5.9) |
| Dancing | Aerobic, low impact | 5.0 | 21 (5.0) |
| Dancing | Aerobic, high impact | 7.0 | 29 (6.9) |
| Dancing | General | 4.5 | 19 (4.5) |
| Dancing | Ballroom, fast (e.g. disco, folk, square) | 5.5 | 23 (5.5) |
| Dancing | Ballroom, slow (e.g. waltz, foxtrot, slow dancing) | 3.0 | 13 (3.1) |
| Fishing and hunting | Fishing, general | 5.0 | 21 (5.0) |
| Fishing and hunting | Digging worms with shovel | 4.0 | 17 (4.0) |
| Fishing and hunting | Fishing from river bank and walking | 5.0 | 21 (5.0) |
| Fishing and hunting | Fishing from boat, sitting | 2.5 | 10 (2.4) |
| Fishing and hunting | Fishing from river bank, standing | 3.5 | 15 (3.6) |
| Fishing and hunting | Fishing in stream, in waders | 6.0 | 25 (5.9) |
| Fishing and hunting | Fishing, ice, sitting | 2.0 | 8 (1.9) |
| Fishing and hunting | Hunting, bow and arrow or crossbow | 2.5 | 10 (2.4) |
| Fishing and hunting | Hunting, deer, elk, large game | 6.0 | 25 (5.9) |
| Fishing and hunting | Hunting, duck, wading | 2.5 | 10 (2.4) |
| Fishing and hunting | Hunting, general | 5.0 | 21 (5.0) |
| Fishing and hunting | Hunting, pheasants or grouse | 6.0 | 25 (5.9) |
| Fishing and hunting | Hunting, rabbit, squirrel, prairie chick, racoon, small game | 5.0 | 21 (5.0) |
| Fishing and hunting | Pistol shooting or trap shooting, standing | 2.5 | 10 (2.4) |
| Home activities | Carpet sweeping, sweeping floors | 2.5 | 10 (2.4) |
| Home activities | Cleaning, heavy or major (e.g. washing car, washing windows, mopping, cleaning garage), vigorous effort | 4.5 | 19 (4.5) |
| Home activities | Cleaning, house or cabin, general | 3.5 | 15 (3.6) |
| Home activities | Cleaning, light (dusting, straightening up, vacuuming, changing linen, carrying out rubbish), moderate effort | 2.5 | 10 (2.4) |
| Home activities | Washing dishes, standing or in general (not broken into stand/walk components) | 2.3 | 9 (2.1) |

| Activity category | Specific activity | METs | kJ·h⁻¹·kg⁻¹ (kcal·h⁻¹·kg⁻¹) body wt |
|---|---|---|---|
| Home activities | Washing dishes, clearing dishes from table (walking) | 2.3 | 9 (2.1) |
| Home activities | Cooking or preparing food, standing or sitting or in general (not broken into stand/walk components) | 2.5 | 10 (2.4) |
| Home activities | Serving food, setting table (implied walking or standing) | 2.5 | 10 (2.4) |
| Home activities | Cooking or food preparation, walking | 2.5 | 10 (2.4) |
| Home activities | Putting away groceries (e.g. carrying groceries, shopping without a trolley) | 2.5 | 10 (2.4) |
| Home activities | Carrying groceries upstairs | 8.0 | 33 (7.8) |
| Home activities | Food shopping, with trolley | 3.5 | 15 (3.6) |
| Home activities | Shopping (non-grocery shopping), standing | 2.0 | 8 (1.9) |
| Home activities | Shopping (non-grocery shopping), walking | 2.3 | 9 (2.1) |
| Home activities | Ironing | 2.3 | 9 (2.1) |
| Home activities | Sitting, knitting, sewing, light wrapping (presents) | 1.5 | 6 (1.4) |
| Home activities | Laundry, folding or hanging clothes, putting clothes in washer or dryer, packing suitcase (implied standing) | 2.0 | 8 (1.9) |
| Home activities | Putting away clothes, gathering clothes to pack, putting away laundry (implied walking) | 2.3 | 9 (2.1) |
| Home activities | Making beds | 2.0 | 8 (1.9) |
| Home activities | Making maple syrup (tapping trees, carrying buckets, carrying wood, etc.) | 5.0 | 21 (5.0) |
| Home activities | Moving furniture, household | 6.0 | 25 (5.9) |
| Home activities | Scrubbing floors on hands and knees | 5.5 | 23 (5.5) |
| Home activities | Sweeping garage, pavement or outside of house | 4.0 | 17 (4.0) |
| Home activities | Moving household items, carrying boxes | 7.0 | 29 (6.9) |
| Home activities | Packing/unpacking boxes, occasional lifting of household items, light–moderate effort (standing) | 3.5 | 15 (3.6) |
| Home activities | Putting away household items, moderate effort (implied walking) | 3.0 | 13 (3.1) |
| Home activities | Move household items upstairs, carrying boxes or furniture | 9.0 | 38 (9.0) |
| Home activities | Light (e.g. pumping gas, changing light bulb, etc.), standing | 2.5 | 10 (2.4) |
| Home activities | Light, non-cleaning (e.g. getting ready to leave, shutting/locking doors, closing windows, etc.), walking | 3.0 | 13 (3.1) |
| Home activities | Playing with child(ren), light effort (sitting) | 2.5 | 10 (2.4) |
| Home activities | Playing with child(ren), light effort (standing) | 2.8 | 12 (2.8) |
| Home activities | Playing with child(ren), moderate effort (walking/running) | 4.0 | 17 (4.0) |
| Home activities | Playing with child(ren), vigorous effort (walking/running) | 5.0 | 21 (5.0) |
| Home activities | Child care: sitting/kneeling—dressing, bathing, grooming, feeding, occasional lifting of child, light effort | 3.0 | 13 (3.1) |
| Home activities | Child care: standing—dressing, bathing, grooming, feeding, occasional lifting of child, light effort | 3.5 | 15 (3.6) |
| Home activities | Weaving at a loom, sitting | 2.0 | 8 (1.9) |
| Home repair | Car body work | 4.5 | 19 (4.5) |
| Home repair | Car repair | 3.0 | 13 (3.1) |
| Home repair | Carpentry, general, workshop | 3.0 | 13 (3.1) |
| Home repair | Carpentry, outside house, installing rain gutters | 6.0 | 25 (5.9) |
| Home repair | Carpentry, finishing or refinishing cabinets or furniture | 4.5 | 19 (4.5) |
| Home repair | Carpentry, sawing hardwood | 7.5 | 31 (7.4) |
| Home repair | Caulking, chinking log cabin | 5.0 | 21 (5.0) |
| Home repair | Caulking, except log cabin | 4.5 | 19 (4.5) |
| Home repair | Cleaning, gutters | 5.0 | 21 (5.0) |

| Activity category | Specific activity | METs | kJ·h⁻¹·kg⁻¹ (kcal·h⁻¹·kg⁻¹) body wt |
|---|---|---|---|
| Home repair | Excavating garage | 5.0 | 21 (5.0) |
| Home repair | Hanging storm windows | 5.0 | 21 (5.0) |
| Home repair | Laying or removing carpet | 4.5 | 19 (4.5) |
| Home repair | Laying tile or linoleum | 4.5 | 19 (4.5) |
| Home repair | Painting, outside house | 5.0 | 21 (5.0) |
| Home repair | Painting, papering, plastering, scraping, inside house, hanging sheet rock, remodelling | 4.5 | 19 (4.5) |
| Home repair | Putting on and removing of sailboat tarpaulin | 3.0 | 13 (3.1) |
| Home repair | Roofing | 6.0 | 25 (5.9) |
| Home repair | Sanding floors with a power sander | 4.5 | 19 (4.5) |
| Home repair | Scraping and painting sailboat or power boat | 4.5 | 19 (4.5) |
| Home repair | Spreading dirt with a shovel | 5.0 | 21 (5.0) |
| Home repair | Washing and waxing hull of sailboat, car, powerboat, airplane | 4.5 | 19 (4.5) |
| Home repair | Washing fence | 4.5 | 19 (4.5) |
| Home repair | Wiring, plumbing | 3.0 | 13 (3.1) |
| Inactivity, quiet | Lying quietly, reclining (watching television), lying quietly in bed—awake | 1.0 | 4 (0.9) |
| Inactivity, quiet | Sitting quietly (riding in a car, listening to a lecture or music, watching television or a film) | 1.0 | 4 (0.9) |
| Inactivity, quiet | Sleeping | 0.9 | 4 (0.9) |
| Inactivity, quiet | Standing quietly (standing in a line) | 1.2 | 5 (1.2) |
| Inactivity, light | Writing, reclining | 1.0 | 4 (0.9) |
| Inactivity, light | Talking or talking on phone, reclining | 1.0 | 4 (0.9) |
| Inactivity, light | Reading, reclining | 1.0 | 4 (0.9) |
| Lawn and garden | Carrying, loading or stacking wood, loading/unloading or carrying lumber | 5.0 | 21 (5.0) |
| Lawn and garden | Chopping wood, splitting logs | 6.0 | 25 (5.9) |
| Lawn and garden | Clearing land, hauling branches | 5.0 | 21 (5.0) |
| Lawn and garden | Digging sandpit | 5.0 | 21 (5.0) |
| Lawn and garden | Digging, spading, filling garden | 5.0 | 21 (5.0) |
| Lawn and garden | Gardening with heavy power tools, tilling a garden (see Occupation, Shovelling) | 6.0 | 25 (5.9) |
| Lawn and garden | Laying crushed rock | 5.0 | 21 (5.0) |
| Lawn and garden | Laying sod | 5.0 | 21 (5.0) |
| Lawn and garden | Mowing lawn, general | 5.5 | 23 (5.5) |
| Lawn and garden | Mowing lawn, riding mower | 2.5 | 10 (2.4) |
| Lawn and garden | Mowing lawn, walk, hand mower | 6.0 | 25 (5.9) |
| Lawn and garden | Mowing lawn, walking, power mower | 4.5 | 19 (4.5) |
| Lawn and garden | Operating snow blower, walking | 4.5 | 19 (4.5) |
| Lawn and garden | Planting seedlings, shrubs | 4.0 | 17 (4.0) |
| Lawn and garden | Planting trees | 4.5 | 19 (4.5) |
| Lawn and garden | Raking lawn | 4.0 | 17 (4.0) |
| Lawn and garden | Raking roof with snow rake | 4.0 | 17 (4.0) |
| Lawn and garden | Riding snow blower | 3.0 | 13 (3.1) |
| Lawn and garden | Collecting grass/leaves | 4.0 | 17 (4.0) |
| Lawn and garden | Shovelling snow by hand | 6.0 | 25 (5.9) |
| Lawn and garden | Trimming shrubs or trees, manual cutter | 4.5 | 19 (4.5) |
| Lawn and garden | Trimming shrubs or trees, power cutter | 3.5 | 15 (3.6) |
| Lawn and garden | Walking, applying fertilizer or seeding a lawn | 2.5 | 10 (2.4) |
| Lawn and garden | Watering lawn or garden, standing or walking | 1.5 | 6 (1.4) |

| Activity category | Specific activity | METs | kJ·h⁻¹·kg⁻¹ (kcal·h⁻¹·kg⁻¹) body wt |
|---|---|---|---|
| Lawn and garden | Weeding, cultivating garden | 4.5 | 19 (4.5) |
| Lawn and garden | Gardening, general | 5.0 | 21 (5.0) |
| Lawn and garden | Tidying up yard, light effort (implied walking/standing) | 3.0 | 13 (3.1) |
| Miscellaneous | Card playing, playing board games (sitting) | 1.5 | 6 (1.4) |
| Miscellaneous | Drawing or writing, casino gambling (standing) | 2.0 | 8 (1.9) |
| Miscellaneous | Reading, book, newspaper, etc. (sitting) | 1.3 | 5 (1.2) |
| Miscellaneous | Writing, desk work (sitting) | 1.8 | 7.5 (1.8) |
| Miscellaneous | Talking or talking on the phone (standing) | 1.8 | 7.5 (1.8) |
| Miscellaneous | Talking or talking on the phone (sitting) | 1.5 | 6 (1.4) |
| Miscellaneous | Studying, general, including reading and/or writing (sitting) | 1.8 | 7.5 (1.8) |
| Miscellaneous | In class, general, including note-taking or class discussion (sitting) | 1.8 | 7.5 (1.8) |
| Miscellaneous | Reading (standing) | 1.8 | 7.5 (1.8) |
| Music playing | Accordion | 1.8 | 7.5 (1.8) |
| Music playing | Cello | 2.0 | 8 (1.9) |
| Music playing | Conducting | 2.5 | 10 (2.4) |
| Music playing | Drums | 4.0 | 17 (4.0) |
| Music playing | Flute (sitting) | 2.0 | 8 (1.9) |
| Music playing | Horn | 2.0 | 8 (1.9) |
| Music playing | Piano or organ | 2.5 | 10 (2.4) |
| Music playing | Trombone | 3.5 | 15 (3.6) |
| Music playing | Trumpet | 2.5 | 10 (2.4) |
| Music playing | Violin | 2.5 | 10 (2.4) |
| Music playing | Woodwind | 2.0 | 8 (1.9) |
| Music playing | Guitar, classical, folk (sitting) | 2.0 | 8 (1.9) |
| Music playing | Guitar, rock and roll band (standing) | 3.0 | 13 (3.1) |
| Music playing | Marching band, playing an instrument, baton twirling (walking) | 4.0 | 17 (4.0) |
| Music playing | Marching band, drum major (walking) | 3.5 | 15 (3.6) |
| Occupation | Bakery, general | 4.0 | 17 (4.0) |
| Occupation | Bookbinding | 2.3 | 9 (2.1) |
| Occupation | Building road (including hauling debris, driving heavy machinery) | 6.0 | 25 (5.9) |
| Occupation | Building road, directing traffic (standing) | 2.0 | 8 (1.9) |
| Occupation | Carpentry, general | 3.5 | 15 (3.6) |
| Occupation | Carrying heavy loads, such as bricks | 8.0 | 33 (7.8) |
| Occupation | Carrying moderate loads up stairs, moving boxes (7–18 kg) | 8.0 | 33 (7.8) |
| Occupation | Chambermaid | 2.5 | 10 (2.4) |
| Occupation | Coal mining, drilling coal, rock | 6.5 | 27 (6.4) |
| Occupation | Coal mining, erecting supports | 6.5 | 27 (6.4) |
| Occupation | Coal mining, general | 6.0 | 25 (5.9) |
| Occupation | Coal mining, shovelling coal | 7.0 | 29 (6.9) |
| Occupation | Construction, outside, remodelling | 5.5 | 23 (5.5) |
| Occupation | Electrical work, plumbing | 3.5 | 15 (3.6) |
| Occupation | Farming, baling hay, cleaning barn, poultry work | 8.0 | 33 (5.5) |
| Occupation | Farming, chasing cattle, non-strenuous | 3.5 | 15 (3.6) |
| Occupation | Farming, driving harvester | 2.5 | 10 (2.4) |
| Occupation | Farming, driving tractor | 2.5 | 10 (2.4) |
| Occupation | Farming, feeding small animals | 4.0 | 17 (4.0) |
| Occupation | Farming, feeding cattle | 4.5 | 19 (4.5) |

| Activity category | Specific activity | METs | kJ·h⁻¹·kg⁻¹ (kcal·h⁻¹·kg⁻¹) body wt |
|---|---|---|---|
| Occupation | Farming, forking straw bales | 8.0 | 33 (5.5) |
| Occupation | Farming, milking by hand | 3.0 | 13 (3.1) |
| Occupation | Farming, milking by machine | 1.5 | 6 (1.4) |
| Occupation | Farming, shovelling grain | 5.5 | 23 (5.5) |
| Occupation | Fire fighter, general | 12.0 | 50 (11.9) |
| Occupation | Fire fighter, climbing ladder with full gear | 11.0 | 46 (10.9) |
| Occupation | Fire fighter, hauling hoses on ground | 8.0 | 33 (7.8) |
| Occupation | Forestry, chopping with axe, fast | 17.0 | 71 (16.9) |
| Occupation | Forestry, chopping with axe, slow | 5.0 | 21 (5.0) |
| Occupation | Forestry, removing bark from trees | 7.0 | 29 (6.9) |
| Occupation | Forestry, carrying logs | 11.0 | 46 (10.9) |
| Occupation | Forestry, felling trees | 8.0 | 33 (7.8) |
| Occupation | Forestry, general | 8.0 | 33 (7.8) |
| Occupation | Forestry, hoeing | 5.0 | 21 (5.0) |
| Occupation | Forestry, planting by hand | 6.0 | 25 (5.9) |
| Occupation | Forestry, sawing by hand | 7.0 | 29 (6.9) |
| Occupation | Forestry, sawing, power | 4.5 | 19 (4.5) |
| Occupation | Forestry, trimming trees | 9.0 | 38 (9.0) |
| Occupation | Forestry, weeding | 4.0 | 17 (4.0) |
| Occupation | Furriery | 4.5 | 19 (4.5) |
| Occupation | Horse grooming | 6.0 | 25 (5.9) |
| Occupation | Locksmith | 3.5 | 15 (3.6) |
| Occupation | Machine tooling, machining, working sheet metal | 2.5 | 10 (2.4) |
| Occupation | Machine tooling, operating lathe | 3.0 | 13 (3.1) |
| Occupation | Machine tooling, operating punch press | 5.0 | 21 (5.0) |
| Occupation | Machine tooling, tapping and drilling | 4.0 | 17 (4.0) |
| Occupation | Machine tooling, welding | 3.0 | 13 (3.1) |
| Occupation | Masonry, concrete | 7.0 | 29 (6.9) |
| Occupation | Masseur, masseuse (standing) | 4.0 | 17 (4.0) |
| Occupation | Moving, pushing heavy objects, 40 kg or more (desks, moving van work) | 7.0 | 29 (6.9) |
| Occupation | Operating heavy duty equipment/automated, not driving | 2.5 | 10 (2.4) |
| Occupation | Orange grove work | 4.5 | 19 (4.5) |
| Occupation | Printing (standing) | 2.3 | 9 (2.1) |
| Occupation | Police, directing traffic (standing) | 2.5 | 10 (2.4) |
| Occupation | Police, driving a squad car (sitting) | 2.0 | 8 (1.9) |
| Occupation | Police, riding in a squad car (sitting) | 1.3 | 5 (1.2) |
| Occupation | Police, making an arrest (standing) | 8.0 | 33 (7.8) |
| Occupation | Shoe repair, general | 2.5 | 10 (2.4) |
| Occupation | Shovelling, digging ditches | 8.5 | 35 (8.3) |
| Occupation | Shovelling, heavy (more than 7 kg·min⁻¹) | 9.0 | 38 (9.0) |
| Occupation | Shovelling, light (less than 4.5 kg·min⁻¹) | 6.0 | 25 (5.9) |
| Occupation | Shovelling, moderate (4.5–7 kg·min⁻¹) | 7.0 | 29 (6.9) |
| Occupation | Light office work, in general (chemistry lab work, light use of hand tools, watch repair or microassembly, light assembly/repair) (sitting) | 1.5 | 6 (1.4) |
| Occupation | Meetings, general, and/or with talking involved (sitting) | 1.5 | 6 (1.4) |
| Occupation | Moderate (e.g. heavy levers, riding mower/forklift, crane operation), sitting | 2.5 | 10 (2.4) |
| Occupation | Light (e.g. bartending, store clerk, assembling, filing, photocopying, putting up Christmas tree), standing | 2.5 | 10 (2.4) |

| Activity category | Specific activity | METs | kJ·h⁻¹·kg⁻¹ (kcal·h⁻¹·kg⁻¹) body wt |
|---|---|---|---|
| Occupation | Light/moderate (e.g. assemble/repair heavy parts, welding, stocking, car repair, packing boxes for moving, etc.), patient care (as in nursing), standing | 3.0 | 13 (3.1) |
| Occupation | Moderate (e.g. assembling at fast rate, lifting 20 kg, hitching/twisting ropes), standing | 3.5 | 15 (3.6) |
| Occupation | Moderate/heavy (e.g. lifting more than 20 kg, masonry, painting, paper hanging), standing | 4.0 | 17 (4.0) |
| Occupation | Steel mill, fettling | 5.0 | 21 (5.0) |
| Occupation | Steel mill, forging | 5.5 | 23 (5.5) |
| Occupation | Steel mill, hand rolling | 8.0 | 33 (7.8) |
| Occupation | Steel mill, merchant mill rolling | 8.0 | 33 (7.8) |
| Occupation | Steel mill, removing slag | 11.0 | 46 (10.9) |
| Occupation | Steel mill, tending furnace | 7.5 | 31 (7.4) |
| Occupation | Steel mill, tipping molds | 5.5 | 23 (5.5) |
| Occupation | Steel mill, working in general | 8.0 | 33 (7.8) |
| Occupation | Tailoring, cutting | 2.5 | 10 (2.4) |
| Occupation | Tailoring, general | 2.5 | 10 (2.4) |
| Occupation | Tailoring, hand sewing | 2.0 | 8 (1.9) |
| Occupation | Tailoring, machine sewing | 2.5 | 10 (2.4) |
| Occupation | Tailoring, pressing | 4.0 | 17 (4.0) |
| Occupation | Truck driving, loading and unloading truck (standing) | 6.5 | 27 (6.4) |
| Occupation | Typing, electric, manual or computer | 1.5 | 6 (1.4) |
| Occupation | Using heavy power tools such as pneumatic tools (jackhammers, drills, etc.) | 6.0 | 25 (5.9) |
| Occupation | Using heavy tools (not power) such as shovel, pick, tunnel bar, spade | 8.0 | 33 (7.8) |
| Occupation | Walking on job, less than 3 km·h⁻¹ (in office or lab area), very slow | 2.0 | 8 (1.9) |
| Occupation | Walking on job, 5 km·h⁻¹, in office, moderate speed, not carrying anything | 3.5 | 15 (3.6) |
| Occupation | Walking on job, 6 km·h⁻¹, in office, brisk speed, not carrying anything | 4.0 | 17 (4.0) |
| Occupation | Walking, 4 km·h⁻¹, slowly and carrying light objects less than 10 kg | 3.0 | 13 (3.1) |
| Occupation | Walking, 5 km·h⁻¹, moderately and carrying light objects less than 10 kg | 4.0 | 17 (4.0) |
| Occupation | Walking, 6 km·h⁻¹, briskly and carrying objects less than 10 kg | 4.5 | 19 (4.5) |
| Occupation | Walking or walking downstairs or standing, carrying objects about 10–22 kg | 5.0 | 21 (5.0) |
| Occupation | Walking or walking downstairs or standing, carrying objects about 23–33 kg | 6.5 | 27 (6.4) |
| Occupation | Walking or walking downstairs or standing, carrying objects about 34–44 kg | 7.5 | 31 (7.4) |
| Occupation | Walking or walking downstairs or standing, carrying objects about 45 kg and over | 8.5 | 35 (8.3) |
| Occupation | Working in scene shop, theatre actor, backstage, employee | 3.0 | 13 (3.1) |
| Running | Jog/walk combination (jogging component of less than 10 min) | 6.0 | 25 (5.9) |
| Running | Jogging, general | 7.0 | 29 (6.9) |
| Running | 8 km·h⁻¹ (7.5 min·km⁻¹) | 8.0 | 33 (7.8) |

| Activity category | Specific activity | METs | kJ·h⁻¹·kg⁻¹ (kcal·h⁻¹·kg⁻¹) body wt |
|---|---|---|---|
| Running | 9.6 km·h⁻¹ (6.25 min·km⁻¹) | 10.0 | 42 (10.0) |
| Running | 10.8 km·h⁻¹ (5.5 min·km⁻¹) | 11.0 | 46 (10.9) |
| Running | 11.3 km·h⁻¹ (5.3 min·km⁻¹) | 11.5 | 48 (11.4) |
| Running | 12 km·h⁻¹ (5.0 min·km⁻¹) | 12.5 | 52 (12.4) |
| Running | 12.8 km·h⁻¹ (4.7 min·km⁻¹) | 13.5 | 56 (13.3) |
| Running | 13.8 km·h⁻¹ (4.3 min·km⁻¹) | 14.0 | 59 (14.0) |
| Running | 14.5 km·h⁻¹ (4.1 min·km⁻¹) | 15.0 | 63 (15.0) |
| Running | 16.1 km·h⁻¹ (3.7 min·km⁻¹) | 16.0 | 67 (15.9) |
| Running | 17.5 km·h⁻¹ (3.4 min·km⁻¹) | 18.0 | 75 (17.8) |
| Running | Running, cross-country | 9.0 | 38 (9.0) |
| Running | Running, general | 8.0 | 33 (7.8) |
| Running | Running, in place | 8.0 | 33 (7.8) |
| Running | Running upstairs | 15.0 | 63 (15.0) |
| Running | Running on a track, team practice | 10.0 | 42 (10.0) |
| Running | Running, training, pushing wheelchair, marathon wheeling | 8.0 | 33 (7.8) |
| Running | Running, wheeling, general | 3.0 | 13 (3.1) |
| Self-care | Getting ready for bed, in general (standing) | 2.5 | 10 (2.4) |
| Self-care | Sitting on toilet | 1.0 | 4 (0.9) |
| Self-care | Bathing, sitting | 2.0 | 8 (1.9) |
| Self-care | Dressing, undressing, standing or sitting | 2.5 | 10 (2.4) |
| Self-care | Eating, sitting | 1.5 | 6 (1.4) |
| Self-care | Talking and eating or eating only, standing | 2.0 | 8 (1.9) |
| Self-care | Grooming (e.g. washing, shaving, brushing teeth, urinating, washing hands, putting on make-up), sitting or standing | 2.5 | 10 (2.4) |
| Self-care | Showering, towelling off, standing | 4.0 | 17 (4.0) |
| Sexual activity | Active, vigorous effort | 1.5 | 6 (1.4) |
| Sexual activity | General, moderate effort | 1.3 | 5 (1.2) |
| Sexual activity | Passive, light effort, kissing, hugging | 1.0 | 4 (0.9) |
| Sports | Archery (non-hunting) | 3.5 | 15 (3.6) |
| Sports | Badminton, competitive | 7.0 | 29 (6.9) |
| Sports | Badminton, social singles and doubles, general | 4.5 | 19 (4.5) |
| Sports | Basketball, game | 8.0 | 33 (7.8) |
| Sports | Basketball, non-game, general | 6.0 | 25 (5.9) |
| Sports | Basketball, officiating | 7.0 | 29 (6.9) |
| Sports | Basketball, shooting baskets | 4.5 | 19 (4.5) |
| Sports | Basketball, wheelchair | 6.5 | 27 (6.4) |
| Sports | Billiards | 2.5 | 10 (2.4) |
| Sports | Bowling | 3.0 | 13 (3.1) |
| Sports | Boxing, in ring, general | 12.0 | 50 (11.9) |
| Sports | Boxing, punching bag | 6.0 | 25 (5.9) |
| Sports | Boxing, sparring | 9.0 | 38 (9.0) |
| Sports | Broomball | 7.0 | 29 (6.9) |
| Sports | Children's games (hopscotch, 4-square, dodgeball, playground apparatus, t-ball, tetherball, marbles, jacks, arcade games) | 5.0 | 21 (5.0) |
| Sports | Coaching: football, soccer, basketball, baseball swimming, etc. | 4.0 | 17 (4.0) |
| Sports | Cricket (batting, bowling) | 5.0 | 21 (5.0) |
| Sports | Croquet | 2.5 | 10 (2.4) |
| Sports | Curling | 4.0 | 17 (4.0) |
| Sports | Darts, wall or lawn | 2.5 | 10 (2.4) |
| Sports | Drag racing, pushing or driving a car | 6.0 | 25 (5.9) |

| Activity category | Specific activity | METs | $kJ \cdot h^{-1} \cdot kg^{-1}$ $(kcal \cdot h^{-1} \cdot kg^{-1})$ body wt |
|---|---|---|---|
| Sports | Fencing | 6.0 | 25 (5.9) |
| Sports | Football, competitive | 9.0 | 38 (9.0) |
| Sports | Football, touch, flag, general | 8.0 | 33 (7.8) |
| Sports | Football or baseball, playing catch | 2.5 | 10 (2.4) |
| Sports | Frisbee playing, general | 3.0 | 13 (3.1) |
| Sports | Frisbee, ultimate | 3.5 | 15 (3.6) |
| Sports | Golf, general | 4.5 | 19 (4.5) |
| Sports | Golf, carrying clubs | 5.5 | 23 (5.5) |
| Sports | Golf, miniature, driving range | 3.0 | 13 (3.1) |
| Sports | Golf, pulling clubs | 5.0 | 21 (5.0) |
| Sports | Golf, using power cart | 3.5 | 15 (3.6) |
| Sports | Gymnastics, general | 4.0 | 17 (4.0) |
| Sports | Handball, competitive | 12.0 | 50 (11.9) |
| Sports | Handball, team | 8.0 | 33 (7.8) |
| Sports | Hang gliding | 3.5 | 15 (3.6) |
| Sports | Hockey, field | 8.0 | 33 (7.8) |
| Sports | Hockey, ice | 8.0 | 33 (7.8) |
| Sports | Horseback riding, general | 4.0 | 17 (4.0) |
| Sports | Horseback riding, saddling horse | 3.5 | 15 (3.6) |
| Sports | Horseback riding, trotting | 6.5 | 27 (6.4) |
| Sports | Horseback riding, walking | 2.5 | 10 (2.4) |
| Sports | Horseshoe pitching, quoits | 3.0 | 13 (3.1) |
| Sports | Jai alai | 12.0 | 50 (11.9) |
| Sports | Judo, jujitsu, karate, kick boxing, tae kwan do | 10.0 | 42 (10.0) |
| Sports | Juggling | 4.0 | 17 (4.0) |
| Sports | Kickball | 7.0 | 29 (6.9) |
| Sports | Lacrosse | 8.0 | 33 (7.8) |
| Sports | Moto-cross | 4.0 | 17 (4.0) |
| Sports | Orienteering | 9.0 | 38 (9.0) |
| Sports | Paddleball, competitive | 12.0 | 50 (11.9) |
| Sports | Paddleball, casual, general | 6.0 | 25 (5.9) |
| Sports | Polo | 8.0 | 33 (7.8) |
| Sports | Racketball, competitive | 12.0 | 50 (11.9) |
| Sports | Racketball, casual, general | 7.0 | 29 (6.9) |
| Sports | Rock climbing, ascending rock | 11.0 | 46 (10.9) |
| Sports | Rock climbing, rapelling | 8.0 | 33 (7.8) |
| Sports | Rope jumping, fast | 12.0 | 50 (11.9) |
| Sports | Rope jumping, moderate, general | 10.0 | 42 (10.0) |
| Sports | Rope jumping, slow | 8.0 | 33 (7.8) |
| Sports | Rugby | 10.0 | 42 (10.0) |
| Sports | Shuffleboard, lawn bowling | 3.0 | 13 (3.1) |
| Sports | Skateboarding | 5.0 | 21 (5.0) |
| Sports | Skating, roller | 7.0 | 29 (6.9) |
| Sports | In-line skating, $16 km \cdot h^{-1}$ | 7.5 | 31 (7.4) |
| Sports | In-line skating, $18 km \cdot h^{-1}$ | 8.5 | 35 (8.3) |
| Sports | In-line skating, $19 km \cdot h^{-1}$ | 10.0 | 42 (10.0) |
| Sports | Rollerskiing, $16 km \cdot h^{-1}$, no grade | 8.0 | 33 (7.8) |
| Sports | Rollerskiing, $18 km \cdot h^{-1}$, no grade | 10.0 | 42 (10.0) |
| Sports | Rollerskiing, $19 km \cdot h^{-1}$, no grade | 11.0 | 46 (10.9) |
| Sports | Rollerskiing, $14.5 km \cdot h^{-1}$, 6% grade | 12.0 | 50 (11.9) |
| Sports | Sky diving | 3.5 | 15 (3.6) |
| Sports | Soccer, competitive | 10.0 | 42 (10.0) |

| Activity category | Specific activity | METs | kJ·h⁻¹·kg⁻¹ (kcal·h⁻¹·kg⁻¹) body wt |
|---|---|---|---|
| Sports | Soccer, casual, general | 7.0 | 29 (6.9) |
| Sports | Softball or baseball, fast or slow pitch general | 5.0 | 21 (5.0) |
| Sports | Softball, officiating | 4.0 | 17 (4.0) |
| Sports | Softball, pitching | 6.0 | 25 (5.9) |
| Sports | Squash | 12.0 | 50 (11.9) |
| Sports | Table tennis, ping-pong | 4.0 | 17 (4.0) |
| Sports | Tai chi | 4.0 | 17 (4.0) |
| Sports | Tennis, general | 7.0 | 29 (6.9) |
| Sports | Tennis, doubles | 6.0 | 25 (5.9) |
| Sports | Tennis, singles | 8.0 | 33 (7.8) |
| Sports | Trampoline | 3.5 | 15 (3.6) |
| Sports | Volleyball, competitive, in gymnasium | 4.0 | 17 (4.0) |
| Sports | Volleyball, non-competitive; 6–9 member team, general | 3.0 | 13 (3.1) |
| Sports | Volleyball, beach | 8.0 | 33 (7.8) |
| Sports | Wrestling (one match = 5 min) | 6.0 | 25 (5.9) |
| Transportation | Driving car or light truck (not a semi) | 2.0 | 8 (1.9) |
| Transportation | Flying airplane | 2.0 | 8 (1.9) |
| Transportation | Motor scooter, motor cycle | 2.5 | 10 (2.4) |
| Transportation | Pushing plane in and out of hangar | 6.0 | 25 (5.9) |
| Transportation | Driving heavy truck, tractor, bus | 3.0 | 13 (3.1) |
| Walking | Backpacking, general | 7.0 | 29 (6.9) |
| Walking | Carrying infant or 7-kg load (e.g. suitcase), on level ground or downstairs | 3.5 | 15 (3.6) |
| Walking | Carrying load upstairs, general | 9.0 | 38 (9.0) |
| Walking | Carrying 0.5–7-kg load upstairs | 5.0 | 21 (5.0) |
| Walking | Carrying 7.5–10.5-kg load upstairs | 6.0 | 25 (5.9) |
| Walking | Carrying 11–22-kg load upstairs | 8.0 | 33 (7.8) |
| Walking | Carrying 22.5–34-kg load upstairs | 10.0 | 42 (10.0) |
| Walking | Carrying >34-kg load upstairs | 12.0 | 50 (11.9) |
| Walking | Climbing hills with 0–4-kg load | 7.0 | 29 (6.9) |
| Walking | Climbing hills with 4.5–9-kg load | 7.5 | 31 (7.4) |
| Walking | Climbing hills with 9.5–19-kg load | 8.0 | 33 (7.8) |
| Walking | Climbing hills with >19-kg load | 9.0 | 38 (9.0) |
| Walking | Downstairs | 3.0 | 13 (3.1) |
| Walking | Hiking, cross-country | 6.0 | 25 (5.9) |
| Walking | Marching, rapidly, military | 6.5 | 27 (6.4) |
| Walking | Pushing or pulling buggy with child | 2.5 | 10 (2.4) |
| Walking | Race walking | 6.5 | 27 (6.4) |
| Walking | Rock or mountain climbing | 8.0 | 33 (7.8) |
| Walking | Upstairs, using or climbing up ladder | 8.0 | 33 (7.8) |
| Walking | Using crutches | 4.0 | 17 (4.0) |
| Walking | Less than 3 km·h⁻¹ on level ground, strolling, household walking, very slow | 2.0 | 8 (1.9) |
| Walking | 3 km·h⁻¹ on level ground, slow pace, firm surface | 2.5 | 10 (2.4) |
| Walking | 4 km·h⁻¹, firm surface | 3.0 | 13 (3.1) |
| Walking | 4 km·h⁻¹, downhill | 3.0 | 13 (3.1) |
| Walking | 5 km·h⁻¹, on level ground, moderate pace, firm surface | 3.5 | 15 (3.6) |
| Walking | 5.5 km·h⁻¹, on level ground, brisk pace, firm surface | 4.0 | 17 (4.0) |
| Walking | 5.5 km·h⁻¹, uphill | 6.0 | 25 (5.9) |
| Walking | 6 km·h⁻¹, on level ground, firm surface, very brisk pace | 4.0 | 17 (4.0) |
| Walking | 7 km·h⁻¹, on level ground, firm surface, very brisk pace | 4.5 | 19 (4.5) |
| Walking | For pleasure, work break, walking the dog | 3.5 | 15 (3.6) |

| Activity category | Specific activity | METs | kJ·h⁻¹·kg⁻¹ (kcal·h⁻¹·kg⁻¹) body wt |
|---|---|---|---|
| Walking | On grass track | 5.0 | 21 (5.0) |
| Walking | To work or school | 4.0 | 17 (4.0) |
| Water activities | Boating, power | 2.5 | 10 (2.4) |
| Water activities | Canoeing, on camping trip | 4.0 | 17 (4.0) |
| Water activities | Canoeing, portaging | 7.0 | 29 (6.9) |
| Water activities | Canoeing, rowing, 3–6 km·h⁻¹, light effort | 3.0 | 13 (3.1) |
| Water activities | Canoeing, rowing, 6.5–9 km·h⁻¹, moderate effort | 7.0 | 29 (6.9) |
| Water activities | Canoeing, rowing, >9 km·h⁻¹, vigorous effort | 12.0 | 50 (11.9) |
| Water activities | Canoeing, rowing, for pleasure, general | 3.5 | 15 (3.6) |
| Water activities | Canoeing, rowing, in competition, or crew or sculling | 12.0 | 50 (11.9) |
| Water activities | Diving, springboard or platform | 3.0 | 13 (3.1) |
| Water activities | Kayaking | 5.0 | 21 (5.0) |
| Water activities | Paddleboat | 4.0 | 17 (4.0) |
| Water activities | Sailing, boat and board sailing, wind-surfing, ice sailing, general | 3.0 | 13 (3.1) |
| Water activities | Sailing, in competition | 5.0 | 21 (5.0) |
| Water activities | Sailing, Sunfish/Laser/Hobby Cat, keel boats, ocean sailing, yachting | 3.0 | 13 (3.1) |
| Water activities | Skiing, water | 6.0 | 25 (5.9) |
| Water activities | Skindiving or scuba diving as frogman | 12.0 | 50 (11.9) |
| Water activities | Skindiving, fast | 16.0 | 67 (15.9) |
| Water activities | Skindiving, moderate | 12.5 | 52 (12.4) |
| Water activities | Skindiving, scuba diving, general | 7.0 | 29 (6.9) |
| Water activities | Snorkeling | 5.0 | 21 (5.0) |
| Water activities | Surfing, body or board | 3.0 | 13 (3.1) |
| Water activities | Swimming laps, freestyle, fast, vigorous effort | 10.0 | 42 (10.0) |
| Water activities | Swimming laps, freestyle, slow, moderate or light effort | 8.0 | 33 (7.8) |
| Water activities | Swimming, backstroke, general | 8.0 | 33 (7.8) |
| Water activities | Swimming, breaststroke, general | 10.0 | 42 (10.0) |
| Water activities | Swimming, butterfly, general | 11.0 | 46 (10.9) |
| Water activities | Swimming, crawl, fast (75 m·min⁻¹), vigorous effort | 11.0 | 46 (10.9) |
| Water activities | Swimming, crawl, slow (50 m·min⁻¹), moderate or light effort | 8.0 | 33 (7.8) |
| Water activities | Swimming, lake, ocean, river | 6.0 | 25 (5.9) |
| Water activities | Swimming, leisurely, not lap swimming, general | 6.0 | 25 (5.9) |
| Water activities | Swimming, sidestroke, general | 8.0 | 33 (7.8) |
| Water activities | Swimming, synchronized | 8.0 | 33 (7.8) |
| Water activities | Swimming, treading water, fast, vigorous effort | 10.0 | 42 (10.0) |
| Water activities | Swimming,treading water, moderate effort, general | 4.0 | 17 (4.0) |
| Water activities | Swimming, underwater, 1.5 km·h⁻¹ | 7.0 | 29 (6.9) |
| Water activities | Water polo | 10.0 | 42 (10.0) |
| Water activities | Water volleyball | 3.0 | 13 (3.1) |
| Water activities | Whitewater rafting, kayaking, or canoeing, non-competitive | 5.0 | 21 (5.0) |
| Winter activities | Moving ice house (set up/drill holes, etc.) | 6.0 | 25 (5.9) |
| Winter activities | Skating, ice, 15 km·h⁻¹ or less | 5.5 | 23 (5.5) |
| Winter activities | Skating, ice, general | 7.0 | 29 (6.9) |
| Winter activities | Skating, ice, rapidly, more than 9 km·h⁻¹ | 9.0 | 38 (9.0) |
| Winter activities | Skating, speed, competitive | 15.0 | 63 (15.0) |
| Winter activities | Skating, figure | 9.0 | 38 (9.0) |
| Winter activities | Ski jumping (climbing up carrying skis) | 7.0 | 29 (6.9) |
| Winter activities | Skiing, general | 7.0 | 29 (6.9) |

| Activity category | Specific activity | METs | kJ·h⁻¹·kg⁻¹ (kcal·h⁻¹·kg⁻¹) body wt |
|---|---|---|---|
| Winter activities | Skiing, cross-country, 4 km·h⁻¹, slow or light effort, ski walking | 7.0 | 29 (6.9) |
| Winter activities | Skiing, cross-country, 6–8 km·h⁻¹, moderate speed and effort, general | 8.0 | 33 (7.8) |
| Winter activities | Skiing, cross-country, 8.1–13 km·h⁻¹, brisk speed, vigorous effort | 9.0 | 38 (9.0) |
| Winter activities | Skiing, cross-country, 13 km·h⁻¹, racing | 14.0 | 59 (14.0) |
| Winter activities | Skiing, cross-country, hard snow, uphill, maximum effort | 16.5 | 69 (16.4) |
| Winter activities | Skiing, downhill, light effort | 5.0 | 21 (5.0) |
| Winter activities | Skiing, downhill, moderate effort, general | 6.0 | 25 (5.9) |
| Winter activities | Skiing, downhill, vigorous effort, racing | 8.0 | 33 (7.8) |
| Winter activities | Sledding, tobogganing, bobsledding, luge | 7.0 | 29 (6.9) |
| Winter activities | Snow shoeing | 8.0 | 33 (7.8) |
| Winter activities | Snowmobiling | 3.5 | 15 (3.6) |

# Chapter 5

# Dietary Carbohydrates

LOUISE M. BURKE

## Introduction

Dietary carbohydrates (CHOs) provide the major energy source in the diets of most people and include a range of compounds which share the common basic elements of carbon, hydrogen and oxygen, and an empirical formula of $(CH_2O)_n$. CHOs occurring naturally in foods, or more recently, manufactured by special chemical techniques and added during food processing, are generally classified according to their chemical structure. However, this system does not account for the variety and overlap of functional, metabolic and nutritional characteristics of 'CHO foods'. This chapter will describe briefly the types of CHOs in our diets, and then focus on the features of CHO-rich foods that may be of interest to athletes and physically active people, justifying the recommendations of many expert nutrition bodies that we should further increase our dietary CHO intake.

## Structural classification of CHOs

Carbohydrates are classified according to the degree of polymerization, or number of saccharide units, in the CHO molecule. Table 5.1 lists the various saccharide categories along with examples of commonly consumed CHOs. The main monosaccharides, glucose and fructose, are present in fruits and vegetables, while fructose is now provided in processed foods in increasing amounts due to the use of high-fructose sweeteners derived from the chemical treatment of corn starch. Sucrose is generally the most abundant disaccharide in Westernized diets, with foods providing naturally occurring and/or added sources of this sugar, while lactose is provided primarily by dairy foods such as milk, yoghurt and ice cream. Oligosaccharides make up only a small amount of dietary CHO intake; for example, raffinose, stachyose and verbascose are unusual CHOs found in legumes, while fructo-oligosaccharides appear in other vegetables. Glucose polymers, short chains of 3–15 glucose units commercially produced by the chemical or enzymatic breakdown of starch, have found a small dietary niche in processed foods, including sports foods such as sports drinks.

Starch is quantitatively the most important food CHO, and may occur as amylose in which the saccharide linkages are almost entirely straight α-1,4 or linear bonds, or as amylopectin in which a mixture of α-1,4 and α-1,6 bonds gives a highly branched structure. Starch is the plant storage CHO, and is found predominantly in grains, legumes and some vegetables and fruit. The non-starch polysaccharides (NSPs) include structural cell wall components (hemicellulose and cellulose, and pectins) as well as storage polysaccharides, gums and mucilages. These NSPs share the characteristic of being largely undigested in the small intestine, and together with lignin comprise 'dietary fibre'. For further review, see Asp (1995).

**Table 5.1** Classification of carbohydrates.

| Type | Examples |
| --- | --- |
| Monosaccharides (1 unit) | Glucose |
| | Fructose |
| | Galactose |
| Disaccharides (2 units) | Sucrose |
| | Lactose |
| | Maltose |
| Oligosaccharides (3–20 units) | Raffinose (3 units) |
| | Stachyose (4 units) |
| | Verbascose (5 units) |
| | Fructo-oligosaccharides |
| | Commercially derived glucose polymers/maltodextrins (5–15 units) |
| Polysaccharides (20–1000 units) | |
| Starch | Amylose |
| | Amylopectin |
| Non-starch polysaccharides | Cellulose |
| | Hemicellulose |
| | Pectins |
| | $\beta$-glucans |
| | Fructans |
| | Gums |
| | Mucilages |
| | Algal polysaccharides |

## Functional characteristics of CHOs in foods

CHOs are responsible for a wide range of the functional characteristics of the foods in which they appear (for review, see Chinachoti 1995). Sweetness is the feature most linked with mono- and di-saccharides, with the relative sweetness of these sugars being fructose > sucrose > glucose > lactose. However, in addition to sweetness, sucrose and corn syrups provide other favourable characteristics such as mouth-feel and viscosity. Sugars also act as a thickening agent, whipping agent, stabilizer, fermenting agent, or emulsifier in various processed foods. The browning of baked foods is produced by the Maillard reaction between a CHO and an amine group, while the caramelization of sugars through intense heat provides characteristic flavouring and colouring in a large variety of foods. Starches provide bulk and texture to foods, and their gelatinization is responsible for many desirable characteristics of viscosity, texture and clarity. In addition to their function in the cell wall structure of naturally occurring foods, gums and other NSPs are used as thickeners, stabilizers and gelling agents in food processing. These non-digestible CHOs may greatly add to the bulk and structure of foods in which they are present.

These functional characteristics of CHOs are important to appreciate since they influence the appeal and ease of consumption of both naturally occurring and manufactured foods. Such practical considerations will influence the success of the athlete in consuming adequate CHO at specific times, or will influence the convenience or attractiveness of certain CHO-rich foods and drinks in specific situations related to training or competition. They are also of interest to the manufacturers of special sports foods which aim to provide a source of CHO that is easy to access and consume in these situations.

## Limitations of the 'simple' vs. 'complex' classification of CHO foods

Traditionally, foods containing significant amounts of CHOs have been categorized according to the structural classification of the principally occurring CHO. This has led to a simplistic division of CHO-containing foods into 'simple' CHOs (containing mono-, di- and oligosaccharides) or 'complex' CHOs (containing polysaccharides). A variety of beliefs about the metabolic and nutritional characteristics of CHO foods have been apportioned to these categories:

**1** 'Simple' CHO foods cause large and rapid excursions of blood glucose levels on ingestion (a rapid rise followed by a rapid and often greater fall). They are prized for their sweetness but are generally not nutritious. 'Simple' CHOs are completely digested and are a cause of dental caries.

**2** 'Complex' CHO foods are nutritious foods which contain significant amounts of other nutrients, including dietary fibre. The digestion and absorption of complex CHO foods are complete but slower, producing a flatter and more sustained blood glucose and insulin response to their ingestion.

**3** Dietary fibre is an inert substance found in nutritious or complex CHO foods. It is undigested, and plays a major role in maintaining bowel function and regularity.

While this classification system may have been developed as a simple nutrition education tool for the lay person, it encompasses many erroneous beliefs which have, in fact, confused both nutrition science and practice. Such misconceptions have spilled over into the area of sports nutrition.

An oversimplification which underpins many of these misconceptions is the labelling of foods according to a significant nutrient in their composition. To describe bananas, bread or lasagne as 'CHO foods' is to undervalue the complex nature of foods and the cocktail of chemicals of which each is composed. Most naturally occurring foods contain a mixture of CHO types, often of both simple and complex structure, as well as other macro- and micronutrients, and a large array of non-nutrient chemicals. This mixture is even more intricate in the case of processed foods, and composite foods and dishes (e.g. lasagne, pizza). Therefore it is preferable to use a description such as 'CHO-rich' or 'CHO-containing', which better recognizes the heterogeneity of characteristics of each food, and the presence of other nutrients. As shown in Table 5.2, many CHO-rich foods containing mostly simple CHOs are also good sources of protein, fibre and micronutrients, and conform to dietary guidelines that promote moderation of the intake of fats and oils. On the other hand, there are a number of examples of CHO-rich foods containing mostly complex CHOs which have low nutrient density and/or a high fat content, and might be considered less 'nutritious'. Clearly, a judgement of the nutritional value of a food based on the structural nature of its CHOs is invalid, and is further confused by the occurrence of foods that contain significant amounts of both simple and complex CHO types (Table 5.2).

Notwithstanding this difficulty of dividing foods cleanly into two categories, there is little correlation between the structural type of CHOs in foods and their actual effect on blood glucose and insulin levels. Data collected since the 1970s have shown overwhelmingly that postprandial responses to various CHO-rich foods vary from that predicted by the simple vs. complex CHO model. Several CHO-rich foods containing predominantly sugars (e.g. fruit and sweetened dairy products) produce a flattened blood glucose curve when ingested, while other foods high in complex carbohydrates (e.g. bread and potatoes) produce a high blood glucose response, similar to that following the ingestion of glucose itself. Furthermore, the presence of dietary fibre in foods does not always seem to delay absorption and flatten the postprandial blood glucose curve; blood glucose responses to wholemeal bread are similar to those following the consumption of white bread.

The availability of carbohydrate types must also be readdressed. A number of simple CHOs are not well digested and absorbed by all people; lactose is poorly digested by a small percentage

**Table 5.2** Examples of the overlap between the nutritional and structural classification of CHO-rich foods.

| | 'Nutritious'* | 'Less nutritious' |
|---|---|---|
| 'Simple' CHO-rich foods | Fruit<br>Fruit juice<br>Canned fruit<br>Dried fruit<br>Flavoured milk, yoghurt and other sweetened dairy foods (especially low-fat types)<br>Liquid meal supplements<br>Some sports bars | Sugar (sucrose)<br>Honey, jam, syrups<br>Soft drinks, flavoured mineral water<br>Sports drinks<br>'Carbohydrate loading' supplements<br>Sweets, chocolates<br>Jelly, mousses and high-fat desserts<br>Ice cream |
| 'Complex' CHO-rich foods | Bread, muffins, bagels<br>Breakfast cereals<br>Pasta and noodles<br>Rice and other grains<br>Starchy vegetables (e.g. potatoes, corn)<br>Legumes and pulses<br>Pizza bases | Pastry<br>Potato crisps<br>Chips/fries<br>Croissants |
| CHO-rich foods with mixture of 'simple' and 'complex' CHOs | Low-fat cake and dessert recipes<br>Sweetened and fruit-containing breakfast cereal<br>Baked beans<br>Some fruits and vegetables (e.g. bananas, pumpkin)<br>Some sports bars | High-fat cakes, pastries, biscuits, desserts<br>Granola/muesli bars<br>Some sports bars |

* In this chapter, 'nutritious' foods are defined as those providing significant amounts of protein and macronutrients, and contributing less than 30% of energy from fat. 'Less nutritious' foods are those providing insignificant amounts of other nutrients, and/or having a fat content of more than 30% of total energy.

of Western populations and the majority of Asian and native populations (e.g. Australian aboriginals) due to a deficiency of the enzyme lactase, whereas fructose is best absorbed in the presence of other carbohydrates in the intestine, and is poorly absorbed when consumed in large amounts on its own (for review, see Gudmand-Hoyer 1994; Southgate 1995). The incomplete digestion of starch is now also recognized. The term *resistant starch* has been coined to describe starch fractions in food that pass undigested into the large bowel. These include particles that are indigestible due to lack of physical contact with digestive enzymes (such as only partially chewed or milled grains and legumes, or whole seeds), or starch found in ungelatinized granules such as in raw bananas, uncooked potatoes, or high amylose-content cereals. Finally, some starch is made resistant by cooking or processing. Foods that have been baked at high temperatures (e.g. bread, cornflakes), or cooled after being cooked to make the starch soluble or gelatinized (e.g. cold baked potato) may contain significant amounts of starch that has retrograded (had the water-bound structure disturbed). For review, see Englyst *et al.* (1992). There is an argument to include resistant starch as a component of dietary fibre.

In any case, the view of dietary fibre needs to be updated to recognize it as a group of diverse compounds which are far from inert. Although they may be undigested in the small intestine, many are fermented by bacteria in the large bowel and may provide a number of their health benefits via this process and the subsequent release of short chain fatty acids. While some components of dietary fibre are responsible for adding faecal bulk and enhancing regularity, various types of dietary fibre offer other apparent health benefits related to glycaemic control, lipid metabolism, weight control and reduced risk of colonic cancer (for review, see Baghurst *et al.* 1996).

Finally, the issue of dental caries is also complex and cannot be entirely explained by the consumption of sucrose and foods rich in simple CHOs. Starch also provides a source of fermentable CHO for the development of caries, and the frequency of intake of CHOs and the physical form of the CHO food/drink which determines the length of time of adhesion to the teeth are important factors in the aetiology of dental decay. Other aetiological factors include fluoride, oral hygiene practices and salivary flow (for review, see Navia 1994).

## Glycaemic index

In recognition of the lack of uniformity and the inability to predict blood glucose responses to the consumption of various CHO-rich foods, the concept of the glycaemic index was introduced by Jenkins in the early 1980s (Jenkins *et al.* 1981). The glycaemic index is a ranking of foods based on their actual postprandial blood glucose response compared to a reference food, either glucose or white bread. The glycaemic index is calculated by measuring the incremental area under the blood glucose curve following the ingestion of a portion of the test food providing 50 g of CHO, compared with the area under the blood glucose curve following an equal CHO intake from the reference food, with all tests being conducted after an overnight fast. Tables of the measured glycaemic index of various CHO-rich foods have now been published internationally (Foster-Powell & Brand-Miller 1995). Thorough research in this area has shown that the glycaemic index has acceptable reproducibility within and between individuals and can be applied to a mixed meal containing CHO-rich

foods (for reviews, see Wolever 1990; Truswell 1992).

Many factors influence the glycaemic index of CHO-rich foods including the food form (e.g. particle size due to degree of milling or processing, texture and viscosity including the presence of soluble fibres) and the degree of food processing and cooking (e.g. degree of gelatinization or retrograding of starch, disruption to the cell structure). The presence of fructose or lactose, and the ratio of amylopectin to amylose in starch are important, as are the presence of starch–protein or starch–fat interactions, or compounds known as 'antinutrients' (e.g. phytates, lectins). Finally, even the ripeness of some fruits such as bananas (i.e. degree of conversion of starches to sugars) may affect their glycaemic index (see Wolever 1990).

Table 5.3 summarizes the glycaemic index of some common CHO-rich foods, and illustrates the impossibility of predicting the glycaemic index of a food based simply on its composition. The glycaemic index concept has been used to manipulate the glucose and insulin response to diets of equal CHO content; lowering the glycaemic index has been shown to improve the metabolic profiles of individuals with diabetes and hyperlipidaemia (Wolever *et al.* 1991) and to increase postmeal satiety (Holt *et al.* 1992). Thus the glycaemic index has gained recognition as a useful education tool in the management of diabetes and hyperlipidaemias.

More recently, it has been suggested that the manipulation of the glycaemic index of meals or the diet may have application in the area of sports nutrition to optimize CHO availability for exercise; high glycaemic index CHO-rich meals have been reported to enhance the storage of muscle glycogen during recovery from prolonged exercise compared with CHO-rich foods of low glycaemic index (Burke *et al.* 1993). CHO-rich drinks or foods with moderate to high glycaemic index have been suggested as the most appropriate source of CHO intake during prolonged exercise (Coyle 1991); whereas there has been some publicity (Thomas *et al.* 1991), but not universal agreement (Febbraio & Stewart 1996),

**Table 5.3** Examples of the glycaemic index (GI) of CHO-rich foods.

|  | Food | GI |
|---|---|---|
| High GI (>70) | Glucose | 100 |
|  | Cornflakes | 84 |
|  | Cocopops | 77 |
|  | Instant mashed potato | 83 |
|  | Baked potato | 85 |
|  | Sports drink | 95 |
|  | Jelly beans | 80 |
|  | White bread | 70 |
|  | Weetbix | 70 |
|  | Watermelon | 72 |
|  | Honey | 73 |
| Moderate GI (55–70) | Wholemeal bread | 69 |
|  | One-minute oats | 66 |
|  | Muesli flake cereal | 68 |
|  | Muffins (cake style) | 62 |
|  | Soft drink | 68 |
|  | Brown/white rice | 59 |
|  | Arrowroot biscuit | 66 |
|  | Ice-cream | 61 |
|  | Mangoes | 55 |
|  | Orange juice | 57 |
|  | Sucrose | 65 |
| Low GI (<55) | Ripe banana | 52 |
|  | Porridge | 49 |
|  | Mixed grain bread | 45 |
|  | All Bran | 42 |
|  | Parboiled rice | 47 |
|  | Milk | 27 |
|  | Flavoured yoghurt | 33 |
|  | Chocolate | 49 |
|  | Unripe banana | 30 |
|  | Apple | 36 |
|  | Orange | 43 |
|  | Pasta | 41 |
|  | Baked beans | 40 |
|  | Kidney beans | 27 |
|  | Red lentils | 26 |
|  | Fructose | 20 |

GI has been based on glucose as a reference food. Where white bread is used as a reference food, GI values are higher by approximately 1.4. See Foster-Powell & Brand-Miller (1995).

that the intake of a pre-exercise meal composed of low glycaemic index CHO-rich foods may enhance endurance or performance during such exercise events. Clearly, the use of the glycaemic index may have implications for the athlete and deserves further attention. However, it is not intended to provide a universal system to rank the virtues of CHO-rich foods. There are a number of other attributes of foods which may be of value to the athlete; these are often specific to the individual and the exercise situation.

## Other valuable characteristics of CHO-rich foods for athletes

### Nutrient density and alignment with goals of healthy eating

The guidelines for healthy eating, and for athletes in particular, recommend that CHO and CHO-rich foods should provide the majority of dietary energy. However, for optimal health and performance, athletes must also achieve their requirements for protein and micronutrients, including any increase in requirement that may result from a heavy exercise programme (see Chapters 10, 21, 23–25). Thus, CHO-rich foods which also provide significant sources of other nutrients are of value in allowing the athlete to meet a number of nutritional goals simultaneously. This is an important consideration in the everyday or training diet of the athlete, particularly for those individuals with very high carbohydrate needs and/or restricted energy intake. In other words, as CHO increases its importance in the total food base, particularly a food base of small size, so should there be an increase in the focus on nutrient-dense types of CHO-rich foods.

Many CHO-rich foods provide valuable amounts of other nutrients, or at least can be constructed into a nutritious CHO-rich meal using typical food combinations. Breads, rice, pasta, breakfast cereals and other grain-based foods provide significant amounts of B vitamins and smaller amounts of some minerals, especially in cases such as breakfast cereals where fortification has occurred. Legumes, pulses and soya products are also valuable sources of these nutrients. Protein provided by legumes and grain foods is significant, even in a non-vegetarian diet, with complementation of amino acids occurring via other foods eaten over the day. Fruits and vegetables provide fair to excellent sources of β-carotenes, some B vitamins and ascorbic acid, in addition to other non-nutrient chemicals that may confer health advantages. Legumes and soya products also provide such phytochemicals. Sweetened dairy foods (e.g. flavoured yoghurts and milk drinks) provide an excellent source of calcium, protein and riboflavin. The potential for nutritional value increases in the case of composite dishes and food combinations; for example, milk eaten with breakfast cereal, fillings added to sandwiches and rolls, or the toppings and sauces added to rice, pasta or pizza can all optimize the nutrient profile of CHO-rich meals. Special sports foods which are nutrient-rich include liquid meal supplements and some (fortified) sports bars.

Most naturally occurring CHO-rich foods are low in fat, in keeping with general health guidelines. However, the athlete may also find low-fat and reduced fat options among processed CHO-rich foods or dishes, ranging from low-fat sweetened dairy products to special recipes for bakery products and composite dishes with minimal added fats/oils. Moderation of fat intake will be an important strategy for athletes who have limited energy budgets; for example, athletes trying to achieve or maintain a lower body fat level, or athletes in aesthetic/skill-based sports such as gymnastics and figure skating who must remain small and lean without the contribution of a high-energy expenditure training programme.

### Practical issues

The athlete is often encouraged to eat CHO at special times, or in quantities greater than that which would be provided in an everyday diet or dictated by their appetite and hunger. Therefore, CHO-rich foods and drinks that are appealing, available or able to be easily consumed will have value in helping the athlete to meet CHO intake recommendations. Sweet-tasting foods and drinks are generally appealing to people; indeed,

the flavour of a CHO-containing drink may encourage greater intake of fluid during and after exercise, thus promoting better hydration as well as achieving CHO intake goals at these times. Sports drinks provide an example of a food that is tailor-made for athletes, providing CHO at a concentration suitable for optimal delivery of both fluid and CHO during and after exercise. The taste profile is manipulated towards preferences experienced while exercising or dehydrated; excessive sweetness in these products is avoided by using a mixture of glucose polymers along with mono- and disaccharides, with a little sodium being added to enhance the palatability. Sports bars are another convenience food in a compact form that can be easily carried and consumed 'on the run', either literally during exercise, or as a general part of an athlete's busy day. Other sports products, such as high CHO powders and drinks, CHO-rich gels and nutrient-dense liquid meal supplements, also offer the advantages of compactness, minimal preparation and known CHO composition. Since CHO intake guidelines may specify a recommended amount of CHO to be consumed in a given situation, foods of known or standardized CHO content such as these specialized sports products are often popular among athletes. However, food tables and ready reckoners of the CHO content of food can make everyday foods more 'user friendly'.

Compactness and ease of consumption are food attributes that are important to an athlete with very high energy and CHO requirements, or in the choice of a pre-exercise or postexercise meal. CHO-rich foods that are high in fibre, particularly in combination with a high water content and an intact, rigid structure, are bulky; they involve greater volumes of food, longer eating time, and greater stomach fullness to provide a given amount of CHO (Table 5.4). This may prevent the athlete from reaching their CHO intake targets, or may be a cause of gastrointestinal discomfort, particularly during exercise. CHO-rich foods that are less fibrous, require less chewing, or have a greater CHO (lower water) density, may be more practical when CHO has to

**Table 5.4** Practical characteristics of CHO-rich foods which may promote or deter their consumption.

| Food | | Serve size for 100 g CHO | Energy (MJ and kcal) |
|---|---|---|---|
| Water content | | | |
| High | Green beans | 4500 g (30 cups) | 3.1 MJ (740 kcal) |
| High | Sports drink | 1.4 l | 1.6 MJ (400 kcal) |
| Low | Jelly beans | 100 g | 1.6 MJ (400 kcal) |
| Fibre content | | | |
| High | Boiled brown rice | 310 g (2 cups) | 1.9 MJ (450 kcal) |
| Low | Boiled white rice | 310 g (2 cups) | 1.9 MK (450 kcal) |
| Fat content | | | |
| High | Croissants | 290 g (4–5) | 4.6 MJ (1100 kcal) |
| Low | Bread rolls | 210 g (2–3) | 2.2 MJ (530 kcal) |

CHO-rich drinks can be consumed in large amounts since they are rapidly emptied and absorbed, and contribute to fluid requirements. However, CHO-rich foods with a high water content particularly in a high-fibre matrix, require chewing and a large volume to provide similar amounts of CHO. Even in low-water-content foods a high-fibre content can limit intake by increasing the time needed to chew and eat them, and by increasing gastric fullness. High-fat CHO-rich foods may not be suitable for athletes with restricted energy intakes.

be consumed in large amounts. For example, 'white' or refined bread and cereal products may be chosen over wholemeal products, and processed fruit and juices may be more easily eaten than fresh fruit. Sugars, jams and syrups may be added to foods or meals to provide an additional low-bulk CHO source, while confectionery items and CHO-rich drinks (e.g. from soft drinks to nutrient-rich milk shakes and fruit smoothies) are also compact forms of dietary CHO. In the postexercise situation, an athlete's CHO intake may be challenged by fatigue and loss of appetite. CHO-containing drinks, or CHO-rich foods with fluid-like appearance (e.g. flavoured yoghurt and other sweetened dairy foods) may have appeal to an athlete who is dehydrated. Food that can be presented in small portions (e.g. sandwich fingers and fruit pieces) may encourage continued nibbling, and be more attractive to an athlete with a depressed appetite, than large food volumes or whole foods with a rigid structure. Conversely, for an athlete who needs to restrict energy intake, CHO-rich foods providing long eating times, large volume and stomach fullness, and high satiety value may assist with this goal.

Finally, the athlete may be required to eat CHO in situations where access to food or facilities for food preparation are poor. This may include the post-training or competition situation, or the 'grazing' pattern of frequent intake during a busy day that is characteristic of athletes with high-energy intakes. Thus, CHO-rich foods which require minimal preparation, are portable, or have good storage properties may be of practical value. These include naturally occurring foods (e.g. fruit) as well as processed and convenience foods such as bars, confectionery items, bakery items and special sports foods.

## Recommendations for CHO intake for athletes

Historically, population dietary guidelines have considered CHO as an 'energy filler', making up energy requirements after protein requirements have been met and fat intake has been moderated. Population guidelines in Westernized countries generally recommend an increase in CHO intake, particularly from nutritious CHO-rich foods, to provide at least 50–55% of total dietary energy (US Department of Agriculture 1990; National Health and Medical Research Council 1992). This tradition of providing guidelines as a percentage of dietary energy reflects the desire to encourage a relative decrease in fat intake and increase in CHO intake across the various energy intakes of individuals in a popu-

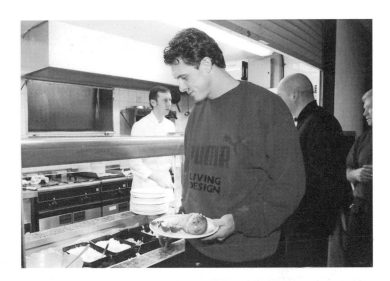

**Fig. 5.1** Athletes making food choices may need guidance to ensure that dietary goals are met. Photo courtesy of Raymond Besant.

lation. However, recent research into CHO and fibre has suggested that CHO intake recommendations might be made on their own accord. Athletes are one group who merit specific CHO intake goals, in order to meet the fuel needs of training, competition and recovery (see Chapters 7 and 8) including the following.

**1** To maximize muscle glycogen recovery after exercise to enhance daily training, or to 'load' the muscle with glycogen before a prolonged exercise competition, the athlete should consume a diet providing 7–10 g CHO per kilogram of body mass (BM) per 24 h (see Chapter 7).

**2** To enhance early recovery after exercise, the athlete should consume at least 1 g $CHO \cdot kg^{-1}$ BM within 30 min after the session is completed (see Chapter 7).

**3** To enhance fuel availability for a prolonged exercise session (particularly competition), the athlete should consume a CHO-rich meal providing 1–4 g $CHO \cdot kg^{-1}$ BM during the 1–4 h before the session (see Chapter 7).

**4** To provide an additional source of CHO during prolonged moderate and high intensity events, the athlete should consume 30–60 g $CHO \cdot h^{-1}$ during exercise (see Chapter 8).

These guidelines are generally directed towards athletes undertaking endurance exercise, and need to be modified according to the individual needs of the athlete and their sport.

Since athletes may range considerably in body size (e.g. from a 35-kg gymnast to a 130-kg rugby player), it is convenient to provide CHO intake guidelines on the basis of BM and allow these to be scaled accordingly. It has been relatively easy to develop and validate the benefits of guidelines addressing acute intake of CHO; for example, a large number of studies have shown that the ingestion of CHO during prolonged moderate- to high-intensity exercise enhances endurance and performance (see Chapter 8), and muscle biopsy studies have determined the rate of muscle glycogen storage following various amounts and types of CHO intake (see Chapter 7).

The development of CHO intake guidelines for the everyday diet of the athlete has been more problematic. This is partly due to terminology, and partly due to the failure of studies to provide unequivocal evidence to support the recommendations. Population dietary guidelines recommending a CHO intake of at least 50–55% of total energy are appropriate to address the health needs and fuel requirements of athletes undertaking a moderate training load. However, the CHO needs of athletes with a heavy training or competition schedule have been a recent source of conflict. Firstly, some authorities have suggested that athletes undertaking prolonged daily exercise sessions should increase CHO intakes to

65–70% of dietary energy (American Dietetic Association 1993). However, the rigid interpretation of this guideline may prove unnecessary and unfeasible for some athletes. Athletes with very high energy intakes (e.g. >16–20 MJ·day⁻¹ or >4000–5000 kcal·day⁻¹) will achieve absolute carbohydrates of over 700–800 g CHO·day⁻¹ with such a dietary prescription. This may exceed their combined requirement for daily glycogen storage and training fuel and, furthermore, be bulky to consume. Athletes with such high energy intakes may be able to meet their daily needs for glycogen recovery with a diet of 50–60% of energy. Therefore, it is preferable to provide CHO intake recommendations in grams (relative to the BM of the athlete) and allow flexibility for the athlete to meet their requirements within the context of their energy needs and other dietary goals. Some athletes, principally females, appear to have lower energy intakes than might be expected. These athletes may need to devote a greater proportion of their dietary intake (e.g. up to 65–70% of energy) to CHO intake, and even then may fail to meet the absolute CHO intakes suggested for optimal daily glycogen recovery (for review, see Burke 1995).

The most interesting point of debate about current CHO intake recommendations, however, lies with the failure of longitudinal studies to show clear-cut benefits to training adaptation and performance with high CHO intakes compared to moderate CHO diets (Table 5.5). Although studies show that higher CHO intakes,

**Table 5.5** Longitudinal studies comparing high CHO intakes (HCHO) and moderate CHO intakes (MCHO) on the training adaptation and performance of athletes in intensive training.

| Reference | Athletes | Duration of study (days) | Daily CHO intake* (g·kg⁻¹ BM) | Muscle glycogen | Effects on performance |
|---|---|---|---|---|---|
| Costill et al. 1988 | Swimmers | 10 | 8.2 vs. 5.3 | Declined in MCHO, maintained in HCHO | Training performance impaired in MCHO group, but swim trials unchanged |
| Kirwan et al. 1988 | Runners | 5 | 8.0 vs. 3.9 | Declined in both groups, but greater reductions in MCHO | Reduction in running economy and increase in perception of effort during training sessions in MCHO |
| Lamb et al. 1990 | Swimmers | 9 | 12.1 vs. 6.5 | NA | No difference in performance of interval training |
| Simonsen et al. 1991 | Rowers | 28 | 10 vs. 5 | Maintained in MCHO, increased in HCHO | Power output maintained during ergometer trials in MCHO; trend toward small improvement at end of study in HCHO |
| Sherman et al. 1993 | Runners | 7 | 10 vs. 5 | Declined in MCHO, maintained in HCHO | No impairment of high-intensity run to exhaustion in either group |
| Sherman et al. 1993 | Cyclists | 7 | 10 vs. 5 | Declined in MCHO, maintained in HCHO | No impairment of high-intensity cycle to exhaustion in either group |

BM, body mass; NA, not available.
*High intake vs. moderate intake of CHO compared in each study.

consistent with the guidelines above, allow better recovery/maintenance of muscle glycogen levels during periods of heavy training, there does not appear to be consistent and significant enhancement of performance in the high CHO group at the end of the study period, nor impairment of performance in the moderate CHO group (for review, see Sherman & Wimer 1991; Sherman *et al.* 1993). It has been suggested that athletes may adapt to the lower CHO intake and muscle glycogen depletion. However, it is also possible that the protocols used to measure performance in these studies were not sufficiently sensitive to detect the differences between the groups, that the studies were not conducted over sufficiently long periods to elicit clear differences in performance, and that the area is confused by some overlap between what is considered 'moderate' and 'high' CHO intakes (Sherman *et al.* 1993). In any case, there is clear proof from studies of acute dietary manipulation that endurance and performance are enhanced when body CHO stores are optimized, and that carbohydrate depletion causes an impairment of performance (see Chapters 6–8). Furthermore, there is anecdotal evidence, including comments from the studies above, that athletes complain of 'tiredness' and 'muscle fatigue' during training when dietary carbohydrate is insufficient. Therefore, the recommendation that athletes should consume a high CHO diet to cover the fuel cost of their training loads and recovery remains prudent, and further long-term studies are awaited to adequately test the benefit of this strategy.

## Conclusion

Dietary CHO is provided by a wide variety of CHO-rich foods and drinks. There is no universal system that can adequately describe the diverse metabolic, functional and nutritional features of these various foods. Dietary guidelines for athletes make recommendations for everyday intake of CHO as well as CHO intake for specific situations pre, during and postexercise sessions. Athletes are encouraged to meet these guidelines by choosing CHO-rich foods and drinks that offer appropriate characteristics such as nutrient-density, desirable glycaemic index, appeal and practicality according to the requirements of the situation.

## References

American Dietetic Association and Canadian Dietetic Association (1993) Position stand on nutrition for physical fitness and athletic performance for adults. *Journal of the American Dietetic Association* **93**, 691–696.

Asp, N.G.L. (1995) Classification and methodology of food carbohydrates as related to nutritional effects. *American Journal of Clinical Nutrition* **61** (Suppl.), 930S–937S.

Baghurst, P.A., Baghurst, K.I. & Record, S.J. (1996) Dietary fibre, non-starch polysaccharides and resistant starch: a review. *Food Australia* **48** (Suppl.), S1–S36.

Burke, L.M. (1995) Nutrition for the female athlete. In *Nutrition in Women's Health* (ed. D. Krummel & P. Kris-Etherton), pp. 263–298. Aspen Publishers, Gaithersburg, MD.

Burke, L.M., Collier, G.R. & Hargreaves, M. (1993) Muscle glycogen storage after prolonged exercise: effect of the glycemic index of carbohydrate feedings. *Journal of Applied Physiology* **75**, 1019–1023.

Chinachoti, P. (1995) Carbohydrates: functionality in foods. *American Journal of Clinical Nutrition* **61** (Suppl.), 922S–929S.

Costill, D.L., Flynn, M.G., Kirwan, J.P. *et al.* (1988) Effects of repeated days of intensified training on muscle glycogen and swimming performance. *Medicine and Science in Sports and Exercise* **20**, 249–254.

Coyle, E.F. (1991) Timing and method of increased carbohydrate intake to cope with heavy training, competition and recovery. *Journal of Sports Science* **9** (Suppl.), 29–52.

Englyst, H.N., Kingman, S.M. & Cummings, J.H. (1992) Classifications and measurement of nutritionally important starch fractions. *European Journal of Clinical Nutrition* **46** (Suppl. 2), S33–S50.

Febbraio, M.A. & Stewart, K.L. (1996) CHO feeding before prolonged exercise: effect of glycemic index on muscle glycogenolysis and exercise performance. *Journal of Applied Physiology* **81**, 1115–1120.

Foster-Powell, K. & Brand-Miller, J. (1995) International tables of glycemic index. *American Journal of Clinical Nutrition* **62** (Suppl.), 871S–893S.

Gudmand-Hoyer, E. (1994) The clinical significance of disaccharide maldigestion. *American Journal of Clinical Nutrition* **59** (Suppl.), 735S–741S.

Holt, S., Brand, J., Soveny, C. & Hansky, J. (1992) Relationship of satiety to postprandial glycaemic, insulin and cholecystokinin responses. *Appetite* **18**, 129–141.

Jenkins, D.J.A., Wolever, T.M.S., Taylor, R.H. *et al.* (1981) Glycemic index of foods: a physiological basis for carbohydrate exchange. *American Journal of Clinical Nutrition* **34**, 362–366.

Kirwan, J.P., Costill, D.L., Mitchell, J.B. *et al.* (1988) Carbohydrate balance in competitive runners during successive days of intense training. *Journal of Applied Physiology* **65**, 2601–2606.

Lamb, D.R., Rinehardt, K.R., Bartels, R.L., Sherman, W.M. & Snook, J.T. (1990) Dietary carbohydrate and intensity of interval swim training. *American Journal of Clinical Nutrition* **52**, 1058–1063.

National Health and Medical Research Council (1992) *Dietary Guidelines for Australians*. Australian Government Publishing Service, Canberra.

Navia, J.M. (1994) Carbohydrates and dental health. *American Journal of Clinical Nutrition* **59** (Suppl.), 719S–727S.

Sherman, W.M. & Wimer, G.S. (1991) Insufficient dietary carbohydrate during training: does it impair athletic performance? *International Journal of Sport Nutrition* **1**, 28–44.

Sherman, W.M., Doyle, J.A., Lamb, D. & Strauss, H. (1993) Dietary carbohydrate, muscle glycogen, and exercise performance during 7 d of training. *American Journal of Clinical Nutrition* **57**, 27–31.

Simonsen, J.C., Sherman, W.M., Lamb, D.R., Dernbach, A.R., Doyle, J.A. & Strauss, R. (1991) Dietary carbohydrate, muscle glycogen and power output during rowing training. *Journal of Applied Physiology* **70**, 1500–1505.

Southgate, D.A.T. (1995) Digestion and metabolism of sugars. *American Journal of Clinical Nutrition* **62** (Suppl.), 203S–211S.

Thomas, D.E., Brotherhood, J.R. & Brand, J.C. (1991) Carbohydrate feeding before exercise: effect of glycemic index. *International Journal of Sports Medicine* **12**, 180–186.

Truswell, A.S. (1992) Glycaemic index of foods. *European Journal of Clinical Nutrition* **46** (Suppl. 2), S91–S101.

US Department of Agriculture and Health and Human Services (1990) *Dietary Guidelines for Americans*. Home and Garden Bulletin no. 232. United States Department of Agriculture and Health and Human Services, Washington, DC.

Wolever, T.M.S. (1990) The glycemic index. *World Review of Nutrition and Dietetics* **62**, 120–185.

Wolever, T.M., Jenkins, D.J., Jenkins, A.L. & Josse, R.G. (1991) The glycemic index: methodology and clinical implications. *American Journal of Clinical Nutrition* **54**, 846–854.

# Chapter 6

# Carbohydrate Metabolism in Exercise

ERIC HULTMAN AND PAUL L. GREENHAFF

## Introduction

During exercise, the energy demands of muscle contraction will fluctuate enormously. For muscle contraction to occur, chemical energy stored in the form of adenosine triphosphate (ATP) must be converted into mechanical energy at rates appropriate to the needs of the muscle. However, the muscle store of ATP is relatively small and therefore for exercise to continue beyond a few seconds ATP must be resynthesized from phosphocreatine, carbohydrate and fat. It is generally accepted that carbohydrate is the major substrate for ATP resynthesis during intense exercise. The carbohydrate stores of the body are principally located in skeletal muscle and liver, with small amounts also being found in the form of circulating glucose. The amount of energy stored as glycogen amounts to approximately 6000 kJ (1430 kcal) and 1500 kJ (360 kcal) in muscle and liver, respectively, which is very small compared with the body store of triacylglycerol (340 MJ, 81 200 kcal), the alternative fuel for ATP resynthesis. Triacylglycerol is the preferred substrate for energy production in resting muscle and can cover the energy demands of exercise up to 50% of maximal oxygen consumption. At higher exercise intensities, the relative contribution of fat to total energy production falls and carbohydrate oxidation increases, such that carbohydrate is the sole fuel oxidized at the highest exercise intensities. This is due to an increasing recruitment of the glycolytic type II muscle fibres and an activa-

tion of glycolytic enzymes when ATP turnover rate is increased. The maximal rate of ATP production from lipid is lower than that of carbohydrate. In addition, the ATP yield per mole of oxygen utilized is lower for lipid compared with carbohydrate. In contrast with lipid, carbohydrate can be metabolized anaerobically via glycolysis. The lactate accumulation that occurs almost instantaneously at the onset of contraction demonstrates that the activation of this pathway is extremely rapid. It should be noted that the anaerobic utilization of carbohydrate will be indispensable during the transition from rest to steady-state exercise and during maximal exercise. Furthermore, the relatively small store of body carbohydrate will limit exercise performance during prolonged intense exercise due to the depletion of muscle and liver glycogen stores.

The body store and maximal rates of ATP resynthesis from phosphocreatine, carbohydrate and lipid are shown in Table 6.1.

## Regulation of muscle carbohydrate utilization during exercise

Glycogenolysis is the hydrolysis of muscle glycogen to glucose-1-phosphate, which is transformed to glucose-6-phosphate via a phosphoglucomutase reaction. The glucose-6-phosphate formed, together with that derived from the phosphorylation of blood glucose by hexokinase at the muscle cell membrane, enters the glycolytic pathway which is a series of

**Table 6.1** The amounts of substrate available and the maximal rates of energy production from phosphocreatine, carbohydrate and lipid in a 70-kg man (estimated muscle mass, 28 kg).

|  | Amount available (mol) | Production rate (mol · min$^{-1}$) |
|---|---|---|
| ATP, PCr → ADP, Cr | 0.67 | 4.40 |
| Muscle glycogen → Lactate | 6.70* | 2.35 |
| Muscle glycogen → $CO_2$ | 84 | 0.85–1.14 |
| Liver glycogen → $CO_2$ | 19 | 0.37 |
| Fatty acids → $CO_2$ | 4000* | 0.40 |

*These pathways of substrate utilization will not be fully utilized during exercise.

reactions involved in the degradation of glucose-6-phosphate to pyruvate.

## Glycogenolysis

The integrative nature of energy metabolism ensures that the activation of muscle contraction by $Ca^{2+}$ and the accumulation of the products of ATP and phosphocreatinine (PCr) hydrolysis (ADP, AMP, IMP, $NH_3$ and $P_i$) act as stimulators of glycogenolysis, and in this way attempt to match the ATP production to the demand. The control of glycogenolysis during muscle contraction is a highly complex mechanism which can no longer be considered to centre only around the degree of $Ca^{2+}$ induced transformation of less active glycogen phosphorylase *b* to the more active *a* form, as is suggested in many textbooks. For some time it has been known that glycogenolysis can proceed at a negligible rate, despite almost total transformation of phosphorylase to the *a* form; for example, following adrenaline infusion (Chasiotis *et al.* 1983). Conversely, an increase in glycogenolytic rate has been observed during circulatory occlusion, despite a relatively low mole fraction of the phosphorylase *a* form (Chasiotis 1983). From this and other related work, it was concluded that inorganic phosphate ($P_i$) accumulation arising from ATP and PCr hydrolysis played a key role in the regulation of the glycogenolytic activity of phosphorylase *a*, and by doing so served as a link between the energy demand of the contraction and the rate of carbohydrate utilization

(Chasiotis 1983). However, the findings that high rates of glycogenolysis can occur within 2 s of the onset of muscle contraction in conjunction with only a small increase in $P_i$ and, more recently, that glycogenolysis can proceed at a low rate despite a high phosphorylase *a* form and $P_i$ concentration, suggest that factors other than the degree of $Ca^{2+}$ induced phosphorylase transformation and $P_i$ availability are involved in the regulation of glycogenolysis (Ren & Hultman 1989, 1990).

Classically, both inosine monophosphate (IMP) and adenosine monophosphate (AMP) have been associated with the regulation of glycogenolysis during exercise (Lowry *et al.* 1964; Aragon *et al.* 1980). IMP is thought to exert its effect by increasing the activity of phosphorylase *b* during contraction (the apparent Km (Michaeli's constant) of phosphorylase *b* for IMP is about 1.2 mmol · l$^{-1}$ intracellular water). AMP has also been shown to increase the activity of phosphorylase *b*, but it is thought to require an unphysiological accumulation of free AMP to do so (the apparent Km of phosphorylase *b* for AMP is about 1.0 mmol · l$^{-1}$ intracellular water). *In vitro* experiments have demonstrated that AMP can bring about a more marked effect on glycogenolysis by increasing the glycogenolytic activity of phosphorylase *a* (Lowry *et al.* 1964). Because 90% or more of the total cell content of AMP may be bound to cell proteins *in vivo*, it has in the past been questioned whether the increase in free AMP during contraction is of a sufficient magnitude to affect the kinetics of phosphorylase *a*. More recent work, however, demonstrates that a small increase in AMP concentration ($10 \mu mol \cdot l^{-1}$) can markedly increase the *in vitro* activity of phosphorylase *a* (Ren & Hultman 1990). Furthermore, *in vivo* evidence demonstrating a close relationship between muscle ATP turnover and glycogen utilization suggests that an exercise-induced increase in free AMP and inorganic phosphate may be the key regulators of glycogen degradation during muscle contraction (Ren & Hultman 1990).

## Glycolysis

From the preceding discussions it can be seen that the rate of glycogenolysis is determined by the activity of glycogen phosphorylase. However, it is the activity of phosphofructokinase (PFK) that dictates the overall rate of glycolytic flux (Tornheim & Lowenstein 1976). PFK acts as a gate to the flow of hexose units through glycolysis and there is no other enzyme subsequent to PFK that is capable of matching flux rate with the physiological demand for ATP. Stimulation of glycogen phosphorylase by adrenaline and/or exercise results in the accumulation of glucose-6-phosphate demonstrating that PFK is the rate limiting step in the degradation of hexose units to pyruvate (Richter *et al.* 1986).

ATP is known to be the most potent allosteric inhibitor of PFK. The most important activators or deinhibitors of PFK are adenosine diphosphate (ADP), AMP, $P_i$, fructose-6-phosphate, glucose 1–6 bisphosphate, fructose 1–6 and 2–6 bisphosphates and, under extreme conditions, ammonia. Removal of the ATP-mediated inhibition of PFK during contraction, together with the accumulation of the positive modulators of PFK, is responsible for the increase in flux through the enzyme during exercise and thereby is responsible for matching glycolytic flux with the energy demand of contraction.

Hydrogen ion and citrate accumulation during contraction have been suggested to be capable of decreasing the activity of PFK and, thereby, the rate of glycolysis during intense exercise. However, it is now generally accepted that the extent of this inhibition of glycolysis during exercise is overcome in the *in vivo* situation by the accumulation of PFK activators (Spriet *et al.* 1987).

## Pyruvate oxidation

It has been accepted for some time that the rate limiting step in carbohydrate oxidation is the decarboxylation of pyruvate to acetyl-coenzyme A (CoA), which is controlled by the pyruvate dehydrogenase complex (PDC), and is essentially an irreversible reaction committing pyruvate to entry into the tricarboxylic acid (TCA) cycle and oxidation (Wieland 1983). The PDC is a conglomerate of three enzymes located within the inner mitochondrial membrane. Adding to its complexity, PDC also has two regulatory enzymes: a phosphatase and a kinase which regulate an activation–inactivation cycle. Increased ratios of ATP/ADP, acetyl-CoA/CoA and NADH/NAD+ activate the kinase, resulting in the inactivation of the enzyme. Conversely, decreases in the above ratios and the presence of pyruvate will inactivate the kinase, whilst increases in calcium will activate the phosphatase, together resulting in the activation of PDC. Thus, it can be seen that the increases in calcium and pyruvate availability at the onset of contraction will result in the rapid activation of PDC. These factors, together with the subsequent decrease in the ATP/ADP ratio as contraction continues, will result in continued flux through the reaction (Constantin-Teodosiu *et al.* 1991).

Following decarboxylation of pyruvate by the PDC reaction, acetyl-CoA enters the TCA cycle, resulting in the formation of citrate, in a reaction catalysed by citrate synthase. The rate of flux through the TCA cycle is thought to be regulated by citrate synthase, isocitrate dehydrogenase, and α-ketoglutarate dehydrogenase. The activity of these enzymes is controlled by the mitochondrial ratios of ATP/ADP and NADH/NAD+. Good agreement has been found between the maximal activity of α-ketoglutarate dehydrogenase and flux through PDC and the TCA cycle.

The last stage in pyruvate oxidation involves NADH and FADH generated in the TCA cycle entering the electron transport chain. In the electron transport chain, NADH and FADH are oxidized and the energy generated is used to rephosphorylate ADP to ATP. The rate of flux through the electron transport chain will be regulated by the availability of NADH, oxygen and ADP (Chance & Williams 1955). Finally, the translocation of ATP and ADP across the mitochondrial membrane is thought to be effected by creatine by way of the mitochondrial creatine kinase reaction (Moreadith & Jacobus 1982), thereby linking mitochondrial ATP production to the ATPase activity in the contractile system.

### Lactate production

Considerable controversy exists concerning the mechanism responsible for lactate accumulation during intense muscle contraction. The most widely accepted theory attributes this to a high rate of energy demand coupled with an inadequate oxygen supply. In short, when tissue oxygen supply begins to limit oxidative ATP production, resulting in the accumulation of mitochondrial and cytosolic NADH, flux through glycolysis and a high cytosolic $NAD^+/NADH$ ratio are maintained by the reduction of pyruvate to lactate. However, it has been suggested that the reduction in mitochondrial redox state during contraction is insignificant, thereby indicating that reduced oxygen availability is not the only cause of lactate accumulation during contraction (Graham & Saltin 1989). In addition, there are data to indicate that it is the activation of the PDC and the rate of acetyl group production, and not oxygen availability, which primarily regulates lactate production during intense muscle contraction (Timmons et al. 1996). Furthermore, it has also been shown that for any given workload, lactate accumulation can be significantly altered by pre-exercise dietary manipulation (Jansson 1980; Putman et al. 1993). Taken together, these findings suggest that an imbalance between pyruvate formation and decarboxylation to acetyl-CoA will dictate the extent of lactate formation during exercise as

seen, for example, during the transition period from rest to steady-state exercise.

## Glycogen utilization with respect to exercise intensity

### Maximal exercise

During submaximal (steady-state) exercise, ATP resynthesis can be adequately achieved by oxidative combustion of fat and carbohydrate stores. However, during high-intensity (non-steady state) exercise, the relatively slow activation and rate of energy delivery of oxidative phosphorylation cannot meet the energy requirements of contraction. In this situation, anaerobic energy delivery is essential for contraction to continue. Typically, oxidative energy delivery requires several minutes to reach a steady state, due principally to the number and complexity of the reactions involved. Once achieved, the maximal rate of ATP production is in the region of approximately $2.5 \, \text{mmol} \cdot \text{kg}^{-1}$ dry matter $(dm) \cdot s^{-1}$. On the other hand, anaerobic energy delivery is restricted to the cytosol, its activation is almost instantaneous and it can deliver ATP at a rate in excess of $11 \, \text{mmol} \cdot \text{kg}^{-1} \, \text{dm} \cdot s^{-1}$. The downside, however, is that this can be maintained for only a few seconds before beginning to decline. Of course, oxidative and anaerobic ATP resynthesis should not be considered to function independently of one another. It has been demonstrated that as the duration of exercise increases, the contribution from anaerobic energy delivery decreases, whilst that from aerobic is seen to increase.

Figure 6.1 shows that maximal rates of ATP resynthesis from PCr and glycogen degradation can only be maintained for short time periods during maximal contraction in man (Hultman et al. 1991). The rate of PCr degradation is at its maximum immediately after the initiation of contraction and begins to decline after only 1.3 s. Conversely, the corresponding rate of glycolysis does not peak until after approximately 5 s of contraction and does not begin to decline until

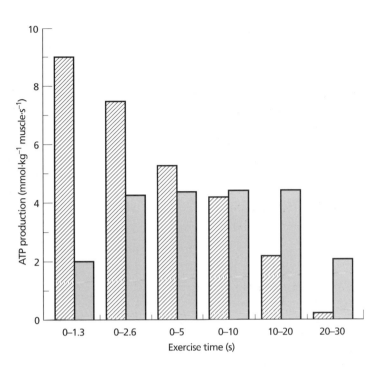

**Fig. 6.1** Rates of anaerobic ATP formation from phosphocreatine and glycolysis during maximal intermittent electrically evoked isometric contraction in man (see Hultman *et al.* 1991). Note that the reference base for the muscle data in the figures and text is dry muscle. This is because the muscle samples were freeze-dried prior to biochemical analysis. To convert to wet weight, values should be divided by 4.3. This assumes 1 kg of wet muscle contains 70 ml of extracellular water and 700 ml of intracellular water. ◨, phosphocreatine; ▨, glycolysis.

after 20 s of contraction. This suggests that the rapid utilization of PCr may buffer the momentary lag in energy provision from glycolysis, and that the contribution of the latter to ATP resynthesis rises as exercise duration increases and PCr availability declines. This point exemplifies the critical importance of PCr at the onset of contraction. Without this large hydrolysis of PCr, it is likely that muscle force production would almost instantaneously be impaired, which is indeed the case in muscles in which the PCr store has been replaced with a Cr analogue (Meyer *et al.* 1986). It is also important to note that ultimately there is a progressive decline in the rate of ATP resynthesis from both substrates during this type of exercise. For example, during the last 10 s of exercise depicted in Fig. 6.1, the rate of ATP production from PCr hydrolysis had declined to approximately 2% of the peak rate. Similarly, the corresponding rate of ATP resynthesis from glycogen hydrolysis had fallen to approximately 40%.

The above example concerns exercise of maximal intensity lasting about 30 s. However, non-steady-state exercise, albeit less intense, can be sustained for durations approaching 5–15 min before fatigue is evident. Under these conditions, carbohydrate oxidation can make a major contribution to ATP production and therefore its importance should not be underestimated.

It has been demonstrated that during 3.2 min of fatiguing exercise, oxidative phosphorylation can contribute as much as 55% of total energy production (Bangsbo *et al.* 1990). This indicates the importance of substrate oxidation during high-intensity exercise, a point which is often overlooked. Under these conditions, muscle glycogen is the principal fuel utilized as muscle glucose uptake is inhibited by glucose 6-phosphate accumulation and adipose tissue lipolysis is inhibited by lactate accumulation.

### Submaximal exercise

The term *submaximal exercise* is typically used to define exercise intensities which can be sustained for durations falling between 30 and 180 min.

In practice, this is usually exercise intensities between 60% and 85% of maximal oxygen consumption. Continuous exercise of any longer duration (i.e. an intensity of less than 60% of maximal oxygen consumption) is probably not limited by substrate availability and, providing adequate hydration is maintained, can probably be sustained for several hours or even days! Unlike maximal intensity exercise, the rate of muscle ATP production required during prolonged exercise is relatively low ($<2.5 \, \text{mmol} \cdot \text{kg}^{-1} \, \text{dm} \cdot \text{s}^{-1}$) and therefore PCr, carbohydrate and fat can all contribute to ATP resynthesis. However, carbohydrate is without question the most important fuel source.

It can be calculated that the maximum rate of ATP production from carbohydrate oxidation will be approximately $2.0–2.8 \, \text{mmol} \cdot \text{kg}^{-1} \, \text{dm} \cdot \text{s}^{-1}$ (based upon a maximum oxygen consumption of $3–4 \, \text{l} \cdot \text{min}^{-1}$), which corresponds to a glycogen utilization rate of approximately $4 \, \text{mmol} \cdot \text{kg}^{-1} \, \text{dm} \cdot \text{min}^{-1}$. Therefore, it can be seen that carbohydrate could meet the energy requirements of prolonged exercise. However, because the muscle store of glycogen is in the region of $350 \, \text{mmol} \cdot \text{kg}^{-1} \, \text{dm}$, under normal conditions, it can be calculated that it could only sustain in the region of 80 min of exercise. This was demonstrated in the 1960s by Bergström and Hultman (1967). The authors also demonstrated that if the glycogen store of muscle was increased by dietary means, exercise duration increased in parallel (Bergström *et al.* 1967). Of course, carbohydrate is also delivered to skeletal muscle from hepatic stores in the form of blood glucose and this can generate ATP at a maximum rate of approximately $1 \, \text{mmol} \cdot \text{kg}^{-1} \, \text{dm} \cdot \text{s}^{-1}$.

The majority of hepatic glucose release during exercise ($1.5–5.5 \, \text{mmol} \cdot \text{min}^{-1}$) is utilized by skeletal muscle. Only $0.5 \, \text{mmol} \cdot \text{min}^{-1}$ is utilized by extramuscular tissue during exercise. Muscle glucose utilization is dependent on glucose supply, transport and metabolism. If blood glucose is unchanged, as in the majority of exercise conditions, glucose supply to muscle is dictated by muscle blood flow, which increases linearly with exercise intensity and can increase by 20-fold from rest to maximal exercise. The increase in muscle glucose delivery as a result of the exercise-mediated increase in blood flow is probably more important for muscle glucose uptake during exercise than the insulin and contraction-induced increase in membrane glucose transport capacity (see Richter & Hespel 1996). As exercise continues, plasma insulin concentration declines, which facilitates hepatic glucose release and reduces glucose utilization by extramuscular tissue. However, insulin supply to muscle probably remains elevated above basal supply due to the contraction-induced elevation in muscle blood flow.

Hexokinase is responsible for the phosphorylation of glucose by ATP when it enters the muscle cell. The enzyme is allosterically inhibited by glucose-6-phosphate, the product of the hexokinase reaction and an intermediate of glycolysis. Thus, during short-term high-intensity exercise and at the onset of prolonged submaximal exercise, glucose phosphorylation by hexokinase will be inhibited by glucose-6-phosphate accumulation. This will increase the concentration of glucose in the extra- and intracellular water and will contribute to the increase in blood glucose observed during high-intensity exercise. However, as submaximal exercise continues, the decline in muscle glucose-6-phosphate results in an increase in glucose phosphorylation.

In comparison with muscle glycogen metabolism, relatively little is known about the interaction between exercise and *hepatic glycogen metabolism* in man. This is not because of a lack of interest but because of the invasive nature of the liver biopsy technique. The few studies that have been performed in healthy volunteers using this technique have demonstrated that the rate of liver glucose release in the postabsorptive state is in the region of $0.8 \, \text{mmol glucose} \cdot \text{min}^{-1}$, which is sufficient to meet the carbohydrate demands of the brain and obligatory glucolytic tissues. Approximately 60% of this release ($0.5 \, \text{mmol} \cdot \text{min}^{-1}$) is derived from liver glycogen stores and the remainder is synthesized by gluconeogenesis in the liver using lactate, pyruvate, glycerol and

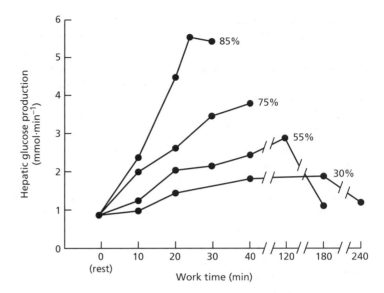

**Fig. 6.2** Hepatic glucose release during exercise at 30%, 55%, 75% and 85% of maximal oxygen consumption in men. From Ahlborg *et al.* (1974), Ahlborg and Felig (1982), Wahren *et al.* (1971) and Hultman (1967).

amino acids as substrates (Hultman & Nilson 1971; Nilsson & Hultman 1973).

The rate of hepatic glucose release during exercise in the postabsorptive state has been shown to be mainly a function of exercise intensity (Fig. 6.2) (Hultman 1967; Wahren *et al.* 1971; Ahlborg *et al.* 1974; Ahlborg & Felig 1982). The uptake of gluconeogenic precursors by the liver is only marginally increased during the initial 40 min of submaximal exercise but increases further as exercise continues (Ahlborg *et al.* 1974). Most (more than 90%) of the glucose release is derived from liver glycogenolysis resulting in a decline and ultimately depletion of liver glycogen stores. Direct measurements of liver glycogen concentration in the postabsorptive state and following 60 min of exercise at 75% of maximal oxygen consumption showed a 50% decrease in the liver glycogen concentration with exercise (Fig. 6.3). This corresponded to a glycogen degradation rate of 4.2 mmol·min⁻¹ (assuming 1.8 kg of liver) and suggested that the liver glycogen store would have been depleted within 120 min of exercise at this intensity.

The exact mechanisms responsible for the regulation of liver glucose release at the onset and during exercise are still unresolved. However, it is known that the decline in blood

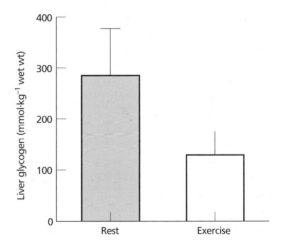

**Fig. 6.3** Hepatic glycogen concentration in men at rest following an overnight fast ($n = 33$) and following an overnight fast and 60 min of exercise at approximately 75% of maximal oxygen consumption in a second group of subjects ($n = 14$). Biopsy samples were obtained at the same time of day in both groups of subjects. From Hultman and Nilsson (1971).

insulin concentration and increases in adrenaline and glucagon with increasing exercise duration together with afferent nervous feedback from contracting muscle will stimulate liver glucose release (for more complete information, see Kjaer 1995).

## Muscle fibre type responses

The conclusions presented so far have been based on metabolite changes measured in biopsy samples obtained from the quadriceps femoris muscle group. However, it is known that human skeletal muscle is composed of at least two functionally and metabolically different fibre types. Type I fibres are characterized as being slow contracting, fatigue resistant, having a low peak power output and favouring aerobic metabolism for ATP resynthesis during contraction. Conversely, in comparison, type II fibres are fast contracting, fatigue rapidly, have a high peak power output and favour mainly anaerobic metabolism for ATP resynthesis (Burke & Edgerton 1975).

### Maximal exercise

Evidence from animal studies performed on muscles composed of predominantly type I or type II fibres and from one study performed using bundles of similar human muscle fibre types, suggest that the rapid and marked rise and subsequent decline in maximal power output observed during intense muscle contraction in man may be closely related to activation and rapid fatigue of type II fibres during contraction (Faulkner *et al.* 1986).

Figure 6.4 demonstrates glycogen degradation in type I and type II muscle fibres during maximal exercise under four different experimental conditions. Notice that during intense contraction the rates of glycogenolysis are higher in type II than in type I fibres. This is true for both dynamic exercise (Greenhaff *et al.* 1994; treadmill sprinting) and electrically induced isometric contractions (Greenhaff *et al.* 1991, 1993). The rates of glycogenolysis observed in both fibre types during treadmill sprinting and intermittent isometric contraction with circulation occluded, are in good agreement with the $\dot{V}_{max.}$ of phosphorylase measured in both fibre types (Harris *et al.* 1976), suggesting that glycogenoly-

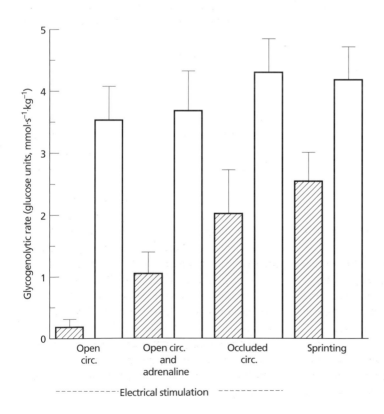

**Fig. 6.4** Glycogenolytic rates in type I (▨) and type II (□) human muscle fibres during 30 s of intermittent electrically evoked maximal isometric contraction with intact circulation (circ.), intact circulation with adrenaline infusion, occluded circulation and during 30 s of maximal sprint running. Adapted from Greenhaff *et al.* (1991, 1993, 1994).

sis is occurring at a near maximal rate during intense exercise. Surprisingly, during intermittent isometric contraction with circulation intact, when the rest interval between contractions is of the order of 1.6s, the rate of glycogenolysis in type I fibres is almost negligible. The corresponding rate in type II fibres is almost maximal and similar to that seen during contraction with circulatory occlusion. This suggests that during maximal exercise glycogenolysis in type II fibres is invariably occurring at a maximal rate, irrespective of the experimental conditions, while the rate in type I fibres is probably very much related to cellular oxygen availability.

### Submaximal exercise

In contrast to maximal exercise, the rate of glycogenolysis during submaximal exercise is greatest in type I fibres, especially during the initial period of exercise (Ball-Burnett et al. 1990). This phenomenon is likely to be the result of differences in the recruitment pattern between muscle fibre types. If exercise is continued, glycogen utilization occurs in both fibre types but depletion is observed first in the type I muscle fibres. The consumption of carbohydrate during exhaustive submaximal exercise has been shown to offset the depletion of glycogen specifically in type I fibres (Tsintzas et al. 1996).

### Fatigue mechanisms related to carbohydrate metabolism

What is clear from the literature is that glycogen availability per se is not usually considered to be responsible for fatigue development during maximal exercise, providing the pre-exercise glycogen store is not depleted to below $100 \, mmol \cdot kg^{-1}$ dm. It is even unlikely that glycogen availability will limit performance during repeated bouts of exercise, due to the decline in glycogenolysis and lactate production that occurs under these conditions. It is more probable that fatigue development during maximal exercise will be caused by a gradual decline in anaerobic ATP production caused by the depletion of PCr and a fall in the rate of glycogenolysis.

Lactic acid accumulation during high-intensity exercise is considered to produce muscle fatigue as a result of $H^+$ and $P_i$ accumulation. An increase in hydrogen ion concentration will negatively affect phosphorylase activity, thereby delaying the rate of glycogenolysis, by delaying transformation of the b form to the a form (Danforth 1965; Chasiotis 1983) and by decreasing the $HPO_4^{2+}$, the dibasic form of $P_i$, which is the substrate for phosphorylase. The inhibition of PFK discussed previously seems to be at least partly offset by an increase in the activators of PFK, especially ADP, AMP and $P_i$, when the rate of ATP utilization is higher than the rate of oxidative ATP resynthesis. The increase in ADP and $P_i$, especially the $H_2PO_4^-$ form, in acidotic muscle is known to have inhibitory effects on contractile function (Cook & Pate 1985; Nosek et al. 1987). However, there is no evidence of a direct relationship between the decline in muscle force during contraction and $H^+$ accumulation. For example, studies involving human volunteers have demonstrated that muscle-force generation following fatiguing exercise can recover rapidly, despite having a very low muscle pH value (Sahlin & Ren 1989). The general consensus at the moment appears to be that the initial generation of muscle force production is dependent on the capacity to generate ATP but the maintenance of force generation is also pH dependent.

Despite the wealth of information showing that carbohydrate availability is essential to performance during submaximal exercise, the biochemical mechanism(s) by which fatigue is brought about in the carbohydrate depleted state are still unclear. Recent evidence suggests that carbohydrate depletion will result in an inability to rephosphorylate ADP to ATP at the required rate, possibly because of a decrease in the rate of flux through the TCA cycle as a result of a decline in muscle TCA cycle intermediates (Sahlin et al. 1990). The consequent rise in ADP concentration will bring about fatigue, perhaps as a direct inhibitory effect of ADP and/or $P_i$ on contraction coupling.

## Conclusion

The carbohydrate stores of the body, liver and muscle glycogen, are utilized immediately at start of exercise. Glucose output from the liver closely matches the increased glucose requirement of the contracting muscles, keeping the blood glucose concentration unchanged during submaximal exercise. Blood glucose levels are normally seen only to increase in the initial period of intense exercise and to fall when the hepatic glycogen store is depleted near to exhaustion. The regulation of the hepatic glucose release is a complex process dependent on both hormonal control and feedback signals from contracting muscles.

Glucose uptake by exercising muscle is directly related to exercise intensity and regulated by muscle blood flow and facilitated by increased glucose transport capacity of the plasma membrane of the contracting muscle. The maximal rate of glucose uptake at a normal blood glucose concentration is about $0.4\,\text{mmol}\cdot\text{min}^{-1}\cdot\text{kg}^{-1}$ exercising muscle. Glucose utilization is also dependent on the glucose phosphorylation capacity mediated by the activity of hexokinase.

The major carbohydrate store of the body is muscle glycogen, which is used in concert with the hepatic glycogen store to provide the exercising muscle with energy.

The rate of utilization is low at rest and during low-intensity exercise, when blood-borne glucose and free fatty acids are the major sources of fuel for ATP resynthesis. With increasing exercise intensity, the use of carbohydrate as an energy substrate increases gradually to cover almost all the energy demand of contraction at exercise intensities near the subject's maximal oxygen uptake. The maximal rate of oxidative energy production from muscle glycogen is of the order of $35\,\text{mmol ATP}\cdot\text{min}^{-1}\cdot\text{kg}^{-1}$ exercising muscle, corresponding to a glycogen degradation rate of $1\,\text{mmol}\cdot\text{min}^{-1}\cdot\text{kg}^{-1}$ wet muscle. The mechanism(s) controlling the integration of fat and carbohydrate utilization during exercise are poorly understood and, as yet, unresolved.

The muscle glycogen store can also produce ATP anaerobically and at a rate that is twice that of oxidative ATP regeneration. Anaerobic energy delivery can be activated within milliseconds, while the aerobic energy production needs several minutes to reach a steady state. Thus, anaerobic carbohydrate utilization will be important as an energy provider during the transition period between rest and exercise and during periods of intense exercise when the energy demand of contraction exceeds the capacity of oxidative ATP regeneration.

It can be concluded that carbohydrate is used as fuel at onset of exercise at all intensities and is an obligatory fuel for the continuation of exercise at intensities above 50–60% of the subject's maximal oxygen uptake. Depletion of the muscle carbohydrate stores will impair exercise performance at this range of exercise intensities. Exhaustion of the liver glycogen store during prolonged exercise results in hypoglycaemia which also impairs continued exercise performance.

Carbohydrate metabolism in exercising muscle is initiated by $Ca^{2+}$ release from the sarcoplasmic reticulum and thereafter is regulated by the rate of ATP degradation via the phosphorylation state of the high-energy phosphate pool (ATP, ADP, AMP, PCr) and $P_i$. AMP and $P_i$ concentrations regulate the flux through the glycolytic pathway while $Ca^{2+}$ and pyruvate concentrations are the main regulators of PDH activity which, together with the intramitochondrial concentration of ADP, determines the rate of carbohydrate oxidation. The result is a tight matching of ATP generation from carbohydrate sources with the ATP demand of contracting muscle.

Other influences on carbohydrate metabolism during exercise include diet, training status and hormonal balance.

## References

Ahlborg, G. & Felig, P. (1982) Lactate and glucose exchange across the forearm, legs and splanchnic bed during and after prolonged leg exercise. *Journal of Clinical Investigation* **69**, 45–54.

Ahlborg, G., Felig, P., Hagenfeldt, L., Hendler, R. &

Wahren, J. (1974) Substrate turnover during prolonged exercise in man: splanchnic and leg metabolism of glucose, free fatty acids and amino acids. *Journal of Clinical Investigation* **53**, 1080–1090.

Aragon, J.J., Tornheim, K. & Lowenstein, J.M. (1980) On a possible role of IMP in the regulation of phosphorylase activity in skeletal muscle. *FEBS Letters* **117**, K56–K64.

Ball-Burnett, M., Green, H.J. & Houston, M.E. (1990) Energy metabolism in slow and fast twitch muscle fibres during prolonged cycle exercise. *Journal of Physiology* **437**, 257–267.

Bangsbo, J., Gollnick, P.D., Graham, T.E. *et al.* (1990) Anaerobic energy production and $O_2$ deficit–debt relationship during exhaustive exercise in humans. *Journal of Physiology* **422**, 539–559.

Bergström, J. & Hultman, E. (1967) A study of glycogen metabolism during exercise in man. *Scandinavian Journal of Clinical Laboratory Investigation* **19**, 218–228.

Bergström, J., Hermansson, L., Hultman, E. & Saltin, B. (1967) Diet, muscle glycogen and physical performance. *Acta Physiologica Scandinavica* **71**, 140–150.

Burke, R.W. & Edgerton, V.R. (1975) Motor unit properties and selective involvement in movement. *Exercise and Sports Science Reviews* **3**, 31–81.

Chance, B. & Williams, G.R. (1955) Respiratory enzymes in oxidative phosphorylation. I. Kinetics of oxygen utilisation. *Journal of Biological Chemistry* **217**, 383–393.

Chasiotis, D. (1983) The regulation of glycogen phosphorylase and glycogen breakdown in human skeletal muscle. *Acta Physiologica Scandinavica* **518** (Suppl.), 1–68.

Chasiotis, D., Sahlin, K. & Hultman, E. (1983) Regulation of glycogenolysis in human muscle in response to epinephrine infusion. *Journal of Applied Physiology* **54**, 45–50.

Constantin-Teodosiu, D., Carlin, J.J., Cederblad, G., Harris, R.C. & Hultman, E. (1991) Acetyl group accumulation and pyruvate dehydrogensae activity in human muscle during incremental exercise. *Acta Physiologica Scandinavica* **143**, 367–372.

Cook, R. & Pate, E. (1985) The effects of ADP and phosphate on the contraction of muscle fibres. *Biophysics Journal* **48**, 789–798.

Danforth, W.H. (1965) Activation of glycolytic pathway in muscle. In *Control of Energy Metabolism* (ed. B. Chance & R.W. Estabrook), pp. 287–296. Academic Press, New York.

Faulkner, J.A., Claflin, D.R. & McCully, K.K. (1986) Power output of fast and slow fibres from human skeletal muscles. In *Human Power Output* (ed. N.L. Jones, N. McCartney & A.J. McComas), pp. 81–89. Human Kinetics, Champaign, IL.

Graham, T.E. & Saltin, B. (1989) Estimation of the mitochondrial redox state in human skeletal muscle during exercise. *Journal of Applied Physiology* **66**, 561–566.

Greenhaff, P.L., Ren, J.-M., Soderlund, K. & Hultman, E. (1991) Energy metabolism in single human muscle fibres during contraction without and with epinephrine infusion. *American Journal of Physiology* **260**, E713–E718.

Greenhaff, P.L., Soderlund, K., Ren, J.-M. & Hultman, E. (1993) Energy metabolism in single human muscle fibres during intermittent contraction with occluded circulation. *Journal of Physiology* **460**, 443–453.

Greenhaff, P.L., Nevill, M.E., Soderlund, K. *et al.* (1994) The metabolic responses of human type I and II muscle fibres during maximal treadmill sprinting. *Journal of Physiology* **478**, 149–155.

Harris, R.C., Essen, B. & Hultman, E. (1976) Glycogen phosphorylase in biopsy samples and single muscle fibres of musculus quadriceps femoris of man at rest. *Scandinavian Journal of Clinical Laboratory Investigation* **36**, 521–526.

Hultman, E. (1967) Studies on muscle glycogen and active phosphate in man with special reference to exercise and diet. *Scandinavian Journal of Clinical Laboratory Investigation* **19** (Suppl. 94), 1–63.

Hultman, E. & Nilsson, L.H. son (1971) Liver glycogen in man, effects of different diets and muscular exercise. In *Muscle Metabolism during Intense Exercise* (ed. B. Pernow & B. Saltin), pp. 143–151. Plenum Press, London.

Hultman, E., Greenhaff, P.L., Ren, J.-M. & Soderlund, K. (1991) Energy metabolism and fatigue during intense muscle contraction. *Biochemical Society Transactions* **19**, 347–353.

Jansson, E. (1980) Diet and muscle metabolism in man. *Acta Physiologica Scandinavica* **487** (Suppl.), 1–24.

Kjaer, M. (1995) Hepatic fuel metabolism during exercise. In *Exercise Metabolism* (ed. M. Hargreaves), pp. 73–97. Human Kinetics, Champaign, IL.

Lowry, O.H., Schulz, D.W. & Passoneau, J.V. (1964) Effects of adenylic acid on the kinetics of muscle phosphorylase a. *Journal of Biological Chemistry* **239**, 1947–1953.

Meyer, R.A., Brown, T.R., Krilowicz, B.L. & Kushmerick, M.J. (1986) Phosphagen and intracellular pH changes during contraction of creatine-depleted rat muscle. *American Journal of Physiology* **250**, C264–C274.

Moreadith, R.W. & Jacobus, W.E. (1982) Creatine kinase of heart mitochondria: functional coupling to ADP transfer to the adenine nucleotide translocase. *Journal of Biological Chemistry* **257**, 899–905.

Nilsson, L.H. son & Hultman, E. (1973) Liver glycogen in man: the effect of total starvation or a carbohydrate-poor diet followed by carbohydrate feedings. *Scandinavian Journal of Clinical Laboratory Investigation* **32**, 325–330.

Nosek, T.M., Fender, K.Y. & Godt, R.E. (1987) It is diprotonated inorganic phosphate that depresses force in skinned skeletal muscle fibres. *Science* **236**, 191–193.

Putman, C.T., Spriet, L.L., Hultman, E., Lindinger, M.I., Lands, L.C., McKelvie, R.S., Cederblad, G., Jones, N.L. & Heigenhauser, G.J.F. (1993) Pyruvate dehydrogenase activity and acetyl group accumulation during exercise after different diets. *American Journal of Physiology* **265**, E752–E760.

Ren, J.-M. & Hultman, E. (1989) Regulation of glycogenolysis in human skeletal muscle. *Journal of Applied Physiology* **67**, 2243–2248.

Ren, J.-M. & Hultman, E. (1990) Regulation of phosphorylase a activity in human skeletal muscle. *Journal of Applied Physiology* **69**, 919–923.

Richter, E.R. & Hespel, P. (1996) Determinants of glucose uptake in contracting muscle. In *Biochemistry of Exercise IX* (ed. R. Maughan & S. Shirreffs), pp. 51–60. Human Kinetics, Champaign.

Richter, E.R., Sonne, B., Ploug, T., Kjaer, M., Mikines, K. & Galbo, H. (1986) Regulation of carbohydrate metabolism in exercise. In *Biochemistry of Exercise IV* (ed. B. Saltin), pp. 151–166. Human Kinetics, Champaign, IL.

Sahlin, K. & Ren, J.-M. (1989) Relationship of contraction capacity to metabolic changes during recovery from fatigueing contraction. *Journal of Applied Physiology* **67**, 648–654.

Sahlin, K., Katz, A. & Broberg, S. (1990) Tricarboxylic cycle intermediates in human muscle during submaximal exercise. *American Journal of Physiology* **259**, C834–C841.

Spriet, L.L., Soderlund, K., Bergstrom, M. & Hultman, E. (1987) Skeletal muscle glycogenolysis, glyxcolysis and pH during electrical stimulation in man. *Journal of Applied Physiology* **62**, 611–615.

Timmons, J.A., Poucher, S.M., Constantin-Teodosiu, D., Worrall, V., Macdonald, I.A. & Greenhaff, P.L. (1996) Increased acetyl group availability enhances contractile function of canine skeletal muscle during ischemia. *Journal of Clinical Investigation* **97**, 879–883.

Tornheim, K. & Lowenstein, J.M. (1976) Control of phosphofructokinase from rat skeletal muscle. *Journal of Biological Chemistry* **251**, 7322–7328.

Tsintzas, O.-K., Williams, C., Boobis, L. & Greenhaff, P.L. (1996) Carbohydrate ingestion and single muscle fibre glycogen metabolism during prolonged running in man. *Journal of Applied Physiology* **81**, 801–809.

Wahren, J., Felig, P., Ahlborg, G. & Jorfelt, L. (1971) Glucose metabolism during leg exercise in man. *Journal of Clinical Investigation* **50**, 2715–2725.

Wieland, O.H. (1983) The mammalian pyruvate dehydrogenase complex, structure and regulation. *Reviews in Physiology Biochemistry and Pharmacology* **96**, 123–170.

# Chapter 7

# Optimization of Glycogen Stores

JOHN L. IVY

## Introduction

The importance of carbohydrates as a fuel source during physical activity has been recognized for many years (Krogh & Lindhard 1920; Levine *et al.* 1924; Dill *et al.* 1932). Krogh and Lindhard (1920) reported that subjects placed on a high fat diet complained of feeling tired and had difficulty performing a standardized 2-h exercise protocol on a cycle ergometer. However, 3 days on a high carbohydrate diet relieved their symptoms of tiredness and the subjects were able to complete the 2-h exercise task without undue stress. Similarly, Christensen and Hansen (1939a, 1939b) found that the capacity for prolonged exercise was three times greater after 3–7 days on a high carbohydrate diet as opposed to a high fat-protein diet. They also reported that exhaustion was accompanied by hypoglycaemia, and that ingestion of a carbohydrate supplement during recovery rapidly returned the blood glucose concentration back to normal and allowed considerable additional exercise to be performed. These results were in agreement with the earlier observations of Levine *et al.* (1924), who found that blood glucose levels of runners fell to very low levels during a marathon. They also noted that in conjunction with this hypoglycaemic state, the participants were physically fatigued and displayed neuroglucopenia symptoms such as muscular twitching and disorientation. Based on these observations, it was generally accepted that hypoglycaemia resulting from liver glycogen depletion was responsible for fatigue dur-

ing prolonged strenuous exercise. However, this view would be modified as technical advances allowed the direct investigation of muscle metabolism during and following prolonged strenuous exercise.

Based on the findings of several Scandinavian research groups, it became apparent that there is an increased reliance on muscle glycogen as a fuel source as exercise intensity increases, and that perception of fatigue during prolonged strenuous exercise parallels the declining muscle glycogen stores. It was also found that aerobic endurance is directly related to the initial muscle glycogen stores, and that strenuous exercise could not be maintained once these stores are depleted (Hermansen *et al.* 1965; Ahlborg *et al.* 1967a; Bergström *et al.* 1967; Hultman 1967).

The amount of glycogen stored in skeletal muscle, however, is limited. If muscle glycogen was the only fuel source available, it could be completely depleted within 90 min of moderate intensity exercise. Therefore, because of the limited availability of muscle glycogen and its importance during prolonged strenuous exercise, methods for increasing its concentration above normal prior to exercise and for its rapid restoration after exercise have been extensively investigated. This chapter discusses our current understanding of the regulation of muscle glycogen synthesis, the effect of diet and exercise on the muscle glycogen concentration prior to exercise, and methods for muscle glycogen restoration immediately after exercise. The chapter concludes with recommendations for increasing and maintaining muscle glycogen stores for competition and training.

## Regulation of muscle glycogen synthesis

Figure 7.1 illustrates the metabolic reactions controlling glycogen synthesis. Upon crossing the sarcolemma, glucose is rapidly converted to glucose-6-phosphate (G6P) by the enzyme hexokinase. The G6P is then converted to glucose-1-phosphate (G1P) by phosphoglucomutase. Next, uridine triphosphate and G1P are combined to form uridine diphosphate (UDP)-glucose, which serves as a glycosyl carrier. The glucose attached to the UDP-glucose is then transferred to the terminal glucose residue at the non-reducing end of a glucan chain to form an $\alpha(1\rightarrow4)$ glycosidic linkage. This reaction is catalysed by the enzyme glycogen synthase. The initial formation of the glucan chain, however, is controlled by the protein glycogenin, which is a UDP-glucose-requiring glucosyltransferase. The first step involves the covalent attachment of glucose to a single tyrosine residue on glycogenin. This reaction is brought about autocatalytically by glycogenin itself. The next step is the extension of the glucan chain which involves the sequential addition of up to seven further glucosyl residues. The glucan primer is elongated by glycogen synthase, but only when glycogenin and glycogen synthase are complexed together. Finally, amylo

$(1,4\rightarrow1,6)$ transglycosylase catalyses the transfer of a terminal oligosaccharide fragment of six or seven glucosyl residues from the end of the glucan chain to the 6-hydroxyl group of a glucose residue of the same or another chain. This occurs in such a manner as to form an $\alpha(1\rightarrow6)$ linkage and thus create a compact molecular structure. The synthesis of the glycogen molecule is terminated by the dissociation of glycogen synthase from glycogenin (Smythe & Cohen 1991; Alonso et al. 1995).

Following its depletion by exercise, muscle glycogen synthesis occurs in a biphasic manner (Bergström & Hultman 1967b; Piehl 1974; Ivy 1977; Maehlum et al. 1977; Price et al. 1994). Initially, there is a rapid synthesis of muscle glycogen that does not require the presence of insulin (Ivy 1977; Maehlum et al. 1977; Price et al. 1994). In normal humans, the rate of synthesis during this insulin-independent phase has been found to range between 12 and $30\,\mu mol\cdot g^{-1}$ wet weight $\cdot h^{-1}$ and to last for about 45–60 min. The second phase is insulin dependent (Ivy 1977; Maehlum et al. 1977; Price et al. 1994) and in the absence of carbohydrate supplementation occurs at a rate that is approximately seven- to 10-fold slower than that of the rapid phase (Price et al. 1994). If supplemented immediately after exercise with carbohydrates, however, the rate of synthesis during the slow phase can be increased several-fold, and if supplementation persists, the muscle glycogen level can be increased above

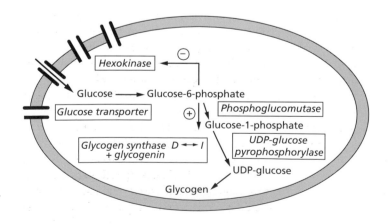

**Fig. 7.1** The metabolic reactions and the enzymes controlling the reactions that are responsible for the synthesis of muscle glycogen. Enzymes are in italic. See text for details.

normal (Bergström *et al.* 1967). This elevation in muscle glycogen above normal is referred to as *glycogen supercompensation*. Interestingly, the effectiveness of the carbohydrate supplement to speed muscle glycogen recovery during the slow phase is directly related to the plasma insulin response to the supplement (Ivy 1991).

### Rapid phase of glycogen synthesis after exercise

After exercise that is of sufficient intensity and duration to deplete the muscle glycogen stores, the activity of glycogen synthase is increased. Glycogen synthase is the rate-limiting enzyme in the glycogen synthesis pathway. Its activity is strongly influenced by the muscle glycogen concentration (Danforth 1965; Bergström *et al.* 1972; Adolfsson 1973). Generally, the percentage of glycogen synthase in its active I-form is inversely related to the muscle glycogen concentration. That is, as the muscle glycogen concentration declines the percentage of glycogen synthase in the I-form increases. Conversely, as the glycogen concentration increases the percentage of glycogen synthase in its inactive D-form increases.

An exercise-induced increase in glycogen synthase activity can catalyse the rapid restoration of glycogen only if adequate substrate is available. Thus, an additional factor that makes possible the rapid increase in muscle glycogen after exercise is a protracted increase in the permeability of the muscle cell membrane to glucose (Holloszy & Narahara 1965; Ivy & Holloszy 1981; Richter *et al.* 1982). The increase in glucose transport induced by muscle contractile activity, however, reverses rapidly in the absence of insulin, with most of the effect lost within several hours (Cartee *et al.* 1989). This rapid decline in muscle glucose transport appears to be inversely related to the muscle glycogen concentration (Cartee *et al.* 1989; Richter *et al.* 1984). Thus, the increase in membrane permeability to glucose, together with the activation of glycogen synthase, allows for an initial rapid insulin-independent resynthesis of muscle glycogen following exercise.

### Slow phase of muscle glycogen synthesis after exercise

After the direct, insulin-independent effect of exercise on glucose transport subsides, it is rapidly replaced by a marked increase in the sensitivity of muscle glucose transport and glycogen synthesis to insulin (Garetto *et al.* 1984; Richter *et al.* 1984; Cartee *et al.* 1989). The magnitude of the increased insulin sensitivity induced by exercise can be extremely high, and result in muscle glucose uptake and glycogen synthesis with insulin concentrations that normally have no detectable effect on either process (Cartee *et al.* 1989; Price *et al.* 1994). Furthermore, this increase in sensitivity can be sustained for a very long period of time, and does not appear to reverse completely until glycogen supercompensation has occurred (Garetto *et al.* 1984; Cartee *et al.* 1989). These findings therefore suggest that an increase in muscle insulin sensitivity is a primary component of the slow phase of glycogen synthesis.

Although the percentage of glycogen synthase in the I-form may be as high as 80% immediately after exercise-induced glycogen depletion, as glycogen levels are normalized the percentage of glycogen synthase I decreases back to the pre-exercise level or lower in a negative feedback manner (Danforth 1965; Bergström *et al.* 1972; Adolfsson 1973; Terjung *et al.* 1974). However, during the slow synthesis phase of glycogen, glycogen synthase appears to be transformed into an intermediate form which has a depressed activity ratio, but enhanced sensitivity to activation by G6P (Kochan *et al.* 1981). Thus, a second important component of the slow phase of glycogen synthase appears to be an increase in the sensitivity of glycogen synthase to G6P.

Another possible mechanism that might contribute to an increase in glycogen synthesis during the slow insulin-dependent phase of recovery is an increase in GLUT-4 concentration. Recently, Ren *et al.* (1994) reported an increase in GLUT-4 protein in skeletal muscle of rats after a single prolonged exercise session. The increase in GLUT-4 protein was accompanied by a proportional increase in insulin-stimulated glucose transport and glycogen synthesis. Ren *et al.* (1994) concluded that a rapid increase in GLUT-4 expression is an early adaptation of muscle to exercise to enhance replenishment of muscle glycogen stores.

### Effect of carbohydrate supplementation

It is evident that the exercise-induced increase in muscle permeability to glucose, insulin sensitivity, and glycogen synthase activity are, together, not sufficient to result in the rapid repletion and supercompensation of the glycogen stores, since only a small increase in muscle glycogen occurs following exercise in the absence of carbohydrate feeding (Bergström *et al.* 1967; Bergström & Hultman 1967b; Maehlum & Hermansen 1978; Ivy *et al.* 1988b). Probable factors that prevent the rapid repletion of muscle glycogen in the fasted state are a depressed circulating insulin concentration, and an increase in plasma free fatty acids and fatty acid oxidation by muscle (Ivy *et al.* 1988a). These conditions are actually advantageous during fasting as they serve to slow muscle glucose uptake and conserve blood glucose for use by the nervous system until sufficient carbohydrate is available.

Carbohydrate feeding after exercise probably stimulates glycogen synthesis by increasing arterial plasma insulin and glucose concentrations. The increase in circulating insulin not only functions to increase muscle glucose uptake, but also functions to keep glycogen synthase activity elevated. It may also play a role in increasing GLUT-4 expression which would facilitate insulin-stimulated glucose transport (Ren *et al.* 1993; Hansen *et al.* 1995; Brozinick *et al.* 1996). With increasing plasma glucose concentration, glucose transport increases regardless of the level of muscle permeability to glucose (Nesher *et al.* 1985). Therefore, the increase in arterial plasma glucose concentration functions to increase the rate of glucose transport, further increasing substrate availability, and providing sufficient G6P for activation of glycogen synthase.

It has also been demonstrated that the insulin response to carbohydrate supplementation increases over subsequent days while glucose tolerance remains the same or actually improves (Ivy *et al.* 1985). This increase in insulin response to carbohydrate loading is thought to be the result of an increase in the pancreatic response to glucose (Szanto & Yudkin 1969). Since insulin is required for normal glycogen repletion and supercompensation, it is possible that the hyperinsulinaemic response following several days of high carbohydrate consumption is responsible for the increased sensitivity of glycogen synthase to G6P. The elevated plasma insulin may also serve to increase the rate of muscle glucose transport, thus increasing the availability of glucose to glycogen synthase, as well as possibly increasing the intracellular concentration of G6P. Hexokinase activity in muscle is also increased during subsequent days of carbohydrate loading (Ivy *et al.* 1983). This too could be of functional significance since an increase in hexokinase activity would prevent the rate-limiting step in glucose uptake from shifting from transport to glucose phosphorylation as the G6P concentration increased.

## Glycogen supercompensation regimens

The discovery by Bergström and Hultman (1967b) that a high carbohydrate diet following the depletion of muscle glycogen by exercise would result in an above normal muscle glycogen concentration led to a series of studies to identify the regimen of exercise and diet that would best supercompensate the muscle glycogen stores. Bergström *et al.* (1967) had subjects exercise to exhaustion to deplete their muscle glycogen stores. Six of the subjects then received a high fat–protein diet for 3 days. This was followed by another exhaustive exercise bout and 3 days of a high carbohydrate diet. The remaining three subjects followed the same protocol as above except the order of administration of the diets was reversed. When the high carbohydrate diet followed the high fat–protein diet, the muscle glycogen concentration was $205.5\,\mu mol\cdot g^{-1}$ wet weight. This represented a 100% increase above the initial muscle glycogen concentration. When the high carbohydrate diet preceded the high fat–protein diet, the muscle glycogen concentration was $183.9\,\mu mol\cdot g^{-1}$ wet weight following the high carbohydrate diet. It was suggested that a period of carbohydrate-free diet further stimulated glycogen synthesis when carbohydrates were given following exercise. Based on this study and several similar studies (Ahlborg et al. 1967b; Bergström & Hultman 1967a), it was recommended that the best way to glycogen supercompensate was, first, to deplete the muscle glycogen stores with an exhaustive exercise bout; second, to eat a carbohydrate-free diet for 3 days; third, to deplete the glycogen stores once more with an exhaustive exercise bout; and fourth, to consume a high carbohydrate diet for 3 days.

Because of the strenuous nature of this regimen, many athletes have found it impractical, even though it has been used successfully by very elite performers. The 3 days of low carbohydrate diet may cause hypoglycaemia, irritability and chronic fatigue. The two bouts of exhaustive exercise prior to competition may result in injury, soreness and fatigue, and prevents a proper taper before competition. To address this problem, Sherman et al. (1981) studied three types of muscle glycogen supercompensation regimens on six trained runners. Over a 6-day period, the subjects ran at approximately 75% of $\dot{V}o_{2max.}$ for 90 min, 40 min, 40 min, 20 min, 20 min, and rested, respectively. During each taper, the subjects received one of three dietary treatments:

**1** a mixed diet composed of 50% carbohydrate (control diet),

**2** a low carbohydrate diet (25% carbohydrate) for the first 3 days and a high carbohydrate diet (70% carbohydrate) for the last 3 days (classic diet), and

**3** a mixed diet (50% carbohydrate) for the first 3 days and a high carbohydrate diet (70% carbohydrate) the last 3 days (modified diet).

Muscle biopsies were obtained on the morning of the 4th and 7th days of each trial. During the

control treatment, muscle glycogen concentrations of the gastrocnemius were 135 and $163\,\mu mol\cdot g^{-1}$ wet weight on days 4 and 7, respectively. During the classic treatment, the corresponding muscle glycogen concentrations were 80 and $210\,\mu mol\cdot g^{-1}$ wet weight, and during the modified treatment they were 135 and $204\,\mu mol\cdot g^{-1}$ wet weight (Fig. 7.2). These results suggest that a normal training taper in conjunction with a moderate carbohydrate–high carbohydrate diet sequence is as effective as the classic glycogen supercompensation regimen for highly trained endurance athletes.

## Enhancement of glycogen synthesis after exercise

### Long-term recovery

The amount of carbohydrate consumed has a significant effect on the rate of glycogen storage after exercise. Unless sufficient carbohydrate is ingested, muscle glycogen will not be normalized on a day-to-day basis between training bouts, nor will efforts to supercompensate muscle glycogen stores be successful. In general, with an increase in carbohydrate ingestion there is an increase in muscle glycogen storage. Costill et al. (1981) reported that consuming 150–650 g carbohydrate·day$^{-1}$ resulted in a proportionately greater muscle glycogen synthesis during the initial 24 h after exercise, and that consumption of more than 600 g carbohydrate·day$^{-1}$ was of no additional benefit (Fig. 7.3). It has also been demonstrated that when the carbohydrate concentration of the diet was inadequate, successive days of intense, prolonged exercise resulted in a gradual reduction in the muscle glycogen stores and a deterioration in performance (Costill et al. 1971; Sherman et al. 1993). For example, Sherman et al. (1993) fed endurance athletes either 5 or 10 g carbohydrate·kg$^{-1}$·day$^{-1}$ over 7 days of controlled training. The lower carbohydrate diet contained 42% of energy from carbohydrate and the higher carbohydrate diet contained 84% of energy from carbohydrate. Both diet and exercise were controlled during the 7 days prior to the

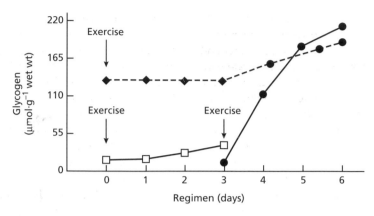

**Fig. 7.2** A comparison of the classic Bergström *et al.* (1967) glycogen supercompensation method and a modification of that method by Sherman *et al.* (1983). The classic method (—) consisted of depleting the glycogen stores with an exhaustive exercise bout, followed by 3 days on a low carbohydrate diet. This was followed with another glycogen-depleting exercise and 3 days on a high carbohydrate diet. The modifications by Sherman (- - - -) included a hard exercise bout that was followed by 6 days of exercise tapering. During the first 3 days of the taper, a mixed diet consisting of 50% carbohydrates was consumed. During the last 3 days, a high carbohydrate diet was consumed. The two values for the classic regimen on day 3 represent before and after an exhaustive exercise bout. □, low carbohydrate diet; ◆, mixed diet; ●, high carbohydrate diet. From Sherman *et al.* (1983), with permission.

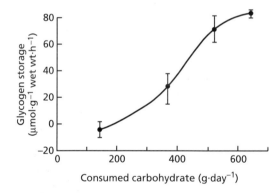

**Fig. 7.3** The relationship between the amount of carbohydrate consumed and the rate of muscle glycogen storage during a 24-h period after glycogen depletion by exercise. From Costill *et al.* (1981), with permission.

experimental period to ensure that subjects started with similar muscle glycogen levels. The lower carbohydrate diet produced a significant 30% decline in muscle glycogen by day 5 of training, which was then maintained through day 7. However, there was no decline in muscle glycogen during the 7 days of training when the athletes consumed the higher carbohydrate diet.

The type of carbohydrate consumed also appears to have an effect on the rate of glycogen resynthesis following exercise. Costill *et al.* (1971) fed glycogen-depleted runners a starch or glucose diet (650 g carbohydrate·day$^{-1}$) during the 2 days following depletion. During the first 24 h there was no difference in the synthesis of muscle glycogen between the two diets, but after the 2nd day, the starch diet resulted in a significantly greater glycogen synthesis than the glucose diet. A difference in glycogen storage between simple and complex carbohydrates, however, was not demonstrated by Roberts *et al.* (1988). Following glycogen-depleting exercise, their subjects were fed diets consisting of either 88% simple and 12% complex carbohydrates or 15% simple and 85% complex carbohydrates. After 3 days of recovery, it was found that the two diets had produced equivalent increases in muscle glycogen storage. The difference between studies is not immediately clear, but may be due to differences in the glycaemic indexes of the different carbohydrates provided.

The only study that appears to have investigated the impact of the glycaemic index of carbohydrate on muscle glycogen storage after exercise was conducted by Burke *et al.* (1993). Subjects were exercised to deplete the muscle glycogen stores on two separate occasions and provided a diet composed of carbohydrate with a high glycaemic index on one occasion, and a diet composed of carbohydrate with a low glycaemic index on the other. Total carbohydrate intake over the 24-h recovery period was $10\,g\cdot kg^{-1}$ body weight, evenly distributed between meals eaten at 0, 4, 8 and 21 h after exercise. The increase in muscle glycogen averaged $106\,\mu mol\cdot g^{-1}$ wet weight for the high glycaemic index carbohydrate and $71.5\,\mu mol\cdot g^{-1}$ wet weight for the low glycaemic index. The difference in glycogen storage was significant. This finding suggests that the increase in muscle glycogen content during long-term recovery is affected by the amount and glycaemic index of the carbohydrate consumed.

### Short-term recovery

While procedures for increasing muscle glycogen above normal levels in preparation for competition and maintaining normal glycogen levels on a day-to-day basis have been defined, these procedures do not address the problem of athletic competitions that require the rapid resynthesis of muscle glycogen within hours. Although it is unlikely that muscle glycogen stores could be completely resynthesized within a few hours by nutritional supplementation alone, it would be of benefit to the athlete if supplementation procedures which maximized the rate of muscle glycogen storage after exercise were defined. Factors that influence the rate of muscle glycogen storage immediately following exercise are the timing, amount and type of carbohydrate supplement consumed, the frequency of feeding, and the type of exercise performed.

#### TIMING OF CARBOHYDRATE CONSUMPTION AFTER EXERCISE

The time elapsed between competition or a prolonged exercise bout and the consumption of a carbohydrate supplement will critically influence the rate of muscle glycogen resynthesis (Ivy

*et al.* 1988a). When carbohydrate supplements are provided immediately after exercise, they generally result in a rate of glycogen resynthesis of between 5 and $6\,\mu mol\cdot g^{-1}$ wet weight $\cdot h^{-1}$ (Maehlum *et al.* 1977; Blom *et al.* 1987; Ivy *et al.* 1988a, 1988b). This rate is maintained for approximately 2 h and then declines by approximately 50% over the next 2 h as the blood glucose and insulin levels decline to after-exercise levels (Ivy *et al.* 1988a). If the supplement is delayed for 2 h, the rate of glycogen resynthesis during the 2 h immediately after consumption ranges between 3 and $4\,\mu mol\cdot g^{-1}$ wet weight $\cdot h^{-1}$, or about 50% as fast as when the supplement is provided immediately after exercise (Fig. 7.4). This lower rate of glycogen resynthesis occurs despite normal increases in blood glucose and insulin levels. It appears that when the carbohydrate supplement is delayed for several hours after exercise, the muscle becomes insulin resistant, reducing the rate of muscle glucose uptake and glycogen

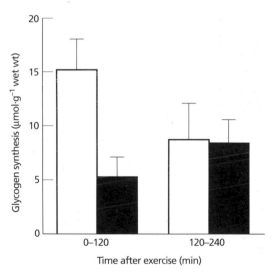

**Fig. 7.4** Muscle glycogen storage during the first 2 h and second 2 h of recovery from exercise. The open bar represents the glycogen storage when the carbohydrate supplement was provided immediately after exercise, and the black bar represents the glycogen storage when the supplement was delayed until 2 h into recovery. The carbohydrate supplement consisted of a 23% solution of glucose polymers ($2\,g\cdot kg^{-1}$ body weight). From Ivy *et al.* (1988a), with permission.

resynthesis. Once developed, this state of insulin resistance persists for several hours. Providing a carbohydrate supplement soon after exercise therefore appears to benefit the muscle glycogen recovery process by preventing the development of muscle insulin resistance. Furthermore, during the time between the end of exercise and the consumption of a carbohydrate supplement, there is very little muscle glycogen resynthesis (approximately $1–2\,\mu mol \cdot g^{-1}$ wet weight $\cdot h^{-1}$) (Ivy *et al.* 1988a). Therefore, providing a carbohydrate supplement soon after exercise has the added benefit of starting the muscle glycogen recovery process immediately.

## FREQUENCY AND AMOUNT OF CARBOHYDRATE CONSUMPTION AFTER EXERCISE

The frequency of carbohydrate supplementation as well as the amount of carbohydrate in each supplement is also of importance in the regulation of muscle glycogen resynthesis. When an adequate carbohydrate supplement is provided immediately after exercise, its effect on muscle glycogen recovery eventually declines as blood glucose and insulin levels decline. However, Blom *et al.* (1987) reported that providing a carbohydrate supplement immediately after exercise

and at 2-h intervals for the next 4 h maintained an elevated blood glucose level and a rapid rate of muscle glycogen resynthesis during a 6-h recovery period. Blom *et al.* (1987) also found that a critical amount of carbohydrate must be consumed if the rate of muscle glycogen resynthesis was to be maximized. When carbohydrate supplements of 0.7 or $1.4\,g$ glucose $\cdot kg^{-1}$ body weight were provided at 2-h intervals, the rate of glycogen storage did not differ between treatments and averaged $5.7\,\mu mol \cdot g^{-1}$ wet weight $\cdot h^{-1}$. However, when Blom *et al.* (1987) provided $0.35\,g$ glucose $\cdot kg^{-1}$ body weight at 2-h intervals, the rate of muscle glycogen resynthesis was reduced by 50%.

To better evaluate the critical level of carbohydrate supplementation required for maximal glycogen resynthesis, we tested the effects of supplements with different concentrations of carbohydrate during 4 h of recovery from exercise (Fig. 7.5). Very little muscle glycogen resynthesis was found when carbohydrate was withheld from the subjects (approximately $0.6\,\mu mol \cdot g^{-1}$ wet weight $\cdot h^{-1}$). With increasing concentration of carbohydrate supplementation, however, the rate of muscle glycogen resynthesis increased in a curvilinear pattern and then plateaued at a rate of $5.5\,\mu mol \cdot g^{-1}$ wet weight $\cdot h^{-1}$ as the carbohydrate concentration

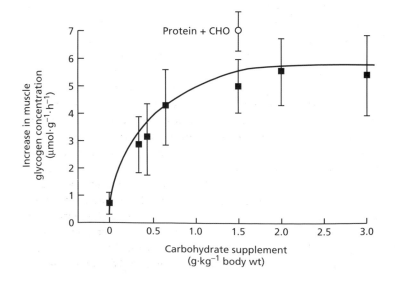

**Fig. 7.5** The average rate of muscle glycogen resynthesis during a 4-h exercise recovery period after oral consumption of different concentrations of carbohydrate (CHO) from a liquid supplement ($\approx 21\%$ wt/vol). Supplements were provided immediately after exercise and 2 h after exercise. Protein + CHO represents the average muscle glycogen resynthesis rate when $1.5\,g$ CHO $\cdot kg^{-1}$ body weight plus $0.53\,g$ protein $\cdot kg^{-1}$ body weight (milk and whey protein isolate mixture, 7.6% wt/vol) was provided.

approached $1–1.5 g \cdot kg^{-1}$ body weight. These results imply that when carbohydrate supplements are provided at 2-h intervals in amounts below $1 g \cdot kg^{-1}$ body weight, the rate of muscle glycogen resynthesis will be submaximal. The reduced rate of resynthesis is probably due to the inability of a small carbohydrate supplement to adequately increase and maintain blood glucose and insulin levels for a 2-h interval, as smaller supplements taken more frequently have been found to be adequate (Doyle *et al.* 1993).

The reason for similar glycogen resynthesis rates when carbohydrate supplements exceed $1 g \cdot kg^{-1}$ body weight was not immediately clear. Estimates of gastric emptying rates, based on the research of Hunt *et al.* (1985), suggest that carbohydrate available to the muscle was far in excess of the amount actually converted to glycogen. This would indicate that under conditions of high carbohydrate supplementation, the rate-limiting step in glycogen resynthesis is either glucose transport or the processing of glucose through the glycogen synthetic pathway. To test this hypothesis, Reed *et al.* (1989) continuously infused glycogen-depleted subjects with $3 g$ glucose $\cdot kg^{-1}$ body weight during the first 3.75 h of a 4-h exercise recovery period. The rate of muscle glycogen resynthesis during infusion was then compared with that which occurred when a liquid supplement containing $1.5 g$ glucose $\cdot kg^{-1}$ body weight was consumed immediately after and 2 h after exercise. During infusion, blood glucose increased to 10 mM, whereas the blood glucose level only reached 6 mM when the liquid glucose supplement was consumed orally. Despite this large difference in blood glucose, the rates of muscle glycogen resynthesis were virtually identical at the end of the recovery periods. The results of Reed *et al.* (1989) therefore support the hypothesis that glycogen resynthesis is not limited by glucose availability when adequate carbohydrate is consumed.

Prior research studies employing glucose infusion (Ahlborg *et al.* 1967b; Bergström & Hultman 1967c; Roch-Norlund *et al.* 1972), however, have generally demonstrated greater rates of glycogen synthesis than those reported by Reed *et al.*

(1989). Possibly accounting for the difference in synthesis rates are the different rates of glucose infusion. The rates of glucose infusion in the earlier studies were much faster and plasma glucose concentrations two to three times higher than those reported by Reed *et al.* (1989). It is likely that plasma insulin concentrations in the earlier studies were greater as well, although these results were not reported.

It was of interest to note that in the study by Reed *et al.* (1989) the plasma insulin response during the infusion treatment was similar to that produced by the liquid supplement, and therefore could account for the similar rates of glycogen storage for these two treatments. The blood insulin concentration plays a major role in determining the rate of muscle glycogen storage. Insulin stimulates both muscle glucose transport and activation of glycogen synthase. The results raised the possibility that increasing the insulin response to a carbohydrate supplement could increase the rate of muscle glucose uptake and glycogen storage.

## PROTEIN PLUS CARBOHYDRATE

Certain amino acids are effective secretagogues of insulin and have been found to synergistically increase the blood insulin response to a carbohydrate load when administered in combination (Floyd *et al.* 1966; Fajans *et al.* 1967). Of the 20 amino acids normally found in protein, the most effective insulin secretagogue is arginine (Fajans *et al.* 1967). When infused with carbohydrate, arginine has been found to increase the insulin response fivefold above that produced by the carbohydrate or arginine alone. However, we have found the use of amino acids to be impractical when added to a carbohydrate supplement because they produce many unwanted side-effects such as mild borborygmus and diarrhoea.

Protein meals and supplements also have been found to enhance the insulin response to a carbohydrate load and do not produce the unwanted side-effects of the amino acids (Rabinowitz *et al.* 1966; Pallota & Kennedy 1968; Spiller *et al.* 1987). For example, Spiller *et al.* (1987) demonstrated an increased blood insulin response and decreased blood glucose response with the addition of protein to a 58 g carbohydrate supplement. The insulin response was found to be directly proportional and the glucose response inversely proportional to the protein content of the carbohydrate–protein supplement. No adverse side-effects were reported.

We therefore investigated the effects of a carbohydrate–protein supplement on muscle glycogen resynthesis after exercise (Zawadzki *et al.* 1992). The supplements tested consisted of 112 g carbohydrate or 112 g carbohydrate plus 40.7 g protein (21% wt/vol mixture). The supplements were administered immediately after exercise and 2 h after exercise. It was found that the combination of carbohydrate plus protein resulted in a synergistic insulin response. In conjunction with the greater insulin response was a significantly lower blood glucose response and a 38% faster rate of muscle glycogen storage compared with carbohydrate supplementation alone. Rates of muscle glycogen resynthesis averaged 7.1 $\mu$mol·g$^{-1}$ wet weight·h$^{-1}$ for the carbohydrate–protein treatment and 5.0 $\mu$mol·g$^{-1}$ wet weight·h$^{-1}$ for the carbohydrate treatment during the 4-h recovery period (see Fig. 7.5). It was also found that carbohydrate oxidation rates and blood lactate concentrations for the carbohy-

drate–protein and carbohydrate treatments were similar. These results suggested that the increased rate of muscle glycogen resynthesis during the carbohydrate–protein treatment was the result of an increased clearance of glucose by the muscle due to the increased blood insulin response. Since the carbohydrate–protein supplement was palatable and there were no unwanted side-effects, it would appear to be a viable supplement for postexercise glycogen recovery.

### DIFFERENCES IN SIMPLE CARBOHYDRATES

The effect of supplements composed of predominately glucose, fructose and sucrose have also been investigated (Blom *et al.* 1987). Glucose and fructose are metabolized differently. They have different gastric emptying rates and are absorbed into the blood at different rates. Furthermore, the insulin response to a glucose supplement is generally much greater than that of a fructose supplement. Blom *et al.* (1987) found that ingestion of glucose or sucrose was twice as effective as fructose for restoration of muscle glycogen (Fig. 7.6). They suggested that the differences between the glucose and fructose supplementations were the result of the way the body metabolized these

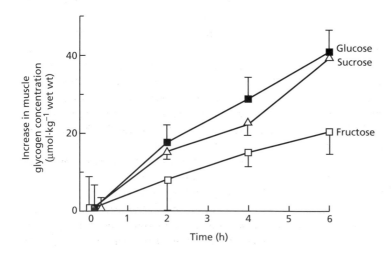

**Fig. 7.6** Increases in muscle glycogen concentration when glucose, fructose and sucrose are provided in amounts of 0.7 g·kg$^{-1}$ body weight immediately after exercise and at 2-h intervals. From Blom *et al.* (1987), with permission.

sugars. Fructose metabolism takes place pre-dominantly in the liver (Zakin *et al.* 1969), whereas the majority of glucose appears to bypass the liver and be stored or oxidized by the muscle (Maehlum *et al.* 1978). When infused, fructose has been found to result in a four times greater liver glycogen storage than glucose (Nilsson & Hultman 1974). On the other hand, a considerably higher glycogen storage rate has been demonstrated in skeletal muscle after glucose than after fructose infusion (Bergström & Hultman 1967c).

The similar rates of glycogen storage for the sucrose and glucose supplements could not be accounted for by Blom *et al.* (1987). Sucrose contains equimolar amounts of glucose and fructose. If muscle glycogen storage was chiefly dependent on the glucose moiety of the disaccharide, one should expect a lower rate of glycogen storage from sucrose than from a similar amount of glucose. One possible explanation provided by Blom *et al.* (1987) was that fructose, by virtue of its rapid metabolism in the liver, compared with that of glucose, inhibits the postexercise hepatic glucose uptake, thereby rendering a large proportion of absorbed glucose available for muscle glycogen resynthesis.

## SOLID VS. LIQUID SUPPLEMENTS

The form in which the carbohydrate is provided has also been investigated. Keizer *et al.* (1986) found that providing approximately 300 g of carbohydrate in either liquid or solid form after exercise resulted in a glycogen storage rate of approximately 5 $\mu$mol · g$^{-1}$ wet weight · h$^{-1}$ over the first 5 h of recovery. However, these solid feedings contained a substantial amount of fat and protein that is typically not found in liquid supplements. Therefore, Reed *et al.* (1989) compared the postexercise glycogen storage rates following liquid and solid carbohydrate supplements of similar compositions. Again there were no differences noted between the two treatments. The average glycogen storage rates for the liquid and solid supplements were 5.1 and 5.5 $\mu$mol · g$^{-1}$ wet weight · h$^{-1}$, respectively.

## INFLUENCE OF TYPE OF EXERCISE

As previously indicated, during prolonged bouts of exercise in which muscle and liver glycogen concentrations are reduced and hypoglycaemia results, muscle glycogen synthesis is typically 5–6 $\mu$mol · g$^{-1}$ wet weight · h$^{-1}$, provided an adequate carbohydrate supplement is consumed. However, if the exercise rapidly reduces the muscle glycogen concentration, resulting in elevated blood and muscle lactate, synthesis of glycogen can be very rapid even in the absence of a carbohydrate supplement. Hermansen and Vaage (1977) depleted the muscle glycogen levels of their subjects by multiple 1-min maximal exercise bouts on a cycle ergometer. During the first 30 min of recovery, the rate of muscle glycogen synthesis averaged 33.6 $\mu$mol · g$^{-1}$ wet weight · h$^{-1}$. The increase in muscle glycogen was found to parallel the decline in muscle lactate, which had increased to 26.4 $\mu$mol · g$^{-1}$ wet weight after the last exercise bout. MacDougall *et al.* (1977) also found a relatively rapid rate of storage after muscle glycogen depletion when subjects performed 1-min cycling sprints at 150% of $\dot{V}o_{2max.}$ to exhaustion. The difference in storage rates following prolonged exercise, as opposed to high-intensity exercise, can probably be explained by the availability of substrate for muscle glycogen synthesis. With multiple high-intensity sprints, glycogen depletion is accompanied by hyperglycaemia and elevated blood and muscle lactate concentrations, which can be used immediately as substrate for glycogen synthesis. By contrast, prolonged sustained exercise severely reduces the endogenous precursors of muscle glycogen, thereby requiring an exogenous carbohydrate source for rapid muscle glycogen synthesis.

Exercise that results in muscle damage also affects muscle glycogen synthesis. Sherman *et al.* (1983) found that after a marathon, restoration of muscle glycogen was delayed and that this delay was related to muscle damage caused by the run (Hikida *et al.* 1983; Sherman *et al.* 1983). Eccentric exercise which involves the forced lengthening of active muscles and the transfer of external power from the environment to the muscle causes severe muscle damage. O'Reilly *et al.* (1987) reported that muscle glycogen stores reduced by eccentric exercise were still significantly below normal levels after 10 days of recovery. Costill *et al.* (1990) also found that the rate of muscle glycogen resynthesis was significantly reduced following glycogen depletion by exercise that incorporated a substantial eccentric component, and that the reduced rate of resynthesis was associated with muscle damage. More recently, Asp *et al.* (1995) demonstrated that muscle damage induced by eccentric exercise resulted in a down regulation of GLUT-4 protein that lasted for several days. In addition, it was not until the GLUT-4 protein returned to the pre-exercise concentration that normal muscle glycogen levels were restored. These results suggest that muscle damage following exercise can limit glucose uptake due to a reduced GLUT-4 protein concentration, and that this limits the restoration of muscle glycogen.

## Recommendations

From a dietary position, the first concern of the endurance athlete is that energy consumption and energy expenditure be in balance (Sherman 1995). The endurance athlete may expend 15–30 MJ·day$^{-1}$ when training. If consumption is inadequate and not balanced with expenditure, the athlete's training and competitive abilities will eventually be adversely affected. It is also important that a substantial percentage of the diet consist of carbohydrate. It was suggested by Sherman and Lamb (1988) that the endurance athelete's diet consists of approximately 65% carbohydrate during strenuous training. However, this percentage can be modified according to actual energy consumption. What is important is the amount of carbohydrate consumed. Costill *et al.* (1981) recommended that endurance trained athletes consume approximately 8 g carbohydrate·kg$^{-1}$ body weight·day$^{-1}$ to maintain a normal muscle glycogen concentration during training. Similarly, a recommendation of 7 g carbohydrate·kg$^{-1}$ body weight·day$^{-1}$ was provided by Sherman (1995).

Prior to competition, the muscle and liver glycogen stores should be maximized. For the best results with the least amount of stress, it is recommended that a hard training bout be performed 7 days prior to competition to reduce the muscle glycogen stores. During the next 3 days, training should be of moderate intensity and duration and a well-balanced mixed diet composed of about 45–50% carbohydrate consumed. During the next 3 days, training should be gradually tapered and the carbohydrate content of the diet should be increased to 70%. This should result in muscle glycogen stores similar to that normally produced by the classic glycogen supercompensation regimen, but with much less stress and fatigue.

For the rapid replenishment of muscle glycogen stores, one should consume a carbohydrate supplement in excess of 1 g·kg$^{-1}$ body weight immediately after competition or after a training bout. Continuation of supplementation every 2 h will maintain a maximal rate of storage up to 6 h after exercise; smaller supplements taken more frequently are also effective. Increasing the amount of carbohydrate consumption above 1.0–1.5 g·kg$^{-1}$ body weight·supplement$^{-1}$ appears to provide no additional benefit, and may have the adverse effects of causing nausea and diarrhoea. Supplements composed of glucose or glucose polymers are more effective for the replenishment of muscle glycogen stores after exercise than supplements composed of predominantly fructose. However, some fructose is recommended because it is more effective than glucose in the replenishment of liver glycogen. It might also be of benefit to include some protein with the carbohydrate supplement as this will enhance the rate of glycogen resynthesis. Finally, carbohydrates in solid or liquid form can be consumed immediately after exercise with similar results. However, a liquid supplement immediately after exercise is recommended because it is easier to digest and less filling, and therefore will not tend to adversely affect one's normal appetite. A liquid supplement also provides a source of fluid for rapid rehydration.

# References

Adolfsson, S. (1973) Effect of contraction *in vitro* on glycogen content and glycogen synthetase activity in muscle. *Acta Physiologica Scandinavica* **88**, 189–197.

Ahlborg, B., Bergström, J., Ekelund, L.G. & Hultman, E. (1967a) Muscle glycogen and muscle electrolytes during prolonged physical exercise. *Acta Physiologica Scandinavica* **70**, 129–142.

Ahlborg, B.G., Bergström, J., Brohult, J., Ekelund, L.G., Hultman, E. & Maschio, G. (1967b) Human muscle glycogen content and capacity for prolonged exercise after different diets. *Foersvarsmedicin* **3**, 85–99.

Alonso, M.D., Lomako, J. & Lomako, W.M. (1995) A new look at the biogenesis of glycogen. *FASEB Journal* **9**, 1126–1137.

Asp, S., Daugaard, J.R. & Richter, E.A. (1995) Eccentric exercise decreases glucose transporter GLUT4 protein in human skeletal muscle. *Journal of Physiology* **482**, 705–712.

Bergström, J. & Hultman, E. (1967a) A study of the glycogen metabolism during exercise in man. *Scandinavian Journal of Clinical and Laboratory Investigation* **19**, 218–226.

Bergström, J. & Hultman, E. (1967b) Muscle glycogen synthesis after exercise: an enhancing factor localized to the muscle cells in man. *Nature* **210**, 309–310.

Bergström, J. & Hultman, E. (1967c) Synthesis of muscle glycogen in man after glucose and fructose infusion. *Acta Medica Scandinavica* **182**, 93–107.

Bergström, J., Hermansen, L., Hultman, E. & Saltin, B. (1967) Diet, muscle glycogen and physical performance. *Acta Physiologica Scandinavica* **71**, 140–150.

Bergström, J., Hultman, E. & Roch-Norlund, A.E. (1972) Muscle glycogen synthetase in normal subjects. *Scandinavian Journal of Clinical and Laboratory Investigation* **29**, 231–236.

Blom, P.C.S., Høstmark, A.T., Vaage, O., Kardel, K.R. & Maehlum, S. (1987) Effect of different post-exercise sugar diets on the rate of muscle glycogen synthesis. *Medicine and Science in Sports and Exercise* **19**, 491–496.

Brozinick, J.T. Jr, Yaspelkis, B.B. III, Wilson, C.M. *et al.* (1996) Glucose transport and GLUT4 distribution in skeletal muscle of GLUT4 transgenic mice. *Biochemistry Journal* **313**, 133–140.

Burke, L.M., Collier, G.R. & Hargreaves, M. (1993) Muscle glycogen storage after prolonged exercise: effect of the glycaemic index of carbohydrate feedings. *Journal of Applied Physiology* **75**, 1019–1023.

Cartee, G.D., Young, D.A., Sleeper, M.D., Zierath, J., Wallberg-Henriksson, H. & Holloszy, J.O. (1989) Prolonged increase in insulin-stimulated glucose transport in muscle after exercise. *American Journal of Physiology* **256**, E494–E499.

Christensen, E.H. & Hansen, O. (1939a) Arbeits-
fähigkeit und Ernünhrung. *Skandinavisches Archiv für Physiologie* **81**, 160–171.

Christensen, E.H. & Hansen, O. (1939b) Hypoglykämie, Arbeitsfähigkeit und Ernührung. *Skandinavisches Archiv für Physiologie* **81**, 172–179.

Costill, D.L., Bowers, R., Branam, G. & Sparks, K. (1971) Muscle glycogen utilization during prolonged exercise on successive days. *Journal of Applied Physiology* **31**, 834–838.

Costill, D.L., Sherman, W.M., Fink, W.J., Maresh, C., Witten, M. & Miller, J.M. (1981) The role of dietary carbohydrate in muscle glycogen resynthesis after strenuous running. *American Journal of Clinical Nutrition* **34**, 1831–1836.

Costill, D.L., Pascol, D.D., Fink, W.J., Roberts, R.A., Barr, S.I. & Pearson, D. (1990) Impaired muscle glycogen resynthesis after eccentric exercise. *Journal of Applied Physiology* **69**, 46–50.

Danforth, W.H. (1965) Glycogen synthetase activity in skeletal muscle: interconversion of two forms and control of glycogen synthesis. *Journal of Biological Chemistry* **240**, 588–593.

Dill, D.B., Edwards, H.T. & Talbott, J.H. (1932) Studies in muscular activity. VII. Factors limiting the capacity for work. *Journal of Physiology* **77**, 49–62.

Doyle, J.A., Sherman, W.M. & Strauss, R.L. (1993) Effects of eccentric and concentric exercise on muscle glycogen replenishment. *Journal of Applied Physiology* **74**, 1848–1855.

Fajans, S.S., Floyd, J.C. Jr, Knopf, R.F. & Conn, J.W. (1967) Effect of amino acids and proteins on insulin secretion in man. *Recent Progress in Hormone Research* **23**, 617–662.

Floyd, J.C. Jr, Fajans, S.S., Conn, J.W., Knopf, R.F. & Rull, J. (1966) Stimulation of insulin secretion by amino acids. *Journal of Clinical Investigation* **45**, 1487–1502.

Garetto, L.P., Richter, E.A., Goodman, M.N. & Ruderman, N.B. (1984) Enhanced muscle glucose metabolism after exercise in the rat: the two phases. *American Journal of Physiology* **246**, E471–E475.

Hansen, P.A., Gulve, E.A., Marshall, B.A. *et al.* (1995) Skeletal muscle glucose transport and metabolism are enhanced in transgenic mice overexpressing the Glut4 glucose transporter. *Journal of Biological Chemistry* **270**, 1679–1684.

Hermansen, L. & Vaage, O. (1977) Lactate disappearance and glycogen synthesis in human muscle after maximal exercise. *American Journal of Physiology* **233**, E422–E429.

Hermansen, L., Hultman, E. & Saltin, B. (1965) Muscle glycogen during prolonged severe exercise. *Acta Physiologica Scandinavica* **71**, 334–346.

Hikida, R., Staron, R., Hagerman, F., Sherman, W. & Costill, D. (1983) Muscle fiber necrosis associated with human marathon running. *Journal of Neurological Science* **59**, 185–203.

Holloszy, J.O. & Narahara, H.T. (1965) Studies of tissue permeability. X. Changes in permeability to 3-methylglucose associated with contraction of isolated frog muscle. *Journal of Biological Chemistry* **240**, 3493–3500.

Hultman, E. (1967) Studies on muscle metabolism of glycogen and active phosphate in man with special reference to exercise and diet. *Scandinavian Journal of Clinical and Laboratory Investigation* **19** (Suppl. 94), 1–63.

Hunt, J.N., Smith, J.L. & Jiang, C.L. (1985) Effect of meal volume and energy density on the gastric emptying of carbohydrate. *Gastroenterology* **89**, 1326–1330.

Ivy, J.L. (1977) Role of insulin during exercise-induced glycogenesis in muscle: effect on cyclic AMP. *American Journal of Physiology* **236**, E509–E513.

Ivy, J.L. (1991) Muscle glycogen synthesis before and after exercise. *Sports Medicine* **11**, 6–19.

Ivy, J.L. & Holloszy, J.O. (1981) Persistent increase in glucose uptake by rat skeletal muscle following exercise. *American Journal of Physiology* **241**, C200–C203.

Ivy, J.L., Sherman, W.M., Miller, W., Farrall, S. & Frishberg, B. (1983) Glycogen synthesis: effect of diet and training. In *Biochemistry of Exercise* (eds H.G. Knuttgen, J.A. Vogel & J. Poortmans), pp. 291–296. Human Kinetics, Champaign, IL.

Ivy, J.L., Frishberg, B.A., Farrell, S.W., Miller, W.J. & Sherman, W.M. (1985) Effects of elevated and exercise-reduced muscle glycogen levels on insulin sensitivity. *Journal of Applied Physiology* **59**, 154–159.

Ivy, J.L., Katz, A.L., Cutler, C.L., Sherman, W.M. & Coyle, E.F. (1988a) Muscle glycogen synthesis after exercise: effect of time of carbohydrate ingestion. *Journal of Applied Physiology* **64**, 1480–1485.

Ivy, J.L., Lee, M.C., Brozinick, J.T. & Reed, M.J. (1988b) Muscle glycogen storage after different amounts of carbohydrate ingestion. *Journal of Applied Physiology* **65**, 2018–2023.

Keizer, H.A., vanKuipers, H., Kranenburg, G. & Guerten, P. (1986) Influence of lipid and solid meals on muscle glycogen resynthesis, plasma fuel hormone response, and maximal physical work capacity. *International Journal of Sports Medicine* **8**, 99–104.

Kochan, R.G., Lamb, D.R., Reimann, E.M. & Schlender, K.K. (1981) Modified assays to detect activation of glycogen synthase following exercise. *American Journal of Physiology* **240**, E197–E202.

Krogh, A. & Lindhard, J. (1920) Relative value of fat and carbohydrate as a source of muscular energy: with appendices on the correlation between standard metabolism and the respiratory quotient during rest and work. *Biochemistry Journal* **14**, 290–298.

Levine, S.A., Gordon, B. & Derrick, C.L. (1924) Some changes in the chemical constituents of the blood following a marathon race: with special reference to the development of hypoglycemia. *Journal of the American Medical Association* **82**, 1778–1779.

MacDougall, J.D., Ward, G.R., Sale, D.G. & Sutton, J.R. (1977) Muscle glycogen repletion after high-intensity intermittent exercise. *Journal of Applied Physiology* **42**, 129–132.

Maehlum, S. & Hermansen, L. (1978) Muscle glycogen during recovery after prolonged severe exercise in fasting subjects. *Scandinavian Journal of Clinical and Laboratory Investigation* **38**, 557–560.

Maehlum, S., Høstmark, A.T. & Hermansen, L. (1977) Synthesis of muscle glycogen during recovery after prolonged severe exercise in diabetic and non-diabetic subjects. *Scandinavian Journal of Clinical and Laboratory Investigation* **37**, 309–316.

Maehlum, S., Felig, P. & Wahren, J. (1978) Splanchnic glucose and muscle glycogen metabolism after glucose feeding post-exercise recovery. *American Journal of Physiology* **235**, E255–E260.

Nesher, R., Karl, S.E. & Kipnis, D.M. (1985) Dissociation of effects of insulin and contraction on glucose transport ion rat epitrochlearis muscle. *American Journal of Physiology* **249**, C226–C232.

Nilsson, L.H. & Hultman, E. (1974) Liver and muscle glycogen in man after glucose and fructose infusion. *Scandinavian Journal of Clinical and Laboratory Investigation* **33**, 5–10.

O'Reilly, K.P., Warhol, M.J., Fielding, R.A., Frontera, W.A., Meredith, C.N. & Evans, W.J. (1987) Eccentric exercise-induced muscle damage impairs muscle glycogen repletion. *Journal of Applied Physiology* **63**, 252–256.

Pallotta, J.A. & Kennedy, P.J. (1968) Response of plasma insulin and growth hormone to carbohydrate and protein feeding. *Metabolism* **17**, 901–908.

Piehl, K. (1974) Time-course for refilling of glycogen stores in human muscle fibers following exercise-induced glycogen depletion. *Acta Physiologica Scandinavica* **90**, 297–302.

Price, T.B., Rothman, D.L., Taylor, R., Avison, M.J., Shulman, G.I. & Shulman, R.G. (1994) Human muscle glycogen resynthesis after exercise: insulin-dependent and -independent phases. *Journal of Applied Physiology* **76**, 104–111.

Rabinowitz, D., Merimee, T.J., Maffezzoli, R. & Burgess, J.A. (1966) Patterns of hormonal release after glucose, protein, and glucose plus protein. *Lancet* **2**, 454–457.

Reed, M.J., Brozinick, J.T., Lee, M.C. & Ivy, J.L. (1989) Muscle glycogen storage postexercise: effect of mode of carbohydrate administration. *Journal of Applied Physiology* **66**, 720–726.

Ren, J.-M., Marshall, B.A., Gulve, E.A. *et al.* (1993) Evidence from transgenic mice that glucose transport is rate-limiting for glycogen deposition and glycolysis in skeletal muscle. *Journal of Biological Chemistry* **268**, 16113–16115.

Ren, J.-M., Semenkovich, C.F., Gulve, E.A., Gao, J. & Holloszy, J.O. (1994) Exercise induces rapid increases in GLUT4 expression, glucose transport capacity, and insulin-stimulated glycogen storage in muscle. *Journal of Biological Chemistry* **269**, 14396–14401.

Richter, E.A., Garetto, L.P., Goodman, N.M. & Ruderman, N.B. (1982) Muscle glycogen metabolism following exercise in the rat. Increased sensitivity to insulin. *Journal of Clinical Investigation* **69**, 785–793.

Richter, E.A., Garetto, L.P., Goodman, N.M. & Ruderman, N.B. (1984) Enhanced muscle glycogen metabolism after exercise: modulation by local factors. *American Journal of Physiology* **246**, E476–E482.

Roberts, K.M., Noble, E.G., Hayden, D.B. & Taylor, A.W. (1988) Simple and complex carbohydrate-rich diets and muscle glycogen content of marathon runners. *European Journal of Applied Physiology* **57**, 70–74.

Roch-Norlund, A.E., Bergström, J. & Hultman, E. (1972) Muscle glycogen and glycogen synthetase in normal subjects and in patients with diabetes mellitus: effect of intravenous glucose and insulin administration. *Scandinavian Journal of Clinical and Laboratory Investigation* **30**, 77–84.

Sherman, W.M. (1995) Metabolism of sugars and physical performance. *American Journal of Clinical Nutrition* **62** (Suppl.), 228s–241s.

Sherman, W.M. & Lamb, D.R. (1988) Nutrition and prolonged exercise. In *Perspectives in Exercise Science and Sports Medicine: Prolonged Exercise* (ed. D.R. Lamb), pp. 213–277. Benchmark Press, Indianapolis, IN.

Sherman, W.M., Costill, D.L., Fink, W.J. & Miller, J.M. (1981) The effect of exercise and diet manipulation on muscle glycogen and its subsequent utilization during performance. *International Journal of Sports Medicine* **2**, 114–118.

Sherman, W.M., Doyle, J.A., Lamb, D.R. & Strauss, R.H. (1993) Dietary carbohydrate, muscle glycogen, and exercise performance during 7 d of training. *American Journal of Clinical Nutrition* **57**, 27–31.

Sherman, W.M., Costill, D.L., Fink, W., Hagerman, F., Armstrong, L. & Murray, T. (1983) Effect of a 42.2-km footrace and subsequent rest or exercise on muscle glycogen and enzymes. *Journal of Applied Physiology* **55**, 1219–1224.

Smythe, C. & Cohen, P. (1991) The discovery of glycogenin and the priming mechanism for glycogen biogenesis. *European Journal of Biochemistry* **200**, 625–631.

Spiller, G.A., Jensen, C.D., Pattison, T.S., Chuck, C.S., Whittam, J.H. & Scala, J. (1987) Effect of protein dose on serum glucose and insulin response to sugars. *American Journal of Clinical Nutrition* **46**, 474–480.

Szanto, S. & Yudkin, J. (1969) The effect of dietary sucrose on blood lipids, serum insulin, platelet adhesiveness and body weight in human volunteers. *Postgraduate Medical Journal* **45**, 602–607.

Terjung, R.L., Baldwin, K.M., Winder, W.W. & Holloszy, J.O. (1974) Glycogen in different types of muscle and in liver after exhausting exercise. *American Journal of Physiology* **226**, 1387–1391.

Zakin, D., Herfman, R.H. & Gordon, W.C. (1969) The conversion of glucose and fructose to fatty acids in the human liver. *Biochemical Medicine* **2**, 427–437.

Zawadzki, K.M., Yaspelkis, B.B. & Ivy, J.L. (1992) Carbohydrate-protein complex increases the rate of muscle glycogen storage after exercise. *Journal of Applied Physiology* **72**, 1854–1859.

# Chapter 8

# Carbohydrate Replacement during Exercise

MARK HARGREAVES

## Introduction

Muscle glycogen depletion and/or hypoglycaemia are associated with fatigue during prolonged strenuous exercise (Hermansen *et al.* 1967; Coyle *et al.* 1986), highlighting the critical importance of carbohydrate (CHO) availability for intramuscular adenosine triphosphate supply (Norman *et al.* 1987; Sahlin *et al.* 1990; Spencer *et al.* 1991). In the early part of this century, the benefit of CHO ingestion during prolonged exercise was recognized in a classic field study (Gordon *et al.* 1925). Over the years since, numerous controlled, laboratory studies have demonstrated that ingestion of CHO during prolonged, strenuous exercise results in enhanced exercise performance. Many studies have used exercise time to fatigue as their measure of endurance capacity and this is increased by CHO ingestion (Coyle *et al.* 1983, 1986; Björkman *et al.* 1984; Coggan & Coyle 1987, 1989; Sasaki *et al.* 1987; Spencer *et al.* 1991; Davis *et al.* 1992; Wilber & Moffatt 1992; Tsintzas *et al.* 1996a, 1996b). Recently it has been argued that time to fatigue is not a reliable test of endurance performance (Jeukendrup *et al.* 1996); however, in well-motivated subjects, who have been familiarized with the testing procedures, it remains a useful laboratory test for elucidating mechanisms of fatigue. Nevertheless, there are no Olympic events in 'exercise time to fatigue', and it is perhaps more appropriate to assess endurance performance by tests that measure the time taken to complete a standard task or the work output in

a certain amount of time. Using such tests, CHO ingestion has been shown to improve performance as measured by enhanced work output or reduced exercise time (Neufer *et al.* 1987; Coggan & Coyle 1988; Mitchell *et al.* 1989; Williams *et al.* 1990; Murray *et al.* 1991; Tsintzas *et al.* 1993; Below *et al.* 1995; McConell *et al.* 1996; Jeukendrup *et al.* 1997). The increases in exercise performance with CHO ingestion are believed to be due to maintenance of a high rate of CHO oxidation and increased CHO availability within contracting skeletal muscle (Coyle *et al.* 1986; Coggan & Coyle 1987; Tsintzas *et al.* 1996a). In addition, the prevention of neuroglucopenia and effects on central nervous system function may play a role (Davis *et al.* 1992). Interestingly, several recent studies have observed improved high-intensity and intermittent exercise performance with CHO ingestion when, under normal circumstances, CHO availability is not thought to be limiting (Anantaraman *et al.* 1995; Ball *et al.* 1995; Below *et al.* 1995; Nicholas *et al.* 1995; Davis *et al.* 1997; Jeukendrup *et al.* 1997). The mechanisms underlying the ergogenic benefit of CHO ingestion under these circumstances remain to be determined, but may involve small increases in intramuscular CHO availability under conditions of high CHO utilization. Performance in a 20-km cycle time trial, lasting about 30 min, was not affected by CHO ingestion (Palmer *et al.* 1998).

## Metabolic responses to CHO ingestion during exercise

Ingestion of CHO during prolonged, strenuous exercise results in higher blood glucose levels and rates of CHO oxidation late in exercise (Fig. 8.1) (Coyle *et al.* 1986; Coggan & Coyle 1987). Liver glucose output is reduced by CHO ingestion (Fig. 8.2) (Bosch *et al.* 1994; McConell *et al.* 1994) and while the tracer method used cannot distinguish between liver glycogenolysis and gluconeogenesis, it is likely that there is a significant liver glycogen sparing effect of CHO ingestion. A reduction in splanchnic gluconeogenic precursor and oxygen uptake during prolonged, low-intensity exercise following CHO ingestion

suggests a lower rate of gluconeogenesis (Ahlborg & Felig 1976) and this has recently been confirmed in experiments using tracers to estimate rates of gluconeogenesis (Jeukendrup *et al.* 1999). Muscle glucose uptake during exercise, as measured by tracer-determined glucose Rd, is increased by CHO ingestion (McConell *et al.* 1994). This is consistent with previous observations of increased leg glucose uptake during low-intensity exercise (Ahlborg & Felig 1976) and elevated rates of glucose disposal and oxidation during strenuous exercise when blood glucose availability is increased (Coggan *et al.* 1991; Coyle *et al.* 1991; Bosch *et al.* 1994; Hawley *et al.* 1994; Howlett *et al.* 1998).

Most, if not all, studies utilizing prolonged

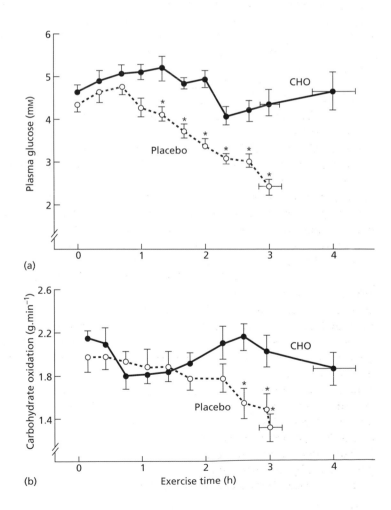

**Fig. 8.1** (a) Plasma glucose and (b) rates of carbohydrate (CHO) oxidation during exercise to fatigue at 70–74% $\dot{V}o_{2peak}$ with ingestion of either a placebo (○) or CHO (●) solution every 20 min. Values are means ± SEM ($n=7$). *, difference from CHO, $P<0.05$. Adapted from Coyle *et al.* (1986).

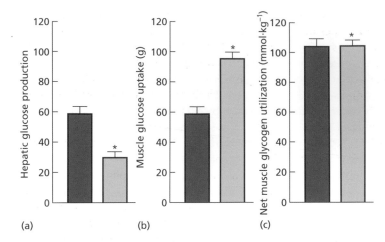

**Fig. 8.2** (a) Total hepatic glucose production, (b) muscle glucose uptake, and (c) net muscle glycogen utilization during 2 h of exercise at 70–74% $\dot{V}o_{2peak}$ with (▢) and without (▨) ingestion of CHO. Values are means ± SEM ($n = 6 - 7$). *, difference from no ingestion of CHO, $P < 0.05$. Data from Coyle *et al.* (1986) and McConell *et al.* (1994).

strenuous, continuous cycling exercise have observed no effect of increased blood glucose availability on net muscle glycogen utilization, either measured directly from biopsy samples (Fig. 8.2) (Fielding *et al.* 1985; Coyle *et al.* 1986, 1991; Flynn *et al.* 1987; Hargreaves & Briggs 1988; Mitchell *et al.* 1989; Widrick *et al.* 1993; Bosch *et al.* 1994) or estimated from total CHO oxidation and tracer-determined glucose uptake (Jeukendrup *et al.* 1998). Decreases in glycogen use during cycling have been reported (Erikson *et al.* 1987), during the latter stages of prolonged exercise (Bosch *et al.* 1996), with a large increase in blood glucose (Bergström & Hultman 1967) and during intermittent exercise protocols (Hargreaves *et al.* 1984; Yaspelkis *et al.* 1993). In two of these studies (Hargreaves *et al.* 1984; Erikson *et al.* 1987), the results are potentially confounded by higher pre-exercise muscle glycogen levels in the control trial which influences the subsequent rate of degradation (Hargreaves *et al.* 1995). It is possible that during intermittent exercise with periods of rest or low-intensity exercise, CHO ingestion may result in glycogen synthesis (Kuipers *et al.* 1987) and a reduction in net muscle glycogen use. On balance, however, the effects of CHO ingestion on muscle glycogen use during prolonged, strenuous cycling exercise appear relatively small. In contrast, recent studies during treadmill running indicate that CHO ingestion reduces net muscle glycogen use, specifically in the type I fibres (Tsintzas *et al.* 1995, 1996a), and that the

increase in muscle glycogen availability late in exercise contributed to the enhanced endurance capacity that was observed (Tsintzas *et al.* 1996a).

The ingestion of CHO results in lower plasma free fatty acid levels during prolonged exercise (Coyle *et al.* 1983, 1986; Murray *et al.* 1989a, 1989b, 1991; Davis *et al.* 1992; Tsintzas *et al.* 1996a). The effects of CHO ingestion during exercise on fat oxidation do not appear to be as great as those observed with pre-exercise CHO ingestion, most likely as a consequence of the smaller increases in plasma insulin levels which, while still blunting lipolysis and the exercise-induced increase in plasma free fatty acid levels (De Glisezinski *et al.* 1998; Horowitz *et al.* 1998), may result in a smaller initial increase in muscle glucose uptake and relatively less inhibition of intramuscular lipid oxidation (Horowitz *et al.* 1998).

## Practical aspects of CHO ingestion during exercise

### Type of CHO

There appear to be relatively few, if any, differences between glucose, sucrose and malto-dextrins in their effects on metabolism and performance when ingested during exercise (Massicotte *et al.* 1989; Murray *et al.* 1989a; Hawley *et al.* 1992; Wagenmakers *et al.* 1993). In contrast, fructose alone is not as readily oxidized as other CHO sources (Massicotte *et al.* 1989) due to its slower rate of absorption, which may cause gastrointestinal distress and impaired performance (Murray *et al.* 1989a). Interestingly, the combination of fructose and glucose results in higher rates of exogenous CHO oxidation than ingestion of either sugar alone (Adopo *et al.* 1994). This may be a consequence of activation of two intestinal transport mechanisms, resulting in greater appearance of ingested CHO from the gastrointestinal tract. Such a finding is consistent with observations of greater fluid absorption from rehydration beverages containing more than one CHO (Shi *et al.* 1995). Whether the increased exogenous CHO oxidation results in enhanced exercise performance has not been tested. Galactose is less available for oxidation when ingested during exercise (Leijssen *et al.* 1995) and soluble corn starch is oxidized to a greater extent than insoluble starch during exercise due to its higher amylopectin/amylose ratio (Saris *et al.* 1993). The physical form of the ingested CHO does not exert a major influence since liquid and solid CHO supplements elicit similar metabolic responses during exercise (Lugo *et al.* 1993; Mason *et al.* 1993).

### Amount of CHO

There is no clear dose–response relationship between the amount of CHO ingested during exercise and subsequent exercise performance (Mitchell *et al.* 1989; Murray *et al.* 1989b, 1991). Ingestion of CHO at a rate of $13\,g \cdot h^{-1}$ is insufficient to alter the glucoregulatory hormone response to prolonged exercise or time to fatigue (Burgess *et al.* 1991). The addition of a small amount of CHO to a rehydration beverage was shown to increase exercise time to fatigue, compared with water alone, and to be more effective than a larger amount of CHO (Maughan *et al.* 1996). This may be the result of better rehydration, due to the stimulatory effect of a hypotonic glucose solution on intestinal fluid absorption, and subsequent maintenance of a higher plasma volume, rather than a metabolic effect of the ingested CHO. Ingestion of CHO at a rate of 26 and $78\,g \cdot h^{-1}$ increased 4.8-km cycle performance to a similar extent, following 2 h of exercise at

65–75% $\dot{V}o_{2peak}$ (Murray *et al.* 1991). No differences in physiological responses to exercise were observed between ingestion of 6%, 8% and 10% sucrose solutions, but performance was only enhanced with 6% (Murray *et al.* 1989b). There is likely to be little benefit in ingesting CHO solutions more concentrated than 6–8% because this does not result in increased rates of exogenous glucose oxidation (Wagenmakers *et al.* 1993) and increases the risk of impaired gastrointestinal function and reduced fluid delivery. The absorption of ingested CHO could potentially limit exogenous CHO oxidation which is observed to peak at $1–1.3\,g \cdot min^{-1}$ (Hawley *et al.* 1992). Such values are similar to those reported for gastric emptying and intestinal absorption of glucose from a 6% glucose–electrolyte solution under resting conditions (Duchman *et al.* 1997). Obviously, the important goal of CHO replacement is to provide sufficient CHO to maintain blood glucose and CHO oxidation without causing impaired fluid delivery. Ingesting CHO at a rate of $30–60\,g \cdot h^{-1}$ has been repeatedly shown to improve exercise performance. This CHO intake can be achieved by ingesting commercially available sports drinks, at a rate of $600–1200\,ml \cdot h^{-1}$, with the added benefit of providing fluid and reducing the negative effects of dehydration (Coyle & Montain 1992; American College of Sports Medicine Position Stand 1996).

## Timing of CHO ingestion

The beneficial effects of CHO ingestion are likely to be most evident during the latter stages of prolonged exercise when endogenous CHO reserves are depleted. Indeed, ingestion of CHO late in exercise, approximately 30 min prior to the point of fatigue, produced increases in exercise time to fatigue similar in magnitude to those seen with ingestion of CHO early or throughout exercise or with intravenous infusion of glucose at the point of fatigue (Coggan & Coyle 1989; Coggan *et al.* 1991; Tsintzas *et al.* 1996b). In contrast, ingestion of CHO at the point of fatigue is not as effective in enhancing endurance capacity (Coggan & Coyle 1987, 1991); however, delaying CHO intake until late in exercise, despite increasing blood glucose availability and CHO oxidation, does not always enhance exercise performance (McConell *et al.* 1996). From a practical perspective, because athletes are unable to assess the level of their carbohydrate reserves and their likely point of fatigue, CHO (and fluid) replacement should commence early and continue throughout exercise.

## Conclusion

In view of the importance of CHO for contracting skeletal muscle during strenuous exercise, CHO should be ingested to maintain CHO availability and high rates of CHO oxidation. Such a strategy results in enhanced endurance performance. There appear to be few differences between glucose, sucrose and maltodextrins, as sources of CHO, in their effects on exercise metabolism and performance, while fructose alone is not an effective CHO supplement. Enough CHO should be ingested to supply CHO to contracting muscle at about $30-60\,g \cdot h^{-1}$, without negative effects on fluid bioavailability.

## References

Adopo, E., Péronnet, F., Massicotte, D., Brisson, G.R. & Hillaire-Marcel, C. (1994) Respective oxidation of exogenous glucose and fructose given in the same drink during exercise. *Journal of Applied Physiology* **76**, 1014–1019.

Ahlborg, G. & Felig, P. (1976) Influence of glucose ingestion on fuel–hormone response during prolonged exercise. *Journal of Applied Physiology* **41**, 683–688.

American College of Sports Medicine Position Stand (1996) Exercise and fluid replacement. *Medicine and Science in Sports and Exercise* **28**, i–vii.

Anantaraman, R., Carmines, A.A., Gaesser, G.A. & Weltman, A. (1995) Effects of carbohydrate supplementation on performance during 1 hour of high-intensity exercise. *International Journal of Sports Medicine* **16**, 461–465.

Ball, T.C., Headley, S.A., Vanderburgh, P.M. & Smith, J.C. (1995) Periodic carbohydrate replacement during 50 min of high-intensity cycling improves subsequent sprint performance. *International Journal of Sport Nutrition* **5**, 151–158.

Below, P.R., Mora-Rodríguez, R., González-Alonso, J. & Coyle, E.F. (1995) Fluid and carbohydrate ingestion independently improve performance during 1 h of

intense exercise. *Medicine and Science in Sports and Exercise* **27**, 200–210.

Bergström, J. & Hultman, E. (1967) A study of the glycogen metabolism during exercise in man. *Scandinavian Journal of Clinical and Laboratory Investigation* **19**, 218–228.

Björkman, O., Sahlin, K., Hagenfeldt, L. & Wahren, J. (1984) Influence of glucose and fructose ingestion on the capacity for long-term exercise in well-trained men. *Clinical Physiology* **4**, 483–494.

Bosch, A.N., Dennis, S.C. & Noakes, T.D. (1994) Influence of carbohydrate ingestion on fuel substrate turnover and oxidation during prolonged exercise. *Journal of Applied Physiology* **76**, 2364–2372.

Bosch, A.N., Weltan, S.M., Dennis, S.C. & Noakes, T.D. (1996) Fuel substrate turnover and oxidation and glycogen sparing with carbohydrate ingestion in non-carbohydrate loaded cyclists. *Pflügers Archives* **432**, 1003–1010.

Burgess, W.A., Davis, J.M., Bartoli, W.P. & Woods, J.A. (1991) Failure of low dose carbohydrate feeding to attenuate glucoregulatory hormone responses and improve endurance performance. *International Journal of Sport Nutrition* **1**, 338–352.

Coggan, A.R. & Coyle, E.F. (1987) Reversal of fatigue during prolonged exercise by carbohydrate infusion or ingestion. *Journal of Applied Physiology* **63**, 2388–2395.

Coggan, A.R. & Coyle, E.F. (1988) Effect of carbohydrate feedings during high-intensity exercise. *Journal of Applied Physiology* **65**, 1703–1709.

Coggan, A.R. & Coyle, E.F. (1989) Metabolism and performance following carbohydrate ingestion late in exercise. *Medicine and Science in Sports and Exercise* **21**, 59–65.

Coggan, A.R. & Coyle, E.F. (1991) Carbohydrate ingestion during prolonged exercise: effects on metabolism and performance. *Exercise and Sports Sciences Reviews* **19**, 1–40.

Coggan, A.R., Spina, R.J., Kohrt, W.M., Bier, D.M. & Holloszy, J.O. (1991) Plasma glucose kinetics in a well-trained cyclist fed glucose throughout exercise. *International Journal of Sport Nutrition* **1**, 279–288.

Coyle, E.F. & Montain, S.J. (1992) Benefits of fluid replacement with carbohydrate during exercise. *Medicine and Science in Sports and Exercise* **24**, S324–S330.

Coyle, E.F., Hagberg, J.M., Hurley, B.F., Martin, W.H., Ehsani, A.A. & Holloszy, J.O. (1983) Carbohydrate feeding during prolonged strenuous exercise can delay fatigue. *Journal of Applied Physiology* **55**, 230–235.

Coyle, E.F., Coggan, A.R., Hemmert, M.K. & Ivy, J.L. (1986) Muscle glycogen utilization during prolonged strenuous exercise when fed carbohydrate. *Journal of Applied Physiology* **61**, 165–172.

Coyle, E.F., Hamilton, M.T., González-Alonso, J., Montain, S.J. & Ivy, J.L. (1991) Carbohydrate metabolism during intense exercise when hyperglycemic. *Journal of Applied Physiology* **70**, 834–840.

Davis, J.M., Bailey, S.P., Woods, J.A., Galiano, F.J., Hamilton, M.T. & Bartoli, W.P. (1992) Effects of carbohydrate feedings on plasma free tryptophan and branched-chain amino acids during prolonged cycling. *European Journal of Applied Physiology* **65**, 513–519.

Davis, J.M., Jackson, D.A., Broadwell, M.S., Queary, J.L. & Lambert, C.L. (1997) Carbohydrate drinks delay fatigue during intermittent, high-intensity cycling in active men and women. *International Journal of Sport Nutrition* **7**, 261–273.

De Glisezinski, I., Harant, I., Crampes, F., Trudeau, F., Felez, A., Cottet-Emard, J.M., Garrigues, M. & Riviere, D. (1998) Effect of carbohydrate ingestion on adipose tissue lipolysis during long-lasting exercise in trained men. *Journal of Applied Physiology* **84**, 1627–1632.

Duchman, S.M., Ryan, A.J., Schedl, H.P., Summers, R.W., Bleiler, T.L. & Gisolfi, C.V. (1997) Upper limit for intestinal absorption of a dilute glucose solution in men at rest. *Medicine and Science in Sports and Exercise* **29**, 482–488.

Erikson, M.A., Schwarzkopf, R.J. & McKenzie, R.D. (1987) Effects of caffeine, fructose, and glucose ingestion on muscle glycogen utilization during exercise. *Medicine and Science in Sports and Exercise* **19**, 579–583.

Fielding, R.A., Costill, D.L., Fink, W.J., King, D.S., Hargreaves, M. & Kovaleski, J.E. (1985) Effect of carbohydrate feeding frequencies and dosage on muscle glycogen use during exercise. *Medicine and Science in Sports and Exercise* **17**, 472–476.

Flynn, M.G., Costill, D.L., Hawley, J.A., Fink, W.J., Neufer, P.D., Fielding, R.A. & Sleeper, M.D. (1987) Influence of selected carbohydrate drinks on cycling performance and glycogen use. *Medicine and Science in Sports and Exercise* **19**, 37–40.

Gordon, B., Kohn, L.A., Levine, S.A., de Matton, M.M., Scriver, W. & Whiting, W.B. (1925) Sugar content of the blood in runners following a marathon race. With especial reference to the prevention of hypoglycaemia: further observations. *Journal of the American Medical Association* **85**, 508–509.

Hargreaves, M. & Briggs, C.A. (1988) Effect of carbohydrate ingestion on exercise metabolism. *Journal of Applied Physiology* **65**, 1553–1555.

Hargreaves, M., Costill, D.L., Coggan, A., Fink, W.J. & Nishibata, I. (1984) Effect of carbohydrate feedings on muscle glycogen utilization and exercise performance. *Medicine and Science in Sports and Exercise* **16**, 219–222.

Hargreaves, M., McConell, G.K. & Proietto, J. (1995) Influence of muscle glycogen on glycogenolysis and glucose uptake during exercise. *Journal of Applied Physiology* **78**, 288–292.

Hawley, J.A., Dennis, S.C. & Noakes, T.D. (1992) Oxidation of carbohydrate ingested during prolonged endurance exercise. *Sports Medicine* **14**, 27–42.

Hawley, J.A., Bosch, A.N., Weltan, S.M., Dennis, S.C. & Noakes, T.D. (1994) Glucose kinetics during prolonged exercise in euglycemic and hyperglycemic subjects. *Pflügers Archives* **426**, 378–386.

Hermansen, L., Hultman, E. & Saltin, B. (1967) Muscle glycogen during prolonged severe exercise. *Acta Physiologica Scandinavica* **71**, 129–139.

Horowitz, J.F., Mora-Rodríguez, R., Byerley, L.O. & Coyle, E.F. (1998) Carbohydrate ingestion during exercise reduces fat oxidation when glucose uptake increases. *FASEB Journal* **10**, A143.

Howlett, K., Angus, D., Proietto, J. & Hargreaves, M. (1998) Effect of increased blood glucose availability on glucose kinetics during exercise. *Journal of Applied Physiology* **84**, 1413–1417.

Jeukendrup, A., Saris, W.H.M., Brouns, F. & Kester, A.D.M. (1996) A new validated endurance performance test. *Medicine and Science in Sports and Exercise* **28**, 266–270.

Jeukendrup, A., Brouns, F., Wagenmakers, A.J.M. & Saris, W.H.M. (1997) Carbohydrate-electrolyte feedings improve 1h time trial cycling performance. *International Journal of Sports Medicine* **18**, 125–129.

Jeukendrup, A., Raben, A., Gijsen, A., Stegen, J.H.C.H., Brouns, F., Saris, W.H.M. & Wagenmakers, A.J.M. (1999) Glucose kinetics during prolonged exercise in highly trained subjects: effect of glucose ingestion. *Journal of Physiology* **515**, 579–589.

Kuipers, H., Keizer, H.A., Brouns, F. & Saris, W.H.M. (1987) Carbohydrate feeding and glycogen synthesis during exercise in man. *Pflügers Archives* **410**, 652–656.

Leijssen, D.P.C., Saris, W.H.M., Jeukendrup, A.E. & Wagenmakers, A.J.M. (1995) Oxidation of exogenous [13C]galactose and [13C]glucose during exercise. *Journal of Applied Physiology* **79**, 720–725.

Lugo, M., Sherman, W.M., Wimer, G.S. & Garleb, K. (1993) Metabolic responses when different forms of carbohydrate energy are consumed during cycling. *International Journal of Sport Nutrition* **3**, 398–407.

McConell, G.K., Fabris, S., Proietto, J. & Hargreaves, M. (1994) Effect of carbohydrate ingestion on glucose kinetics during exercise. *Journal of Applied Physiology* **77**, 1537–1541.

McConell, G., Kloot, K. & Hargreaves, M. (1996) Effect of timing of carbohydrate ingestion on endurance exercise performance. *Medicine and Science in Sports and Exercise* **28**, 1300–1304.

Mason, W.L., McConell, G. & Hargreaves, M. (1993) Carbohydrate ingestion during exercise: liquid vs. solid feedings. *Medicine and Science in Sports and Exercise* **25**, 966–969.

Massicotte, D., Péronnet, F., Brisson, G., Bakkouch, K. & Hillaire-Marcel, C. (1989) Oxidation of a glucose polymer during exercise: comparison with glucose and fructose. *Journal of Applied Physiology* **66**, 179–183.

Maughan, R.J., Bethell, L.R. & Leiper, J.B. (1996) Effects of ingested fluids on exercise capacity and on cardiovascular and metabolic responses to prolonged exercise in man. *Experimental Physiology* **81**, 847–859.

Mitchell, J.B., Costill, D.L., Houmard, J.A., Fink, W.J., Pascoe, D.D. & Pearson, D.R. (1989) Influence of carbohydrate dosage on exercise performance and glycogen metabolism. *Journal of Applied Physiology* **67**, 1843–1849.

Murray, R., Paul, G.L., Seifert, J.G., Eddy, D.E. & Halaby, G.A. (1989a) The effects of glucose, fructose, and sucrose ingestion during exercise. *Medicine and Science in Sports and Exercise* **21**, 275–282.

Murray, R., Seifert, J.G., Eddy, D.E., Paul, G.L. & Halaby, G.A. (1989b) Carbohydrate feeding and exercise: effect of beverage carbohydrate content. *European Journal of Applied Physiology* **59**, 152–158.

Murray, R., Paul, G.L., Seifert, J.G. & Eddy, D.E. (1991) Responses to varying rates of carbohydrate ingestion during exercise. *Medicine and Science in Sports and Exercise* **23**, 713–718.

Neufer, P.D., Costill, D.L., Flynn, M.G., Kirwan, J.P., Mitchell, J.B. & Houmard, J. (1987) Improvements in exercise performance: effects of carbohydrate feedings and diet. *Journal of Applied Physiology* **62**, 983–988.

Nicholas, C.W., Williams, C., Lakomy, H.K.A., Phillips, G. & Nowitz, A. (1995) Influence of ingesting a carbohydrate-electrolyte solution on endurance capacity during intermittent, high intensity shuttle running. *Journal of Sports Sciences* **13**, 283–290.

Norman, B., Sollevi, A., Kaijser, L. & Jansson, E. (1987) ATP breakdown products in human skeletal muscle during prolonged exercise to exhaustion. *Clinical Physiology* **7**, 503–509.

Palmer, G.S., Clancy, M.C., Hawley, J.A., Rodger, I.M., Burke, L.M. & Noakes, T.D. (1998) Carbohydrate ingestion immediately before exercise does not improve 20 km time trial performance in well trained cyclists. *International Journal of Sports Medicine* **19**, 415–418.

Sahlin, K., Katz, A. & Broberg, S. (1990) Tricarboxylic acid cycle intermediates in human muscle during prolonged exercise. *American Journal of Physiology* **259**, C834–C841.

Saris, W.H.M., Goodpaster, B.H., Jeukendrup, A.E., Brouns, F., Halliday, D. & Wagenmakers, A.J.M. (1993) Exogenous carbohydrate oxidation from different carbohydrate sources during exercise. *Journal of Applied Physiology* **75**, 2168–2172.

Sasaki, H., Maeda, J., Usui, S. & Ishiko, T. (1987) Effect of sucrose and caffeine ingestion on performance of prolonged strenuous running. *International Journal of Sports Medicine* **8**, 261–265.

Shi, X., Summers, R.W., Schedl, H.P., Flanagan, S.W., Chang, R. & Gisolfi, C.V. (1995) Effects of carbohydrate type and concentration and solution osmolality on water absorption. *Medicine and Science in Sports and Exercise* **27**, 1607–1615.

Spencer, M.K., Yan, Z. & Katz, A. (1991) Carbohydrate supplementation attenuates IMP accumulation in human muscle during prolonged exercise. *American Journal of Physiology* **261**, C71–C76.

Tsintzas, O.K., Liu, R., Williams, C., Campbell, I. & Gaitanos, G. (1993) The effect of carbohydrate ingestion on performance during a 30-km race. *International Journal of Sport Nutrition* **3**, 127–139.

Tsintzas, O.K., Williams, C., Boobis, L. & Greenhaff, P. (1995) Carbohydrate ingestion and glycogen utilization in different muscle fibre types in man. *Journal of Physiology* **489**, 242–250.

Tsintzas, O.K., Williams, C., Boobis, L. & Greenhaff, P. (1996a) Carbohydrate ingestion and single muscle fibre glycogen metabolism during prolonged running in men. *Journal of Applied Physiology* **81**, 801–809.

Tsintzas, O.-K., Williams, C., Wilson, W. & Burrin, J. (1996b) Influence of carbohydrate supplementation early in exercise in endurance running capacity. *Medicine and Science in Sports and Exercise* **28**, 1373–1379.

Wagenmakers, A.J.M., Brouns, F., Saris, W.H.M. & Halliday, D. (1993) Oxidation rates of orally ingested carbohydrates during prolonged exercise in men. *Journal of Applied Physiology* **75**, 2774–2780.

Widrick, J.J., Costill, D.L., Fink, W.J., Hickey, M.S., McConell, G.K. & Tanaka, H. (1993) Carbohydrate feedings and exercise performance: effect of initial muscle glycogen concentration. *Journal of Applied Physiology* **74**, 2998–3005.

Wilber, R.L. & Moffatt, R.J. (1992) Influence of carbohydrate ingestion on blood glucose and performance in runners. *International Journal of Sport Nutrition* **2**, 317–327.

Williams, C., Nute, M.G., Broadbank, L. & Vinall, S. (1990) Influence of fluid intake on endurance running performance. *European Journal of Applied Physiology* **60**, 112–119.

Yaspelkis, B.B., Patterson, J.G., Anderla, P.A., Ding, Z. & Ivy, J.L. (1993) Carbohydrate supplementation spares muscle glycogen during variable-intensity exercise. *Journal of Applied Physiology* **75**, 1477–1485.

# Chapter 9

# Amino Acid Metabolism in Exercise

ANTON J.M. WAGENMAKERS

## Introduction

The body of a 70-kg man contains about 12 kg of protein (amino acid polymers) and 200–220 g of free amino acids. There is a continuous exchange of amino acids between these pools as proteins are constantly being synthesized and simultaneously being degraded (protein turnover). Skeletal muscle accounts for some 40–45% of total body mass and contains some 7 kg of protein, primarily in the form of the contractile (myofibrillar) proteins. About 120 g of the free amino acids are present intracellularly in skeletal muscle, while only 5 g of free amino acids are present in the circulation. In the 1840s the German physiologist Von Liebig hypothesized that muscle protein was the main fuel used to achieve muscular contraction. After this view had been invalidated around 1870 by experimental data, many exercise physiologists took the opposite stand and disregarded the amino acid pool in muscle as playing any role of significance in exercise and energy metabolism. For over a century the amino acid pool in skeletal muscle has been considered as an inert reservoir from which the building blocks are obtained for the synthesis of contractile proteins and enzymes. A review is given here to show that resting skeletal muscle actively participates in the handling of amino acids in the overnight fasted state and following ingestion of a protein-containing meal and that muscle actively collaborates with other tissues in these situations. Major and rapid changes occur in the muscle free amino acid pool during exercise. Evidence will be presented indicating that changes in the size of the muscle pool of some amino acids and in amino acid metabolism play an important role in the establishment and maintenance of a high concentration of tricarboxylic acid (TCA)-cycle intermediates and via this mechanism in the maintenance of a high aerobic capacity during prolonged exercise. Amino acids also seem to play a role in the failure to maintain high concentrations of TCA-cycle intermediates during prolonged exercise, an event which potentially plays a role in the development of fatigue in glycogen-depleted muscles. The conclusion therefore of this chapter will be that muscle amino acid metabolism occupies a central place in energy metabolism during exercise not as a direct fuel competing with fatty acids, blood glucose and glycogen, but as a precursor for the synthesis of TCA-cyle intermediates and glutamine.

## Muscle amino acid metabolism at rest

As an introduction to the changes that occur during exercise, we will first have a look at the resting state. In contrast to the liver, which is able to oxidize most of the 20 amino acids that are present in proteins, rat and human skeletal muscle when incubated *in vitro* can oxidize only six amino acids (Chang & Goldberg 1978a, 1978b; Wagenmakers *et al.* 1985). These are the branched-chain amino acids (BCAA—leucine, isoleucine and valine), glutamate, aspartate and asparagine (Fig. 9.1).

119

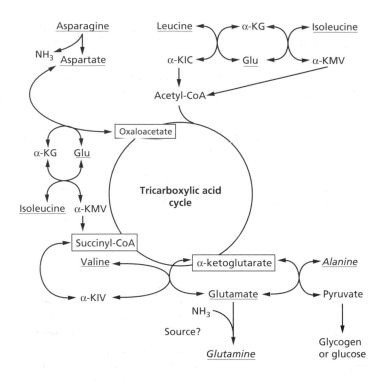

**Fig. 9.1** Amino acid metabolism in muscle. α-KG, α-ketoglutarate; α-KIC, α-ketoisocaproate; α-KIV, α-ketoisovalerate; α-KMV, α-keto-β-methylvalerate; CoA, coenzyme A.

### *In vitro* muscle amino acid metabolism

Rat muscles incubated *in vitro* are in net protein breakdown (protein synthesis < protein degradation) and release amounts of glutamine and alanine in excess by far of the relative occurrence of these amino acids in muscle protein. This suggests that *de novo* synthesis of these amino acids occurs (Chang & Goldberg 1978b). Ruderman and Lund (1972) were the first to observe that addition of BCAA to the perfusion medium of rat hindquarters increased the release of alanine and glutamine. The relationship between the metabolism of BCAA on the one hand and the release of alanine and glutamine has since been the subject of many studies (for reviews, see Goldberg & Chang 1978; Wagenmakers & Soeters 1995). Most of this relationship today has been firmly established. In the BCAA aminotransferase reaction, the amino group is donated to α-ketoglutarate to form glutamate and a branched-chain α-keto acid (Fig. 9.1). In the reaction catalysed by glutamine synthase, glutamate reacts with ammonia to form glutamine. Alternatively, glutamate may

donate the amino group to pyruvate to form alanine and regenerate α-ketoglutarate. These reactions provide a mechanism for the elimination of amino groups from muscle in the form of the non-toxic nitrogen carriers alanine and glutamine (Fig. 9.1).

### Arteriovenous difference studies in postabsorptive man

Muscle amino acid metabolism has also been investigated in man *in vivo* in the resting state and during exercise by measuring the exchange of amino acids across a forearm or a leg (arteriovenous difference multiplied by blood flow gives the net exchange of amino acids; e.g. Felig & Wahren 1971; Marliss *et al.* 1971; Wahren *et al.* 1976; Eriksson *et al.* 1985; Van Hall *et al.* 1995b; Van Hall 1996). As muscle is the largest and most active tissue in the limbs, the assumption that limb exchange primarily reflects muscle metabolism seems reasonable. After overnight fasting there is net breakdown of muscle proteins as protein synthesis is slightly lower than protein degradation (Rennie *et al.* 1982; Cheng *et al.* 1987; Pacy *et al.* 1994). This implies that those amino acids that are not metabolized in muscle will be released in proportion to their relative occurrence in muscle protein, while a discrepancy will be found when amino acids are transaminated, oxidized or synthesized. Human limbs release much more glutamine (48% of total amino acid release) and alanine (32%) than would be anticipated from the relative occurrence in muscle protein (glutamine 7% and alanine 9%; Clowes *et al.* 1980). This implies that glutamine with two N-atoms per molecule is dominant for the amino acid N-release from human muscle. The BCAA (19% relative occurrence in muscle protein), glutamate (7%), aspartate and asparagine (together, 9%), on the other hand, are not released or in lower amounts than their relative ocurrence. Glutamate, in fact, is constantly taken up from the circulation by skeletal muscle. This suggests that the BCAA, glutamate, aspartate and asparagine originating from net breakdown of muscle proteins and glutamate taken up from the circulation are metabolized in muscle and used for *de novo* synthesis of glutamine and alanine after overnight starvation. All other amino acids are released in proportion to their relative occurrence in muscle protein, implying that little or no metabolism occurs in muscle.

## Source of alanine and glutamine carbon and nitrogen

The next issue to address is whether the carbon and nitrogen atoms from the six amino acids that can be degraded in muscle (Fig. 9.1) can be used for complete synthesis of both glutamine and alanine or whether other precursors help to provide some of the required building blocks. Studies with [15N]-leucine have shown that the amino group of the BCAA is indeed incorporated in humans *in vivo* in the α-amino nitrogen of alanine (Haymond & Miles 1982) and of glutamine (Darmaun & Déchelotte 1991). As glutamate is central in all aminotransferase reactions in muscle (Fig. 9.1), this implies that the amino group of all six amino acids is interchangeable

and can be incorporated in the α-amino nitrogen of alanine and of glutamine. The source of ammonia in glutamine synthesis (incorporated in the amide nitrogen) forms one of the puzzles in muscle amino acid metabolism remaining today. A small part is derived from the uptake of ammonia from the circulation. The positive femoral arteriovenous difference for ammonia in man is between 5% and 10% of the glutamine release in postabsorptive subjects at rest (Eriksson *et al.* 1985; Van Hall *et al.* 1995b). Two intracellular enzymatic reactions are main candidates for the production of the remainder of the required ammonia. The adenosine monophosphate (AMP)-deaminase reaction is not only involved in the breakdown of adenine nucleotides to inosine monophosphate (IMP), but, as proposed by Lowenstein and colleagues, also in the deamination of aspartate via the reactions of the purine nucleotide cycle (Lowenstein & Goodman 1978). A second possible source of ammonia production in muscle is the reaction catalysed by glutamate dehydrogenase:

$$\text{glutamate} + NAD^+ \leftrightarrow \alpha\text{-ketoglutarate} + NH_4^+ + NADH$$

The BCAA indirectly can also be deaminated by these reactions after transfer via transamination of the amino group to glutamate and aspartate. However, both AMP deaminase and glutamate dehydrogenase have been suggested to have very low activities in muscle both *in vivo* and *in vitro* (Lowenstein & Goodman 1978). Estimates of limb production rates in the fed and fasted state nevertheless indicate that between 10 and 25 g of glutamine is synthesized in the combined human skeletal muscles per 24 h, much more than any other amino acid. This also implies that there must be a corresponding rate of ammonia production in muscle.

*In vitro* muscle incubations and perfusions with [U-14C]-amino acids have led to the general consensus that the carbon skeletons of the six indicated amino acids (Fig. 9.1) are used for *de novo* synthesis of glutamine (Chang & Goldberg 1978b; Wagenmakers *et al.* 1985; Lee & Davis 1986). This has been confirmed more recently in rats *in vivo* by Yoshida *et al.* (1991), who showed that leucine C-2 was incorporated into glutamine after giving L-[1,2-¹³C]leucine. No, or very little, radioactivity was found in lactate, pyruvate and alanine during incubation of rat diaphragms (Wagenmakers *et al.* 1985) and perfusion of rat hindquarters (Lee & Davis 1986) with [U-¹⁴C]valine. This implies that there is no active pathway in muscle for conversion of TCA-cycle intermediates into pyruvate. It also implies that the carbon skeleton of the five amino acids that are converted to TCA-cycle intermediates (Fig. 9.1) cannot be used for complete oxidation (which is only possible when carbon enters the TCA-cycle as a 2-carbon acetyl group linked to coenzyme A (acetyl-CoA) as is the case for leucine and for part of the isoleucine molecule) or for pyruvate and alanine synthesis. Therefore,

the only fate of these carbon skeletons is synthesis of TCA-cycle intermediates and glutamine (Fig. 9.1). The question then is what is the source of the carbon atoms of alanine? The remaining sources are muscle glycogen and blood glucose converted by glycolysis into pyruvate (Fig. 9.1). In agreement with this conclusion Chang and Goldberg (1978a) reported that over 97% of the carbons of the alanine, pyruvate and lactate released by incubated diaphragms were derived from exogenous glucose.

### Glucose–alanine cycle revisited

The conclusion of the above section slightly changes the concept of the glucose–alanine cycle (Fig. 9.2) (Felig *et al.* 1970) which by now has become generally accepted textbook knowledge.

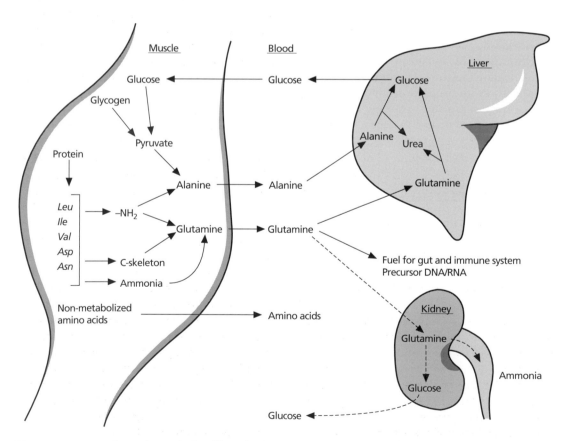

**Fig. 9.2** Interorgan relationship in the handling of amino acids. Dashed arrow, prolonged starvation only.

According to the original formulation of the glucose–alanine cycle, the pyruvate used for alanine production in muscle either was derived from glycolysis of blood glucose or from pyruvate derived from metabolism of other muscle protein-derived amino acids. The alanine is then released to the blood and converted to glucose via gluconeogenesis in the liver. Carbon derived from muscle protein in this way was suggested to help maintain blood glucose concentrations after overnight fasting and during prolonged starvation. The implication, however, of the above conclusions is that all pyruvate is either derived from glycolysis of blood glucose or from breakdown of muscle glycogen followed by glycolysis. In a recent tracer study in man (Perriello *et al.* 1995), 42% of the alanine released by muscle was reported to originate from blood glucose. This implies that more than half of the alanine released by muscle is formed from pyruvate derived from muscle glycogen. This route provides a mechanism to slowly mobilize the sitting muscle glycogen stores during starvation, such that these stores can be used to help and maintain the blood glucose concentrations (Fig. 9.2) and function as fuel in tissues that critically depend on glucose such as brain, red blood cells and kidney cortex. The amino acids liberated during starvation by increased net rates of protein degradation (Rennie *et al.* 1982; Cheng *et al.* 1987; Pacy *et al.* 1994) are instead converted to glutamine, which also is a precursor for gluconeogenesis in the liver in the postabsorptive state (Ross *et al.* 1967). Glutamine also is a precursor for gluconeogenesis in the kidney (Wirthensohn & Guder 1986), but renal gluconeogenesis only starts to be significant (>10% of total glucose output) in man after 60 h starvation (Björkman *et al.* 1980) and is at its highest rate after prolonged (4–6 weeks) starvation (Owen *et al.* 1969). Protein-derived amino acids metabolized in muscle thus still can help maintain blood glucose concentration during starvation but by a different route from that suggested in the original formulation of the glucose alanine cycle. Recent tracer studies in man also suggest that glutamine is more important than alanine as a gluco-neogenic precursor after overnight starvation (Nurjhan *et al.* 1995), and that glutamine is more important than alanine as a vehicle for transport of muscle protein-derived carbon and nitrogen through plasma to the sites of gluconeogenesis or further metabolism (Perriello *et al.* 1995).

## Effect of ingestion of protein or a mixed meal

Following ingestion of a mixed protein-containing meal, small amounts of most amino acids are taken up by muscle and most other tissues as there is net protein deposition in the fed state (protein synthesis > protein degradation), which compensates for the net losses in the overnight fasting period (Rennie *et al.* 1982; Cheng *et al.* 1987; Pacy *et al.* 1994). An excessively large uptake of BCAA and glutamate is seen in the 4-h period after ingestion of a mixed meal (Elia *et al.* 1989) and after ingestion of a large steak (Elia & Livesey 1983). BCAA and glutamate then together cover more than 90% of the muscle amino acid uptake. The BCAA originate from dietary protein. After digestion of dietary protein most of the resulting BCAA escape from uptake and metabolism in gut and liver due to the low BCAA aminotransferase activity in these tissues (Wagenmakers & Soeters 1995; Hoerr *et al.* 1991). The source of the glutamate is not clear today. The diet only seems to deliver a minor proportion as both a [15N] and [13C] glutamate tracer were almost quantitatively removed in the first pass through the splanchnic area (gut and liver; Matthews *et al.* 1993; Batezzati *et al.* 1995). Marliss *et al.* (1971) showed that the splanchnic area (gut and liver) in man constantly produces glutamate both after overnight and after prolonged starvation. After ingestion of a large steak the muscle release of glutamine more than doubles, while the alanine release is reduced to 10% of the overnight fasted value. In the 4-h period after ingestion of a mixed meal (Elia *et al.* 1989), the dominance of glutamine in carrying nitrogen out of skeletal muscle was even more clear than after overnight fasting. Glutamine then accounted for 71% of the amino acid release and 82% of the N-release from muscle. In summary, these data suggest that after consumption of protein-containing meals, BCAA and glutamate are taken up by muscle and their carbon skeletons are used for *de novo* synthesis of glutamine.

### Function of muscle glutamine synthesis and release

In the previous sections it has become clear that glutamine is the main end product of muscle amino acid metabolism both in the overnight fasted state and during feeding. Alanine only serves to export part of the amino groups. Glutamine is the most abundant amino acid in human plasma (600–700 μM) and in the muscle free amino acid pool (20 mM; 60% of the intramuscular pool excluding the nonprotein amino acid taurine). The synthesis rate of glutamine in muscle is higher than that of any other amino acid. Extrapolations of limb production rates in the fed and fasted state suggest that between 10 and 25 g of glutamine is synthesized in the combined human skeletal muscles per day. Tracer dilution studies even indicate that 80 g of glutamine is produced per day (Darmaun *et al.* 1986), but this may be a methodological overestimation due to slow mixing of the glutamine tracer with the large endogenous glutamine pool in muscle (Van Acker *et al.* 1998). Furthermore, although muscle is the main glutamine-producing tissue, other tissues (e.g. adipose tissue, liver and brain) may also contribute to the rate of appearance of glutamine in the plasma pool that is measured by tracer dilution techniques.

The reason for this high rate of glutamine production in muscle probably is that glutamine plays an important role in human metabolism in other organs. Sir Hans Krebs (1975) has already written:

> Maybe the significance of glutamine synthesis is to be sought in the role of glutamine in other organs, as a precursor of urinary ammonia and as a participant in the biosynthesis of purines, NAD+, amino sugars and proteins. Glutamine is an important blood constituent, present in higher concentrations than any other amino

acid, presumably to serve these various functions. Muscle may play a role in maintaining the high plasma concentration of glutamine.

Glutamine has been shown to be an important fuel for cells of the immune system (Ardawi & Newsholme 1983) and for mucosal cells of the intestine (Windmueller & Spaeth 1974; Souba 1991). Low muscle and plasma glutamine concentrations are observed in patients with sepsis and trauma (Vinnars *et al.* 1975; Rennie *et al.* 1986; Lacey & Wilmore 1990), conditions that also are attended by mucosal atrophy, loss of the gut barrier function (bacterial translocation) and a weakened immune response. Although the link between the reduced glutamine concentrations and these functional losses has not been fully underpinned by experimental evidence, the possibility should seriously be considered that it is a causal relationship. Due to its numerous metabolic key functions and a potential shortage in patients with sepsis and trauma, glutamine has recently been proposed to be a conditionally essential amino acid (Lacey & Wilmore 1990), which should especially be added to the nutrition of long-term hospitalized critically ill and depleted patients. These patients have a reduced muscle mass due to continuous muscle wasting and therefore probably also a reduced capacity for glutamine production.

### Glutamine–glutamate cycle

The existence of the glutamine–glutamate cycle was first demonstrated by Marliss *et al.* (1971). In muscle there is a continuous glutamate uptake and glutamine release with the glutamate uptake accounting for about half of the glutamine release. Most of the glutamine produced by muscle is extracted by the splanchnic bed, most probably partly by the gut (Souba 1991) and partly by the liver (Ross *et al.* 1967). This glutamine is converted to glutamate and ammonia by glutaminase. When generated in the gut, the ammonia is transported via the portal vein to the liver and disposed of as urea; the same holds for ammonia generated in the liver. About half of the glutamate is retained in the splanchnic area and used as a fuel in the gut (Souba 1991) or for gluconeogenesis in the liver (Ross *et al.* 1967), and the other half is released and transported back to the muscle. This glutamine–glutamate cycle provides a means to transport ammonia produced in muscle in the form of a non-toxic carrier (glutamine) through the blood to the splanchnic area where it can be removed as urea.

## Muscle amino acid metabolism during exercise

### Anaplerotic role of the alanine aminotransferase reaction

During one- and two-legged cycling exercise at intensities between 50% and 70% of $W_{max}$ only two amino acids change substantially in concentration in the muscle free amino acid pool, i.e. glutamate and alanine (Bergström *et al.* 1985; Sahlin *et al.* 1990; Van Hall *et al.* 1995b). Glutamate decreases by 50–70% within 10 min of exercise, while alanine at that point in time is increased by 50–60%. The low concentration of glutamate is maintained when exercise is continued for periods up to 90 min or until exhaustion, while alanine slowly returns to resting levels. Substantial amounts of alanine, furthermore, are released into the circulation during the first 30 min of exercise (Van Hall *et al.* 1995b). Alanine release is reduced again when exercise is continued and the muscle glycogen stores are gradually emptied (Van Hall *et al.* 1995b). The functionality of the rapid fall in muscle glutamate concentration most likely is conversion of its carbon skeleton into α-ketoglutarate and TCA-cycle intermediates. The sum concentration of the most abundant TCA-cycle intermediates in skeletal muscle has been shown to increase rapidly by about 10-fold after the start of exercise (Essen & Kaijser 1978; Sahlin *et al.* 1990). Although the mechanisms of metabolic control of the flux in the TCA cycle are not exactly understood today because of the complexity of this multienzyme system, both allosteric activation mechanisms (increases in the concentration of mitochondrial free ADP and calcium among

others activate α-ketoglutarate dehydrogenase) and increases in the concentration of some of the TCA-cycle intermediates (the substrates of the TCA-cycle enzymes) most likely both contribute to the increased TCA-cycle flux during exercise. The increase in the sum concentration of the most abundant TCA-cycle intermediates, in other words, may be needed for an optimal aerobic energy production and to meet the increased energy demand for contraction.

The high rate of alanine production during the first 30 min of exercise (Van Hall *et al.* 1995b) and the temporary increase in muscle alanine concentration after 10 min of exercise indicate that the alanine aminotransferase reaction (Fig. 9.3) is used for the rapid conversion of glutamate carbon into TCA-cycle intermediates. The alanine aminotransferase reaction is a near equilibrium reaction. At the start of exercise the rate of glycolysis and thus of pyruvate formation is high, as indicated by a temporary increase of the muscle pyruvate concentration (Dohm *et al.* 1986; Sahlin *et al.* 1990; Spencer *et al.* 1992) and an increased release of pyruvate and lactate from the exercising muscle during the first 30 min (Van Hall 1996). The increase in muscle pyruvate automatically forces the alanine aminotrans-

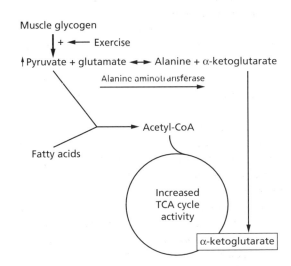

**Fig. 9.3** The alanine aminotransferase reaction feeds carbon into the tricarboxylic acid (TCA) cycle during the first minutes of exercise.

ferase reaction towards a new equilibrium with production of α-ketoglutarate and alanine from pyruvate (continuously supplied by glycolysis) and glutamate (falling in concentration). Felig and Wahren (1971) have shown that the rate of release of alanine from muscle depended on the exercise intensity (see also Eriksson *et al.* 1985) and suggested a direct relation between the rate of formation of pyruvate from glucose and the rate of alanine release. This led to the suggestion that the glucose–alanine cycle also operated during exercise: glucose taken up by muscle from the blood is converted via glycolysis to pyruvate and then via transamination to alanine to subsequently serve as substrate for gluconeogenesis in the liver and to help maintain blood glucose concentration during exercise. Here we propose that the alanine aminotransferase reaction primarily functions for *de novo* synthesis of α-ketoglutarate and TCA-cycle intermediates at the start of exercise. The augmented glycolysis during exercise thus appears to serve a dual function (Fig. 9.3). More pyruvate is generated to function (i) as a substrate for pyruvate dehydrogenase and subsequent oxidation and (ii) to force the alanine aminotransferase reaction towards production of α-ketoglutarate and TCA-cycle intermediates and thus to increase TCA-cycle activity and the capacity to oxidize acetyl-CoA derived from pyruvate and fatty acid oxidation.

### Carbon drain of the BCAA aminotransferase reaction in glycogen-depleted muscles: its potential role in fatigue mechanisms

After the early increase in the concentration of TCA-cycle intermediates during exercise, Sahlin *et al.* (1990) observed a subsequent gradual decrease in human subjects exercising until exhaustion at 75% $\dot{V}o_{2max}$. We (Wagenmakers *et al.* 1990, 1991; Van Hall *et al.* 1995b, 1996; Wagenmakers & Van Hall 1996) have hypothesized that the increased oxidation of the BCAA plays an important role in that subsequent decrease. The branched-chain α-keto acid dehydrogenase (BCKADH; the enzyme catalysing the rate determining step in the oxidation of BCAA

in muscle) is increasingly activated during prolonged exercise leading to glycogen depletion (Wagenmakers *et al.* 1991; Van Hall *et al.* 1996). After prolonged exercise, the muscle also begins to extract BCAA from the circulation in gradually increasing amounts (Ahlborg *et al.* 1974; Van Hall *et al.* 1995b, 1996). Ahlborg *et al.* (1974) suggested that these BCAA were released from the splanchnic bed. An increase in oxidation of the BCAA by definition will increase the flux through the BCAA aminotransferase step. In the case of leucine this reaction will put a net carbon drain on the TCA cycle as the carbon skeleton of leucine is oxidized to three acetyl-CoA molecules and the aminotransferase step uses α-ketoglutarate as the amino group acceptor (Fig. 9.4). Increased oxidation of valine and isoleucine will not lead to net removal of TCA-cycle intermediates as the carbon skeleton of valine is oxidized to succinyl-CoA and that of isoleucine to both succinyl-CoA and acetyl-CoA (Fig. 9.1). Net removal of α-ketoglutarate via leucine transamination (Fig. 9.4) can be compensated for by regeneration of α-ketoglutarate in the alanine aminotransferase reaction as long as muscle

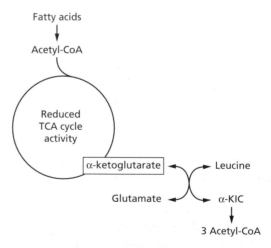

**Fig. 9.4** Increased rates of leucine transamination remove α-ketoglutarate from the tricarboxylic acid (TCA) cycle during prolonged exercise. The subsequent decrease in TCA-cycle flux limits the maximal rate of fat oxidation in glycogen-depleted muscles. α-KIC, α-ketoisocaproate.

glycogen is available and the muscle pyruvate concentration is kept high (Fig. 9.3). However, as activation of the BCKADH complex is highest in glycogen-depleted muscle (Van Hall et al. 1996), this mechanism eventually is expected to lead to a decrease in the concentration of TCA-cycle intermediates. This again may lead to a reduction of the TCA-cycle activity, inadequate adenosine triphosphate turnover rates and, via increases in the known cellular mediators, to muscle fatigue (Fitts 1994).

## BCAA supplementation and performance

After oral ingestion, BCAA escape from hepatic uptake and are rapidly extracted by the leg muscles (Aoki et al. 1981; MacLean et al. 1996; Van Hall et al. 1996) and this is accompanied by activation of the BCKADH complex at rest and increased activation during exercise (Van Hall et al. 1996). This could imply that the indicated carbon drain on the TCA cycle is larger after BCAA ingestion and that BCAA ingestion by this mechanism leads to premature fatigue during prolonged exercise, leading to glycogen depletion. Evidence in support of this hypothesis has been obtained (Wagenmakers et al. 1990) in patients with McArdle's disease, who have no access to muscle glycogen due to glycogen phosphorylase deficiency and therefore can be regarded as an 'experiment of nature' from which we can learn what happens during exercise with glycogen-depleted muscles. BCAA supplementation increased heart rate and led to premature fatigue during incremental exercise in these patients. This may contain the message that BCAA supplementation has a negative effect on performance by the proposed mechanism in healthy subjects in conditions where the glycogen stores have been completely emptied by highly demanding endurance exercise. However, with coingestion of carbohydrate, BCAA ingestion did not change time to exhaustion in healthy subjects (Blomstrand et al. 1995; Van Hall et al. 1995a; Madsen et al. 1996). As BCAA ingestion increases ammonia production by the muscle and plasma ammonia concentra-

tion during exercise (Wagenmakers 1992; Van Hall et al. 1995a, 1996; MacLean et al. 1996; Madsen et al. 1996), and as ammonia has been suggested to lead to central fatigue and loss of motor coordination (Banister & Cameron 1990), great care seems to be indicated with the use of BCAA supplements during exercise, especially in sports that critically depend on motor coordination. The hypothesis of Newsholme and colleagues (see Chapter 11 for details) (Blomstrand et al. 1991) that BCAA supplements improve endurance performance via a reduction of central fatigue by serotoninergic mechanisms has not been confirmed in recent controlled studies (Blomstrand et al. 1995; Van Hall et al. 1995a; Madsen et al. 1996).

## Importance of TCA-cycle anaplerosis for the maximal rate of substrate oxidation during exercise

Muscle glycogen is the primary fuel during prolonged high-intensity exercise such as practised by elite marathon runners. High running speeds ($\geq 20\,\text{km}\cdot\text{h}^{-1}$) are maintained by these athletes for periods of 2 h. However, they have to reduce the pace when the muscle glycogen concentration is falling and glycolytic rates cannot be maintained. This either indicates that there is a limit in the maximal rate at which fatty acids can be mobilized from adipose tissue and intramuscular stores and oxidized or that there is a limitation in the maximal rate of the TCA cycle when glycolytic rates are falling as a consequence of glycogen depletion. It is proposed here that the decrease in muscle pyruvate concentration which occurs when the glycogen stores are reduced leads to a decrease of the anaplerotic capacity of the alanine aminotransferase reaction and thus leads to a decrease in the concentration of TCA-cycle intermediates (due to insufficient counterbalance of the carbon-draining effect of the BCAA aminotransferase reaction). This again will lead to a reduction of TCA-cycle activity and the need to reduce the pace (fatigue). The following observation seems to support this hypothesis. Patients with McArdle's disease cannot substantially increase the glycolytic rate during exercise due to the glycogen breakdown defect in muscle and they therefore do not increase muscle pyruvate. The arterial alanine concentration does not increase in these patients during exercise (Wagenmakers et al. 1990) and the muscle only produces alanine by means of protein degradation and not via the alanine aminotransferase reaction (Wagenmakers et al. 1990). This implies that the anaplerotic capacity of these patients is substantially reduced compared with that of healthy subjects. The maximal work rate and oxygen consumption of these patients during cycling exercise is between 40% and 50% of the maximum predicted for their age and build. In ultra-endurance exercise without carbohydrate ingestion, healthy subjects have to reduce the work rate to about the same level when the glycogen stores have been emptied, suggesting that muscle glycogen indeed is needed to maintain high work rates, potentially by means of its ability to establish and maintain high concentrations of TCA-cycle intermediates.

## Alternative anaplerotic reactions in glycogen-depleted muscles

From the previous sections it has become clear that the alanine aminotransferase reaction plays an important role in the establishment and maintenance of adequate concentrations of TCA-cycle intermediates during exercise. In the glycogen-depleted state, glucose released from the liver by glycogenolysis and gluconeogenesis and glucose absorbed from the gut following oral ingestion of carbohydrates may provide another source of pyruvate to serve as a driving force for synthesis of TCA-cycle intermediates via the alanine aminotransferase reaction. This, in fact, may explain why higher exercise intensities can be maintained for prolonged periods when athletes ingest carbohydrates during exercise. Other mechanisms that may generate TCA-cycle intermediates are increased deamination rates of amino acids in muscle. Increased deamination of amino acids indeed has been observed during prolonged one-leg exercise by Van Hall et

al. (1995b). Deamination of valine, isoleucine, aspartate, asparagine and glutamate in contrast to transamination does not use $\alpha$-ketoglutarate as amino group acceptor. Deamination therefore leads to net production of ammonia and net synthesis of TCA-cycle intermediates (see Fig. 9.1). During prolonged one-leg exercise at 60–65% of the maximal one-leg-power output, we also observed an excessive net breakdown rate of muscle protein (Wagenmakers et al. 1996a). During one-leg exercise, the workload per kilogram of muscle in the small muscle group used (maximally 3 kg) is exceedingly high and this may be the reason why one-leg exercise leads to net protein degradation (protein synthesis < protein degradation) in muscle. The amino acid exchange observed under these conditions indicated that BCAA and glutamate released by the net breakdown of muscle protein and taken up from the circulation were used for net synthesis of TCA-cycle intermediates and glutamine. Removal of amino groups from muscle in the form of glutamine provides another mechanism for net synthesis of TCA-cycle intermediates (Wagenmakers et al. 1996b) as illustrated by the following net reactions (see Fig. 9.1 for the complete metabolic pathways):

2 glutamate > glutamine + $\alpha$-ketoglutarate

valine + isoleucine > succinyl-CoA + glutamine

aspartate + isoleucine > oxaloacetate + glutamine

An excessive release of ammonia and glutamine and excessive net breakdown of muscle protein (severalfold more than in one-leg exercise in healthy subjects) also was observed during two-legged cycling in patients with McArdle's disease (Wagenmakers et al. 1990), indicating that deamination of amino acids and synthesis of glutamine and TCA-cycle intermediates from glutamate and BCAA also provided alternative mechanisms of TCA-cycle anaplerosis in this muscle disease with zero glycogen availability and low pyruvate concentrations. The fact that high exercise intensities cannot be maintained by these patients and in glycogen-depleted muscles seems to indicate that these alternative anaplerotic reactions are not as effective as the alanine aminotransferase reaction and only allow muscular work at 40–50% of $W_{max}$.

It is far from clear whether dynamic whole-body exercise as practised by athletes during competition (cycling or running) leads to net protein breakdown in muscle and helps to provide carbon skeletons for synthesis of TCA-cycle intermediates. Different stable isotope tracers used to measure protein synthesis and degradation in laboratory conditions give different answers (for reviews, see Chapter 10 and Rennie 1996). Whole-body measurements with L-[1-$^{13}$C] leucine suggest that there is net protein breakdown during exercise, but is not clear whether this occurs in muscle or in the gut. Furthermore, carbohydrate ingestion during exercise as practised by endurance athletes during competition reduces net protein breakdown and amino acid oxidation.

## Conclusion

Six amino acids are metabolized in resting muscle: leucine, isoleucine, valine, asparagine, aspartate and glutamate. These amino acids provide the aminogroups and probably the ammonia required for synthesis of glutamine and alanine, which are released in excessive amounts in the postabsorptive state and during ingestion of a protein-containing meal. Only leucine and part of the isoleucine molecule can be oxidized in muscle as they are converted to acetyl-CoA. The other carbon skeletons are used solely for *de novo* synthesis of TCA-cycle intermediates and glutamine. The carbon atoms of the released alanine originate primarily from glycolysis of blood glucose and of muscle glycogen (about half each in resting conditions). After consumption of a protein-containing meal, BCAA and glutamate are taken up by muscle and their carbon skeletons are used for *de novo* synthesis of glutamine. About half of the glutamine release from muscle originates from glutamate taken up from the blood both after overnight starvation, prolonged starvation and after consumption of a mixed meal. Glutamine produced by muscle is

an important fuel and regulator of DNA and RNA synthesis in mucosal cells and immune system cells and fulfils several other important functions in human metabolism.

The alanine aminotransferase reaction functions to establish and maintain high concentrations of TCA-cycle intermediates in muscle during the first 10 min of exercise. The increase in concentration of TCA-cycle intermediates probably is needed to increase the rate of the TCA-cycle and meet the increased energy demand of exercise. A gradual increase in leucine oxidation subsequently leads to a carbon drain on the TCA cycle in glycogen-depleted muscles and may thus reduce the maximal flux in the TCA cycle and lead to fatigue. Deamination of amino acids and glutamine synthesis present alternative anaplerotic mechanisms in glycogen-depleted muscles but only allow exercise at 40–50% of $W_{max}$. One-leg exercise leads to net breakdown of muscle protein. The liberated amino acids are used for synthesis of TCA-cycle intermediates and glutamine. Today it is not clear whether and how important this process is in endurance exercise in the field (running or cycling) in athletes who ingest carbohydrates. It is proposed that the maximal flux in the TCA cycle is reduced in glycogen-depleted muscles due to insufficient TCA-cycle anaplerosis and that this presents a limitation for the maximal rate of fatty acid oxidation. Interactions between the amino acid pool and the TCA cycle are suggested to play a central role in the energy metabolism of the exercising muscle.

## References

Ahlborg, G., Felig, P., Hagenfeldt, L., Hendler, R. & Wahren, J. (1974) Substrate turnover during prolonged exercise in man: splanchnic and leg metabolism of glucose, free fatty acids, and amino acids. *Journal of Clinical Investigation* **53**, 1080–1090.

Aoki, T.T., Brennan, M.F., Fitzpatrick, G.F. & Knight, D.C. (1981) Leucine meal increases glutamine and total nitrogen release from forearm muscle. *Journal of Clinical Investigation* **68**, 1522–1528.

Ardawi, M.S.M. & Newsholme, E.A. (1983) Glutamine metabolism in lymphocytes of the rat. *Biochemical Journal* **212**, 835–842.

Banister, E.W. & Cameron, B.J. (1990) Exercise-induced hyperammonemia: peripheral and central effects. *International Journal of Sports Medicine* **11**, S129–142.

Battezzati, A., Brillon, D.J. & Matthews, D.E. (1995) Oxidation of glutamic acid by the splanchnic bed in humans. *American Journal of Physiology* **269**, E269–E276.

Bergström, J., Fürst, P. & Hultman, E. (1985) Free amino acids in muscle tissue and plasma during exercise in man. *Clinical Physiology* **5**, 155–160.

Björkman, O., Felig, P. & Wahren, J. (1980) The contrasting responses of splanchnic and renal glucose output to gluconeogenic substrates and to hypoglucagonemia in 60 h fasted humans. *Diabetes* **29**, 610–616.

Blomstrand, E., Hassmén, P., Ekblom, B. & Newsholme, E.A. (1991) Administration of branched-chain amino acids during sustained exercise-effects on performance and on plasma concentration of some amino acids. *European Journal of Applied Physiology* **63**, 83–88.

Blomstrand, E., Andersson, S., Hassmén, P., Ekblom, B. & Newsholme, E.A. (1995) Effect of branched-chain amino acid and carbohydrate supplementation on the exercise induced change in plasma and muscle concentration of amino acids in human subjects. *Acta Physiologica Scandinavica* **153**, 87–96.

Chang, T.W. & Goldberg, A.L. (1978a) The origin of alanine produced in skeletal muscle. *Journal of Biological Chemistry* **253**, 3677–3684.

Chang, T.W. & Goldberg, A.L. (1978b) The metabolic fates of amino acids and the formation of glutamine in skeletal muscle. *Journal of Biological Chemistry* **253**, 3685–3695.

Cheng, K.N., Pacy, P.J., Dworzak, F., Ford, G.C. & Halliday, D. (1987) Influence of fasting on leucine and muscle protein metabolism across the human forearm determined using L-[1–13C, 15N]leucine as the tracer. *Clinical Science* **73**, 241–246.

Clowes, G.H.A., Randall, H.T. & Cha, C.-J. (1980) Amino acid and energy metabolism in septic and traumatized patients. *Journal of Parenteral and Enteral Nutrition* **4**, 195–205.

Darmaun, D. & Déchelotte, P. (1991) Role of leucine as a precursor of glutamine α-amino nitrogen *in vivo* in humans. *American Journal of Physiology* **260**, E326–E329.

Darmaun, D., Matthews, D. & Bier, D. (1986) Glutamine and glutamate kinetics in humans. *American Journal of Physiology* **251**, E117–E126.

Dohm, G.L., Patel, V. & Kasperek, G.J. (1986) Regulation of muscle pyruvate metabolism during exercise. *Biochemical Medicine and Metabolic Biology* **35**, 26–266.

Elia, M. & Livesey, G. (1983) Effects of ingested steak and infused leucine on forearm metabolism in man and the fate of amino acids in healthy subjects. *Clinical Science* **64**, 517–526.

Elia, M., Schlatmann, A., Goren, A. & Austin, S. (1989) Amino acid metabolism in muscle and in the whole body of man before and after ingestion of a single mixed meal. *American Journal of Clinical Nutrition* **49**, 1203–1210.

Eriksson, L.S., Broberg, S., Björkman, O. & Wahren, J. (1985) Ammonia metabolism during exercise in man. *Clinical Physiology* **5**, 325–336.

Essen, B. & Kaijser, L. (1978) Regulation of glycolysis in intermittent exercise in man. *Journal of Physiology* **281**, 499–511.

Felig, P. & Wahren, J. (1971) Amino acid metabolism in exercising man. *Journal of Clinical Investigation* **50**, 2703–2714.

Felig, P., Pozefsky, T., Marliss, E. & Cahill, G.F. (1970) Alanine: a key role in gluconeogenesis. *Science* **167**, 1003–1004.

Fitts, R.H. (1994) Cellular mechanisms of muscle fatigue. *Physiological Reviews* **74**, 49–94.

Goldberg, A.L. & Chang, T.W. (1978) Regulation and significance of amino acid metabolism in skeletal muscle. *Federation Proceedings* **37**, 2301–2307.

Haymond, M.W. & Miles, J.M. (1982) Branched-chain amino acids as a major source of alanine nitrogen in man. *Diabetes* **31**, 86–89.

Hoerr, R.A., Matthews, D.E., Bier, D.M. & Young, V.R. (1991) Leucine kinetics from [2H3]- and [13C]leucine infused simultaneously by gut and vein. *American Journal of Physiology* **260**, E111–E117.

Krebs, H.A. (1975) The role of chemical equilibria in organ function. *Advances in Enzyme Regulation* **15**, 449–472.

Lacey, J.M. & Wilmore, D.W. (1990) Is glutamine a conditionally essential amino acid? *Nutrition Reviews* **48**, 297–309.

Lee, S.-H.C. & Davis, E.J. (1986) Amino acid catabolism by perfused rat hindquarter: the metabolic fates of valine. *Biochemical Journal* **233**, 621–630.

Lowenstein, J.M. & Goodman, M.N. (1978) The purine nucleotide cycle in skeletal muscle. *Federation Proceedings* **37**, 2308–2312.

MacLean, D.A., Graham, T.E. & Saltin, B. (1996) Stimulation of muscle ammonia production during exercise following branched-chain amino acid supplementation in humans. *Journal of Physiology* **493**, 909–922.

Madsen, K., MacLean, D.A., Kiens, B. & Christensen, D. (1996) Effects of glucose, glucose plus branched-chain amino acids or placebo on bike performance over 100 km. *Journal of Applied Physiology* **81**, 2644–2650.

Marliss, E.B., Aoki, T.T., Pozefsky, T., Most, A.S. & Cahill, G.F. (1971) Muscle and splanchnic glutamine and glutamate metabolism in postabsorptive and starved man. *Journal of Clinical Investigation* **50**, 814–817.

Matthews, D.E., Marano, M.A. & Campbell, R.G. (1993) Splanchnic bed utilization of glutamine and glutamic acid in humans. *American Journal of Physiology* **264**, E848–E854.

Nurjhan, N., Bucci, A., Perriello, G., Stumvoll, N., Dailey, G., Bier, D.M., Toft, I., Jenssen, T.G. & Gerich, J.E. (1995) Glutamine: a major gluconeogenic precursor and vehicle for interorgan carbon transport in man. *Journal of Clinical Investigation* **95**, 272–277.

Owen, O.E., Felig, P., Morgan, A.P., Wahren, J. & Cahill, G.F. (1969) Liver and kidney metabolism during prolonged starvation. *Journal of Clinical Investigation* **48**, 574–583.

Pacy, P.J., Price, G.M., Halliday, D., Quevedo, M.R. & Millward, D.J. (1994) Nitrogen homeostasis in man: the diurnal responses of protein synthesis and degradation and amino acid oxidation to diets with increasing protein intakes. *Clinical Science* **86**, 103–118.

Perriello, G., Jorde, R., Nurjhan, N. *et al.* (1995) Estimation of glucose–alanine–lactate–glutamine cycles in postabsorptive humans: role of skeletal muscle. *American Journal of Physiology* **269**, E443–E450.

Rennie, M.J. (1996) Influence of exercise on protein and amino acid metabolism. In *Handbook of Physiology. Section 12, Exercise: Regulation and Integration of Multiple Systems* (ed. L.B. Rowell & J.T. Shepherd), pp. 995–1035. Oxford University Press, Oxford.

Rennie, M.J., Edwards, R.H.T., Halliday, D., Matthews, D.E., Wolman, S.L. & Millward, D.J. (1982) Muscle protein synthesis measured by stable isotope techniques in man: the effects of feeding and fasting. *Clinical Science* **63**, 519–523.

Rennie, M.J., Babij, P., Taylor, P.M. *et al.* (1986) Characteristics of a glutamine carrier in skeletal muscle have important consequences for nitrogen loss in injury, infection and chronic disease. *Lancet* **2**, 1008–1012.

Ross, B.D., Hems, R. & Krebs, H.A. (1967) The rates of gluconeogenesis from various precursors in the perfused rat liver. *Biochemical Journal* **102**, 942–951.

Ruderman, N.B. & Lund, P. (1972) Amino acid metabolism in skeletal muscle: regulation of glutamine and alanine release in the perfused rat hindquarter. *Israel Journal Medical Sciences* **8**, 295–302.

Sahlin, K., Katz, A. & Broberg, S. (1990) Tricarboxylic acid cycle intermediates in human muscle during prolonged exercise. *American Journal of Physiology* **259**, C834–C841.

Spencer, M.K., Yan, Z. & Katz, A. (1992) Effect of glycogen on carbohydrate and energy metabolism in human muscle during exercise. *American Journal of Physiology* **262**, C975–C979.

Souba, W.W. (1991) Glutamine: a key substrate for the splanchnic bed. *Annual Reviews of Nutrition* **11**, 285–308.

Van Acker, B.A.C., Hulsewé, K.W.E., Wagenmakers, A.J.M. *et al.* (1998) Absence of glutamine isotopic steady state: implications for studies on glutamine metabolism. *Clinical Science* **95**, 339–346.

Van Hall, G. (1996) *Amino acids, ammonia and exercise in man.* Thesis, Maastricht University, The Netherlands.

Van Hall, G., Raaymakers, J.S.H., Saris, W.H.M. & Wagenmakers, A.J.M. (1995a) Ingestion of branched-chain amino acids and tryptophan during sustained exercise: failure to affect performance. *Journal of Physiology* **486**, 789–794.

Van Hall, G., Saltin, B., van der Vusse, G.J., Söderlund, K. & Wagenmakers, A.J.M. (1995b) Deamination of amino acids as a source for ammonia production in human skeletal muscle during prolonged exercise. *Journal of Physiology* **489**, 251–261.

Van Hall, G., MacLean, D.A., Saltin, B. & Wagenmakers, A.J.M. (1996) Mechanisms of activation of muscle branched-chain α-keto acid dehydrogenase during exercise in man. *Journal of Physiology* **494**, 899–905.

Vinnars, E., Bergström, J. & Fürst, P. (1975) Influence of the postoperative state on the intracellular free amino acids in human muscle tissue. *Annals of Surgery* **182**, 665–671.

Wagenmakers, A.J.M. (1992) Role of amino acids and ammonia in mechanisms of fatigue. In *Muscle Fatigue Mechanisms in Exercise and Training, Medicine and Sport Science*, Vol. 34 (ed. P. Marconnet, P.V. Komi, B. Saltin & O.M. Sejersted), pp. 69–86. Karger, Basel, Switzerland.

Wagenmakers, A.J.M. & Soeters, P.B. (1995) Metabolism of branched-chain amino acids. In *Amino Acid Metabolism and Therapy in Health and Nutritional Disease* (ed. L.A. Cynober), pp. 67–83. CRC Press, New York.

Wagenmakers, A.J.M. & Van Hall, G. (1996) Branched-chain amino acids: nutrition and metabolism in exercise. In *Biochemistry of Exercise IX* (ed. R.J. Maughan & S.M. Shirreffs), pp. 431–443. Human Kinetics, Champaign, IL.

Wagenmakers, A.J.M., Salden, H.J.M. & Veerkamp, J.H. (1985) The metabolic fate of branched-chain amino acids and 2-oxo acids in rat muscle homogenates and diaphragms. *International Journal of Biochemistry* **17**, 957–965.

Wagenmakers, A.J.M., Coakley, J.H. & Edwards, R.H.T. (1990) Metabolism of branched-chain amino acids and ammonia during exercise: clues from McArdle's disease. *International Journal of Sports Medicine* **11**, S101–S113.

Wagenmakers, A.J.M., Beckers, E.J., Brouns, F., Kuipers, H., Soeters, P.B., van der Vusse, G.J. & Saris, W.H.M. (1991) Carbohydrate supplementation, glycogen depletion, and amino acid metabolism during exercise. *American Journal of Physiology* **260**, E883–E890.

Wagenmakers, A.J.M., Van Hall, G. & Saltin, B. (1996a) Excessive muscle proteolysis during one leg exercise is exclusively attended by increased de novo synthesis of glutamine, not of alanine. *Clinical Nutrition* **15** (Suppl. 1), 1.

Wagenmakers, A.J.M., Van Hall, G. & Saltin, B. (1996b) High conversion rates of glutamate and branched-chain amino acids to glutamine during prolonged one leg exercise: an alternative mechanism for synthesis of tricarboxylic acid cycle intermediates. *The Physiologist* **39**, A-73.

Wahren, J., Felig, P. & Hagenfeldt, L. (1976) Effect of protein ingestion on splanchnic and leg metabolism in normal man and patients with Diabetes Mellitus. *Journal of Clinical Investigation* **57**, 987–999.

Windmueller, H.G. & Spaeth, A.E. (1974) Uptake and metabolism of plasma glutamine by the small intestine. *Journal of Biological Chemistry* **249**, 5070–5079.

Wirthensohn, G. & Guder, W. (1986) Renal substrate metabolism. *Physiological Reviews* **66**, 469–497.

Yoshida, S., Lanza-Jacoby, S. & Stein, T.P. (1991) Leucine and glutamine metabolism in septic rats. *Biochemical Journal* **276**, 405–409.

# Chapter 10

# Effects of Exercise on Protein Metabolism

PETER W.R. LEMON

## Introduction

For at least 150 years, scientists have studied fuel use during various types of physical exercise. Over this time, there has been considerable debate relative to the importance of dietary protein for individuals who exercise regularly. In fact, the understanding of protein's role in exercise metabolism has changed dramatically several times since the middle of the 19th century. In the mid-1800s it was thought that protein was the major fuel for muscle contraction (von Liebig 1842) and, consequently, it is understandable that large amounts of protein were consumed by the athletes of that time. However, a number of studies completed later in the 19th century and during the first part of the 20th century (reviewed in Cathcart 1925) indicated that protein played a much smaller role in terms of exercise fuel (contributing less than 10% of the energy expended during exercise). As a result, at least in the scientific community, the belief regarding the importance of protein in exercise metabolism was essentially totally reversed (going from the major contributor to virtually no contribution). Based on these data, it was believed that exercise did not increase one's need for dietary protein. It is unknown why the observed protein contribution was considered unimportant, but likely it was an over-reaction to the new information which was so vastly different from the prevailing view of the time or perhaps simply the belief that the amount of protein typically consumed was sufficient to cover this small increased need. In any event, the understanding that dietary protein needs were unaffected by physical exercise became so dominant that the vast majority of the exercise metabolic work throughout the first three-quarters of the 20th century concentrated on carbohydrate and fat and, as a result, almost totally ignored the role of protein (Åstrand & Rodahl 1977).

Beginning in the 1970s, first sporadically (Felig & Wahren 1971; Poortmans 1975; Haralambie & Berg 1976; Dohm et al. 1977; Lemon & Mullin 1980; Lemon & Nagle 1981; White & Brooks 1981; Lemon et al. 1982), but recently more regularly (for review, see Lemon 1997), studies began to appear which suggested that protein intakes in excess of sedentary recommendations may be beneficial for those who regularly engage in strenuous physical exercise. However, the issue of exercise effects on protein need is extremely complex and still there is no absolute consensus (Lemon 1987, 1991, 1996; Butterfield 1991; Evans 1993; Millward et al. 1994; Rennie et al. 1994; Wagenmakers & van Hall 1996). Further complicating this issue is the fact that the current dietary recommendations for protein in several countries do not adequately address this topic because they are based primarily on studies of subjects who were essentially sedentary. Moreover, some recommendations have not been kept up to date. For example, not only were the current recommendations in the United States published a number of years ago but, in addition, they do not contain a single reference relating to the possible influence of chronic exercise on

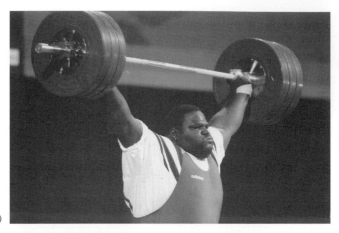

(a)

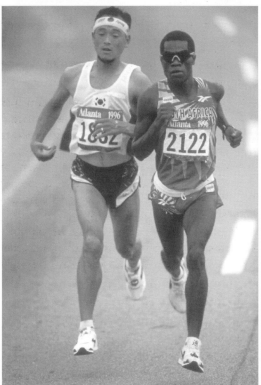

(b)

**Fig. 10.1** Athletes in both strength and endurance events have a greater dietary protein requirement than sedentary individuals. (a) Photo © Allsport / J. Jacobsohn. (b) Photo © Allsport / G.M. Prior.

protein requirements after 1977 (US Food and Nutrition Board 1989). As a great many studies have examined the question of exercise effects on dietary protein needs since then, the rationale for this strategy is unclear. Interestingly, over this entire time period (in fact, going as far back as there are records), regardless of the scientific opinion, many athletes, especially those involved in heavy resistance (strength/power) activities, have consumed routinely vast amounts (300–775% of the recommended daily allowance (RDA)) of dietary protein (Steen 1991; Kleiner *et al.* 1994).

With this background in mind, this chapter reviews some of the more recent experimental results, outlines several methodological concerns that may compromise some of the experimental data, examines the limited information on whether supplemental protein can enhance exercise performance, and considers a variety of potential underlying mechanisms responsible, in an attempt to understand how physical exercise affects dietary protein needs.

## Protein metabolism simplified

A brief outline of how the body metabolizes protein is shown in Fig. 10.2. Although the free amino acid pool(s) contain(s) only a very small percentage of the body's amino acids (the vast majority are in tissue protein), the important role of the body's free amino acid pool(s) (through which all amino acids must pass) is indicated by the size and central location of its sphere in Fig. 10.2. Physiologically, there are only three ways amino acids can enter the free pool(s) (from dietary protein during digestion, from tissue protein breakdown, or as dispensable—that is, non-essential—amino acids formed in the body from $NH_3$ and a carbon source; numbers 1, 2 and 3, respectively, in Fig. 10.2). Of course, some consumed amino acids are never absorbed (lost in faeces) and a fourth method of input is possible, at least in the laboratory (via intravenous infusion of amino acids). When studying indispensible (essential) amino acids, route 3 is eliminated, as these amino acids cannot be formed in the body. Once in the free pool(s), there are also four ways amino acids can leave (secretion into the gut, incorporation into tissue protein, oxidation—amino acid nitrogen lost in urine or sweat; carbon in breath—or incorporation into carbohydrate or fat for storage energy—amino nitrogen lost in urine; letters a, b, c and d, respectively, in Fig. 10.2). During exercise, routes a (due to blood redistribution) and d (due to the overall catabolic stimulus) are considered unimportant. Over time, following constant infusion or repeated ingestion of a labelled representative indicator amino acid (tracer), an isotopic equilibrium can be obtained, i.e. input into the free pool(s) equals output, and movement of the tracer amino acid through the system (turnover

or flux) can be measured. This requires only minimal invasiveness because tissue values (enrichment) can be estimated from blood (reciprocal pool model; Matthews *et al.* 1982; Horber *et al.* 1989) or urine samples (assumption is that the urinary enrichment is representative of the end product of protein breakdown). By combining these data with dietary intake (and infusion rate, if applicable), and/or measures of oxidation (requires breath sampling), it is possible to estimate whole-body protein degradation rates (Picou & Taylor-Roberts 1969):

turnover (or flux) − intake + infusion
    = degradation

or whole-body protein synthetic rates (i.e. non-oxidative loss):

turnover − oxidation or urinary excretion
    = synthesis

Traditionally, whole-body nitrogen status has been evaluated by a technique known as nitrogen balance. This involves measuring duplicate meals to those consumed by the experimental subjects in order to accurately quantify nitrogen intake (protein intake is estimated by assuming that the average nitrogen content of food protein is 16%, i.e. multiplying the nitrogen intake by 6.25), all routes of nitrogen excretion (typically only urine and faeces are measured and miscellaneous losses, including through the skin, are

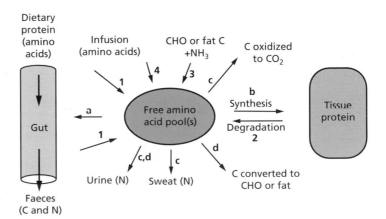

**Fig. 10.2** Simplified diagram of protein metabolism. Amino acid entry into the free pool is shown by numbers and exit from the free pool by letters. Nitrogen status (balance) measures involve quantifying the difference between all nitrogen intake and excretion while protein turnover measures allow estimates of the component process involved, i.e. whole-body protein synthesis and degradation. Adapted from Lemon (1996).

estimated), and then calculating the difference between the two. Estimating the miscellaneous nitrogen losses is usually appropriate because in sedentary individuals they are small, quite consistent and extremely difficult to measure completely. However, with exercise, dermal nitrogen loss via sweating should be quantified, as it can be substantial (Consolazio *et al.* 1963; Lemon & Mullin 1980). When intake of nitrogen exceeds the total excreted, one is in positive nitrogen balance (negative nitrogen balance if excretion exceeds intake). This latter situation cannot continue for very long without losses of essential body components because, unlike carbohydrate and fat, the body does not contain an energy reserve as protein (all body protein has a structural or functional role). Although 'negative' and 'positive' as descriptors of balance are commonplace in the literature, it is recommended that 'status' be used instead of 'balance', to avoid the terms 'positive balance' or 'negative balance', which seem nonsensical.

Nitrogen balance (status) is a classic technique which has been used in the vast majority of studies considered by the expert committees in many countries when determining the recommended dietary allowance for protein (US Food and Nutrition Board 1989). However, it should be understood that this method has a number of limitations (inconvenient for the subjects, labour intensive for the investigators, tends to overestimate the nitrogen that is actually retained, i.e. generally overestimates intake and underestimates excretion), and due to its 'black box' nature cannot provide specific information about the various component parts of protein metabolism (Lemon *et al.* 1992; Fuller & Garlick 1994). Also, nitrogen status (balance) is affected by energy balance (Munro 1951), which can confound the data, especially in exercise studies where this is not always tightly controlled. Further, a number of potential confounders frequently exist, including: inadequate adaptation time to changing experimental diets (Scrimshaw *et al.* 1972), exercise-induced changes in the time course and/or relative importance of the various

routes of nitrogen excretion (Austin *et al.* 1921; Lemon & Mullin 1980; Dolan *et al.* 1987), technical problems making complete collections of nitrogen excretion difficult (Lutwak & Burton 1964; Bingham & Cummings 1983; Lemon *et al.* 1986; Dolny & Lemon 1988), and the inappropriate use of linear regression to estimate protein need with either very high or very low protein diets, i.e. when the response is curvilinear (Rennie *et al.* 1994). As a result, the literature must be examined very critically.

More recently, investigators have utilized the metabolic tracer technique, where the component parts of the protein metabolism 'black box' can be investigated (Waterlow 1995). As alluded to above, this means one can estimate wholebody protein synthetic rates, if oxidation rates or urinary excretion are measured, and whole-body protein degradation rates, if dietary/infusion rates are measured. Although this technique has great promise to help elucidate how exercise affects protein metabolism, it too has several limitations, including expense, invasiveness and the validity of its various assumptions (Young *et al.* 1989; Wolfe 1992; Garlick *et al.* 1994; Rennie *et al.* 1994; Tessari *et al.* 1996). Although technically more difficult, muscle protein synthesis, which represents about 25–30% of whole-body protein synthesis, can also be measured by quantifying isotope enrichment in muscle samples obtained via the needle biopsy technique (Nair *et al.* 1988; Chesley *et al.* 1992; Biolo *et al.* 1995; MacDougall *et al.* 1995).

## Evidence that protein needs are increased with physical exercise

In recent years, a variety of experimental data which suggest that exercise has dramatic effects on protein metabolism have begun to accumulate. For example, several investigators have measured losses in rodent muscle (Varrik *et al.* 1992) and/or liver protein (Dohm *et al.* 1978; Kasperek *et al.* 1980) following exercise, especially with prolonged endurance exercise (Fig. 10.3). Consistent with these observations, we have measured a 113% increase in the active muscle urea nitrogen content ($268\pm68$ to $570\pm89$ $\mu g \cdot g^{-1}$ muscle wet mass) of rodents immediately following 1 h of running exercise at $25\,m \cdot min^{-1}$ (unpublished data). Moreover, increased rates of muscle protein degradation (Kasperek & Snider 1989) and significant muscle damage (Armstrong *et al.* 1983; Newman *et al.* 1983; Friden *et al.* 1988; Evans & Cannon 1991; Kuipers 1994) with exercise are well documented in several mammalian species (including humans), especially when the exercise has a significant eccentric component. Lysosomal proteases, i.e. cathepsins, have been implicated in this exercise catabolic response (Seene & Viru 1982; Tapscott *et al.* 1982; Salminen *et al.* 1983; Salminen & Vihko 1984) but some believe (Kasperek & Snider 1989) these do not play a major role. Recently it has been suggested (Belcastro *et al.* 1996) that non-lysosomal proteases, perhaps a calcium-activated neutral protease (calpain), stimulated by an exercise-induced increased intracellular calcium may be primarily responsible for the initial damage which occurs immediately after exercise. Evidence for this comes not only from the observation that isozymes of calpain increase 22–30% with exercise (Belcastro 1993) but also because the pattern of exercise-induced myofibrillar damage is similar to that induced by calpain (Goll *et al.* 1992). Lysosomal protease

activity may play an more important role in the muscle damage that is seen later (several days) following exercise (Evans & Cannon 1991; MacIntyre *et al.* 1995). Whether increased protein intake can reduce this damage or speed the subsequent repair processes are interesting questions.

Together, the large efflux of the amino acids alanine (Felig & Wahren 1971) and glutamine (Ruderman & Berger 1974) from active muscle, as well as the frequently observed accumulation/ excretion of protein metabolism end products, urea (Refsum & Stromme 1974; Haralambie & Berg 1976; Lemon & Mullin 1980; Dohm *et al.* 1982) and ammonia (Czarnowski & Gorski 1991; Graham & MacLean 1992; Graham *et al.* 1995) provide strong indirect evidence that significant increases in branched-chain amino acid (BCAA) metabolism occur with endurance exercise (Fig. 10.4). Further, this has been confirmed using direct oxidation measures (Fig. 10.5) by a number of independent investigations (White & Brooks 1981; Hagg *et al.* 1982; Lemon *et al.* 1982; Babij *et al.* 1983; Meredith *et al.* 1989; Phillips *et al.* 1993). This is likely the result of an exercise intensity-dependent activation of the limiting enzyme (branched-chain oxoacid dehydrogenase) in the oxidation pathway of the BCAA (Kasperek & Snider 1987). This response is apparently directly proportional to BCAA availability (Knapik *et al.*

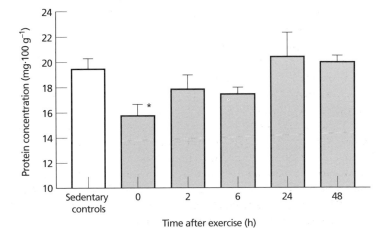

**Fig. 10.3** Effect of prolonged endurance exercise (10 h swimming in rodents) on protein concentration in the red portion of the quadriceps muscle. Note the decrease immediately following the exercise bout. *, $P<0.05$. Adapted from Varrik *et al.* (1992).

1991; Layman *et al.* 1994) and inversely proportional to glycogen availability (Lemon & Mullin 1980; Wagenmakers *et al.* 1991), although other factors may also be important (Jackman *et al.* 1997). This suggests that dietary protein, dietary carbohydrate, prior exercise and time since the previous meal are probably all important determinants of BCAA oxidation during exercise.

The magnitude of this increased BCAA oxidation could be important relative to daily BCAA requirements because a single bout of moderate exercise (2 h at 55% $\dot{V}_{O_{2max.}}$) can produce an oxidation rate equivalent to almost 90% of the daily requirement for at least one of the BCAA (Evans *et al.* 1983). In addition, it is possible that this oxidation rate could be even higher in endurance-trained individuals because at least two studies

with rodents have shown that the endurance training process results in further increases in BCAA oxidation both at rest and during endurance exercise (Dohm *et al.* 1977; Henderson *et al.* 1985). With endurance exercise, this increase is proportional to exercise intensity (Babij *et al.* 1983) but, despite the extremely intense nature of strength exercise, BCAA oxidation appears to be largely unaffected by this exercise stimulus (Fig. 10.6) (Tarnopolsky *et al.* 1991). This is likely due to the fact that strength exercise is so intense that a major portion of the necessary energy must be derived via anaerobic metabolism, i.e. stored phosphagens and muscle glycogen, rather than via oxidative pathways.

Interesting data are also available from several elegant nitrogen status (balance) experiments

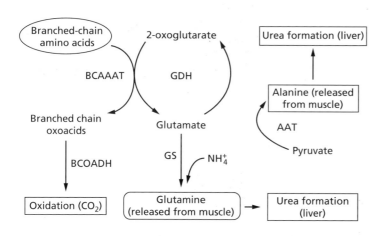

**Fig. 10.4** Overview of branched-chain amino acid metabolism showing the production of alanine and glutamine in muscle, as well as the formation of urea in the liver. AAT, alanine amino transferase; BCAAAT, branched-chain amino acid amino transferase; BCOADH, branched-chain oxoacid dehydrogenase; GDH, glutamate dehydrogense; GS, glutamine synthetase; $NH_4^+$, ammonium.

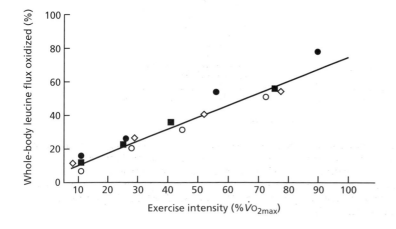

**Fig. 10.5** Effect of endurance exercise intensity ($\dot{V}_{O_{2max.}}$) on the oxidation of one of the branched-chain amino acids (leucine) in four human subjects. Note the linear increase in oxidation with increasing exercise intensity. $r = 0.93$; $y = 0.71x + 8.44$. Adapted from Babij *et al.* (1983).

suggesting that dietary protein needs are elevated with both endurance and strength exercise. The data of Gontzea *et al.* (1974) suggest that dietary protein needs are elevated with an aerobic exercise programme (Fig. 10.7) but subsequent work by the same group (Gontzea *et al.* 1975) indicates that this might be true only transiently during the first few weeks of an endurance exercise programme (Fig. 10.8).

However, the data in this second investigation may have been confounded by an exercise training effect because the exercise stimulus remained constant over the 3-week period when nitrogen status was assessed. In other words, the improved endurance capacity ($\dot{V}o_{2max}$) likely experienced as the study progressed by these previously untrained subjects would mean that the same absolute exercise bout represented a

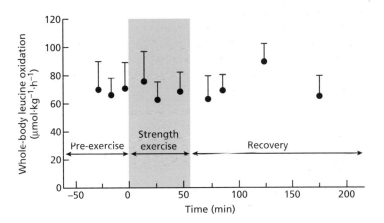

**Fig. 10.6** Effect of a strenuous, whole-body heavy resistance exercise bout on oxidation of the branched-chain amino acid leucine in humans. Note that despite the vigorous nature of the training session, there is little effect on leucine oxidation either during the exercise or during 2 h of recovery. Adapted from Tarnopolsky *et al.* (1991).

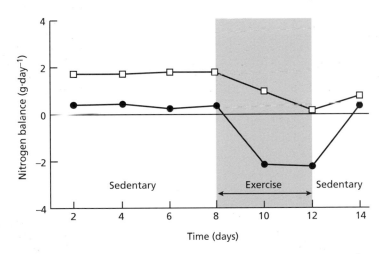

**Fig. 10.7** Effect of an acute endurance exercise bout on nitrogen status (balance) while consuming differing protein intake in humans. Note that the overall pattern of nitrogen status with exercise is similar with both protein intakes and that with the lower protein intake (125% of the recommended dietary intake for protein) nitrogen status becomes negative with the exercise programme, suggesting that this amount of dietary protein, while adequate for the sedentary individual, is inadequate for exercise. ●, 1 g protein · kg⁻¹ body mass · day⁻¹; □, 1.5 g protein · kg⁻¹ body mass · day⁻¹. Adapted from Gontzea *et al.* (1974).

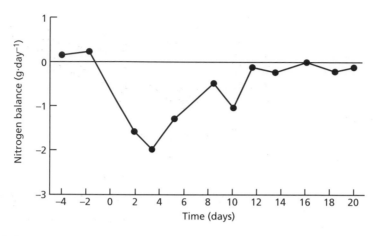

**Fig. 10.8** Effect of adaptation to an exercise programme on nitrogen status while consuming 1 g protein·kg$^{-1}$·day$^{-1}$ (125% of the recommended protein intake) in humans. Note that nitrogen status (balance) appears to recover over several weeks of the same exercise stimulus. These data have been interpreted to mean that this protein intake, although inadequate for a few days at the beginning of an endurance exercise programme, becomes adequate over a few weeks as a result of some adaptation. However, this apparent improved nitrogen status could also be an artifact of a decreased exercise stimulus due to an increasing endurance capacity over the several weeks of training. Adapted from Gontzea *et al.* (1975).

lower relative exercise intensity, and perhaps as a result, an improved nitrogen status. To examine this possibility, we decided to repeat the initial investigation of Gontzea *et al.* (1974) with a few minor but significant changes. First, we studied experienced endurance runners (>5 years' training experience, 94±21 km·week$^{-1}$, $\dot{V}o_{2max.}$ =71±5 ml·kg$^{-1}$·min$^{-1}$) and, second, we used an exercise bout which simulated their daily training load. We observed a negative nitrogen status in the trained runners when they consumed 0.9 g protein·kg$^{-1}$·day$^{-1}$ and a positive nitrogen status when they consumed 1.5 g· kg$^{-1}$·day$^{-1}$ (Friedman & Lemon 1989). The fact that these experienced endurance runners responded similarly to the untrained subjects who were unaccustomed to the exercise stimulus in the Gontzea *et al.* (1974) study indicates that the negative nitrogen status in the endurance runners on the diet of 0.9 g protein·kg$^{-1}$·day$^{-1}$ reflects an inadequate protein diet rather than a transient response to the initiation of an exercise programme.

In another study, Tarnopolosky *et al.* (1988), using various protein intakes (1.0–2.7 g·kg$^{-1}$· day$^{-1}$) and the nitrogen status (balance) technique, not only observed an increased protein need in the endurance athletes studied, agreeing with the other studies mentioned above, but also in a group of strength athletes (see discussion of strength studies below; Fig. 10.9). Typically, regression procedures, i.e. protein intake that elicits nitrogen balance plus a safety margin (twice the standard deviation of the subject sample) to cover the needs of 97.5% of the population of interest (US Food and Nutrition Board 1989), are used with these kinds of data to determine a recommended dietary allowance (RDA). In this study the investigators used this procedure but utilized only 1 SD to arrive at recommended protein intakes of 1.6 g·kg$^{-1}$·day$^{-1}$ for endurance athletes and 1.2 g·kg$^{-1}$·day$^{-1}$ for strength athletes (167% and 112% of the current RDA in the United States, respectively). This conservative approach was used because they wanted to minimize any overestimation that might result when extrapolating from protein intakes as high as 2.7 g·kg$^{-1}$·day$^{-1}$ to those

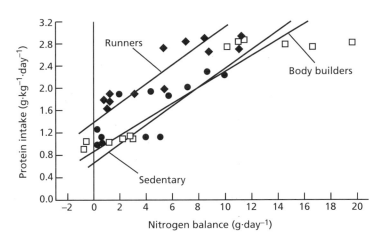

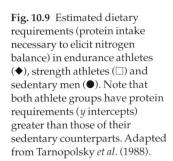

**Fig. 10.9** Estimated dietary requirements (protein intake necessary to elicit nitrogen balance) in endurance athletes (◆), strength athletes (□) and sedentary men (●). Note that both athlete groups have protein requirements (y intercepts) greater than those of their sedentary counterparts. Adapted from Tarnopolsky *et al.* (1988).

required for nitrogen balance. Finally, inclusion of the sedentary group in this study is noteworthy because any methodological errors would be similar across all three groups and therefore the differences in protein intake necessary to elicit nitrogen balance (0.73, 0.82 and 1.37 g·kg⁻¹·day⁻¹ for sedentary, strength athlete and endurance athlete groups, respectively) should reflect true differences in the dietary protein need of these groups.

Shortly thereafter, Meredith *et al.* (1989) used both the traditional nitrogen status (balance) technique and protein turnover measures (oral doses of $^{15}$N-glycine every 3 h for 60 h) to assess dietary protein needs in young (26.8±1.2 years) and middle-aged (52.0±1.9 years) endurance-trained men (>11 years' training). These nitrogen status data indicate that protein needs were elevated similarly in both age groups (by 37%) relative to the data of a previously published study on sedentary individuals from the same laboratory. When these data were used to calculate a recommended dietary allowance for protein based on regression procedures (as described above, except here, twice the sample SD was added because the protein intakes used were near the requirement, i.e. 0.61, 0.91 and 1.21 g protein·kg⁻¹·day⁻¹) the obtained value was 1.26 g protein·kg⁻¹·day⁻¹ (157% of the current RDA in the United States). In addition,

further support for the advantage of the higher protein intake was found in the protein turnover data which showed that the protein synthetic rate was higher in both age groups when 1.21 vs. 0.61 g protein·kg⁻¹·day⁻¹ was consumed.

The subsequent data of Phillips *et al.* (1993), who found a negative nitrogen status (balance) in endurance runners (>5 years' training experience, 43–50 km·week⁻¹, $\dot{V}O_{2max.} = 66$–68 ml·kg⁻¹ fat free mass·min⁻¹), adapted to a protein intake of 0.8–0.94 g·kg⁻¹·day⁻¹ provide further support that protein needs are elevated in trained endurance athletes. In addition, a greater negative nitrogen status (balance) in the male vs. the female subjects was noted in this study and this apparent gender difference in protein use was confirmed by greater leucine oxidation rates (Fig. 10.10) in the men both at rest and during exercise (Phillips *et al.* 1993). Apparently, this gender difference is related to reduced glycogen and/or enhanced fat use in women, perhaps as a result of differing hormonal responses (Tarnopolsky *et al.* 1995). These observations, if confirmed with subsequent work, provide another example where data derived on male subjects may not be directly applicable to women.

At least two groups (Lemon *et al.* 1992; Tarnopolsky *et al.* 1992) have observed even higher protein needs in strength athletes (Fig. 10.11) and based on nitrogen balance data have

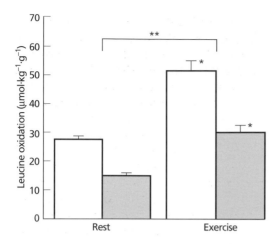

**Fig. 10.10** Effect of gender on oxidation of the amino acid leucine both at rest and during an endurance exercise bout in humans. Note that exercise increases leucine oxidation (*, $P < 0.01$, exercise vs. rest) and that both at rest and during exercise the leucine oxidation rate is greater in the men (**, $P < 0.01$, men vs. women). □, men; ▨, women. Adapted from Phillips *et al.* (1993).

recommended intakes of 1.7 and 1.8 g protein·kg⁻¹·day⁻¹, respectively. Moreover, Fern *et al.* (1991) found a greater gain in mass over 4 weeks of training in body builders who consumed 3.3 vs. 1.3 g protein·kg⁻¹·day⁻¹. This study is fascinating because it supports the age-old (but poorly documented) belief of strength athletes that very large amounts of dietary protein (and the resulting highly positive nitrogen balance) in combination with the anabolic stimulus of strength exercise may be able to stimulate muscle growth (Lemon 1991). However, amino acid oxidation also increased by 150% in this study, suggesting that the optimum protein intake was likely exceeded. Subsequently, Tarnopolsky *et al.* (1992) observed an increase in whole-body protein synthesis (Fig. 10.12) when athletes participating in a strength training programme increased their protein intake from 0.9 to 1.4 g·kg⁻¹·day⁻¹. Interestingly, there was no additional increase when they consumed a diet

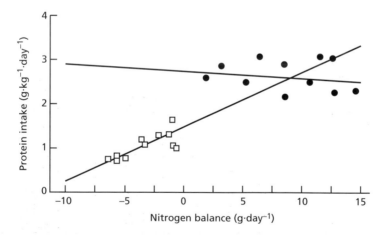

**Fig. 10.11** Estimated dietary requirements (protein intake necessary to elicit nitrogen balance) in novice body-building men. Note that while consuming 0.99 g protein·kg⁻¹ body mass·day⁻¹ (125% of the recommended dietary intake for protein) (□), all subjects had a negative nitrogen status and a strong linear relationship between protein intake and nitrogen status ($r = 0.82$, $P < 0.01$, $y = 0.13x + 1.43$). Using these data, the estimated dietary requirement for protein ($y$ intercept) is 1.43 g protein·kg⁻¹·day⁻¹. Typically, recommendations for protein are equal to this value ($y$ intercept) plus a safety buffer equal to 2 SD of the sample mean (in order to account for the variability in the population relative to the sample studied). Here, the recommendation would be 1.63 g protein·kg⁻¹·day⁻¹ (204% of the current recommendation). The linear relationship between protein intake and nitrogen status is lost at the high protein intake studied (2.62 g protein·kg⁻¹·day⁻¹) (●) and the nitrogen status was highly positive indicating that this intake exceeded protein need ($r = 0.11$; $P < 0.05$; $y = -0.93x + 2.76$). For both treatments combined, $r = 0.86$; $P < 0.01$; $y = -0.11x + 1.53$. Adapted from Lemon *et al.* (1992).

containing 2.4 g protein·kg⁻¹·day⁻¹. Further, amino acid oxidation increased with the 1.4 and 2.4 g·kg⁻¹·day⁻¹ diet in the sedentary group but only with the 2.4 g·kg⁻¹·day⁻¹ diet in the strength athletes. This suggests that at an intake of 1.4 g protein·kg⁻¹·day⁻¹, the amino acids consumed in excess of needs were removed from the body via oxidation in the sedentary subjects but were used to support an enhanced protein synthesis rate in the strength group. Obviously with time this should lead to increases in muscle mass and potentially in strength. These results confirm the Fern *et al.* (1991) data (that increased dietary protein combined with strength exercise enhances muscle growth over training alone) and further indicate that 2.4 g protein·kg⁻¹·day⁻¹ is excessive. These data and the nitrogen balance data (Lemon *et al.* 1992; Tarnopolsky *et al.* 1992) indicate that optimal protein intakes for male strength athletes are likely about 1.4–1.8 g protein·kg⁻¹·day⁻¹ (175–225% of current recommendations). Finally, it should be understood that these studies all involved men who were not taking any anabolic substances. Although not condoned due the potential adverse side-effects, it is possible that the ceiling effect relative to muscle growth observed in the vicinity of 1.4–1.8 g protein·kg⁻¹·day⁻¹ might be extended to higher intakes if combined with pharmacologic manipulations known to enhance muscle development (Bhasin *et al.* 1996). If so, this could explain why the athletes' beliefs about the benefits of very high protein diets differ from the scientific data. Finally, these studies need to be repeated in women to assess whether there are gender differences in the protein needed to enhance muscle growth.

Campbell *et al.* (1995) studied protein turnover and nitrogen status (balance) in older men and women (ages, 56–80 years) consuming either 1.62 or 0.8 g protein·kg⁻¹·day⁻¹ while participating in a 12-week, whole-body, heavy resistance training programme. They observed a negative nitrogen status and a tendency for whole-body protein

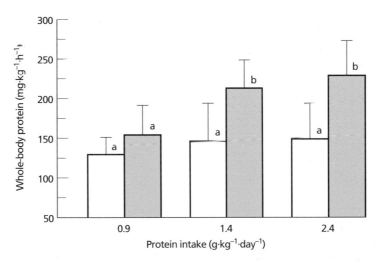

**Fig. 10.12** Whole-body protein synthesis in sedentary (□) vs. strength-trained (▨) men consuming 0.9, 1.4 or 2.4 g protein·kg⁻¹·day⁻¹ (112%, 175% and 300% of the current recommended protein intake). Note that the protein synthetic rate increased in the strength-trained men when going from 112% to 175% of the current recommended protein intake, indicating that this latter protein intake would facilitate mass and strength development. However, there was no additional increase when protein intake was further increased to 300%, suggesting that this quantity exceeded the optimal protein intake. Note also that strength training is necessary to increase the protein synthetic rate with additional dietary protein, as no increase was observed in the sedentary men. Unlike letters, $P < 0.05$. Adapted from Tarnopolsky *et al.* (1992).

plus mineral mass to decrease (−3.5%) on the lower protein diet. In contrast, subjects (no gender difference was apparent) on the higher protein diet had a greater protein synthetic rate and a tendency to increase whole-body protein plus mineral mass (+1.9%). These data agree with the findings in younger subjects (discussed above) and further suggest that higher protein diets are beneficial for older individuals who strength train. This is especially important because as the benefits of strength training for seniors become more apparent (Fiatarone *et al.* 1990; Fiatarone *et al.* 1994), the number of older individuals adding this type of exercise training to their fitness/wellness programmes is growing significantly.

There is other supportive evidence for the suggestion that physically active individuals need additional dietary protein (Consolazio *et al.* 1963, 1975; Celejowa & Homa 1970; Laritcheva *et al.* 1978; Marable *et al.* 1979; Dragan *et al.* 1985; Meredith *et al.* 1992) and, taking these together with the recent nitrogen balance and protein turnover results, it is difficult to deny that protein intakes in excess of the current recommendations ($0.8\,g \cdot kg^{-1} \cdot day^{-1}$ in most countries) are beneficial for those who are physically active. It appears that the optimal protein intake for strength athletes may be as high as $1.7–1.8\,g \cdot kg^{-1} \cdot day^{-1}$ and for endurance athletes slightly less, perhaps $1.2–1.4\,g$ protein $\cdot kg^{-1} \cdot day^{-1}$. However, as mentioned, these data have been collected primarily on men. The limited data available on female endurance athletes suggest that dietary protein needs for women may be somewhat less but this is not well documented. Moreover, there are almost no data on female body builders. Consequently, these nitrogen balance and tracer studies need to be repeated with female subjects to confirm the apparent gender differences with endurance exercise and to establish protein intake recommendations for female strength athletes.

Currently, despite anecdotal claims to the contrary, there is little good evidence that high protein intakes (>$1.3–1.4\,g$ protein $\cdot kg^{-1} \cdot day^{-1}$)

actually enhance muscle performance (Dragan *et al.* 1985; Brouns *et al.* 1989; Vukovich *et al.* 1992; Fry *et al.* 1993). Moreover, we did not observe an enhanced endurance running performance with supplemental protein in rodents undergoing endurance training (Cortright *et al.* 1993) nor could we document greater muscle strength or mass gains in strength athletes with supplemental protein ($2.6\,g \cdot kg^{-1} \cdot day^{-1}$) despite improved nitrogen status (Lemon *et al.* 1992). Further, our studies with differing protein types (soy, casein, whey) and strength training have not revealed any obvious performance advantage of any particular type of protein (Appicelli *et al.* 1995). However, our studies have only investigated the initial response (4–8 weeks) to training and it is possible that over longer time periods an advantage could become apparent. Given the fantastic claims and the obvious potential monetary benefits in the athletic arena, it is somewhat surprising that this area has received such little attention among scientists.

## Are these moderately high protein recommendations healthy?

Many believe high protein diets are hazardous but it is difficult to document an adverse effect except in patients with impaired kidney function (Brenner *et al.* 1982). Clearly, high dietary protein increases the work of the kidneys because of the additional nitrogen load that must be excreted, but this does not seem to be a problem for healthy individuals. In addition, serious adverse effects have not been observed in rodents that consumed extremely high protein diets (80% of energy intake) for more than half their lifespan (Zaragoza *et al.* 1987). These data are particularly interesting not only because of their longitudinal nature but also because this diet represents at least three times the protein percentage observed in the highest protein diets of athletes. Finally, the absence of reports of kidney problems in middle-aged weight lifters/body builders suggests that the dangers of high protein diets in healthy individuals have probably been overestimated because many of these athletes have consumed high protein diets regularly for 20–30 years or more.

Similarly, the association between high protein diets and atherogenesis is likely overstated. For example, it appears that the well-documented positive relationship between animal protein and plasma cholesterol observed in animals doesn't apply to humans (West & Beynen 1985) and, as a result, the association between dietary fat and blood fats is much weaker than once thought (McNamara *et al.* 1987; Clifton & Nestel 1996). Furthermore, even if these relationships are strong in sedentary individuals, the fate of ingested fat may be substantially different in physically active individuals (used as a fuel rather than stored in blood vessel walls or adipose tissue; Muoio *et al.* 1994; Leddy *et al.* 1997).

At one time it appeared that high protein diets resulted in an obligatory loss of calcium in the urine (Allen *et al.* 1979) and, if so, this could be problematic, especially for women, because of the potential to accelerate the development of osteoporosis. However, this appears to be a concern only with purified protein supplements because the phosphate content of protein food apparently negates this accelerated calcium loss (Flynn 1985).

There are, however, at least two areas of concern with high protein diets. First, the additional water excretion associated with the nitrogen loss via the kidneys could be detrimental in physically active individuals (especially endurance athletes) because of their already increased fluid losses as sweat. The resulting dehydration could adversely affect exercise performance (Armstrong *et al.* 1985) and, if severe enough, even threaten health (Adolph 1947; Bauman 1995). For this reason, it is critical that rehydration be adequate in athletes who ingest high protein diets. The best way to do this is by regularly monitoring changes in body mass. Dramatic acute weight changes in athletes consuming high protein diets indicate that additional rehydration is required. Second, the intake of megadoses of individual amino acids (which has only become possible in recent years with the widespread commercial development of individual amino acid supplements) could potentially be detrimental. The ergogenic benefits of these food supplements are promoted to athletes very successfully because of the intense desire of most athletes to excell. Although many of the theoretical benefits sound convincing (especially to the non-scientist), few are documented, despite considerable investigation (Brodan *et al.* 1974; Kasai *et al.* 1978; Isidori *et al.* 1981; Maughan & Sadler 1983; Segura & Ventura 1988; Wessen *et al.* 1988; Bucci *et al.* 1990; Blomstrand *et al.* 1991; Kreider *et al.* 1992, 1996; Fogelholm *et al.* 1993; Lambert *et al.* 1993; Newsholme & Parry-Billings 1994; Bigard *et al.* 1996; Wagenmakers & van Hall 1996; Suminski *et al.* 1997), and substantial potential complications exist (Harper *et al.* 1970; Benevenga & Steele 1984; Yokogoshi *et al.* 1987; Tenman & Hainline 1991). As a result, it is recommended that these supplements be avoided until such time as their safety as well as their ergogenic benefits are proven.

## Protein supplementation: is it necessary?

Protein supplementation is probably not necessary for the vast majority of physically active individuals because the amounts of protein found to be necessary ($1.2–1.8\,g \cdot kg^{-1} \cdot day^{-1}$) can be obtained in one's diet assuming total energy intake is adequate. For example, a sedentary individual consuming about $10.5\,MJ \cdot day^{-1}$ ($2500\,kcal \cdot day^{-1}$), of which 10% is protein, would be consuming about 63 g protein daily. Assuming a body mass of 70 kg, this would be about $0.9\,g$ $protein \cdot kg^{-1} \cdot day^{-1}$ or about 112% of the current protein RDA in most countries. Should this individual begin an exercise programme and, consequently, double his/her energy intake to 21 MJ (5000 kcal) while maintaining 10% protein intake, the resulting protein intake would also double to $1.8\,g \cdot kg^{-1} \cdot day^{-1}$. This would be sufficient to cover the increased needs of all the studies mentioned in this review. Moreover, despite the emphasis on carbohydrate in the diet of most athletes, maintaining 10% (2100 kJ or 500 kcal) of energy intake as protein should not pose a problem because, if fat intake was 30% (6300 kJ or 1500 kcal), 12.6 MJ (3000 kcal) would remain, enabling this hypothetical athlete to consume about 750 g of carbohydrate ($10.7 \mathrm{g \cdot kg^{-1}}$). This quantity of carbohydrate is certainly more than sufficient for any carbohydrate loading programme.

Inadequate protein intake in active individuals is most likely to occur in those who have other pre-existing conditions that interact with the exercise effect to increase the quantity of dietary protein required—for example, during periods of rapid growth, e.g. in adolescents, children, women who are pregnant, etc.; in situations where total energy intake is inadequate, e.g. dieters, those in body mass-restricted activities, etc.; or in those who do not consume a diet from a wide variety of food sources, e.g. many adolescents, vegetarians, women, seniors, etc. For some athletes, insufficient energy intake occurs (and therefore perhaps protein, as well) because of the sheer bulk of food and fluids required to maintain energy and fluid balance. In such situations, the use of a liquid meal replacement formula may be advantageous.

If dietary inadequacies are suspected it is best to complete a diet analysis (typically a 3–7-day food record is analysed with commercially available software) in order to verify that there is in fact a problem. Unfortunately, in free living humans these analyses can be grossly inadequate not only because the subjects are sometimes given poor instructions but also because some subjects modify their diet in an attempt to please the investigator. In addition, use of inadequate methods to accurately quantify serving size is a common problem (weigh scales must be used), as is simply forgetting to record all food consumed. Finally, 3 days may not be representative of one's true diet especially if weekends are excluded (food intake may differ substantially between week and weekend days) and 7-day records are not always better because less-motivated subjects can become bored with the process and, consequently, fail to report accurately. For all these reasons, extreme care must be used in the interpretation of this kind of information.

Assuming that care has been taken to obtain an accurate representation of an individual's diet and an insufficient protein intake is found, one can usually correct the problem with a few minor adjustments in the individual's food selections. This means that, despite the fact that regular participation in an exercise programme (either strength or endurance) will apparently increase protein requirements, special protein supplements (which are considerably more expensive than food protein per kilogram of protein mass) are rarely necessary. Further, if it is determined that it is not possible to consume sufficient protein in food and a decision is made to use a supplement, one of the best and most cost-effective approaches would be to fortify one's food with a high-quality, low-cost protein such as skim milk powder. Finally, there is even less support for the commonly used practice of individual amino acid supplementation. Until such time as it is clear that one or a few individual amino acids in high dosages are both beneficial and safe, this latter strategy is definitely contraindicated.

## Conclusion

After reviewing the literature, it is possible to make a case that protein needs are elevated in physically active individuals, apparently to a greater extent with those actively engaged in regular strength exercise than with endurance exercise. The limited available information suggests that the exercise effect on protein needs may be greater in men than in women. In addition, the increased protein need is likely greatest in situations where other factors compound the exercise effect. However, there is still considerable debate regarding the magnitude of this exercise effect on protein requirements. This debate centres on a variety of methodological concerns which compromise a significant amount of the experimental data that have been collected. As a result, it is likely that a definite answer to the question of the optimal quantities of protein necessary for athletes must await the arrival of more definitive measures to assess protein requirements. Until that time, it appears that the increased protein needs (perhaps 50–125% of the current recommended intakes in many countries) can be met via appropriate food selections without consuming expensive protein supplements. Finally, few data exist to support the fantastic performance effects frequently attributed to extremely high protein diets and this is an area that needs much more attention.

## Acknowledgements

The ongoing support of the author's laboratory by the Joe Weider Foundation is gratefully acknowledged.

## References

Adolf, E.F. (ed.) (1947) *Physiology of Man in the Desert*. Interscience, New York.

Allen, L.H., Oddoye, E.A. & Margen, S. (1979) Protein-induced hypercalciuria: a longer term study. *American Journal of Clinical Nutrition* **32**, 741–749.

Armstrong, R.B., Ogilivie, R.W. & Schwane, J.A. (1983) Eccentric exercise induced injury in rat skeletal muscle. *Journal of Applied Physiology* **54**, 80–93.

Åstrand, P.-O. & Rodahl, K. (1977) *Textbook of Work Physiology*. McGraw-Hill, New York.

Austin, J.H., Stillman, E. & Van Slyke, D.D. (1921) Factors governing the excretion of urea. *Journal of Biological Chemistry* **46**, 91–112.

Babij, P., Matthews, S.M. & Rennie, M.J. (1983) Changes in blood ammonia, lactate and amino acids in relation to workload during bicycle ergometer exercise in man. *European Journal of Applied Physiology* **50**, 405–411.

Bauman, A. (1995) The epidemiology of heat stroke and associated thermoregulatory disorders. In *Exercise and Thermoregulation* (ed. J.R. Sutton, M.W. Thompson and M.E. Torode), pp. 203–208. The University of Sydney, Sydney.

Belcastro, A.N. (1993) Skeletal muscle calcium-activated neutral protease (calpain) with exercise. *Journal of Applied Physiology* **74**, 1381–1386.

Belcastro, A.N., Albisser, T.A. & Littlejohn, B. (1996) Role of calcium-activated neutral protease (calpain)

with diet and exercise. *Canadian Journal of Applied Physiology* **21**, 328–346.

Benevenga, N.J. & Steele, R.D. (1984) Adverse effects of excessive consumption of amino acids. *Annual Review of Nutrition* **4**, 157–181.

Bhasin, S., Storer, T.W., Berman, N. *et al.* (1996) The effects of supraphysiologic doses of testosterone on muscle size and strength in normal men. *New England Journal of Medicine* **335**, 1–7.

Bigard, A.X., Laviet, P., Ullmann, L., Legrand, H., Douce, P. & Guezennec, C.Y. (1996) Branched-chain amino acid supplementation during repeated prolonged skiing exercises at altitude. *International Journal of Sports Nutrition* **6**, 295–306.

Bingham, S. & Cummings, J.H. (1983) The use of 4-aminobenzoic acid as a marker to validate completeness of 24 h urine collections in man. *Clinical Science* **64**, 629–635.

Biolo, G., Maggi, S.P., Williams, B.D., Tipton, K.D. & Wolfe, R.R. (1995) Increased rates of muscle protein turnover and amino acid transport after resistance exercise in humans. *American Journal of Physiology* **268**, E514–E520.

Blomstrand, E., Hackmen, P., Kebob, B. & Newsholme, E.A. (1991) Administration of branched-chain amino acids during prolonged exercise effects on performance and on plasma concentration of some amino acids. *European Journal of Applied Physiology* **63**, 83–88.

Brenner, B.M., Meter, T.W. & Hosteler, D. (1982) Protein intake and the progressive nature of kidney disease: the role of hemodynamically mediated glomerular sclerosis in aging, renal ablation, and intrinsic renal disease. *New England Journal of Medicine* **307**, 652–657.

Brodan, V., Kuhn, E., Pechar, J., Placer, Z. & Slabochova, Z. (1974) Effects of sodium glutamate infusion on ammonia formation during intense physical exercise. *Nutrition Reports International* **9**, 223–232.

Brouns, F., Saris, W.H.M., Beckers, E. *et al.* (1989) Metabolic changes induced by sustained exhaustive cycling and diet manipulation. *International Journal of Sports Medicine* **10** (Suppl. 1), S49–S62.

Bucci, L.R., Hickson, J.F., Pivarnik, J.M., Wolinsky, I., McMahon, J.S. & Turner, S.D. (1990) Ornithine ingestion and growth hormone release in bodybuilders. *Nutrition Research* **10**, 239–245.

Butterfield, G.E. (1991) Amino acids and high protein diets. In *Perspectives in Exercise Science and Sports Medicine*. Vol. 4. *Ergogenics: The Enhancement of Exercise and Sport Performance* (ed. M. William & D. Lamb), pp. 87–122. Benchmark Press, Indianapolis, IN.

Campbell, W.W., Crim, M.C., Young, V.R., Joseph, L.J. & Evans, W.J. (1995) Effects of resistance training and dietary protein intake on protein metabolism in older adults. *American Journal of Physiology* **268**, E1143–E1153.

Cathcart, E.P. (1925) Influence of muscle work on protein metabolism. *Physiological Reviews* **5**, 225–243.

Celejowa, I. & Homa, M. (1970) Food intake, nitrogen and energy balance in Polish weightlifters during a training camp. *Nutrition and Metabolism* **12**, 259–274.

Chesley, A., MacDougall, J.D., Tarnopolsky, M.A., Atkinson, S.A. & Smith, K. (1992) Changes in human muscle protein synthesis following resistance exercise. *Journal of Applied Physiology* **73**, 1383–1388.

Clifton, P.M. & Nestel, P.J. (1996) Effect of dietary cholesterol on postprandial lipoproteins in three phenotypic groups. *American Journal of Clinical Nutrition* **64**, 361–367.

Consolazio, C.F., Nelson, R.A., Matoush, L.O., Harding, R.S. & Canham, J.E. (1963) Nitrogen excretion is sweat and its relation to nitrogen balance experiments. *Journal Nutrition* **79**, 399–406.

Consolazio, C.F., Johnson, H.L., Nelson, R.A., Dramise, J.G. & Skala, J.H. (1975) Protein metabolism during intensive physical training in the young adult. *American Journal of Clinical Nutrition* **28**, 29–35.

Cortright, R.N., Rogers, M.E. & Lemon, P.W.R. (1993) Does protein intake during endurance training affect growth, nitrogen balance, or exercise performance? *Canadian Journal of Applied Physiology* **18**, 403.

Czarnowski, D. & Gorski, J. (1991) Sweat ammonia excretion during submaximal cycling exercise. *Journal of Applied Physiology* **70**, 371–374.

Dohm, G.L., Hecker, A.L., Brown, W.E. *et al.* (1977) Adaptation of protein metabolism to endurance training. *Biochemical Journal* **164**, 705–708.

Dohm, G.L., Puente, F.R., Smith, C.P. & Edge, A. (1978) Changes in tissue protein levels as a result of exercise. *Life Science* **23**, 845–850.

Dohm, G.L., William, R.T., Kasperek, G.J. & van Rij, A.M. (1982) Increased urea and Nt-methylhistidine by rats and humans after a bout of exercise. *Journal of Applied Physiology* **52**, 27–33.

Dolan, P.L., Hackney, A.C. & Lemon, P.W.R. (1987) Improved exercise protein utilization estimates by forced hydration. *Medicine and Science in Sports and Exercise* **19**, S33.

Dolny, D.G. & Lemon, P.W.R. (1988) Effect of ambient temperature on protein breakdown during prolonged exercise. *Journal of Applied Physiology* **64**, 550–555.

Dragan, G.I., Vasiliu, A. & Georgescu, E. (1985) Effect of increased supply of protein on elite weight lifters. In *Milk Proteins '84* (ed. T.E. Galesloot & B.J. Tinbergen), pp. 99–103. Pudoc, Wageningen.

Evans, W.J. (1993) Exercise and protein metabolism. In *Nutrition and Fitness for Athletes* (ed. A.P. Simopoulos & K.N. Pavlou), pp. 21–33. World Review of Nutrition and Dietetics, Karger, Basel.

Evans, W.J. & Cannon, J.G. (1991) The metabolic effects of exercise-induced muscle damage. In *Exercise and Sport Science Reviews*, Vol. 19 (ed. J.O. Holloszy), pp. 99–125. William & Wilkins, Baltimore, MD.

Evans, W.C., Fisher, E.C., Hoerr, R.A. & Young, V.R. (1983) Protein metabolism and endurance exercise. *Physician and Sportsmedicine* **11**, 63–72.

Felig, P. & Wahren, J. (1971) Amino acid metabolism in exercising man. *Journal of Clinical Investigation* **50**, 2703–2714.

Fern, E.B., Bielinski, R.N. & Schutz, Y. (1991) Effects of exaggerated amino acid and protein supply in man. *Experientia* **47**, 168–172.

Fiatarone, M.A., Marks, E.C., Ryan, N.D., Meredith, C.N., Lipstiz, L.A. & Evans, W.J. (1990) High intensity strength training in nonagenarians: effects on skeletal muscle. *Journal of the American Medical Association* **263**, 3029–3034.

Fiatarone, M.A., O'Neill, E.F., Ryan, N.D. *et al.* (1994) Exercise training and nutritional supplementation for physical frailty in very elderly people. *New England Journal of Medicine* **330**, 1769–1775.

Flynn, A. (1985) Milk proteins in the diets of those of intermediate years. In *Milk Proteins '84* (ed. T.E. Galesloot & B.J. Tinbergen), pp. 154–157. Pudoc, Wageningen.

Fogelholm, G.M., Naveri, H.K., Kiilavuori, K.T.K. & Harkonen, M.H.K. (1993) Low dose amino acid supplementation: no effects on serum growth hormone and insulin in male weightlifters. *International Journal of Sport Nutrition* **3**, 290–297.

Friden, J., Sfakianos, P.N., Hargens, A.R. & Akeson, W.H. (1988) Residual swelling after repetitive eccentric contractions. *Journal of Orthopaedic Research* **6**, 493–498.

Friedman, J.E. & Lemon, P.W.R. (1989) Effect of chronic endurance exercise on retention of dietary protein. *International Journal of Sports Medicine* **10**, 118–123.

Fry, A.C., Kraemer, W.J., Stone, M.H. *et al.* (1993) Endocrine and performance responses to high volume training and amino acid supplementation in elite junior weightlifters. *International Journal of Sport Nutrition* **3**, 306–322.

Fuller, M.F. & Garlick, P.J. (1994) Human amino acid requirements: can the controversy be resolved? *Annual Review of Nutrition* **14**, 217–241.

Garlick, P.J., McNurlan, M.A., Essen, P. & Wernerman, J. (1994) Measurement of tissue protein synthesis rates *in vivo*: critical analysis of contrasting methods. *American Journal of Physiology* **266**, E287–E297.

Goll, D.E., Thompson, V.F., Talyor, R.G. & Zalewska, T. (1992) Is calpain activity regulated by membranes and autolysis or by calcium and capastatin? *Bioessays* **14**, 549–556.

Gontzea, I., Sutzescu, P. & Dumitrache, S. (1974) The influence of muscular activity on the nitrogen balance and on the need of man for proteins. *Nutrition Reports International* **10**, 35–43.

Gontzea, I., Sutzescu, P. & Dumitrache, S. (1975) The influence of adaptation of physical effort on nitrogen balance in man. *Nutrition Reports International* **11**, 231–234.

Graham, T.E. & MacLean, D.A. (1992) Ammonia and amino acid metabolism in human skeletal muscle during exercise. *Canadian Journal of Physiology and Pharmacology* **70**, 132–141.

Graham, T.E., Turcotte, L.P., Kiens, B. & Richter, E.A. (1995) Training and muscle ammonia amino acid metabolism in humans during prolonged exercise. *Journal of Applied Physiology* **78**, 725–735.

Hagg, S.A., Morse, E.L. & Adibi, S.A. (1982) Effect of exercise on rates of oxidation, turnover, and plasma clearance of leucine in human subjects. *American Journal of Physiology* **242**, E407–E410.

Haralambie, G. & Berg, A. (1976) Serum urea and amino nitrogen changes with exercise duration. *European Journal of Applied Physiology* **36**, 39–48.

Harper, A.E., Benevenga, N.J. & Wohleuter, R.M. (1970) Effects of ingestion of disproportionate amounts of amino acids. *Physiological Reviews* **50**, 428–557.

Henderson, S.A., Black, A.L. & Brooks, G.A. (1985) Leucine turnover in trained rats during exercise. *American Journal of Physiology* **249**, E137–E144.

Horber, F.F., Haiber-Feyder, C.M., Krayer, S., Schwenk, W.F. & Haymond, M.W. (1989) Plasma reciprocal pool specific activity predicts that of intracellular free leucine for protein synthesis. *American Journal of Physiology* **257**, E385–E399.

Isidori, A., Lo Monaco, A. & Cappa, M. (1981) A study of growth hormone release in man after oral administration of amino acids. *Current Medical Research Opinion* **7**, 475–481.

Jackman, M.L., Gibala, M.J., Hultman, E. & Graham, T.E. (1997) Nutritional status affects branched-chain oxoacid dehydrogenase activity during exercise in humans. *American Journal of Physiology* **272**, E233–E238.

Kasai, K., Kobayashi, M. & Shimoda, S. (1978) Stimulatory effect of glycine on human growth hormone secretion. *Metabolism* **27**, 201–208.

Kasperek, G.J. & Snider, R.D. (1987) Effect of exercise intensity and starvation on the activation of branched-chain keto acid dehydrogenase by exercise. *American Journal of Physiology* **252**, E33–E37.

Kasperek, G.J. & Snider, R.D. (1989) Total and myofibrillar protein degradation in isolated soleus muscles after exercise. *American Journal of Physiology* **257**, E1–5.

Kasperek, G.J., Dohm, G.L., Tapscott, E.B. & Powell, T. (1980) Effect of exercise on liver protein loss and lyso-somal enzyme levels in fed and fasted rats. *Proceedings of the Society of Biological Medicine* **164**, 430–434.

Kleiner, S.M., Bazzarre, T.L. & Ainsworth, B.E. (1994) Nutritional status of nationally ranked elite body-builders. *International Journal of Sport Nutrition* **4**, 54–69.

Knapik, J., Meredith, C., Jones, B., Fielding, R., Young, V. & Evans, W. (1991) Leucine metabolism during fasting and exercise. *Journal of Applied Physiology* **70**, 43–47.

Kreider, R.B., Miller, G.W., Mitchell, M. *et al.* (1992) Effects of amino acid supplementation on ultraendurance triathlon performance. In *Proceedings of the First World Congress on Sports Nutrition* (ed. A. Mariné, M. Rivero & R. Segura), pp. 490–536. Enero, Barcelona.

Kreider, R.B., Klesges, R., Harmon, K. *et al.* (1996) Effects of ingesting supplements designed to promote lean tissue accretion on body composition during resistance training. *International Journal of Sports Nutrition* **6**, 234–246.

Kuipers, H. (1994) Exercise-induced muscle damage. *International Journal of Sports Medicine* **15**, 132–135.

Lambert, M.I., Hefer, J.A., Millar, R.P. & Macfarlane, P.W. (1993) Failure of commercial oral amino acid supplements to increase serum growth hormone concentrations in male body-builders. *International Journal of Sport Nutrition* **3**, 298–305.

Laritcheva, K.A., Yalavaya, N.I., Shubin, V.I. & Smornov, P.V. (1978) Study of energy expenditure and protein needs of top weight lifters. In *Nutrition, Physical Fitness and Health* (ed. J. Parizkova & V.A. Rogozkin), pp. 155–163. University Park Press, Baltimore, MD.

Layman, D.K., Paul, G.L. & Olken, M.H. (1994) Amino acid metabolism during exercise. In *Nutrition in Exercise and Sport*, 2nd edn (ed. I. Wolinsky & J.F. Hickson), pp. 123–137. CRC Press, Boca Raton, LA.

Leddy, J., Horvath, P., Rowland, J. & Pendergast, D. (1997) Effect of a high or low fat diet on cardiovascular risk factors in male and female runners. *Medicine and Science in Sports and Exercise* **29**, 17–25.

Lemon, P.W.R. (1987) Protein and exercise: update 1987. *Medicine and Science in Sports and Exercise* **19** (No. 5, Suppl.): S179–S190.

Lemon, P.W.R. (1991) Protein and amino acid needs of the strength athlete. *International Journal of Sport Nutrition* **1**, 127–145.

Lemon, P.W.R. (1996) Is increased dietary protein necessary or beneficial for individuals with a physically active lifestyle? *Nutrition Reviews* **54** (4, part II), S169–S175.

Lemon, P.W.R. (1997) Dietary protein requirements in athletes. *Nutritional Biochemistry* **8**, 52–60.

Lemon, P.W.R. & Mullin, J.P. (1980) Effect of initial

muscle glycogen levels on protein catabolism during exercise. *Journal of Applied Physiology* **48**, 624–629.

Lemon, P.W.R. & Nagle, F.J. (1981) Effects of exercise on protein and amino acid metabolism. *Medicine and Science in Sports and Exercise* **13**, 141–149.

Lemon, P.W.R., Nagle, F.J., Mullin, J.P. & Benevenga, N.J. (1982) In vivo leucine oxidation at rest and during two intensities of exercise. *Journal of Applied Physiology* **53**, 947–954.

Lemon, P.W.R., Yarasheski, K.E. & Dolny, D.G. (1986) Validity/reliability of sweat analysis by whole body washdown vs. regional collections. *Journal of Applied Physiology* **61**, 1967–1971.

Lemon, P.W.R., Tarnopolsky, M.A., MacDougall, J.D. & Atkinson, S.A. (1992) Protein requirements and muscle mass/strength changes during intensive training in novice bodybuilders. *Journal of Applied Physiology* **73**, 767–775.

Lutwak, L. & Burton, B.T. (1964) Fecal dye markers in metabolic balance studies: the use of brilliant blue and methylcellulose for accurate separation of stool periods. *American Journal of Clinical Nutrition* **14**, 109–111.

MacDougall, J.D., Gibala, M.J., Tarnopolosky, M.A., MacDonald, J.R., Interisano. & Yarasheski, K.E. (1995) The time course of elevated muscle protein synthesis following heavy resistance exercise. *Canadian Journal of Applied Physiology* **20**, 480–486.

MacIntyre, D.L., Reid, W.D. & Mackenzie, D.C. (1995) Delayed muscle soreness: the inflammatory response to muscle injury and its clinical implications. *Sports Medicine* **20**, 24–40.

McNamara, D.J., Kolb, P., Parker, T.S. *et al.* (1987) Heterogeneity of cholesterol homeostasis in man: response to changes in dietary fat quality and cholesterol quantity. *Journal of Clinical Investigation* **79**, 1729–1739.

Marable, N.L., Hickson, J.F., Korslund, M.K., Herbert, W.G., Desjardins, R.F. & Thye, F.W. (1979) Urinary nitrogen excretion as influenced by a muscle-building exercise program and protein intake variation. *Nutritional Reports International* **19**, 795–805.

Matthews, D.E., Schwarz, H.P., Yang, R.D., Motil, K.J. & Young, V.R. (1982) Relationship of plasma leucine and alpha-ketoisocaproate during L[1-13C] leucine infusion in man: a method for measuring human intracellular tracer enrichment. *Metabolism* **31**, 1105–1112.

Maughan, R.J. & Sadler, D.J.M. (1983) The effects of oral administration of salts of aspartic acid on the metabolic response to prolonged exhausting exercise in man. *International Journal of Sports Medicine* **4**, 119–123.

Meredith, C.N., Frontera, W.R., O'Reilly, K.P. & Evans,

W.J. (1992) Body composition in elderly men: effect of dietary modification during strength training. *Journal of the American Geriatrics Society* **40**, 155–162.

Meredith, C.N., Zackin, M.J., Frontera, W.R. & Evans, W.J. (1989) Dietary protein requirements and protein metabolism in endurance-trained men. *Journal of Applied Physiology* **66**, 2850–2856.

Millward, D.J., Bowtell, J.L., Pacy, P. & Rennie, M.J. (1994) Physical activity, protein metabolism and protein requirements. *Proceedings of the Nutrition Society* **53**, 223–240.

Munro, H.N. (1951) Carbohydrate and fat as factors in protein utilization and metabolism. *Physiological Reviews* **31**, 449–488.

Muoio, D.M., Leddy, J.J., Horvath, P.J., Awad, A.B. & Pendergast, D.R. (1994) Effect of dietary fat on metabolic adjustments to maximal $VO_2$ and endurance in runners. *Medicine and Science in Sports and Exercise* **26**, 81–88.

Nair, K.S., Halliday, D. & Griggs, R.C. (1988) Leucine incorporation into mixed skeletal muscle protein in humans. *American Journal of Physiology* **254**, E208–E213.

Newman, D.J., McPhail, G., Mills, K.R. & Edwards, R.H.T. (1983) Ultrastructural changes after concentric and eccentric contractions of human muscle. *Journal of Neurological Sciences* **61**, 109–122.

Newsholme, E.A. & Parry-Billings, M. (1994) Effects of exercise on the immune system. In *Physical Activity, Fitness, and Health* (ed. C. Bouchard, R.J. Shephard & T. Stephens), pp. 451–455. Human Kinetics, Champaign, IL.

Phillips, S.M., Atkinson, S.A., Tarnopolsky, M.A. & MacDougall, J.D. (1993) Gender differences in leucine kinetics and nitrogen balance in endurance athletes. *Journal of Applied Physiology* **75**, 2134–2141.

Picou, D. & Taylor-Roberts, T. (1969) The measurement of total protein synthesis and catabolism and nitrogen turnover in infants in different nutritional states and receiving different amounts of dietary protein. *Clinical Science London* **36**, 283–301.

Poortmans, J.R. (1975) Effect of long lasting physical exercise and training on protein metabolism. In *Metabolic Adaptations to Prolonged Physical Exercise* (ed. H.H. Howald & J.R. Poortmans), pp. 212–228. Birkhäuser, Basel.

Refsum, H.E. & Stromme, S.B. (1974) Urea and creatinine production and excretion in urine during and following prolonged heavy exercise. *Scandinavian Journal of Clinical Laboratory Investigation* **33**, 247–254.

Rennie, M.J., Bowtell, J.L. & Millward, D.J. (1994a) Physical activity and protein metabolism. In *Physical Activity, Fitness, and Health* (ed. C. Bouchard, R.J.

Shephard & T. Stephens), pp. 432–450. Human Kinetics, Champaign, IL.

Rennie, M.J., Smith, K. & Watt, P.W. (1994b) Measurement of human protein synthesis: an optimal approach. *American Journal of Physiology* **266**, E298–E307.

Ruderman, N.B. & Berger, M. (1974) The formation of glutamine and alanine in skeletal muscle. *Journal of Biological Chemistry* **249**, 5500–5506.

Salminen, A. & Vihko, V. (1984) Autophagic response to strenuous exercise in mouse skeletal muscle fibers. *Virchows Archives [Cell Pathology]* **45**, 97–106.

Salminen, A., Komulainen, J., Ahomaki, E., Kainulainen, H., Takala, T. & Vihko, V. (1983) Effect of endurance training on alkaline protease activities in rat skeletal muscles. *Acta Physiologica Scandinavica* **119**, 261–265.

Scrimshaw, N.S., Hussein, M.A., Murray, E., Rand, W.M. & Young, V.R. (1972) Protein requirements of man: variations in obligatory and fecal nitrogen losses in young men. *Journal of Nutrition* **102**, 1595–1604.

Seene, T. & Viru, A. (1982) The catabolic effect of glucocorticoids on different types of skeletal muscle fibers and its dependence upon muscle activity and interaction with anabolic steroids. *Journal of Steroid Biochemistry* **16**, 349–352.

Segura, R. & Ventura, J. (1988) Effect of L-tryptophan supplementation on exercise performance. *International Journal of Sports Medicine* **9**, 301–305.

Steen, S.N. (1991) Precontest strategies of a male bodybuilder. *International Journal of Sports Nutrition* **1**, 69–78.

Suminski, R.R., Robertson, R.J., Goss, F.L. *et al.* (1997) Acute effect of amino acid ingestion and resistance exercise on plasma growth hormone concentration in young men. *Journal of Sport Nutrition* **7**, 48–60.

Tapscott, E.B., Kasperek, G.J. & Dohm, G.L. (1982) Effect of training on muscle protein turnover in male and female rats. *Biochemical Medicine* **27**, 254–259.

Tarnopolsky, M.A., MacDougall, J.D. & Atkinson, S.A. (1988) Influence of protein intake and training status on nitrogen balance and lean body mass. *Journal of Applied Physiology* **64**, 187–193.

Tarnopolsky, M.A., Atkinson, S.A., MacDougall, J.D., Senor, B.B., Lemon, P.W.R. & Schwarcz, H. (1991) Whole body leucine metabolism during and after resistance exercise in fed humans. *Medicine and Science in Sports and Exercise* **23**, 326–333.

Tarnopolsky, M.A., Atkinson, S.A., MacDougall, J.D., Chesley, A., Phillips, S. & Schwarcz, H. (1992) Evaluation of protein requirements for trained strength athletes. *Journal of Applied Physiology* **73**, 1986–1995.

Tarnopolsky, M.A., Atkinson, S.A., Phillips, S.M. &

MacDougall, J.D. (1995) Carbohydrate loading and metabolism during exercise in men and women. *Journal of Applied Physiology* **78**, 1360–1368.

Tenman, A.J. & Hainline, B. (1991) Eosinophilia–myalgia syndrome. *Physician and Sportsmedicine* **19**, 81–86.

Tessari, P., Barazzoni, R., Zanetti, M. *et al.* (1996) Protein degradation and synthesis measured with multiple amino acid tracers *in vivo*. *American Journal of Physiology* **271**, E733–E741.

US Food and Nutrition Board (1989) *Recommended Dietary Allowances*. National Academy Press, Washington, DC.

Varrik, E., Viru, A., Ööpik, V. & Viru, M. (1992) Exercise-induced catabolic responses in various muscle fibers. *Canadian Journal of Sport Sciences* **17**, 125–128.

von Liebig, J. (1842) *Animal Chemistry or Organic Chemistry in Its Application to Physiology* (transl. G. Gregory). Taylor & Walton, London.

Vukovich, M.D., Sharp, R.L., King, D.S. & Kershishnik, K. (1992) The effect of protein supplementation on lactate accumulation during submaximal and maximal exercise. *International Journal of Sport Nutrition* **2**, 307–316.

Wagenmakers, A.J.M. & van Hall, G. (1996) Branched-chain amino acids: nutrition and metabolism in exercise. In *Biochemistry of Exercise* Vol. IX (ed. R.J. Maughan & S.M. Shirreffs), pp. 431–443. Human Kinetics, Champaign, IL.

Wagenmakers, A.J.M., Beckers, E.J., Brouns, F. *et al.* (1991) Carbohydrate supplementation, glycogen depletion, and amino acid metabolism during exercise. *American Journal of Physiology* **260**, E883–E890.

Waterlow, J.C. (1995) Whole-body protein turnover in humans: past, present, and future. *Annual Review of Nutrition* **15**, 57–92.

Wessen, M., McNaughton, L., Davies, P. & Tristram, S. (1988) Effects of oral administration of aspartic acid salts on the endurance capacity of trained athletes. *Research Quarterly in Exercise and Sport* **59**, 234–239.

West, C.E. & Beynen, A.C. (1985) Milk protein in contrast to plant protein: effects on plasma cholesterol. In *Milk Proteins '84* (ed. T.E. Galesloot & B.J. Tinbergen), pp. 80–87. Pudoc, Wageningen.

White, T.P. & Brooks, G.A. (1981) [U-14C] glucose, -alanine, -leucine oxidation in rats at rest and during two intensities of running. *American Journal of Physiology* **240**, E155–E165.

Wolfe, R.R. (1992) *Radioactive and Stable Isotope Tracers in Biomedicine: Principles and Practice of Kinetic Analysis*. Wiley-Liss, New York.

Yokogoshi, H., Iwata, T., Ishida, K. & Yoshida, A. (1987) Effect of amino acid supplementation to low protein diet on brain and plasma levels of tryptophan and brain 5-hydroxyinodoles in rats. *Journal of Nutrition* **117**, 42–47.

Young, V.R., Bier, D.M. & Pellet, P.L. (1989) A theoretical basis for increasing current estimates of the amino acid requirements in adult man with experimental support. *American Journal of Clinical Nutrition* **50**, 80–92.

Zaragoza, R., Renau-Piqueras, J., Portoles, M., Hernandez-Yago, J., Jorda, A. & Grisolia, G.S. (1987) Rats fed prolonged high protein diets show an increase in nitrogen metabolism and liver megamitochondria. *Archives of Biochemistry and Biophysics* **258**, 426–435.

# Chapter 11

# Amino Acids, Fatigue and Immunodepression in Exercise

ERIC A. NEWSHOLME AND LINDA M. CASTELL

## Introduction

### Amino acids and the athlete

This chapter discusses the importance of some amino acids in relation to exercise, in particular to prolonged, exhaustive exercise. Protein metabolism and the protein requirements of the athlete have already been discussed in Chapter 10. Nevertheless, it is worth mentioning here that consideration of daily protein requirements is complicated by the fact that not all proteins in the diet have the same nutritional value, since they contain different amounts of essential amino acids. First-class proteins (e.g. in eggs, milk and meat) contain enough of each essential amino acid to allow protein synthesis to occur without the need to eat extra protein (Fig. 11.1).

By contrast, proteins of plant origin are termed 'second class' because they are deficient in the same amino acids. Adequate amounts of each of the essential amino acids can be obtained from a vegetarian diet by eating a wide range of plant foods, e.g. cereals and legumes. This does mean, however, that the extra protein consumed takes the place in the diet of the all-important carbohydrate. The athlete must therefore seek a balance: too much protein and the diet is distorted; too little and recovery after intensive training might be slowed. This problem leads to a consideration of supplementation of the diet with essential amino acids, especially during peak training. Furthermore, from studies on individual cells

*in vitro*, knowledge is becoming available of the individual nutritional requirements of particular cells and how these change under different conditions. Transfer of this knowledge to clinical situations has occurred over the past 10 years with considerable success. Consequently, it is now possible to provide nutrients designed to deliver fuels to particular cells, tissues and organs that are involved in the response to injury or illness, and this will enhance the natural healing process.

This information can be extended to include the athlete. Furthermore, a specific response to exercise, and to physical and mental fatigue, can provide information that could be applied in the clinic. In addition, it is possible to suggest some amino acids with which athletes might consider supplementing their diet (Table 11.1). Some of the acquired non-dispensable amino acids that might be of benefit to athletes if taken as a supplement have been discussed elsewhere (Newsholme *et al.* 1994). In this chapter discussion will centre on glutamine and the branched chain amino acids, for which evidence of benefit in the athletic field is available.

## Fatigue in physical activity

Fatigue in physical activity can be considered at physiological or biochemical levels. Potential mechanisms for fatigue at a physiological level are as follows (see Fitts 1994).

1 Central fatigue:
   (a) excitatory input to higher motor centres;

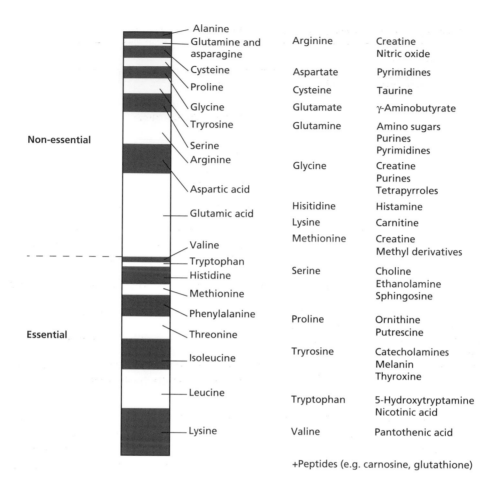

**Fig. 11.1** The amino acid composition of myosin, one of the two major proteins in muscle—and, therefore, in lean meat—and the biosynthetic role of some of these amino acids. From Newsholme *et al.* (1994), with permission.

(b) excitatory drive to lower motor neurones;

(c) motor neurone excitability.

In these three mechanisms there is a decrease in neural drive. This can be detected by showing that fatiguing muscle can still maintain power output if the nerve is stimulated artificially or the brain is stimulated.

2 Peripheral fatigue:

(a) neuromuscular transmission;

(b) sarcolemma excitability;

(c) excitation–contraction coupling.

Biochemical mechanisms for fatigue can also be put forward:

- depletion of phosphocreatine in muscle;
- accumulation of protons in muscle;
- accumulation of phosphate in muscle;
- depletion of glycogen in muscle;
- hypoglycaemia;
- changes in the concentrations of key amino acids in the blood leading to changes in the concentrations of neurotransmitters in the brain.

Some of these mechanisms have been discussed elsewhere (Newsholme *et al.* 1994). The first four are explanations for peripheral fatigue and the last two are explanations of central fatigue. The advantage of proposing a biochemical mechanism is that, from this knowledge, ideas can be put forward for manipulations to delay fatigue. A hypothesis is suggested that links all of the latter three biochemical mecha-

Table 11.1 A 'contemporary' view of dispensable and non-dispensable amino acids.

| Category | Amino acid |
|---|---|
| Totally non-dispensable | Lysine, threonine |
| Oxoacid non-dispensable* | Branched-chain amino acids[†], methionine, phenylalanine, tryptophan |
| Conditionally non-dispensable[‡] | Cysteine, tyrosine |
| Acquired non-dispensable[§] | Arginine, cysteine, glutamine, glycine, histidine, serine |
| Dispensable[¶] | Alanine, asparagine, aspartate, glutamate |

*The carbon skeleton of these amino acids cannot be synthesized by the body. However, if the oxo(keto) acids are provided, the amino acids can be synthesized from the oxoacids via the process of transamination. The oxoacids can be provided artificially.
[†] The branched-chain amino acids may play a role in fatigue but, to place them in context, it is important to outline various explanations for fatigue (see text).
[‡] These are produced from other amino acids—cysteine from methionine and tyrosine from phenylalanine— provided that these amino acids are present in excess.
[§] The demand for these amino acids can increase markedly under some conditions, e.g. infection, severe trauma, burns and in some premature babies.
[¶] It is assumed that all these amino acids can be synthesized at sufficient rates in the body to satisfy all requirements. It is now beginning to be appreciated that this may not always be the case for glutamine.

nisms into one mechanism involving the central serotoninergic pathway in central fatigue.

There is considerable evidence that depletion of muscle glycogen results in fatigue. In middle-distance events, aerobic and anaerobic metabolism both contribute to adenosine triphosphate (ATP) generation. The athlete can use the aerobic system towards its maximum capacity, i.e. that which is limited by oxygen supply to the muscle but, in addition, further ATP can be produced from the conversion of glycogen to lactate. So what causes fatigue in this situation? It is suggested that it is either depletion of glycogen or the accumulation of protons in the muscle; whichever occurs will depend upon the distance of the event, the class of the athlete and his/her fitness. If the rate of conversion of glycogen to lactate is greater than the capacity to lose protons from the muscle, protons will eventually accumulate sufficiently to cause fatigue (Newsholme et al. 1994). However, it is also possible that depletion of glycogen before the end of the event can result in fatigue. As glycogen levels fall, fatty

acid mobilization will occur and increase the plasma fatty acid level. In a prolonged event such as the marathon, fatty acids must be mobilized since there is not enough glycogen to provide the energy required for the whole event. For an optimum performance, the marathon runner must oxidize both glycogen and fat simultaneously, but the rate of utilization of the latter should be such as to allow glycogen to be used for the whole of the distance—and for depletion to occur at the finishing post. Consequently, precision in control of the rates of utilization of the two fuels, fat and glycogen, is extremely important.

An interesting question is why glycogen depletion should result in fatigue. If, as is already known, it were possible to switch to the enormous store of fat as a fuel, this would delay fatigue dramatically: theoretically, the runner should then be able to maintain a good pace for a considerable period of time—possibly several days. At least two explanations have been put forward to account for the fact that this does not occur. First, there is a limitation in the rate of fatty acid oxidation so that a high rate of ATP generation cannot be supported by fatty acid oxidation alone so that, once fat becomes the dominant fuel, the pace must slow. Secondly, and these are not mutually exclusive, fatty acids must be mobilized from adipose tissue to be oxidized and mobilization of fatty acids can result in central fatigue. A mechanism for this is described below.

## Plasma levels of tryptophan, branched-chain amino acids and the 5-HT hypothesis for central fatigue

The branched-chain amino acids (leucine, isoleucine and valine), unlike other amino acids, are taken up largely by muscle and adipose tissue. Like most amino acids, tryptophan is taken up and metabolized by the liver. However, a small amount of tryptophan is taken up by the brain, where it is converted to the neurotransmitter 5-hydroxytryptamine (5-HT). Once this neurotransmitter is released in the synapses of some neurones, it can influence a variety of behaviours, including tiredness, sleep, mood and possibly mental fatigue. It is suggested that an increase in 5-HT level in these neurones makes it harder mentally to maintain the same pace of running, cycling, etc.

The basic tenets of the hypothesis are as follows.

**1** Both branched-chain amino acids and tryptophan (and other aromatic amino acids) enter the brain upon the same amino acid carrier so that there is competition between the two groups of amino acids for entry (for review, see Fernstrom 1990).

**2** Tryptophan is converted via two enzymes in the brain to 5-HT. However, an increased level of brain tryptophan can increase the rate of formation and hence the level of 5-HT in some areas of the brain (Blomstrand *et al.* 1989).

**3** A high 5-HT level could result in increased amount of this neurotransmitter being released into the synaptic cleft during neuronal firing, therefore leading to a greater postsynaptic stimulation in some 5-HT neurones.

**4** It is proposed that some of these neurones are involved in fatigue.

**5** Tryptophan is unique amongst the amino acids in that it is bound to albumin, so that it exists in the plasma and interstitial space in bound and free forms, which are in equilibrium. This equilibrium changes in favour of free tryptophan as the plasma fatty acid level increases, since the latter also binds to albumin and this decreases the affinity for tryptophan.

**6** It is considered that the plasma concentration of free tryptophan governs, in competition with branched chain amino acids, the rate of entry of tryptophan into the brain, the level of tryptophan in the brain and hence that of 5-HT (Fernstrom 1990).

As a consequence of these basic tenets, it is proposed that either an increase in the plasma fatty acid level and/or a decrease in that of branched-chain amino acids would increase the plasma concentration ratio of free tryptophan to branched chain amino acids. This would then favour the entry of tryptophan into the brain, and increase the level of 5-HT which would lead to a decrease in motor drive and a fall in power output. Hence a marked increase in the plasma fatty acid level could lead, via changes in the plasma level of free tryptophan, to fatigue. This could occur in both the middle-distance or marathon runner as the muscle and liver glycogen stores are depleted and the fatty acid is mobilized from adipose tissue.

## Importance of precision in the mobilization and oxidation of fatty acids

The precise balance between the use of the two fuels, glycogen and fatty acids, may be extremely important for the athlete, since too high or too low a rate of fatty acid mobilization/oxidation could cause problems (Newsholme *et al.* 1994). After 20–30 min of exercise, mobilization of fatty acids from adipose tissue increases, probably as a result of sympathetic stimulation. However, despite increased rates of mobilization, the plasma concentration of fatty acids may be only slightly increased: this is because the rates of fatty acid uptake and oxidation by the active muscle are increased (Winder 1996).

It is possible that the plasma fatty acid concentration and therefore the free tryptophan level increases markedly in exercise only in some conditions:
• when the muscle (and liver) glycogen store are totally depleted;
• in unfit subjects, when control of fatty acid mobilization may not be precisely regulated in relation to demand and control of oxidation within the muscle;
• when the rate of fatty acid oxidation by muscle is somewhat restricted by the intermittent nature of the exercise that occurs, in games such as soccer, rugby, tennis, or squash;
• in obese individuals, in whom precision of release may be restricted by the amount of adipose tissue.

If the rate of fatty acid mobilization from adipose tissue is higher than that of oxidation by muscle, the plasma concentration of fatty acids will increase, increasing the free tryptophan level in the plasma, which will result in central fatigue as described above. If the rate of fatty acid oxidation is too low (e.g. if the rate of mobilization is too low), the rate of glycogen oxidation will be high, and the athlete may deplete glycogen stores before the end of the race, resulting in a very poor performance. Thus, the endurance athlete appears to have to run on a metabolic tightrope of fatty acid mobilization/oxidation during the race, and the precise rate of mobilization/oxidation for each athlete must be learnt by training.

A summary of experimental findings which support the hypothesis is as follows.
1 The plasma concentration ratio of free tryptophan/branched-chain amino acids is increased in humans after prolonged exhaustive exercise and, in the rat, the brain levels of tryptophan and 5-HT are increased (Blomstrand *et al.* 1989, 1991a).
2 Administration of a 5-HT agonist impairs running performance, whereas a 5-HT antago-

nist improved running performance in rats (Bailey *et al.* 1992).
3 Administration of a 5-HT re-uptake blocker to human subjects decreased physical performance—exercise time to exhaustion during standardized exercise was decreased in comparison with a control condition (Wilson & Maughan 1992).
4 The secretion of prolactin from the hypothalamus is controlled, in part, by 5-HT neurones, and 5-HT stimulates the rate of secretion. During exercise, there is a correlation between the plasma levels of prolactin and free tryptophan, supporting the view that increased free tryptophan level in the blood can influence the 5-HT level in the hypothalamus (Fischer *et al.* 1991).
5 The blood prolactin level increased to a much smaller extent in well-trained endurance athletes, compared with controls, in response to an agent that increased 5-HT levels in the hypothalamus (e.g. fenfluramine). This could be caused by down-regulation of 5-HT receptors as a result of chronic elevation of the 5-HT level in this part of the brain (Jakeman *et al.* 1994).

In the past few years, supplementary feeding with branched-chain amino acids has produced some results supporting the hypothesis and some which show no effect. The latter are described in more detail by Davis in Chapter 12. Table 11.2 gives a brief comparison of the results from supplementation studies in exercise of which the authors are aware. In one of the most recent studies, a laboratory-based, cross-over study, seven endurance cyclists were monitored for perceived effort and mental fatigue (using the Borg scale), with and without branched-chain amino acid supplementation. When subjects received the branched-chain amino acids, compared with the placebo, there was a lower perception of effort required to sustain the level of exercise required (Blomstrand *et al.* 1997). Mittleman *et al.* (1998) have reported a positive effect of branched-chain amino acids on performance in moderate exercise during heat stress in men and women.

In rats, injection of branched-chain amino acids not only increased the time to fatigue of

**Table 11.2** A comparison of studies on branched-chain amino acid (BCAA) supplementation in humans during endurance exercise.

| No. of subjects | Exercise | $\dot{V}o_{2max.}$ (%) | Duration (min) | Amount of BCAA ingested | p[BCAA] | Effect on $NH_3$ | Effect on performance Mental | Effect on performance Physical | Reference |
|---|---|---|---|---|---|---|---|---|---|
| 13 | Cycling | 40 | c. 137–153 | 12.8 g | 1250 μM | None | None | Improved[a] | Mittleman et al. (1998) |
| 10 | Cycling | 70–75 | c. 122 | 23.4 g | 2400 μM | Rise | N/M | None[b] | van Hall et al. (1995) |
| 10 | Cycling | 70–75 | | 7.8 g | 950 μM | Rise | N/M | None[b] | van Hall et al. (1995) |
| 193ᶜ | Marathon[d] | N/M | c. >210 | 16 g | 1250 μM | N/M | Improved | Improved[e] | Blomstrand et al. (1991a) |
| 25ᶜ | 30-km run[d] | | | | | | | | |
| 5 | Cycling | 75 | 60–80 | 6.3 g.l⁻¹ | 1000 μM | N/M | N/M | None | Blomstrand et al. (1995) |
| 10 | Cycling | 72.7 | 50–60 | 16 g.day⁻¹ᵍ | N/M | N/M | N/M | Improved | Hefler et al. (1995) |
| 7 | Cycling | 65–75 | c. 30 | 30 g | 3000 μM | Rise | N/M | None | Wagenmakers (1992) |
| 6 | Soccer[d] | N/M | | 10 gᶠ | 1200 μM | N/M | Improved | N/M | Blomstrand et al. (1991b) |
| 52 | 30-km run[d] | N/M | 145 | 5.3 gʰ | 650 μM | N/M | Improved | N/M | Hassmen et al. (1994) |
| 10 | Cycling | 70 | c. 230 | 0.74 g.l⁻¹ᶠ | 420 μM | N/M | N/M | None | Galiano et al. (1991) |
| 7 | Cycling | 70 | 60 | 6–9 g | 1050 μM | None | Improved | Improved | Blomstrand et al. (1997) |
| 9 | Cycling[i] | 63.1 | c. 159 | 18 gʲ | 1026 μM | Rise | N/M | None | Madsen et al. (1996) |
| 10 | Cycling | N/M | c. 125–212 | 21 g | c.1250 μM | Rise | Improved | None | Struder et al. (1998) |

N/M, not measured; p[BCAA], the peak plasma concentration of branched-chain amino acids observed in each study.
a Subjects experienced heat stress.
b Very high day-to-day intraindividual variation in time to fatigue for some subjects.
c Not all subjects gave blood samples.
d Field study.
e In subset of slower runners.
f 6% carbohydrate added.
g 14-day study.
h 7% carbohydrate added.
i 100-km trials.
j 5% carbohydrate added.

exercising rats but also prevented the normal increase in brain tryptophan level caused by exhaustive exercise (T. Yamamoto, personal communication). Calders *et al.* (1997) observed an increase in the time to fatigue, as well as an increase in plasma ammonia, in fasting rats injected with 30 mg of branched-chain amino acids 5 min before exercise, compared to those injected with placebo.

The data in Table 11.2 indicate that administration of branched-chain amino acids alone appears to have a more beneficial effect than when added to carbohydrate. It also seems that the higher the dose of branched-chain amino acids, the more likely it is that plasma ammonia levels will be elevated. This suggests that lower doses are more likely to be beneficial. In the majority of studies, the branched-chain amino acids have been administered before exercise. It may be that administration during exercise was the reason that Blomstrand *et al.* (1997) and Mittleman *et al.* (1998) failed to observe a change in plasma ammonia. Whether a bolus dose is given or whether separate doses are given during exercise could be important for the release of ammonia from muscle.

In conclusion, beneficial effects of branched-chain amino acids have been seen on aspects of both mental and physical fatigue in exhaustive exercise. Most studies have not investigated effects on mental fatigue. However, the mental exertion necessary to maintain a given power output is an integral feature of central fatigue.

## Cellular nutrition in the immune system

For many years, it was thought that both lymphocytes and macrophages obtained most of their energy from the oxidation of glucose. However, it has now been shown that these cells also use glutamine and that its rate of utilization is either similar to or greater than that of glucose. There are clear lines of evidence which support the view that glutamine is used at a very high rate by lymphocytes and by macrophages *in vivo*.
1 The maximal catalytic activity of glutaminase,

the key enzyme in the glutamine utilization pathway, is high in freshly isolated resting lymphocytes and macrophages (Ardawi & Newsholme 1983, 1985).
2 The rates of utilization of glutamine are high: (i) in freshly isolated lymphocytes and macrophages (Ardawi & Newsholme 1983, 1985) and (ii) in cultured lymphocytes and macrophages, and in T- and B-lymphocyte-derived cell lines (Ardawi & Newsholme 1983, 1985; Newsholme *et al.* 1988).
3 A high rate of glutamine utilization by lymphocytes *in vitro* maintains unusually high intracellular concentrations of glutamine, glutamate, aspartate and lactate. Very similar levels of these intermediates are seen in intact lymph nodes removed from anaesthetized rats and frozen rapidly prior to extraction of the tissues (T. Piva and E.A. Newsholme, unpublished data).

In addition, although various lymphocyte subsets have not been studied, the available evidence suggests that B- and T-lymphocytes utilize glutamine at similar rates (Ardawi & Newsholme 1983, 1985; Newsholme *et al.* 1988).

Surprisingly, little of the carbon of glucose (<10%) and only some of that of glutamine (10–30%) is oxidized completely by these cells: glucose is converted almost totally into lactate, glutamine into glutamate, aspartate, alanine and $CO_2$. The partial oxidation of these fuels is known as glycolysis and glutaminolysis, respectively. From these simple metabolic characteristics several questions arise.
1 What is the significance of these high rates?
2 Why is the oxidation only partial?
3 What are the consequences for the whole organism?
4 Does the plasma glutamine level ever decrease sufficiently to decrease the rate of such utilization by these cells, and hence decrease their ability to respond to an immune challenge?

High rates of glycolysis and glutaminolysis will provide energy for these cells. In addition, glutamine provides nitrogen for synthesis of several important compounds, e.g. purine and pyrimidine nucleotides, which are needed for the synthesis of new DNA and RNA during proliferation of lymphocytes and for mRNA synthesis and DNA repair in macrophages. This will also be important for the production of these and other cells in the bone marrow, especially when stimulated to increase their production during trauma, infection, burns and if white cells are damaged, for example, during exercise. However, when it has been quantitatively studied — so far, only in lymphocytes — the rate of glutaminolysis is very markedly in excess of the rates of synthesis of these compounds. For example, the rate of utilization of glutamine by lymphocytes is very much greater than the measured rate of synthesis of uridine nucleotides and much higher than the maximum activity of the rate limiting enzyme, carbamoyl phosphate synthase II (Newsholme & Leech 1999).

A theory has been proposed which accounts both for these high rates of glutamine utilization and the fact that its oxidation is partial. The synthetic pathways for *de novo* nucleotide synthesis require specific and precise increases in the rate of synthesis of these nucleotides during the proliferative process. This theory is known as *branched point sensitivity* and has been discussed in detail elsewhere (Newsholme *et al.* 1985). The important point to emerge from this is that glutamine (and glucose) must be used at a high rate by some of the cells of the immune system even when they are quiescent, since an immune challenge can occur at any time so that cells must be 'primed' to respond whenever there is an invasion by a foreign organism. This requires glutamine to be available in the bloodstream at a fairly constant level. Furthermore, if pyruvate produced from glutamine were fully oxidized via the Krebs cycle, the cells might produce too much ATP, and this could lead to inhibition of the rates of glutaminolysis and branched-point sensitivity would be lost. Consistent with the branched-point sensitivity theory, it has been shown that a decrease in the glutamine concentration in culture medium below that normally present in plasma decreases the maximum rate of proliferation and slows the response to a mitogenic signal in both human and rat lymphocytes, even though they are provided with all other nutrients and growth factors in excess (Parry-Billings *et al.* 1990b). In addition, a decrease in glutamine concentration also decreased phagocytosis and the rate of cytokine production by macrophages.

Several tissues, including liver, muscle, adipose and lung, can synthesize and release glutamine into the bloodstream. This is important, since 50–60% of the glutamine that enters the body via protein in the diet is utilized by the intestine. Thus, the glutamine required by other tissues, including the immune system, must be synthesized within the body. Quantitatively, the most important tissue for synthesis, storage and release of glutamine is thought to be skeletal muscle. As much glutamine is stored in muscle as glycogen is stored in liver, and the rate of release across the plasma membrane, which occurs via a specific transporter, appears to be controlled by various hormones (Newsholme & Parry-Billings 1990). Because of the importance of glutamine for cells of the immune system, it is suggested that immune cells may communicate with skeletal muscle to regulate the rate of glutamine release. This may also involve some cytokines and glucocorticoids.

The plasma concentration of glutamine is decreased in conditions such as major surgery (Powell *et al.* 1994); burns (Stinnett *et al.* 1982; Parry-Billings *et al.* 1990b); starvation (Marliss *et al.* 1971); sepsis (Clowes *et al.* 1980; Roth *et al.* 1982). There is also evidence that the immune system is suppressed in clinical trauma (Baker *et al.* 1980; Green & Faist 1988). The requirement for glutamine, synthesized within muscle and other cells, will therefore be increased in these conditions, since there will be increased activity of the immune system, and an increased number of cells involved in proliferation and repair. Similarly, damage caused to muscle by prolonged, exhaustive exercise will also lead to a greater demand for glutamine. Although the plasma glutamine concentration is increased in athletes undertaking short-term exercise (Decombaz *et al.* 1979), it is decreased in prolonged, exhaustive exercise (Poortmans *et al.* 1974; Castell *et al.* 1996) and in overtraining (Parry-Billings 1989; Parry-

Billings *et al.* 1990a; Rowbottom *et al.* 1996; see also Budgett *et al.* 1998).

In a study on athletes with the overtraining syndrome (Parry-Billings 1989), the plasma concentrations of alanine and branched-chain amino acids were similar in trained and overtrained athletes. However, the plasma concentration of glutamine was lower in overtrained athletes compared with that in trained athletes and the concentration in trained subjects was lower than in recreational runners (Parry-Billings *et al.* 1990a). Moreover, after a 6-week recovery period, despite a significant improvement in the exercise performance of these subjects, the plasma glutamine concentration remained below control values. This suggests that immunodepression due to overtraining may persist for longer periods than indicated by the decrease in physical performance.

Exercise-induced immunodepression has been demonstrated in a large number of different types of athletes, including runners, swimmers, skiers (Noakes 1992) and ballet dancers (Sun *et al.* 1988). It is therefore suggested that intense, prolonged exercise, particularly if it is undertaken regularly, can cause a marked decrease in the plasma glutamine level, and that this might result in immunodepression. Can muscle, together with other tissues, always respond sufficiently to release enough glutamine to maintain the normal blood concentration? This may be a particularly relevant question if muscle is damaged due to excessive exercise. However, the reason for the decrease in the plasma glutamine concentration in longer term, strenuous exercise is not understood.

Enzymes which are normally localized in muscle fibres appear in the blood and are assumed to be evidence of disruption or increased permeability of the muscle cell membranes (Altland & Highman 1961; Newham *et al.* 1983). The occurrence of muscle damage after prolonged exercise has been reported by Appell *et al.* (1992), who observed increased levels of circulating complement anaphylotoxin, which is a likely result of tissue damage. Tiidus and Ianuzzo (1983) observed that the extent of injury

is proportional to the intensity of exercise. Muscle injuries have been found to be widespread in military personnel during strenuous training (Greenberg & Arneson 1967; Armstrong 1986).

Although it might be hypothesized that the marked decrease in plasma glutamine after prolonged exhaustive exercise could be due to an inhibition of the glutamine release mechanism, it seems unlikely, since increased non-specific permeability of muscle cell membranes would be expected to lead to greater release of glutamine from muscle. The possibility arises that muscle damage caused by prolonged exercise presents an area of tissue which is larger than normal, to which immune cells might migrate (see Galun *et al.* 1987; Pabst & Binns 1989, 1992). As the numbers of these cells increase, activity increases and/or proliferation of some cells may result which, in turn, increases the local demand for glutamine. It is suggested that failure of muscle to provide enough glutamine could result in an impairment of the function of the immune system via lack of precision for the regulation of, for example, the rates of purine and pyrimidine nucleotide synthesis for DNA and RNA formation in lymphocytes (Newsholme 1994). It can be speculated that excessive damage could produce resistance to the proposed stimulatory effect of cytokines and glucocorticoids on glutamine release, e.g. by a reduction in the number of cytokine receptors and/or glucocorticoid receptors on muscle.

## Glutamine feeding in clinical situations

Over many years, there has been considerable physiological interest in the phenomenon of hypoglycaemia, since this can cause abnormal function of the brain, which is normally dependent upon glucose as a fuel. Similar considerations should be applied to the maintenance of the plasma glutamine level, which can be considered to be as important a plasma fuel as that of glucose, but for different cells. Furthermore, the requirement for glutamine, synthesized within muscle and other cells, will increase after prolonged exhaustive exercise, since there will be increased activity of the immune system, and an increased number of cells involved in proliferation to carry out the necessary repair. The question therefore arises as to whether extra glutamine should be provided after exhaustive exercise.

Evidence that both parenteral and enteral glutamine feeding can have beneficial effects comes from several clinical studies: of particular relevance to this chapter is the evidence that glutamine has a beneficial effect upon some cells of the immune system in the patients investigated (Table 11.3).

## Exercise, infections and immunodepression

### Strenuous exercise and upper respiratory tract infections

Upper respiratory tract infections (URTI) occur frequently in athletes after prolonged, exhaustive exercise compared with the normal seden-

**Table 11.3** Some beneficial effects of glutamine feeding upon the immune system.

| Recipients | Clinical situation | Method of feeding | Beneficial effects | Reference |
|---|---|---|---|---|
| Humans | Bone marrow transplant | TPN (L-glutamine) | Decreased number of positive microbial cultures | Ziegler et al. 1992, 1998 |
| | | | Decreased number of clinical infections | |
| | | | Enhanced recovery of circulating lymphocytes, total T-lymphocytes, CD4 helper, CD8 suppressor | |
| Humans | Colorectal cancer | TPN (glycyl-glutamine dipeptide) | Enhanced postoperative T-lymphocyte DNA synthesis | O'Riordain et al. 1994 |
| Humans | Severe, acute pancreatitis | TPN (glycyl-glutamine dipeptide) | Enhanced T-cell response, decreased interleukin 8 production | O'Riordain et al. 1996 |
| Rats | Healthy, suppressed biliary immunoglobulin A | TPN (L-glutamine) | Increased biliary concentration of immunoglobulin A normally suppressed by TPN | Burke et al. 1989 |
| Rats | Tumour-bearing | TPN (alanyl-glutamine dipeptide) | Increased phagocytic activity of alveolar macrophages | Kweon et al. 1991 |
| Rats | Tumour-bearing | Oral | Increased mitogenic response in splenocytes, increased NK cell numbers in spleen but not activity | Shewchuk et al. 1997 |
| Rats | Sepsis | TPN (alanyl-glutamine dipeptide) | Increased rate of lymphocyte proliferation and increased number of lymphocytes | Yoshida et al. 1992 |
| Rats | Chemotherapy | Oral | Decreased sepsis defined as decreased white blood cell count plus decreased positive blood cultures | Klimberg et al. 1992 |

TPN, total parenteral nutrition.

tary population or with non-competing athletes (Linde 1987; Fitzgerald 1991; Brenner *et al.* 1994; Nieman 1994a; Weidner 1994). For example, in a study on participants in the Los Angeles marathon who did not have an infection before the race, the number of runners who became ill during the week after the race was almost sixfold higher than that of the control group. The control group comprised endurance athletes who had undergone a similar level of training but who did not participate in the marathon (Nieman *et al.* 1990). A high incidence of infections has also been observed in military personnel undergoing prolonged and repeated intensive training (Lee 1992; Gray *et al.* 1994).

It has been suggested that moderate, regular exercise helps to reduce the level of infection in sedentary individuals but that, in individuals who undertake intensive or excessive training, the incidence of infection can increase sharply. An overall view of this situation has been graphically described by a 'J-curve' (Fig. 11.2) which is emphasized as being descriptive, rather than quantitative (Nieman 1994a).

RISK FACTORS FOR
UPPER RESPIRATORY TRACT INFECTION

Weidner (1994) critically evaluated 10 epi-

demiological studies which have investigated the incidence of URTI in different sports. The majority of the studies which showed an increased incidence of URTI after physical activity have been performed on runners. A longitudinal study on 530 male and female runners suggested that an URTI was more likely to occur with higher training mileage (Heath *et al.* 1991). Similarly, the risk of illness increased in endurance runners when training exceeded 97 $km \cdot week^{-1}$ (Nieman 1994b). Another study, on marathon runners, demonstrated that the stress of competition more than doubled the risk of getting an URTI (O'Connor *et al.* 1979). A low body mass may be another risk factor for infections (Heath *et al.* 1991).

One problem associated with prolonged exercise is that athletes start at some point to breathe through the mouth rather than through the nose, thus bypassing the nasal filter mechanism (Niinima *et al.* 1980). This dries up bronchial secretions, thus impeding the protective activity of the cilia which cover the cell surface with mucous (Rylander 1968). The high incidence of infections after prolonged, exhaustive exercise suggests therefore that immunodepression may occur in some athletes due to the stress of hard training and/or competition.

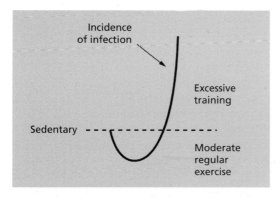

**Fig. 11.2** The incidence of infection in sedentary individuals can be decreased with moderate exercise but increases sharply in individuals who undertake excessive amounts of exercise, or who suffer from over-training. From Nieman (1994a), with permission.

### Immune response to exhaustive exercise

There is evidence that numbers of circulating white blood cells and subsets, together with cytokine levels, are markedly altered as a result of prolonged, exhaustive exercise. A substantial increase in numbers of circulating white blood cells, mainly due to a large increase in circulating neutrophils, was first observed by Larrabee (1902). Despite earlier reports of leucocytosis and, particularly, an increase in circulating numbers of neutrophils, relatively little work has been undertaken on this phenomenon until the past few years. Recently, however, several publications have reported not only that the total number of white blood cells in the circulation are substantially increased during the recovery period immediately after a marathon or intensive training session but that numbers of lymphocytes in the circulation decrease below pre-exercise levels during the recovery period and lymphocyte proliferation is impaired (*see* Fry *et al.* 1992; Haq *et al.* 1993; Nieman 1994a, 1994b; Castell & Newsholme 1998). There is now also considerable evidence that prolonged, exhaustive exercise is associated with adverse effects on immune function (for reviews, see Brenner *et al.* 1994; Shinkai *et al.* 1994; Nieman 1997; Pedersen *et al.* 1998).

These effects include:
• decreased cytolytic activity of natural killer cells;
• lower circulating numbers of T-lymphocytes for 3–4 h after exercise;
• a decrease in the proliferative ability of lymphocytes;
• impaired antibody synthesis;
• decreased immunoglobulin levels in blood and saliva;
• a decreased ratio of CD4 to CD8 cells.

In contrast, it has been suggested that low-intensity exercise is beneficial for the immune system (Fitzgerald 1988; Nieman 1994a, 1994b). Nehlsen-Cannarella *et al.* (1991) reported a 20% increase in serum immunoglobulins and a decrease in circulating T-cell numbers in mildly obese women after 6 weeks of brisk walking. Natural killer cell activity is enhanced by moderate exercise (Pedersen & Ullum 1994).

Hack *et al.* (1997) reported a correlation between a decreased plasma glutamine concentration and circulating levels of CD4 cells after 8 weeks of anaerobic training. Rohde *et al.* (1996), in *in vitro* studies on T-cell derived cytokines, found that glutamine influenced the production of the cytokines interleukin 2 and γ-interferon. In a study on triathletes, they also found that a time course of changes in serum glutamine correlated with changes in lymphokine-activated killer cell activities.

If, as indicated above, glutamine is important for the immune system, then provision of glutamine might be beneficial for athletes at particular times during their training.

## GLUTAMINE FEEDING AFTER PROLONGED EXHAUSTIVE EXERCISE

Since the plasma concentration of glutamine is decreased by approximately 25% in endurance runners after a marathon as well as in clinical conditions, a series of studies was undertaken in which glutamine was administered. The first study established a suitable glutamine dose and timing in resting, normal subjects (Castell & Newsholme 1997). The results showed that glutamine (at concentrations of $0.1\,g \cdot kg^{-1}$ body weight and 5 g per subject), given as a drink, significantly increased the plasma glutamine concentration within 30 min in healthy humans. This level returned to close to baseline levels after approximately 2 h.

The effect of giving glutamine or a placebo after exercise was subsequently investigated in full and ultramarathon runners. Glutamine (5 g L-glutamine (GlutaminOx5, Oxford Nutrition Ltd) in 330 ml mineral water) or placebo (maltodextrin) was given to athletes on a double-blind basis after prolonged, exhaustive exercise. Athletes were asked to take two drinks (glutamine/placebo), the first drink immediately after exercise and the second drink 1 or 2 h after exercise. This timing was chosen as a result of information obtained from the glutamine feeding studies in normal subjects. Blood samples were also taken after exercise, before and after a glutamine or placebo drink. In addition to measurement of plasma glutamine and cytokine concentrations and acute phase markers, numbers of leucocytes and lymphocytes (for details, see Castell *et al.* 1996) were measured before and after the drinks, as well as CD4 and CD8 cells (Castell & Newsholme 1997). The plasma concentrations of glutamine and branched-chain amino acids were decreased (23% and 26%, respectively) 1 h after the marathon but had returned to normal the next morning (Castell *et al.* 1997). The number of leucocytes tripled in the blood samples taken from runners immediately after the marathon. This leucocytosis, due mainly to a substantial increase in numbers of neutrophils, was sustained in the sample taken at 1 h postexercise. A substantial decrease, to below baseline, was observed in numbers of circulating T-cells 1 h after exhaustive exercise. However, there was a 30% decrease in total lymphocytes at the same time point. There was no significant difference in leucocyte or lymphocyte numbers between the glutamine and the placebo group. The provision of glutamine appeared to have a beneficial effect upon the ratio of CD4 to CD8 T-cells (Castell & Newsholme 1997). A decrease in this ratio has been suggested as being a possible cause and indicator of immunosuppression in athletes (Nash 1986; Keast et al. 1988; Shepherd et al. 1991).

Questionnaires were given during the studies to establish the incidence of infection for 7 days after exercise (for details, see Castell et al. 1996). Completed questionnaires on the incidence of infection were received from more than 200 individuals in 14 studies, who participated in rowing, or endurance or middle-distance running. The levels of infection were lowest in middle-distance runners, and were highest in runners after a full or ultramarathon and in elite rowers after a period of intensive training (Table 11.4). The majority of the infections reported were URTIs. Athletes who consumed two drinks, containing either glutamine or a placebo, immediately after and 2 h after a marathon, also completed 7-day questionnaires ($n=151$). Overall, the level of infections reported by the glutamine group was considerably less than that reported

by the placebo group (Table 11.5). A simple explanation for the effects of glutamine observed in these studies may be the fact that its provision after prolonged exercise might make more glutamine available for key cells of the immune system at a critical time for induction of infection.

This series of studies provide more evidence for the fact that prolonged, exhaustive exercise such as a marathon produces a response which is analogous to some aspects of the acute phase response. Increases were demonstrated in acute phase response markers, such as C-reactive protein, interleukin 6 and complement C5a in blood samples taken after a marathon race (Castell et al. 1997). An increase in the activation of complement indicates enhanced macrophage activity which may be involved in clearance of fragments from damaged muscle tissue. The fourfold increase in the plasma concentration of C-reactive protein, observed 16 h after the race, is consistent with damage to muscle after prolonged, exhaustive exercise.

The studies also confirm observations made by others (for reviews, see Brenner et al. 1994; Nieman 1994a; Shinkai et al. 1994), viz. that, after marathon running, decreases occurred in the numbers of some circulating immune cells which were sustained until at least the next day (Castell et al. 1997). In one glutamine feeding study in this series, the numbers of circulating lymphocytes,

**Table 11.4** Incidence of infections in athletes during 7 days after different types of exercise (mean values ±SEM). After Castell et al. (1996a), with permission.

| Event | No. of studies | No. of participants | Infections (%) |
|---|---|---|---|
| Marathon | 5 | 88 | 46.8±4.8 |
| Ultramarathon | 2 | 40 | 43.3±4.8 |
| Mid-distance race | 3 | 41 | 24.7±4.0 |
| Rowing | 4 | 45 | 54.5±7.8 |

**Table 11.5** Overall incidence of infections during 7 days for athletes given either glutamine or placebo after running a marathon (mean values ±SEM). After Castell et al. (1996a), with permission.

| | No. of participants | No. of participants with no reported infections | Participants with no reported infections (%) |
|---|---|---|---|
| Glutamine | 72 | 57 | 80.8±4.2* |
| Placebo | 79 | 31 | 48.8±7.4 |

*Statistical significance between glutamine and placebo groups ($P<0.001$).

which decreased 1h after a marathon, were restored next morning to baseline levels in the glutamine group, compared with the placebo group (Castell *et al.* 1997). In another of these studies, white blood cells and neutrophils were elevated after a marathon, but were closer to baseline levels ($P < 0.05$ and $< 0.001$, respectively) the next morning in the glutamine group compared with the placebo group. For future studies, it would be of interest to take samples at daily intervals after a marathon in order to monitor immune cell function, since the effect of a viral attack should be manifest within 2–3 days of running a marathon.

No increase in the plasma concentration of glutamine was observed in samples from those marathon runners who received glutamine drinks after the race. However, for logistical reasons, blood samples were not taken until an hour after glutamine feeding, whereas the peak concentration of plasma glutamine after a bolus dose at rest occurred at 30min (Castell & Newsholme 1997). Glutamine supplementation in the doses used, and at the times ingested after this series of marathon studies, appeared to modify the incidence of URTI and to effect two or three changes in concentrations of acute phase response markers or in circulating cell populations.

An important issue is whether measurements of the numbers and activities of leucocytes in the blood properly reflect the performance of the immune system in the whole body. In human studies, it is the only measurable link we have with the much larger number of cells in the whole immune system but the authors are aware of the dangers of overinterpretation of these data. The safety and efficacy of glutamine feeding have been discussed by Ziegler *et al.* (1990). There are now more than 120 published reports on glutamine feeding studies: no problems of toxicity have been reported. It is suggested that, in situations where plasma glutamine levels in individuals are low, provision of exogenous glutamine is a safe and simple method of restoring physiological levels. This might enhance the functional ability of cells of the immune system, as well as improving the digestive and defence mechanisms of the intestine, both for the patient and the athlete.

## Conclusion

In summary, the picture which emerges from these studies is that infection levels are higher in athletes undergoing exhaustive exercise of long duration than in those undertaking shorter or more moderate exercise. Glutamine concentration in the blood is decreased more by prolonged, exhaustive exercise than by anaerobic/aerobic or moderate exercise. More marked leucocytosis and subsequent decrease in lymphocytes occurs as a result of prolonged, exhaustive exercise than anaerobic/aerobic or moderate exercise. The decreases tend to occur at similar times and within 3–4h after prolonged, exhaustive exercise: this creates an opportunity for apparent immunosuppression to occur, which may coincide with exposure to viral or bacterial agents. The net result is an increase in the number of infections, which appears to be modified by glutamine feeding.

Much more work needs to be done, preferably in well-controlled field studies, to obtain a more accurate picture of precisely how glutamine might be affecting the levels of infection perceived in athletes after prolonged, exhaustive exercise.

## Acknowledgements

The authors are indebted to the subjects for their willing participation in the studies, and to Professor Jacques Poortmans for his helpful comments on this chapter.

## References

Altland, P.D. & Highman, B. (1961) Effects of exercise on serum enzyme values and tissues of rats. *American Journal of Physiology* **201**, 393–395.

Appell, H.J., Soares, J.M.C. & Duarte, J.A.R. (1992) Exercise, muscle damage and fatigue. *Sports Medicine* **13**, 108–115.

Ardawi, M.S.M. & Newsholme, E.A. (1983) Glutamine

metabolism in lymphocytes of the rat. *Biochemical Journal* **212**, 835–842.

Ardawi, M.S.M. & Newsholme, E.A. (1985) Metabolism in lymphocytes and its importance in the immune response. *Essays in Biochemistry* **21**, 1–44.

Armstrong, R.B. (1986) Muscle damage and endurance events. *Sports Medicine* **3**, 370–381.

Bailey, S.P., Davis, J.M. & Ahlborn, E.N. (1992) Effect of increased brain serotonergic activity on endurance performance in the rat. *Acta Physiologica Scandinavica* **145**, 75–76.

Baker, C.C., Oppenheimer, L., Stephens, B., Lewis, F.R. & Trunkey, D.D. (1980) Epidemiology of trauma deaths. *American Journal of Surgery* **140**, 144–150.

Blomstrand, E., Perrett, D., Parry-Billings, M. & Newsholme, E.A. (1989) Effect of sustained exercise on plasma amino acid concentrations and on 5-hydroxytryptamine metabolism in six different brain regions in the rat. *Acta Physiologica Scandinavica* **136**, 473–481.

Blomstrand, E., Hassmen, P. & Newsholme, E.A. (1991a) Administration of branched-chain amino acids during sustained exercise: effects on performance and on the plasma concentration of some amino acids. *European Journal of Applied Physiology* **63**, 83–88.

Blomstrand, E., Hassmen, P. & Newsholme, E.A. (1991b) Effects of branched-chain amino acid supplementation on mental performance. *Acta Physiologica Scandinavica* **143**, 225–226.

Blomstrand, E., Andersson, S., Hassmen, P., Ekblom, B. & Newsholme, E.A. (1995) Effect of branched-chain amino acid and carbohydrate supplementation on the exercise-induced change in plasma and muscle concentration of amino acids in human subjects. *Acta Physiologica Scandinavica* **153**, 87–96.

Blomstrand, E., Hassmen, P., Ek, S., Ekblom, B. & Newsholme, E.A. (1997) Influence of ingesting a solution of branched-chain amino acids on perceived exertion during exercise. *Acta Physiologica Scandinavica* **159**, 41–49.

Brenner, I.K.M., Shek, P.N. & Shephard, R.J. (1994) Infection in athletes. *Sports Medicine* **17**, 86–107.

Budgett, R., Castell, L.M. & Newsholme, E.A. (1998) The overtraining syndrome. In *Oxford Textbook for Sports Medicine* (ed. M. Harries), pp. 367–377. Oxford University Press, Oxford.

Burke, D.J., Alverdy, J.A., Aoys, E. & Moss, G.S. (1989) Glutamine-supplemented total parenteral nutrition improves gut immune function. *Archives of Surgery* **124**, 1396–1399.

Calders, P., Pannier, J.-L., Matthys, D.M. & Lacroix, E.M. (1997) Pre-exercise branched-chain amino acid administration increases endurance performance in rats. *Medicine and Science in Sports and Exercise* **29**, 1182–1186.

Castell, L.M. & Newsholme, E.A. (1997) The effects of oral glutamine supplementation upon athletes after prolonged, exhaustive exercise. *Nutrition* **13**, 738–742.

Castell, L.M. & Newsholme, E.A. (1998) Glutamine and the effects of exhaustive exercise upon the immune response. *Canadian Journal of Physiology and Pharmacology* **76**, 524–532.

Castell, L.M., Poortmans, J. & Newsholme, E.A. (1996) Does glutamine have a role in reducing infections in athletes? *European Journal of Applied Physiology* **73**, 488–491.

Castell, L.M., Poortmans, J.R., Leclercq, R., Brasseur, M., Duchateau, J. & Newsholme, E.A. (1997) Some aspects of the acute phase response after a marathon race, and the effects of glutamine supplementation. *European Journal of Applied Physiology* **75**, 47–53.

Clowes, G.A., Heiderman, M., Lundberg, B. *et al.* (1980) Effects of parenteral alimentation on amino acid metabolism in septic patients. *Surgery* **88**, 531–543.

Decombaz, J., Reinhardt, P., Anantharaman, K., von Glutz, G. & Poortmans, J.R. (1979) Biochemical changes in a 100 km run: free amino acids, urea and creatinine. *European Journal of Applied Physiology* **41**, 61–72.

Fernstrom, J.D. (1990) Aromatic amino acids and monamine synthesis in the CNS: influence of the diet. *Journal of Nutrition and Biochemistry* **1**, 508–517.

Fischer, H.G., Hollman, W. & De Meirleir, K. (1991) Exercise changes in plasma tryptophan fractions and relationship with prolactin. *International Journal of Sports Medicine* **12**, 487–489.

Fitts, R.H. (1994) Cellular mechanisms of muscle fatigue. *Physiological Reviews* **74**, 49–94.

Fitzgerald, L. (1988) Exercise and the immune system. *Immunology Today* **9**, 337–339.

Fitzgerald, L. (1991) Overtraining increases the susceptibility to infection. *International Journal of Sports Medicine* **12**, 55–58.

Fry, R.W., Morton, A.R., Crawford, G.P.M. & Keast, D. (1992) Cell numbers and *in vitro* responses of leucocytes and lymphocyte subpopulations following maximal exercise and interval training sessions of different intensities. *European Journal of Applied Physiology* **64**, 218–227.

Galiano, F.J., Davis, J.M., Bailey, S.P., Woods, J.A. & Hamilton, M. (1991) Physiologic, endocrine and performance effects of adding branch chain amino acids to a 6% carbohydrate-electrolyte beverage during prolonged cycling. *Medicine and Science in Sports and Exercise* **23**, S14.

Galun, E., Burstein, R. & Assia, E. (1987) Changes of white blood cell count during prolonged exercise. *International Journal of Sports Medicine* **8**, 253–255.

Gray, G.C., Mitchell, B.S., Tueller, J.E. *et al.* (1994) Adult pneumonia hospitalizations in the US Navy: rates and risk factors for 6522 admissions, 1981–91. *American Journal of Epidemiology* **139**, 793–802.

Green, D.R. & Faist, E. (1988) Trauma and the immune response. *Immunology Today* **9**, 253–255.

Greenberg, J. & Arneson, L. (1967) Exertional rhabdomyolosis with myoglobinuria in a large group of military trainees. *Neurology* **17**, 216–222.

Hack, V., Weiss, C., Friedmann, B. *et al.* (1997) Decreased plasma glutamine level and $CD_4^+$ T cell number in response to 8 wk of anaerobic training. *American Journal of Physiology* **272**, E788–E795.

Haq, A., Al-Hussein, K., Lee, J. & Al-Sedairy, S. (1993) Changes in peripheral blood lymphocyte subsets associated with marathon running. *Medicine and Science in Sports and Exercise* **25**, 186–190.

Hassmen, P., Blomstrand, E., Ekblom, B. & Newsholme, E.A. (1994) Branched-chain amino acid supplementation during 30-km competitive run: mood and cognitive performance. *Nutrition* **10**, 405–410.

Heath, G.W., Ford, E.S., Craven, T.E., Macera, C.A., Jackson, K.L. & Pate, R.R. (1991) Exercise and the incidence of upper respiratory tract infections. *Medicine and Science in Sports and Exercise* **23**, 152–157.

Hefler, S.K., Wideman, L., Gaesser, G.A. & Weltman, A. (1995) Branched-chain amino acid supplementation improves endurance performance in competitive cyclists. *Medicine and Science in Sports and Exercise* **27** (Suppl.), S5.

Jakeman, P.M., Hawthorne, J.E., Maxwell, S.R., Kendall, M.J. & Holder, G. (1994) Evidence for downregulation of hypothalamic 5-hydroxytryptamine receptor function in endurance-trained athletes. *Experimental Physiology* **79**, 461–464.

Keast, D., Cameron, K. & Morton, A.R. (1988) Exercise and immune response. *Sports Medicine* **5**, 248–267.

Klimberg, V.S., Nwokedi, E., Hutchins, L.F. *et al.* (1992) Glutamine facilitates chemotherapy while reducing toxicity. *Journal of Parenteral and Enteral Nutrition* **16**, 83–87S.

Kweon, M.N., Moriguchi, S., Mukai, K. & Kishino, Y. (1991) Effect of alanylglutamine-enriched infusion on tumor growth and cellular immune function in rats. *Amino Acids* **1**, 7–16.

Larrabee, R.C. (1902) Leucocytosis after violent exercise. *Journal of Medicine Research* **2**, 76–82.

Lee, D.J. (1992) Immune responsiveness and risk of illness in US Air Force Academy recruits during basic recruit training. *Aviation Space and Environmental Medicine* **63**, 517–523.

Linde, F. (1987) Running and upper respiratory tract infections. *Scandinavian Journal of Sports Science* **9**, 21–23.

Madsen, K., MacLean, D.A., Kiens, B. & Christensen, D. (1996) Effects of glucose, glucose plus branchedchain amino acids, or placebo on bike performance over 100 km. *Journal of Applied Physiology* **81**, 2644–2650.

Marliss, E.B., Aoki, T.T., Pozefsky, T., Most, A.S. & Cahill, G.F. (1971) Muscle and splanchnic glutamine metabolism in postabsorptive and starved men. *Journal of Clinical Investigation* **50**, 814–817.

Mittleman, K.D., Ricci, M.R. & Bailey, S.P. (1998) Branched-chain amino acids prolong exercise during heat stress in men and women. *Medicine and Science in Sports and Exercise* **30**, 83–91.

Nash, H.L. (1986) Can exercise make us immune to disease? *Physician and Sportsmedicine* **14**, 251–253.

Nehlsen-Cannarella, S.L., Nieman, D., Balk-Lamberton, A.J. *et al.* (1991) The effects of moderate exercise training on immune response. *Medicine and Science in Sports and Exercise* **23**, 64–70.

Newham, D.H., Jones, D.A. & Edwards, R.H.T. (1983) Large delayed plasma creatine kinase changes after stepping exercise. *Muscle and Nerve* **6**, 380–385.

Newsholme, E.A. (1994) Biochemical mechanisms to explain immunosuppression. *International Journal of Sports Medicine* **15**, S142–S147.

Newsholme, E.A. & Leech, A.R. (1999) *Biochemistry for the Medical Sciences*. John Wiley & Sons, Chichester (in press).

Newsholme, E.A. & Parry-Billings, M. (1990) Properties of glutamine release from muscle and its importance for the immune system. *Journal of Parenteral and Enteral Nutrition* **14**, 63–67S.

Newsholme, E.A., Crabtree, B. & Ardawi, M.S.M. (1985) Glutamine metabolism in lymphocytes: its biochemical, physiological and clinical importance. *Quarterly Journal of Experimental Physiology* **70**, 473–489.

Newsholme, E.A., Newsholme, P., Curi, R. *et al.* (1988) A role for muscle in the immune system and its importance in surgery, trauma, sepsis and burns. *Nutrition* **4**, 261–268.

Newsholme, E.A., Leech, A.R. & Duester, G. (1994) *Keep on Running*. Wiley, Chichester.

Nieman, D. (1994a) Exercise, infection, and immunity. *International Journal of Sports Medicine* **15**, S131–141.

Nieman, D. (1994b) Exercise, upper respiratory tract infection and the immune system. *Medicine and Science in Sports and Exercise* **26**, 128–139.

Nieman, D. (1997) Immune response to heavy exertion. *Journal of Applied Physiology* **82**, 1385–1394.

Nieman, D., Johanssen, L.M., Lee, J.W. & Arabatzis, K. (1990) Infectious episodes before and after the Los Angeles marathon. *Journal of Sports Medicine and Physical Fitness* **30**, 289–296.

Niinima, V., Cole, P., Mintz, S. & Shephard, R.J. (1980) The switching point from nasal to oronasal breathing. *Respiration Physiology* **42**, 61–71.

Noakes, T.D. (1992) *The Lore of Running*, 2nd edn. Oxford University Press, Oxford.

O'Connor, S.A., Jones, D.P., Collins, J.V., Heath, R.B., Campbell, M.J. & Leighton, M.H. (1979) Changes in pulmonary function after naturally acquired respiratory infection in normal persons. *American Review of Respiratory Disease* **120**, 1087–1093.

O'Riordain, M.G., Fearon, K.C.H., Ross, J.A. *et al.* (1994) Glutamine-supplemented total parenteral nutrition enhances T-lymphocyte response in surgical patients undergoing colorectal resection. *Annals of Surgery* **220**, 212–221.

O'Riordain, M.G., De Beaux, A. & Fearon, K. (1996) Effect of glutamine on immune function in the surgical patient. *Nutrition* **12**, S82–S84.

Pabst, R. & Binns, R.M. (1989) Heterogeneity of lymphocyte homing physiology: several mechanisms operate in the control of migration to lymphoid and non-lymphoid organs *in vivo*. *Immunological Reviews* **108**, 83–109.

Pabst, R. & Binns, R.M. (1992) Lymphocyte trafficking. In *Encyclopaedia of Immunology* (ed. I. Roitt & P.S. Delves), Vol. 2, pp. 1003–1005. Academic Press, London.

Parry-Billings, M. (1989) *Studies of glutamine release from skeletal muscle*. D.Phil. thesis, University of Oxford.

Parry-Billings, M., Blomstrand, E., McAndrew, N. & Newsholme, E.A. (1990a) A communicational link between skeletal muscle, brain, and cells of the immune system. *International Journal of Sports Medicine* **11**, S122.

Parry-Billings, M., Evans, J., Calder, P.C. & Newsholme, E.A. (1990b) Does glutamine contribute to immunosuppression? *Lancet* **336**, 523–525.

Pedersen, B.K. & Ullum, H. (1994) NK cell response to physical activity: possible mechanisms of action. *Medicine and Science in Sports and Exercise* **26**, 140–146.

Pedersen, B.K., Rohde, T. & Ostrowski, K. (1998) Recovery of the immune system after exercise. *Acta Physiologica Scandinavica* **162**, 325–332.

Poortmans, J.R., Siest, G., Galteau, M.M. & Houot, O. (1974) Distribution of plasma amino acids in humans during submaximal prolonged exercise. *European Journal of Applied Physiology* **32**, 143–147.

Powell, H., Castell, L.M., Parry-Billings, M. *et al.* (1994) Growth hormone suppression and glutamine flux associated with cardiac surgery. *Clinical Physiology* **14**, 569–590.

Rohde, T., MacLean, D.A., Hartkopp, A. & Pedersen, B.K. (1996) The immune system and serum glutamine during a triathlon. *European Journal of Applied Physiology* **74**, 428–434.

Roth, E., Karner, J., Ollenschlager, G. *et al.* (1982) Metabolic disorders in severe abdominal sepsis: glutamine deficiency in skeletal muscle. *Clinical Nutrition* **1**, 25–41.

Rowbottom, D.G., Keast, D. & Morton, A.R. (1996) The emerging role of glutamine as an indicator of exercise stress and overtraining. *Sports Medicine* **21**, 80–97.

Rylander, R. (1968) Pulmonary defence mechanism to airborne bacteria. *Acta Physiologica Scandinavica* **72** (Suppl. 306), 6–85.

Shepherd, R.J., Verde, T.J., Thomas, S.G. & Shek, P. (1991) Physical activity and the immune system. *Canadian Journal of Sports Science* **16**, 163–185.

Shewchuk, L.D., Baracos, V.E. & Field, C.J. (1997) Dietary L-glutamine supplementation reduces the growth of the Morris Hepatoma 7777 in exercise-trained and sedentary rats. *Journal of Nutrition* **127**, 158–166.

Shinkai, S., Shore, S., Shek, P.N. & Shepherd, R.J. (1994) Acute exercise and immune function. *International Journal of Sports Medicine* **13**, 452–461.

Soppi, E., Varjo, P., Eskola, J. *et al.* (1982) Effect of strenuous physical stress on circulating lymphocyte number and function before and after training. *Journal of Clinical and Laboratory Immunology* **8**, 43–46.

Stinnet, J.D., Alexander, J.W., Watanabe, C. *et al.* (1982) Plasma and skeletal muscle amino acids following severe burn injury in patients and experimental animals. *Annals of Surgery* **195**, 75–89.

Struder, H.K., Hollman, W.K., Platen, P., Donike, M., Gotzmann, A. & Weber, K. (1998) Influence of paroxetine, branched-chain amino acids and tyrosine on neuroendocrine system responses and fatigue in humans. *Hormone and Metabolic Research* **30**, 188–194.

Sun, X., Xu, Y., Zhu, R. & Li, S. (1988) Preliminary study on immunity in ballet dancers. *Canadian Journal of Sports Science* **13**, 33.

Tiidus, P.M. & Ianuzzo, C.D. (1983) Effects of intensity and duration of muscular exercise on delayed soreness and serum enzyme activities. *Medicine and Science in Sports and Exercise* **15**, 461–465.

Van Hall, G., Raaymakers, J.S.H., Saris, W.H.M. & Wagenmakers, A.J.M. (1995) Ingestion of branched-chain amino acids and tryptophan during sustained exercise in man: failure to affect performance. *Journal of Physiology* **486**, 789–794.

Wagenmakers, A.J.M. (1992) Role of amino acids and ammonia in mechanisms of fatigue. *Medicine and Sport Science* **34**, 69.

Weidner, T.G. (1994) Literature review: upper respiratory tract illness and sport and exercise. *International Journal of Sports Medicine* **15**, 1–9.

Wilson, W.M. & Maughan, R.J. (1992) Evidence for a possible role of 5-hydroxytryptamine in the genesis of fatigue in man: administration of paroxetine, a 5-HT re-uptake inhibitor, reduces the capacity to perform prolonged exercise. *Experimental Physiology* **77**, 921–924.

Winder, W.W. (1996) Malonyl CoA as a metabolic regulator. In *Biochemistry of Exercise* (ed. R.J. Maughan &

S.M. Sherriffs), Vol. 9, pp. 173–184. Human Kinetics: Champaign, IL.

Yoshida, S., Hikida, S., Tanaka, Y. *et al.* (1992) Effect of glutamine supplementation on lymphocyte function in septic rats. *Journal of Parenteral and Enteral Nutrition* **16** (Suppl. 1).

Ziegler, T.R., Benfell, K., Smith, R.J. *et al.* (1990) Safety and metabolic effects of L-glutamine administration in humans. *Journal of Parenteral and Enteral Nutrition* **14**, S137–146.

Ziegler, T.R., Young, L.S., Benfell, K. *et al.* (1992) Clinical and metabolic efficacy of glutamine supplemented parenteral nutrition after bone marrow transplantation. *Annals of Internal Medicine* **116**, 821–828.

Ziegler, T.R., Bye, R.L., Persinger, R.L., Young, L.S., Antin, J.H. & Wilmore, D.W. (1998) Effects of glutamine supplementation on circulating lymphocytes after bone marrow transplantation: a pilot study. *American Journal of Medical Sciences* **315**, 4–10.

# Chapter 12

# Nutrition, Neurotransmitters and Central Nervous System Fatigue

J. MARK DAVIS

## Introduction

Physical, and perhaps mental, training, along with adequate nutrition, is generally thought to decrease fatigue and optimize physical performance. However, the specific mechanisms of such strategies are not fully understood because not much is known about the specific causes of fatigue. The problem is complex because fatigue can be caused by peripheral muscle weakness (peripheral fatigue) or by a failure to initiate or sustain voluntary drive to the muscle by the central nervous system (CNS fatigue). It may also vary with the type, duration and intensity of the work, the individual level of fitness and numerous environmental factors (Davis & Fitts 1998). Even the specific definition of fatigue is often debated. For the purpose of this review, fatigue is defined as the loss of force or power output in response to voluntary effort that leads to reduced performance of a given task. *CNS fatigue* is the progressive reduction in voluntary drive to motor neurones during exercise, whereas *peripheral fatigue* is the loss of force and power that occurs independent of neural drive.

Peripheral mechanisms of fatigue could include impaired electrical transmission via the sarcolemma and T-tubule, disruption of calcium release and uptake within the sarcoplasmic reticulum, substrate depletion and other metabolic events that impair energy provision and muscle contraction (Davis & Fitts 1998). Much less is known about CNS mechanisms, even though it is well known that 'mental factors' can affect physi-

cal performance. In fact, inadequate CNS drive to the working muscles is the most likely explanation of fatigue in most people during normal activities. Most people stop exercising because the exercise starts to feel too hard (i.e. there is increased perceived effort) which almost always precedes an inability of the muscle to produce force. Therefore, CNS fatigue may include neurobiological mechanisms of altered subjective effort, motivation, mood and pain tolerance, as well as those that directly inhibit central motor drive in the upper most regions of the brain (Gandevia 1998).

Evidence for specific inhibition of motor drive within the brain during fatiguing exercise has only recently appeared in the scientific literature. The best evidence comes from recent studies in humans using a new technique called transcranial magnetic stimulation (TMS). This technique has been used to assess the magnitude of the motor responses elicited in the muscle by magnetic stimulation of neurones in the motor cortex. Recent reports show that the electrical stimulus reaching the muscle following magnetic stimulation of the motor cortex (motor-evoked potential) is suppressed following fatiguing exercise (Brasil-Neto *et al.* 1993; Samii *et al.* 1996). Gandevia and colleagues (Gandevia *et al.* 1996; Taylor *et al.* 1996) also showed that fatigue was accompanied by a prolonged silent period in response to TMS that likely results from inadequate neural drive by the motor cortex. These data suggest strongly that specific mechanisms within the brain are involved in fatigue during exercise.

LIVERPOOL
JOHN MOORES UNIVERSITY
AVRIL ROBARTS LRC
TITHEBARN STREET

CNS fatigue is also thought to be the most likely explanation of fatigue that accompanies viral or bacterial infections, recovery from injury or surgery, chronic fatigue syndrome, depression, 'jet lag' and meal-induced sleepiness and fatigue (Davis & Bailey 1997). However, a full understanding of the causes of fatigue in these situations will await future studies designed to provide plausible neurobiological mechanisms to explain the fatigue.

Progress in this area is minimal, but much recent interest has focused on hypotheses involving exercise-induced alterations in neurotransmitter function as possible explanations for central fatigue. Alterations in serotonin (5-hydroxytryptamine, 5-HT), noradrenaline, dopamine and acetylcholine (ACh) have all been implicated as possible mediators of central fatigue during stressful situations, including strenuous physical exercise. These neurotransmitters are known to play a role in arousal, motivation, mood, sleepiness and other behaviours/perceptions that, if adversely affected, could impair physical and mental performance. These neurotransmitter hypotheses also provide the basis of new intriguing nutritional strategies designed to improve performance by offsetting exercise-induced alterations in these neurotransmitters. This chapter will briefly review the evidence for a possible role of 5-HT, noradrenaline, dopamine and ACh in central fatigue and then provide a more detailed discussion of possible nutritional strategies that may limit CNS fatigue.

## Brain 5-HT and CNS fatigue

The neurotransmitter serotonin (5-HT) has received the most attention with respect to CNS fatigue during prolonged exercise. Eric Newsholme *et al.* (1987) were the first to hypothesize such a role for brain 5-HT, and present some of their findings in Chapter 11. It was argued that regional increases in brain 5-HT activity could cause central fatigue because of its well-known role in sensory perception, arousal, lethargy, sleepiness and mood. This hypothesis was of

particular interest because both exercise and nutrition could influence brain 5-HT metabolism by affecting the uptake of tryptophan from the blood into the brain. Subsequent studies have confirmed certain aspects of this hypothesis, as well as to test the potential role of carbohydrate (CHO) and/or branched-chain amino acid (BCAA) feedings as a way to limit CNS fatigue involving 5-HT.

Increased brain 5-HT synthesis and metabolism typically occurs in response to an increase in the delivery of blood-borne tryptophan (TRP) to the brain because the enzyme tryptophan hydroxylase (rate limiting enzyme in 5-HT synthesis) is largely unsaturated under physiological conditions. Most of the TRP in blood plasma circulates loosely bound to albumin, but it is the unbound or free tryptophan (f-TRP) that is transported across the blood–brain barrier. This transport occurs via a specific mechanism that TRP shares with other large neutral amino acids, most notably the BCAAs leucine, isoleucine and valine. Thus, brain 5-HT synthesis will increase when there is an increase in the ratio of f-TRP to BCAAs in blood plasma (i.e. when f-TRP/BCAA rises; Chaouloff *et al.* 1986a). There are two primary reasons for this increase during exercise. Note that clear differences in this mechanism may exist at rest, during periods of stress and in various clinical conditions (Curzon 1996). During exercise, large increases in plasma free fatty acids (FFAs) cause a parallel increase in plasma f-TRP because FFAs displace TRP from its usual binding sites on albumin. Small decreases in plasma BCAAs also occur as they are taken up into working muscle and oxidized for energy (Fig. 12.1).

Studies in both rats and humans provide good evidence that brain 5-HT metabolism increases during prolonged exercise and that this is associated with fatigue (Davis & Bailey 1996). Chaouloff's initial work in rats demonstrated that prolonged treadmill running increases the plasma f-TRP/BCAA ratio, and brain and cerebrospinal fluid levels of tryptophan, 5-HT and 5-hydroxyindole acetic acid (primary metabolite of 5-HT, 5-HIAA) (Chaouloff *et al.* 1985, 1986a,

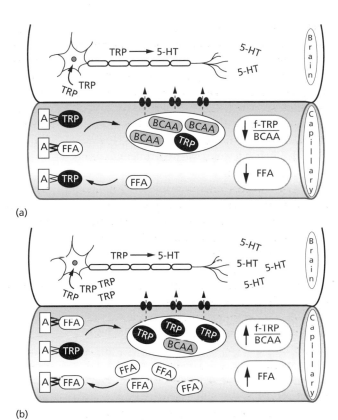

**Fig. 12.1** The primary components of the central fatigue hypothesis. (a) At rest, plasma concentration of BCAA, FFA and TRP (bound and unbound to albumin (A)) and their proposed effects on transport of TRP across the blood–brain barrier for the synthesis of serotonin (5-HT) in serotonergic neurones. (b) Reflects the increases in FFA, f-TRP and f-TRP/BCAA that occur during prolonged exercise. The resulting increase in brain 5-HT synthesis can cause central fatigue.

1986b). Bailey *et al.* (1992, 1993a) further established the relationship between fatigue and increased concentrations of 5-HT and 5-HIAA in various brain regions during treadmill running. These data, however, cannot differentiate between intra- and extracellular concentrations of these substances and therefore are not sufficient to conclude that fatigue is necessarily associated with increased release of 5-HT from serotonergic neurones. Techniques involving microdialysis are necessary for this purpose (Meeusen & De Meirleir 1995). Good evidence using microdialysis is now available to show that 5-HT release from serotonergic nerve terminals does increase during treadmill running and that this is increased further by tryptophan administration (Meussen *et al.* 1996, 1997). However, no such studies have been done during exercise to fatigue.

Other studies have addressed the potential functional role of altered brain 5-HT activity on exercise fatigue. Bailey *et al.* (1992, 1993a, 1993b) did a series of experiments involving drug-induced alterations in brain 5-HT activity during exercise to fatigue in rats. It was hypothesized that administration of drugs known to specifically increase brain 5-HT activity (5-HT agonists) would result in early fatigue, whereas drugs that decrease brain 5-HT activity (5-HT antagonists) would delay it. The results show that run time to fatigue was decreased following administration of the 5-HT receptor agonists m-chlorophenyl piperazine and quipazine dimaleate, whereas run time was increased with a 5-HT receptor antagonist (LY-53857). The supposition that these drug-induced effects resulted from altered neurotransmitter function in the brain is supported by the observation that fatigue could not be explained by alterations in body temperature, blood glucose, muscle and liver glycogen, or various stress hormones. Similar results were also found in human subjects in which brain 5-HT activity was increased by the administration of paroxetine (Paxil; Wilson & Maughan 1992) or fluoxetine (Prozac; Davis *et al.* 1993) prior to running or cycling. These results clearly support the hypothesized relationship between increased brain 5-HT activity and central fatigue. However, as with all pharmacological experiments, it is not possible to rule out possible crossover effects of the drug on other neurotransmitter systems or other side-effects.

## Nutritional effects on brain 5-HT and CNS fatigue

An interesting aspect of the neurotransmitter hypotheses of CNS fatigue is the fact that nutrition can alter brain neurochemistry in ways that might offset CNS fatigue. With respect to brain 5-HT and fatigue, the focus has been on two main nutritional strategies. These strategies involve feedings of BCAA and/or CHO during exercise. Intake of BCAA would lower plasma f-TRP/BCAA (by increasing plasma BCAA concentration) and presumably 5-HT due to decreased f-TRP transport across the blood–brain barrier (mechanisms explained earlier in this chapter). The postulated benefits of CHO feedings is based primarily on the premise that the normally large exercise-induced increase in circulating FFAs would be attenuated by the maintenance of blood glucose and slightly elevated insulin (Davis *et al.* 1992). Since FFAs have a higher affinity for albumin than the loosely bound TRP, this would attenuate the normally large increase in f-TRP and therefore f-TRP/BCAA would remain lower (Fig. 12.2). This is unlike the situation at rest, in which a high CHO meal would elicit a large increase in plasma insulin and a correspondingly large decrease in BCAA levels that have been linked to meal-induced sleepiness and fatigue (Fernstrom 1994). The insulin response is substantially blunted during exercise to the extent that little or no decrease in plasma BCAA occurs (Davis *et al.* 1992).

Blomstrand *et al.* (1991) focused primarily on administration of BCAAs to delay central fatigue during activities such as marathon racing and 30-km running. Upon administration of 7.5–16 g BCAAs prior to and during exercise, small improvements were reported in both physical and mental performance in some subjects. However, it should be noted that while field studies such as these are designed to mimic the real world situation in which athletes find themselves, they are often limited in scientific value. This is because the subject groups are often not appropriately matched for performance or 'blinded' to the treatment they are receiving, and there is little or no control over important variables such as exercise intensity, food and water intake, and environmental conditions. This increases the likelihood that a potential nutritional benefit may have actually resulted from inherent differences in the groups of subjects, subject bias and/or uncontrolled variables.

This is perhaps illustrated by the fact that well-controlled laboratory experiments have generally not confirmed the benefit of BCAA on exercise performance. Varnier *et al.* (1994) found no differences in performance of a graded incremental exercise test to fatigue following infusion of approximately 20 g BCAA or saline over 70 min prior to exercise using a double-blinded, cross-over design. Verger *et al.* (1994) also reported in rats that feeding relatively large amounts of BCAAs actually caused early fatigue during prolonged treadmill running as compared to rats fed glucose.

Recent well-controlled laboratory studies involving endurance cycling in humans also fail to confirm a performance benefit of BCAA administration. Blomstrand *et al.* (1995) studied five endurance trained male cyclists during a ride to fatigue at 75% $\dot{V}o_{2max}$, which was preceded by a muscle glycogen-depleting regimen, presumably to increase the likelihood that an effect would occur. All subjects were given in random order one of the following drinks during the ride: a 6% CHO solution, a 6% CHO solution containing $7 g \cdot l^{-1}$ BCAA, or a flavoured water placebo. Increases in performance were seen in both CHO and CHO+ BCAA treatments when

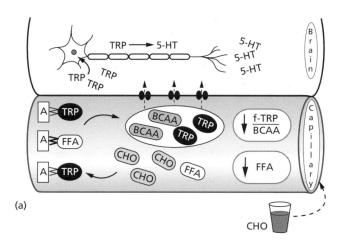

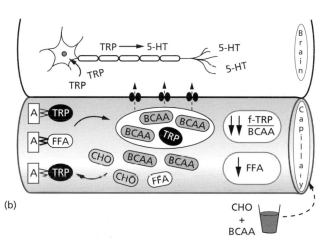

**Fig. 12.2** The proposed nutritional effects on the central fatigue hypothesis during prolonged exercise. (a) The proposed effects of CHO ingestion on the mechanisms of central fatigue with regard to the attenuation of FFA and f-TRP during prolonged exercise. (b) The proposed effects of CHO and BCAA ingestion on the mechanisms of central fatigue with regard to the larger decrease in the plasma f-TRP/BCAA ratio during prolonged exercise. A, albumin.

compared with the placebo. However, there was no added benefit of BCAA despite increases in plasma (120%) and muscle (35%) concentrations of BCAA. Van Hall *et al.* (1995) used more subjects ($n=10$) and tested a low ($6\,g \cdot l^{-1}$) and high ($18\,g \cdot l^{-1}$) dose of BCAAs added to a 6% CHO solution on cycling time to fatigue at 70–75% of maximal power output. Despite large changes in plasma concentrations of BCAA, exercise time to exhaustion ($\approx 122\,min$) was again not different from the control treatment (6% CHO). This study also included a treatment condition in which tryptophan ($3\,g \cdot l^{-1}$) was added to the 6% CHO solution. However, this also failed to affect fatigue. The authors concluded that these nutritional manipulations either had no additional

effect upon brain 5-HT activity or that the change in 5-HT did not contribute significantly to mechanisms of fatigue. It is also possible that the effects were lessened by the fact that they were given in a solution with CHO. The CHO would have suppressed the normally large increase in circulating levels of stress hormones that is known to alter TRP transport kinetics.

This brings up the fundamental question of whether CHO or BCAA supplementation actually produces the hypothesized effects on brain 5-HT during exercise. This, of course, cannot be answered in human subjects during exercise. We recently completed a preliminary study which partially addressed this issue (Welsh *et al.* 1997). Solutions containing BCAA, CHO or pure water were infused into the stomach of rats at regular intervals during treadmill running. Subgroups of rats in each group were killed at 60, 90 and 120 min of exercise for determination of 5-HT and 5-HIAA in the brainstem and striatum regions of the brain. The results showed that neither BCAA nor CHO feedings affected brain 5-HT or 5-HIAA at 60 and 90 min of exercise. However, at 120 min, both BCAA and CHO feedings lowered 5-HT and 5-HIAA in the brainstem and CHO lowered 5-HT in the striatum. Therefore, at least in this preliminary study, BCAA and CHO feedings were able to influence brain 5-HT metabolism in a presumably positive direction during exercise. However, since exercise time to fatigue was not measured in this study, the question of whether a direct link exists between these nutritional strategies, lower brain 5-HT metabolism and fatigue during exercise remains to be firmly established.

Even if BCAA supplementation is found to alter brain 5-HT during exercise, there is still a question of potential negative side-effects. For BCAA to be physiologically effective in reducing brain 5-HT metabolism, relatively large doses are likely to be required and this increases the likelihood that plasma ammonia will result (van Hall et al. 1995). Ammonia is known to be toxic to the brain and may also impair muscle metabolism. The buffering of ammonia could cause fatigue in working muscles by depleting glycolytically derived carbon skeletons (pyruvate) and by draining intermediates of the Krebs cycle that are coupled to glutamine production by transamination reactions (Wagenmakers et al. 1990). Elevated plasma ammonia can also increase brain TRP uptake and 5-HT metabolism in various brain regions (Mans et al. 1987). Other potential side-effects include slower water absorption across the gut, gastrointestinal disturbances and decreased drink palatability. It should be noted, however, that when these potential side-effects were minimized by providing a small, more palatable, dose of BCAA in a sports drink ($0.5 \mathrm{g} \cdot \mathrm{h}^{-1}$ consumed in a CHO–electrolyte drink), no benefits were found

during cycling to fatigue at 70% $\dot{V}o_{2\mathrm{max.}}$ in trained cyclists. No measurable side-effects were reported, but ride time to fatigue, perceived exertion and various cardiovascular, metabolic and endocrine responses were similar in the BCAA and placebo groups (Galiano et al. 1991). In fact, to the author's knowledge there is only one recent controlled laboratory study that shows a performance benefit of BCAA supplementation (Mittleman et al. 1998). In this study, BCAA were given during a 2-h pre-exercise exposure to high heat that was followed by a ride to fatigue at 40% $\dot{V}o_{2\mathrm{peak}}$. As expected, the f-TRP/BCAA ratio was significantly lower during the 2-h period prior to exercise and during exercise when subjects received the BCAA supplement. However, in this case fatigue was apparently delayed by the supplement. It is possible that administration of BCAA during the rest period in the heat prior to exercise may have provided a beneficial effect that would otherwise not occur, or be offset by other negative side-effects, if the supplements are given only during exercise. However, support for this hypothesis from other physiological and psychological data in this paper were equivocal.

This led us to consider another, perhaps more reasonable nutritional approach involving CHO feedings alone to offset the increase in 5-HT and CNS fatigue. The literature is consistent in showing that CHO feedings can delay fatigue in a variety of exercise protocols, which is not surprising given the well-known benefit of CHO feedings in maintaining blood glucose and muscle glycogen as important sources of energy for the working muscle (Coyle 1998). However, it now appears possible that CHO feedings may also delay CNS fatigue as well as peripheral fatigue (Davis et al. 1992).

This effect is based on the premise that CHO feedings suppress normally large rises in FFA and therefore f-TRP and f-TRP/BCAA during exercise without the potential negative consequences of administering large doses of BCAA. This hypothesis was tested in a double-blinded, placebo-controlled laboratory study in which subjects drank $5\,ml\cdot kg^{-1}\cdot h^{-1}$ of either a water placebo, a 6% CHO drink or a 12% CHO drink during prolonged cycling at 70% $\dot{V}o_{2max.}$ to fatigue (Davis *et al.* 1992). When subjects consumed the water placebo, plasma f-TRP increased dramatically (in direct proportion to plasma FFAs), while total TRP and BCAA changed very little during the ride. When subjects consumed either the 6% or 12% CHO solution, the increases in plasma f-TRP were greatly reduced and fatigue was delayed by approximately 1 h. The CHO feedings caused a slight reduction in plasma BCAA (19% and 31% in the 6% and 12% CHO groups, respectively), but this decrease was probably inconsequential with respect to the very large attenuation (five- to sevenfold) of plasma f-TRP. Although it was not possible to distinguish between the beneficial effects of CHO feedings on central vs. peripheral mechanisms of fatigue in this study, it was interesting that the substantial delay in fatigue could not be explained by typical markers of peripheral muscle fatigue involving cardiovascular, thermoregulatory and metabolic function.

## Brain catecholamines and CNS fatigue

The primary catecholamine neurotransmitters in the brain are dopamine and noradrenaline. Both neurotransmitters are formed from the amino acid tyrosine in similar metabolic pathways, but they are released from different neurones found in different regions of the brain. The rate-limiting step in their biosynthesis is the hydroxylation of tyrosine to dihydroxyphenylalanine (L-dopa) by the enzyme tyrosine hydroxylase. L-Dopa is then decarboxylated to dopamine. In noradrenaline neurones, dopamine is then converted to noradrenaline by the enzyme dopamine β-hydroxylase.

Dopamine and noradrenaline neurones modulate a wide variety of functions in the CNS. Dopaminergic neurones arise primarily from cell bodies in the ventral tegmental area (VTA) and pars compacta of the substantia nigra (CSN). The VTA gives rise to neurones of the mesolimbic and mesocortical pathways that project to many components of the limbic system. These neurones are involved in various emotions, memory and especially behaviours related to motivation, reward, wakefulness and attention (Olds & Fobes 1981). The CSN gives rise to the nigrostriatal pathway that projects to the putamen and caudate nuclei of the striatum and is intimately involved in motor behaviour. Noradrenaline neurones primarily arise in the locus coeruleus and lateral brain stem tegmentum and project to various areas of the limbic system, cortex, cerebellum and spinal cord. These neurones are involved in control of sympathetic nervous system activity, anxiety and arousal. Both neurotransmitter systems, along with 5-HT, have been implicated in the aetiology of depression (Dunn & Dishman 1991; Cabib & Puglisi-Allegra 1996).

Brain catecholamine metabolism is dramatically increased during periods of stress, including physical exercise (Meeusen & De Meirleir 1995). This often leads to partial depletion of catecholamines in various brain regions of rodents. Although direct evidence of brain catecholamine depletion is lacking in human subjects, it is generally believed that alterations in brain noradrenaline and dopamine are involved in the neurochemical manifestations of acute stress. These include behavioural deficits like fatigue, distress, helplessness, inattention and impaired motor and cognitive performance. The military has been very interested in these effects that have been attributed to deficits in physical and mental performance that occur in soldiers during the stress of battle (Owasoyo *et al.* 1992).

The possibility that depletion of these neurotransmitters, especially dopamine, may specifically relate to CNS fatigue during exercise has also been put forth by several investigators (Heyes *et al.* 1988; Chaouloff *et al.* 1989; Davis & Bailey 1997). Dopamine was probably the first neurotransmitter to be linked to CNS fatigue due to its well-known role in motor behaviour and motivation. The specific mechanisms underlying an effect of dopamine on CNS fatigue remains to be elucidated. It is hypothesized that decreased dopamine activity would lead to a reduction in motivation, arousal and/or motor control that would contribute to CNS fatigue.

It is clear that drug-induced increases in dopamine activity as well as electrical brain stimulation of the primary dopamine system in the brain can motivate various exercise tasks in rats and can delay fatigue during treadmill running. For example, pretreatment of rats with amphetamine, a dopamine releaser with powerful rewarding properties, or apomorphine, a dopamine agonist, has been shown to delay fatigue (Gerald 1978; Heyes *et al.* 1988). There are also numerous reports of amphetamine use to control fatigue and improve performance in athletes and soldiers (Ivy 1983). Electrical stimulation of the VTA or other areas of the mesolimbic dopamine pathway mediate reinforcement and reward (Olds & Fobes 1981). It has recently been shown to motivate rats to lift weights (Garner *et al.* 1991), run on a motorized treadmill (Burgess *et al.* 1991) and run in running wheels (Schwarzberg & Roth 1989). We did a series of studies in which activation of this dopaminergic reward system was used to motivate rats to run on a treadmill (Burgess *et al.* 1991, 1993a, 1993b). In one of the studies we compared run time to fatigue on a motorized treadmill in rats that ran for rewarding VTA stimulation vs. those in which the fear of an electric shock grid placed at the back of the treadmill was used as motivation. We found that rats ran significantly longer (25 m·min$^{-1}$, 5% grade) while receiving VTA stimulation (63±10 min) that when they received the electric shocks (42±10 min). We did not measure neurotransmitters in this study to confirm a presumed role of elevated dopamine in delayed fatigue in this experiment, but in other experiments it was determined that this delay in fatigue was not likely related to cardiovascular or metabolic function.

There is also good evidence that increased dopamine metabolism occurs normally during exercise. Regional brain analysis shows that dopamine metabolism is enhanced during treadmill exercise in the midbrain, hippocampus, striatum and hypothalamus (Chaouloff *et al.* 1987; Bailey *et al.* 1993a). Increased dopamine metabolism has been shown to be a good marker for speed, direction and posture of moving animals (Freed & Yamamoto 1985). Conversely, endurance performance was impaired following destruction of dopaminergic neurones by 6-hydroxydopamine, an effect diminished by giving back a drug that increases dopamine activity (i.e. apomorphine; Heyes *et al.* 1988).

Bailey *et al.* (1993a) demonstrated a relationship between decreased brain dopamine metabolism and fatigue during prolonged treadmill running in rats. Fatigue was associated with specific decreases in dopamine in the brain stem and midbrain. These data, along with other data showing a phasic inhibitory control of 5-HT over dopamine-dependent forms of behaviour (Soubrie *et al.* 1984), led to the hypothesis that elevated 5-HT, also associated with fatigue, may inhibit dopamine activity (Davis & Bailey 1997). Further support for this comes from studies that show an inverse relationship between brain 5-HT and dopamine in association with fatigue following administration of drugs that affect brain 5-HT and dopamine systems. When a 5-HT agonist (quipizine dimalate) was administered to rats prior to treadmill running, it appeared to block the increase in dopamine at 1 h and fatigue occurred early. Alternatively, a 5-HT antagonist (LY53857) partially blocked the decrease in dopamine and fatigue was delayed. Also, when amphetamine is given to rats in doses known to delay fatigue, brain 5-HT metabolism is decreased (Chaouloff *et al.* 1987). These data add support to our hypothesis that central fatigue occurs when dopamine is reduced in association with elevated 5-HT (Davis & Bailey 1997).

## Nutrition, brain catecholamines and CNS fatigue

Tyrosine is a non-essential, large, neutral, amino acid found in dietary proteins and is the precursor of the neurotransmitters noradrenaline and dopamine. Researchers, especially those employed by the US Army, have been interested in the possibility that tyrosine supplementation may protect against the adverse behavioural effects of prolonged periods of stress by preventing the depletion of brain catecholamines that may counteract mood and performance degradation in soldiers (Owasoyo et al. 1992). Most of this work has focused on noradrenaline depletion, even though good evidence in animals show that both dopamine and noradrenaline synthesis can be increased by tyrosine administration (see Owasoyo et al. 1992). It is thought that noradrenaline neurones in the locus coeruleus regulate, in part, behavioural functions like anxiety (tension), vigilance and attention that are apparently improved following administration of tyrosine. However, it is also possible that some of the beneficial effects of tyrosine can be attributed to prevention of dopamine depletion, especially in the case of motivation, wakefulness, motor control and overall fatigue.

Unlike tryptophan, however, catecholaminergic neurones are not sensitive to the presence of excess tyrosine while at rest, but become sensitive when the neurones are activated by stress (Milner & Wurtman 1986). This theory is consistent with work from both human (Growden et al. 1982) and animal research (Lehnert et al. 1984).

Research on the possible beneficial effects of tyrosine on adverse behavioural responses to stress in humans comes primarily from one group of investigators headed by H.R. Lieberman and associates at Massachusetts Institute of Technology and the US Army Research Institute of Environmental Medicine. They initially showed that tyrosine decreased some of the adverse consequences of a 4.5-h exposure to cold and hypoxia (Banderet & Lieberman 1989). Tyrosine $(100\,mg\cdot kg^{-1})$ returned mood, cognitive performance, vigilance and feelings of fatigue and sleepiness to baseline levels in subjects who were most affected by the environmental stressors. They also found that tyrosine increased tolerance to lower body negative pressure with an accompanying decrease in depression, tension and anxiety (Dollins et al. 1995) and lessened the impairments of learning and memory during

severe hypoxia (Shukitt-Hale et al. 1996). There is also one report from another group that showed that tyrosine improved performance in perceptual motor tasks during lower body negative pressure (Deijen & Orlebeke 1994).

There are no studies that specifically focus on the possible effects of tyrosine as a means of delaying fatigue during exercise. This is unfortunate, since there is reasonable information to hypothesize a possible beneficial effect of tyrosine in preventing a depletion of noradrenaline and dopamine that appears to be essential to optimal physical performance. It is reasonable to suspect that tyrosine could limit some of the negative behavioural consequences of prolonged stressful exercise including reductions in alertness, attention, motivation (drive), positive mood and motor control that would be expected to limit optimal performance perhaps though an effect on central fatigue. Special attention needs to be focused on the possible role of dopamine since this has essentially not been addressed in the literature to date.

## Acetylcholine and CNS fatigue

Acetylcholine is the most abundant neurotransmitter in the body. It is essential for the generation of muscular force at the neuromuscular junction, and within the CNS is generally associated with memory, awareness, and temperature regulation.

As with 5-HT and the catecholamines, the rate of synthesis of acetylcholine is determined by the availability of its precursor, choline, which is normally obtained from the diet. ACh is synthesized in the cytoplasm from choline and acetyl coenzyme A via the enzyme choline acetyltransferase that is not saturated with choline at physiological concentrations, and ACh does not 'feed-back' to inhibit its own synthesis. There is also some evidence in animals to suggest that depletion of ACh may contribute to fatigue during sustained electrical activity. However, no studies have investigated the relationship between modified plasma choline levels and concentrations of ACh in skeletal muscle, although synthesis of ACh was found to be increased in electrically stimulated hemidiaphragm perfused with choline *in vitro* (Bierkamper & Goldberg 1980).

Wurtman and colleagues hypothesized that fatigue during prolonged exercise may be initiated by a reduction in ACh activity subsequent to depletions in availability of choline (Conley *et al.* 1986; Sandage *et al.* 1992). This group recently showed that plasma choline levels were reduced approximately 40% in runners following completion of the Boston Marathon (Conley *et al.* 1986). They also reported that performance of a 32-km run was improved when plasma choline was maintained or elevated by consumption of a beverage supplemented with choline citrate (Sandage *et al.* 1992). However, there is still no evidence that decreased plasma choline is associated with ACh depletion at the neuromuscular junction, or in the brain for that matter, and that this leads to fatigue. In addition, as described earlier in this chapter, relatively uncontrolled field studies such as these are often misleading because it is difficult to know for sure whether the effect ascribed to choline was not due to a number of other uncontrolled variables.

Results of the only well-controlled laboratory study of the effects of choline supplementation on exercise performance do not support a beneficial effect of choline supplementation (Spector *et al.* 1995). Neither low- nor high-intensity exercise performance was improved with choline supplementation. Choline was given (2.43 g, 1 h before exercise) prior to either a prolonged cycling bout to fatigue at 70% $\dot{V}o_{2max.}$ ($\approx$73 min) or a shorter term, high-intensity cycling bout at 150% of $\dot{V}o_{2max.}$ ($\approx$2 min). In addition, serum choline levels were not reduced by either of these exercise conditions. The authors did suggest that the duration of exercise protocols might have to be extended to allow for the hypothesized benefit of choline administration to be realized.

## Conclusion

It is unfortunate that so little is known about the mechanisms underlying a CNS effect on fatigue. This area of investigation has largely been

ignored due in large part to difficulty in studying brain function in humans, a lack of good theories to explain such an occurrence, and a lack of good methodologies to directly measure central fatigue. However, in recent years, new methodologies and viable theories have sparked renewed interest in the development of hypotheses, which can be tested in a systematic fashion, that may help to explain the role of the CNS in fatigue.

Nutritional interventions are a common aspect of recent studies on CNS fatigue. Nutritional strategies designed to alter brain 5-HT metabolism have received the most attention in this regard. While 5-HT is almost certainly not the only neurotransmitter involved in central fatigue during prolonged exercise, review of the mechanisms involved in the control of brain serotonin synthesis and turnover make it a particularly attractive candidate. It is well known that increases in brain 5-HT can have important effects on arousal, lethargy, sleepiness and mood that could be linked to altered perception of effort and feelings of fatigue. Increases in 5-HT metabolism appear to increase in several brain regions due to an increase in plasma f-TRP during prolonged exercise and reach a peak at fatigue. Drugs that increase and decrease brain 5-HT activity have predictable effects on run times to fatigue in the absence of any apparent peripheral markers of muscle fatigue.

The evidence for a benefit of nutrition on central fatigue during exercise is more tenuous. Studies involving BCAA supplementation usually show no performance benefit even though preliminary evidence in rats suggests that it may suppress brain 5-HT metabolism during exercise. Perhaps negative effects of ammonia accumulation on muscle and brain function offset the potentially beneficial effect of BCAA on brain 5-HT. CHO supplementation, on the other hand, is associated with a large suppression of plasma f-TRP and f-TRP/BCAA and decreased brain 5-HT metabolism, and fatigue is delayed by this strategy. In this case, however, it is not possible to distinguish with certainty the effects of CHO feedings on CNS fatigue mechanisms and the well-established beneficial effects of CHO supplementation on the contracting muscle.

The potential role of tyrosine supplementation to increase or maintain noradrenaline and dopamine as a way to offset CNS fatigue is theoretically feasible, but there is essentially no direct evidence to support this hypothesis at this time. The potential role of choline supplementation to prevent ACh depletion and neuromuscular transmission failure is even more tenuous.

Future research on possible relationships among nutrition, brain neurochemistry and fatigue is likely to lead to important discoveries that may enhance physical and mental performance during sports participation and, although not addressed in any depth in this review, during activities of normal daily life. It may also help to understand and better treat the debilitating fatigue that often occurs in patients with chronic fatigue syndrome, fibromyalgia, viral illness and depression, among others.

# References

Bailey, S.P., Davis, J.M. & Ahlborn, E.N. (1992) Effect of increased brain serotonergic (5-HT1C) activity on endurance performance in the rat. *Acta Physiologica Scandinavica* **145**, 75–76.

Bailey, S.P., Davis, J.M. & Ahlborn, E.N. (1993a) Neuroendocrine and substrate responses to altered brain 5-HT activity during prolonged exercise to fatigue. *Journal of Applied Physiology* **74**, 3006–3012.

Bailey, S.P., Davis, J.M. & Ahlborn, E.N. (1993b) Brain serotonergic activity affects endurance performance in the rat. *International Journal of Sports Medicine* **6**, 330–333.

Banderet, L.B. & Lieberman, H.R. (1989) Treatment with tyrosine, a neurotransmitter precursor, reduces environmental stress in humans. *Brain Research Bulletin* **22**, 759–762.

Bierkamper, G.G. & Goldberg, A.M. (1980) Release of acetylcholine from the vascular perfused rat phrenic nerve hemidiaphragm. *Brain Research* **202**, 234–237.

Blomstrand, E., Hassmen, P., Ekblom, B. & Newsholme, E.A. (1991) Administration of branched-chain amino acids during sustained exercise-effects on performance and on plasma concentration of some amino acids. *European Journal of Applied Physiology* **63**, 83–88.

Blomstrand, E., Andersson, S., Hassmen, P., Ekblom, B. & Newsholme, E.A. (1995) Effect of branched-chain amino acid and carbohydrate supplementation on the exercise-induced change in plasma and muscle concentration of amino acids in human subjects. *Acta Physiologica Scandinavica* **153**, 87–96.

Brasil-Neto, J.P., Pascual-Leone, A., Valls-Sole, J., Cammarota, A., Cohen, L.G. & Hallett, M. (1993) Post-exercise depression of motor evoked potentials: a measure of central nervous system fatigue. *Experimental Brain Research* **93**, 181–184.

Burgess, M.L., Davis, J.M., Borg, T.K. & Buggy, J. (1991) Intracranial self-stimulation motivates treadmill running in rats. *Journal of Applied Physiology* **71** (4), 1593–1597.

Burgess, M.L., Davis, J.M., Borg, T.K., Wilson, S.P., Burgess, W.A. & Buggy, J. (1993a) Exercise training alters cardiovascular and hormonal responses to intracranial self-stimulation. *Journal of Applied Physiology* **75**, 863–869.

Burgess, M.L., Davis, J.M., Wilson, S.P., Borg, T.K., Burgess, W.A. & Buggy, J. (1993b) Effects of intracranial self-stimulation on selected physiological variables in rats. *American Journal of Physiology* **264**, R149–R155.

Cabib, S. & Puglisi-Allegra, S. (1996) Stress, depression and the mesolimbic dopamine system. *Psychopharmacology* **128**, 331–342.

Chaouloff, F., Elghozi, J.L., Guezennec, Y. & Laude, D. (1985) Effects of conditioned running on plasma, liver and brain tryptophan and on brain 5-hydroxytryptamine metabolism of the rat. *British Journal of Pharmacology* **86**, 33–41.

Chaouloff, F., Kennett, G.A., Serrurier, B., Merina, D. & Curson, G. (1986a) Amino acid analysis demonstrates that increased plasma free tryptophan causes the increase of brain tryptophan during exercise in the rat. *Journal of Neurochemistry* **46**, 1647–1650.

Chaouloff, F., Laude, D., Guezennec, Y. & Elghozi, J.L. (1986b) Motor activity increases tryptophan, 5-hydroxyindoleacetic acid, and homovanillic acid in ventricular cerebrospinal fluid of the conscious rat. *Journal of Neurochemistry* **46**, 1313–1316.

Chaouloff, F., Laude, D., Merino, D., Serrurier, B., Guezennec, Y. & Elghozi, J.L. (1987) Amphetamine and alpha-methyl-p-tyrosine affect the exercise induced imbalance between the availability of tryptophan and synthesis of serotonin in the brain of the rat. *Neuropharmacology* **26**, 1099–1106.

Chaouloff, F., Laude, D. & Elghozi, J.L. (1989) Physical exercise: evidence for differential consequences of tryptophan on 5-HT synthesis and metabolism in central serotonergic cell bodies and terminals. *Journal of Neural Transactions* **78**, 121–130.

Coggan, A.R. & Coyle, E.F. (1991) Carbohydrate ingestion during prolonged exercise: effects on metabolism and performance. In *Exercise and Sports Sciences*

*Reviews* (ed. J.O. Holloszy), pp. 1–40. Williams and Wilkins, Baltimore.

Conley, L., Wurtman, R.J., Blusztain, J.K., Coviella, I., Maher, T.J. & Evoniuk, G.E. (1986) Decreased plasma choline concentration in marathon runners. *New England Journal of Medicine* **175**, 892.

Coyle, E.F. (1998) Fuels for sport performance. In *Perspectives in Exercise Science and Sports Medicine*. Vol. 10. *Optimizing Sport Performance* (eds D.R. Lamb & R. Murray), pp. 95–137. Cooper Publishing, Carmel, IN.

Curzon, G. (1996) Brain tryptophan: normal and disturbed control. In *Recent Advances in Tryptophan Research* (eds G.A. Filippini, C.V.L. Costa & A. Bertazzo), pp. 27–34. Plenum Press, New York.

Davis, J.M. & Bailey, S.P. (1997) Possible mechanisms of central nervous system fatigue during exercise. *Medicine and Science in Sports and Exercise* **29**, 45–45.

Davis, J.M. & Fitts, R. (1998) mechanisms of muscular fatigue. In *ACSM's Resource Manual for Guidelines for Exercise Testing and Prescription* (ed. J.L. Roitman), pp. 182–188. Williams & Wilkins, Baltimore, MD.

Davis, J.M., Bailey, S.P., Woods, J.A., Galiano, F.J., Hamilton, M. & Bartoli, W.P. (1992) Effects of carbohydrate feedings on plasma free-tryptophan and branched-chain amino acids during prolonged cycling. *European Journal of Applied Physiology* **65**, 513–519.

Davis, J.M., Bailey, S.P., Jackson, D.A., Strasner, A.B. & Morehouse, S.L. (1993) Effects of a serotonin (5-HT) agonist during prolonged exercise to fatigue in humans. *Medicine and Science in Sports and Exercise* **25**, S78.

Deijen, J.B. & Orlebeke, J.F. (1994) Effect of tyrosine on cognitive function and blood pressure under stress. *Brain Research Bulletin* **33**, 319–323.

Dollins, A.B., Krock, J.L., Storm, W.F., Wurtman, R.J. & Lieberman, H.R. (1995) L-tyrosine ameliorates some of the effect of lower body negative pressure stress. *Physiological Behavior* **57**, 223–230.

Dunn, A.L. & Dishman, R.K. (1991) Exercise and the neurobiology of depression. In *Exercise and Sports Science Reviews* (ed. J.D. Holloszy), pp. 41–98. Williams and Wilkins, Baltimore, MD.

Fernstrom, J.D. (1994) Dietary amino acids and brain function. *Journal of the American Dietetic Association* **94**, 71–77.

Freed, C.R. & Yamamoto, B.K. (1985) Regional brain dopamine metabolism: a marker for speed, direction, and posture of moving animals. *Science* **229**, 62–65.

Galiano, F.J., Davis, J.M., Bailey, S.P., Woods, J.A. & Hamilton, M. (1991) Physiologic, endocrine and performance effects of adding branch chain amino acids to a 6% carbohydrate–electrolyte beverage during prolonged cycling. *Medicine and Science in Sports and Exercise* **23**, S14.

Gandevia, S.C. (1998) Neural control in human muscle

fatigue: changes in muscle afferents, motoneurones and motor cortical drive. *Acta Physiologica Scandinavica* **162**, 275–284.

Gandevia, S., Gabrielle, M.A., Butler, J.E. & Taylor, J.L. (1996) Supraspinal factors in human muscle fatigue: evidence for suboptimal output from the motor cortex. *Journal of Applied Physiology* **490**, 520–536.

Garner, R.P., Terracio, L., Borg, T.K. & Buggy, J. (1991) Cardiac hypertrophy after weight lifting exercise motivated by intracranial self-stimulation. *Journal of Applied Physiology* **71**, 1672–1631.

Gerald, M.C. (1978) Effect of (+)-amphetamine on the treadmill endurance performance of rats. *Neuropharmacology* **17**, 703–704.

Growden, J.H., Melamed, E., Logue, M., Hefti, F. & Wurtman, R.J. (1982) Effects of oral L-tyrosine administration on CSF tyrosine and homovanillic acid levels in patients with Parkinson's Disease. *Life Science* **30**, 827–832.

Heyes, M.P., Garnett, E.S. & Coates, G. (1988) Nigrostriatal dopaminergic activity increased during exhaustive exercise stress in rats. *Life Science* **42**, 1537–1542.

Ivy, J.L. (1983) Amphetamines. In *Ergogenic Aids in Sport* (ed. M.H. Williams), pp. 101–127. Human Kinetics, Champaign, IL.

Lehnert, H., Reinstein, D.K., Strowbridge, B.W. & Wurtman, R.J. (1984) Neurochemical and behavioural consequences of acute uncontrollable stress: effects of dietary tyrosine. *Brain Research* **303**, 215–219.

Mans, A.M., Beibuyck, J.F. & Hawkins, R.A. (1987) Brain tryptophan abnormalities in hyperammonaemia and liver disease. In *Progress in Tryptophan and Serotonin Research* (ed. D.A. Bender, M.H. Joseph, W. Kochen & H. Steinhart), pp. 207–212. De Gruyter, Berlin.

Meeusen, R. & De Meirleir, K. (1995) Exercise and brain neurotransmission. *Sports Medicine* **20**, 160–188.

Meussen, R., Thorre, K., Chaouloff, F. *et al.* (1996) Effects of tryptophan and/or acute running on extracellular 5-HT and 5-HIAA levels in the hippocampus of food deprived rats. *Brain Research* **740**, 245–254.

Meussen, R., Smolders, I., Sarre, S. *et al.* (1997) Endurance training effects on neurotransmitter release in rat striatum: an in vivo microdialysis study. *Acta Physiologica Scandinavica* **159**, 335–341.

Milner, J.D. & Wurtman, R.J. (1986) Commentary: Catecholamine synthesis: physiological coupling to precursor supply. *Biochemistry and Pharmacology* **35**, 875–881.

Mittleman, K.D., Ricci, M.R. & Bailey, S.P. (1998) Branched-chain amino acids prolong exercise during heat stress in men and women. *Medicine and Science in Sports and Exercise* **30**, 83–91.

Newsholme, E.A., Acworth, I.N. & Blomstrand, E.

(1987) Amino acids, brain neurotransmitters and a functional link between muscle and brain that is important in sustained exercise. In *Advances in Myochemistry* (ed. G. Benzi), pp. 127–133. John Libbey Eurotext, London.

Olds, M.E. & Fobes, J.L. (1981) The central basis of motivation: intracranial self-stimulation studies. *Annual Reviews of Psychology* **32**, 23–74.

Owasoyo, J.O., Neri, D. & Lamberth, J.G. (1992) Tyrosine and its potential use as a contermeasure to performance decrement in military sustained operations. *Aviation and Space Environmental Medicine* **63**, 364–369.

Samii, A., Wasserman, E.M., Ikoma, K., Mercuri, B. & Hallett, M. (1996) Characterization of postexercise facilitation and depression of motor evoked potentials to transcranial magnetic stimulation. *Neurology* **46**, 1376–1382.

Sandage, B.W., Sabounjian, L., White, R. & Wurtman, R.J. (1992) Choline citrate may enhance athletic performance. *Physiologist* **35**, 236.

Schwarzberg, H. & Roth, N. (1989) Increased locomotor activity of rats by self-stimulation in a running wheel. *Physiological Behavior* **46**, 767–769.

Shukitt-Hale, B., Stillman, M.J. & Leiberman, H.R. (1996) Tyrosine administration prevents hypoxia-induced decrements in learning and memory. *Physiological Behavior* **59**, 867–871.

Soubrie, P., Reisine, T.D. & Glowinski, J. (1984) Functional aspects of serotonin transmission in the basal ganglia: a review and an in vivo approach using push-pull cannula technique. *Neuroscience* **13**, 605–625.

Spector, S.A., Jackman, M.R., Sabounjian, L.A., Sakkas, C., Landers, D.M. & Willis, W.T. (1995) Effect of choline supplementation on fatigue in trained cyclists. *Medicine and Science in Sports and Exercise* **27**, 668–673.

Taylor, J.L., Butler, J.E., Allen, G.M. & Gandevia, S. (1996) Changes in motor cortical excitability during human muscle fatigue. *Journal of Applied Physiology* **490**, 519–528.

van Hall, G., Raaymakers, J.S.H., Saris, W.H.M. & Wagenmakers, A.J.M. (1995) Ingestion of branched-chain amino acids and tryptophan during sustained exercise-failure to affect performance. *Journal of Applied Physiology* **486**, 789–794.

Varnier, M., Sarto, P. & Martines, D. (1994) Effect of infusing branched-chain amino acid during incremental exercise with reduced muscle glycogen content. *European Journal of Applied Physiology* **69**, 26–31.

Verger, P.H., Aymard, P., Cynobert, L., Anton, G. & Luigi, R. (1994) Effects of administration of branched-chain amino acids vs. glucose during acute exercise in the rat. *Physiological Behavior* **55**, 523–526.

Wagenmakers, A.J.M., Coakley, J.H. & Edwards, R.H.T. (1990) Metabolism of branched-chain amino acids and ammonia during exercise: clues from McArdle's disease. *International Journal of Sports Medicine* **11**, S101–S113.

Welsh, R.S., Waskovich, M., Alderson, N.L. & Davis, J.M. (1997) Carbohydrate and branched-chain amino acid feedings suppress brain 5-HT during prolonged exercise. *Medicine and Science in Sports and Exercise* **29**, S192.

Wilson, W.M. & Maughan, R.J. (1992) Evidence for a possible role of 5-hydroxytryptamine in the genesis of fatigue in man: administration of paroxetine, a 5-HT re-uptake inhibitor, reduces the capacity to perform prolonged exercise. *Experimental Physiology* **77**, 921–924.

# Fat Metabolism during Exercise

JOHN A. HAWLEY, ASKER E. JEUKENDRUP AND FRED BROUNS

## Introduction

In the search for strategies to improve athletic performance, recent interest has focused on several nutritional procedures which may, theoretically, promote fatty acid (FA) oxidation, attenuate the rate of muscle glycogen utilization and improve exercise capacity (for reviews, see Chapter 14 and Lambert *et al.* 1997; Hawley *et al.* 1998). The aim of this chapter is to provide the reader with a general overview of the role of endogenous fat as an energy source for muscular contraction, to discuss the effects of exercise intensity and duration on the regulation of fat metabolism, and to give a synopsis of some of the factors which may potentially limit FA mobilization, uptake and oxidation by human skeletal muscle during exercise.

## Fat as an energy source for physical activity

The human body utilizes carbohydrate (CHO), fat and, to a lesser, extent protein as fuel for muscular work. Fat as an energy source has several advantages over CHO: the energy density of fat is higher ($37.5\,kJ \cdot g^{-1}$ ($9\,kcal \cdot g^{-1}$) for stearic acid vs. $16.9\,kJ \cdot g^{-1}$ ($4\,kcal \cdot g^{-1}$) for glucose), therefore the relative weight as stored energy is lower. FAs provide more adenosine triphosphate (ATP) per molecule than glucose (147 vs. 38 ATP). However, in order to produce the equivalent amount of ATP, the complete oxidation of FA requires more oxygen than the oxidation of CHO

(6 vs. 26 molecules of oxygen per molecule of substrate for the complete oxidation of glucose and stearic acid, respectively). Using CHO as a fuel, $21\,kJ$ ($5\,kcal$) of energy are available for each litre of oxygen used, whereas only $19.7\,kJ$ ($4.7\,kcal$) per litre of oxgyen are available when fat is the sole fuel oxidized: this may be important when the oxygen supply is limited.

On the other hand, for every gram of CHO stored as glycogen, approximately $2\,g$ of water are stored (Holloszy 1990). Consequently, the amount of glycogen stored in muscle and liver is limited to about $450\,g$ in an average-sized adult. Of interest is that although skeletal muscle comprises up to 40% of body mass in well-trained individuals, CHO utilization by muscle in the resting or postabsorptive state is minimal, accounting for less than 10% of total glucose turnover (Felig & Wahren 1975).

Fat can be stored in much greater amounts. In a healthy, untrained male, up to $20\,kg$ of fat can be stored, mainly in adipose tissue: in the obese individual, the fat store may exceed $100\,kg$. Even in highly trained athletes with much lower levels of adipose tissue, endogenous fat stores still far exceed the requirements of all athletic pursuits.

Both FA stored in adipose tissue and fat entering the circulation after a meal can serve as potential energy sources for the muscle cell (Fig. 13.1). For humans ingesting a typical Western diet (approximately 35% of energy from fat), FAs are comprised of approximately 40% oleate, 25% palmitate, 15% stearate and 10% linoleate. The remainder is thought to be a mixture of both

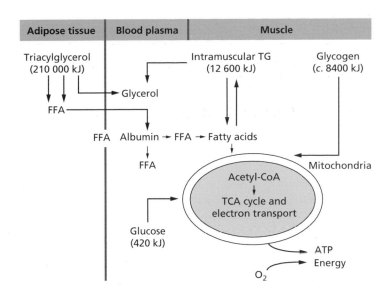

**Fig. 13.1** The storage and mobilization of peripheral adipose and intramuscular triacylglycerol (TG). TG from peripheral adipose tissue can be broken down to glycerol and free fatty acids (FFAs). FFAs can be mobilized by binding to plasma albumin for transport into the systemic circulation to skeletal muscle. Intramuscular TG can also be broken down to glycerol plus fatty acids, which can enter the mitochondria for oxidation during exercise. TCA, tricarboxylic acid. From Coyle (1997), with permission.

saturated and unsaturated FAs with chain lengths of 12–20 carbon atoms (Havel *et al.* 1964).

Small but physiologically important amounts of FA are also stored as triacylglycerols (TG) inside the muscle cells: the total muscle mass may contain up to 300 g of fat of which the major part is stored within the myocyte as small lipid droplets (Björkman 1986). FAs liberated from TG stored in adipocytes are released to blood, where they are bound to albumin. The albumin concentration of blood is about 6 mM, while the concentration of FA is about 0.2–1.0 mM. As albumin can bind up to eight FAs, the albumin transport capacity is far in excess of the amount of FAs bound under physiological circumstances and therefore cannot be the limiting factor for FA oxidation by muscle.

FA can also be derived from the triacylglycerol core of circulating chylomicrons and very low density lipoproteins (VLDL), which are both formed from dietary fat in the postabsorptive state. Chylomicrons are formed in the epithelial wall of the intestine and reach the blood stream after passage through the lymphatic system. VLDLs are synthesized in the liver after which they are released directly into the blood stream.

## Effects of exercise intensity and duration of fat metabolism

More than 50 years ago, Christensen and Hansen (1939) provided evidence from respiratory gas exchange measurements that fat was a major fuel for exercise metabolism. Since that time, a number of investigations have provided evidence that plasma FAs contribute a significant portion to the energy demands of mild-to-moderate exercise. However, until recently the rates of whole-body lipolysis had only been measured during very low-intensity exercise, and in untrained or moderately active individuals.

Our understanding of the regulation of endogenous fat and CHO metabolism in relation to exercise intensity and duration has been advanced considerably by modern-day studies which have used a combination of stable isotope techniques in association with conventional indirect calorimetry (Romijn *et al.* 1993, 1995; Sidossis & Wolfe 1996; Siddossis *et al.* 1996, 1997). As the three most abundant FAs are oxidized in proportion to their relative presence in the total plasma FA pool (Havel *et al.* 1964), total plasma FA kinetics can be reliably estimated from stable isotope studies using infusions of either palmitate or oleate (when the concentrations of total FAs and palmitate and oleate are known). Palmitate is a saturated 16-C FA ($CH_3(CH_2)_{14}COOH$) whose kinetics closely resemble those of most other long-chain FAs (Havel *et al.* 1964). As such, the rate of appearance (Ra) of palmitate gives an index of the release of FAs into the plasma. The Ra of glycerol, on the other hand, gives an index of whole-body lipolysis. Rates of total fat and CHO oxidation are determined by indirect calorimetry. The use of these methods has allowed estimates to be made of the rates of lipid kinetics, including the contribution to energy expenditure from peripheral lipolysis occurring in the adipocytes and from intramuscular lipolysis.

During low-intensity exercise (25% of maximum oxygen uptake ($\dot{V}o_{2max}$)), peripheral lipolysis is strongly stimulated, with little lipolysis of intramuscular TG (Fig. 13.2). Similarly, CHO oxidation appears to be met exclusively by blood glucose with little or no muscle glycogen utilization. Ra of FA into the plasma and their oxidation are highest during exercise at 25% of $\dot{V}o_{2max}$, and decline progressively as the exercise intensity

increases. Conversely, although intramuscular TG (and glycogen) do not contribute significantly to energy production during low-intensity work, fat oxidation is highest during exercise at about 65% of $\dot{V}o_{2max}$. (Fig. 13.2). At this intensity, lipolysis in both peripheral adipocytes and intramuscular TG stores attains its highest rates, and these two sources contribute about equally to the rate of total fat oxidation. With an increase in exercise intensity to 85% of $\dot{V}o_{2max}$, total fat oxidation falls. This is mainly due to a suppression in the Ra of FA into the plasma, presumably caused by the increases in circulating plasma catecholamines, which stimulate muscle glycogenolysis and glucose uptake. Lipolysis of intramuscular TG does not increase substantially with an increase in exercise intensity from 65% to 85% of $\dot{V}o_{2max}$, indicating that lipolysis of peripheral adipose tissue and lipolysis of intramuscular TG are regulated differently. Further evidence for this hypothesis comes from studies which have increased FA delivery (by intravenous infusion of lipid and heparin) during intense (85% of $\dot{V}o_{2max}$) exercise in well-trained subjects (Romijn *et al.* 1995). These data reveal that even when plasma FA concentration is artificially maintained above 1 mM, this only partly restores fat oxidation to those (higher) levels seen at more moderate intensity (65% of $\dot{V}o_{2max}$) exercise. Taken collectively, these observations indicate that factors other than FA availability play an important role in the regulation of FA oxidation during high-intensity exercise (see following sections).

With regard to the effects of exercise duration on fat metabolism, there is little change in either the rates of total fat or total CHO oxidation after 2h compared with the first 30 min of exercise at 25% of $\dot{V}o_{2max}$. However, at an intensity of 65% of $\dot{V}o_{2max}$, there is a progressive increase in the Ra of FA into the plasma (and presumably their oxidation) and glucose availability over time. After 2h of cycling at this intensity, there is no change in either the rates of total fat and total CHO oxidation compared with the situation after 30 min of exercise. Thus, it is likely that the contribution of intramuscular substrates (TG and glycogen)

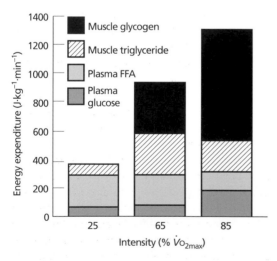

**Fig. 13.2** The maximal contribution to energy expenditure from endogenous fat and carbohydrate, expressed as a function of increasing exercise intensity. FFA, free fatty acids; $\dot{V}o_{2max}$, maximal oxygen uptake. From Romijn *et al.* (1993), with permission from the American Physiological Society.

to total energy expenditure decreases with increasing exercise duration during prolonged (>90 min) moderate-intensity (65% of $\dot{V}o_{2max.}$) exercise.

## Factors limiting fat oxidation by muscle

### Factors limiting fatty acid uptake by muscle cells

As previously discussed, the metabolism of FA derived from adipose tissue lipolysis constitutes a major substrate for oxidative metabolism, especially during prolonged, low-intensity exercise. The metabolism of long-chain FA is a complex and integrated process that involves a number of events: FA mobilization from peripheral adipose tissue, transport in the plasma, transport and permeation across muscle cell membranes and interstitium, cytoplasmic transport, and intracellular metabolism. The first stage in this process, the mobilization of lipids, plays a key role in the subsequent regulation of FA utilization during both the resting state and exercise.

During perfusion of the muscle capillaries, FA bound to albumin or stored in the core of chylomicrons and VLDL have to be released prior to transport across the vascular membrane. In the case of VLDL and chylomicrons, this is achieved by the action of the enzyme lipoprotein lipase (LPL). LPL is synthesized within the muscle cell and, after an activation process, is translocated to the vascular endothelial cell membrane where it exerts its enzymatic action on TG. LPL also expresses phospholipase $A_2$ activity which is necessary for the breakdown of the phospholipid surface layer of the chylomicrons and lipoproteins.

LPL activity is upregulated by caffeine, catecholamines and adrenocorticotrophic hormone (ACTH), and downregulated by insulin (for review, see Jeukendrup 1997). After TG hydrolysis, most of the FA will be taken up by muscle, whereas glycerol will be taken away via the bloodstream to the liver, where it may serve as a gluconeogenic precursor. During the postabsorptive state, the concentration of circulating TG in plasma is usually higher than that of FA, in contrast to the fasting state when chylomicrons are practically absent from the circulation. Nevertheless, the quantitative contribution of circulating TG to FA oxidation by the exercising muscle cells in humans is somewhat uncertain. Due to technical limitations, no reliable data are available to determine whether FA derived from the TG core of VLDL or chylomicrons substantially contribute to overall FA utilization. However, it is interesting to note that even a small extraction ratio of the order of 2–3% of FA/TG could potentially cover over up to 50% of total exogenous FA uptake and subsequent oxidation (Havel et al. 1967).

The arterial concentration of FA strongly affects FA uptake into muscle both at rest and during low-intensity exercise (for review, see Bulow 1988). This implies an FA gradient from blood to muscle in these conditions, which is achieved by a relatively rapid conversion of FA, taken up by the muscle cell, to fatty acyl-CoA. The rate of the latter reaction step is controlled by fatty acyl-CoA synthetase. During transport of FA from blood to muscle, several barriers may limit FA uptake, including the membranes of the vascular endothelial cell, the interstitial space between endothelium and muscle cell, and finally the muscle cell membrane (for review, see van der Vusse & Reneman 1996).

Uptake by endothelial cells is most likely protein mediated. Both albumin-binding protein and membrane-associated FA-binding proteins (FABP) may play a role. After uptake, most FAs will diffuse from the luminal to the abluminal membrane of the endothelial cells as free molecules. Although small amounts of FABP are present at this site, their role in transmembrane FA transport is assumed to be unimportant. Once in the interstitial space, albumin will bind the FAs for transport to the muscle cell membrane. Here the FAs are taken over by a fatty-acid-transporting protein, or will cross the membrane directly because of their lipophilic nature. In the sarcoplasm, FABP, which is present in relatively high concentrations, is crucial for FA transport to the mitochondria. This transport is assumed not to ultimately limit FA oxidation.

As indicated earlier, an alternative source of FA are TGs present inside the skeletal muscle cells. For the storage of FA, glycerol is obtained from glycolysis (as glycerol-3-phosphate) which reacts with fatty acyl-CoA, after which further condensation to and storage as TG take place in small fat droplets, mainly located in the proximity of the mitochondrial system. It has been suggested that adipocytes, positioned between muscle cells may also supply FA for oxidation, although the physiological significance of this has never been accurately quantified. During periods of increased muscle contractile activity, muscle lipase is activated by hormonal actions which leads to the release of FA from the intramuscular TG. Noradrenaline infusion has been observed to cause a significant reduction in muscle TG, and insulin counteracts this effect. Apart from hormonal stimuli, there is also local muscular control of lipase activity, shown by the observation that electrical stimulation of muscle enhances TG breakdown.

Compared to fast twitch (type II) muscle fibres, slow twitch (type I) fibres have a high lipase activity (Gorski 1992) as well as TG content (Essen 1977). Interestingly, TG storage within the muscle cell can be increased by regular endurance training (Morgan *et al.* 1969; Howald *et al.* 1985; Martin 1996). However, whereas some studies report an increased utilization of intramuscular triacylglycerol after endurance training (Hurley *et al.* 1986; Martin *et al.* 1993), others (Kiens 1993) find no change. These conflicting results may simply be a reflection of the different type of exercise modes employed (cycling vs. dynamic knee-extension exercise), which result in marked differences in circulating catecholamine levels. On the other hand, an inability to detect exercise-induced perturbations in intramuscular TG content does not exclude the possibility that while FAs are being hydrolysed from the intramuscular TG pool, TG is also being synthesized, with the net result that there is no change in concentration (Turcotte *et al.*

1995). If indeed the intramuscular TG pool is in a state of constant turnover, a net decline in stores would only be observed when the rate of utilization of intramuscular TG is greater than the rate of TG synthesis.

### Factors limiting fatty acid oxidation by muscle cells

As previously discussed, a relatively high percentage of the total energy production is derived from FA oxidation at rest and during low-intensity exercise. However, with increasing exercise intensities, particularly above 70–80% of $\dot{V}o_{2max}$, there is a progressive shift from fat to CHO (Gollnick 1985), indicating a limitation to the rate of FA oxidation. Several explanations for this shift from fat to CHO have been proposed, including an increase in circulating catecholamines, which stimulates glycogen breakdown in both the muscle and liver. However, the increased lactate formation (and accompanying hydrogen ion accumulation) which occurs when glycogen breakdown and glycolytic flux are increased also suppresses lipolysis. The net result will be a decrease in plasma FA concentration and hence in the supply of FA to muscle cells. As a consequence, enhanced CHO oxidation will most likely compensate for the reduced FA oxidation.

Another reason for this substrate shift is the lower ATP production rate per unit of time from fat compared with that from CHO, combined with the fact that more oxygen is needed for the production of any given amount of ATP from fat than from CHO, as previously noted. Finally, limitations in the FA flux from blood to mitochondria might explain the shift from fat to CHO at higher exercise intensities. This flux is dependent on the concentration of FA in the blood, capillary density, transport capacity across vascular and muscle cell membranes, mitochondrial density and mitochondrial capacity to take up and oxidize FA. The latter depends on the action of the carnitine transport system across the mitochondrial membrane which is regulated by malonyl-CoA (Winder *et al.* 1989). During exercise, malonyl-CoA formation is reduced and therefore the capacity to transport FAs across the mitochondrial inner membrane is enhanced.

The rate of oxidation of FA is the result of three processes:

1 Lipolysis of TG in adipose tissue and circulating TG and transport of FA from blood plasma to the sarcoplasm.

2 Availability and rate of hydrolysis of intramuscular TG.

3 Activation of the FA and transport across the mitochondrial membrane.

It is likely that the first two processes pose the ultimate limitations to fat oxidation observed during conditions of maximal FA flux. This is most evident during both short-term intense exercise or during the initial phase of a long-term exercise. In this condition, lipolysis in adipose tissue and in muscle TG is insufficiently upregulated to result in enhanced FA supply. The result will be that the rate of FA oxidation exceeds the rate at which FAs are mobilized, leading to a fall in plasma FAs and intracellular FAs in muscle. As a consequence, the use of CHO from glycogen must be increased to cover the increased energy demand.

Direct evidence that the rate of FA oxidation can be limited by a suppression of lipolysis, at least during low-to-moderate intensity (44% of $\dot{V}o_{2max.}$) exercise, comes from a recent investigation by Horowitz *et al.* (1997). They showed that CHO ingestion ($0.8\,g\cdot kg^{-1}$ body mass) *before* exercise, which resulted in a $10–30\,\mu U\cdot ml^{-1}$ elevation in plasma insulin concentration, was enough to reduce fat oxidation *during* exercise, primarily by a suppression of lipolysis. They also showed that fat oxidation could be elevated (by about 30%) when plasma FA concentration was increased via Intralipid and heparin infusion, even when CHO was ingested. However, the increase in lipolysis was not sufficient to restore fat oxidation to those levels observed after fasting. Taken collectively, these results suggest that CHO ingestion (and the concomitant eleva-

tion in plasma insulin concentration) has another (additional) effect on reducing the rates of FA oxidation by exercising skeletal muscle.

## Conclusion

In contrast to body CHO reserves, fat stores are abundant in humans and represent a vast source of fuel for exercising muscle. FAs stored both in peripheral adipose tissue and inside the muscle cells serve as quantitatively important energy sources for exercise metabolism. During low-intensity work (25% of $\dot{V}o_{2max.}$), plasma FA liberated from adipose tissue represents the main source of fuel for contracting muscle, with little or no contribution from intramuscular lipolysis to total energy metabolism. On the other hand, during moderate-intensity exercise (65% of $\dot{V}o_{2max.}$), fat metabolism is highest, with the contribution of lipolysis from peripheral adipocytes and of intramuscular TG stores contributing about equally to total fat oxidation. During high-intensity exercise (85% of $\dot{V}o_{2max.}$), there is a marked reduction in the rate of entry of FA into the plasma, but no further increase in intramuscular TG utilization. At such workrates, muscle glycogenolysis and the accompanying increased lactate concentration suppress the rates of whole-body lipolysis.

The major hormonal changes which promote lipolysis during exercise are an increase in catecholamine concentration and a decline in insulin levels, both of which facilitate activation of LPL. The rate of FA oxidation is also regulated indirectly by the oxidative capacity of the working muscles and the intramuscular concentration of malonyl-CoA. The muscle tissue level of malonyl-CoA is dependent on the prevailing concentrations of plasma glucose and insulin: elevated circulating levels of these two compounds is associated with elevated concentrations of malonyl-CoA. Any increase in glycolytic flux therefore may directly inhibit long-chain FA oxidation, possibly by inhibiting its transport into the mitochondria (Sidossis & Wolfe 1996; Sidossis *et al.* 1996; Coyle *et al.* 1997).

# References

Björkman, O. (1986) Fuel utilization during exercise. In *Biochemical Aspects of Physical Exercise* (ed. O. Björkman), pp. 245–260. Elsevier, Amsterdam.

Bulow, J. (1988) Lipid mobilization and utilization. In *Principles of Exercise Biochemistry: Medicine and Sports Science* (ed. J.R. Poortmans), pp. 140–163. Karger, Basel.

Christensen, E.H. & Hansen, O. (1939) Respiratorischer quotient und $O_2$-aufnahme (Respiratory quotient and $O_2$ uptake). *Scandinavian Archives of Physiology* **81**, 180–189.

Coyle, E.F. (1997) Fuels for sport performance. In *Perspectives in Exercise Science and Sports Medicine*. Vol. 10. *Optimizing Sport Performance* (ed. D.R. Lamb & R. Murray), pp. 95–137. Cooper Publishing, Carmel, IN.

Coyle, E.F., Jeukendrup, A.E., Wagenmakers, A.J.M. & Saris, W.H.M. (1997) Fatty acid oxidation is directly regulated by carbohydrate metabolism during exercise. *American Journal of Physiology* **273**, E268–E275.

Essen, B. (1977) Intramuscular substrate utilization during prolonged exercise. In *The Marathon: Physiological, Medical, Epidemiological, and Psychological Studies* (ed. P. Milvy), pp. 30–44. New York Academy of Sciences, New York.

Felig, P. & Wahren, J. (1975) Fuel homeostasis in exercise. *New England Journal of Medicine* **293**, 1078–1084.

Gollnick, P.D. (1985) Metabolism of substrates: energy substrate metabolism during exercise and as modified by training. *Federation Proceedings* **44**, 353–357.

Gorski, J. (1992) Muscle triglyceride metabolism during exercise. *Canadian Journal of Physiology and Pharmacology* **70**, 123–131.

Havel, R.J., Carlson, L.A., Ekelund, L.G. & Holmgren, A. (1964) Turnover rate and oxidation of different fatty acids in man during exercise. *Journal of Applied Physiology* **19**, 613–619.

Havel, R.J., Pernow, B. & Jones, N.L. (1967) Uptake and release of free fatty acids and other metabolites in the legs of exercising men. *Journal of Applied Physiology* **23**, 90–99.

Hawley, J.A., Brouns, F. & Jeukendrup, A.E. (1998) Strategies to enhance fat utilisation during exercise. *Sports Medicine* **25**, 241–257.

Holloszy, J.O. (1990) Utilization of fatty acids during exercise. In *Biochemistry of Exercise*. Vol. VII (ed. A.W. Taylor, P.D. Gollnick & H.J. Green *et al.*), pp. 319–327. Human Kinetics, Champaign, IL.

Horowitz, J.F., Mora-Rodriguez, R., Byerley, L.O. & Coyle, E.F. (1997) Lipolytic suppression following carbohydrate ingestion limits fat oxidation during exercise. *American Journal of Physiology* **273**, E768–E775.

Howald, H., Hoppeler, H. & Claassen, H. (1985) Influences of endurance training on the ultrastructural composition of the different muscle fiber types in humans. *Pflugers Archives* **403**, 369–376.

Hurley, B.F., Nemeth, P.M., Martin, W.H., Hagberg, J.M., Dalsky, G.P. & Holloszy, J.O. (1986) Muscle triglyceride utilization during exercise: effect of training. *Journal of Applied Physiology* **60**, 562–567.

Jeukendrup, A.E. (1997) Fat metabolism during exercise, a review. In *Aspects of Carbohydrate and Fat Metabolism*, pp. 21–71. De Vrieseborch: Haarlem.

Kiens, B., Essen-Gustavsson, B., Christensen, N.J. & Saltin, B. (1993) Skeletal muscle substrate utilisation during submaximal exercise in man: effect of endurance training. *Journal of Physiology (London)* **469**, 459–478.

Lambert, E.V., Hawley, J.A., Goedecke, J., Noakes, T.D. & Dennis, S.C. (1997) Nutritional strategies for promoting fat utilization and delaying the onset of fatigue during prolonged exercise. *Journal of Sports Science* **15**, 315–324.

Martin, W.H. (1996) Effects of acute and chronic exercise on fat metabolism. In *Exercise and Sports Science Reviews*, Vol. 24 (ed. J.O. Holloszy), pp. 203–231. Williams & Wilkins, Baltimore.

Martin, W.H., Dalsky, G.P. & Hurley, B.F. (1993) Effect of endurance training on plasma free fatty acid turnover and oxidation during exercise. *American Journal of Physiology* **265**, E708–E714.

Morgan, T.E., Short, F.A. & Cobb, L.A. (1969) Effect of long-term exercise on skeletal muscle lipid composition. *American Journal of Physiology* **216**, 82–86.

Romijn, J.A., Coyle, E.F., Sidossis, L.S. *et al.* (1993) Regulation of endogenous fat and carbohydrate metabolism in relation to exercise intensity and duration. *American Journal of Physiology* **265**, E380–E391.

Romijn, J.A., Coyle, E.F., Sidossis, L.S., Zhang, X.J. & Wolfe, R.R. (1995) Relationship between fatty acid delivery and fatty acid oxidation during strenuous exercise. *Journal of Applied Physiology* **79**, 1939–1945.

Sidossis, L.S. & Wolfe, R.R. (1996) Glucose and insulin-induced inhibition of fatty acid oxidation: the glucose fatty-acid cycle reversed. *American Journal of Physiology* **270**, E733–E738.

Sidossis, L.S., Stuart, C.A., Schulman, G.I., Lopaschuk, G.D. & Wolfe, R.R. (1996) Glucose plus insulin regulate fat oxidation by controlling the rate of fatty acid entry into the mitochondria. *Journal of Clinical Investigation* **98**, 2244–2250.

Sidossis, L.S., Gastaldelli, A., Klien, S. & Wolfe, R.R. (1997) Regulation of plasma free fatty acid oxidation during low- and high-intensity exercise. *American Journal of Physiology* **272**, E1065–E1070.

Turcotte, L.P., Richter, E.A. & Kiens, B. (1995) Lipid metabolism during exercise. In *Exercise Metabolism* (ed. M. Hargreaves), pp. 99–130. Human Kinetics, Champaign, IL.

van der Vusse, G.J. & Reneman, R.S. (1996) Lipid metabolism in muscle. In *Handbook of Physiology. Section 12. Exercise: Regulation and integration of multiple systems* (ed. L.B. Rowell & J.T. Shepherd), pp. 952–994. American Physiological Society, Oxford Press, New York.

Winder, W.W., Arogyasami, J., Barton, R.J., Elayan, I.M. & Vehrs, P.R. (1989) Muscle malonyl-CoA decreases during exercise. *Journal of Applied Physiology* **67**, 2230–2233.

# Chapter 14

# Adaptations to a High Fat Diet

BENTE KIENS AND JØRN W. HELGE

## Historical perspective

It is known from practical experience, obtained from the large number of polar expeditions occurring from the middle of the last century, that the dietary intake of indigenous people and their domestic animals (sledge dogs) had a very high fat content. As early as 1908, August and Marie Krogh studied the metabolism of the Greenland Eskimo where food consumption was calculated, based on observations made by the Danish explorer Rink in 1855 (Krogh & Krogh 1913). Despite such a fat-rich diet, these indigenous people and their dogs seemed to maintain normal work capacity and normal body function.

In the laboratory, several groups of scientists from the turn of the century have tried to elucidate what substrate is oxidized in muscle during exercise. Short-term dietary changes, mostly to fat-rich and carbohydrate-rich diets, were applied. Zuntz *et al.* (1901) demonstrated that respiratory quotient (RQ) values during mild exercise after a fat-rich diet were of a magnitude that suggested an almost exclusive oxidation of fat. This was later supported by Krogh and Lindhard (1920) and Marsh and Murlin (1928). In the studies by Krogh and Lindhard (1920), the subjects were asked to describe their food intake and the perception of daily living chores and exercise sessions while eating a fat-rich or a carbohydrate-rich diet for 3–5 days. The subjects almost uniformly described that exercise was performed easily after consumption of the carbo-

hydrate diet, while exercise was performed with severe difficulty after consumption of the fat diet. Krogh and Lindhard (1920) also demonstrated that the muscular efficiency, measured on a Krogh bicycle ergometer positioned within a Jaquet respiration chamber, was some 10–11% more effective while carbohydrates were oxidized than while fat was oxidized. These findings were later supported by Hill (1924) and Marsh and Murlin (1928).

The work by Christensen and Hansen (1939) revealed a lower respiratory exchange ratio (RER) during exercise and a shorter endurance performance time at a submaximal exercise intensity after 3–5 days' adaptation to a fat diet than after 3–5 days' adaptation to a carbohydrate diet. Thus, interest in the influence of diet on work capacity is not new, but during the last 50 years, focus has mainly been on the role of dietary carbohydrates for enhancing physical performance. However, because athletes today participate in physically demanding events of ever-increasing duration, it has been speculated whether habitually eating a high-fat diet could provide some of the adaptations that are produced by habitual physical exercise and thus improve physical performance.

## Endurance performance in rats

In animals, the effect of adaptation to a fat-rich diet on endurance performance has mostly been investigated in rodents and less often in dogs and other animals. Studies in rats adapted to a fat-rich diet have shown a positive effect on endurance performance. However, in most studies, fat-rich diets that are practically carbohydrate free have been used. For instance, in the study by Miller *et al.* (1984), endurance performance was evaluated after rats were exposed to a diet consisting of 78% of total energy intake (E%) as fat, 1 E% carbohydrate and 15 E% protein, or a diet containing 69 E% carbohydrate, 11 E% fat and 20 E% protein for 1 and 5 weeks. They demonstrated that rats ran for a longer time after adaptation to the fat diet than on the normal diet already after only 1 week's adaptation to the diet (45±5 min vs. 42±4 min) and this difference was even larger after 5 weeks' adaptation (47±4 min vs. 35±3 min). These findings are in contrast to those of Conlee *et al.* (1990), who report unchanged endurance performance time when rats had been exposed for 4–5 weeks to either a fat- or carbohydrate-rich diet, similar in composition to those diets utilized in the study by Miller *et al.* (1984). In both of these studies, training status of the rats was not altered during the dietary intervention period. However, if both training and a fat diet induce adaptations that increase the fat oxidative capacity, then it might be reasoned that combining the two interventions could result in an additive effect and in turn could optimize endurance capacity. In the study by Simi *et al.* (1991), where 12 weeks of training in combination with the intake of either a fat-rich diet (no carbohydrates included) or a carbohydrate-rich diet (no fat included), rats ran for a longer time after adaptation to training and the fat-rich diet than those on a carbohydrate-rich diet. Rats fed the carbohydrate diet were all exhausted before 7 h of exercise, whereas half of the fat-fed rats had to be stopped after 7.5 h of running before becoming exhausted. However, in that study untrained rats fed the fat-rich diet also ran longer (68±5 min) than those fed the carbohydrate diet (42±4 min).

In the study by Lapachet *et al.* (1996), rats were trained 5 days per week, for 2 h at a time on a treadmill for 8 weeks while fed either a fat diet (79 E% fat, 0 E% carbohydrates) or a carbohydrate diet (69 E% carbohydrates, 10 E% fat). They found a 31% longer endurance performance time in the fat-adapted rats than in the rats adapted to the carbohydrate diet.

In summary, it appears that endurance performance time in rats is not shorter but mostly longer in fat-fed than in carbohydrate-fed rats, both in rats adapted to training and in sedentary rats. In these studies, the fat diets contained no carbohydrates and a very high proportion of fat. In a recent study, however, findings demonstrated that after 4 weeks of training and adaptation to a fat-rich diet containing 15 E% carbohydrates, endurance performance was similarly enhanced compared with that of rats which had been exposed to a carbohydrate-rich diet (Helge *et al.* 1998). This study demonstrated no effect of dietary composition on exercise time to exhaustion in either sedentary (mean running time to exhaustion, 50±3 min) or trained rats (153±8 min). In the study by Tollenar (1976), similar findings were obtained. In that study, rats were initially fed a stock diet for 4 months, followed by 3 weeks on a 40 E% fat diet. Then the rats were trained on a treadmill for 16 weeks while fed *ad libitum* one of three different diets consisting of 20 E%, 40 E% or 70 E% of fat. Data revealed that dietary fat content had no effect on running time to exhaustion. These findings lead to the conclusion that the relative proportion of carbohydrate–fat content in the diet is of significance in the adaptation to dietary fat and thus on running time to exhaustion in rats. Enhanced performance is apparently only observed when the fat-rich diet is virtually free from carbohydrates.

An interesting idea to investigate is whether prolonged exposure to a fat-rich diet followed by brief exposure to a carbohydrate-rich diet *per se* could improve endurance performance further. The reasoning behind such a speculation is that a prolonged fat-diet regimen might induce a high-fat oxidative capacity. Then after switching to a carbohydrate-rich diet, muscle glycogen stores are maximized and thus the muscle is provided with both a high-fat oxidative capacity and with large muscle glycogen stores. This approach was first addressed by Conlee *et al.* (1990), who investigated whether animals adapted to a prolonged high-fat diet could tolerate a second bout of exercise following 3 days of recovery consuming a carbohydrate-rich diet compared with animals adapted to a prolonged high-carbohydrate diet after consuming a fat-rich diet. Even though Conlee and co-workers (1990) found that fat-fed rats ran equally long as carbohydrate-fed rats, switching the diet for the last 3 days resulted in better endurance performance by fat-adapted animals switched to the carbohydrate diet for 3 days than carbohydrate-fed animals continued on the carbohydrate diet for 3 more days. Also, in the study by Lapachet et al. (1996), when training was combined with diet for 8 weeks, rats ran approximately 40% longer when the rats, after fat adaptation, switched to the carbohydrate diet for 3 days than when the rats were fed only a carbohydrate diet. Thus, in rats endurance performance time was increased after prolonged fat adaptation and a subsequent brief exposure to a carbohydrate-rich diet.

In rats the literature reveals a fairly uniform positive effect of fat-rich, virtually carbohydrate-free diet on endurance performance in rats, whereas there is an apparent discrepancy regarding the effect of dietary fats on endurance performance in man.

## Endurance performance in man

It is well known from the classic literature that increasing the dietary fat relative to carbohydrates results in increased fat and decreased carbohydrate utilization during submaximal exercise (Christensen & Hansen 1939). Thus, it has been hypothesized that increasing the availability of fatty acids for oxidation might increase the oxidation of fat and spare carbohydrate and furthermore increase performance. Due to this hypothesis, acute dietary and pharmacological methods have been used to enhance the availability of fatty acids for oxidation. In the study by Griffiths et al. (1996), eight subjects consumed either a fat-rich meal (65 E% fat, 28 E% carbohydrate, 7 E% protein) or a carbohydrate meal (2 E% fat, 80 E% carbohydrate, 18 E% protein) and

were followed over the next 6 h, while resting. Prior to the fat meal the plasma concentration of free fatty acids (FFAs) amounted to $400 \mu mol \cdot l^{-1}$. One hour after ingestion of the fat meal, the plasma concentration of FFA had decreased to $200 \mu mol \cdot l^{-1}$, whereafter plasma FFA increased continuously to $500 \mu mol \cdot l^{-1}$ at 4 h and approximately $550 \mu mol \cdot l^{-1}$ at 6 h. Thus, the intake of 80 g fat, as in this study, was not associated with any particular increase in circulating fatty acids during the following 6 h. Studies have established that glucose feeding prior to exercise produces hyperglycaemia, inducing stimulation of insulin secretion, which in turn depresses the exercise-induced lipolysis and increases RQ, indicating an increased participation of carbohydrates in the total energy expenditure. The question is whether fat feeding prior to exercise would enhance the oxidation of fat at the expense of carbohydrate during exercise. This question was addressed in the study by Satabin et al. (1987). Nine trained male subjects either were fasting or ingested a pre-exercise meal (1.7 MJ, 400 kcal) 1 h prior to a submaximal exercise test (60% of $\dot{V}o_{2max.}$) to exhaustion. The meals contained either medium-chain triacylglycerols, long-chain triacylglycerols or glucose. During exercise, plasma insulin concentrations were decreased in all conditions. The FFA concentrations were increased similarly after the two lipid meals and in the fasting situation and markedly higher than that in the glucose trial, and RQ was significantly lower in the lipid trials and in the fasting condition than in the glucose trial. Despite the enhanced fat oxidation during exercise, after the consumption of a fat meal, no differences in endurance time (approximately 110 min) between any of the four dietary trials were seen. Also, in studies in which intralipid-heparin was infused during exercise, the availability of fatty acids was markedly increased. In the study by Hargreaves et al. (1991), a sparing of muscle glycogen during exercise was not seen, whereas a decreased rate of glycogen degradation was found in another study (Dyck et al. 1993). Endurance performance was, however, not measured in any of these studies. Also, the ingestion of caffeine appears to stimulate the release of fatty acids from the fat stores, at least in well-trained athletes, thus increasing the plasma concentration of FFA. However, studies have provided a conflicting picture of the effect on endurance performance in man (Spriet 1995).

With regard to all these attempts to increase the plasma concentration of fatty acids, one must bear in mind that during submaximal exercise only a small percentage (7–15%) of the arterial plasma FFA concentration is extracted (Turcotte *et al.* 1992). Moreover, from the literature it seems as if there is a fairly linear relationship between FFA availability and FFA uptake and oxidation until a FFA concentration of approximately $700\,\mu mol \cdot l^{-1}$. Beyond this concentration, no further uptake and oxidation of FFA appears in non-trained subjects despite a further increase in circulating FFA availability (Turcotte *et al.* 1992; Kiens *et al.* 1993). It seems, however, that the concentration at which saturation occurs is somewhat higher in trained subjects (Fig. 14.1) (Kiens *et al.* 1993). By using stable isotopes, Romijn *et al.* (1995) evaluated the relationship between fatty acid availability and oxidation in six endurance-trained cyclists. They were studied during 30 min of exercise at 84% of $\dot{V}o_{2max.}$ on two different occasions: once during a control trial when plasma FFA concentrations were normally low (0.2–0.3 mmol·l⁻¹) and again when plasma FFA concentration was maintained between 1 and 2 mmol·l⁻¹ by intravenous infusion of lipid-heparin. In the control trial, total fat oxidation amounted to $27 \pm 3\,\mu mol \cdot kg^{-1} \cdot min^{-1}$. Even though the availability of FFA in the lipid-heparin infusion trial was increased severalfold, the total fat oxidation only increased to an average of $34 \pm 4\,\mu mol \cdot kg^{-1} \cdot min^{-1}$ (Fig. 14.2). Thus, the contribution of fat oxidation to energy expenditure increased from approximately 27% during control to approximately 35% during lipid-heparin infusion ($P < 0.05$).

Summarizing these findings, it appears that in those studies in which the plasma FFA concentration was succesfully elevated, no clear effects on endurance performance were demonstrated. A reason for this could be that the FFA uptake

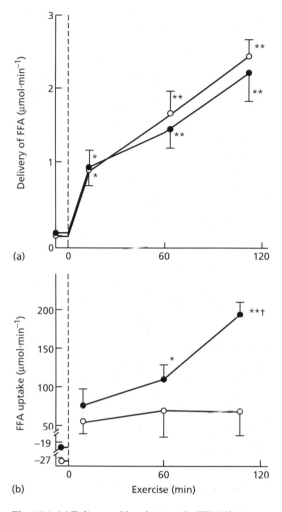

**Fig. 14.1** (a) Delivery of free fatty acids (FFA) (fatty acid concentration times plasma flow), and (b) net uptake of FFA during 2 h of dynamic knee-extensor exercise with either the non-trained (○) or the endurance-trained (●) thigh. *, $P < 0.05$ compared with resting values; **, $P < 0.05$ compared with previous measurements; †, $P < 0.05$ between non-trained and trained. Adapted from Kiens *et al.* (1993).

plateaus around $700-1000\,\mu mol \cdot l^{-1}$. Another explanation might be that increasing the fatty acid oxidation at a given power output is not of importance for endurance.

In dietary intervention studies lasting 3–5 days, the prevailing concept is that endurance performance after consuming a carbohydrate-

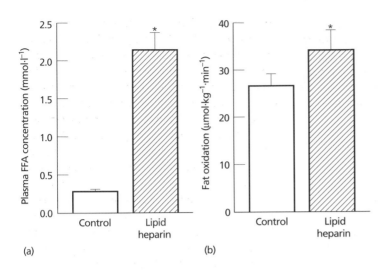

**Fig. 14.2** (a) Plasma free fatty acid (FFA) concentrations, and (b) total fat oxidation during a 20–30-min exercise period for six subjects during a control trial and during intralipid infusion. Subjects exercised for 30 min at 85% of maximal oxygen uptake. *, $P < 0.05$ compared with control trial. Adapted from Romijn *et al.* (1995).

rich diet is superior to that when a fat-rich diet is consumed. Thus, in the classic study by Christensen and Hansen from 1939, three trained subjects consumed either a fat-rich diet (containing only 5 E% carbohydrates) or a carbohydrate-rich diet (90 E% carbohydrates) for 3–5 days. Exercise to exhaustion at approximately 65–70% of maximal oxygen uptake revealed an average endurance time on the carbohydrate diet of 210 min, which was markedly longer than when on the fat diet (90 min). Also, when intermittent exercise (30 min running followed by 10 min rest) at 70% of maximal oxygen uptake was performed in trained men, endurance performance time to exhaustion was significantly impaired after consuming a fat diet, consisting of 76 E% fat, 13.5 E% protein, for 4 days (62±6 min) compared with when a carbohydrate-rich diet (77 E% carbohydrate, 13.5 E% protein) was consumed for 4 days (106±5 min) (Galbo *et al.* 1979). Also, the short-term studies by Bergström *et al.* (1967) and Karlsson and Saltin (1971) suggested that 3–7 days of fat diet were detrimental to exercise performance. Thus, it is evident from these brief dietary manipulations that 'fat-loading' impairs endurance performance. However, in these short-term dietary studies, the primary goal was to determine the extent to which muscle glycogen content could be altered by varying the dietary regimen after depletion of the glycogen

stores and subsequently to ascertain the relation between the individual muscle glycogen content and the capacity for prolonged exercise. Thus, these short-term carbohydrate-restricted diets probably reflect rather acute responses to changes in diet.

Longer-term adaptation to fat-rich diets may, on the other hand, induce skeletal muscle adaptations, metabolic as well as morphological, which in turn could influence exercise performance. It has been known for a long time that endurance training induces several adaptations in skeletal muscle such as increased capillarization, increased mitochondrial density, increased activity of several oxidative enzymes (Saltin & Gollnick 1983) and, furthermore, as recently shown, an increased content of fatty acid binding protein in the sarcolemma (FABPpm) (Kiens *et al.* 1997), parameters that all are suggested to play a significant role in enhancing lipid oxidation.

It might be speculated that a way to influence the fat oxidative system further, is to increase the substrate flux of fatty acids through the system by increasing the fat content of the diet. This might result in further adaptations in the fat oxidative capacity, providing possibilities for an increased fat oxidation, a sparing of carbohydrates and an increasing endurance performance. Thus, in the study by Muoio *et al.* (1994), five well-trained runners followed a dietary regimen lasting 7 days. The runners performed two different treadmill tests after consuming either a normal diet, a mixed diet, a moderate fat diet (38 E% fat, 50 E% carbohydrates) or a carbohydrate-rich diet (73 E% carbohydrates, 15 E% fat) assigned in this order. Running time, at 85% of $\dot{V}o_{2max.}$ for 30 min and then at 75–80% of $\dot{V}o_{2max.}$ until exhaustion, was longer following the fat diet (91±10 min) than after both the normal, mixed (69±7 min) and the carbohydrate-rich diet (76±8 min). Although these findings suggest that a 7-day fat diet improves endurance performance in trained males, several flaws in the design of the study are obvious. For example, the diets were not administered randomly and there was no separation between the different dietary periods. The fat diet only contained 38 E% fat and can therefore hardly be characterized as a fat-rich diet. Besides, a dietary carbohydrate intake of 50 E% resulted in a daily intake of a fairly high amount of carbohydrates (approximately 430 g·day⁻¹). Furthermore, a maximal exercise test was performed before the submaximal endurance test only separated by a short break, and this inevitably confounds the interpretation of dietary effects on endurance performance. Moreover, during exercise the R-values were similar in all three diets and although the concentration of plasma fatty acids was highest in the fat diet, plasma glycerol concentrations were lower than in the two other diets. Thus, the metabolic responses during exercise do not give support to the concept that the longer running time was induced by the diet.

Lambert *et al.* (1994) extended the dietary intervention period to 14 days. They studied five endurance-trained cyclists consuming, in a random order, either a 74 E% carbohydrate diet (HC) or a 76 E% fat diet (HF), separated by 2 weeks on *ad libitum* or normal diet, during which they continued their normal training. The study revealed that maximal power output (862±94 W vs. 804±65 W for HF and HC, respectively) and high-intensity bicycle exercise to exhaustion at approximately 90% of $\dot{V}o_{2max.}$ (8.3±2 vs. 12.5± 4 min for HF and HC, respectively) were not impaired after the fat diet. Moreover, during a subsequent prolonged submaximal exercise test at approximately 60% $\dot{V}o_{2max.,}$ endurance performance was significantly enhanced on the fat diet compared with when on the carbohydrate diet. This improvement in submaximal endurance capacity occurred despite an initial muscle glycogen content twofold lower (32±6 mmol·kg⁻¹ wet weight) than in the carbohydrate-adapted trial (78±5 mmol·kg⁻¹ wet weight). However, the subjects performed three consecutive tests on the same day only separated by short rest intervals and the submaximal endurance test to exhaustion was always performed as the last test. This design confounds the interpretation of dietary effects on endurance performance. In contrast, in the study by Pruett (1970), relatively well-trained subjects performed intermittent exercise tests (45-min bouts followed each time by a 15-min rest period) until exhaustion after consuming either a standard diet (31 E% fat, 59 E% carbohydrate, 10 E% protein), a fat diet (64 E% fat, 26 E% carbohydrate, 10 E% protein) or a carbohydrate diet (8 E% fat, 82 E% carbohydrate, 9 E% protein) for at least 14 days. Nine subjects participated in the study and each subject was placed on one of the three different diets; four of the subjects consumed all three diets. The exercise experiments were performed with 2-week intervals at power outputs equal to 50% and 70% of $\dot{V}o_{2max.}$ The subjects maintained their training throughout the 2 months required to complete a series of experiments. It was reported that exercising at 50% $\dot{V}o_{2max.}$ time to exhaustion was not different between the three diets. However, maximal possible work time was 270 min and due to that, several of the subjects were stopped before they were exhausted. At 70% $\dot{V}o_{2max.,}$ exercise time to exhaustion was not different between the standard (175±15 min) and the fat diet (164±19 min), whereas a longer work time was observed when on the carbohydrate diet (193±12 min) than when on the fat diet (164±19 min).

An even longer period of adaptation to a fat diet was studied by Phinney *et al.* (1983). Submaximal endurance performance was studied in five well-trained bicyclists fed a eucaloric balanced diet (EBD) for 1 week, providing 147–

$210 \, kJ \cdot kg^{-1} \cdot day^{-1}$ ($35–50 \, kcal \cdot kg^{-1} \cdot day^{-1}$), $1.75 \, g$ protein $\cdot kg^{-1} \cdot day^{-1}$ and the remainder of calories as two-thirds carbohydrates and one-third fat. This was followed by 4 weeks of a eucaloric ketogenic diet (EKD), isocaloric and isonitrogenous with the EBD diet, but providing fewer than $20 \, g$ carbohydrates daily. The subjects continued their normal training throughout the study. Endurance time to exhaustion, at $60–65\% \, \dot{V}o_{2max}$, was longer in three subjects (57%, 30%, 2%) and shorter in two (36%, 28%) after 4 weeks' adaptation to EKD, resulting in no statistical difference in the mean exercise time after the two dietary trials ($147 \pm 13 \, min$ for EBD vs. $151 \pm 25 \, min$ for EKD). However, the big variability in performance time of the subjects makes the results difficult to interpret. A highly significant decrease in RQ values during the endurance test was found and in agreement with this a threefold drop in glucose oxidation and a fourfold reduction in muscle glycogen use were demonstrated.

To summarize, so far the literature has provided a conflicting picture when the effect of dietary fat on endurance performance is investigated in man. These disparate results could be explained by the varied research designs used, making firm conclusions impossible. Moreover, dietary manipulations for only 4 weeks may not be long enough to induce adaptations in skeletal muscle of importance for endurance exercise capacity. Also, one might speculate whether training status, as indicated by maximal oxygen uptake of the subjects, could be of any significance. In the study by Helge *et al.* (1998), the interaction between training and diet was investigated. Fifteen initially non-trained male subjects were randomly assigned to consume a fat diet (62 E% fat, 21 E% carbohydrate, 17 E% protein) or a carbohydrate diet (20 E% fat, 65 E% carbohydrate, 15 E% protein) while following a supervised training programme for 4 weeks. Training was performed four times weekly and each training session alternated between short and long-lasting intervals at $60–85\%$ of $\dot{V}o_{2max}$, lasting $60 \, min$. After the 4-week intervention period, $\dot{V}o_{2max}$ was similarly increased by 9% in both dietary groups ($P < 0.05$). Endurance perfor-

mance time to exhaustion, measured on a Krogh bicycle ergometer, at 72% of $\dot{V}o_{2max}$ (same absolute power output as in the initial non-trained trial), was similarly and significantly increased in both dietary groups both after 2 and 4 weeks of training and dieting (Table 14.1). Thus, comparing the trained subjects in the fat group with those in the carbohydrate group after 4 weeks, exercising at the same relative workload (72% of $\dot{V}o_{2max}$), no differences in exercise time to exhaustion were found between the two dietary groups ($79 \pm 8 \, min$ in the fat group vs. $79 \pm 15 \, min$ in the carbohydrate group). Thus, it appears that adaptation to a fat diet in combination with training up to 4 weeks, exercising at a submaximal intensity ($60–70\%$ of $\dot{V}o_{2max}$), does not impair endurance performance (Phinney *et al.* 1983; Helge *et al.* 1998). However, in the study by Helge *et al.* (1996), two groups of non-trained male subjects underwent a 7-week supervised training programme while consuming either a fat diet (62 E% fat, 21 E% carbohydrate, 17 E% protein) or a carbohydrate diet (20 E% fat, 65 E% carbohydrate, 15 E% protein). Maximal oxygen uptake increased similarly in the two groups by 11% ($P < 0.05$). Time to exhaustion, exercising on a Krogh bicycle ergometer at 82% of pretraining $\dot{V}o_{2max}$, was significantly increased, from initial mean values for the two groups of $35 \pm 4 \, min$ to $65 \pm 7 \, min$ in the fat group, but significantly more in the carbohydrate group ($102 \pm 5 \, min$). Thus, combining these findings it is apparent that the

**Table 14.1** Endurance performance (mean $\pm$ SE, measured in minutes) until exhaustion before and after 2 weeks' and after 4 weeks' adaptation to training and a fat-rich or a carbohydrate-rich diet.

|  | Before | After 2 weeks | After 4 weeks |
|---|---|---|---|
| Fat-rich diet | $29.5 \pm 4.3$ | $47.8 \pm 8.1$* | $78.5 \pm 8.2$* |
| Carbohydrate-rich diet | $31.7 \pm 4.3$ | $59.5 \pm 10.6$* | $79.3 \pm 15.1$* |

From Helge *et al.* (1998).
*$P < 0.05$ compared to before values.

training-induced increase in endurance performance is less when a major part of daily energy intake is covered by fat for a period longer than 4 weeks than when carbohydrates made up the major part of daily energy intake (Fig. 14.3). Furthermore, comparing the trained subjects, exercising at the same relative exercise intensity, time to exhaustion is significantly shorter when a fat diet has been consumed for a longer period than when a carbohydrate diet has been consumed. Summarizing these studies, it appears that a further increase in endurance performance will be impaired when a fat diet is continued beyond 4 weeks.

It is not clear why prolonged elevated dietary

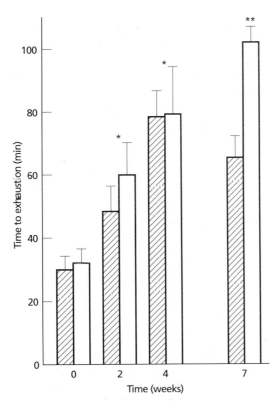

**Fig. 14.3** Endurance performance to exhaustion measured on a Krogh bicycle ergometer before and after 2, 4 and 7 weeks of endurance training when consuming a fat-rich diet (▨) or a carbohydrate-rich diet (□). *, $P < 0.05$ compared with 0 week in both diets; **, $P < 0.05$ compared with the fat-rich diet after 7 weeks. Adapted from Helge *et al.* (1996, 1998).

fat intake attenuates the improvement in endurance performance in man. One aspect of significance in the adaptation to dietary fat could be the capacity of enzymes involved in the fat oxidation as a strong correlation between β-hydroxy-acyl-CoA-dehydrogenase (HAD) activity and fatty acid uptake and oxidation has been demonstrated in man (Kiens 1997). In the study by Helge and Kiens (1997), the activity of HAD was increased by 25% after 7 weeks' adaptation to a fat-rich diet, irrespective of whether subjects were trained or not. Furthermore, after 4 weeks' adaptation to a fat-rich diet, carnitine palmitoyl transferase (CPT I) activity was increased by 35% and hexokinase activity was decreased by 46% (Fisher *et al.* 1983). Putman *et al.* (1993) demonstrated that the PDHa activity, the active form of pyruvate dehydrogenase (Reed & Yeaman 1987), was higher after 3 days' adaptation to a high-fat diet than after adaptation to a high-carbohydrate diet. Preliminary data from our laboratory (unpublished data) also reveal that a fat-rich diet *per se*, consumed for 4 weeks, induces a significant increase in the FABPpm. Thus, allowing for the complexity of this issue, it seems fair to conclude that a fat-rich diet consumed for a longer period increases the capacity for fatty acid transport and oxidation. Despite this adaptation, training-induced increases in endurance performance are nevertheless impaired compared with when a carbohydrate diet is consumed during training. Thus, the fat oxidative capacity does not by itself seem to be decisive for endurance. Other explanations have to be found. Possible mechanisms could be increasing sympathetic activity with time when a fat-rich diet is consumed or changes in phospholipid fatty acid membrane composition induced by dietary fat intake over a longer time (Helge *et al.* 1996).

The relation between muscle glycogen content and the capacity for prolonged submaximal exercise is evident in the brief dietary studies. The question is whether content of muscle glycogen is of the same significance for endurance performance during prolonged dietary adaptations. In the study by Phinney *et al.* (1983), endurance performance, at 60–65% of $\dot{V}o_{2max.}$, was similar (averaging approximately 2.5 h) after consuming a fat or a balanced diet even though initial muscle glycogen levels amounted to only $76 \pm 4$ mmol · $kg^{-1}$ wet weight on the fat diet vs. $143 \pm 10$ mmol · $kg^{-1}$ wet weight on the balanced diet. In the study by Lambert et al. (1994), where the endurance test to exhaustion, at 60% of $\dot{V}o_{2max},$ was performed as the last of three consecutive tests, muscle glycogen stores on the carbohydrate diet amounted to $77 \pm 5$ mmol · $kg^{-1}$ wet weight prior to the endurance test, and exercise time to exhaustion lasted only $43 \pm 9$ min, whereas when on the fat diet, exercise time to exhaustion was $80 \pm 8$ min, when muscle glycogen levels averaged $32 \pm 6$ mmol · $kg^{-1}$ wet weight prior to the test. In these studies, endurance time to exhaustion after consumption of a fat diet was not impaired but in fact even improved despite an initial glycogen content fourfold and twofold lower, respectively, than in the carbohydrate trials. Also, in the study by Helge et al. (1996), muscle glycogen levels prior to exercise were significantly different after 7 weeks' adaptation to the fat diet ($128 \pm 6$ mmol · $kg^{-1}$ wet weight) and the carbohydrate diet ($153 \pm 7$ mmol · $kg^{-1}$ wet weight). However, the rate of muscle glycogen breakdown during exercise was similar in both trials and muscle glycogen stores were not depleted in either group at exhaustion. This was even more conspicuous after 8 weeks, when a carbohydrate diet had been consumed for 1 week after 7 weeks' adaptation to a fat diet. In this case muscle glycogen concentrations at exhaustion were as high as resting values before initiating the dietary intervention period. These observations indicate that content of muscle glycogen prior to an endurance test does not seem to be closely correlated to submaximal performance time when adaptation to a fat diet for more than 14 days has been induced, whereas after acute or a few days' dietary manipulation, exercise time to exhaustion seems more closely related to initial muscle glycogen content (Christensen & Hansen 1939; Bergström et al. 1967; Galbo et al. 1979).

The hypothesis that manipulation of dietary fat can improve endurance performance by increasing fat oxidation and decreasing carbohydrate oxidation can probably be true for the rat. However, in man there are no scientific data to support this notion inasmuch as those few laboratory studies purporting to show a benefit suffer from serious methodological flaws. It has also been hypothesized that if a combination of training and the intake of a fat-rich diet was performed, then a subsequent brief switch to a carbohydrate-rich diet should create optimal conditions for increased endurance because a high-fat oxidative capacity is combined with large glycogen stores. This hypothesis may arise from studies in rats which have demonstrated, as mentioned earlier, that endurance performance time was increased after prolonged fat adaptation and a subsequent brief exposure to a carbohydrate-rich diet (Conlee et al. 1990; Lapachet et al. 1996). However, these findings are not supported in man. In the study by Helge et al. (1996), trained subjects switched to a carbohydrate diet (65 E% CHO, 20 E% fat) for another week, after 7 weeks' adaptation to a fat diet, while continuing their supervised training programme (T-FAT/ CHO group). Another group, also participating in the same training programme, followed a carbohydrate diet through all 8 weeks (T-CHO group). An endurance test to exhaustion performed after the 8th week revealed that exercise time, at the same relative exercise intensity (70% $\dot{V}o_{2max}$) as at the 7-week endurance test was modestly increased by 18%, from $65 \pm 7$ min at 7 weeks to $77 \pm 9$ min in the T-FAT/CHO group. This exercise time was, however, 26% shorter than endurance time to exhaustion in the T-CHO group (Fig. 14.4). It is of note that in the T-FAT/ CHO group the muscle glycogen stores were significantly higher initially ($738 \pm 53$ mmol · $kg^{-1}$ dry weight) than in the T-CHO group ($561 \pm 22$ mmol · $kg^{-1}$ dry weight). Moreover, blood glucose concentrations were significantly higher during exercise and at exhaustion in the T-FAT/CHO group than in the T-CHO group. Even so, endurance performance was still shorter in the T-FAT/CHO group. These data give no support to the belief that several weeks' adaptation to a fat diet followed by a few days on

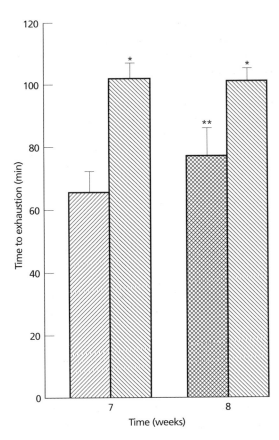

**Fig. 14.4** Endurance performance to exhaustion measured on a Krogh bicycle ergometer after 7 weeks' training on a fat-rich diet (▨) or a carbohydrate-rich diet (▨) followed by an additional week of training during which both groups consumed the carbohydrate-rich diet. *, $P<0.05$ compared with the fat-rich and combined diets, respectively; **, $P<0.05$ compared with the fat-rich diet. Adapted from Helge *et al.* (1996).

a carbohydrate-rich diet is of benefit for the athlete before an event.

## Conclusion

From the available literature, based on human studies, it seems fair to conclude the following.

1 An acute increase in the availability of circulating fatty acids does not result in any clear effects on endurance performance.

2 Short-term ingestion of a fat-rich diet (3–5 days) leads to a deterioration of endurance performance when compared with ingestion of a carbohydrate-rich diet.

3 Adaptation to a fat-rich diet, in combination with training, for a period of 1–4 weeks does not attenuate endurance performance compared with adaptation to a diet rich in carbohydrates, but when dieting and training are continued for 7 weeks, endurance performance is markedly better when a carbohydrate-rich diet is consumed.

4 No benefit is obtained when switching to a carbohydrate-rich diet after long-term adaptation to a fat-rich diet, compared with when a carbohydrate-rich diet is consumed all along.

## References

Bergström, J., Hermansen, L., Hultman, E. & Saltin, B. (1967) Diet, muscle glycogen and physical performance. *Acta Physiologica Scandinavica* **71**, 140–150.

Christensen, E.H. & Hansen, O. (1939) Arbeitsfähigkeit und ernärung (Work capacity and diet). *Skandinavishes Archiv für Physiologie* **81**, 160–171.

Conlee, R., Hammer, R., Winder, W., Bracken, M., Nelson, A. & Barnett, D. (1990) Glycogen repletion and exercise endurance in rats adapted to a high fat diet. *Metabolism* **39**, 289–294.

Dyck, D.J., Putman, C.T., Heigenhauser, G.J.F., Hultman, E. & Spriet, L.L. (1993) Regulation of fat-carbohydrate interaction in skeletal muscle during intense aerobic cycling. *American Journal of Physiology* **265**, E852–E859.

Fisher, E.C., Evans, W.J., Phinney, S.D., Blackburn, G.L., Bistrian, B.R. & Young, V.R. (1983) Changes in skeletal muscle metabolism induced by a eucaloric ketogenic diet. In *Biochemistry of Exercise*, Vol. 13 (ed. H.G. Knuttgen, J.A. Vogel & J. Portman), pp. 497–501. Human Kinetics, Champaign, IL.

Galbo, H., Holst, J.J. & Christensen, N.J. (1979) The effect of different diets and of insulin on the hormonal response to prolonged exercise. *Acta Physiologica Scandinavica* **107**, 19–32.

Griffiths, J., Humphreys, S.M., Clark, M.L., Fielding, B.A. & Frayn, K.N. (1996) Immediate metabolic availability of dietary fat in combination with carbohydrate. *American Journal of Clinical Nutrition* **59**, 53–59.

Hargreaves, M., Kiens, B. & Richter, E.A. (1991) Effect of increased plasma free fatty acid concentrations on muscle metabolism in exercising men. *Journal of Applied Physiology* **70**, 194–201.

Helge, J.W. & Kiens, B. (1997) Muscle enzyme activity in man: role of substrate availability and training. *American Journal of Physiology* **272**, R1620–R1624.

Helge, J.W., Richter, E.A. & Kiens, B. (1996) Interaction of training and diet on metabolism and endurance during exercise in man. *Journal of Physiology (London)* **292**, 293–306.

Helge, J.W., Wulff, B. & Kiens, B. (1998) Impact of a fat-rich diet on endurance in man: role of the dietary period. *Medicine and Science in Sports and Exercise* **30**, 456–461.

Hill, A.V. (1924) Muscular activity and carbohydrate metabolism. *Science* **60**, 505–514.

Karlsson, J. & Saltin, B. (1971) Diet, muscle glycogen, and endurance performance. *Journal of Applied Physiology* **31**, 203–206.

Kiens, B. (1997) Effect of endurance training on fatty acid metabolism: local adaptations. *Medicine in Science, Sports and Exercise* **29**, 640–645.

Kiens, B., Essen-Gustavsson, B., Christensen, N.J. & Saltin, B. (1993) Skeletal muscle substrate utilization during submaximal exercise in man: effect of endurance training. *Journal of Physiology (London)* **469**, 459–478.

Kiens, B., Kristiansen, S., Jensen, P., Richter, E.A. & Turcotte, L.P. (1997) Membrane associated fatty acid binding protein (FABPpm) in human skeletal muscle is increased by endurance training. *Biochemical and Biophysical Research Communications* **231**, 463–465.

Krogh, A. & Krogh, M. (1913) A study of the diet and metabolism of eskimos. *Meddelelser om Grønland* **51**, 3–52.

Krogh, A. & Lindhard, J. (1920) The relative value of fat and carbohydrate as sources of muscular energy. *Biochemistry Journal* **14**, 290–363.

Lambert, E.V., Speechly, D.P., Dennis, S.C. & Noakes, T.D. (1994) Enhanced endurance in trained cyclists during moderate intensity exercise following 2 weeks' adaptation to a high fat diet. *European Journal of Applied Physiology* **69**, 287–293.

Lapachet, R.A.B., Miller, W.C. & Arnall, D.A. (1996) Body fat and exercise endurance in trained rats adapted to a high fat diet and/or a high carbohydrate diet. *Journal of Applied Physiology* **80**, 1173–1179.

Marsh, E. & Murlin, J.R. (1928) Muscular efficiency on high carbohydrate and high fat diets. *Journal of Nutrition* **1**, 105–137.

Miller, W.C., Bryce, G.R. & Conlee, R.K. (1984) Adaptations to a high-fat diet that increase exercise endurance in male rats. *Journal of Applied Physiology* **56**, 78–83.

Muoio, D.M., Leddy, J.J., Horvath, P.J., Awad, A.B. & Pendergast, D.R. (1994) Effects of dietary fat on metabolic adjustments to maximal VO₂ and endurance in runners. *Medicine and Science in Sports and Exercise* **26**, 81–88.

Phinney, S.D., Bistrian, B.R., Evans, W.J., Gervino, E. & Blackburn, G.L. (1983) The human metabolic response to chronic ketosis without caloric restriction: preservation of submaximal exercise capability with reduced carbohydrate oxidation. *Metabolism* **32**, 769–776.

Pruett, E.D.R. (1970) Glucose and insulin during prolonged work stress in men living on different diets. *Journal of Applied Physiology* **2**, 199–208.

Putman, C.T., Spriet, L.L., Hultman, E. *et al.* (1993) Pyruvate dehydrogenase activity and acetyl group accumulation during exercise after different diets. *American Journal of Physiology* **265**, E752–E760.

Reed, L.J. & Yeaman, S.J. (1987) Pyruvate dehydrogenase. In *Enzymes* (ed. P.D. Boyer & E.G. Krebs), pp. 77–95. Academic Press, Toronto.

Romijn, J.A., Coyle, E.F., Sidossis, L.S., Zhang, X.J. & Wolfe, R.R. (1995) Relationship between fatty acid delivery and fatty acid oxidation during strenuous exercise. *Journal of Applied Physiology* **79**, 1939–1945.

Saltin, B. & Gollnick, P. (1983) Skeletal muscle adaptability: significance for metabolism and performance. In *Handbook of Physiology*, Section 10 (eds L.D. Peachy, R.H. Adrian & S.R. Geiger), pp. 555–631. American Physiological Society, Bethesda.

Satabin, P., Portero, P., Defer, G., Bricout, J. & Guezennec, C.Y. (1987) Metabolic and hormonal responses to lipid and carbohydrate diets during exercise in man. *Medicine and Science in Sports and Exercise* **19**, 218–223.

Simi, B., Sempore, B., Mayet, M.-H. & Favier, R.J. (1991) Additive effects of training and high-fat diet on energy metabolism during exercise. *Journal of Applied Physiology* **71**, 197–203.

Spriet, L.L. (1995) Caffeine and performance. *International Journal of Sports Nutrition* **5**, S84–S99.

Tollenar, D. (1976) Dietary fat level as affecting running performance and other performance-related parameters of rats restricted or nonrestricted in food intake. *Journal of Nutrition* **106**, 1539–1546.

Turcotte, L.P., Richter, E.A. & Kiens, B. (1992) Increased plasma FFA uptake and oxidation during prolonged exercise in trained vs. untrained humans. *American Journal of Physiology* **262**, E791–E799.

Zuntz, N. (1901) Über die bedeutung der verschiedenen nahrstoffe als erzeuger der muskelkraft. *Pflügers Archives* **83**, 557–571.

# Chapter 15

# Temperature Regulation and Fluid and Electrolyte Balance

RONALD J. MAUGHAN AND ETHAN R. NADEL

## Introduction

Hard physical exercise poses a formidable challenge to the body's ability to maintain its internal environment within the range that allows optimum function. In sport, however, both in training and competition, these homeostatic mechanisms are under constant threat, and fatigue is the result of a failure to stay within the zone of optimum functioning. It may be an excess acidosis resulting from lactic acid formation, a change in the extracellular potassium concentration causing a decrease in the muscle excitability or a rise in the temperature of the tissues as a result of a high rate of metabolic heat production. Some increase in body temperature is normally observed during exercise, and may even have beneficial effects by increasing the rate of key chemical reactions and altering the elastic modulus of tissues, but high temperatures are detrimental to exercise performance and may be harmful to health. Sweating is the normal physiological response invoked to limit the rise in body temperature by increasing evaporative heat loss, but the loss of significant amounts of sweat results in dehydration and electrolyte depletion if the losses are not replaced. Some understanding of the regulatory processes involved in the control of body temperature and of fluid and electrolyte balance is therefore fundamental to the design of drinks intended for use during exercise and to an understanding of how and when these drinks should be used.

## Temperature regulation in exercise

The temperature of the skin can vary widely, depending on the environmental temperature, but the temperature of the deep tissues must be maintained within only a few degrees of the normal resting level of about 37°C. For this to be the case, the rate of heat gain by the body must be balanced by the rate of heat loss: any imbalance will result in a change in body temperature. All chemical reactions occurring in the body are relatively inefficient, resulting in a large part of the chemical energy involved appearing as heat. The rate of heat production is therefore directly proportional to the metabolic rate. The resting metabolic rate for a healthy adult with a body mass of 70 kg is about 60 W. In a warm climate, this is sufficient to balance the rate of heat loss, but in cold weather the insulative layer surrounding the body must be increased to reduce the rate of heat loss. In other words, more or thicker clothes are worn when it is cold. Alternative strategies are to raise the ambient temperature (by turning up the thermostat on the heating system if indoors) or to increase the metabolic rate, thus increasing the rate of heat production.

The metabolic rate increases in proportion to the rate of energy turnover during exercise: in activities such as walking, running, swimming or cycling at a constant speed, the energy demand is a function of the rate of movement. In walking or running, where the body mass is moved against gravity at each step, body mass and speed will together determine the energy cost. Air resistance becomes a factor at the higher speeds involved in cycling, and reducing the energy needed to overcome air resistance is a crucial factor in improving performance. In swimming, more so than in the other types of activity, technique is important in determining the energy cost of covering a fixed distance or moving at a fixed speed. In most sporting situations, as in most daily activities, the exercise intensity is not constant, but consists of intermittent activity of varying intensity and duration.

Elite marathon runners can sustain speeds that result in rates of heat production in the order of 1200 W for a little over 2 h, which is the time it takes for the top performers to complete a marathon race (Maughan 1994a). In spite of this, however, the rise in body temperature that is observed seldom exceeds 2–3°C, indicating that the rate of heat loss from the body has been increased to match the increased rate of heat production. In general, the rise in body temperature during exercise is proportional to the exercise intensity, whether this is expressed in absolute terms as a power output or in relative terms as a proportion of each individual's aerobic capacity. This observation indicates that the balance between heat production and heat loss is not perfect, but the relationship is none the less rather precise.

Heat exchange between the body surface and the environment occurs by conduction, convection and radiation (Fig. 15.1), and each of these physical processes can result in either heat gain or heat loss: in addition, evaporation can cause heat to be lost from the body (Leithead & Lind 1964). Air has a low thermal conductivity, but the thermal conductivity of water is high, which is why an air temperature of, say, 28°C feels warm but water at the same temperature feels cool or even cold. The pool temperature is therefore of critical importance for swimmers. Convection and radiation are effective methods of heat loss when the temperature gradient between the skin and the environment is large and positive, i.e. when the skin temperature is much higher than the ambient temperature. Under such conditions, these two processes will account for a major part of the heat loss even during intense exercise. As ambient temperature rises, however, the gradient from skin to environment falls, and above about 35°C, the temperature gradient from skin to environment is reversed so that heat is gained by the body. In these conditions, evaporation is therefore the only means of heat loss.

The heat balance equations are described by Kenney (1998) and are usually described by the following equation:

$$S = M \pm R \pm K \pm C - E \pm Wk$$

This indicates that the rate of body heat storage (S) is equal to the metabolic heat production (M) corrected for the net heat exchange by radiation (R), conduction (K), convection (C) and evaporation (E). A further correction must be applied to allow for work (Wk) done: this may be negative in the case of external work done, or positive when eccentric exercise is performed.

A high rate of evaporative heat loss is clearly essential when the rate of metabolic heat production is high and when physical transfer is limited or actually results in a net heat gain by the body. Evaporation of water from the skin surface will result in the loss from the body of about 2.6 MJ (620 kcal) of heat energy for each litre of water evaporated. If we again use our marathon runner as an example, and again assume a rate of heat production of 1200 W, the effectiveness of evaporation is readily apparent. Assuming no other mechanisms of heat exchange, body temperature would rise rapidly and would reach an intolerable level within only about 20 min of exercise.

Evaporation of sweat at a rate of 1 l·h⁻¹ would result in heat loss by evaporation occurring at a rate of 2.6 MJ·h⁻¹ (620 kcal·h⁻¹), which is equivalent to 722 J·s⁻¹ (172 cal·s⁻¹), or 722 W. The entire metabolic heat load would therefore be balanced by the evaporation of about 1.7 l sweat·h⁻¹, and this is well within the range of sweat rates normally observed in various sports during exercise (Rehrer & Burke 1997).

Although the potential for heat loss by evaporation of water from the skin is high, this will only be the case if the skin surface is kept wet by constant replacement of the sweat that evapo-

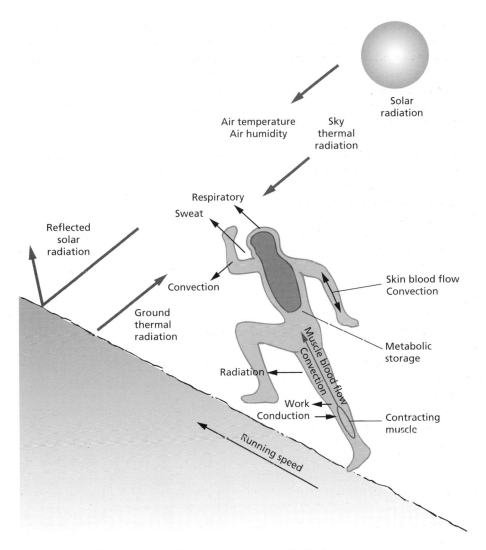

**Fig. 15.1** Main avenues of heat gain or heat loss in the exercising individual.

rates or drips off the skin. Effective evaporation is also prevented if the vapour pressure gradient between the skin and the environment is low. This latter situation will arise if the skin temperature is low or if the ambient water vapour pressure is high: clothing that restricts air flow will allow the air close to the skin to become saturated with water vapour and will therefore restrict the evaporation of water from the skin surface. A large body surface area and a high rate of air movement over the body surface are also factors that will have a major impact on evaporative heat loss, but these same factors may be a disadvantage in that they will promote heat gain from the environment by radiation and convection when the ambient temperature is higher than skin temperature (Leithead & Lind 1964). Smaller individuals will have a high surface area relative to their body mass, and may be at an advantage in hot conditions, but this will depend on the relative rates of evaporative heat loss and heat gain by physical transfer.

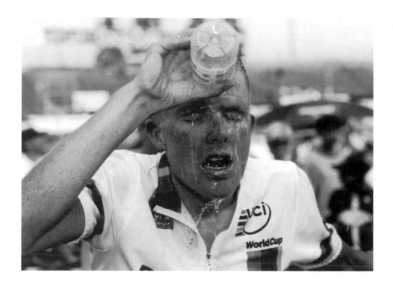

**Fig. 15.2** Water may be less effective for dehydration but effective for cooling. Photo © Cor Vos.

The ability of athletes to complete events such as the marathon, even in adverse climatic conditions, with relatively little change in body temperature, indicates that the thermoregulatory system is normally able to dissipate the associated heat load (Sutton 1990). Nielsen (1996) calculated that a marathon runner competing in a hot climate would be seriously disadvantaged: her calculations suggested that a marathon runner with a best time of 2 h 10 min, competing in conditions typical of the south-eastern United States at the time of the 1996 Summer Olympic Games, would not be able to run faster than about 3 h 20 min because of the limited heat loss that would be possible. The winner of the men's race at those Games actually finished in a time of 2 h 12 min 36 s compared with his previous best time of 2 h 11 min 46 s. This apparently minor effect on performance was in part due to the environmental conditions being less severe than expected, but also indicated that the body is remarkably able to perform even in adverse environmental conditions. It is also worth noting that many of the spectacular collapses that have occurred in the history of marathon running have occurred in hot weather. Famous examples include those of Dorando Pietri at the 1908 Olympic marathon in London, Jim Peters at the

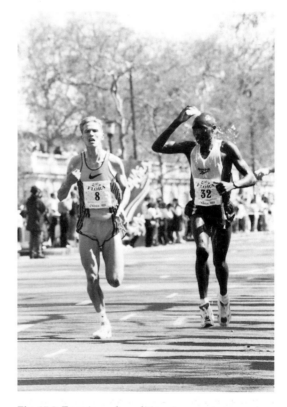

**Fig. 15.3** Even in cool conditions temperature regulation is a big factor in endurance events. Photo courtesy of Ron Maughan.

1954 Empire Games marathon in Vancouver, and Gabriella Andersen-Scheiss at the 1984 Los Angeles Olympics. Such problems are rarely encountered in cooler conditions. None the less, high rates of evaporation require high rates of sweat secretion onto the skin surface, and the price to be paid for the maintenance of core temperature is a progressive loss of water and electrolytes in sweat. If not corrected, this dehydration will impair exercise performance (Chapter 16) and may itself become life-threatening.

## Water balance

The body's hydration status is determined by the balance between water input and water losses from the body. As with all nutrients, a regular intake of water is required for the body to maintain health, and deficiency symptoms and overdosage symptoms can both be observed. Water is the largest single component of the normal human body, accounting for about 50–60% of the total body mass. Lean body tissues contain about 75% water by mass, whereas adipose tissue consists mostly of fat, with little water content. The body composition, and specifically the fat content, therefore largely determines the normal body water content. For a healthy lean young male with a body mass of 70 kg, total body water will be about 42 l. Losses of only a few per cent of total body water will result in an impaired exercise tolerance and an increased risk of heat illness, and yet the sweating rate can reach $2–3 l \cdot h^{-1}$ in extreme situations.

Sweat losses for various sporting and occupational activities are well categorized, but the variability is large because of the different factors that affect the sweating response (Rehrer & Burke 1996). Even at low ambient temperatures, high sweat rates are sometimes observed when the energy demand is high, as in marathon running, so it cannot be concluded that dehydration is a problem only when the ambient temperature and humidity are high: marathon runners competing in cool temperatures (10–12°C) typically lose between 1% and 5% of body mass during a race (Maughan 1985). The sweat loss is, however, closely related to the environmental conditions, and large fluid deficits are much more common in the summer months and in tropical climates. Body mass losses of 6 l or more have been reported for marathon runners in warm weather competition (Costill 1977). This corresponds to a water deficit of about 8% of body mass, or about 12–15% of total body water, and this is sufficient to give cause for concern.

It is well established that women tend to sweat less than men under standardized conditions, even after a period of acclimatization (Wyndham et al. 1965). It is likely, however, that a large part of the apparent sex difference can be accounted for by differences in training and acclimation status. There is a limited amount of information on the effects of age on the sweating response, and again levels of fitness and acclimation are confounding factors, but the sweating response to a standardized challenge generally decreases with age (Kenney 1995). These observations should not, however, be interpreted as suggesting an inability of older people to exercise in the heat, nor should they be taken to indicate a decreased need for women or older individuals to pay attention to fluid intake during exposure to heat stress. Rather, because of the reduced sensitivity of the thirst mechanism in older individuals (Kenney 1995), there is a need for a greater conscious effort to increase fluid intake. There are some differences between children and adults in the sweating response to exercise and in sweat composition. The sweating capacity of children is low, when expressed per unit surface area, and the sweat electrolyte content is low relative to that of adults (Meyer et al. 1992), but the need for fluid and electrolyte replacement is no less important than in adults. Indeed, in view of the evidence that core temperature increases to a greater extent in children than in adults at a given level of dehydration, the need for fluid replacement may well be greater in children (Bar-Or 1989). There may also be a need to limit the duration of children's sports events, or to provide for specified rest periods, when the temperature and humidity are high.

## Water losses

The turnover rate of water exceeds that of most other body components: for the individual who lives in a temperate climate and takes no exercise, daily water losses are about 2–4 l, or 5–10% of the total body water content. Urine, faeces, sweat, expired air and through the skin are the major avenues of water loss, and the approximate size of these different routes of water loss are shown in Table 15.1. In spite of its relative abundance, however, there is a need to maintain the body water content within narrow limits, and the body is much less able to cope with restriction of water intake than with restriction of food intake. A few days of total fasting has relatively little impact on functional capacity, provided fluids are allowed, and even longer periods of abstinence from food are well tolerated. In contrast, cessation of water intake results in serious debilitation after times ranging from as little as an hour or two to a few days at most.

Environmental conditions will affect the basal water requirement by altering the losses that occur by the various routes. Water requirements for sedentary individuals living in a hot climate may be two- or threefold higher than the requirement when living in a temperate climate, even when this is not accompanied by obvious sweating (Adolph & Associates 1947). Transcutaneous and respiratory losses will be markedly influenced by the humidity of the ambient air, and

this may be a more important factor than the ambient temperature. Respiratory water losses are incurred because of the humidification of the inspired air. These losses are relatively small in the resting individual in a warm, moist environment (amounting to about 200 ml·day$^{-1}$), but will be increased approximately twofold in regions of low humidity, and may be as high as 1500 ml·day$^{-1}$ during periods of hard work in the cold, dry air at altitude (Ladell 1965).

The nature of the diet has some effect on water requirements because of the requirement for excretion of excess electrolytes and the products of metabolism. An intake of electrolytes in excess of the amounts lost in sweat and faeces must be corrected by excretion in the urine, with a corresponding increase in the volume and osmolality of urine formed. The daily intake of electrolytes varies widely between individuals, and there are also regional variations. Daily dietary sodium chloride intakes for 95% of the young male UK population fall between 3.8 and 14.3 g, with a mean of 8.4 g; the corresponding values for young women are 2.8–9.4 g, with a mean value of 6.0 g (Gregory et al. 1990). A high-protein diet requires a greater urine output to allow excretion of water-soluble nitrogenous waste (LeMagnen & Tallon 1967). Although this effect is relatively small compared with other losses, it can become meaningful when water availability is limited, and may be a factor to be considered in some athletes who habitually consume diets with a very high protein content. When a high-protein diet is used in combination with fluid restriction and dehydration practices as part of the making-weight process in weight category sports, there are real dangers. The water content of the food ingested will also be influenced greatly by the nature of the diet, and water associated with food will make some contribution to the total fluid intake.

## Electrolyte losses in sweat

The sweat which is secreted onto the skin contains a wide variety of organic and inorganic solutes, and significant losses of some of these

**Table 15.1** Avenues of water loss from the body for sedentary adult men and women. From Bender & Bender (1997).

|  | Water loss (ml·day$^{-1}$) | |
|---|---|---|
|  | Men | Women |
| Urine | 1400 | 1000 |
| Expired air | 320 | 320 |
| Transcutaneous loss | 530 | 280 |
| Sweat loss | 650 | 420 |
| Faecal water | 100 | 90 |
| Total | 3000 | 2100 |

components will occur where large volumes of sweat are produced. The electrolyte composition of sweat is variable, and the concentration of individual electrolytes as well as the total sweat volume will influence the extent of losses. The normal concentration ranges for the main ionic components of sweat are shown in Table 15.2, along with their plasma and intracellular concentrations for comparison. A number of factors contribute to the variability in the composition of sweat: methodological problems in the collection procedure, including evaporative loss, incomplete collection and contamination with skin cells account for at least part of the variability, but there is also a large biological variability (Shirreffs & Maughan 1997).

The sweat composition undoubtedly varies between individuals, but can also vary within the same individual depending on the rate of secretion, the state of training and the state of heat acclimation (Leithead & Lind 1964), and there seem also to be some differences between different sites on the body. In response to a standard heat stress, there is an earlier onset of sweating and an increased sweat rate with training and acclimation, but the electrolyte content decreases although it would normally be expected to increase with increasing sweat rate, at least for sodium. These adaptations allow improved thermoregulation by increasing the evaporative capacity while conserving electrolytes. The con-

servation of sodium in particular may be important in maintaining the plasma volume and thus maintaining the cardiovascular capacity.

The major electrolytes in sweat, as in the extracellular fluid, are sodium and chloride (Table 15.2), although the sweat concentrations of these ions are invariably substantially lower than those in plasma, indicating a selective reabsorption process in the sweat duct. Contrary to what might be expected, Costill (1977) reported an increased sodium and chloride sweat content with increased flow, but Verde et al. (1982) found that the sweat concentration of these ions was unrelated to the sweat flow rate. Acclimation studies have shown that elevated sweating rates are accompanied by a decrease in the concentration of sodium and chloride in sweat (Allan & Wilson 1971). The potassium content of sweat appears to be relatively unaffected by the sweat rate, and the magnesium content is also unchanged or perhaps decreases slightly. These apparently conflicting results demonstrate some of the difficulties in interpreting the literature in this area. Differences between studies may be due to differences in the training status and degree of acclimation of the subjects used as well as difference in methodology: some studies have used whole-body washdown techniques to collect sweat, whereas others have examined local sweating responses using ventilated capsules or collection bags.

Because sweat is hypotonic with respect to body fluids, the effect of prolonged sweating is to increase the plasma osmolality, which may have a significant effect on the ability to maintain body temperature. A direct relationship between plasma osmolality and body temperature has been demonstrated during exercise (Greenleaf et al. 1974; Harrison et al. 1978). Hyperosmolality of plasma, induced prior to exercise, has been shown to result in a decreased thermoregulatory effector response; the threshold for sweating is elevated and the cutaneous vasodilator response is reduced (Fortney et al. 1984). In short-term (30 min) exercise, however, the cardiovascular and thermoregulatory response appears to be independent of changes in osmolality induced

**Table 15.2** Normal concentration ranges of the major electrolytes in sweat, plasma and intracellular water. From Maughan (1994b).

| | Sweat $(mmol \cdot l^{-1})$ | Plasma $(mmol \cdot l^{-1})$ | Intracellular water $(mmol \cdot l^{-1})$ |
|---|---|---|---|
| Sodium | 20–80 | 130–155 | 10 |
| Potassium | 4–8 | 3.2–5.5 | 150 |
| Calcium | 0–1 | 2.1–2.9 | 0 |
| Magnesium | <0.2 | 0.7–1.5 | 15 |
| Chloride | 20–60 | 96–110 | 8 |
| Bicarbonate | 0–35 | 23–28 | 10 |
| Phosphate | 0.1–0.2 | 0.7–1.6 | 65 |
| Sulphate | 0.1–2.0 | 0.3–0.9 | 10 |

during the exercise period (Fortney et al. 1988). The changes in the concentration of individual electrolytes are more variable, but an increase in the plasma sodium and chloride concentrations is generally observed in response to both running and cycling exercise. Exceptions to this are rare and occur only when excessively large volumes of drinks low in electrolytes are consumed over long periods; these situations are discussed further below.

The plasma potassium concentration has been reported to remain constant after marathon running (Meytes et al. 1969; Whiting et al. 1984), although others have reported small increases, irrespective of whether drinks containing large amounts of potassium (Kavanagh & Shephard 1975) or no electrolytes (Costill et al. 1976) were given. Much of the inconsistency in the literature relating to changes in the circulating potassium concentration can be explained by the variable time taken to obtain blood samples after exercise under field conditions; the plasma potassium concentration rapidly returns to normal in the postexercise period (Stansbie et al. 1982). Laboratory studies where an indwelling catheter can be used to obtain blood samples during exercise commonly show an increase in the circulating potassium concentration in the later stages of prolonged exercise. The potassium concentration of extracellular fluid ($4–5\,mmol \cdot l^{-1}$) is small relative to the intracellular concentration ($150–160\,mmol \cdot l^{-1}$), and release of potassium from liver, muscle and red blood cells will tend to elevate plasma potassium levels during exercise in spite of the losses in sweat.

The plasma magnesium concentration is generally unchanged after moderate intensity exercise, and although a modest fall has been reported after extreme exercise, it seems likely that this reflects a redistribution of the available magnesium between body compartments rather than a net loss from the body (Maughan 1991). A larger fall in the serum magnesium concentration has, however, been observed during exercise in the heat than at neutral temperatures (Beller et al. 1972), supporting the idea that losses in sweat are responsible, and further studies with more reliable methodologies are required to clarify this issue. Although the concentration of potassium and magnesium in sweat is high relative to that in the plasma, the plasma content of these ions represents only a small fraction of the whole body stores; Costill and Miller (1980) estimated that only about 1% of the body stores of these electrolytes was lost when individuals were dehydrated by 5.8% of body weight.

## Control of water intake and water loss

The excretion of some of the waste products of metabolism and the regulation of the body's water and electrolyte balance are the primary functions of the kidneys. Excess water or solute is excreted, and where there is a deficiency of water or electrolytes, these are conserved until the balance is restored. Under normal conditions, the osmolality of the extracellular fluid is maintained within narrow limits; since this is strongly influenced by the sodium concentration, sodium and water balance are closely linked. At rest, approximately 15–20% of the renal plasma flow is continuously filtered out by the glomeruli, resulting in the production of about 170 l filtrate · $day^{-1}$. Most (99% or more) of this is reabsorbed in the tubular system, leaving about 1–1.5 l to appear as urine. The volume of urine produced is determined primarily by the action of antidiuretic hormone (ADH) which regulates water reabsorption by increasing the permeability of the distal tubule of the nephron and the collecting duct to water. ADH is released from the posterior lobe of the pituitary in response to signals from the supraoptic nucleus of the hypothalamus: the main stimuli for release of ADH, which is normally present only in low concentrations, are an increased signal from the osmoreceptors located within the hypothalamus, a decrease in blood volume, which is detected by low-pressure receptors in the atria, and by high-pressure baroreceptors in the aortic arch and carotid sinus. An increased plasma angiotensin concentration will also stimulate ADH output.

The sodium concentration of the plasma is regulated by the renal reabsorption of sodium from the glomerular filtrate. Most of the reabsorption occurs in the proximal tubule, but active absorption also occurs in the distal tubules and collecting ducts. A number of factors influence the extent to which reabsorption occurs, and among these is the action of aldosterone, which promotes sodium reabsorption in the distal tubules and enhances the excretion of potassium and hydrogen ions. Aldosterone is released from the kidney in response to a fall in the circulating sodium concentration or a rise in plasma potassium: aldosterone release is also stimulated by angiotensin which is produced by the renin-angiotensin system in response to a decrease in the plasma sodium concentration. Angiotensin thus has a two-fold action, on the release of aldosterone as well as ADH. Atrial natriuretic factor (ANF) is a peptide synthesized in and released from the atria of the heart in response to atrial distension. It increases the glomerular filtration rate and decreases sodium and water reabsorption leading to an increased loss: this may be important in the regulation of extracellular volume, but it seems unlikely that ANF plays a significant role during exercise. Regulation of the body's sodium balance has profound implications for fluid balance, as sodium salts account for more than 90% of the osmotic pressure of the extracellular fluid.

Loss of hypotonic fluid as sweat during prolonged exercise usually results in a fall in blood volume and an increased plasma osmolality: both these changes act as stimuli for the release of ADH (Castenfors 1977). The plasma ADH concentration during exercise has been reported to increase as a function of the exercise intensity (Wade & Claybaugh 1980). Renal blood flow is also reduced in proportion to the exercise intensity and may be as low as 25% of the resting level during strenuous exercise (Poortmans 1984). These factors combine to result in a decreased urine flow during, and usually for some time after, exercise (Poortmans 1984). It has been pointed out, however, that the volume of water conserved by this decreased urine flow during exercise is small, probably amounting to no more than $12-45\,\text{ml}\cdot\text{h}^{-1}$ (Zambraski 1990).

The effect of exercise is normally to decrease the renal excretion of sodium and to increase the excretion of potassium, although the effect on potassium excretion is rather variable (Zambraski 1990). These effects appear to be largely due to an increased rate of aldosterone production during exercise (Poortmans 1984). Although the concentrations of sodium and more especially of potassium in the urine are generally high relative to the concentrations in extracellular fluid, the extent of total urinary losses in most exercise situations is small.

The daily water intake in the form of food and drink is usually in excess of obligatory water loss, with the kidneys being responsible for excretion of any excess and the regulation of body water content. The kidneys can only function effectively, however, if the fluid intake is in excess of the requirement. Drinking is a complex behaviour which is influenced by a number of physiological, psychological and social events. The sensation of thirst is only one of the factors involved, and short-term studies suggest that it is a poor indicator of acute hydration status in man (Adolph *et al.* 1947). The overall stability of the total body water content, however, indicates that the desire to drink is a powerful regulatory factor over the long term (Ramsay 1989).

The urge to drink, which is perceived as thirst, may not be directly involved with a physiological need for water intake, but can be initiated by habit, ritual, taste or desire for nutrients, stimulants, or a warm or cooling effect. A number of the sensations associated with thirst are learned, with signals such as dryness of the mouth or throat inducing drinking, while distension of the stomach can stop ingestion before a fluid deficit has been restored. There are clearly changes in the sensitivity of the thirst mechanism associated with the ageing process, with older individuals showing a reduced response to mild levels of dehydration (Kenney 1995).

Notwithstanding the various factors that modulate the subjective perception of thirst, there is an underlying physiological basis involving both chemical and pressure sensors. The sensation of thirst is controlled separately by both the osmotic pressure of the body fluids and the central venous volume. The same mechanisms are involved in water and solute reabsorption in the kidneys and in the control of blood pressure. The thirst control centres are located in the hypothalamus and forebrain, and appear to play a key role in the regulation of both thirst and diuresis. Receptors in the thirst control centres respond directly to changes in osmolality, volaemia and blood pressure, while others are stimulated by the fluid balance hormones which also regulate renal excretion (Phillips *et al.* 1985). These regions of the brain also receive afferent input from systemic receptors monitoring osmolality and circulating sodium concentration, and from alterations in blood volume and pressure. There may also be a direct neural link from the thirst control centres to the kidneys which would allow a greater degree of integration between the control of fluid intake and excretion. Changes in the balance of neural activity in the thirst control centres regulated by the different monitoring inputs determine the relative sensations of thirst and satiety, and influence the degree of diuresis. Input from the higher centres of the brain, however, can override the basic biological need for water to some extent and cause inappropriate drinking responses.

A rise of between 2% and 3% in plasma osmolality is sufficient to evoke a profound sensation of thirst coupled with an increase in the circulating concentration of ADH (Hubbard *et al.* 1990). The mechanisms that respond to changes in intravascular volume and pressure appear to be less sensitive than those that monitor plasma osmolality, with hypovolaemic thirst being evident only following a 10% decrease in blood volume (Fitzsimons 1990). As fairly large variations in blood volume and pressure occur during normal daily activity, this lack of sensitivity presumably prevents excessive activity of the volaemic control mechanisms. Prolonged exercise, especially in the heat, is associated with a decrease in plasma volume and a tendency for an increase in plasma osmolality, but fluid intake during and immediately following exercise is often less than that required to restore normal

hydration status (Ramsay 1989). This appears not to be due to a lack of initiation of the drinking response but rather to a premature termination of the drinking response (Rolls *et al.* 1980).

When a water deficit is present and volunteers are allowed free access to fluids, the normal drinking response involves an initial period of avid drinking during which more than 50% of the total volume is consumed; this is followed by a longer period of intermittent consumption of relatively small volumes (Verbalis 1990). The initial alleviation of thirst occurs before significant amounts of the beverage have been absorbed and entered the body pools. Therefore, although decreasing osmolality and increasing extracellular volume promote a reduction in the perception of thirst, other preabsorptive factors also affect the volume of fluid ingested. Receptors in the mouth, oesophagus and stomach are thought to meter the volume of fluid ingested, while distension of the stomach tends to reduce the perception of thirst. These preabsorptive signals appear to be behavioural, learned responses and may be subject to disruption in situations which are essentially novel to the individual. This may partly explain the inappropriate voluntary fluid intake in individuals exposed to an acute increase in environmental temperature or to exercise-induced dehydration.

In addition to the water consumed in the form of drinks, some water is obtained from solid foods, and water is also available as a result of the oxidation of nutrients. The amount of water available from these sources will depend on the amount and type of food eaten and on the total metabolic rate. Oxidation of the components of a mixed diet, with an energy content of 12.6 MJ (3000 kcal) per day, will give about 400 ml water · day$^{-1}$. The contribution of this water of oxidation to water requirements is appreciable when water turnover is low, but becomes rather insignificant when water losses are high.

## Role of the kidney

The excretion of some of the waste products of metabolism and the regulation of the body's water and electrolyte balance are the primary functions of the kidneys. Excess water or solute is excreted, and where there is a deficiency of water or electrolytes an attempt is made to conserve these until the balance is restored. Blood volume, plasma osmolality and plasma sodium concentration seem to be the primary factors regulated. Under normal conditions, the osmolality of the extracellular fluid is maintained within narrow limits. As the major ion of the extracellular space is sodium, which accounts for about 50% of the total osmolality, maintenance of osmotic balance requires that both sodium and water intake and loss are closely coupled.

At rest, about 20% of the cardiac output goes to the two kidneys, and approximately 15–20% of the renal plasma flow is continuously filtered out by the glomeruli, resulting in the production of about 170 l filtrate $\cdot$ day$^{-1}$. Most (99% or more) of this is reabsorbed in the tubular system, leaving about 1–1.5 l to appear as urine. The volume of urine produced is determined primarily by the action of ADH which regulates water reabsorption by increasing the permeability of the distal tubule of the nephron and the collecting duct to water. ADH is released from the posterior lobe of the pituitary in response to signals from the supraoptic nucleus of the hypothalamus: the main stimuli for release of ADH, which is normally present only in low concentrations, are an increased signal from the osmoreceptors located within the hypothalamus, a decrease in blood volume, which is detected by low-pressure receptors in the atria, and by high-pressure baroreceptors in the aortic arch and carotid sinus. An increased plasma angiotensin concentration will also stimulate ADH output.

The sodium concentration of the plasma is regulated by the reabsorption of sodium from the glomerular filtrate, with most of the reabsorption occurring in the proximal renal tubule. Several factors influence the extent to which reabsorption occurs: of particular importance is the action of aldosterone, which promotes sodium reabsorption in the distal tubules and enhances the excretion of potassium and hydrogen ions. Aldosterone is released from the kidney in

response to a fall in the circulating sodium concentration or a rise in plasma potassium: aldosterone release is also stimulated by angiotensin which is produced by the renin–angiotensin system in response to a decrease in the plasma sodium concentration. Angiotensin thus has a twofold action, on the release of aldosterone as well as ADH. ANF is a peptide synthesized in and released from the heart in response to atrial distension. It increases the glomerular filtration rate and decreases sodium and water reabsorption leading to an increased loss: this may be important in the regulation of extracellular volume, but probably does not play a significant role during exercise. Regulation of the body's sodium balance has profound implications for fluid balance, as sodium salts account for more than 90% of the osmotic pressure of the extracellular fluid.

Loss of hypotonic fluid as sweat during prolonged exercise usually results in a fall in blood volume and an increased plasma osmolality: these changes in turn act as stimuli for the release of ADH (Castenfors 1977). The plasma ADH concentration during exercise has been reported to increase as a function of the exercise intensity (Wade & Claybaugh 1980). Renal blood flow is also reduced in proportion to the exercise intensity and may be as low as 25% of the resting level during strenuous exercise (Poortmans 1984). These factors combine to result in a decreased urine flow during, and usually for some time after, exercise. The volume of water conserved by this decreased urine flow during exercise is small, probably amounting to no more than 12–45 ml $\cdot$ h$^{-1}$ (Zambraski 1990): compared with water losses in sweat, this volume is trivial.

Exercise normally results in a decrease in the renal excretion of sodium and an increased excretion of potassium, although the effect on potassium excretion is rather variable (Zambraski 1990). These effects appear to be largely due to an increased rate of aldosterone production during exercise. Although the concentrations of sodium, and more especially of potassium, in the urine are generally high relative to the concentrations in extracellular fluid, the extent of total urinary electrolyte losses in most exercise situations is small.

# References

Adolph, A. & Associates (1947) *Physiology of Man in the Desert*. Wiley, New York.

Allan, J.R. & Wilson, C.G. (1971) Influence of acclimatization on sweat sodium secretion. *Journal of Applied Physiology* **30**, 708–712.

Bar-Or, O. (1989) Temperature regulation during exercise in children and adolescents. In *Perspectives in Exercise Science and Sports Medicine. Vol. 2. Youth, Exercise, and Sport* (ed. C.V. Gisolfi & D.R. Lamb), pp. 335–362. Benchmark Press, Indianapolis, IN.

Beller, G.A., Maher, J.T., Hartley, L.H., Bass, D.E. & Wacker, W.E.C. (1972) Serum Mg and K concentrations during exercise in thermoneutral and hot conditions. *Physiologist* **15**, 94.

Castenfors, J. (1977) Renal function during prolonged exercise. *Annals of the New York Academy of Sciences* **301**, 151–159.

Costill, D.L. (1977) Sweating: its composition and effects on body fluids. *Annals of the New York Academy of Science* **301**, 160–174.

Costill, D.L. & Miller, J.M. (1980) Nutrition for endurance sport. *International Journal of Sports Medicine* **1**, 2–14.

Costill, D.L., Branam, G., Fink, W. & Nelson, R. (1976) Exercise induced sodium conservation: changes in plasma renin and aldosterone. *Medicine and Science in Sports and Exercise* **8**, 209–213.

Fitzsimons, J.T. (1990) Evolution of physiological and behavioural mechanisms in vertebrate body fluid homeostasis. In *Thirst: Physiological and Psychological Aspects* (ed. D.J. Ramsay & D.A. Booth), pp. 3–22. ILSI Human Nutrition Reviews. Springer-Verlag, London.

Fortney, S.M., Wenger, C.B., Bove, J.R. & Nadel, E.R. (1984) Effect of hyperosmolality on control of blood flow and sweating. *Journal of Applied Physiology* **57**, 1688–1695.

Fortney, S.M., Vroman, N.B., Beckett, W.S., Permutt, S. & LaFrance, N.D. (1988) Effect of exercise hemoconcentration and hyperosmolality on exercise responses. *Journal of Applied Physiology* **65**, 519–524.

Greenleaf, J.E., Castle, B.L. & Card, D.H. (1974) Blood electrolytes and temperature regulation during exercise in man. *Acta Physiologica Polonica* **25**, 397–410.

Gregory, J., Foster, K., Tyler, H. & Wiseman, M. (1990) *The Dietary and Nutritional Survey of British Adults*. HMSO, London.

Harrison, M.H., Edwards, R.J. & Fennessy, P.A. (1978) Intravascular, volume and tonicity as factors in the regulation of body temperature. *Journal of Applied Physiology* **44**, 69–75.

Hubbard, R.W., Szlyk, P.C. & Armstrong, L.E. (1990) Influence of thirst and fluid palatability on fluid ingestion. In *Perspectives in Exercise Science and Sports Medicine. Vol. 3. Fluid Homeostasis during Exercise* (ed. C.V. Gisolfi & D.R. Lamb), pp. 39–95. Benchmark Press, Indianapolis, IN.

Kavanagh, T. & Shephard, R.J. (1975) Maintenance of hydration in 'post-coronary' marathon runners. *British Journal of Sports Medicine* **9**, 130–135.

Kenney, W.L. (1995) Body fluid and temperature regulation as a function of age. In *Perspectives in Exercise Science and Sports Medicine. Vol. 8. Exercise in Older Adults* (ed. D.R. Lamb, C.V. Gisolfi & E.R. Nadel), pp. 305–352. Benchmark Press, Indianapolis, IN.

Kenney, W.L. (1998) Heat flux and storage in hot environments. *International Journal of Sports Medicine* **19**, S92–S95.

Ladell, W.S.S. (1965) Water and salt (sodium chloride) intakes. In *The Physiology of Human Survival* (ed. O. Edholm & A. Bacharach), pp. 235–299. Academic Press, New York.

Leithead, C.S. & Lind, A.R. (1964) *Heat Stress and Heat Disorders*. Casell, London.

LeMagnen, J. & Tallon, S.A. (1967) Les determinants quantitatif de la prise hydratique dans ses relations avec la prise d'aliments chez le rat. *Comptes Rendues Society of Biology* **161**, 1243–1246.

Maughan, R.J. (1985) Thermoregulation and fluid balance in marathon competition at low ambient temperature. *International Journal of Sports Medicine* **6**, 15–19.

Maughan, R.J. (1991) Effects of CHO–electrolyte solution on prolonged exercise. In *Perspectives in Exercise Science and Sports Medicine. Vol. 4. Ergogenics: Enhancement of Performance in Exercise and Sport* (ed. D.R. Lamb & M.H. Williams), pp. 35–85. Benchmark Press, Carmel, CA.

Maughan, R.J. (1994a) Physiology and nutrition for middle distance and long distance running. In *Perspectives in Exercise Science and Sports Medicine. Vol. 7. Physiology and Nutrition in Competitive Sport* (ed. D.R. Lamb, H.G. Knuttgen & R. Murray), pp. 329–371. Cooper, Carmel, CA.

Maughan, R.J. (1994b) Fluid and electrolyte loss and replacement in exercise. In *Oxford Textbook of Sports Medicine* (ed. M. Harries, G. Williams, W.D. Stanish & L.L. Micheli), pp. 82–93. Oxford University Press, New York.

Meyer, F., Bar-Or, O., MacDougall, D. & Heigenhauser, G.J.F. (1992) Sweat electrolyte loss during exercise in the heat: effects of gender and maturation. *Medicine and Science in Sports and Exercise* **24**, 776–781.

Meytes, I., Shapira, Y., Magazanik, A., Meytes, D. & Seligsohn, U. (1969) Physiological and biochemical changes during a marathon race. *International Journal of Biometeorology* **13**, 317.

Nielsen, B. (1996) Olympics in Atlanta: a fight against physics. *Medicine and Science in Sports and Exercise* **28**, 665–668.

Phillips, P.A., Rolls, B.J., Ledingham, J.G.G., Forsling, M.L. & Morton, J.J. (1985) Osmotic thirst and vasopressin release in humans: a double-blind crossover study. *American Journal of Physiology* **248**, R645–R650.

Poortmans, J. (1984) Exercise and renal function. *Sports Medicine* **1**, 125–153.

Ramsay, D.J. (1989) The importance of thirst in the maintenance of fluid balance. In *Clinical Endocrinology and Metabolism*. Vol. 3, No. 2. *Water and Salt Homeostasis in Health and Disease*, pp. 371–391. Baillicre Tindall, London.

Rehrer, N.J. & Burke, L.M. (1996) Sweat losses during various sports. *Australian Journal of Nutrition and Dietetics* **53** (Suppl. 4), S13–S16.

Rolls, B.J., Wood, R.J., Rolls, E.T., Lind, W. & Ledingham, J.G.G. (1980) Thirst following water deprivation in humans. *American Journal of Physiology* **239**, R476–R482.

Shirreffs, S.M. & Maughan, R.J. (1997) Whole body sweat collection in man: an improved method with some preliminary data on electrolyte composition. *Journal of Applied Physiology* **82**, 336–341.

Stansbie, D., Tomlinson, K., Potman, J.M. & Walters, E.G. (1982) Hypothermia, hypokalaemia and marathon running. *Lancet* ii, 1336.

Sutton, J.R. (1990) Clinical implications of fluid imbalance. In *Perspectives in Exercise Science and Sports Medicine*. Vol. 3. *Fluid Homeostasis during Exercise* (ed. C.V. Gisolfi & D.R. Lamb), pp. 425–448. Benchmark Press, Indianapolis, IN.

Verbalis, J.G. (1990) Inhibitory controls of drinking: satiation of thirst. In *Thirst: Physiological and Psychological Aspects* (ed. D.J. Ramsay & D.A. Booth), pp. 313–334. ILSI Human Nutrition Reviews. Springer-Verlag, London,

Verde, T., Shephard, R.J., Corey, P. & Moore, R. (1982) Sweat composition in exercise and in heat. *Journal of Applied Physiology* **53**, 1540–1545.

Wade, C.E. & Claybaugh, J.R. (1980) Plasma renin activity, vasopressin concentration and urinary excretory responses to exercise in men. *Journal of Applied Physiology* **49**, 930–936.

Whiting, P.H., Maughan, R.J. & Miller, J.D.B. (1984) Dehydration and serum biochemical changes in runners. *European Journal of Applied Physiology* **52**, 183–187.

Wyndham, C.H., Morrison, J.F. & Williams, C.G. (1965) Heat reactions of male and female Caucasians. *Journal of Applied Physiology* **20**, 357–364.

Zambraski, E.J. (1990) Renal regulation of fluid homeostasis during exercise. In *Perspectives in Exercise Science and Sports Medicine*. Vol. 3. *Fluid Homeostasis during Exercise* (ed. C.V. Gisolfi & C.V. Lamb), pp. 247–280. Benchmark Press, Carmel, CA.

# Chapter 16

# Effects of Dehydration and Rehydration on Performance*

MICHAEL N. SAWKA, WILLIAM A. LATZKA
AND SCOTT J. MONTAIN

## Introduction

Athletes encounter heat stress from climatic conditions (e.g. temperature, humidity, solar load) and body heat production. Depending on the climatic conditions, the relative contributions of evaporative and dry (radiative and conductive) heat exchange to the total heat loss will vary. The hotter the climate, the greater the dependence on evaporative heat loss and, thus, on sweating. Therefore, a substantial volume of body water may be lost via sweating to enable evaporative cooling in hot environments. In addition, physical exercise will elevate metabolic rate above resting levels, and thus increase the rate at which heat must be dissipated to the environment to keep core temperature from rising to dangerous levels. Environmental heat stress and physical exercise interact synergistically and may push physiological systems to their limits (Sawka *et al.* 1996b).

Climatic heat stress and physical exercise will cause both fluid and electrolyte imbalances that need to be re-established (Marriott 1993, 1994; Convertino *et al.* 1996). Athletes performing exercise in the heat often incur body water deficits. Generally, athletes dehydrate during exercise because of fluid non-availability or a mismatch between thirst and body water

requirements (Greenleaf 1992). In these instances, the athlete starts exercise euhydrated, but incurs an exercise-heat-mediated dehydration over a prolonged period. This scenario is common for many athletic and occupational settings; however, there are several sports (e.g. boxing, power lifting, wrestling) where athletes will purposely achieve hypohydration prior to competition.

This chapter reviews fluid balance in the heat and the effects of hydration status on temperature regulation and physical exercise performance. Throughout this chapter, *euhydration* refers to normal body water content, *hypohydration* refers to body water deficit, and *hyperhydration* refers to increased body water content.

## Fluid and electrolyte balance

An athlete's sweating rate is dependent upon the climatic conditions, clothing worn and exercise intensity (Molnar *et al.* 1946; Shapiro *et al.* 1982). Figure 16.1 provides a range of sweating rates expected from running in different climatic conditions (Sawka & Pandolf 1990). Athletes performing high-intensity exercise commonly have sweating rates of $1.0–2.5 l \cdot h^{-1}$ while in the heat. These high sweating rates, however, are not maintained continuously and are dependent upon the person's need to dissipate body heat. Daily fluid requirements range (for sedentary to active persons) from 2 to $4 l \cdot day^{-1}$ in temperate climates and from 4 to $10 l \cdot day^{-1}$ in hot climates (Greenleaf 1994). Clearly, hot weather and

---

*The views, opinions and/or findings contained in this chapter are those of the authors and should not be construed as an official Department of Army position or decision, unless so designated by other official documentation.

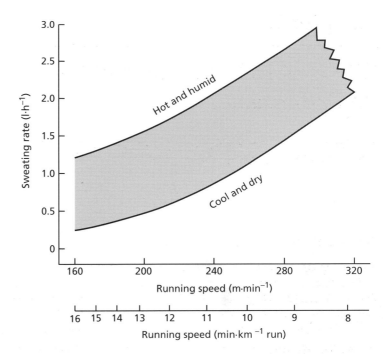

**Fig. 16.1** An approximation of hourly sweating rates as a function of climate and running speed. From Sawka and Pandolf (1990).

intense training can greatly increase daily fluid requirements.

Electrolytes, primarily sodium chloride and, to a lesser extent, potassium, calcium and magnesium, are contained in sweat. Sweat sodium concentration averages approximately $35\,mmol \cdot l^{-1}$ (range, $10–70\,mmol \cdot l^{-1}$) and varies depending upon diet, sweating rate, hydration and heat acclimation level (Allan & Wilson 1971; Brouns 1991). Sweat glands reabsorb sodium by active transport, and the ability to reabsorb sodium does not increase with the sweating rate, so at high sweating rates the concentration of sweat sodium increases. Heat acclimation improves the ability to reabsorb sodium so acclimated persons have lower sweat sodium concentrations (>50% reduction) for any sweating rate (Dill *et al.* 1933; Bass *et al.* 1955; Allan & Wilson 1971). Sweat potassium concentration averages $5\,mmol \cdot l^{-1}$ (range, $3–15\ mmol \cdot l^{-1}$), calcium averages $1\,mmol \cdot l^{-1}$ (range, $0.3–2\,mmol \cdot l^{-1}$) and magnesium averages $0.8\,mmol \cdot l^{-1}$ (range, $0.2–1.5\,mmol \cdot l^{-1}$) (Brouns 1991). Electrolyte supplementation is not necessary, except occasionally for their first several days of heat exposure where

evidence indicates that this is warranted (Marriott 1994; Convertino *et al.* 1996), as normal dietary sodium intake will replenish sweat electrolyte losses (Marriott 1994; Convertino *et al.* 1996).

During exercise in the heat, a principal problem is to avoid hypohydration by matching fluid consumption to sweat loss. This is a difficult problem because thirst does not provide a good index of body water requirements (Adolph & Associates 1947; Hubbard *et al.* 1984; Engell *et al.* 1987). Thirst is probably not perceived until an individual has incurred a water deficit of approximately 2% body weight loss (BWL) (Adolph & Associates 1947; Hubbard *et al.* 1984; Armstrong *et al.* 1985b). In addition, *ad libitum* water intake during exercise in the heat results in an incomplete replacement of body water losses (Adolph & Associates 1947; Hubbard *et al.* 1984). Heat-acclimated persons will usually only replace less than one half of their fluid deficit when replacing fluid *ad libitum* (Adolph & Associates 1947). As a result, it is likely that unless forced hydration is stressed, some dehydration will occur during exercise in the heat. Humans will usually fully rehydrate at mealtime, when fluid consumption is stimulated by consuming food (Adolph & Associates 1947; Marriott 1993). Therefore, active persons need to stress drinking at mealtime in order to avoid persistent hypohydration.

Persons will hypohydrate by 2–6% BWL during situations of stress and prolonged high sweat loss. Water is the largest component of the human body, comprising 45–70% of body weight (Sawka 1988). The average male (75 kg) is composed of about 45 l of water, which corresponds to about 60% of body weight. Since adipose tissue is about 10% water and muscle tissue is about 75% water, a person's total body water depends upon their body composition. In addition, muscle water and glycogen content parallel each other probably because of the osmotic pressure exerted by glycogen granules within the muscle's sarcoplasm (Neufer et al. 1991). As a result, trained athletes have a relatively greater total body water than their sedentary counterparts, by virtue of a smaller percentage body fat and perhaps a higher skeletal muscle glycogen concentration.

The water contained in body tissues is distributed between the intracellular and extracellular fluid spaces. Hypohydration mediated by sweating will influence each fluid space as a consequence of free fluid exchange. Nose and colleagues (1983) determined the distribution of BWL among the fluid spaces as well as among different body organs. They thermally dehydrated rats by 10% BWL, and after the animals regained their normal core temperature, the body water measurements were obtained. The water deficit was apportioned between the intracellular (41%) and extracellular (59%) spaces; and among the organs: 40% from muscle, 30% from skin, 14% from viscera and 14% from bone. Neither the brain nor liver lost significant water content. They concluded that hypohydration results in water redistribution largely from the intra- and extracellular spaces of muscle and skin in order to defend blood volume.

Sweat-induced hypohydration will decrease plasma volume and increase plasma osmotic pressure in proportion to the level of fluid loss (Sawka et al. 1996a). Plasma volume decreases because it provides the precursor fluid for sweat, and osmolality increases because sweat is ordinarily hypotonic relative to plasma. Sodium and chloride are primarily responsible for the elevated plasma osmolality (Senay 1968; Kubica et al. 1983). It is the plasma hyperosmolality which mobilizes fluid from the intracellular to the extracellular space to enable plasma volume defence in hypohydrated subjects. This concept is demonstrated by heat-acclimated persons who, compared with unacclimated persons, have a smaller plasma volume reduction for a given body water deficit (Sawka 1992). By virtue of having a more dilute sweat, heat-acclimated persons retain additional solutes within the extracellular space to exert an osmotic pressure and redistribute fluid from the intracellular space (Mack & Nadel 1996).

Some persons use diuretics for medical purposes or to reduce their body weight. Diuretics increase urine formation and often result in the loss of solutes. Commonly used diuretics include thiazide (e.g. Diuril), carbonic anhydrase inhibitors (e.g. Diamox) and furosemide (e.g. Lasix). Diuretic-induced hypohydration often results in an iso-osmotic hypovolaemia, with a much greater ratio of plasma loss to body water loss than either exercise or heat-induced hypohydration. Relatively less intracellular fluid is lost after diuretic administration, since there is not an extracellular solute excess to stimulate redistribution of body water.

## Exercise performance and temperature regulation

Numerous studies have examined the influence of hypohydration on maximal aerobic power and physical exercise capacity. In temperate climates, a body water deficit of less than 3% BWL does not alter maximal aerobic power (Sawka et al. 1996a). Maximal aerobic power has been reported as being decreased (Buskirk et al. 1958; Caldwell et al. 1984; Webster et al. 1990) when hypohydration equalled or exceeded 3% BWL. Therefore, a critical water deficit (3% BWL) might exist before

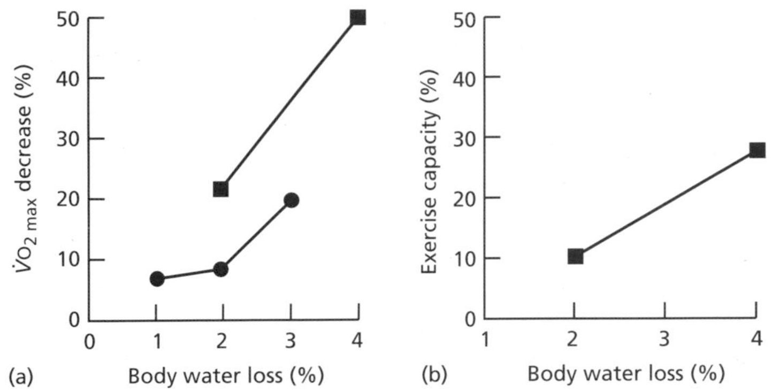

**Fig. 16.2** Relationship between hypohydration level and (a) $\dot{V}o_{2max.}$ decrement, and (b) physical exercise capacity decrement during heat exposure. ■, from Craig and Cummings (1966); ●, from Pinchan *et al.* (1988).

hypohydration reduces maximal aerobic power in temperate climates. In hot climates, Craig and Cummings (1966) demonstrated that small (2% BWL) to moderate (4% BWL) water deficits resulted in a large reduction of maximal aerobic power. Likewise, their data indicate a disproportionately larger decrease in maximal aerobic power with an increased magnitude of body water deficit. It seems environmental heat stress has a potentiating effect on the reduction of maximal aerobic power elicited by hypohydration.

The physical exercise capacity (exercise to fatigue) for progressive intensity exercise is decreased when hypohydrated. Physical exercise capacity is decreased by marginal (1–2% BWL) water deficits that do not alter $\dot{V}o_{2max.}$ (Caldwell *et al.* 1984; Armstrong *et al.* 1985a), and the decreases are larger with increasing water deficits. Clearly, hypohydration results in larger decrements of physical exercise capacity in hot than in temperate climates (Armstrong *et al.* 1985a). It appears that the thermoregulatory system, perhaps via increased body temperatures, has an important role in the reduced exercise performance mediated by a body water deficit. Figure 16.2 presents the relationship between hypohydration level and $\dot{V}o_{2max.}$ decrement or physical exercise capacity decrement during heat exposure (Craig & Cummings 1966; Pinchan *et al.* 1988). Note that for a given hypohydration level, greater decrements are observed for physical exercise capacity than $\dot{V}o_{2max.}$.

Studies have demonstrated that hypohydration can impair athletic endurance exercise

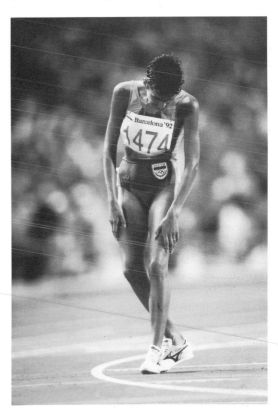

**Fig. 16.3** With many major competitions held in hot environments, the outcome of races may depend on maintaining hydration status. Photo © Allsport / Martin.

performance. Armstrong and colleagues (1985a) studied the effects of a body water deficit on competitive distance running performance. They had athletes compete in 1500-, 5000- and 10 000-m races when euhydrated and when hypohydrated. Hypohydration was achieved by diuretic administration (furosemide), which decreased body weight by 2% and plasma volume by 11%. Running performance was impaired at all race distances, but to a greater extent in the longer races ($\approx$5% for the 5000 and 10 000 m) than the shorter race (3% for the 1500 m). Burge *et al.* (1993) recently examined whether hypohydration (3% BWL) affected simulated 2000 m rowing performance. They found that, on average, it took 22 s longer to complete the task when hypohydrated than when euhydrated. Average power was reduced by 5% in the hypohydrated state.

Two studies have examined the adverse effects of hypohydration on moderate to intense cycle ergometer performance. In both studies, high-intensity performance tests were conducted immediately after 55–60 min of cycling during which volunteers either drank nothing or drank sufficient fluid to replace sweat losses. Walsh *et al.* (1994) reported that time to fatigue when cycling at 90% $\dot{V}_{O_{2max}}$ was 51% longer (6.5 vs. 9.8 min) when subjects drank sufficient fluids to prevent hypohydration. Below *et al.* (1995) found that cyclists completed a performance ride 6.5% faster if they drank fluids during exercise. The results of these studies clearly demonstrate the detrimental effects of hypohydration in submaximal exercise performance.

Investigators have documented the effects of hypohydration on a person's ability to tolerate heat strain during submaximal intensity exercise. These studies demonstrate that persons who drink can continue to exercise in the heat for many hours, whereas those who under-drink discontinue because of exhaustion (Adolph & Associates 1947; Ladell & Shephard 1961; Sawka *et al.* 1992). To address whether hypohydration alters heat tolerance, Sawka and colleagues (1992) had subjects walk to voluntary exhaustion when either euhydrated or hypohydrated (by 8% of total body water). The experiments were designed so that the combined environment ($T_a$, 49°C; rh, 20%) and exercise intensity (47% $\dot{V}_{O_{2max}}$) would not allow thermal equilibrium and heat exhaustion would eventually occur. Hypohydration reduced tolerance time

(121–55 min), but more important, hypohydration reduced the core temperature that a person could tolerate. Heat exhaustion occurred at a core temperature approximately 0.4°C lower when hypohydrated than when euhydrated. These findings indicate that hypohydration not only impairs exercise performance, but also reduces tolerance to heat strain.

Hypohydration increases core temperature responses during exercise in temperate (Grande *et al.* 1959; Cadarette *et al.* 1984) and hot (Sawka *et al.* 1983, 1985) climates. A critical water deficit of 1% body weight elevates core temperature during exercise (Ekblom *et al.* 1970). As the magnitude of water deficit increases, there is a concomitant graded elevation of core temperature during exercise heat stress (Sawka *et al.* 1985; Montain & Coyle 1992). Figure 16.4 illustrates relationships between BWL and core temperature elevations reported by studies (Adolph & Associates 1947; Strydom & Holdsworth 1968; Sawka *et al.* 1985; Montain & Coyle 1992) which examined several hypohydration levels (Sawka *et al.* 1996a). The magnitude of core temperature elevation ranges from 0.1 to 0.23°C for every percentage body weight lost. Hypohydration not

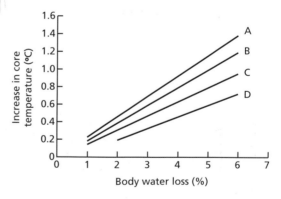

**Fig. 16.4** Relationship between the elevation in core temperature (above euhydration) at a given hypohydration level during exercise with heat stress, according to different studies: A, 65% $\dot{V}_{O_{2max}}$, 33°C db (Montain & Coyle 1992); B, marching in the desert (Adolph & Associates 1947); C, 25% $\dot{V}_{O_{2max}}$, 49°C db (Sawka *et al.* 1985); D, 45 W, 34°C db (Strydom & Holdsworth 1968). From Sawka *et al.* (1996a).

only elevates core temperature responses, but it negates the core temperature advantages conferred by high aerobic fitness and heat acclimation (Buskirk *et al.* 1958; Sawka *et al.* 1983; Cadarette *et al.* 1984).

Hypohydration impairs both dry and evaporative heat loss (or, if the air is warmer than the skin, dehydration aggravates dry heat gain) (Sawka *et al.* 1985, 1989; Kenney *et al.* 1990; Montain *et al.* 1995). Figure 16.5 presents local sweating responses (Sawka *et al.* 1989) and skin blood flow responses (Kenney *et al.* 1990) to hypohydration (5% BWL) during exercise in the heat. This figure indicates that hypohydration reduced both effector heat loss responses for a given core temperature level (Sawka 1992). Hypohydration is usually associated with either reduced or unchanged whole-body sweating rates at a given metabolic rate in the heat (Sawka *et al.* 1984). However, even when hypohydration is associated with no change in sweating rate, core temperature is usually elevated, so that sweating rate for a given core temperature is lower when hypohydrated.

## Hyperhydration

Hyperhydration, increased total body water, has been suggested to improve thermoregulation during exercise-heat stress above euhydration levels (Sawka *et al.* 1996a). The concept that hyperhydration might be beneficial for exercise performance arose from the adverse consequences of hypohydration. Studies examining thermoregulatory effects of hyperhydration during exercise-heat stress have reported disparate results. Some investigators report lower core temperatures during exercise after hyperhydration (Moroff & Bass 1965; Nielsen *et al.* 1971; Gisolfi & Copping 1974; Nielsen 1974; Grucza *et al.* 1987), while other studies do not (Greenleaf & Castle 1971; Nadel *et al.* 1980; Candas *et al.* 1988). Also, several studies (Moroff & Bass 1965; Nielsen 1974; Lyons *et al.* 1990) report higher sweating rates with hyperhydration. In most studies, heart rate was lower during exercise with hyperhydration (Sawka *et al.* 1996a).

We believe that these conflicting results are due to differences in experimental design and not hyperhydration *per se*. For example, studies (Moroff & Bass 1965; Nielsen *et al.* 1971; Lyons *et al.* 1990) reporting that hyperhydration reduces thermal strain have not had subjects fully replace fluid lost during exercise; therefore, the differences reported may be due to dehydration causing increased thermal strain during 'control' conditions. Maintaining euhydration during exercise is essential to determine the effi-

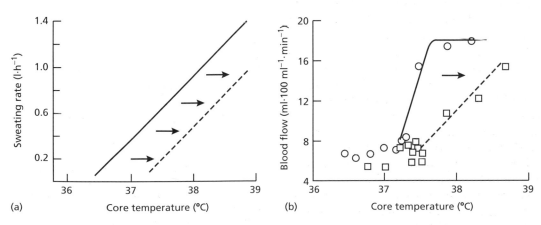

**Fig. 16.5** (a) Local sweating rate (Sawka *et al.* 1989), and (b) forearm skin blood flow (Kenney *et al.* 1990) responses for euhydrated (—) and hypohydrated (5% body water loss) (---) persons during exercise with heat stress. From Sawka (1992).

cacy of hyperhydration on thermoregulation during exercise-heat stress. In addition, some studies (Moroff & Bass 1965; Nielsen *et al.* 1971) report that overdrinking before exercise lowered body core temperature prior to exercise. This was likely due to the caloric cost of warming the ingested fluid. Exercise *per se* did not exacerbate the difference that existed prior to exercise. Hyperhydration in these studies therefore did not improve heat dissipation during the exercise period.

While many studies have attempted to induce hyperhydration by overdrinking water or water-electrolyte solutions, these approaches have produced only transient expansions of body water. One problem often encountered is that much of the fluid overload is rapidly excreted (Freund *et al.* 1995). Some evidence has been accrued that greater fluid retention can be achieved by drinking an aqueous solution containing glycerol while resting in temperate conditions (Riedesel *et al.* 1987; Freund *et al.* 1995). Riedesel *et al.* (1987) first reported that following hyperhydration with a glycerol solution, rather than with water alone, subjects excreted significantly less of the water load. They found that subjects drinking glycerol solutions achieved greater hyperhydration than subjects drinking water while resting in temperate conditions. Freund *et al.* (1995) reported that glycerol increased fluid retention by reducing free water clearance. Exercise and heat stress decrease renal blood flow and free water clearance and therefore both stressors might reduce glycerol's effectiveness as a hyperhydrating agent.

Lyons *et al.* (1990) reported that glycerol/water hyperhydration had dramatic effects on improving a person's ability to thermoregulate during exercise-heat stress. Subjects completed three trials in which they exercised in a hot (42°C) climate. For one trial, fluid ingestion was restricted to $5.4 \, ml \cdot kg^{-1}$ body weight, and in the other two trials subjects ingested water ($21.4 \, ml \cdot kg^{-1}$) with or without a bolus of glycerol ($1 \, g \cdot kg^{-1}$). Subjects began exercise 90 min after this hyperhydration period. Glycerol ingestion increased fluid retention by 30% compared to drinking water alone. During exercise, glycerol hyperhydration produced a higher sweating rate ($300–400 \, ml \cdot h^{-1}$) and substantially lower core temperatures (0.7°C) than those produced in control conditions with water hyperhydration. These thermoregulatory benefits during exercise-heat stress have not been confirmed. Other studies report similar core temperatures and sweating rates between glycerol and water hyperhydration fluids before exercise (Montner *et al.* 1996) in a temperate climate, or as rehydration solutions during exercise in a warm climate (Murray *et al.* 1991).

Recently, Latzka and colleagues (1997) examined the effects of hyperhydration on fluid balance and thermoregulation during exercise-heat stress. Their approach was to determine if pre-exercise hyperhydration with and without glycerol would improve sweating responses and reduce core temperature. The glycerol and water dosages were similar to those employed by Riedesel *et al.* (1987) and Lyons *et al.* (1990). Latzka and colleagues (1997) found that during exercise (45% $\dot{V}o_{2max}$) in the heat (35°C, 45% rh), there was no difference between hyperhydration methods for increasing total body water ($\approx 1.5 l$). In addition, unlike euhydration, hyperhydration did not alter core temperature (rectal or eosophageal), skin temperature, local sweating rate, sweating threshold, sweating sensitivity or heart rate responses. Likewise, no differences were found between water and glycerol hyperhydration methods for these physiological responses. Latzka and colleagues (1997) concluded that hyperhydration provides no thermoregulatory advantage over the maintenance of euhydration.

## Conclusion

During exercise, sweat output often exceeds water intake, producing a body water deficit or hypohydration. The water deficit lowers both intracellular and extracellular volume. It also results in plasma hypertonicity and hypovolaemia. Aerobic exercise tasks are likely to be adversely affected by hypohydration, with the potential affect being greater in warm environments. Hypohydration increases heat storage and reduces one's ability to tolerate heat strain. The increased heat storage is mediated by reduced sweating rate and reduced skin blood flow for a given core temperature. Hyperhydration has been suggested to reduce thermal strain during exercise in the heat; however, data supporting that notion are not robust.

## References

Adolph, E.F. & Associates (1947) *Physiology of Man in the Desert*. Intersciences, New York.

Allan, J.R. & Wilson, C.G. (1971) Influence of acclimatization on sweat sodium concentration. *Journal of Applied Physiology* **30**, 708–712.

Armstrong, L.E., Costill, D.L. & Fink, W.J (1985a) Influence of diuretic-induced dehydration on competitive running performance. *Medicine and Science in Sports and Exercise* **17**, 456–461.

Armstrong, L.E., Hubbard, R.W., Szlyk, P.C., Matthew, W.T. & Sils, I.V. (1985b) Voluntary dehydration and electrolyte losses during prolonged exercise in the heat. *Aviation and Space Environmental Medicine* **56**, 765–770.

Bass, D.E., Kleeman, C.R., Quinn, M., Henschel, A. & Hegnauer, A.H. (1955) Mechanisms of acclimatization to heat in man. *Medicine* **34**, 323–380.

Below, P.R., Mora-Rodríguez, R., González-Alonso, J. & Coyle, E.F. (1995) Fluid and carbohydrate ingestion independently improve performance during 1 h of exercise. *Medicine and Science in Sports and Exercise* **27**, 200–210.

Brouns, F. (1991) Heat–sweat–dehydration–rehydration: a praxis oriented approach. *Journal of Sports Science* **9**, 143–152.

Burge, C.M., Carey, M.F. & Payne, W.R. (1993) Rowing performance, fluid balance, and metabolic function following dehydration and rehydration. *Medicine and Science in Sports and Exercise* **25**, 1358–1364.

Buskirk, E.R., Iampietro, P.F. & Bass, D.E. (1958) Work performance after dehydration: effects of physical conditioning and heat acclimatization. *Journal of Applied Physiology* **12**, 189–194.

Cadarette, B.S., Sawka, M.N., Toner, M.M. & Pandolf, K.B. (1984) Aerobic fitness and the hypohydration response to exercise-heat stress. *Aviation and Space Environment Medicine* **55**, 507–512.

Caldwell, J.E., Ahonen, E. & Nousiainen, U. (1984) Differential effects of sauna-, diuretic-, and exercise-induced hypohydration. *Journal of Applied Physiology* **57**, 1018–1023.

Candas, V., Libert, J.P., Brandenberger, G., Sagot, J.C. & Kahn, J.M. (1988) Thermal and circulatory responses during prolonged exercise at different levels of hydration. *Journal of Physiology Paris* **83**, 11–18.

Convertino, V.A., Armstrong, L.E., Coyle, E.F. *et al.* (1996) American College of Sports Medicine Position Stand: exercise and fluid replacement. *Medicine and Science in Sports and Exercise* **28**, i–vii.

Craig, F.N. & Cummings, E.G. (1966) Dehydration and muscular work. *Journal of Applied Physiology* **21**, 670–674.

Dill, D.B., Jones, B.F., Edwards, H.T. & Oberg, S.A. (1933) Salt economy in extreme dry heat. *Journal of Biological Chemistry* **100**, 755–767.

Ekblom, B., Greenleaf, C.J., Greenleaf, J.E. & Hermansen, L. (1970) Temperature regulation during exercise dehydration in man. *Acta Physiologica Scandinavica* **79**, 475–483.

Engell, D.B., Maller, O., Sawka, M.N., Francesconi, R.P., Drolet, L.A. & Young, A.J (1987) Thirst and fluid intake following graded hypohydration levels in humans. *Physiology and Behaviour* **40**, 229–236.

Freund, B.J., Montain, S.J., Young, A.J. *et al.* (1995) Glycerol hyperhydration: hormonal, renal, and vascular fluid responses. *Journal of Applied Physiology* **79**, 2069–2077.

Gisolfi, C.V. & Copping, J.R. (1974) Thermal effects of prolonged treadmill exercise in the heat. *Medicine and Science in Sports* **6**, 108–113.

Grande, F., Monagle, J.E., Buskirk, E.R. & Taylor, H.L. (1959) Body temperature responses to exercise in man on restricted food and water intake. *Journal of Applied Physiology* **14**, 194–198.

Greenleaf, J.E. (1992) Problem: thirst, drinking behavior, and involuntary dehydration. *Medicine and Science in Sports and Exercise* **24**, 645–656.

Greenleaf, J.E. (1994) Environmental issues that influence intake of replacement beverages. In *Fluid Replacement and Heat Stress* (ed. B.M. Marriott), pp. 195–214. National Academy Press, Washington, DC.

Greenleaf, J.E. & Castle, B.L. (1971) Exercise temperature regulation in man during hypohydration and hyperhydration. *Journal of Applied Physiology* **30**, 847–853.

Grucza, R., Szczypaczewska, M. & Kozlowski, S. (1987) Thermoregulation in hyperhydrated men during physical exercise. *European Journal of Applied Physiology* **56**, 603–607.

Hubbard, R.W., Sandick, B.L., Matthew, W.T. *et al.* (1984) Voluntary dehydration and alliesthesia for water. *Journal of Applied Physiology* **57**, 868–875.

Kenney, W.L., Tankersley, C.G., Newswanger, D.L., Hyde, D.E., Puhl, S.M. & Turnera, N.L. (1990) Age and hypohydration independently influence the peripheral vascular response to heat stress. *Journal of Applied Physiology* **8**, 1902–1908.

Kubica, R., Nielsen, B., Bonnesen, A., Rasmussen, I.B., Stoklosa, J. & Wilk, B. (1983) Relationship between plasma volume reduction and plasma electrolyte changes after prolonged bicycle exercise, passive heating and diuretic dehydration. *Acta Physiologica Polonica* **34**, 569–579.

Ladell, W.S.S. & Shephard, R.J (1961) Aldosterone inhibition and acclimatization to heat. *Journal of Physiology* **160**, 19–20.

Latzka, W.A., Sawka, M.N., Montain, S. *et al.* (1997) Hyperhydration: thermoregulatory effects during compensable exercise–heat stress. *Journal of Applied Physiology* **83**, 860–866.

Lyons, T.P., Riedesel, M.L., Meuli, L.E. & Chick, T.W. (1990) Effects of glycerol-induced hyperhydration prior to exercise in the heat on sweating and core temperature. *Medicine and Science in Sports and Exercise* **22**, 477–483.

Mack, G.W. & Nadel, E.R. (1996) Body fluid balance during heat stress in humans. In *Environmental Physiology* (ed. M.J. Fregly & C.M. Blatteis), pp. 187–214. Oxford University Press, New York.

Marriott, B.M. (1993) *Nutritional Needs in Hot Environments: Application for Military Personnel in Field Operations.* National Academy Press, Washington, DC.

Marriott, B.M. (1994) *Fluid Replacement and Heat Stress.* National Academy Press, Washington, DC.

Molnar, G.W., Towbin, E.J., Gosselin, R.E., Brown, A.H. & Adolph, E.F. (1946) A comparative study of water, salt and heat exchanges of men in tropical and desert environments. *American Journal of Hygiene* **44**, 411–433.

Montain, S.J. & Coyle, E.F. (1992) Influence of graded dehydration on hyperthermia and cardiovascular drift during exercise. *Journal of Applied Physiology* **73**, 1340–1350.

Montain, S.J., Latzka, W.A. & Sawka, M.N. (1995) Control of thermoregulatory sweating is altered by hydration level and exercise intensity. *Journal of Applied Physiology* **79**, 1434–1439.

Montner, P., Stark, D.M., Riedesel, M.L. *et al.* (1996) Pre-exercise glycerol hydration improves cycling endurance time. *International Journal of Sports Medicine* **17**, 27–33.

Moroff, S.V. & Bass, D.E. (1965) Effects of overhydration on man's physiological responses to work in the heat. *Journal of Applied Physiology* **20**, 267–270.

Murray, R., Eddy, D.E., Paul, G.L., Seifert, J.G. & Halaby, G.A. (1991) Physiological responses to glycerol ingestion during exercise. *Journal of Applied Physiology* **71**, 144–149.

Nadel, E.R., Fortney, S.M. & Wenger, C.B. (1980) Effect of hydration state on circulatory and thermal regulations. *Journal of Applied Physiology* **49**, 715–721.

Neufer, P.D., Sawka, M.N., Young, A., Quigley, M., Latzka, W.A. & Levine, L. (1991) Hypohydration does not impair skeletal muscle glycogen resynthesis after exercise. *Journal of Applied Physiology* **70**, 1490–1494.

Nielsen, B. (1974) Effects of changes in plasma volume and osmolarity on thermoregulation during exercise. *Acta Physiologica Scandinavica* **90**, 725–730.

Nielsen, B., Hansen, G., Jorgensen, S.O. & Nielsen, E. (1971) Thermoregulation in exercising man during dehydration and hyperhydration with water and saline. *International Journal of Biometeorology* **15**, 195–200.

Nose, H., Morimoto, T. & Ogura, K. (1983) Distribution of water losses among fluid compartments of tissues under thermal dehydration in the rat. *Journal of Physiology* **33**, 1019–1029.

Pinchan, G., Gauttam, R.K., Tomar, O.S. & Bajaj, A.C. (1988) Effects of primary hypohydration on physical work capacity. *International Journal of Biometeorology* **32**, 176–180.

Riedesel, M.L., Allen, D.Y., Peake, G.T. & Al-Qattan, K. (1987) Hyperhydration with glycerol solutions. *Journal of Applied Physiology* **63**, 2262–2268.

Sawka, M.N. (1988) Body fluid responses and hypohydration during exercise-heat stress. In *Human Performance Physiology and Environmental Medicine at Terrestrial Extremes* (ed. K.B. Pandolf, M.N. Sawka & R.R. Gonzalez), pp. 227–266. Cooper Publishing, Indianapolis, IN.

Sawka, M.N. (1992) Physiological consequences of hydration: exercise performance and thermoregulation. *Medicine and Science in Sports and Exercise* **24**, 657–670.

Sawka, M.N. & Pandolf, K.B. (1990) Effects of body water loss on physiological function and exercise performance. In *Perspectives in Exercise Science and Sports Medicine.* Vol. 3. *Fluid Homeostasis during Exercise* (ed. C.V. Gisolfi & D.R. Lamb), pp. 1–38. Benchmark Press, Carmel, IN.

Sawka, M.N., Toner, M.M., Francesconi, R.P. & Pandolf, K.B. (1983) Hydration and exercise: effects of heat acclimation, gender, and environment. *Journal of Applied Physiology* **55**, 1147–1153.

Sawka, M.N., Francesconi, R.P., Young, A.J. & Pandolf, K.B. (1984) Influence of hydration level and body fluids on exercise performance in the heat. *Journal of the American Medical Association* **252**, 1165–1169.

Sawka, M.N., Young, A.J., Francesconi, R.P., Muza, S.R. & Pandolf, K.B. (1985) Thermoregulatory and blood responses during exercise at graded hypohydration levels. *Journal of Applied Physiology* **59**, 1394–1401.

Sawka, M.N., Gonzalez, R.R., Young, A.J., Dennis, R.C., Valeri, C.R. & Pandolf, K.B. (1989) Control of thermoregulatory sweating during exercise in the heat. *American Journal of Physiology* **257**, R311–R316.

Sawka, M.N., Young, A.J., Latzka, W.A., Neufer, P.D., Quigley, M.D. & Pandolf, K.B. (1992) Human tolerance to heat strain during exercise: influence of hydration. *Journal of Applied Physiology* **73**, 368–375.

Sawka, M.N., Montain, S.J. & Latzka, W.A. (1996a) Body fluid balance during exercise: heat exposure. In *Body Fluid Balance: Exercise and Sport* (ed. E.R. Buskirk & S.M. Puhl), pp. 143–161. CRC Press, Boca Raton, FL.

Sawka, M.N., Wenger, C.B. & Pandolf, K.B. (1996b) Thermoregulatory responses to acute exercise-heat stress and heat acclimation. In *Handbook of Physiology*. Section 4. *Environmental Physiology* (ed. M.J Fregly & C.M. Blatteis), pp. 157–185. Oxford University Press, New York.

Senay, L.C. (1968) Relationship of evaporative rates to serum [Na+], [K+], and osmolality in acute heat stress. *Journal of Applied Physiology* **25**, 149–152.

Shapiro, Y., Pandolf, K.B. & Goldman, R.F. (1982) Predicting sweat loss response to exercise, environment and clothing. *European Journal of Applied Physiology* **48**, 83–96.

Strydom, N.B. & Holdsworth, D.L. (1968) The effects of different levels of water deficit on physiological responses during heat stress. *Internationale Zeitschrift für Angewandte Physiologie* **26**, 95–102.

Walsh, R.M., Noakes, T.D., Hawley, J.A. & Dennis, S.C. (1994) Impaired high-intensity cycling performance time at low levels of dehydration. *International Journal of Sports Medicine* **15**, 392–398.

Webster, S., Rutt, R. & Weltman, A. (1990) Physiological effects of a weight loss regimen practiced by college wrestlers. *Medicine and Science in Sports and Exercise* **22**, 229–234.

# Chapter 17

# Water and Electrolyte Loss and Replacement in Exercise

RONALD J. MAUGHAN

## Introduction

As described in the previous chapters, the sweating mechanism is effective in limiting the rise in body temperature that occurs during exercise but, if the exercise is severe and prolonged and the climatic conditions hot and humid, the dehydration that results will inevitably have an adverse effect of exercise capacity. Sweat losses equivalent to 2–5% of body mass are often incurred in the course of endurance events, and if these are not replaced, the dehydration that ensues may precipitate circulatory collapse and heat illness. Fluid replacement is therefore important in situations where some degree of sweating is unavoidable: prolonged hard exercise in extreme conditions may increase the total daily water requirement from about 2.5 l to something in excess of 12–15 l. Even though this amounts to about 25–30% of total body water content for the average individual, such conditions can be tolerated for prolonged periods provided that the sweat losses are replaced. The choice of rehydration beverage will vary, depending on the circumstances, and requires an awareness of the extent of water and electrolyte losses and of substrate utilization by the working muscles as well as some understanding of the psychological and physiological factors that influence the rehydration process.

## Sweat losses in exercise

The physics of heat exchange between the human body and the environment have been described in several excellent reviews (e.g. Nadel 1988). Sweating is an effective mechanism of heat loss when heat loss by physical transfer cannot prevent a rise in core temperature. The heat required to evaporate 1 kg of sweat from the skin surface is approximately 2.6 MJ (620 kcal), allowing high rates of heat loss from the body to be achieved, provided only that sweat secretion is possible and that evaporation can occur. Although high temperature poses a threat to the athlete by adding to the heat load and reducing heat loss by physical transfer, high humidity, which prevents the evaporation of sweat, is more of a challenge: heat loss is limited, leading to hyperthermia, and high sweat rates occur without effective heat loss, leading to dehydration. The combination of hyperthermia and hypohydration will reduce exercise performance and may lead to potentially fatal heat illness (Sutton 1990).

Several different factors will interact to determine the sweat rate during exercise. The major determinants are the metabolic heat load and the environmental conditions of temperature, radiant heat load, humidity and wind speed, but there is a large interindividual variability in the sweating response even in standardized conditions. Although the sweat loss incurred on a daily basis by an athlete during training will be determined largely by the training load (intensity, duration and frequency of training sessions) and weather conditions, there will also be an effect of the amount and type of clothing worn, of activities apart from training, and of the presence or absence of air conditioning in living and sleeping accommodation. The training status of the individual will influence the amount of work that is performed, and thus the total heat load, but also influences the sweating response to a standardized heat stress. It is often reported that the sweating response is enhanced by training, but Piwonka *et al.* (1965) showed that trained runners sweated less than untrained men when they walked at the same speed on a treadmill in the heat (40°C), but that they increased their sweating rate more in response to a rise in core temperature. The usual response to a period of acclimatization to heat is an enhanced sweating response, resulting in an increase, rather than a decrease, in fluid requirements as an individual becomes adapted to living and training in the heat (Sawka 1988).

The daily water requirement of athletes living and training in the heat will be determined primarily by the sweat losses during training, but there may also be substantial losses during the remainder of the day if this is spent outdoors or if air conditioning is not available. Water requirements for sedentary individuals, and this generally includes coaches, doctors, administrators and other team support staff, may be two- or threefold higher than the requirement when living in a temperate climate (Adolph & Associates 1947). Respiratory water losses, while relatively small at sea level (amounting to about $200\,ml \cdot day^{-1}$) will be increased approximately twofold in regions of low humidity, but may be as high as $1500\,ml \cdot day^{-1}$ during periods of hard work in the cold dry air at altitude (Ladell 1965). To these losses must be added insensible loss through the skin (about $600\,ml \cdot day^{-1}$) and urine loss, which will not usually be less than about $800\,ml \cdot day^{-1}$.

Chapter 15 discusses the sex and age differences found in sweating rates and patterns.

The extent of sweat loss during training or competition is easily determined from changes in body mass adjusted for food or fluid intake and for urinary or faecal loss. The relatively small changes in body mass resulting from respiratory

water loss and substrate oxidation are usually neglected in the field situation: respiratory water losses will, in any case, represent a water deficit that should be replaced. There is a large amount of information in the published literature on sweat losses in different sports, and much of that information has recently been collated (Rehrer & Burke 1996). The relationship between exercise intensity and sweat loss is seen most clearly in the simple locomotor sports such as running or cycling. Figure 17.1 shows that, when exercise is carried out in the laboratory under standardized conditions of environment, clothing and exercise intensity, the sweating rate is closely related to ambient temperature, with relatively little variation between individuals. It is clear from Fig. 17.2, however, which shows sweating rate in a heterogeneous group of marathon runners, that the variation between individuals is large, even at the same running speed (Maughan 1985): the total sweat loss for these runners, however, was unrelated to the finishing time.

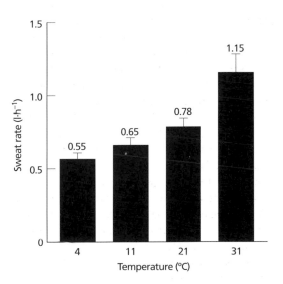

**Fig. 17.1** Mean sweat rate for eight male subjects exercising to the point of exhaustion on a cycle ergometer at an exercise intensity corresponding to about 70% of $\dot{V}o_{2max.}$ at different ambient temperatures. Values are mean ±SEM. Adapted from Galloway and Maughan (1997).

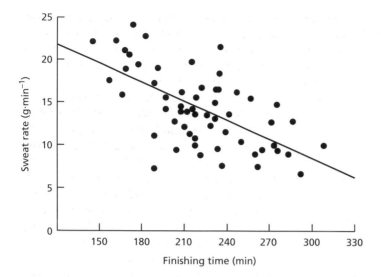

**Fig. 17.2** Sweat rates for subjects who competed in a marathon race held in cool (about 12°C) conditions. The sweat rate was closely related to the running speed, but there was a large variation between individuals, even at the same speed. Total sweat loss was unrelated to finishing time. $r = -0.629$; $P < 0.001$. From Maughan (1985).

## Electrolyte composition of sweat: implications for electrolyte balance

Electrolyte losses in sweat are a function of sweating rate and sweat composition, and both of these vary over time as well as being substantially influenced by the exercise conditions and the physiology of the individual. Added to this variability is the difficulty in obtaining a reliable estimate of sweat composition (Shirreffs & Maughan 1997): as well as problems of contamination of the sample and of ensuring completeness of collection, there are regional variations in electrolyte content, so measurements made at a single site may not reflect whole body losses.

In spite of the variability in the composition of sweat, it is invariably isotonic with respect to plasma, although the major electrolytes are sodium and chloride, as in the extracellular space (Table 17.1). It is usual to present the composition in $mmol \cdot l^{-1}$, and the extent of the sodium losses in relation to daily dietary intake, which is usually expressed in grams, is not widely appreciated. Loss of 1 litre of sweat with a sodium content of $50 \, mmol \cdot l^{-1}$ represents a loss of 2.9 g of sodium chloride: the athlete who sweats 5 l in a daily training session will therefore lose almost 15 g of salt. Daily dietary intakes for the 95% of the young male UK population fall between 3.8

**Table 17.1** Concentration ($mmol \cdot l^{-1}$) of the major electrolytes in sweat, plasma and intracellular water. Values are taken from a variety of sources identified in Maughan (1994).

|  | Sweat | Plasma | Intracellular |
|---|---|---|---|
| Sodium | 20–80 | 130–155 | 10 |
| Potassium | 4–8 | 3.2–5.5 | 150 |
| Calcium | 0–1 | 2.1–2.9 | 0 |
| Magnesium | <0.2 | 0.7–1.5 | 15 |
| Chloride | 20–60 | 96–110 | 8 |
| Bicarbonate | 0–35 | 23–28 | 10 |
| Phosphate | 0.1–0.2 | 0.7–1.6 | 65 |
| Sulphate | 0.1–2.0 | 0.3–0.9 | 10 |

and 14.3 g with a mean of 8.4 g: the corresponding values for young women are 2.8–9.4 g, with a mean value of 6.0 g (Gregory *et al.* 1990). For the same population, mean urinary sodium losses were reported to account for about 175 $mmol \cdot day^{-1}$ (Gregory *et al.* 1990), which is equivalent to about 10.2 g of sodium chloride. Even allowing for a decreased urinary output when sodium losses in sweat are large, it is clear that the salt balance of individuals exercising in the heat is likely to be precarious. The possible need for supplementary salt intake in extreme conditions will be discussed below.

The potassium concentration of sweat is high

relative to that in the extracellular fluid, and this is often quoted to suggest that sweat losses will result in the need for potassium supplementation, but the sweat concentration is low relative to the intracellular potassium concentration (Table 17.1). The potassium loss in sweat (about 4–8 mmol·l⁻¹, or $0.15–0.3\,g\cdot l^{-1}$) is small relative to the typical daily intake of about 3.2 g for men and 2.4 g for women (Gregory *et al.* 1990). In spite of the relatively high concentration of potassium in sweat, the normal response to exercise is for the plasma potassium concentration to increase due to efflux of potassium from the intracellular space, primarily from muscles, liver and red blood cells (Maughan 1994).

There is generally little change in the plasma magnesium concentration during exercise, but a slight fall may occur during prolonged exercise, and this has been attributed to the loss of magnesium in sweat. Some support for the idea that losses in sweat may be responsible comes from the observation of a larger fall in the serum magnesium concentration during exercise in the heat than at neutral temperatures (Beller *et al.* 1972), but a redistribution of the body's labile magnesium seems to be a more likely explanation for any fall in plasma magnesium concentration during exercise (Maughan 1994). Although the concentration of magnesium in sweat is high relative to that in the plasma (Table 17.1), the plasma content represents only a small fraction of the whole body store; Costill and Miller (1980) estimated that only about 1% of the body stores of these electrolytes was lost when individuals were dehydrated by about 6% of body mass.

Magnesium loss in sweat is considered by some athletes and coaches to be a potentially serious problem and to be a contributing factor to exercise-induced muscle cramp, resulting in suggestions that magnesium salts should be included in the formulation of drinks intended for consumption during exercise, but there is little evidence to substantiate this belief. Addition of magnesium to intravenous fluids administered to athletes with cramp after a triathlon was shown not to be effective in relieving the cramp (O'Toole *et al.* 1993). The causes of

exercise-induced muscle cramp are not well understood, and descriptive studies measuring changes in blood or plasma electrolyte concentrations or sweat losses of electrolytes are unlikely to provide any answers.

The sweating response to exercise is influenced by the hydration status of the individual, and sweat rates and thus thermoregulatory capacity, will fall if a fluid deficit is incurred (Sawka 1988). Less sweat is secreted for any given increase in core temperature. For reasonably well hydrated individuals, however, drinking during exercise seems to have little (Cage *et al.* 1970) or no (Davis & Yousef 1987) effect on sweating rate and to have no effect on sweat composition, even when plain water or electrolyte-containing solutions are consumed. Senay and Christensen (1965), however, observed that fluid ingestion in dehydrated subjects exposed for prolonged periods to hot (43°C) dry (<40% rh) conditions stimulated a prompt sweating response and increased skin blood flow, suggesting that fluid ingestion may restore thermoregulatory capacity in dehydrated individuals. It is clear that most of the benefits in terms of physiological responses and performance capacity that accrue from a period of acclimatization are lost if an individual becomes dehydrated (Sawka 1988).

## Gastrointestinal function and availability of ingested fluids

The available evidence suggests that most athletes do not ingest sufficient fluid to replace losses (Murray 1996). In some situations, opportunities for replacement are limited by the rules of sport, with drinks being available only during scheduled breaks in play, but even when there is unlimited access to fluids, intake is generally less than loss.

The first physical barrier to the availability of ingested fluids is the rate of gastric emptying, which controls the rate at which fluids are delivered to the small intestine and the extent to which they are influenced by the gastric secretions. The rate of emptying is determined by the volume and composition of fluid consumed, although there is again a large variability between individuals. The volume of the stomach contents is a major factor in regulating the rate of emptying, and the rate of emptying of any solution can be increased by increasing the volume present in the stomach; emptying follows an exponential time course, and falls rapidly as the volume remaining in the stomach decreases (Leiper & Maughan 1988). The presence of large volumes in the stomach may cause discomfort during exercise, and is not well tolerated by some individuals, but there is a strong learning process and the athlete can increase the amount that can be consumed with practice. The effects of exercise on gastrointestinal function are described in detail in the following chapter.

Dilute solutions of glucose will leave the stomach almost, but not quite, as fast as plain water; the rate of emptying is slowed in proportion to the glucose content (Fig. 17.3) and concentrated sugar solutions will remain in the stomach for long periods (Vist & Maughan 1994). There has been some debate as to the concentration of carbohydrate at which an inhibitory effect on gastric emptying is first observed: these studies have been reviewed by Maughan (1994). The

conflicting results reported in the literature are caused at least in part by deficiencies in the methodology employed in some studies. It appears that glucose concentrations as low as $40\,g\cdot l^{-1}$ will have some slowing effect on the rate of gastric emptying (Vist & Maughan 1994), but increasing the concentration will increase the carbohydrate delivery. Where a high rate of emptying is desirable, fluid delivery can be promoted by keeping the volume high by repeated drinking (Rehrer 1990), although repeated ingestion of concentrated carbohydrate solutions is likely to result in a progressive increase in the volume of fluid in the stomach (Noakes *et al.* 1991).

An increasing osmolality of the gastric contents will tend to delay emptying, and there is some evidence that substitution of glucose polymers for free glucose, which will result in a decreased osmolality for the same carbohydrate content, may be effective in achieving a higher rate of delivery of both fluid and substrate to the intestine. This has led to the inclusion of glucose polymers of varying chain length in the formulation of sports drinks. Vist and Maughan (1995) have shown that there is an acceleration of emptying when glucose polymer solutions are substituted for free glucose solutions with the same

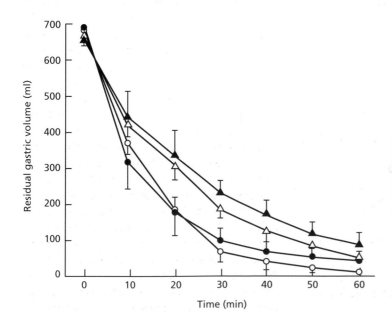

**Fig. 17.3** Increasing the glucose concentration in ingested solutions slows the rate of gastric emptying in proportion to the glucose concentration. This figure shows the total volume in the stomach after ingestion of 600 ml of water (○) or of drinks containing 2% (●), 4% (△) or 6% glucose (▲). A significant slowing is observed at a concentration of 4%. From Vist and Maughan (1994).

energy density: at low (about 4%) concentrations, this effect is small, but it becomes appreciable at higher (18%) concentrations; where the osmolality is the same (as in the 4% glucose solution and 18% polymer solution), the energy density is shown to be of far greater significance in determining the rate of gastric emptying (Fig. 17.4). This effect may therefore be important when large amounts of energy must be replaced after exercise, but is unlikely to be a major factor during exercise where more dilute drinks are taken. There may be benefits in including a number of different carbohydrates, including free glucose, sucrose and maltodextrin: this has taste implications, which may influence the amount consumed, and may maximize the rate of sugar and water absorption in the small intestine (Shi *et al.* 1995).

The temperature of ingested drinks has been reported to have an influence on the rate of emp-

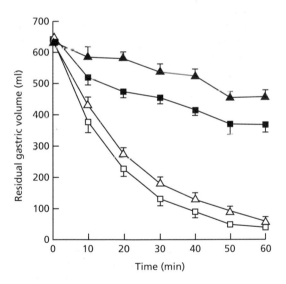

**Fig. 17.4** Substituting glucose polymers for free glucose reduces the inhibitory effect on gastric emptying. This figure shows the total volume in the stomach after ingestion of 600 ml of drinks containing glucose at concentrations of 4% (△) or 18.8% (▲) or of glucose polymer at concentrations of 4% (□) or 18.8% (■). The difference between isoenergetic solutions is small at low concentrations but becomes meaningful at high carbohydrate concentrations. Adapted from Vist and Maughan (1995).

tying, and it has been recommended that drinks should be chilled to promote gastric emptying (American College of Sports Medicine 1984). The balance of the available evidence, however, indicates that there is not a large effect of temperature on the rate of gastric emptying of ingested liquids (Maughan 1994). Lambert and Maughan (1992) used a deuterium tracer technique to show that water ingested at high temperature (50°C) appears in the circulation slightly faster than if the drink is chilled (4°C) before ingestion. The temperature will, of course, affect palatability, and drinks that are chilled are likely to be preferred and therefore consumed in greater volumes (Hubbard *et al.* 1990). Other factors, such as pH, may have a minor role to play. Although there is some evidence that emptying is hastened if drinks are carbonated, more recent results suggest that carbonation has no effect (Lambert *et al.* 1993): it is probable that light carbonation as used in most sports drinks does not influence the gastric emptying rate, but a greater degree of carbonation, as used in many soft drinks, may promote emptying of the gastric contents by raising the intragastric pressure. Zachwieja *et al.* (1992) have shown that carbonated and non-carbonated carbohydrate (10%) solutions were equally effective in improving cycling performance relative to water administration: there was no effect of carbonation on the rate of gastric emptying or on the reported prevalence of gastrointestinal symptoms. Lambert *et al.* (1993) did report a greater sensation of stomach fullness in exercising subjects drinking a carbonated 6% carbohydrate solution relative to the same drink without carbonation, but there was no apparent effect on physiological function.

No net absorption of carbohydrate, water or electrolytes occurs in the stomach, but rapid absorption of glucose occurs in the small intestine, and is an active, energy-consuming process linked to the transport of sodium. There is no active transport mechanism for water, which will cross the intestinal mucosa in either direction depending on the local osmotic gradients. The factors which govern sugar and water absorption have been extensively reviewed (Schedl *et al.*

1994). The rate of glucose uptake is dependent on the luminal concentrations of glucose and sodium, and dilute glucose electrolyte solutions with an osmolality which is slightly hypotonic with respect to plasma will maximize the rate of water uptake (Wapnir & Lifshitz 1985). Solutions with a very high glucose concentration will not necessarily promote an increased glucose uptake relative to more dilute solutions, but, because of their high osmolality, will cause a net movement of fluid into the intestinal lumen (Fig. 17.5). This results in an effective loss of body water and will exacerbate any pre-existing dehydration. This effect is sufficiently marked to be apparent during exercise in laboratory conditions (Fig. 17.6): ingestion of a dilute glucose–electrolyte solution can be shown to be more effetive than an equal volume of concentrated glucose solution in reversing the exercise-induced decrease in plasma volume that normally occurs. Other sugars, such as sucrose or glucose polymers, can be substituted for glucose without impairing glucose or water uptake. In contrast, the absorp-

tion of fructose is not an active process in man: it is absorbed less rapidly than glucose, is not associated with sodium cotransport, and promotes less water uptake.

Several studies have shown that exercise at intensities of less than about 70% of $\dot{V}o_{2max.}$ has little or no effect on intestinal function, although both gastric emptying and intestinal absorption may be reduced when the exercise intensity exceeds this level. Some more recent results, using an isotopic tracer technique to follow ingested fluids, have suggested that there may be a decreased availability of ingested fluids even during low intensity exercise: a decreased rate of appearance in the blood of a tracer for water added to the ingested drinks indicated a decreased rate of appearance of the tracer at an exercise intensity of 40% of $\dot{V}o_{2max.}$ (Maughan *et al.* 1990). These studies have been reviewed and summarized by Brouns *et al.* (1987) and Schedl *et al.* (1994). The results generally imply that the absorptive capacity of the intestinal tract is not seriously compromised by exercise at an inten-

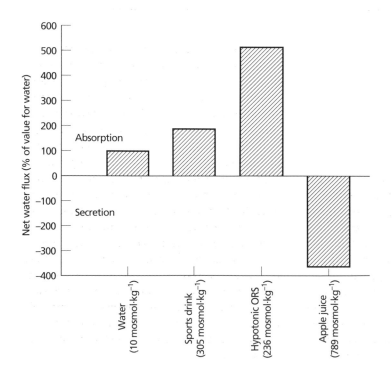

**Fig. 17.5** Dilute glucose electrolyte solutions stimulate water absorption in the small intestine, with hypotonic solutions being more effective than sports drinks, although the latter will be more effective in supplying energy in the form of carbohydrate. Concentrated solutions—such as fruit juices—will reverse the movement of water because of the high intraluminal osmotic pressure and will exacerbate any dehydration in the short term. The initial osmolality of each drink is given in brackets.

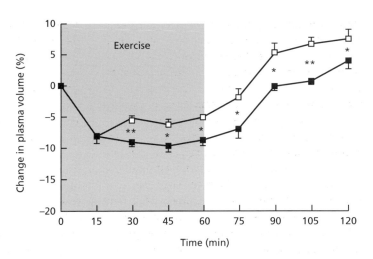

**Fig. 17.6** Because of the faster gastric emptying and faster intestinal absorption of water, ingestion of dilute carbohydrate–electrolyte solutions (□) is more effective in restoring plasma volume during and after exercise compared with ingestion of an equal volume of concentrated glucose solution (■). Values are mean ±SEM; *, $P<0.05$; **, $P<0.01$. Adapted from Maughan et al. (1987).

**Table 17.2** Composition of some of the most widely used commercial sports drinks.

|  | Carbohydrate (g · 100 ml$^{-1}$) | Sodium (mmol · l$^{-1}$) | Potassium (mmol · l$^{-1}$) | Osmolality (mosmol · kg$^{-1}$) |
| --- | --- | --- | --- | --- |
| Allsport | 8.0 | 10 | 6 | |
| Gatorade | 6.0 | 18 | 3 | 330–340 |
| Isostar | 6.5 | 17 | 5 | |
| Lucozade Sport | 6.9 | 23 | 5 | 260–280 |
| Powerade | 8.0 | 10 | 4 | |

sity that can be sustained for long enough (about 40 min or more) for fluid intake to be seriously considered.

## Electrolyte replacement during exercise

Commercially available sports drinks intended for use by athletes in training and competition are generally rather similar in their electrolyte content, suggesting a consensus, at least among the manufacturers, as to the requirements for electrolyte replacement (Table 17.2). It is clear that the major requirement is for addition of sodium, which is important in improving palatability and maintaining the drive to drink (Hubbard et al. 1990), for the absorption of glucose and of water in the small intestine (Maughan 1994), and for the maintenance of the extracellular volume (Hubbard et al. 1990).

In spite of the need to replace sodium, the main requirement is for replacement after exercise (see Chapter 19). During exercise, the plasma sodium concentration normally rises as water is lost in excess of sodium. When the exercise duration is likely to exceed 3–4 h, there may be advantages in adding sodium to drinks to avoid the danger of hyponatraemia, which has been reported to occur when excessively large volumes of drinks with a low sodium content are taken (Noakes et al. 1990). This condition, however, is rather rare, and does not in itself justify the inclusion of sodium in drinks intended for use in exercise where sweat losses do not exceed a few litres. The optimum sodium concentration for use in sports drinks intended for consumption during exercise has not been established, as this will vary depending on the conditions and on the individual, but is likely to be between about 20 and 40 mmol · l$^{-1}$.

Potassium is normally present in commercial sports drinks in concentrations similar to those in plasma and in sweat (see Tables 17.1, 17.2), but there is little evidence to support its inclusion. Although there is some loss of potassium in sweat, an increase in the circulating potassium concentration is the normal response to exercise: increasing this further by ingestion of potassium does not seem useful. Compared with the total daily intake of potassium (about 80 mmol for men and 60 mmol for women; Gregory *et al.* 1990), the amounts present in sports drinks are small. Replacement of losses will normally be achieved after exercise: 1 litre of orange juice will provide about 30 mmol of potassium, and tomato juice contains about twice this amount. A similar situation applies with magnesium replacement, and there seems to be no good reason for its addition to drinks consumed during exercise.

## Choice of rehydration fluids

The aim of ingesting drinks during exercise is to enhance performance, and the choice of drinks will therefore be dictated by the need to address the potential causes of fatigue. Provision of substrate, usually in the form of carbohydrate, to supplement the body's endogenous stores, and replacement of water lost in sweat are the primary concerns. In some situations, replacement of the electrolytes lost in sweat also becomes important. Because of the interactions among the different components of a drink, however, it is difficult to analyse these requirements separately. There are also many different situations in sport which will dictate the composition of drinks to be taken. The final formulation must also take account of the taste characteristics and palatability of the drink: not only will this influence the amount of fluid that the athlete consumes, but it will also have a major effect on how he or she feels.

The duration and intensity of exercise will be the main determinant of the extent of depletion of the body's carbohydrate reserves, and the same factors, together with the climatic conditions, will determine the extent of sweat loss.

There will however, always be a large variability between individuals in their response and therefore in their requirements. The requirements for rehydration and substrate provision will also be influenced by activity in the preceding hours and days. In a tournament competition in soccer, hockey or rugby, which may involve more than one game in a single day, or in a multistage cycle race with events on successive days, there is unlikely to be complete recovery from the previous round, and the requirements will be different from those in a single event for which proper preparation has been possible.

These difficulties are immediately apparent when any of the published guidelines for fluid intake during exercise is examined. Guidelines are generally formulated to include the needs of most individuals in most situations, with the results that the outer limits become so wide as to be, at best meaningless, and at worst positively harmful. The American College of Sports Medicine published a Position Statement in 1984 on the prevention of heat illness in distance running: the recommendations for fluid replacement during running events were more specific than an earlier (1975) version of these guidelines. It was suggested that marathon runners should aim for an intake of 100–200 ml of fluid every 2–3 km, giving a total intake of 1400–4200 ml at the extremes. For the elite runner, who takes only a little over 2 h to complete the distance, this could mean an intake of about $2 \, l \cdot h^{-1}$, which would not be well tolerated; it is equally unlikely that an intake of $300 \, ml \cdot h^{-1}$ would be adequate for the slowest competitors, except perhaps when the ambient temperature was low. These same guidelines also recommended that the best fluid to drink during prolonged exercise is cool water: in view of the accumulated evidence on the performance-enhancing effects of adding glucose and electrolytes, this recommendation seems even less acceptable than it was in 1984. This has now been recognized and a further updated version of the Guidelines (American College of Sports Medicine 1996) is in accord with the current mainstream thinking: for events lasting more than 60 min, the use of drinks containing 'proper amounts of carbohydrates and/or electrolytes' is recommended. The evolution of this series of American College of Sports Medicine Position Stands demonstrates the progress made in our understanding of this complex area.

Because of the difficulty in making specific recommendations that will meet the needs of all individuals in all situations, the only possible way forward is to formulate some general guidelines, to suggest how these might be adapted to suit the individual, and to indicate how these should be modified in different circumstances. Assuming that athletes are willing and able to take fluids during training, the recommendations for fluid use in training will not be very different from those for competition, except in events of very short duration. The sprinter or pursuit cyclist, whose event lasts a few seconds or minutes, has no opportunity or need for fluid intake during competition, but should drink during training sessions which may stretch over 2 h or more. The body does not adapt to repeated bouts of dehydration: training in the dehydrated state will impair the quality of training, and confers no advantage. Training is also the time to experiment with different rehydration strategies and to identify likes and dislikes among the variety of drinks available. Drinking in training will also allow the individual to become habituated to the sensation of exercising with fluid in the stomach: most athletes cite abdominal discomfort and a sensation of fullness as the reason for not drinking more during exercise (Brouns *et al.* 1987).

The choice of the fluid to be used is again a decision for the individual. Water ingestion is better than fluid restriction, but adding carbohydrate is also beneficial: Below *et al.* (1994) showed that the effects of fluid and carbohydrate provision on exercise performance are independent and additive (Fig. 17.7). Dilute carbohydrate–electrolyte drinks will provide greater benefits than water alone (Fig. 17.8) (Maughan *et al.* 1989, 1996; Maughan 1994). The optimum carbohydrate concentration in most situations will be in the range of about 2–8%, and a variety of differ-

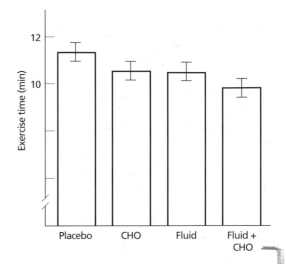

**Fig. 17.7** Ingestion of water and carbohydrate (CHO) have independent and additive effects in improving exercise performance. A time trial was performed at the end of a prolonged exercise test in which either a small or large fluid volume with a small or large amount of carbohydrate was given. A faster exercise time indicates a better performance. Values are mean ± SEM. Data from Below *et al.* (1994).

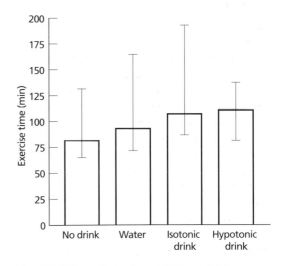

**Fig. 17.8** Effects of ingestion of different drinks on exercise capacity during a cycle ergometer test to exhaustion at a power output requiring about 70% of maximum oxygen uptake. Ingestion of water gave a longer time to exhaustion than the no drink trial, but the two dilute carbohydrate–electrolyte drinks gave the longest exercise times. Values are mean ± SEM. Data from Maughan *et al.* (1996).

ent carbohydrates, either alone or in combination, are effective. Glucose, sucrose, maltose and glucose oligomers are all likely to promote improved performance: addition of small amounts of fructose to drinks containing other carbohydrates seems to be acceptable, but high concentrations of fructose alone are best avoided because of a risk of gastrointestinal distress. Fructose is poorly absorbed, and an osmotic diarrhoea may occur after large doses. Some sodium should probably be present, with the optimum concentration somewhere between 10 and 60 mmol·l⁻¹, but there is also a strong argument that, in events of short duration, this may not be necessary. Adding sodium will have several consequences, the most important of which are a stimulation of water absorption and the maintenance of plasma volume. In events of longer duration, replacement of sweat sodium losses and maintenance of plasma sodium concentration and osmolality become important considerations. Sodium chloride, in high concentrations, may have a negative impact on taste, and home-made sports drinks generally score badly in this respect. There is little evidence to suggest that small variations in the concentration of these components of ingested fluids will significantly alter their efficacy. There is not at present any evidence to support the addition of other components (potassium, magnesium, other minerals or vitamins) to drinks intended to promote or maintain hydration status.

In most situations, the volume of fluid ingested is insufficient to match the sweat loss, and some degree of dehydration is incurred (Sawka & Pandolf 1990), and this suggests an important role for palatability and other factors that encourage consumption. It also indicates the need for an education programme to make athletes, coaches and officials aware of the need for an adequate fluid intake: a conscious effort is needed to avoid dehydration. Noakes *et al.* (1993) reported that the voluntary fluid intake of athletes in endurance running events seldom exceeds about 0.5 l·h⁻¹, even though the sweat losses are generally substantially higher than this. Even in relatively cool conditions and in

sports that are less physically demanding than marathon running, sweat rates of more than 1 l·h⁻¹ are not uncommon (Rehrer & Burke 1996).

## Pre-exercise hydration

Because of the need to minimize the impact of sweat loss and volume depletion on exercise performance, it is important to ensure that exercise begins with the individual fully hydrated. On the basis that a further increase in the body water content may be beneficial, there have been many attempts to induce overhydration prior to the commencement of exercise, but these attempts have usually been thwarted by the prompt diuretic response that ensues when the body water content is increased. Because this is largely a response to the dilution of blood sodium concentration and plasma osmolality, attempts have been made to overcome this. Some degree of temporary hyperhydration can be induced if drinks with sodium concentrations of 100 mmol·l⁻¹ or more are ingested, but this seems unlikely to be beneficial for performance carried out in the heat, as a high plasma osmolality will ensue with negative implications for thermoregulatory capacity (Fortney *et al.* 1984).

An alternative strategy which has recently been the subject of interest has attempted to induce an expansion of the blood volume prior to exercise by the addition of glycerol to ingested fluids. Glycerol in high concentrations has little metabolic effect, but exerts an osmotic action with the result that some of the water ingested with the glycerol will be retained rather than being lost in the urine, although there must be some concern that the elevated osmolality of the extracellular space will result in some degree of intracellular dehydration. The implications of this are at present unknown (Waldegger & Lang 1998), but it might again be expected that the raised plasma osmolality will have negative consequences for thermoregulatory capacity. The available evidence at the present time seems to indicate that this is not the case, but the results of studies investigating the effects on exercise performance of glycerol feeding before or during exercise have shown mixed results (Miller *et al.* 1983; Latzka *et al.* 1996). There have been some suggestions of improved performance after administration of glycerol and water prior to prolonged exercise (Montner *et al.* 1996) but some earlier work clearly indicated that it did not improve the capacity to perform prolonged exercise (Burge *et al.* 1993).

## Postexercise rehydration

Rehydration and restoration of sweat electrolyte losses are both crucial parts of the recovery process after exercise where significant sweat losses have occurred, and these issues are covered in detail in Chapter 19. In most sports, there is a need to recover as quickly and as completely as possibly after training or competition to begin preparation for the next event or training session. The need for replacement will obviously depend on the volume of sweat lost and on its electrolyte content, but will also be influenced by the amount of time available before the next exercise bout. Rapid rehydration may also be important in events where competition is by weight category, including weightlifting and the combat sports. It is common for competitors in these events to undergo acute thermal and exercise-induced dehydration to make weight, with weight losses of 10% of body mass sometimes being achieved within a few days: the time interval between the weigh-in and competition is normally about 3 h, although it may be longer, and is not sufficient for full recovery when significant amounts of weight have been lost, but some recovery is possible. The practice of acute dehydration to make weight has led to a number of fatalities in recent years, usually where exercise has been performed in a hot environment while wearing waterproof clothing to prevent the evaporation of sweat, and should be strongly discouraged, but it will persist and there is a need to maximize rehydration in the time available.

An awareness of the extent of volume and electrolyte loss during exercise will help plan the recovery strategy. Where speed of recovery is essential, a dilute glucose solution with added sodium chloride is likely to be most effective in promoting rapid recovery by maintaining a high rate of gastric emptying and promoting intestinal water absorption: a hypotonic solution is likely to be most effective (Maughan 1994). Complete restoration of volume losses requires that the total amount of fluid ingested in the recovery period exceeds the total sweat loss: the recommendation often made that 1 litre of fluid should be ingested for each kilogram of weight lost neglects to take account of the ongoing loss of water in urine, and it is recommended that the volume of fluid ingested should be at least 50% more than the volume of sweat loss (Maughan & Shirreffs 1997).

It is more difficult, because of the wide interindividual variability in the composition of sweat, to make clear recommendations about electrolyte replacement. It is clear, however, that failure to replace the electrolytes lost (principally sodium, but to some extent also potassium) will result in a fall in the circulating sodium concentration and a fall in plasma osmolality, leading to a marked diuresis. The diuretic effect is observed even when the individual may still be in negative fluid balance. If sufficient salt is ingested together with an adequate volume of water, fluid balance will be restored, and any excess solute will be excreted by the kidneys (Maughan & Leiper 1995). A relatively high sodium content in drinks will also be effective in retaining a large proportion of the ingested fluid in the extracellular space, and maintenance of a high plasma volume is important for maintenance of cardiovascular function (Rowell 1986).

## Conclusion

Water and electrolyte losses in sweat will result in volume depletion and disturbances of electrolyte (especially sodium) balance. Sweat loss depends on many factors, including especially environmental conditions, exercise intensity and duration, and the individual characteristics of the athlete. Replacement of losses will help maintain exercise capacity and reduce the risk of heat illness. Replacement may be limited by the rates of gastric emptying or of intestinal absorption, and dilute carbohydrate–electrolyte solutions can optimize replacement. Electrolyte replacement is not a priority during exercise, but sodium may be needed if sweat losses are very large and are replaced with plain water. Athletes should ensure that, whenever possible, they are fully hydrated at the beginning of exercise. Rehydration after exercise requires that an adequate fluid volume is ingested and that electrolyte losses are replaced.

## References

Adolph, A. & Associates (1947) *Physiology of Man in the Desert*. Wiley, New York.

American College of Sports Medicine (1975) Position statement on prevention of heat injuries during distance running. *Medicine and Science in Sports and Exercise* **7**, vii–ix.

American College of Sports Medicine (1984) Position stand on prevention of thermal injuries during distance running. *Medicine and Science in Sports and Exercise* **16**, ix–xiv.

American College of Sports Medicine (1996) Exercise and fluid replacement. *Medicine and Science in Sports and Exercise* **28**, i–vii.

Beller, G.A., Maher, J.T., Hartley, L.H. *et al.* (1972) Serum Mg and K concentrations during exercise in thermoneutral and hot conditions. *The Physiologist* **15**, 94.

Below, P., Mora-Rodriguez, R., Gonzalez-Alonso, J. & Coyle, E.F. (1994) Fluid and carbohydrate ingestion independently improve performance during 1 h of intense cycling. *Medicine and Science in Sports and Exercise* **27**, 200–210.

Brouns, F., Saris, W.H.M. & Rehrer, N.J. (1987) Abdominal complaints and gastrointestinal function during long-lasting exercise. *International Journal of Sports Medicine* **8**, 175–189.

Burge, C.M., Carey, M.F. & Payne, W.R. (1993) Rowing performance, fluid balance and metabolic function following dehydration and rehydration. *Medicine and Science in Sports and Exercise* **25**, 1358–1364.

Cage, G., Wolfe, S., Thompson, R. & Gordon, R. (1970) Effects of water intake on composition of thermal sweat in normal human volunteers. *Journal of Applied Physiology* **29**, 687–690.

Costill, D.L. & Miller, J.M. (1980) Nutrition for endurance sport. *International Journal of Sports Medicine* **1**, 2–14.

Davis, T.P. & Yousef, M.K. (1987) Sweat loss and voluntary dehydration during work in humid heat. In *Adaptive Physiology to Stressful Environments* (ed. S. Samueloff & M.K. Yousef), pp. 103–110. CRC Press, Boca Raton, FL.

Fortney, S.M., Wenger, C.B., Bove, J.R. & Nadel, E.R. (1984) Effect of hyperosmolality on control of blood flow and sweating. *Journal of Applied Physiology* **57**, 1688–1695.

Galloway, S.D.R. & Maughan, R.J. (1997) Effects of ambient temperature on the capacity to perform prolonged cycle exercise in man. *Medicine and Science in Sports and Exercise* **29**, 1240–1249.

Gregory, J., Foster, K., Tyler, H. & Wiseman, M. (1990) *The Dietary and Nutritional Survey of British Adults*. HMSO, London.

Hubbard, R.W., Szlyk, P.C. & Armstrong, L.E. (1990) Influence of thirst and fluid palatability on fluid ingestion during exercise. In *Perspectives in Exercise Science and Sports Medicine*. Vol. 3. *Fluid Homeostasis during Exercise* (ed. C.V. Gisolfi & D.R. Lamb), pp. 103–110. Benchmark Press, Indianapolis, IN.

Ladell, W.S.S. (1965) Water and salt (sodium chloride) intakes. In *The Physiology of Human Survival* (ed. O. Edholm & A. Bacharach), pp. 235–299. Academic Press, New York.

Lambert, C.P. & Maughan, R.J. (1992) Effect of temperature of ingested beverages on the rate of accumulation in the blood of an added tracer for water uptake. *Scandinavian Journal of Medicine and Science in Sports* **2**, 76–78.

Lambert, G.P., Blieler, T.L., Chang, R.T. *et al.* (1993) Effects of carbonated and noncarbonated beverages at specific intervals during treadmill running in the heat. *International Journal of Sport Nutrition* **2**, 177–193.

Latzka, W.A., Sawka, M.N., Matott, R.P., Staab, J.E., Montain, S.J. & Pandolf, K.B. (1996) *Hyperhydration: Physiologic and Thermoregulatory Effects during Compensable and Uncompensable Exercise-heat Stress*. US Army Technical Report, T96-6.

Leiper, J.B. & Maughan, R.J. (1988) Experimental models for the investigation of water and solute transport in man: implications for oral rehydration solutions. *Drugs* **36** (Suppl. 4), 65–79.

Maughan, R.J. (1985) Thermoregulation and fluid balance in marathon competition at low ambient temperature. *International Journal of Sports Medicine* **6**, 15–19.

Maughan, R.J. (1986) Exercise-induced muscle cramp: a prospective biochemical study in marathon runners. *Journal of Sports Science* **4**, 31–34.

Maughan, R.J. (1994) Fluid and electrolyte loss and replacement in exercise. In *Oxford Textbook of Sports Medicine* (ed. M. Harries, C. Williams, W.D. Stanish & L.L. Micheli), pp. 82–93. Oxford University Press, New York.

Maughan, R.J. & Leiper, J.B. (1995) Effects of sodium content of ingested fluids on post-exercise rehydration in man. *European Journal of Applied Physiology* **71**, 311–319.

Maughan, R.J. & Shirreffs, S.M. (1997) Recovery from prolonged exercise: restoration of water and electrolyte balance. *Journal of Sports Science* **15**, 297–303.

Maughan, R.J., Fenn, C.E., Gleeson, M. & Leiper, J.B. (1987) Metabolic and circulatory responses to the ingestion of glucose polymer and glucose/electrolyte solutions during exercise in man. *European Journal of Applied Physiology* **56**, 365–362.

Maughan, R.J., Fenn, C.E. & Leiper, J.B. (1989) Effects of fluid, electrolyte and substrate ingestion on endurance capacity. *European Journal of Applied Physiology* **58**, 481–486.

Maughan, R.J., Leiper, J.B. & McGaw, B.A. (1990) Effects of exercise intensity on absorption of ingested fluids in man. *Experimental Physiology* **75**, 419–421.

Maughan, R.J., Bethell, L. & Leiper, J.B. (1996) Effects of ingested fluids on homeostasis and exercise performance in man. *Experimental Physiology* **81**, 847–859.

Miller, J.M., Coyle, E.F., Sherman, W.M. *et al.* (1983) Effect of glycerol feeding on endurance and metabolism during prolonged exercise in man. *Medicine and Science in Sports and Exercise* **15**, 237–242.

Montner, P., Stark, D.M., Riedesel, M.L. *et al.* (1996) Pre-exercise glycerol hydration improves cycling endurance time. *International Journal of Sports Medicine* **17**, 27–33.

Murray, R. (1996) Guidelines for fluid replacement during exercise. *Australian Journal of Nutrition and Diet* **53** (Suppl. 4), S17–S21.

Nadel, E.R. (1988) Temperature regulation and prolonged exercise. In *Perspectives in Exercise Science and Sports Medicine*. Vol. 1. *Prolonged Exercise* (ed. D.R. Lamb & R. Murray), pp. 125–152. Benchmark, Indianapolis, IN.

Noakes, T.D. (1993) Fluid replacement during exercise. In *Exercise and Sports Science Reviews*. Vol. 21 (ed. J.O. Holloszy), pp. 297–330. Williams & Wilkins, Baltimore, MD.

Noakes, T.D., Norman, R.J., Buck, R.H., Godlonton, J., Stevenson, K. & Pittaway, D. (1990) The incidence of hyponatraemia during prolonged ultraendurance exercise. *Medicine and Science in Sports and Exercise* **22**, 165–170.

Noakes, T.D., Rehrer, N.J. & Maughan, R.J. (1991) The importance of volume in regulating gastric emptying. *Medicine and Science in Sports and Exercise* **23**, 307–313.

O'Toole, M.L., Douglas, P.S., Lebrun, C.M. *et al.* (1993)

Magnesium in the treatment of exertional muscle cramps. *Medicine and Science in Sports and Exercise* **25**, S19.

Piwonka, R.W., Robinson, S., Gay, V.L. & Manalis, R.S. (1965) Preacclimatization of men to heat by training. *Journal of Applied Physiology* **20**, 379–384.

Rehrer, N.J. (1990) *Limits to Fluid Availability during Exercise*. De Vrieseborsch: Haarlem.

Rehrer, N. & Burke, L.M. (1996) Sweat losses during various sports. *Australian Journal of Nutrition and Diet* **53**, S13–S16.

Rowell, L.B. (1986) *Human Circulation*. Oxford University Press, New York.

Sawka, M.N. (1988) Body fluid responses and hypohydration during exercise-heat stress. In *Human Performance Physiology and Environmental Medicine at Terrestrial Extremes* (ed. K.B. Pandolf, M.N. Sawka & R.R. Gonzalez), pp. 227–266. Benchmark, Indianapolis, IN.

Sawka, M. & Pandolf, K.B. (1990) Effects of body water loss on physiological function and exercise performance. In *Perspectives in Exercise Science and Sports Medicine*. Vol. 3. *Fluid Homeostasis during Exercise* (ed. C.V. Gisolfi & D.R. Lamb), pp. 1–38. Benchmark Press, Indianapolis, IN.

Schedl, H.P., Maughan, R.J. & Gisolfi, C.V. (1994) Intestinal absorption during rest and exercise: implications for formulating oral rehydration beverages. *Medicine and Science in Sports and Exercise* **26**, 267–280.

Senay, L.C. & Christensen, M.L. (1965) Cardiovascular and sweating responses to water ingestion during dehydration. *Journal of Applied Physiology* **20**, 975–979.

Shi, X., Summers, R.W., Schedl, H.P. *et al.* (1995) Effect of carbohydrate type and concentration and solution osmolality on water absorption. *Journal of Applied Physiology* **27**, 1607–1615.

Shirreffs, S.M. & Maughan, R.J. (1997) Whole body sweat collection in man: an improved method with some preliminary data on electrolyte composition. *Journal of Applied Physiology* **82**, 336–341.

Sutton, J.R. (1990) Clinical implications of fluid imbalance. In *Perspectives in Exercise Science and Sports Medicine*. Vol. 3. *Fluid Homeostasis during Exercise* (ed. C.V. Gisolfi & D.R. Lamb), pp. 425–455. Benchmark Press, Indianapolis, IN.

Vist, G.E. & Maughan, R.J. (1994) The effect of increasing glucose concentration on the rate of gastric emptying in man. *Medicine and Science in Sports and Exercise* **26**, 1269–1273.

Vist, G.E. & Maughan, R.J. (1995) The effect of osmolality and carbohydrate content on the rate of gastric emptying of liquids in man. *Journal of Physiology* **486**, 523–531.

Waldegger, S. & Lang, F. (1998) Cell volume-regulated

gene transcription. *Kidney and Blood Pressure Research* **21**, 241–244.

Wapnir, R.A. & Lifshitz, F. (1985) Osmolality and solute concentration: their relationship with oral rehydration solution effectiveness—an experimental assessment. *Pediatric Research* **19**, 894–898.

Zachwieja, J.J., Costill, D.L., Beard, G.C. *et al.* (1992) The effects of a carbonated carbohydrate drink on gastric emptying, gastrointestinal distress, and exercise performance. *International Journal of Sport Nutrition* **2**, 239–250.

# Chapter 18

# Gastrointestinal Function and Exercise

NANCY J. REHRER AND DAVID F. GERRARD

## Introduction

Investigations into the adaptations of the musculoskeletal and cardiovascular systems to exercise training have taken precedence in exercise science research, with very few controlled studies of the effects of exercise on gastrointestinal function. Nevertheless, there is a wealth of knowledge of normal gastrointestinal function which is pertinent to the design of an optimal nutritional plan for those actively engaged in sport. There is also a growing body of knowledge concerning alterations in gastrointestinal function as a result of exercise. The focus of this review is to highlight those aspects of gastrointestinal function and dysfunction to give a basis for nutritional supplementation regimens and to gain an understanding of the causative factors involved in the development of gastrointestinal symptoms as a result of exercise.

## Normal gastrointestinal function and the effects of exercise

### Oesophageal function

The tone of the lower oesophageal sphincter is of primary importance for the maintenance of a unidirectional flow of fluids and nutrients through the digestive tract. Several studies have examined the effects of exercise on this sphincter. In one study by Worobetz and Gerrard (1986), 1 h of treadmill running at 50% of $\dot{V}o_{2max.}$ resulted in an increase of the lower sphincter pressure from a baseline of 24 mmHg to 32 mmHg in asymptomatic, trained individuals. Oesophageal peristalsis, however, remained unchanged. Another study, however, found a decrease in lower oesophageal sphincter pressure and an increase in disordered motility with intensive exercise compared with rest (Peters et al. 1988). This is supported by a more recent study by Soffer et al. (1993), who demonstrated decreasing oesophageal peristalsis with increasing cycling intensity from rest to 60% to 75% to 90% of $\dot{V}o_{2peak}$ in trained subjects. The duration, amplitude and frequency of oesophageal contractions all declined with increasing intensity. The number of gastro-oesophageal reflux episodes and the duration of acid exposure were significantly increased at 90% $\dot{V}o_{2peak}$. Another study by the same authors (Soffer et al. 1994) demonstrated similar results with untrained subjects. Again, subjects cycled at graded intensities from 60% to 90% of $\dot{V}o_{2peak}$ and a decrease in oesophageal peristalsis with increasing intensity was observed. Also, an increase in the number and duration of reflux episodes and acid exposure was observed during cycling at 90% of $\dot{V}o_{2peak}$ as with trained subjects.

The discrepancy between the results obtained by Worobetz and Gerrard (1986) and those of the others may be explained by a differential effect of exercise intensity. It may be that a relatively mild exercise bout, for those accustomed to training at a higher intensity, may decrease the lower oesophageal tone. Beyond a certain relative intensity, an inverse effect may occur. This idea of

241

a U-shaped relationship between exercise intensity and digestive processes is in line with early advice, based on anecdotal evidence, to perform mild exercise after a meal to facilitate digestion. There is some evidence to support the idea that this type of curvilinear relationship also exists between exercise intensity and gastric emptying.

Schoeman and coworkers (1995) also looked at the effects of standardized meals and standardized exercise on lower oesophageal pressure and reflux. It was found that the timing of the meal had a greater effect on the incidence of reflux than did exercise. Sixty-six per cent (81 of 123) of reflux episodes occurred within 3 h after food intake, but only two episodes occurred during exercise. A number of other factors, including fat, alcohol, coffee ingestion and smoking also reduce sphincter pressure.

## Gastric emptying

Early observations of gastric function were made in which an inhibitory effect of emotional stress on gastric emptying rate was documented (Beaumont 1838). In another early study, Campbell *et al.* (1928) demonstrated that physical stress also decreased gastric emptying. Costill and Saltin (1974) showed that 15 min of cycling above 70% of $\dot{V}o_{2max.}$ decreased gastric emptying of a carbohydrate- and electrolyte-containing fluid, but that exercise at a lower intensity did not affect the emptying rate. It is, however, only in the last decade that a larger number of studies have been conducted to assess the effects of exercise on gastric function. In contrast to most of the early work, exercise intensity has been more closely controlled and clearly defined.

There is some disparity in results with regard to the effects of low- to moderate-intensity exercise on the gastric emptying rate. Neufer and colleagues (1989b) found an increased gastric emptying rate with exercise of a low to moderate intensity, with both walking (28%, 41% and 56% of $\dot{V}o_{2max.}$) and running (57% and 65% of $\dot{V}o_{2max.}$) when compared with rest. They also showed a decrease in emptying with intensive exercise

(75% of $\dot{V}o_{2max.}$). Marzio *et al.* (1991) also examined the effects of mild (50% max HR) and strenuous (70% max HR) treadmill exercise on gastric emptying. Their data support those of Neufer in that the gastric emptying was accelerated with mild exercise but delayed with more strenuous exercise. Research by Sole and Noakes (1989) also demonstrated a decreased emptying of water with exercise at 75% of $\dot{V}o_{2max.}$ compared with rest, but there was no effect of exercise on the emptying of a 10% carbohydrate beverage. Since it is known that increasing carbohydrate concentration decreases the gastric emptying rate (Vist & Maughan 1994), one may speculate that this effect overshadowed any exercise-induced inhibition of gastric function. Other researchers have failed to find a significant difference at moderate intensities (50% and 70% of $\dot{V}o_{2max.}$), although trends towards slowing have been observed (Rehrer *et al.* 1989), while others have shown a consistently increasing inhibition with moderate through to intensive (42%, 60% and 80% $\dot{V}o_{2max.}$) exercise (Maughan *et al.* 1990).

Some of the variance in results may be attributed to the testing protocol. In Neufer's work, gastric emptying was measured at a single time point, after 15 min of exercise, by aspirating the amount of beverage remaining. Marzio's experimental design entailed 30 min of exercise followed by ingestion of a beverage and thereafter following emptying with ultrasonography and scintigraphy. Rehrer and coworkers (1989) used a repeated, dye-dilution, sampling technique in which comparisons were made at frequent intervals over a period of 1 h, representing the complete emptying curve of a beverage ingested at the onset of exercise. Maughan and coworkers' research (1990) was also done with multiple measurement points over a complete emptying curve. They, however, measured blood accumulation of a deuterium tracer added to the ingested drink, which represents the effects of both gastric emptying and intestinal absorption. Nevertheless, both methods in which measurements were made at multiple points, over a longer exercise time, with beverage ingestion prior to exercise, show similar effects. It is tempting to speculate that the 15-min time period is not sufficient to give a full picture of the gastric emptying rate of the total volume of fluid ingested and that the chance of error would be greater. However, Costill and Saltin (1974) also only looked at 15 min of exercise and found no significant effect of exercise up to around 70% of $\dot{V}o_{2max.}$. Furthermore, in the experiments in which complete emptying curves were monitored, the 15-min measuring point also showed no significant effect.

The previously cited studies all examined the emptying of water or carbohydrate-containing liquids. One study also investigated the effect of mild exercise (walking at speeds of $3.2\,km \cdot h^{-1}$ and $6.4\,km \cdot h^{-1}$) on the emptying of a solid meal (Moore et al. 1990). An increased emptying was observed during exercise as compared with rest, based upon half-emptying times of radio-labelled meals and gamma camera monitoring. Another fairly recent study, by Brown et al. (1994), demonstrated with ultrasound imaging that the emptying of a semisolid meal was delayed with cycling at 85% of the predicted maximum heart rate compared to rest. In this study, postexercise contraction frequencies and antral areas were also monitored. Both were significantly decreased when compared with measurements made in experiments without exercise. Further, there was closure of the pylorus and a narrowing of the antrum. These changes in gastric function might explain the decreased gastric emptying observed. Another study, performed with dogs, showed that with 2 h of exercise, at 60–70% of the maximum heart rate, the gastric emptying of a mixed (23.5% protein, 3.5% fat, 66.5% carbohydrate) liquid meal was delayed and the migrating motor complex ceased, again indicating that exercise inhibits gastric motility. Gastric acid and pepsin secretion were also inhibited during exercise.

In summary, there appear to be no clear effects on gastric emptying at moderate intensities. High-intensity exercise (>70% of $\dot{V}o_{2max}$) does appear to increase emptying time. The few studies that were done at very low intensities (<42% of $\dot{V}o_{2max.}$), however, do indicate that gastric emptying may be enhanced by mild exercise.

One may speculate that some of the disparity in results of different studies was due to the training status of the subjects or the mode of exercise. However, when two groups, one trained and competitive in bicycling and the other untrained for all endurance activity, were compared, no difference in gastric emptying rate at rest or during cycling was observed (Rehrer et al. 1989). Another study, however, was conducted in which emptying of a radio-labelled egg omelette was compared in distance runners and sedentary subjects (Carrio et al. 1989). The trained runners had an accelerated gastric emptying of the meal at rest (runners, $t_{1/2}=67.7\pm5.9\,min$; sedentaries, $t_{1/2}=85.3\pm4.5\,min$, $P<0.001$).

Two studies have also compared gastric emptying rates of the same subjects cycling and running at similar relative intensities (Rehrer et al. 1990b; Houmard et al. 1991). No difference in gastric emptying rates was observed due to mode of exercise. These results are somewhat unexpected, since the magnitude of accelerations of the body while running are more than double that experienced during bicycling; therefore one might expect that this would result in an increased gastric emptying rate during running (Rehrer & Meijer 1991).

Other consequences of exercise can have an indirect effect on gastric function. Exercise can sometimes result in hypohydration and hyperthermia. When hyperthermia and hypohydration occur during exercise, the rate of gastric emptying is reduced (Neufer et al. 1989b; Rehrer et al. 1990a). The emotional stress that competition can cause may also delay gastric emptying and thus some of the conclusions drawn from data collected in a standardized laboratory setting may not always be applicable to an individual athlete during high-level competition. Further, a large variation in standardized gastric emptying rates between individuals exists (Foster & Thompson 1990; Brunner et al. 1991).

The factors which influence gastric emptying rate to a significant degree have, however, the same relative effect among both 'slow' and 'fast emptiers'. Beverage or meal size and composition, including nutrient concentration, osmolality and particle size, are all strong modulators of gastric emptying. In particular, increasing carbohydrate concentration, osmolality and particle size decrease the gastric emptying rate. For a more complete review of the factors which influence gastric emptying, see Murray (1987), Costill (1990), Maughan (1991) or Rehrer *et al.* (1994).

Bearing in mind the individual differences and situations, it is useful to look at the upper limits to gastric emptying rates during continuous exercise and to compare these with sweat rates when one is attempting to balance fluid losses. Mitchell and Voss (1990) observed increasing gastric emptying rates with increasing gastric volume up to approximately 1000 ml. With ingestion rates of around $1000 \, ml \cdot h^{-1}$, depending upon the composition of the beverage, the volume emptied can reach about 90% of that ingested (Ryan *et al.* 1989; Mitchell & Voss 1990; Rehrer *et al.* 1990b). Similar high rates of gastric emptying have also been observed with intermittent exercise ($1336 \, ml \cdot 2 \, h^{-1}$ ingested; $1306 \pm 76$, $1262 \pm 82$, $1288 \pm 75$, $1278 \pm 77 \, ml \cdot 2 \, h^{-1}$ emptied for water, 5%, 6% and 7.5% carbohydrate, respectively; Beltz 1988). For a review on the effects of volume on gastric emptying, see Noakes *et al.* (1991).

## Intestinal absorption

Net absorption of water and carbohydrates occurs primarily in the small intestine (duodenum and jejunum). To a lesser extent, water absorption also occurs in the large intestine (colon). A large body of research evidence exists which describes the functioning of the intestinal tract and the factors which influence the absorption of fluids and carbohydrates, at rest (Riklis & Quastel 1958; Curran 1960; Crane 1962; Schedl & Clifton 1963; Holdsworth & Dawson 1964; Fordtran 1975; Leiper & Maughan 1988; Gisolfi *et al.* 1990). Relatively little has been published

regarding intestinal absorption during exercise. Herewith only research specifically designed to look at the effects of exercise upon intestinal function will be discussed.

One of the first controlled studies directly measuring intestinal absorption during exercise was conducted by Fordtran and Saltin (1967). Intestinal perfusion of the jejunum and ileum with a triple lumen catheter was done with subjects at rest and during treadmill running at 70% of $\dot{V}o_{2max}$. A 30-min equilibration period was maintained prior to measurement in each condition. No effect of exercise on glucose absorption within the jejunum or ileum was observed. Similarly, no consistent effect of exercise on net water or electrolyte absorption or secretion was observed. It should be noted, however, that only four or five subjects were used in the jejunal perfusion experiments and only two to three in the ileal perfusion experiments. Conflicting results were found in another jejunal perfusion study (Barclay & Turnberg 1988), in which cycling was performed at a constant, absolute exercise intensity ($15 \, km \cdot h^{-1}$, 40–50% above resting heart rate). A significant net decrease in net water and electrolytes was observed. One difference between this study and that of Fordtran and Saltin (1967) is that in the earlier study, the perfusate contained glucose and in the latter study it did not. The stimulatory effect of glucose on water absorption may have masked any inhibitory effects of exercise. Further, the amount of glucose in the perfusate was not constant across subjects. This may have given added variability in results and with the small sample size may have precluded finding a consistent effect.

A more recent study by Maughan *et al.* (1990) has been conducted using deuterium accumulation in the plasma after drinking a $^2H_2O$-labelled beverage to investigate the effects of exercise on absorption. Subjects performed four separate trials at rest and cycling at 42%, 61% and 80% of $\dot{V}o_{2max}$. A consistent effect of exercise to reduce the rate of plasma deuterium accumulation was observed. One must bear in mind that the rate of deuterium accumulation in the plasma is not solely a consequence of the rate of intestinal absorption but also is influenced by the gastric emptying rate. Thus it is impossible to conclude if it is decreased gastric emptying or intestinal absorption which is responsible for the reduction in absorption. Further, deuterium accumulation in the plasma does not give information as to the net absorption. Alterations in intestinal secretion are not represented by deuterium accumulation (Gisolfi *et al.* 1990). However, it is assumed that the osmolality of the intestinal contents, as a function of beverage composition, is primarily responsible for changes in secretion. There is no evidence to suggest that exercise affects intestinal secretion. Thus, in the study by Maughan *et al.* (1990) in which the same beverage was administered during exercise at various intensities, one may expect that the secretion rate is constant.

One other problem with using a tracer to evaluate the appearance of a substance is that one measures the concentration in the plasma which is also influenced by the rate of disappearance, i.e. the rate at which the substance is taken up from the circulation by the tissues. During exercise the rate of mixture of the tracer with the total body water pool is nearly instantaneous and the different body compartments may be treated as one pool (N.J. Rehrer and R.J. Maughan, unpublished observations). This mixing of the tracer into the body water pool is delayed at rest. However, this could not account entirely for the difference in plasma deuterium accumulation during exercise in the study in question (Maughan *et al.* 1990), since during exercise the concentration of the label in the plasma continued to rise throughout the exercise protocol, rather than peaking early and decreasing with exercise duration, as one would expect if a delayed rate of efflux accounted for the reduced rate of plasma accumulation of the deuterium.

In conclusion, no consistent clear picture of the effect of exercise upon intestinal absorption is evident. Beverage composition, in particular carbohydrate concentration and osmolality, has a greater influence on net absorption.

A few studies have looked at intestinal permeability during or after exercise. Both Moses *et al.* (1991) and Oktedalen *et al.* (1992) have shown a decreased functioning of the mucosal barrier with running. More recently, Ryan *et al.* (1996) have shown that intestinal permeability is reduced to a greater degree when exercise and aspirin ingestion are combined than with aspirin ingestion at rest. This apparent lack of maintenance of intestinal membrane integrity may be related to alterations in blood flow to the intestinal region during strenuous exercise.

## Splanchnic blood flow

Rowell *et al.* (1964) and others (Clausen 1977; Qamar & Read 1987; Rehrer *et al.* 1992a; Kenney & Ho 1995; Seto *et al.* 1995) have demonstrated a decrease in blood flow to the intestinal tract as a result of physical exercise. Early studies, with limited exercise, indicated that splanchnic blood flow could be altered with exercise. Bishop *et al.* (1957) showed a decrease in arteriovenous difference in oxygen content over the liver, with supine cycling ergometry. Wade *et al.* (1956) demonstrated reduced bromosulphalein clearance in patients recovering from pulmonary infections, undertaking 'light', supine exercise (7–8 min of leg lifts). Rowell *et al.* (1964) were the first to quantify this decrease during upright treadmill exercise, using indocyanine green (ICG) clearance as an indication of splanchnic flow. They showed decreases of up to 84% with exercise.

A number of the more recent studies have made use of pulsed Doppler ultrasound to measure blood flow. In some cases the superior mesentery artery is measured and in others the portal vein. The measurements of the superior mesenteric artery (SMA) are typically done at rest prior to or after exercise as accurate measurements during exercise are made difficult due to the increased force of contraction of the heart during intensive exercise. This gives large fluctuations in the aortic flow which results in a superimposed flow on top of the true mesentery flow. Nevertheless, the measurements that are taken shortly after exercise has stopped do show a reduction in SMA flow. In one study, in which subjects walked at $5 \, \text{km} \cdot \text{h}^{-1}$ up a 20% incline for

15 min, a reduction in SMA flow of 43% was observed (Qamar & Read 1987).

In other studies, the venous portal flow was monitored by Doppler to give an indication of splanchnic blood flow. In one study in which upright cycling was conducted at 70% $\dot{V}O_{2max.}$, and environmental temperature was 26.8±0.2°C and humidity was 58±2%, a reduction in portal flow after 60 min of exercise of 80±7% was observed (Rehrer *et al.* 1992a). These results are in line with Rowell's earlier work using ICG clearance with intensive upright exercise.

Kenney and Ho (1995) demonstrated a difference in redistribution of blood flow with exercise between old and young subjects, even when matched for $\dot{V}O_{2max.}$ and exercising at the same intensity. Younger (26±2 years) subjects experienced a 45±2% reduction in estimated splanchnic flow (ICG clearance) during cycling at 60% of $\dot{V}O_{2peak}$ at an ambient temperature of 36°C. Older (mean, 64±2 years) subjects only experienced a 33±3% decrease. A decrease in blood supply and relative ischaemia to the splanchnic area decreases the absorption of actively transported nutrients, e.g. glucose (Varro *et al.* 1965). However, a decrease in flow of less than 40% is compensated for by an increase in oxygen extraction, and absorptive capacity is not altered. A greater decrease than this results in a reduced oxygen supply and reduced absorption. This leads one to wonder if the decreased splanchnic flow caused by exercise may inhibit normal absorption of nutrients during exercise.

Relatively few studies have assessed the combined effects of exercise and nutrient ingestion on splanchnic blood flow. It has been known for some time that ingestion and absorption of nutrients results in an increased blood flow to the intestinal tract at rest. The effect of exercise and nutrient ingestion/absorption has been little studied. One early study did look at the blood flow within the SMA in dogs after a meal, at rest and during exercise (Burns & Schenck 1969). Exercise consisted of treadmill running on an incline until panting began (after about 5–10 min). An indwelling electromagnetic flow probe, which was surgically placed several days

prior to experiments, was used to measure flow. A 20% decrease in SMA flow with exercise was observed, and this was lessened (14% decrease) when the exercise was performed 3 h after feeding. Another similar study with dogs was performed in which they were exercised on a treadmill for 4 min at 1.5 km·h⁻¹ (Fronek & Fronek 1970). Although no effect of exercise on SMA flow in the fasted state was observed, exercise immediately following meal ingestion resulted in a relatively reduced blood flow in contrast to that seen with feeding at rest.

Qamar and Read (1987) found that mild exercise (walking, 15 min at 5 km·h⁻¹, 20% incline) reduced the increase in SMA blood flow observed after a meal in man. The flow, however, was still greater than that observed at rest in the fasted state. Strenuous exercise of longer duration (70% of $\dot{V}O_{2max.}$ for 60 min) has been observed to cause an attenuation of the increased flow through the portal vein observed with glucose (100 g·h⁻¹) ingestion (Rehrer *et al.* 1993). Flow increased to 195±19% of the resting, fasted value after glucose ingestion and decreased to 61±15% with glucose ingestion during exercise. Although this type and intensity of exercise with glucose ingestion did result in a significant decrease in portal flow, it is of a lesser magnitude than that observed with similar exercise in the fasted state (Rehrer *et al.* 1992a). Thus, when glucose is ingested during exercise, the reduction in flow is lessened to such a degree that one would not expect glucose absorption to be inhibited.

The redistribution in splanchnic blood flow observed as a result of exercise and meal ingestion is regulated by hormonal and neural stimuli, with the sympathetic nervous system playing a central role. Several studies have demonstrated a relationship between sympathoadrenergic activation and splanchnic blood flow alterations with exercise (Chaudhuri *et al.* 1992; Iwao *et al.* 1995; Kenney & Ho 1995). In particular, an inverse correlation between portal venous flow and plasma noradrenaline concentration has been observed with measurements taken at rest and during mild and intensive exercise in man

($r=-0.54$, $P<0.01$; Iwao *et al.* 1995). In this study, however, exercise was performed on a treadmill, but measurements were made after exercise ceased, with subjects in a supine position. A similar inverse correlation between portal venous flow and plasma noradrenaline concentration in man was observed ($r=-0.65$, $P<0.01$) when data were collected at rest and during cycling exercise at 70% of $\dot{V}o_{2max.}$ with and without glucose ingestion, inhibitory and stimulatory influences, respectively (Rehrer *et al.* 1993). Neuropeptide Y is also known to be released from nerve endings with sympathetic activation and has been observed to be increased during exercise (Ahlborg *et al.* 1992). As it also is a vasoconstrictor in the blood vessels of the kidneys and splanchnic region, it may be implicated in the redistribution of blood flow during exercise.

Other hormones implicated in the regulation of intestinal blood flow include cholecystekinin (CCK) and secretin, both having been observed to increase blood flow within the SMA (Fara & Madden 1975). Although these hormones are of particular relevance with respect to blood supply to the digestive organs after the ingestion of a meal, it is doubtful that they play a role in the regulation of blood flow in response to exercise. Angiotensin II, however, is increased during exercise and it causes vasoconstriction of splanchnic and renal blood vessels (Stebbins & Symons 1995). Similarly, endothelin-1 (ET-1) increases during exercise and an infusion of ET-1 has been shown to decrease the splanchnic blood flow to levels lower than those observed during exercise without ET-1 infusion (Ahlborg *et al.* 1995).

### Gastrointestinal transit

Regular exercise has been observed to increase the rate of gastrointestinal transit. Cordain *et al.* (1986) observed an increased transit as a result of participation in a running training programme. It was thought that the mechanical jarring occurring during running may have caused the increased transit. However, in another study, Koffler *et al.* (1992) have demonstrated that strength training also increases gastrointestinal transit in elderly and middle-aged men. Further in support of these findings is a study showing that a brief period (2 weeks) of relative inactivity decreases transit in elderly individuals (Liu *et al.* 1993). The mechanism responsible for the decreased transit time with exercise is uncertain. Changes in hormones and/or parasympathetic tone, an increased food intake and mechanical effects have been speculated upon.

A positive health effect may be related to this adjustment in gastrointestinal transit time observed with regular exercise. A number of studies indicate an inverse relationship between physical activity and colorectal cancer; among these, one of the most comprehensive is a cohort study of 104 485 Norwegians (Thune & Lund 1996). These authors speculate that it is the increase in gastrointestinal transit, reducing exposure of the gut to potentially carcinogenic components of the diet, which may account for the decrease in colorectal cancer seen with increased levels of exercise participation.

## Exercise and gastrointestinal dysfunction

A number of gastrointestinal symptoms have long been linked to various forms of moderate exercise (Larson & Fisher 1987; Green 1992; Brukner & Kahn 1993). Surveys of runners and multisport athletes have confirmed the frequency with which prolonged physical exertion precipitates significant digestive tract problems which may interrupt training and hinder performance (Moses 1990). Fortunately, such symptoms are most often self-limiting rather than life-threatening, but it is increasingly more common for sports physicians to evaluate gastrointestinal symptoms.

Common explanations for these clinical symptoms include dehydration, altered gastrointestinal blood flow, changes in gut permeability, disturbed gastrointestinal tract motility, psychological influences ('stress') and pharmacological agents (Table 18.1) (Brukner & Khan 1993). Irrespective of the cause, exercise-induced al-

**Table 18.1** Common gastrointestinal symptoms associated with exercise.

| Symptom | Possible contributing factors |
| --- | --- |
| *Upper gastrointestinal* | |
| Nausea | Dehydration |
| Vomiting | Altered gastrointestinal |
| Reflux | blood flow |
| Epigastric pain | Altered gut permeability |
| Bloating | Disturbed gastrointestinal |
| Belching | motility |
| | Psychological |
| *Lower gastrointestinal* | influences |
| Constipation | Pharmacological agents |
| Diarrhoea | |
| Rectal blood loss | |
| Flatulence | |
| Urge to defecate | |
| Abdominal cramps | |
| Faecal incontinence | |

terations to normal gastrointestinal tract function have frequent clinical associates. These include such uppergastrointestinal tract complaints as nausea, vomiting, reflux, epigastric pain, bloating and excessive belching. Lower gastrointestinal tract symptoms include altered bowel habit (constipation or diarrhoea), rectal blood loss, flatulence, the urge to defecate, abdominal cramps and faecal incontinence (Brukner & Kahn 1993).

Various studies have reported the frequency of symptomatic, gastrointestinal tract-affected athletes to range from 50% (Brouns 1991; Wright 1991) to over 80% in a group of New Zealand endurance athletes (Worobetz & Gerrard 1985). It therefore behoves all sports physicians to recognize the exercise-related symptoms of gastrointestinal tract dysfunction and offer appropriate therapy.

This section will discuss some of the more common symptoms related to gastrointestinal tract dysfunction in athletes and describe them on a regional basis.

### Oesophageal symptoms

Symptoms including 'heartburn' and acid reflux are frequent associates of exercise, generally thought to be linked to altered oesophageal sphincter tone. A consequence of lowered oesophageal sphincter pressure is disruption to the unidirectional flow of upper gastrointestinal tract contents. This is frequently reported to be exacerbated by exercise, resulting in altered oesophageal peristalsis, reflux and exposure of the oesophagus to acid gastric contents (Worobetz & Gerrard 1986; Larson & Fisher 1987; Moses 1990; Wright 1991; Green 1992; Peters *et al.* 1993). The local irritant effect gives rise to the unpleasant sensation of retrosternal pain described colloquially as 'heartburn'. It is well recognized that the retrosternal discomfort often precipitated by exercise may have cardiological origins. Clinical wisdom demands a full investigation in cases where the age, family history and risk factors for ischaemic heart disease coexist.

The ingestion of carbohydrate-rich supplements was followed by bouts of cycling and running in a study by Peters *et al.* (1993). This association was found to correlate highly with symptoms of nausea, belching, epigastric fullness (bloating), the urge to defecate, abdominal cramps and flatulence. The mode of exercise as a factor in provoking oesophageal symptoms was investigated by Rehrer *et al.* (1992) in a group of triathletes. These investigators found a higher incidence of gastrointestinal tract symptoms associated with running. Similar conclusions were drawn by Sullivan (1994), who questioned 110 triathletes to find that running was associated with 'a preponderance of gastro-oesophageal and colonic symptoms'. However, given the fact that the running section of a triathlon is always preceded by the swim and cycle phases, the results of these studies should be interpreted with some caution. Factors such as hydration status, fatigue level and posture are possible influences of some significance. In fact, Rehrer *et al.* (1990) identified a body weight loss of 3.5–4.0% by dehydration, to be associated with an increase in gastrointestinal tract symptoms in runners.

Worobetz and Gerrard (1986) found that only

moderate amounts of exercise were associated with altered lower oesophageal sphincter pressure, which was measured using a small manometer placed at the gastro-oesophageal junction. Other studies link symptoms of disordered oesophageal motility to factors which include exercise intensity, the timing of food intake, specific foods such as alcohol and coffee and the influence of smoking (Schoeman *et al.* 1995). However, the latter is an unlikely habitual associate of the athlete.

Measures which reduce the volume of the stomach contents during exercise are likely to reduce the possibility of symptoms associated with reflux. In the same way, the composition of the prerace meal has been found to influence symptoms such as flatulence and side ache. Peters *et al.* (1993) tested different carbohydrate supplements in 32 male triathletes to determine the prevalence, duration and seriousness of gastrointestinal symptoms. Their results suggested possible mechanisms including duration of exercise, altered gastrointestinal tract blood supply, carbohydrate 'spill over' and the postural (vertical) effect of running.

The symptomatic relief of 'heartburn' can be achieved through the use of simple antacids such as aluminium hydroxide, sodium bicarbonate, magnesium carbonate or alignic acid. If such agents alone are insufficient to relieve symptoms then the use of $H_2$-receptor antagonists is indicated. Examples of these agents include cimetidine and ranitidine. Their action is to inhibit both the stimulated basal secretion of gastric acid and to reduce pepsin output by histamine $H_2$-receptor antagonism. Additional therapy may include the use of muscarinic $M_1$-antagonists, prostaglandin analogues or proton pump inhibitors such as omeprazole. Metaclopramide may also provide short-term relief by improving the contractility of the lower oesophageal sphincter tone.

Reports of upper gastrointestinal tract bleeding associated with physical exertion have been well documented, and recently correlated with digestive complaints and clinically demonstrable iron-deficient states (Brouns 1991; Wright 1991; Moses 1993; Rudzki *et al.* 1995). The causes of such blood losses can include a Mallory–Weiss tear from the mechanical trauma of repetitive vomiting to bleeding from a peptic ulcer. Any unaccountable blood loss from the gastrointestinal tract deserves full clinical investigation.

## Gastric symptoms

The commonly reported effects of gastric dysfunction in athletes include nausea, bloating, epigastric pain and belching. In addition, haemorrhagic gastritis is reported as a common cause of gastrointestinal tract bleeding but is most often transient and usually localized to the fundus (Brukner & Kahn 1993). The use of salicylates and non-steroidal anti-inflammatory drugs (NSAIDs) in the athletic population is also recognized as having a potential for gastrointestinal tract irritation leading to gastritis and ulceration. However, in two studies the use of these drugs was not correlated with an increase in upper gastrointestinal tract bleeding (McMahon *et al.* 1984; Baska *et al.* 1990). An additional problem with NSAID ingestion linked with their antiprostaglandin effect is a reduction of renal blood flow, which is considered to be a potential factor in the genesis of renal failure in athletes (Walker *et al.* 1994).

Documented influences upon the rate of gastric emptying in athletes include the temperature, energy content and osmolality of the gastric contents, environmental temperature and exercise conditions (Costill & Saltin 1974; Murray 1987; Neufer 1989a; Moses 1990; Rehrer *et al.* 1990b; Green 1992). Hyperosmolar solutions have been found to empty more slowly from the stomach during exercise and therefore should be avoided. While light exercise is considered a positive stimulus to the gastric emptying of fluids, the passage of solid foods is delayed by vigorous activity (Moses 1990). The clinical significance of this information is the timing and composition of precompetition meals, and advice for those athletes whose choice of event demands that they 'top up' during a race or on long training runs. Gastric retention has been suggested as causing nausea and vomiting after exercise, or the cause of disabling cramps during running (Olivares 1988 cited in Moses 1990). It would seem from the literature that gastric stasis may be avoided by choosing low-volume, isotonic, liquid meals which are low in fat, protein and dietary fibre.

In addition, there appear to be a number of anecdotal references to athletes in whom gastric clearance has been influenced by the psychological stresses of competition (Larson & Fisher 1987). References to the link between psychological stress and gastric function were made over 60 years ago. A delay in gastric emptying was noted by Campbell et al. (1928) and revisited by Beaumont 10 years later. These influences, which are often more difficult to quantify but are no less important to the athlete, represent an area of considerable research potential that can be explored with the aid of contemporary instruments of measurement including radio isotope-labelled meals, gamma cameras and ultrasound.

### Intestinal symptoms

Reported lower gastrointestinal tract symptoms during exercise (particularly running) include abdominal cramps, urgency of bowel movement, diarrhoea, rectal bleeding, flatulence and post-exercise anorexia.

A model for factors associated with gastrointestinal tract symptoms during exercise has been proposed by Peters et al. (1995). There is a strong recognition of the interrelationship between several factors:

* Hydration status.
* Mechanical trauma.
* Neuroendocrine alterations.
* Psychological stress.
* Reduced gastrointestinal tract blood supply.
* Altered gut motility.
* Influence of medication.

### Gastrointestinal tract bleeding

Exercise-associated gastrointestinal bleeding has been reported by several authors (Porter 1983; McMahon et al. 1984; Stewart et al. 1984; Scobie 1985; Robertson et al. 1987; Baska et al. 1990; Moses 1990; Schwartz et al. 1990; Green 1992). Haemorrhage from the gastrointestinal tract is always of concern to the athlete. The presentation may be very dramatic and, irrespective of the source, it is important to evaluate the frequency and significance of the blood loss given that occult blood loss has been frequently reported in endurance athletes (Green 1992). It has become more evident through contemporary methods of endoscopic examination that the intensity of exercise rather than mechanical influences are causative in the loss of blood from the gastrointestinal tract. A proposed mechanism of direct trauma to the gut through running was the basis for the syndrome of 'caecal slap' reported by Porter in 1982. It was postulated that the mechanical effect of running was physically insulting on the ileocaecal junction and produced a localized contusion. However, since then the study of other athletes, including cyclists (Dobbs et al. 1988 cited in Green 1992), suggests that any endurance athletes, and not just runners, may suffer significant occult gastrointestinal blood loss and that the mechanism for this is likely to be the result of endocrine and vascular insults and factors related to hydration status.

The athlete presenting with frank gastrointestinal tract bleeding deserves a full clinical evaluation. Local anorectal causes such as haemorrhoids and fissures are easily ruled out by physical examination, but inflammatory bowel disease and more sinister causes of bleeding including carcinoma will require more extensive endoscopic investigations. In many cases the athlete may present with haematological evidence of anaemia which is often nutritional, or due to the expanded plasma volume of exercise (an apparent or athletes' pseudoanaemia), but might also signal insidious blood loss from an undetermined site. Endoscopic examinations of both upper and lower gastrointestinal tract are mandatory investigations particularly where the age of the athlete, their medical history and the concurrent use of NSAIDs are reported.

Although the aetiology of gastrointestinal bleeding is likely to be multifactorial, the literature frequently implicates two factors. These are dehydration and reduced splanchnic blood flow. The former factor has been associated with generalized hypovolaemia, particularly in endurance athletes, but intestinal ischaemia is the factor most frequently linked with lower gastrointestinal bleeding. The diversion of blood from the splanchnic bed to supply exercising muscles is a well-recognized physiological phenomenon. This is reported to deplete local visceral blood flow by up to 75% and establish the basis of localized ischaemia reported to result in symptoms such as abdominal cramping and diarrhoea (Schwartz *et al.* 1990). Both the upper and lower portions of the gastrointestinal tract may be affected by diminished blood supply with the gastric mucosa appearing to be particularly susceptible to insult. Denied the protective influence of its mucosal layer, the gastric fundus is reported to be the most frequently reported site of gastrointestinal bleeding (Brukner & Kahn 1993). No small bowel sites of haemorrhage appear to have been reported, but bleeding from the colon has been frequently reported in association with exercise (Fogoros 1980). Documented cases have included ischaemic colitis (Porter 1982; Pruett *et al.* 1985; Schaub *et al.* 1985; Heer *et al.* 1986, Moses *et al.* 1988). It has also been proposed that these cases of gut ischaemia represent a more accurate pathogenesis of the earlier report of 'caecal slap'.

## Symptoms of altered gastrointestinal transit

As with the pathogenesis of other exercise-related gastrointestinal symptoms, it is likely that the causes of altered transit, in particular diarrhoea, are several. These include the athlete's diet (including fluid intake), the use of medication, the influence of psychological stresses, the intensity and mechanical effect of exercise, hormonal influences and the relative ischaemia of the gut during exercise.

The term 'runner's trots' was coined by Fogoros in 1980. It has been widely considered that the exercise-induced bloody diarrhoea with antecedent abdominal cramps is the single most debilitating symptom of gastrointestinal tract disturbance to the athlete. There are many anecdotal references to this in both lay and professional publications. The full syndrome includes lower abdominal cramping, the urge to defecate, rectal bleeding, an increased frequency of bowel movements with exercise, and frank diarrhoea (Swain 1994). Clinicians must rule out abnormalities such as irritable bowel syndrome, lactose intolerance, coeliac disease, ulcerative colitis and infective causes of diarrhoea before attributing these symptoms simply to exercise. Such medications as laxatives, $H_2$-antagonists, iron supplements and antibiotics may also induce diarrhoea, and less common causes, including pancreatic disease, exercise-induced anaphylaxis, and diverticular disease are also frequently associated with chronic recurrent symptoms of diarrhoea.

Of greater importance to the symptomatic athlete is the clinical management of this debilitating problem. Clearly the clinician's first responsibility is to eliminate any significant pathology and by so doing reassure the athlete. The pharmacological management of chronic diarrhoea in the athlete may employ antidiarrhoeal agents such as loperamide, or antispasmodics to reduce gastrointestinal motility and thereby enhance absorption. The common antispasmodics include agents from the anticholinergic group of drugs: as these drugs also inhibit sweating, their use must be balanced against an increased risk of heat intolerance. Non-pharmacological interventions include attention to adequate hydration before and during exercise, the avoidance of caffeine because of its diuretic and cathartic effects, and a low-residue meal taken several hours before running. Some authorities also favour the establishment of a predetermined daily ritual of bowel evacuation.

In summary, however, the management of exercise-induced lower gastrointestinal tract symptoms involves the established protocol of accurate history taking, physical examination, diagnosis by exclusion and the initial use of non-pharmacological agents. The use of simple antidiarrhoeal medication is widely accepted on an infrequent basis and must be in accordance with the permitted list of IOC substances.

## Conclusion

For the active athlete, the clinical consequences of disturbed gastrointestinal tract function may limit successful participation in athletic performance. Furthermore, while attention to fluid and carbohydrate ingestion is shown to enhance exercise performance, gastrointestinal dysfunction can significantly limit the assimilation of essential nutrients. An understanding of gastrointestinal function and the aetiology of gastrointestinal symptoms associated with exercise is necessary for the design of appropriate supplementation regimens. Athletes thereby benefit from maximum rates of delivery of nutrients with less risk of gastrointestinal distress.

## References

Ahlborg, G., Weitzberg, E., Sollevi, A. & Lundberg, J.M. (1992) Splanchnic and rental vasoconstrictor and metabolic responses to neuropeptide Y in resting and exercising man. *Acta Physiologica Scandinavica* **145**, 139–149.

Ahlborg, G., Weitzberg, E. & Lundberg, J. (1995) Metabolic and vascular effects of circulating endothelin-1 during moderately heavy prolonged exercise. *Journal of Applied Physiology* **78**, 2294–2300.

Barclay, G.R. & Turnberg, L.A. (1988) Effect of moderate exercise on salt and water transport in the human jejunum. *Gut* **29**, 816–820.

Baska, R.S., Moses, F.M. & Deuster, P.A. (1990) Cimetidine reduces running-associated gastrointestinal bleeding: a prospective observation. *Digestive Diseases and Sciences* **35**, 956–960.

Beaumont, W. (1838, rpt 1983) *Experiments and Observations on the Gastric Juice and the Physiology of Digestion.* Andrew Combe, Edinburgh.

Beltz, J.D. (1988) Effects of carbohydrate ingestion on gastric emptying and exercise performance. *Medicine and Science in Sports and Exercise* **20**, 110–115.

Bishop, J.M., Donald, K.W., Taylor, S.H. & Wormald, P.N. (1957) Changes in arterial-hepatic venous oxygen content difference during and after supine leg exercise. *Journal of Physiology* **137**, 309–317.

Brouns, F. (1991) Etiology of gastrointestinal disturbances during endurance events. *Scandinavian Journal of Medicine and Science in Sports* **1**, 66–77.

Brown, B.P., Ketelaar, M.A., Schulze-Delrieu, K., Abu-Yousef, M.M. & Brown, C.K. (1994) Strenuous exercise decreases motility and cross-sectional area of human gastric antrum: a study using ultrasound. *Digestive Diseases and Sciences* **39**, 940–945.

Brukner, P. & Khan, K. (1993) *Clinical Sports Medicine.* McGraw-Hill, Roseville, NSW.

Brunner, J., Barezat, G.O. & Häcki, W.H. (1991) Die magentleerung verschiedener oraler rehydrationslosungen gemessen mit dem ultraschall (Gastric emptying differences of oral rehydration solutions measured by ultrasound). *Schweizerische Medizinische Wochenschrift* **121**, 881–883.

Burns, G.P. & Schenk, W.G. (1969) Effect of digestion and exercise on intestinal blood flow and cardiac output. *Archives of Surgery* **98**, 790–794.

Campbell, J.M.H., Mitchell, M.D. & Powell, A.T.W. (1928) The influence of exercise on digestion. *Guy's Hospital Reports* **78**, 279–293.

Carrio, I., Estorch, M., Serra-Grima, R. *et al.* (1989) Gastric emptying in marathon runners. *Gut* **30**, 152–155.

Chaudhuri, K.R., Thomaides, T. & Mathias, C.J. (1992) Abnormality of superior mesenteric artery blood flow responses in human sympathetic failure. *Journal of Physiology* **457**, 477–489.

Clausen, J.P. (1977) Effect of physical training on cardiovascular adjustments to exercise in man. *Physiological Reviews* **57**, 779–815.

Cordain, L., Latin, R.W. & Behnke, M.S. (1986) The effects of an aerobic running program on bowel transit time. *Journal of Sports Medicine* **26**, 101–104.

Costill, D.L. (1990) Gastric emptying of fluids during exercise during exercise. In *Fluid Homeostasis during Exercise* (ed. C.V. Gisolfi & D.R. Lamb), pp. 97–127. Benchmark Press, Carmel, IN.

Costill, D.L. & Saltin, B. (1974) Factors limiting gastric emptying. *Journal of Applied Physiology* **37**, 679–683.

Crane, R.K. (1962) Hypothesis for mechanism of intestinal active transport of sugars. *Federation Proceedings* **21**, 891–895.

Curran, P.F. (1960) Na, Cl and water transport by rat ileum *in vitro. Journal of General Physiology* **43**, 1137–1148.

Dobbs, T.W., Atkins, M., Ratliff, R. & Eichner, E.R. (1988) Gastrointestinal bleeding in competitive cyclists. *Medicine and Science in Sports and Exercise* **20**, S178.

Fara, J.W. & Madden, K.S. (1975) Effect of secretin and cholecystokinin on small intestinal blood flow distribution. *American Journal of Physiology* **229**, 1365–1370.

Fogoros, R.N. (1980) 'Runners trots': gastrointestinal disturbances in runners. *Journal of the American Medical Association* **243**, 1743–1744.

Fordtran, J.S. (1975) Stimulation of active and passive

absorption by sugars in the human jejunum. *Journal of Clinical Investigation* **55**, 728–737.

Fordtran, J.S. & Saltin, B. (1967) Gastric emptying and intestinal absorption during prolonged severe exercise. *Journal of Applied Physiology* **23**, 331–335.

Foster, C. & Thompson, N.N. (1990) Serial gastric emptying studies: effect of preceding drinks. *Medicine and Science in Sports and Exercise* **22**, 484–487.

Fronek, K. & Fronek, A. (1970) Combined effect of exercise and digestion on hemodynamics in conscious dogs. *American Journal of Physiology* **218**, 555–559.

Gisolfi, C.V., Summers, R.W., Schedl, H.P., Bleiler, T.L. & Oppliger, R.A. (1990) Human intestinal water absorption: direct vs. indirect measurements. *American Journal of Physiology* **258**, G216–G222.

Green, G. (1992) Gastrointestinal disorders in the athlete. *Clinics in Sports Medicine* **11**, 453–470.

Heer, M., Repond, F., Hany, A. & Sulser, H. (1986) Hemorrhagic colitis, gastritis, hematuria and rhabdomyolysis: manifestations of multisystemic ischemia? *Schweizerische Rundschau für Medizin Praxis* **75**, 1538–1430.

Holdsworth, C.D. & Dawson, A.M. (1964) The absorption of mono saccharides in man. *Clinical Science* **27**, 371–379.

Houmard, J.A., Egan, P.C., Johns, R.A., Neufer, P.D., Chenierm, T.C. & Israel, R.G. (1991) Gastric emptying during 1 h of cycling and running at 75% $\dot{V}o_{2max}$. *Medicine and Science in Sports and Exercise* **23**, 320–325.

Iwao, T., Toyonaga, A., Ikegami, M. *et al.* (1995) Effects of exercise-induced sympathoadrenergic activation on portal blood flow. *Digestive Diseases and Sciences* **40**, 48–51.

Kenney, W.L. & Ho, C. (1995) Age alters regional distribution of blood flow during moderate-intensity exercise. *Journal of Applied Physiology* **79**, 1112–1119.

Koffler, K.H., Menkes, R.A., Redmond, R.A., Whitehead, W.E., Prattley, R.E. & Hurley, B.F. (1992) Strength training accelerates gastrointestinal transit in middle-aged and older men. *Medicine and Science in Sports and Exercise* **24**, 415–419.

Larson, D.C. & Fisher, R. (1987) Management of exercise-induced gastrointestinal problems. *The Physician and Sports Medicine* **15**, 112–126.

Leiper, J.B. & Maughan, R.J. (1988) Experimental models for the investigation of water and solute transport in man: implications for oral rehydration solutions. *Drugs* **36** (Suppl. 4), 65–79.

Liu, F., Kondo, T. & Toda, Y. (1993) Brief physical inactivity prolongs colonic transit time in elderly active men. *International Journal of Sports Medicine* **14**, 465–467.

McMahon, L.F., Ryan, M.J., Larson, D. & Fisher, R.L. (1984) Occult gastrointestinal blood loss associated with running a marathon. *Annals of Internal Medicine* **100**, 836–837.

Marzio, L., Formica, P., Fabiani, F., LaPenna, D., Vecchiett, L. & Cuccurullo, F. (1991) Influence of physical activity on gastric emptying of liquids in normal human subjects. *American Journal of Gastroenterology* **86**, 1433–1436.

Maughan, R.J. (1991) Fluid and electrolyte loss and replacement in exercise. *Journal of Sports Sciences* **9**, 117–142.

Maughan, R.J., Leiper, J.B. & McGaw, B.A. (1990) Effects of exercise intensity on absorption of ingested fluids in man. *Experimental Physiology* **75**, 419–421.

Mitchell, J.B. & Voss, K.W. (1991) The influence of volume on gastric emptying and fluid balance during prolonged exercise. *Medicine and Science in Sports and Exercise* **23**, 314–319.

Moore, J.G., Datz, F.L. & Christian, P.E. (1990) Exercise increase solid meal gastric emptying rates in men. *Digestive Diseases and Sciences* **35**, 428–432.

Moses, F.M. (1988) Running-associated proximal hemorrhagic colitis. *Annals of Internal Medicine* **108**, 385–386.

Moses, F.M. (1990) The effect of exercise on the gastrointestinal tract. *Sports Medicine* **9**, 159–172.

Moses, F.M. (1993) Gastrointestinal bleeding and the athlete. *American Journal of Gastroenterology* **88**, 1157–1159.

Moses, F., Singh, A., Smoak, B., Hollander, D. & Deuster, P. (1991) Alterations in intestinal permeability during prolonged high intensity running. *Gastroenterology* **100**, 472.

Murray, R. (1987) The effects of consuming carbohydrate-electrolyte beverages on gastric emptying and fluid absorption during and following exercise. *Sports Medicine* **5**, 322–351.

Neufer, P.D., Young, A.J. & Sawka, M.N. (1989a) Gastric emptying during exercise: effects of heat stress and hypohydration. *European Journal of Applied Physiology and Occupational Physiology* **58**, 433–439.

Neufer, P.D., Young, A.J. & Sawka, M.N. (1989b) Gastric emptying during walking and running: effects of varied exercise intensity. *European Journal of Applied Physiology and Occupational Physiology* **58**, 440–445.

Noakes, T.D. (1991) The importance of volume in regulating gastric emptying. *Medicine and Science in Sports and Exercise* **23**, 307–313.

Oktedalen, O., Lunde, O.C., Aabakken, P.K. & Kvernebo, K.K. (1992) Changes in the gastrointestinal mucosa after long-distance running. *Scandinavian Journal of Gastroenterology* **27**, 270–274.

Olivares, C.J. (1988) Toughest ironman ever. *Triathlete* **52**, 33–42.

Peters, H.P., Van Schelven, F.W., Verstappen, P.A., De Boer, R.W., Bol, E. & De Vries, W.R. (1993) Gastrointestinal problems as a function of carbohydrate supplements and mode of exercise. *Medicine and Science in Sports and Exercise* **25**, 1211–1224.

Peters, H.P., Akkermans, L.M., Bol, E. & Mosterd, W.L. (1995) Gastrointestinal symptoms during exercise. *Sports Medicine* **20**, 65–76.

Peters, O., Peters, P., Clarys, J.P., DeMeirleir, K. & Devis, G. (1988) Esophageal motility and exercise. *Gastroenterology* **94**, a351.

Porter, A.M.W. (1982) Marathon running and the cecal slap syndrome. *British Journal of Medicine* **16**, 178.

Porter, A.M.W. (1983) Do some marathon runners bleed into the gut? *British Journal of Medicine* **287**, 1427.

Pruett, T.L., Wilkins, M.E. & Gamble, W.G. (1985) Cecal volvulus: a different twist for the serious runner. *New England Journal of Medicine* **312**, 1262–1263.

Qamar, M.I. & Read, A.E. (1987) Effects of exercise on mesenteric blood flow in man. *Gut* **28**, 583–587.

Rehrer, N.J. & Maughan, R.J. (1991) The importance of volume in regulating gastric emptying. *Medicine and Science in Sports and Exercise* **23**, 314–319.

Rehrer, N.J. & Meijer, G.A. (1991) Biomechanical vibration of the abdominal region during running and bicycling. *Journal of Sports Medicine* **31**, 231–234.

Rehrer, N.J., Beckers, E., Brouns, F., ten Hoor, F. & Saris, W.H. (1989) Exercise and training effects on gastric emptying of carbohydrate beverages. *Medicine and Science in Sports and Exercise* **21**, 540–549.

Rehrer, N.J., Beckers, E.J., Brouns, F., ten Hoor, F. & Saris, W.H. (1990a) Effects of dehydration on gastric emptying and gastrointestinal distress while running. *Medicine and Science in Sports and Exercise* **22**, 790–795.

Rehrer, N.J., Brouns, F., Beckers, E.J., ten Hoor, F. & Saris, W.H. (1990b) Gastric emptying with repeated drinking during running and bicycling. *International Journal of Sports Medicine* **11**, 238–243.

Rehrer, N.J., Smets, A., Reynaert, H., Goes, E. & DeMeirleir, K. (1992a) Direct measurement of splanchnic blood flow during exercise in man. *Medicine and Science in Sports and Exercise* **24**, s165.

Rehrer, N.J., van Kemenade, M., Meester, W., Brouns, F. & Saris, W.H.M. (1992b) Gastrointestinal complaints in relation to dietary intake in triathletes. *International Journal of Sport Nutrition* **2**, 48–59.

Rehrer, N.J., Goes, E., DuGgardeyn, C., Reynaert, H. & DeMeirleir, K. (1993) Effects of carbohydrate and fluid ingestion on splanchnic blood flow at rest and during exercise. *Medicine and Science in Sports and Exercise* **25**, s84.

Rehrer, N.J., Brouns, F., Beckers, E.J. & Saris, W.H.M. (1994) The influence of beverage composition and gastrointestinal function on fluid and nutrient availability during exercise. *Scandinavian Journal of Medicine and Science in Sports* **4**, 159–172.

Riklis, E. & Quastel, J.H. (1958) Effects of cations on sugar absorption by isolated surviving guinea pig intestine. *Canadian Journal of Biochemistry and Physiology* **36**, 347–363.

Robertson, J.D., Maughan, R.J. & Davidson, R.J. (1987) Faecal blood loss in response to exercise. *British Journal of Medicine* **295**, 303–305.

Rowell, L.B., Blackmon, J.R. & Bruce, R.A. (1964) Indocyanine green clearance and estimated hepatic blood flow during mild to maximal exercise in upright man. *Journal of Clinical Investigation* **43**, 1677–1690.

Rudzki, S.J., Hazard, H. & Collinson, D. (1995) Gastrointestinal blood loss in triathletes: its etiology and relationship to sports anaemia. *Australian Journal of Science and Medicine in Sport* **27**, 3–8.

Ryan, A.J., Bleiler, T.L., Carter, J.E. & Gisolfi, C.V. (1989) Gastric emptying during prolonged cycling exercise in the heat. *Medicine and Science in Sports and Exercise* **21**, 51–58.

Ryan, A.J., Chang, R.T. & Gisolfi, C.V. (1996) Gastrointestinal permeability following aspirin intake and prolonged running. *Medicine and Science in Sports and Exercise* **28**, 698–705.

Schaub, N., Spichtin, H.P. & Stalder, G.A. (1985) Ischamische kolitis als ursche einer darmblutung bei marathonlauf? (Is ischaemic colitis responsible for intestinal bleeding during marathon running?) *Schweizerische Medizinische Wochenschrift* **115**, 454–457.

Schedl, H.P. & Clifton, J.A. (1963) Solute and water absorption by human small intestine. *Nature* **199**, 1264–1267.

Schoeman, M.N., Tippett, M.D., Akkermans, L.M., Dent, J. & Holloway, R.H. (1995) Mechanisms of gastroesophageal reflux in ambulant healthy human subjects. *Gastroenterology* **108**, 83–91.

Schwartz, A.E., Vanagunas, A. & Kamel, P.L. (1990) Endoscopy to evaluate gastrointestinal bleeding in marathon runners. *Annals of Internal Medicine* **113**, 632–633.

Scobie, B.A. (1985) Recurrent gut bleeding in five long-distance runners. *New Zealand Medical Journal* **98**, 966.

Seto, H., Kageyama, M., Nomura, K. *et al.* (1995) Whole body 201TI scintigraphy during one-leg exercise and at rest in normal subjects: estimation of regional blood flow changes. *Nuclear Medicine Communications* **16**, 661–666.

Soffer, E.E., Merchant, R.K., Duethman, G., Launspach, J., Gisolfi, C. & Adrian, T.E. (1993) Effect of graded exercise on esophageal motility and gastroesophageal reflux in trained athletes. *Digestive Diseases and Sciences* **38**, 220–224.

Soffer, E.E., Wilson, J., Duethman, G., Launspach, J. & Adrian, T.E. (1994) Effect of graded exercise on oesophageal motility and gastroesophageal reflux in nontrained subjects. *Digestive Diseases and Sciences* **39**, 193–198.

Sole, C.C. & Noakes, T.D. (1989) Faster gastric emptying for glucose-polymer and fructose solutions than for glucose in humans. *European Journal of Applied Physiology and Occupational Physiology* **58**, 605–612.

Stebbins, C.L. & Symons, J.D. (1995) Role of angiotensin II in hemodynamic responses to dynamic exercise in miniswine. *Journal of Applied Physiology* **78**, 185–190.

Stewart, J.G., Ahlquist, D.A., McGill, D.B., Ilstrup, D.M., Schwartz, S. & Owen, R.A. (1984) Gastrointestinal blood loss and anemia in runners. *Annals of Internal Medicine* **100**, 843–845.

Sullivan, S.N. (1994) Functional abdominal bloating. *Journal of Clinical Gastroenterology* **19**, 23–27.

Swain, R.A. (1994) Exercise-induced diarrhea: when to wonder. *Medicine and Science in Sports and Exercise* **26**, 523–526.

Thune, I. & Lund, E. (1996) Physical activity and risk of colorectal cancer in men and women. *British Journal of Cancer* **73**, 1134–1140.

Varr, V., Blah, G., Csernay, L., Jung, I. & Szarvas, F. (1965) Effect of decreased local circulation on the absorptive capacity of a small-intestine loop in the dog. *American Journal of Digestive Diseases* **10**, 2.

Vist, G.E. & Maughan, R.J. (1994) Gastric emptying of ingested solutions in man: effect of beverage glucose concentration. *Medicine and Science in Sports Exercise* **26**, 1269–1273.

Wade, O.L., Combes, B., Childs, A.W., Wheeler, H.O., Cournand, A. & Bradley, S.E. (1956) The effect of exercise on the splanchnic blood flow and splanchnic blood volume in normal man. *Clinical Science* **15**, 457–463.

Walker, R.J., Fawcett, J.P., Flannery, E.M. & Gerrard, D.F. (1994) Indomethacin potentiates exercise-induced reduction in renal hemodynamics in athletes. *Medicine and Science in Sports and Exercise* **26**, 1302–1306.

Worobetz, L.J. & Gerrard, D.F. (1985) Gastrointestinal symptoms during exercise in enduro athletes: prevalence and speculations on the aetiology. *New Zealand Medical Journal* **98**, 644–646.

Worobetz, L.J. & Gerrard, D.F. (1986) Effect of moderate exercise on esophageal function in asymptomatic athletes. *American Journal of Gastroenterology* **81**, 1048–1051.

Wright, J.P. (1991) Exercise and the gastro-intestinal tract. *South African Medical Journal* **83**, 50–52.

# Chapter 19

# Rehydration and Recovery after Exercise

SUSAN M. SHIRREFFS

## Introduction

Exercise can lead to a depletion of the body's glycogen stores, particularly those of the liver and in the exercising muscle, and to the development of a body water deficit. This chapter concerns itself with recovery after exercise: carbohydrate replacement during exercise is discussed in Chapter 8, and fluid replacement during exercise is described in detail in Chapter 17.

Glycogen depletion results from the mobilization of the stores to provide energy for the muscular contraction of the exercise, and is a major factor contributing to fatigue. This has been discussed in detail in Chapter 6. Depending on the intensity, frequency and duration of the exercise sessions, an almost complete emptying of the glycogen stores in the exercising muscle is possible.

Dehydration during exercise results largely from activation of the body's temperature-regulating mechanisms, and a state of hypohydration will be incurred if fluid is not ingested to match the seat loss. In an attempt to dissipate the heat produced due to the mechanical inefficiency of exercise, the sweating mechanism may be activated and the subsequent evaporation of the water secreted onto the skin surface removes with it latent heat of evaporation. This has been discussed in more detail in Chapters 15 and 17. Water loss from the respiratory tract, from the gastrointestinal tract and from urine production all will add to the body's water loss. Each of these routes may result in substantial water losses in some situations, but for most individuals and in most exercise situations, sweat production will be the greatest single factor responsible for creating a situation of hypohydration (Chapter 17). Sweat production, however, is not a situation of pure water being secreted onto the skin, but rather a variety of electrolytes and other substances are included in the sweat that is secreted. A general description of the composition of sweat with regard to its electrolyte content is given in Chapter 17.

## Effects of muscle glycogen depletion and hypohydration

### Muscle glycogen depletion

If exercise is undertaken when the muscles are depleted of their glycogen stores, performance will be poorer than when the muscle glycogen stores are optimal. This has been shown to be true for prolonged exercise of 1–2h duration (Costill *et al.* 1988), for high-intensity exercise lasting only a few minutes (Maughan & Poole 1981), and will also result in a reduction in the amount of running done by games players (Jacobs *et al.* 1982; Bangsbo 1994). In most of these situations, performance will be closely related to the size of the glycogen stores at the beginning of exercise. This has been discussed in detail in Chapters 5–8.

### Hypohydration

Exercise undertaken by individuals who begin exercise in a hypohydrated state has been shown to be impaired relative to that possible when fully hydrated at the beginning of exercise (see Chapter 16). However, in addition to these adverse effects on performance, hypohydration increases the likelihood of heat illness, and exercise in this state is only likely to accelerate and exacerbate these effects (Sutton 1990).

## Postexercise carbohydrate replacement

Many of the issues relating to carbohydrate replacement during exercise are relevant to carbohydrate replacement after exercise and a full discussion of this topic can be found in Chapter 8.

The primary aim of carbohydrate ingestion following exercise is to promote glycogen resynthesis and restoration of the muscle and liver glycogen utilized during exercise. This is of particular importance when a further bout of exercise is to be undertaken and therefore is of significance to all athletes in training and in competition where more than one game or round is involved. Several factors will influence the rate at which glycogen resynthesis occurs after exercise. The most important factor is undoubtedly the amount of carbohydrate consumed: the type of carbohydrate and the time of ingestion are less important, but also have an effect.

### Amount of carbohydrate to be ingested

The general pattern for glycogen synthesis after exercise is one of an increasing rate with increasing amount of carbohydrate consumed up to a certain rate of resynthesis after which there is no further increase with increasing quantities of carbohydrate ingestion. This has been demonstrated in studies where subjects were fed different amounts of glucose or maltodextrins every 2 h after exercise (Blom *et al.* 1987; Ivy *et al.* 1988a). The results showed that muscle glycogen synthe-

sis occurred at a rate of $2\,mmol\cdot kg^{-1}\cdot h^{-1}$ when 25 g of carbohydrate was ingested every 2 h, and that the replenishment rate increased to $6\,mmol\cdot kg^{-1}\cdot h^{-1}$ when 50 g was ingested every 2 h. However, muscle glycogen synthesis did increase to more than about $5-6\,mmol\cdot kg^{-1}\cdot h^{-1}$ even when very large amounts (up to 225 g) of carbohydrate were ingested every 2 h.

Further, with intravenous glucose infusion of 100 g every 2 h, a muscle glycogen synthesis of about $7-8\,mmol\cdot kg^{-1}\cdot h^{-1}$ has been reported (Reed *et al.* 1989). This is not significantly greater than the rates achieved with oral intake, and suggests that the failure to keep increasing glycogen synthesis with increasing carbohydrate consumption is not caused by a limitation in substrate availability imposed by the gastrointestinal tract. Also, increasing the amount of carbohydrate ingested will increase the rate of delivery to the intestine for absorption (see Chapter 18).

Therefore, it seems that the maximum rate of muscle glycogen synthesis after exercise is in the region of $5-8\,mmol\cdot kg^{-1}\cdot h^{-1}$, provided that at least 50 g of glucose is ingested every 2 h after exercise.

### Carbohydrate type and form of ingestion

Glucose and sucrose ingestion both give rise to similar glycogen synthesis rates when consumed after exercise. Fructose alone, however, seems only to be able to promote glycogen synthesis after exercise at a much lower rate of approximately $3\,mmol\cdot kg^{-1}\cdot h^{-1}$ (Jenkins *et al.* 1984; Blom *et al.* 1987). This is likely to be because of the relatively slow rate with which the liver converts fructose to blood glucose, and even when fructose is consumed in large amounts, the entry of glucose into the blood does not reach a rate of 50 g every 2 h. Although the use of fructose as a carbohydrate source is often promoted for athletes, it is poorly absorbed in the small intestine relative to many other sugars, and ingestion of large amounts is likely to result in diarrhoea (Maughan *et al.* 1989).

There is some evidence that carbohydrates

with a high glycaemic index—those carbohydrates which result in a large and sustained elevation of the blood glucose concentration after ingestion—are the most effective when rapid glycogen replacement is desired (Coyle 1991). However, the nature in which carbohydrates with a high or moderate glycaemic index are consumed after exercise (i.e. as a solid or liquid) appears to have no influence on glycogen synthesis rates (Keizer *et al.* 1986; Reed *et al.* 1989).

## Timing of carbohydrate intake

The muscle appears to have a particularly high affinity for carbohydrate immediately after exercise, and the greatest rate of muscle glycogen resynthesis occurs over the first 2 h immediately after exercise (i.e. 7–8 mmol·kg⁻¹·h⁻¹ vs. the rate after this time of 5–6 mmol·kg⁻¹·h⁻¹: Fig. 19.1) (Ivy *et al.* 1998b). This increased synthesis rate can only take place, however, if sufficient carbohydrate is ingested and is available to the body. Therefore, to optimize this transient increase in maximal glycogen resynthesis rate, carbohydrate should be consumed as soon as possible after exercise as this will allow the maximum

advantage to be taken by allowing the increased rate to be utilized for as long as possible. As a guide, it is suggested that approximately 0.7 g glucose·kg⁻¹ body mass should be consumed every 2 h for the first 4–6 h after exercise in order to maximize the rate of glycogen resynthesis (Keizer *et al.* 1986; Blom *et al.* 1987). It does not make any difference whether this carbohydrate to be consumed is ingested as a few large meals or as many small, frequent meals (Burke *et al.* 1996).

## Liver glycogen resynthesis

Liver glycogen restoration occurs less rapidly than muscle glycogen restoration and indeed, the fast repletion of muscle glycogen stores may be at the expense of liver glycogen levels (Fell *et al.* 1980). However, whereas fructose does not promote as rapid a muscle glycogen restoration as glucose, fructose infusion has been found to give a greater liver glycogen resynthesis than glucose (Nilsson & Hultman 1974). Some replenishment of the liver glycogen stores may be possible by gluconeogenesis, but this will not be sufficient to maintain carbohydrate homeostasis. After very high intensity exercise, however, such as multiple sprints in training, a substantial part of the muscle glycogen that has been converted to lactate by anaerobic glycolysis will be available as a substrate for hepatic gluconeogenesis.

## Postexercise fluid replacement

It has been pointed out elsewhere in this volume that the athlete who begins exercise in a state of hypohydration will be unable to achieve peak performance and will also be at increased risk of heat illness when the exercise is to be performed in a warm environment. Where substantial sweat losses have been incurred, it is therefore essential that restoration of fluid and electrolyte balance should be as rapid and complete as the circumstances allow. The opportunities for replacement may be limited, as when several rounds of a tournament are scheduled for a single day, or when the time allowed between the weigh-in and com-

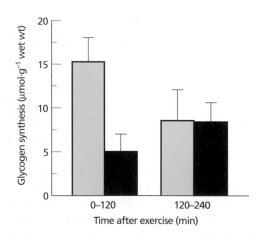

**Fig. 19.1** Muscle glycogen storage during the first 2 h and second 2 h of recovery from exercise. The subjects consumed 2 g glucose polymer·kg⁻¹ body mass (as a 23% solution) either immediately following exercise (☐) or 2 h after exercise (■). Adapted from Ivy *et al.* (1988b).

petition is short in weight category sports where sweating and fluid restriction have been used to achieve an artificially low body mass.

The primary factors influencing the postexercise rehydration process are the volume and composition of the fluid consumed. The volume consumed will be influenced by many factors, including the palatability of the drink and its effects on the thirst mechanism, and many different formulation options are open. The ingestion of solid food, and the composition of that food, will also be an important factor, but there are many situations where solid food is avoided between exercise sessions or immediately after exercise.

### Beverage composition

It is well established that plain water consumed after exercise is not the ideal rehydration beverage when rapid and complete restoration of fluid balance is necessary and where all intake is in liquid form. Costill and Sparks (1973) demonstrated that ingestion of plain water after exercise-induced dehydration caused a large fall in serum osmolality with a subsequent diuresis: the result of this stimulation of urinary water loss was a failure to achieve positive fluid balance by the end of the 4-h study period. However, when an electrolyte-containing solution ($106 g \cdot l^{-1}$ carbohydrate, $22 mmol \cdot l^{-1}$ Na+, $2.6 mmol \cdot l^{-1}$ K+, $17.2 mmol \cdot l^{-1}$ Cl-) was ingested after exercise which caused a loss of 4% of body mass, the urine output was less and net water balance was closer to the pre-exercise level. Nielsen et al. (1986) showed differences in the rate and extent of changes in the plasma volume with recovery from exercise-induced dehydration when different carbohydrate-electrolyte solutions were consumed: the plasma volume increase was greater after drinks with sodium as the only electrolyte (at concentrations of 43 and $128 mmol \cdot l^{-1}$) were consumed than when drinks containing additional potassium (at a concentration of $51 mmol \cdot l^{-1}$) or less electrolytes and more carbohydrate were consumed. González-Alonso et al. (1992) have also confirmed that a dilute carbohydrate-

electrolyte solution ($60 g \cdot l^{-1}$ carbohydrate, $20 mmol \cdot l^{-1}$ Na+, $3 mmol \cdot l^{-1}$ K+, $20 mmol \cdot l^{-1}$ Cl-) is more effective in promoting postexercise rehydration than either plain water or a low-electrolyte diet cola: the difference in rehydration effectiveness between the drinks was a result of differences in the volume of urine produced. In none of these studies, however, could the mechanism of the action be identified, as the drinks used were different from each other in a number of respects. They did, however, establish that, because of the high urine flow that ensued, even drinking large volumes of electrolyte-free drinks did not allow subjects to remain in positive fluid balance for more than a very short time. They also established that the plasma volume was better maintained when electrolytes were present in the fluid ingested, and it seemed likely that this effect was due primarily to the presence of sodium in the drinks.

The first studies to investigate the mechanisms that might be involved showed that the ingestion of large volumes of plain water after exercise-induced dehydration results in a rapid fall in plasma osmolality and in the plasma sodium concentration (Nose et al. 1988a, 1988b, 1988c), and both of these effects will stimulate urine output. In these studies, subjects exercised at low intensity in the heat for 90–110 min, inducing a mean level of dehydration equivalent to 2.3% of the pre-exercise body mass, and then rested for 1 h before beginning to drink. Plasma volume was not restored until after 60 min when plain water was ingested together with placebo (sucrose) capsules. In contrast, when sodium chloride capsules were ingested with water to give a saline solution with an effective concentration of 0.45% ($77 mmol \cdot l^{-1}$), restoration of plasma volume was complete within 20 min. In the NaCl trial, voluntary fluid intake was higher and urine output was less; 29% of the water intake was lost as urine within 3 h compared with 49% in the plain water trial. The delayed rehydration in the water trial was a result of a loss of water as urine caused by a rapid return to control levels of plasma renin activity and aldosterone levels.

Therefore, the addition of sodium to rehydration beverages can be justified on two accounts. Firstly, sodium stimulates glucose absorption in the small intestine (Olsen & Ingelfinger 1968): water absorption from the intestinal lumen is a purely passive process that is determined largely by local osmotic gradients (Parsons & Wingate 1961). The active cotransport of glucose and sodium creates an osmotic gradient that acts to promote net water absorption (Sladen 1972), and the rate of rehydration is therefore greater when glucose–sodium chloride solutions are consumed than when plain water is ingested. This was discussed in detail in Chapter 18. Secondly, replacement of sweat losses with plain water will, if the volume ingested is sufficiently large, lead to haemodilution: the fall in plasma osmolality and sodium concentration that occurs in this situation will reduce the drive to drink and will stimulate urine output (Nose *et al.* 1988b) and has potentially more serious consequences such as hyponatraemia (Noakes *et al.* 1985).

It has been proposed that drinks used for post-exercise rehydration should have a sodium concentration similar to that of sweat (Maughan 1991), but as the electrolyte content of sweat itself shows considerable variation between individuals and over time (see Chapter 17), it would seem impossible to prescribe a single formulation for every individual or every situation. However, a study to investigate the relation between whole-body sweat sodium losses and the rehydration effectiveness of beverages with different sodium concentrations seems to confirm that optimum rehydration is achieved with a drink with a sodium concentration similar to that of sweat (Shirreffs & Maughan 1997b).

Sodium is the major ion in the extracellular fluid but potassium is the major ion in the intracellular fluid (see Table 17.1). It has been suggested therefore that potassium may also be to some degree important in achieving rehydration by aiding the retention of water in the intracellular space. Yawata (1990) undertook experimental work on rats subjected to thermal dehydration of approximately 9% of body mass and then given free access to either tap water, a $150 \, mmol \cdot l^{-1}$

NaCl solution or a $154 \, mmol \cdot l^{-1}$ KCl solution. The results indicated that despite ingestion of a smaller volume of the KCl solution compared to the NaCl solution, there was a tendency for a greater restoration of the intracellular fluid space in the KCl group than in the NaCl group. Maughan *et al.* (1994) undertook a study in which men were dehydrated by approximately 2% of body mass by exercising in the heat, and then ingested a glucose beverage ($90 \, mmol \cdot l^{-1}$), a sodium-containing beverage (NaCl $60 \, mmol \cdot l^{-1}$), a potassium-containing beverage (KCl $25 \, mmol \cdot l^{-1}$) or a beverage consisting of the addition of all three. A smaller volume of urine was excreted following rehydration when the electrolyte-containing beverages were ingested than when the electrolyte-free beverage was consumed (Fig. 19.2). An estimated plasma volume decrease of 4.4% was observed with dehydration over all trials but the rate of recovery was slowest when the KCl beverage was consumed. Although there were differences in the total amount of electrolyte replaced as well as differences in the type of electrolytes present in the drinks, there was no difference in the fraction of ingested fluid retained 6h after finishing drinking the drinks which contained electrolytes. This may be because the beverage volume consumed was equivalent to the volume of sweat lost and subjects were dehydrated, because of the ongoing urine losses, throughout the entire study, even following the drinking period. The volumes of urine excreted were close to basal levels and significant further reductions in output may not have been possible when both sodium and potassium were ingested, over and above the reductions already induced when the sodium and potassium were ingested separately. The importance of potassium in enhancing rehydration by aiding intracellular rehydration over and above that with sodium seems therefore to be realistic but further investigation is required to provide conclusive evidence.

### Drink volume

Obligatory urine losses persist even in the dehy-

**Fig. 19.2** Cumulative urine output over time after rehydration. After exercise-induced dehydration by approximately 2% of body mass, different rehydration drinks in a volume equivalent to the sweat loss were consumed, and all the urine produced was collected. □, glucose 90 mmol·l⁻¹; △, KCl 25 mmol·l⁻¹; ○, NaCl 60 mmol·l⁻¹; ●, mixture of three drinks. See text for full explanation. Adapted from Maughan *et al.* (1994).

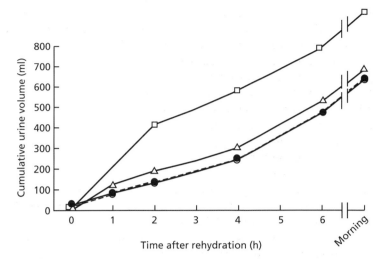

drated state, acting as a vehicle for the elimination of metabolic waste products. It is clear therefore that the total fluid intake after exercise-induced or thermal sweating must amount to a volume greater than the volume of sweat that has been lost if an effective rehydration is to be achieved. Shirreffs *et al.* (1996) investigated the influence of drink volume on rehydration effectiveness following exercise-induced dehydration equivalent to approximately 2% of body mass. Drink volumes equivalent to 50%, 100%, 150% and 200% of the sweat loss were consumed after exercise. To investigate the possible interaction between beverage volume and its sodium content, a relatively low sodium drink (23 mmol·l⁻¹) and a moderately high sodium drink (61 mmol·l⁻¹) were compared.

With both beverages, the urine volume produced was, not surprisingly, related to the beverage volume consumed; the smallest volumes were produced when 50% of the loss was consumed and the greatest when 200% of the loss was consumed. Subjects did not restore their hydration status when they consumed a volume equivalent to, or only half, their sweat loss irrespective of the drink composition. When a drink volume equal to 150% of the sweat loss was consumed, subjects were slightly hypohydrated 6 h after drinking when the test drink had a low sodium concentration, and they were in a similar

condition when they drank the same beverage in a volume of twice their sweat loss. With the high-sodium drink, enough fluid was retained to keep the subjects in a state of hyperhydration 6 h after drink ingestion when they consumed either 150% or 200% of their sweat loss. The excess would eventually be lost by urine production or by further sweat loss if the individual resumed exercise or moved to a warm environment. Calculated plasma volume changes indicated a decrease of approximately 5.3% with dehydration. At the end of the study period, the general pattern was for the increases in plasma volume to be a direct function of the volume of fluid consumed: additionally, the increase tended to be greater for those individuals who ingested the high sodium drink.

## Food and fluid consumption

In some situations, there may be opportunities to consume solid food between exercise bouts, and in most situations it should be encouraged unless it is likely to result in gastrointestinal disturbances. In a study to investigate the role of food intake in promoting rehydration from a hypohydration of approximately 2% of body mass, induced by exercising in the heat, a solid meal plus flavoured water or a commercially available sports drink were consumed (Maughan *et al.*

**Table 19.1** Fluid consumed, quantities of major electrolytes ingested and volume of urine produced. Values in brackets are mean (SEM) or median (range) as appropriate.

|  | Meal + water | Sports drink |
|---|---|---|
| Fluid volume (ml) | 2076 (131) | 2042 (132) |
| Electrolytes ingested (mmol) |  |  |
| Na+ | 63 (4) | 43 (3) |
| K+ | 21 (1) | 7 (1) |
| 6 h urine volume (ml) | 665 (396–1190) | 934 (550–1403) |

1996). The volume of fluid contained within the meal plus water was the same as the volume of sports drink consumed, but the volume of urine produced following food and water ingestion was less than that when the sports drink was consumed (Table 19.1). Although the amount of water consumed with both rehydration methods was the same, the meal had a greater sodium and potassium content and it seems most likely that the greater efficacy of the meal plus water treatment in restoring whole body water balance was a consequence of the greater total cation content.

### Alcohol consumption

Because of the well-known diuretic properties of alcohol and caffeine, it is usual to advise against the consumption of drinks containing these substances when fluid replacement is a priority. However, many people enjoy consuming these beverages, and where large volumes of fluid must be consumed in a relatively short time, a wide choice of drinks will help to stimulate consumption. In many sports, particularly team sports, alcohol intake is a part of the culture of the sport, and athletes are resistant to suggestions that they should abstain completely (see Chapter 30). However, it is now apparent that the diuretic effect expected from alcohol, over and above an alcohol-free beverage having otherwise the same composition, is blunted when consumed by individuals who are moderately hypohydrated from exercise in a warm environment (Shirreffs & Maughan 1997a).

After exercise, subjects consumed beer shandy

(a peculiarly British drink produced by mixing beer with lemonade) containing 0%, 1%, 2% or 4% alcohol. The volume of urine excreted for the 6 h following drink ingestion was related to the quantity of alcohol consumed, but despite a tendency for the urinary output to increase with increasing alcohol intake, only with the 4% beverage did the increased value approach significance. The calculated decrease in plasma volume with dehydration was approximately 7.6% across all trials. With rehydration, the plasma volume increased, but the rate of increase seemed to be related to the quantity of alcohol consumed; 6 h after finishing drinking, the increase in plasma volume relative to the dehydrated value was approximately 8% with 0% alcohol, 7% with 1%, 6% with 2% and 5% with 4%. It may be worth noting that the high sugar content of lemonade (10%) means that beer shandy has a carbohydrate content of about 5%, and this carbohydrate may play an important role in the restoration of muscle and liver glycogen stores after exercise.

### Voluntary fluid intake

The information from the work described above was obtained from studies in which a fixed volume of fluid was consumed. In practice, however, intake will be determined by the interaction of physiological and psychological factors. A second consequence of ingestion of plain water is to remove the drive to drink by causing plasma osmolality and sodium concentration to fall (Nose et al. 1988b). Where a fixed volume of fluid is given, this is not important, but it will tend to prevent complete rehydration when fluid intake is on a volitional basis (Maughan & Leiper 1993).

## Conclusion

Complete restoration of fluid balance after exercise is an important part of the recovery process, and becomes even more important in hot, humid conditions. If a second bout of exercise has to be performed after a relatively short interval, the speed of rehydration accomplishment becomes of crucial importance. Rehydration after exercise requires not only replacement of volume losses, but also replacement of the electrolytes, primarily sodium, lost in the sweat. The electrolyte composition of sweat is highly variable between individuals and although the optimum drink may be achieved by matching electrolyte loss with equal quantities from the drink, this is virtually impossible in a practical situation. Sweat composition not only varies between individuals, but also varies with time during exercise and is further influenced by the state of acclimation (Taylor 1986). Typical values for sodium and potassium concentrations are about $50\,mmol \cdot l^{-1}$ and $5\,mmol \cdot l^{-1}$, respectively. Drinks intended specifically for rehydration should therefore probably have higher electrolyte content than drinks formulated for consumption during exercise, especially where opportunities for ingestion of solid food are restricted.

Where sweat losses are large, the total sodium loss will be high: $10\,l$ of sweat at a sodium concentration of $50\,mmol \cdot l^{-1}$ amounts to about $29\,g$ of sodium chloride. However, a moderate excess of salt intake would appear to be beneficial as far as hydration status is concerned without any detrimental effects on health provided that fluid intake is in excess of sweat loss and that renal function is not impaired.

The Oral Rehydration Solution recommended by the World Health Organization for the treatment of acute diarrhoea has a sodium content of $60–90\,mmol \cdot l^{-1}$ (Farthing 1994), reflecting the high sodium losses which may occur in some types of diarrhoea. In contrast, the sodium content of most sports drinks is in the range of $10–30\,mmol \cdot l^{-1}$ (see Table 17.2) and in some cases is even lower. Most commonly consumed soft drinks contain virtually no sodium and these drinks are therefore unsuitable when the need for rehydration is crucial. The problem with a high sodium concentration in drinks is that some people find the taste undesirable, resulting in reduced consumption. However, drinks with a low sodium content are ineffective at rehydration, and they will also reduce the stimulus to drink.

Addition of an energy source is not necessary for rehydration, although a small amount of carbohydrate may improve the rate of intestinal uptake of sodium and water, and will improve palatability. Where sweat losses are high, rehydration with carbohydrate solutions has implications for energy balance: $10\,l$ of soft drinks will provide approximately $1000\,g$ of carbohydrate, equivalent to about $16.8\,MJ$ (4000 kcal). The volume of beverage consumed should be greater than the volume of sweat lost in order to make a provision for the ongoing obligatory urine losses, and palatability of the beverage is a major issue when large volumes of fluid have to be consumed.

Although water alone is adequate for rehydration, when food is also consumed this replaces the electrolytes lost in sweat. However, there are many situations where intake of solid food is avoided. This is particularly true in weight category sports where the interval between the weigh-in and competition is short, but is also the case in events where only a few hours intervene between succeeding rounds of the competition. It is in these situations that electrolytes must be present in the drinks consumed.

If a body water deficit is incurred during exercise, it is important that this is rectified in the postexercise period if a decrement in performance during a subsequent exercise bout is to be avoided. If no further exercise is planned, there may be no urgency for fluid replacement and the water will generally be replaced over the following day or so by a combination of eating and drinking. If, however, a second bout of exercise is to be undertaken and a decrement in performance is to be avoided, the water lost must be replaced as completely as possible before the exercise commences and further sweat production occurs.

## Prioritizing rehydration and recovery after exercise: carbohydrate vs. water replacement

Drinks consumed during or after exercise are generally intended to replace the water and electrolyte losses incurred as a result of sweat secretion, and also to provide carbohydrate to supplement or replenish the glycogen stores in the liver and the working muscles. The relative importance of providing water or substrate is influenced by many factors. However, disturbances in body fluid balance and temperature not only can impair exercise performance but are potentially life-threatening (Åstrand & Rodahl 1986). In comparison, the depletion of carbohydrate stores in the liver and working muscles will result in fatigue and a reduction in exercise intensity, but on the whole presents no great risk to health. Therefore, except in situations where depletion of body water has not occurred, the first aim of postexercise recovery should be to restore any fluid deficit incurred, followed by repletion of liver and muscle glycogen stores.

It must, of course, be recognized that these aims need not be mutually exclusive. Selection of suitable food and drinks should provide both the carbohydrate necessary for optimization of muscle and liver glycogen resynthesis and the water and electrolytes necessary for replacement of sweat losses and restoration of fluid balance.

## References

Åstrand, P.-O. & Rodahl, K. (1986) *Textbook of Work Physiology: Physiological Bases of Exercise*, 3rd edn. McGraw-Hill, Singapore.

Bangsbo, J. (1994) Physiological demands. In *Football* (ed. B. Ekblom), pp. 43–58. Blackwell Scientific Publications, Oxford.

Blom, P.C.S., Høstmark, A.T., Vaage, O., Kardel, K.R. & Mæhlum, S. (1987) Effect of different post-exercise sugar diets on the rate of muscle glycogen synthesis. *Medicine and Science in Sports and Exercise* **19**, 491–496.

Burke, L.M., Collier, G.R., Davis, P.G., Fricker, P.A., Sanigorski, A.J. & Hargreaves, M. (1996) Muscle glycogen storage after prolonged exercise: effect of the frequency of carbohydrate feedings. *American Journal of Clinical Nutrition* **64**, 115–119.

Costill, D.L. & Sparks, K.E. (1973) Rapid fluid replacement following thermal dehydration. *Journal of Applied Physiology* **34**, 299–303.

Costill, D.L., Sherman, W.M., Fink, W.J., Maresh, C., Witten, M. & Miller, J.M. (1988) Effects of repeated days of intensified training on muscle glycogen and swimming performance. *Medicine and Science in Sports and Exercise* **20**, 249–254.

Coyle, E.F. (1991) Timing and method of increased carbohydrate intake to cope with heavy training, competition and recovery. *Journal of Sports Science* **9** (Special Issue), 29–52.

Farthing, M.J.G. (1994) Oral rehydration therapy. *Pharmacological Therapeutics* **64**, 477–492.

Fell, R.D., McLane, J.A., Winder, W.W. & Holloszy, J.O. (1980) Preferential resynthesis of muscle glycogen in fasting rats after exhaustive exercise. *American Journal of Physiology* **238**, R328–R332.

González-Alonso, J., Heaps, C.L. & Coyle, E.F. (1992) Rehydration after exercise with common beverages and water. *International Journal of Sports Medicine* **13**, 399–406.

Ivy, J.L., Lee, M.C., Brozinick, J.T. & Reed, M.J. (1988a) Muscle glycogen storage after different amounts of carbohydrate ingestion. *Journal of Applied Physiology* **65**, 2018–2023.

Ivy, J.L., Katz, A.L., Cutler, C.L., Sherman, W.M. & Coyle, E.F. (1988b) Muscle glycogen synthesis after exercise: effect of time of carbohydrate ingestion. *Journal of Applied Physiology* **64**, 1480–1485.

Jacobs, I., Westlin, N., Karlsson, J., Rasmusson, M. & Houghton, B. (1982) Muscle glycogen and diet in elite soccer players. *European Journal of Applied Physiology* **48**, 297–302.

Jenkins, D.J.A., Wolever, T.M.S., Jenkins, A.L., Josse, R.G. & Wong, G.S. (1984) The glycaemic response to carbohydrate foods. *Lancet* **18**, 388–391.

Keizer, H.A., Kuipers, H., van Kranenburg, G. & Geurten, P. (1986) Influence of liquid and solid meals on muscle glycogen resynthesis, plasma fuel hormone response, and maximal physical working capacity. *International Journal of Sports Medicine* **8**, 99–104.

Maughan, R.J. (1991) Carbohydrate-electrolyte solutions during prolonged exercise. In *Perspectives in Exercise Science and Sports Science*. Vol. 4. *Ergogenics: The Enhancement of Sport Performance* (ed. D.R. Lamb

& M.H. Williams), pp. 35–85. Benchmark Press, Carmel, CA.

Maughan, R.J. & Leiper, J.B. (1993) Post-exercise rehydration in man: effects of voluntary intake of four different beverages. *Medicine and Science in Sports and Exercise* 25 (Suppl.), S2.

Maughan, R.J. & Poole, D.C. (1981) The effects of a glycogen loading regimen on the capacity to perform anaerobic exercise. *European Journal of Applied Physiology* 46, 211–219.

Maughan, R.J., Fenn, C.E. & Leiper, J.B. (1989) Effects of fluid, electrolyte and substrate ingestion on endurance capacity. *European Journal of Applied Physiology* 58, 481–486.

Maughan, R.J., Owen, J.H., Shirreffs, S.M. & Leiper, J.B. (1994) Post-exercise rehydration in man: effects of electrolyte addition to ingested fluids. *European Journal of Applied Physiology* 69, 209–215.

Maughan, R.J., Leiper, J.B. & Shirreffs, S.M. (1996) Restoration of fluid balance after exercise-induced dehydration: effects of food and fluid intake. *European Journal of Applied Physiology* 73, 317–325.

Nielsen, B., Sjogaard, G., Ugelvig, J., Knudsen, B. & Dohlmann, B. (1986) Fluid balance in exercise dehydration and rehydration with different glucose-electrolyte drinks. *European Journal of Applied Physiology* 55, 318–325.

Nilsson, L.H. & Hultman, E. (1974) Liver and muscle glycogen in man after glucose and fructose infusion. *Scandinavian Journal of Clinical and Laboratory Investigation* 33, 5–10.

Noakes, T.D., Goodwin, N., Rayner, B.L., Branken, T. & Taylor, R.K.N. (1985) Water intoxication: a possible complication during endurance exercise. *Medicine and Science in Sports and Exercise* 17, 370–375.

Nose, H., Mack, G.W., Shi, X. & Nadel, E.R. (1988a) Shift in body fluid compartments after dehydration in humans. *Journal of Applied Physiology* 65, 318–324.

Nose, H., Mack, G.W., Shi, X. & Nadel, E.R. (1988b) Role of osmolality and plasma volume during rehydration in humans. *Journal of Applied Physiology* 65, 325–331.

Nose, H., Mack, G.W., Shi, X. & Nadel, E.R. (1988c) Involvement of sodium retention hormones during rehydration in humans. *Journal of Applied Physiology* 65, 332–336.

Olsen, W.A. & Ingelfinger, F.J. (1968) The role of sodium in intestinal glucose absorption in man. *Journal of Clinical Investigation* 47, 1133–1142.

Parsons, D.S. & Wingate, D.L. (1961) The effect of osmotic gradients on fluid transfer across rat intestine *in vitro*. *Biochemica Biophysica Acta* 46, 170–183.

Reed, M.J., Brozlnick, J.T. Jr, Lee, M.C. & Ivy, J.L. (1989) Muscle glycogen storage post exercise: effect on mode of carbohydrate administration. *Journal of Applied Physiology* 66, 720–726.

Shirreffs, S.M. & Maughan, R.J. (1997a) Restoration of fluid balance after exercise-induced dehydration: effects of alcohol consumption. *Journal of Applied Physiology* 83, 1152–1158.

Shirreffs, S.M. & Maughan, R.J. (1997b) Whole body sweat collection in humans: an improved method with preliminary data on electrolyte content. *Journal of Applied Physiology* 82, 336–341.

Shirreffs, S.M., Taylor, A.J., Leiper, J.B. & Maughan, R.J. (1996) Post-exercise rehydration in man: effects of volume consumed and drink sodium content. *Medicine and Science in Sports and Exercise* 28, 1260–1271.

Sladen, G.E.G. (1972) A review of water and electrolyte absorption in man. In *Transport across the Intestine* (ed. W.L. Burland & P.K. Sammuel), pp. 14–34. Churchill Livingstone, London.

Sutton, J.R. (1990) Clinical implications of fluid imbalance. In *Perspectives in Exercise Science and Sports Science. Vol. 3. Fluid Homeostasis during Exercise* (ed. C.V. Gisolfi & D.R. Lamb), pp. 425–448. Benchmark Press, Carmel, CA.

Taylor, N.A.S. (1986) Eccrine sweat glands. Adaptations to physical training and heat acclimation. *Sports Medicine* 3, 387–397.

Yawata, T. (1990) Effect of potassium solution on rehydration in rats: comparison with sodium solution and water. *Japanese Journal of Physiology* 40, 369–381.

# Chapter 20

# Vitamins: Metabolic Functions

MIKAEL FOGELHOLM

## Introduction

### Vitamins in sports

Vitamin supplements, including especially vitamin C, but also the B-complex vitamins and vitamin E, are frequently used by athletes (Sobal & Marquart 1994). The common motivation for vitamin supplementation is to improve sports performance and enhance recovery (Williams 1986). Reversing the view, many athletes and coaches fear that a normal diet will eventually lead to marginal vitamin supply and to a deterioration in sports performance.

As regards vitamins and optimal physical performance, there are two questions with substantial practical importance. First, if vitamin supply is marginal, would an athlete's functional capacity be less than optimal? Second, if vitamins are given in excess of daily needs, would this improve functional capacity? This chapter reviews the basic metabolic functions of different vitamins (Table 20.1) and aims at giving answers to the two above-mentioned questions. The vitamin requirements of physically active people are reviewed in Chapter 21, and antioxidant functions in Chapter 22.

### What are vitamins?

Vitamins are organic compounds required in very small amounts (from a few micrograms to a few milligrams on a daily basis) to prevent development of clinical deficiency and deterioration in

health, growth and reproduction (McCormick 1986). A distinct feature of vitamins is that the human body is not able to synthesize them. Classification of vitamins is based on their relative solubility (McCormick 1986): fat-soluble vitamins (A, D, E and K) are more soluble in organic solvents, and water-soluble vitamins (B-complex and C) in water.

Ubiquinone and 'vitamin $B_{15}$' are examples of compounds announced as 'vitamins' and as ergogenic substances for athletes. Ubiquinone, an electron carrier in the mitochondrial respiratory chain, is indeed needed for normal body function and health, and it is found in a Western mixed diet (Greenberg & Frishman 1988). Nevertheless, because the body can synthesize ubiquinone, the name 'vitamin Q' is misleading and should not be used.

'Vitamin $B_{15}$', in contrast to ubiquinone, cannot be synthesized by the human body. However, it is not a vitamin, because there are no specific diseases or signs associated with depletion. In fact, 'vitamin $B_{15}$' in products with ergogenic claims does not even have a well-defined chemical identity (Williams 1986). There is no evidence that supplementation with ubiquinone or 'vitamin $B_{15}$' would increase athletic performance (Williams 1986; Laaksonen *et al.* 1995).

### Vitamin supply and functional capacity

Adequate nutritional status means a sufficiency of the host nutriture to permit cells, tissues,

266

**Table 20.1** Summary of the most important effects of vitamins on body functions related to athletic performance.

| | Cofactors for energy metabolism | Nervous function | Haemoglobin synthesis | Immune function | Antioxidant function | Bone metabolism |
|---|---|---|---|---|---|---|
| Water-soluble vitamins | | | | | | |
| Thiamin | X | X | | | | |
| Riboflavin | X | X | (X) | | | |
| Vitamin B$_6$ | X | X | X | X | | |
| Folic acid | | X | X | | | |
| Vitamin B$_{12}$ | | X | X | | | |
| Niacin | X | X | | | | |
| Pantothenic acid | X | | | | | |
| Biotin | X | | | | | |
| Vitamin C | | | (X) | X | X | |
| Fat-soluble vitamins | | | | | | |
| Vitamin A | | | | X | X | |
| Vitamin D | | | | | | X |
| Vitamin E | | | | X | X | |

organs, anatomical systems or the host him/herself to perform optimally the intentioned, nutrient-dependent function (Solomons & Allen 1983). Vitamins—like all micronutrients—are needed directly or indirectly (because of activity on structural integrity) for innumerable functions. Metabolic functions may be viewed from an isolated, molecular viewpoint (i.e. a single biochemical reaction in a single metabolic pathway), or from a perspective of the entire human body.

The metabolic functions of vitamins required in sports are mainly those needed for production of energy and for neuromuscular functions (skills). Physical performance involve several metabolic pathways, all including several biochemical reactions. The relation between vitamin supply and functional capacity is S-shaped or 'bell-shaped', depending on whether the examination is extended to megadoses (Fig. 20.1) (Brubacher 1989). The core in the above relation is that the output (functional capacity) is not improved after the 'minimal requirement for maximal output' is reached (Brubacher 1989).

In contrast, overvitaminosis may in some cases reduce the output below the maximal level.

Different body functions (single biochemical reactions, metabolic pathways, function of anatomical systems, and function of the host him/herself) reach their maximal output at different levels of supply. In other words, the supply needed for optimal function of an anatomical system (e.g. the muscle) may be quite different from the supply needed to maximize the activity of a single enzyme (Solomons & Allen 1983).

Short-term inadequacy of vitamin intake is characterized by lowering of vitamin concentrations in different tissues and lowering of certain enzyme activities (Fig. 20.2) (Piertzik 1986). However, functional disturbances (such as decreased physical performance capacity) appear later (Solomons & Allen 1983; Fogelholm 1995). In the opposite case, very large vitamin intakes increase the body pool and activity of some enzymes, but do not necessarily improve functional capacity (Fogelholm 1995).

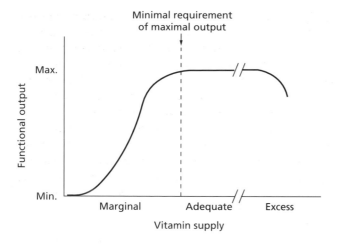

**Fig. 20.1** The association between vitamin supply and functional output.

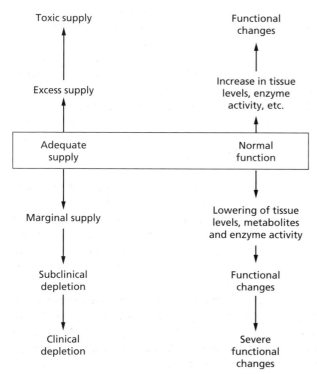

**Fig. 20.2** Dietary micronutrient intake and stages of nutritional status. Adapted from Solomons and Allen (1983), Piertzik (1986) and Brubacher (1989).

## Water-soluble vitamins and functional capacity

### Thiamin

CHEMISTRY AND
BIOCHEMICAL FUNCTIONS

Thiamin or vitamin $B_1$, the former being the accepted chemical name, consists of a pyrimidine ring joined to a thiazole ring (Halsted 1993). The principal, if not sole, cofactor form of thiamin (vitamin $B_1$) is thiaminpyrophosphate (TPP) (McCormick 1986). TPP is needed as a cofactor in muscle metabolism and in the central nervous system. Body stores are small, about 30 mg, almost half of which is stored in the muscles (Johnson Gubler 1984).

Two important enzyme complexes of glycolysis and the citric acid cycle require TPP as a cofactor, namely, pyruvate dehydrogenase (formation of acetyl-coenzyme A from pyruvate) and α-ketoglutarate dehydrogenase (formation of succinyl-coenzyme A from α-ketoglutarate) (Johnson Gubler 1984). If the decarboxylation of pyruvate is inadequate to match the increased speed of glycolysis, pyruvate will accumulate in the tissue (Sauberlich 1967). The accumulation of pyruvate will eventually lead to increased lactic acid production (Johnson Gubler 1984), which is lowered after thiamin supplementation (Sauberlich 1967). By interfering with the citric acid cycle, improper function of α-ketoglutarate dehydrogenase would affect aerobic energy production, and through feedback reactions, also the overall rate of glycolysis.

Although the muscle tissue contains more than 40% of the total body thiamin, the vitamin concentration is much higher in the liver, kidney and brain (Johnson Gubler 1984). Also, the nerves contain a constant and significant amount of TPP (Johnson Gubler 1984), and thiamin is indeed very important for the function of the brain and the nervous system (McCormick 1986; Halsted 1993).

In addition to the two above-mentioned enzyme complexes, thiamin is also needed in the pentose phosphate pathway (PPP) as a cofactor for transketolase (Johnson Gubler 1984). PPP is important for production of pentoses for RNA and DNA synthesis, and nicotinamide adenine dinucleotide phosphate (NADPH) for biosynthesis of fatty acids. The role of PPP in energy production is minor (Johnson Gubler 1984). However, the interesting feature about transketolase is that the activity of erythrocyte transketolase, with and without *in vitro* added TPP, is widely used as an indicator of thiamin status (Bayomi & Rosalki 1976). Several papers have been published on erythrocyte transketolase activity in athletes (for a review, see Fogelholm 1995).

## SUPPLY AND METABOLIC FUNCTIONS

In subclinical thiamin deficiency, the exercise-induced blood lactate concentrations are elevated, especially after a pre-exercise glucose load (Sauberlich 1967). The deterioration of physical capacity in marginal deficiency is less evident. Wood *et al.* (1980) did not find decreased working capacity, neurophysiological changes or adverse psychological reactions in male students, despite a 5-week thiamin-depleted diet. However, the erythrocyte transketolase activity decreased, showing that the activity of this enzyme is affected faster than the activity of the enzymes of glycolysis and the citric acid cycle.

A combined depletion of thiamin, riboflavin, vitamin $B_6$ and ascorbic acid has been found to affect both erythrocyte transketolase activity and aerobic working capacity (van der Beek *et al.* 1988). However, because of the multiple depletion, the independent role of thiamin could not be demonstrated. The uncertainty of the independent role of thiamin was a concern also in studies showing improved shooting accuracy (Bonke & Nickel 1989) or neuromuscular irritability (van Dam 1978) after combined thiamin, riboflavin, vitamin $B_6$ or vitamin $B_{12}$ supplementation.

A 1–3-month vitamin B-complex supplementation ($>7.5 \, mg \cdot day^{-1}$) usually improves the activity of erythrocyte transketolase (van Dam 1978; Guilland *et al.* 1989; Fogelholm *et al.* 1993b). Nevertheless, despite improved erythrocyte transketolase activity or increased blood thiamin concentration, several studies have shown that vitamin supplementation did not improve functional capacity in athletes (Telford *et al.* 1992a, 1992b), young adults (Singh *et al.* 1992a, 1992b; Fogelholm *et al.* 1993b) or in elderly subjects (Suboticanec *et al.* 1989).

## SAFETY OF ELEVATED THIAMIN INTAKE

Adverse reactions of chronic, elevated oral administration of thiamin are virtually unknown (Marks 1989). Hypersensitivity reactions may sometimes occur after very high oral loads (5–10 g), or following much lower doses (5–10 mg) by parenteral administration (Marks 1989). For chronic oral use, the safe dose is at least 50–100 times the recommended daily intake; that is, above 100 mg daily.

## Riboflavin

### CHEMISTRY AND BIOCHEMICAL FUNCTIONS

Riboflavin (correct chemical name) or vitamin $B_2$ is composed of an isoalloxazine ring linked to a ribityl side chain (Halsted 1993). Modification of the side chain yields flavin mononucleotide (FMN). When linked to adenine monophosphate, FMN forms flavin adenine dinucleotide (FAD). FMN and FAD function as coenzymes in numerous oxidation-reduction reactions in glycolysis and the respiratory chain (Cooperman & Lopez 1984). Enzymes requiring FAD are, e.g. pyruvate dehydrogenase complex (glycolysis), $\alpha$-ketoglutarate dehydrogenase complex and succinate dehydrogenase (citric acid cycle). FAD is also needed in fatty acid oxidation, whereas FMN is necessary for the synthesis of fatty acids from acetate (Cooperman & Lopez 1984).

Riboflavin has also indirect effects on body functions by affecting iron utilization (Fairweather-Tait et al. 1992). The mechanism is still unknown in humans, but some results indicate that correction of riboflavin deficiency also raises low blood haemoglobin concentrations (Cooperman & Lopez 1984; Fairweather-Tait et al. 1992). Severe riboflavin deficiency can also affect the status of other B-complex vitamins, mainly by decreased conversion of vitamin $B_6$ to its active coenzyme and of tryptophan to niacin (Cooperman & Lopez 1984).

Like thiamin, the activity of an enzyme isolated from the erythrocytes is widely used as an indicator of riboflavin status (Bayomi & Rosalki 1976; Cooperman & Lopez 1984). The enzyme, glutathione reductase, catalyses the reduction of oxidized glutathione with simultaneous oxidation of NADPH. The enzyme activity *in vitro* is related to activity after saturation by FAD. The better the vitamin status, the smaller the increase in activity after added FAD (Bayomi & Rosalki 1976).

### SUPPLY AND METABOLIC FUNCTIONS

Changes in riboflavin supply have been postulated to affect both muscle metabolism and neuromuscular function. Data on the effects of marginal riboflavin supply are, however, scarce. In three studies (Belko et al. 1984, 1985; Trebler Winters et al. 1992), a 4–5-week period with marginal riboflavin intake resulted in lowering of the erythrocyte glutathione reductase activity, but no relation with aerobic capacity was found. Similarly, Soares et al. (1993) did not find changes in muscular efficiency during moderate-intensity exercise after a 7-week period of riboflavin-restricted diet.

In contrast to the above studies, van der Beek et al. (1988) reported impaired maximal oxygen uptake and increased blood lactate appearance after a 10-week period with marginal thiamin, riboflavin and vitamin $B_6$ intake. The independent role of riboflavin was, however, uncertain.

Decreased urinary riboflavin excretion might be one mechanism in preventing changes in riboflavin-dependent body functions during marginal depletion (Belko et al. 1984, 1985; Soares et al. 1993). More severe riboflavin deficiency is obviously likely to affect both maximal and submaximal aerobic work capacity, as well as neuromuscular function (Cooperman & Lopez 1984).

A 1–3-month vitamin B-complex supplementation improves the activity of erythrocyte glutathione reductase (van Dam 1978; Weight et al. 1988b; Guilland et al. 1989; Fogelholm et al. 1993b) in athletes or trained students, even without indications of impaired vitamin status (Weight et al. 1988b). Two studies have suggested that supplementation and improvement in riboflavin status (judged by changes in erythrocyte glutathione reductase activity) were related to improved neuromuscular function (Haralambie 1976; Bamji et al. 1982).

Riboflavin supplementation, in combination with one or more water-soluble vitamins, has been shown to affect both erythrocyte enzyme activity and maximal oxygen uptake (Buzina et al. 1982; Suboticanec-Buzina et al. 1984) or work efficiency (Powers et al. 1985) in children with known nutritional deficiencies. In contrast, several other studies did not find an association between increased erythrocyte glutathione reductase activity and maximal oxygen uptake (Suboticanec-Buzina *et al.* 1984; Weight *et al.* 1988a, 1988b; Suboticanec *et al.* 1990; Singh *et al.* 1992a, 1992b), exercise-induced lactate appearance in the blood (Weight *et al.* 1988a, 1988b; Fogelholm *et al.* 1993b), work efficiency (Powers *et al.* 1987) or grip strength (Suboticanec *et al.* 1989).

## SAFETY OF ELEVATED RIBOFLAVIN INTAKE

As with thiamin, there is no evidence of any harmful effects even with oral doses exceeding 100 times the recommended daily intake (Marks 1989). Riboflavin in large doses may cause a yellow discoloration of the urine which might obviously cause concern in people not aware of the origin of the colour (Alhadeff *et al.* 1984).

## Vitamin B$_6$

### CHEMISTRY AND BIOCHEMICAL FUNCTIONS

Vitamin B$_6$ is a common name for pyridoxine, pyridoxamine and pyridoxal (McCormick 1986). Pyridoxine hydrochloride is the synthetic pharmaceutical form of vitamin B$_6$ (Halsted 1993). All three chemical forms of vitamin B$_6$ are metabolically active after phosphorylation. The most common cofactor in human body is pyridoxal phosphate (PLP) (Driskell 1984). It is a prosthetic group of transaminases, transferases, decarboxylases and cleavage enzymes needed in many reactions involving for instance protein breakdown (Manore 1994). PLP is also an essential structural component of glycogen phosphorylase, the first enzyme in glycogen breakdown pathway (Allgood & Cidlowski 1991). In fact, muscle-bound PLP represents 80% of the approximately 4-g body pool of vitamin B$_6$ (Coburn *et al.* 1988).

In addition to energy metabolism, vitamin B$_6$ is needed for synthesis and metabolism of many neurotransmitters (e.g. serotonin), and in the development and maintenance of a competent immune system (Allgood & Cidlowski 1991). PLP-dependent enzymes are involved in synthesis of catecholamines (Driskell 1984), and perhaps in regulation of steroid hormone action (Allgood & Cidlowski 1991). Vitamin B$_6$ is also needed for the synthesis of aminolevulic acid, an intermediate compound in the formation of the porphyrin ring in haemoglobin (Manore 1994).

From a physiological viewpoint, vitamin B$_6$ depletion could decrease glycogen breakdown and impair capacity for glycolysis and anaerobic energy production. Because glycogen phosphorylase is not a rate-limiting enzyme in glycogenolysis, small changes in its activity would, however, not affect glycogen metabolism. Severe depletion would also affect haemoglobin synthesis, and impair oxygen transport in the blood. The contribution of amino acids in total energy expenditure is not likely to exceed 10%, even in a glycogen depleted state. Therefore, it is unclear how an impairment in amino acid breakdown would affect physical performance.

The activity of two enzymes involved in erythrocytic protein metabolism, namely aspartate aminotransferase (ASAT) and alanine aminotransferase (ALAT), are used as indicators of vitamin B$_6$ status (Bayomi & Rosalki 1976; Driskell 1984). The principle of the assay, with and without *in vitro* saturation, is similar to that explained earlier for thiamin (transketolase) and riboflavin (glutathione reductase) (Bayomi & Rosalki 1976).

### SUPPLY AND METABOLIC FUNCTIONS

In male wrestlers and judo-athletes, a decrease in the erythrocyte ASAT activity indicated deterioration in vitamin B$_6$ supply during a 3-week weight-loss regimen (Fogelholm *et al.* 1993a). Maximal anaerobic capacity, speed or strength were, however, not affected. Coburn *et al.* (1991) showed that the muscle tissue is, in fact, quite resistant to a 6-week vitamin B$_6$ depletion.

LIVERPOOL
JOHN MOORES UNIVER
AVRIL ROBARTS LRC
TITHEBARN STREET

Marginal vitamin $B_6$ supply has been related to impaired aerobic functions only in combination with a simultaneous thiamin and riboflavin depletion (van der Beek *et al.* 1988).

In an interesting study, indices of vitamin $B_6$ status were examined during a 3-month submarine patrol (Reynolds *et al.* 1988). The results indicated deterioration in status and marginal vitamin $B_6$ supply at the end of the patrol. Psychological tests indicated pronounced depression after submergence and at the midpatrol point. However, the depression measures were neither correlated with indicators of vitamin $B_6$ status nor affected by vitamin supplementation.

Chronic supplementation of vitamin $B_6$ increases the erythrocyte ASAT activity (van Dam 1978; Guilland *et al.* 1989; Fogelholm *et al.* 1993b) and plasma PLP-concentration (Weight *et al.* 1988a; Coburn *et al.* 1991) even in healthy subjects. However, an increase in the above indicators of vitamin $B_6$ status is not necessarily associated with a marked increase in intramuscular vitamin $B_6$ content (Coburn *et al.* 1991).

It appears that vitamin $B_6$, either as an infusion (Moretti *et al.* 1982) or given orally as a $20\,mg \cdot day^{-1}$ supplement (Dunton *et al.* 1993), has a stimulating effect on exercise-induced growth hormone production. The hypothetical mechanism behind this effect is that PLP acts as the coenzyme for dopa decarboxylase, and high concentrations might promote the conversion of L-dopa to dopamine (Manore 1994). The physiological significance of the above effect is not known (Manore 1994). Moreover, the effects of chronic vitamin $B_6$ administration on the 24-h growth hormone concentration of plasma have not been studied.

Supplementation of vitamin $B_6$, alone (Suboticanec *et al.* 1990) or in combination with other B-complex vitamins (van Dam 1978; Bonke & Nickel 1989), has improved maximal oxygen uptake in undernourished children (Suboticanec *et al.* 1990), and shooting performance (Bonke & Nickel 1989) and muscle irritability (van Dam 1978) in male athletes. In contrast, a number of other studies did not find any association between improved indicators of vitamin $B_6$

status and maximal oxygen uptake (Suboticanec-Buzina *et al.* 1984; Weight *et al.* 1988a, 1988b), exercise-induced lactate appearance in blood (Manore & Leklem 1988; Weight *et al.* 1988a, 1988b; Fogelholm *et al.* 1993b), grip strength (Suboticanec *et al.* 1989) or other tests of physical performance (Telford *et al.* 1992a, 1992b).

### SAFETY OF ELEVATED VITAMIN $B_6$ INTAKE

In contrast to thiamin and riboflavin, megadoses of vitamin $B_6$ may have important toxic effects. The most common disorder is sensory neuropathy, sometimes combined with epidermal vesicular dermatosis (Bässler 1989). The safe dose for chronic oral administration of vitamin $B_6$ appears to be around 300–500 mg daily (Bässler 1989). However, it is recommended that long-term supplementation should not exceed $200\,mg \cdot day^{-1}$ — that is, 100 times the recommended dietary allowance (Marks 1989).

## Folic acid and vitamin $B_{12}$

### CHEMISTRY AND BIOCHEMICAL FUNCTIONS

*Folate* and *folic acid* are generic terms for compounds related to pteroic acid. The body pool is 5–10 mg (Herbert 1987), and liver folate is a major part of the total. Folate coenzymes are needed in transportation of single carbon units in, for instance, thymidylate, methionine and purine synthesis (Fairbanks & Klee 1986).

Deficiency of folate results in impaired cell division and alterations in protein synthesis. The effects are most significant in rapidly growing tissues (Herbert 1987). A typical deficiency symptom is megaloblastic anaemia (lowered blood haemoglobin concentration, with increased mean corpuscular volume; Halsted 1993). Decreased oxygen transport capacity would affect submaximal and eventually also maximal aerobic performance. If iron deficiency exists simultaneously with folate deficiency, red cell morphology does not necessarily deviate from reference values (Fairbanks & Klee 1986). Folate is also needed in the nervous system, and depletion during pregnancy might cause lethal neural tube defects (Reynolds 1994).

Vitamin $B_{12}$ and cobalamin refer to a larger group of physiologically active cobalamins (Fairbanks & Klee 1986). Cyanocobalamin is the principal commercial and therapeutic product (Halsted 1993). Cobalamin is a cofactor for two reactions: the synthesis of methionine and the conversion of methylmalonic acid to succinic acid (Halsted 1993). Through these reactions, cobalamin is needed in normal red blood cell synthesis and neuronal metabolism (Fairbanks & Klee 1986).

Cobalamin deficiency leads to megaloblastic anaemia and to neurological disorders. As in anaemia caused by folate deficiency, erythrocyte volume is usually increased, in contrast to frank iron-deficiency anaemia (Fairbanks & Klee 1986). Compared with the daily requirements, the 2–3 mg body pool of cobalamin is very large. Even with no dietary cobalamin, the body pool would suffice for about 3–5 years (Fairbanks & Klee 1986).

SUPPLY AND METABOLIC FUNCTIONS

There are only a few studies linking folic acid or vitamin $B_{12}$ supply to sports-related functional capacity. Folate supplementation and increased serum folate concentration did not affect maximal oxygen uptake (Matter *et al.* 1987), anaerobic threshold (Matter *et al.* 1987), grip strength (Suboticanec *et al.* 1989) or other measures of physical performance (Telford *et al.* 1992a, 1992b). Together with thiamin and vitamin $B_6$ supplementation, elevated intake of vitamin $B_{12}$ was, however, associated with improved shooting performance (Bonke & Nickel 1989).

SAFETY OF ELEVATED FOLIC ACID AND VITAMIN $B_{12}$ INTAKE

The effects of high doses of folic acid have not been studied very much, but some results indicate a possible interference with zinc metabolism (Marks 1989; Reynolds 1994). The current estimate of the safety dose is between 50 and 100 times the daily recommended intake (Marks 1989). The safety margin for vitamin $B_{12}$ appears to be much larger, because even doses as high as $30\,mg \cdot day^{-1}$ (that is, 10000 times the recommended intake) have been used without noticeable toxic effects (Marks 1989).

## Other vitamins of the B-group

### NIACIN

*Niacin* is used as a name for nicotinic acid as well as for its derivatives nicotinamide and nicotinic acid amide (McCormick 1986). About 67% of niacin required by an adult can be converted from the amino acid tryptophan; 60 mg of tryptophan is needed for the formation of 1 mg niacin.

Nicotinamide, as a part of nicotinamide adenine dinucleotide (NAD) and NADPH, participates in hundreds of oxidation-reduction reactions (McCormick 1986; Halsted 1993). NAD is needed as an electron acceptor in glycolysis (enzyme: glyceraldehyde-3-phosphate dehydrogenase) and the citric acid cycle (pyruvate dehydrogenase, isocitrate dehydrogenase, α-ketoglutarate dehydrogenase and malate dehydrogenase), and the reduced form of NADPH as an electron donor in fatty acid synthesis.

Because of its important role in mitochondrial metabolism, niacin deficiency has the potential to affect both muscular and nervous function. Unfortunately, there are no direct studies on the effects of niacin deficiency on physical performance. In contrast, high-dose supplementation (e.g. intravenous administration) of niacin blocks the release of free fatty acids from the adipose tissue, and impairs long-term submaximal endurance (Pernow & Saltin 1971).

Acute oral intake of at least 100 mg of nicotinic acid per day (i.e. at least five times the recommended daily allowance) causes vasodilatation and flushing, which is a rather harmless effect (Marks 1989). Very large, chronic supplementation of niacin has been reported to cause hepatotoxicity, cholestatic jaundice, an increased serum concentration of uric acid, cardiac dysrhythmias and various dermatologic problems (Alhadeff *et al.* 1984). The safe chronic dose appears to be at least 50 times the recommended allowance, i.e. $1\,g\cdot day^{-1}$ (Marks 1989).

### BIOTIN

The main function of biotin is as cofactor in enzymes catalysing transport of carboxyl units (McCormick 1986). In the cytosol, a biotin-dependent enzyme, acetyl-coenzyme A carboxylase, catalyses the formation of malonyl-coenzyme A from acetyl-coenzyme A. Malonyl-coenzyme A is used for fatty acid synthesis. In the mitochondria, biotin is an integral part of pyruvate carboxylase. This enzyme catalyses the conversion of pyruvate to oxaloacetate, which is an intermediate in gluconeogenesis and the citric acid cycle.

Through the function of pyruvate carboxylase, biotin has a critical role in maintaining the level of citric acid cycle intermediates. Although it is likely that aerobic performance would be impaired by biotin deficiency, the physical performance of biotin deficient patients has never been investigated. Moreover, excluding individuals with an excessive intake of raw egg-white (which contains avidin, a biotin-binding glycoprotein), dietary biotin deficiency is almost impossible in practice (McCormick 1986).

There are no reported toxic effects of biotin intake up to $10\,mg\cdot day^{-1}$ ($>100$ times the recommended allowance) (Marks 1989; Halsted 1993).

### PANTOTHENIC ACID

Pantothenic acid functions as a cofactor in coenzyme A, which, as acetyl-coenzyme A, is in a central position for both energy production and fatty acid synthesis (McCormick 1986). Pantothenic acid is also needed in the 4′-phosphopantetheine moiety of acyl carrier protein of fatty acid synthetase.

Pantothenic acid deficiency due to dietary reasons has never been reported. Deficiency symptoms have been induced with a semisynthetic diet practically free of pantothenate. Symptoms include general fatigue and increased heart rate during exertion (McCormick 1986). Relations between pantothenic acid status and physical performance capacity have not been investigated.

Pantothenic acid has not been reported to cause any toxic affects even at doses up to $10\,g$ daily, i.e. 1000 times the recommended intake level (Alhadeff *et al.* 1984; Marks 1989).

## Vitamin C

### CHEMISTRY AND BIOCHEMICAL FUNCTIONS

Vitamin C or ascorbic acid is a strong reducing agent, which is reversibly oxidized to dehydroascorbic acid in numerous biochemical reactions (Padh 1991). By its reducing capacity, ascorbic acid stimulates enzymes involved in, for instance, biosynthesis of collagen, carnitine, pyrimidine and noradrenaline (McCormick 1986; Padh 1991).

In addition to the above biosynthetic pathways, ascorbic acid has a very important role as an extracellular antioxidant against many types of free radical compounds (see Chapter 22). In the gastrointestinal tract, ascorbic acid enhances iron absorption by keeping iron in a reduced ferrous state (Gershoff 1993). In contrast, high doses of ascorbic acid may suppress copper absorption by reducing copper to a less absorbable monovalent state (Finley & Cerklewski 1983).

### SUPPLY AND METABOLIC FUNCTIONS

Ascorbic acid is needed in carnitine synthesis, and therefore indirectly for transfer of long-chain fatty acids across the inner mitochondrial membrane. A substantial decrease in muscle carnitine would theoretically decrease submaximal endurance capacity by increasing the dependence on glycogen instead of fatty acids (Wagenmakers 1991). In one study (van der Beek *et al.* 1990), a vitamin C restricted diet was followed by reduced whole blood ascorbic acid concentration. The marginal vitamin C supply did not produce any significant effects on maximal aerobic capacity or lactate threshold in healthy volunteers. Carnitine, or any other metabolites related to vitamin C status, was not measured.

Vitamin C supplementation has been associated with increased maximal aerobic capacity (Buzina *et al.* 1982; Suboticanec-Buzina *et al.* 1984) and work efficiency (Powers *et al.* 1985) in malnourished children. However, the above positive effects were seen simultaneously with supplementation of one or more vitamins of the B-complex group. Hence, the independent role of ascorbic acid was not shown. The majority of other studies have not shown any measurable effects of vitamin C supplementation on maximal oxygen uptake, lactate threshold or exercise-induced heart-rate in well-nourished subjects (Gerster 1989).

Due to its function as an antioxidant in phagocytic leucocytes, supplementary vitamin C may slightly decrease the duration of common cold episodes (Hemilä 1992). The study of Peters *et al.* (1993) provided evidence that 600 mg vitamin C daily reduced the incidence (33% vs. 68%) and duration (4.2 vs. 5.6 days) of upper-respiratory-tract infection in runners after a 90-km ultra-marathon race. It is not known, however, whether the potential effect of vitamin C supplementation on the common cold in athletes has any significant long-term effects on performance.

In a large epidemiological survey in the US, dietary vitamin C intake was weakly but positively associated with pulmonary function (forced expiratory volume in 1 s) in healthy subjects, but a stronger relationship was found in asthmatic patients (Schwartz & Weiss 1994). The authors postulated that the antioxidant effects of vitamin C have a protective role on pulmonary function. Finally, earlier results suggest that vitamin C supplementation ($\geq$250 mg daily) might reduce heat strain in unacclimatized individuals (Kotze *et al.* 1977) which could theoretically enhance physical performance in certain circumstances.

### SAFETY OF ELEVATED VITAMIN C INTAKE

There are reports suggesting that very high (>1 g daily), chronic doses of vitamin C might lead to formation of oxalate stones, increased uric acid excretion, diarrhoea, vitamin $B_{12}$ destruction and iron overload, and induce a dependency state (Alhadeff *et al.* 1984). However, excluding diarrhoea, the risk for the above toxic effects is likely to be very low in healthy individuals, even with intake of several grams daily (Marks 1989; Rivers 1989).

## Fat-soluble vitamins

### Vitamin E

#### CHEMISTRY AND BIOCHEMICAL FUNCTIONS

Vitamin E consists of a trimethylhydroquinone head and a diterpenoid side chain (Jenkins 1993). The most active biological form of vitamin E is $\alpha$-tocopherol. It is stored in many tissues, with the largest amount in the liver. Vitamin E is transported mainly in very low density lipoproteins.

Vitamin E is one of the most important antioxidants in cellular membranes (see Chapter 22), and it stabilizes the structural integrity of membranes by breaking the chain reaction of lipid peroxidation (Jenkins 1993). Vitamin E is also essential for normal function of the immune system (Meydani 1995).

#### SUPPLY AND METABOLIC FUNCTIONS

It has been hypothesized that free radical damage to mitochondrial membranes in vitamin E depletion would impair the reactions of oxidative phosphorylation, and hence physical work capacity. Vitamin E deficiency is, however, very rare, and the relationship between decreased vitamin E supply and physical capacity has not been investigated (Jenkins 1993).

Supplementation of vitamin E has well-established and rather consistent effects on some metabolic functions even in well-nourished humans: after chronic vitamin E supplementation (typical dose, >100 mg·day⁻¹), indices of exercise-induced lipid peroxidation, mainly serum malondialdehyde concentration and breath pentane exhalation, are reduced (Jenkins 1993; Rokitzki *et al.* 1994; Kanter & Williams 1995; Tiidus & Houston 1995). There are some interpretation problems, however, mainly because of the lack of specificity and/or reliability of most indicators of lipid peroxidation (Kanter & Williams 1995).

In one study (Simon-Schnass & Pabst 1988), vitamin E supplementation helped to maintain aerobic working capacity at very high altitude (>5000 m). Other studies have not conclusively proven that vitamin E intake exceeding daily recommendations would have any beneficial effects on athletic performance (Rokitzki *et al.* 1994; Kanter & Williams 1995; Tiidus & Houston 1995).

## SAFETY OF ELEVATED VITAMIN E INTAKE

Vitamin E, in contrast to two other fat-soluble vitamins (A and D), is apparently not toxic for healthy individuals (Machlin 1989). The safety factor for long-term administration is at least 100 times the recommended daily intake—that is, at least 1 g daily in oral use (Marks 1989). Overdoses of vitamin E are contraindicated only in individuals receiving vitamin K antagonists (Machlin 1989).

## Other fat-soluble vitamins

### VITAMIN A

The two natural forms of vitamin A are retinol and 3-dehydroretinol, of which retinol is the more abundant in the human body (Bates 1995). All higher animals can convert plant-derived carotenes and cryptoxanthin to retinol. The most common and effective provitamin in the human diet is β-carotene. Retinol is transported in chylomicrons from the gut, and later bound to a protein (retinol-binding protein, RBP). Several hundred milligrams of retinol are stored in the liver (McCormick 1986).

The best known function of retinol is as an essential component in vision. In vitamin A deficiency, worsening of night vision is an early clinical sign (McLaren *et al.* 1993). Both retinol and β-carotene are capable of scavenging singlet oxygens and hence act as antioxidants (Bates 1995). Vitamin A is also important for immunity. The literature provides no evident data on relations between vitamin A status and physical performance.

Chronic toxicity of retinol will cause joint or bone pain, hair loss, anorexia and liver damage. The safety level for chronic use is estimated to be 10 times the recommended daily intake—that is, 10 mg retinol daily (Marks 1989). Because of an increased risk for spontaneous abortions and birth defects (Underwood 1989), the safe level during pregnancy might be only four to five times the daily recommendation (Marks 1989). β-carotene, in contrast to retinol, is not toxic. This provitamin is stored under the skin and it is converted to retinol only when needed.

### VITAMIN D

In the diet, vitamin D occurs mainly as cholecalciferol ($D_3$), which can also be synthesized in skin after ultraviolet irradiation (Fraser 1995). In the liver, $D_3$ is hydroxylated to 25-hydroxycholecalciferol (25-OH-$D_3$), and further in the kidneys to 1,25-dihydroxycholecalciferol (1,25-(OH)$_2$-$D_3$, active form) or to 24,25-dihydroxycholecalciferol (24,25-(OH)$_2$-$D_3$, inactive form). Vitamin D is stored in several parts in the body, e.g. in the liver and under the skin.

Vitamin D stimulates calcium absorption in the small intestine and increases calcium reabsorption by the distal renal tubules. Deficiency results in bone demineralization (rickets and osteomalacia), and this may eventually increase the risk for stress fractures (Fraser 1995).

Vitamin D is potentially toxic, especially for young children, causing hypercalcaemia, hypercalciuria, soft-tissue calcification, anorexia and constipation, and eventually irreversible renal and cardiovascular damage (Davies 1989). Intakes of 10 times the recommendation should not be exceeded (Marks 1989). High calcium intakes may enhance the toxicity of vitamin D.

VITAMIN K

Vitamin K is the general name of compounds containing a 2-methyl-1,4-naptho-quinone moiety. Vitamin K is needed for formation of prothrombin in the blood, and defective blood coagulation is the only major sign of deficiency (McCormick 1986). No evident associations between vitamin K and exercise metabolism are to be found. Further, very little is known about the safety of orally administered vitamin K (Marks 1989).

## Conclusion

Vitamins are extremely important for the functional capacity of the human body (see Table 20.1). Many B vitamins participate as enzyme cofactors in pathways of energy metabolism and in neuromuscular functions. Folic acid and vitamins $B_{12}$ and $B_6$ are needed for haemoglobin synthesis, and consequently for optimal oxygen transport from the lungs to the working tissues. Some vitamins (e.g. vitamins A, $B_6$ and C) are required for normal immune function. Finally, vitamins A, C and E have important antioxidant properties.

Studies have clearly shown that the output of many vitamin-dependent functions both *in vivo* (e.g. breath pentane exhalation) and *in vitro* (e.g. erythrocyte enzymes) may increase after supplementation above normal dietary intake. Similarly, the output of many functions is decreased at marginal vitamin supply. However, the output of the entire human body (e.g. athletic performance) was only rarely related to marginal vitamin supply or to supplementation.

The dietary intake of vitamins is not high enough to ensure maximal output of many isolated functions. However, it appears that the vitamin intake, at least in developed countries, is above the minimal requirement for maximal

output of the human body. Consequently, the evidence that vitamin supplementation would increase athletic performance is not very encouraging. On the other hand, the risk for toxic intake also seems to be marginal.

The above conclusions are made with some reservations. First, the results on marginal supply and physical function were mostly extrapolated from nonathletic subjects. Moreover, there were hardly any data on athletes from developing countries. Finally, many studies had a very low statistical power, that is, there were too few subjects to detect anything else than substantial effects.

## References

Alhadeff, L., Gualtieri, T. & Lipton, M. (1984) Toxic effects of water-soluble vitamins. *Nutrition Reviews* **42**, 33–40.

Allgood, V.E. & Cidlowski, J.A. (1991) Novel role for vitamin $B_6$ in steroid hormone action: a link between nutrition and the endocrine system. *Journal of Nutritional Biochemistry* **2**, 523–534.

Bamji, M.S., Arya, S., Sarma, K.V.R. & Radhaiah, G. (1982) Impact of long term, low dose B-complex vitamin supplements on vitamin status and psychomotor performance of rural school boys. *Nutrition Research* **2**, 147–153.

Bässler, K.-H. (1989) Use and abuse of high dosages of vitamin $B_6$. In *Elevated Dosages of Vitamins* (ed. P. Walter, H. Stähelin & G. Brubacher), pp. 120–126. Hans Huber Publishers, Stuttgart.

Bates, C.J. (1995) Vitamin A. *Lancet* **345**, 31–35.

Bayomi, R.A. & Rosalki, S.B. (1976) Evaluation of methods of coenzyme activation of erythrocyte enzymes for detection of deficiency of vitamins B-1, B-2, and B-6. *Clinical Chemistry* **22**, 327–335.

Belko, A.Z., Obarzanec, E., Roach, R. *et al.* (1984) Effects of aerobic exercise and weight loss on riboflavin requirements of moderately obese marginally deficient young women. *American Journal of Clinical Nutrition* **40**, 553–561.

Belko, A.Z., Meredith, M.P., Kalkwarf, H.J. *et al.* (1985) Effects of exercise on riboflavin requirements: biological validation in weight reducing women. *American Journal of Clinical Nutrition* **41**, 270–277.

Bonke, D. & Nickel, B. (1989) Improvement of fine motoric movement control by elevated dosages of vitamin $B_1$, $B_6$, and $B_{12}$ in target shooting. In *Elevated Dosages of Vitamins* (ed. P. Walter, H. Stähelin & G. Brubacher), pp. 198–204. Hans Huber Publishers, Stuttgart.

Brubacher, G.B. (1989) Scientific basis for the estimation of the daily requirements for vitamins. In *Elevated Dosages of Vitamins* (ed. P. Walter, H. Stähelin & G. Brubacher), pp. 3–11. Hans Huber Publishers, Stuttgart.

Buzina, R., Grgic, Z., Jusic, M., Sapunar, J., Milanovic, N. & Brubacher, G. (1982) Nutritional status and physical working capacity. *Human Nutrition: Clinical Nutrition* 36C, 429–438.

Coburn, S.P., Lewis, D.L.N., Fink, W.J., Mahuren, J.D., Schaltenbrand, W.E. & Costill, D.L. (1988) Human vitamin B-6 pools estimated through muscle biopsies. *American Journal of Clinical Nutrition* 48, 291–294.

Coburn, S.P., Ziegler, P.Z., Costill, D.L. *et al.* (1991) Reponse of vitamin B-6 content of muscle to changes in vitamin B-6 intake in men. *American Journal of Clinical Nutrition* 53, 1436–1442.

Cooperman, J.M. & Lopez, R. (1984) Riboflavin. In *Handbook of Vitamins. Nutritional, Biochemical, and Clinical Aspects* (ed. L.J. Machlin), pp. 299–327. Marcel Dekker, New York.

Davies, M. (1989) High-dose vitamin D therapy: indications, benefits and hazards. In *Elevated Dosages of Vitamins* (ed. P. Walter, H. Stähelin & G. Brubacher), pp. 81–86. Hans Huber Publishers, Stuttgart.

Driskell, J.A. (1984) Vitamin $B_6$. In *Handbook of Vitamins: Nutritional, Biochemical, and Clinical Aspects* (ed. L.J. Machlin), pp. 379–401. Marcel Dekker, New York.

Dunton, N., Virk, R., Young, J. & Leklem, J. (1993) The influence of vitamin $B_6$ supplementation and exercise on vitamin $B_6$ metabolism and growth hormone. *FASEB Journal* 7, A727 (abstract).

Fairbanks, V.F. & Klee, G.G. (1986) Biochemical aspects of hematology. In *Textbook of Clinical Chemistry* (ed. N.W. Tietz), pp. 1495–1588. W.B. Saunders, Philadelphia.

Fairweather-Tait, S.J., Powers, H.J., Minski, M.J., Whitehead, J. & Downes, R. (1992) Riboflavin deficiency and iron absorption in adult Gambian men. *Annals of Nutrition and Metabolism* 36, 34–40.

Finley, E.B. & Cerklewski, F.L. (1983) Influence of ascorbic acid supplementation on copper status in young adult men. *American Journal of Clinical Nutrition* 37, 553–556.

Fogelholm, M. (1995) Indicators of vitamin and mineral status in athletes' blood: a review. *International Journal of Sport Nutrition* 5, 267–286.

Fogelholm, M., Koskinen, R., Laakso, J., Rankinen, T. & Ruokonen, I. (1993a) Gradual and rapid weight loss: effects on nutrition and performance in male athletes. *Medicine and Science in Sports and Exercise* 25, 371–377.

Fogelholm, M., Ruokonen, I., Laakso, J., Vuorimaa, T. & Himberg, J.-J. (1993b) Lack of association between indices of vitamin $B_1$, $B_2$ and $B_6$ status and exercise-induced blood lactate in young adults. *International Journal of Sport Nutrition* 3, 165–176.

Fraser, D.R. (1995) Vitamin D. *Lancet* 345, 104–107.

Gershoff, S.N. (1993) Vitamin C (Ascorbic acid): new roles, new requirements? *Nutrition Reviews* 51, 313–326.

Gerster, H. (1989) The role of vitamin C in athletic performance. *Journal of the American College of Nutrition* 8, 636–643.

Greenberg, S.M. & Frishman, W.H. (1988) Coenzyme $Q_{10}$: a new drug for myocardial ischemia? *Medical Clinics of North America* 72, 243–258.

Guilland, J.-C., Penaranda, T., Gallet, C., Boggio, V., Fuchs, F. & Klepping, J. (1989) Vitamin status of young athletes including the effects of supplementation. *Medicine and Science in Sports and Exercise* 21, 441–449.

Halsted, C.H. (1993) Water-soluble vitamins. In *Human Nutrition and Dietetics* (ed. J.S. Garrow & W.P.T. James), pp. 239–263. Churchill Livingstone, Edinburgh.

Haralambie, G. (1976) Vitamin $B_2$ status in athletes and the influence of riboflavin administration on neuromuscular irritability. *Nutrition and Metabolism* 20, 1–8.

Hemilä, H. (1992) Vitamin C and the common cold. *British Journal of Nutrition* 67, 3–16.

Herbert, V. (1987) Recommended dietary intakes (RDI) of folate in humans. *American Journal of Clinical Nutrition* 45, 661–670.

Jenkins, R.R. (1993) Exercise, oxidative stress, and antioxidants: a review. *International Journal of Sport Nutrition* 3, 356–375.

Johnson Gubler, C. (1984) Thiamin. In *Handbook of Vitamins: Nutritional, Biochemical, and Clinical Aspects* (ed. L.J. Machlin), pp. 245–295. Marcel Dekker, New York.

Kanter, M.M. & Williams, M.H. (1995) Antioxidants, carnitine, and choline as putative ergogenic aids. *International Journal of Sport Nutrition* 5, S120–S131.

Kotze, H.F., van der Walt, W.H., Rogers, G.G. & Strydom, N.B. (1977) Effects of plasma ascorbic acid levels on heat acclimatization in man. *Journal of Applied Physiology* 42, 711–716.

Laaksonen, R., Fogelholm, M., Himberg, J.-J., Laakso, J. & Salorinne, Y. (1995) Ubiquinone supplementation and exercise capacity in trained young and older men. *European Journal of Applied Physiology* 72, 95–100.

McCormick, D.B. (1986) Vitamins. In *Textbook of Clinical Chemistry* (ed. N.W. Tietz), pp. 927–964. W.B. Saunders, Philadelphia.

Machlin, L.J. (1989) Use and safety of elevated dosages of vitamin E in adults. In *Elevated Dosages of Vitamins* (ed. P. Walter, H. Stähelin & G. Brubacher), pp. 56–68. Hans Huber Publishers, Stuttgart.

McLaren, D.S., Loveridge, N., Duthie, G. &

Bolton-Smith, C. (1993) Fat-soluble vitamins. In *Human Nutrition and Dietetics* (ed. J.S. Garrow & W.P.T. James), pp. 298–238. Churchill Livingstone, Edinburgh.

Manore, M. (1994) Vitamin $B_6$ and exercise. *International Journal of Sport Nutrition* **4**, 89–103.

Manore, M. & Leklem, J.E. (1988) Effects of carbohydrate and vitamin $B_6$ on fuel substrates during exercise in women. *Medicine and Science in Sports and Exercise* **20**, 233–241.

Marks, J. (1989) The safety of the vitamins: an overview. In *Elevated Dosages of Vitamins* (ed. P. Walter, H. Stähelin & G. Brubacher), pp. 12–20. Hans Huber Publishers, Stuttgart.

Matter, M., Stittfall, T., Graves, J. *et al.* (1987) The effect of iron and folate therapy on maximal exercise performance in female marathon runners with iron and folate deficiency. *Clinical Science* **72**, 415–422.

Meydani, M. (1995) Vitamin E. *Lancet* **345**, 170–175.

Moretti, C., Fabbri, A., Gnessi, L., Bonifacio, V., Fraiolo, F. & Isidori, A. (1982) Pyridoxine (B6) suppresses the rise in prolactin and increases the rise in growth hormone induced by exercise. *New England Journal of Medicine* **307**, 444–445.

Padh, H. (1991) Vitamin C: newer insights into its biochemical functions. *Nutrition Reviews* **49**, 65–80.

Pernow, B. & Saltin, B. (1971) Availability of substrates and capacity for prolonged heavy exercise in man. *Journal of Applied Physiology* **31**, 416–422.

Peters, E.M., Goetzsche, J.M., Grobbelaar, B. & Noakes, T.D. (1993) Vitamin C supplementation reduces the incidence of postrace symptoms of upper-respiratory-tract infection in ultramarathon runners. *American Journal of Clinical Nutrition* **57**, 170–174.

Piertzik, K. (1986) Vitamin deficiency: aetiology and terminology. In *B Vitamins in Medicine: Proceedings of a Symposium held in Helsinki, October 1985* (ed. J.-J. Himberg, W. Tackman, D. Bonke & H. Karppanen), pp. 31–43. Friedr. Wieweg & Sohn, Wiesbaden.

Powers, H.J., Bates, C.J., Lamb, W.H., Singh, J., Gelman, W. & Webb, E. (1985) Effects of multivitamin and iron supplement on running performance in Gambian children. *Human Nutrition: Clinical Nutrition* **39C**, 427–437.

Powers, H.J., Bates, C.J., Eccles, M., Brown, H. & George, E. (1987) Bicycling performance in Gambian children: effects of supplements of riboflavin and ascorbic acid. *Human Nutrition: Clinical Nutrition* **41C**, 59–69.

Reynolds, R.D. (1994) Vitamin supplements: current controversies. *Journal of the American College of Nutrition* **13**, 118–126.

Reynolds, R.D., Styer, D.J. & Schlichting, C.L. (1988) Decreased vitamin B-6 status of submariners during prolonged patrol. *American Journal of Clinical Nutrition* **47**, 463–469.

Rivers, J.M. (1989) Safety of high-level vitamin C ingestion. In *Elevated Dosages of Vitamins* (ed. P. Walter, H. Stähelin & G. Brubacher), pp. 95–102. Hans Huber Publishers, Stuttgart.

Rokitzki, L., Logemann, E., Huber, G., Keck, E. & Keul, J. (1994) α-Tocopherol supplementation in racing cyclists during extreme endurance training. *International Journal of Sports Nutrition* **4**, 253–264.

Sauberlich, H.E. (1967) Biochemical alterations in thiamine deficiency: their interpretation. *American Journal of Clinical Nutrition* **20**, 528–542.

Schwartz, J. & Weiss, S.T. (1994) Relationship between dietary vitamin C intake and pulmonary function in the First National Health and Nutrition Examination Survey (NHANES I). *American Journal of Clinical Nutrition* **59**, 110–114.

Simon-Schnass, I. & Pabst, H. (1988) Influence of vitamin E on physical performance. *International Journal of Vitamin and Nutrition Research* **58**, 49–54.

Singh, A., Moses, F.M. & Deuster, P.A. (1992a) Chronic multivitamin-mineral supplementation does not enhance physical performance. *Medicine and Science in Sports and Exercise* **24**, 726–732.

Singh, A., Moses, F.M. & Deuster, P.A. (1992b) Vitamin and mineral status in physically active men: effects of high-potency supplement. *American Journal of Clinical Nutrition* **55**, 1–7.

Soares, M.J., Satyanaryana, K., Bamji, M.S., Jacob, C.M., Venkata Ramana, Y. & Sudhakar Rao, S. (1993) The effects of exercise on riboflavin status of adult men. *British Journal of Nutrition* **69**, 541–551.

Sobal, J. & Marquart, L.F. (1994) Vitamin/mineral supplement use among athletes: a review of the literature. *International Journal of Sport Nutrition* **4**, 320–334.

Solomons, N.W. & Allen, L.H. (1983) The functional assessment of nutritional status: principles, practise and potential. *Nutrition Reviews* **41**, 33–50.

Suboticanec, K., Stavljenic, A., Bilic-Pesic, L. *et al.* (1989) Nutritional status, grip strength, and immune function in institutionalized elderly. *International Journal of Vitamin and Nutrition Research* **59**, 20–28.

Suboticanec, K., Stavljenic, A., Schalch, W. & Buzina, R. (1990) Effects of pyridoxine and riboflavin supplementation on physical fitness in young adolescents. *International Journal of Vitamin and Nutrition Research* **60**, 81–88.

Suboticanec-Buzina, K., Buzina, R., Brubacher, G., Sapunar, J. & Christeller, S. (1984) Vitamin C status and physical working capacity in adolescents. *International Journal of Vitamin and Nutrition Research* **54**, 55–60.

Telford, R.D., Catchpole, E.A., Deakin, V., Hahn, A.G. & Plank, A.W. (1992a) The effects of 7–8 months of vitamin/mineral supplementation on the vitamin and mineral status of athletes. *International Journal of Sport Nutrition* **2**, 123–134.

Telford, R.D., Catchpole, E.A., Deakin, V., Hahn, A.G. & Plank, A.W. (1992b) The effects of 7–8 months of vitamin/mineral supplementation on athletic performance. *International Journal of Sport Nutrition* **2**, 135–153.

Tiidus, P.M. & Houston, M.E. (1995) Vitamin E status and response to exercise training. *Sports Medicine* **20**, 12–23.

Trebler Winters, L.R., Yoon, J.-S., Kalkwarf, H.J. *et al.* (1992) Riboflavin requirements and exercise adaptation in older women. *American Journal of Clinical Nutrition* **56**, 526–532.

Underwood, B.A. (1989) Teratogenicity of vitamin A. In *Elevated Dosages of Vitamins* (ed. P. Walter, H. Stähelin & G. Brubacher), pp. 42–55. Hans Huber Publishers, Stuttgart.

van Dam, B. (1978) Vitamins and sport. *British Journal of Sports Medicine* **12**, 74–79.

van der Beek, E.J., van Dokkum, W., Schriver, J., Wesstra, A., Kistemaker, C. & Hermus, R.J.J. (1990) Controlled vitamin C restriction and physical performance in volunteers. *Journal of the American College of Nutrition* **9**, 332–339.

van der Beek, E.J., van Dokkum, W., Schrijver, J. *et al.* (1988) Thiamin, riboflavin, and vitamins B-6 and C: impact of combined restricted intake on functional performance in man. *American Journal of Clinical Nutrition* **48**, 1451–1462.

Wagenmakers, A.J.M. (1991) L-Carnitine supplementation and performance in man. In *Advances in Nutrition and Top Sport. Medicine and Sport Science*, Vol. 32 (ed. F. Brouns), pp. 110–127. Karger, Basel.

Weight, L.M., Myburgh, K.H. & Noakes, T.D. (1988a) Vitamin and mineral supplementation: effect on the running performance of trained athletes. *American Journal of Clinical Nutrition* **47**, 192–195.

Weight, L.M., Noakes, T.D., Labadarios, D., Graves, J., Jacobs, P. & Berman, P.A. (1988b) Vitamin and mineral status of trained athletes including the effects of supplementation. *American Journal of Clinical Nutrition* **47**, 186–191.

Williams, M.H. (1986) *Nutritional Aspects of Human Physical and Athletic Performance.* Charles C. Thomas, Springfield, IL.

Wood, B., Gijsbers, A., Goode, A., Davis, S., Mulholland, J. & Breen, K. (1980) A study of partial thiamin restriction in human volunteers. *American Journal of Clinical Nutrition* **33**, 848–861.

# Chapter 21

# Vitamins: Effects of Exercise on Requirements

JIDI CHEN

## Introduction

Vitamins are a group of organic compounds required in tiny amounts in the diet of humans for proper biological functioning and maintenance of health. Vitamins do not supply energy, but act mainly as regulators of the numerous and diverse physiological processes in the human body including vision, skin integrity, bone ossification, DNA formation, metabolism of carbohydrate, fat, and proteins, mitochondrial metabolism, utilization of oxygen in the cells, red blood cell (RBC) formation and other functions which are closely related to energy production and resultant physical performance (see Chapter 20). The human body is not able to synthesize the majority of the vitamins or the amount synthesized in the body cannot meet the needs. It is clear that a certain amount of each of the vitamins is essential in the diet and that lack of a specific vitamin can cause a specific deficiency disease (Williams 1985; Daniel 1991; Chen & Wu 1996). Due to the many and varied roles of vitamins, they are probably the most widespread nutrients taken as supplements by both the general and athletic population. Furthermore, vitamins meet with great interest in the world of sports because of their supposed role in enhancing physical performance (Williams 1989; van der Beek 1991, 1994; Singh *et al.* 1992b; Weight *et al.* 1998a, 1998b).

Exercise enhances energy metabolism and increases the total energy expenditure which gives rise to a number of concerns:

- Does exercise training result in increased needs or deficiencies of vitamins?
- Is the vitamin status of athletes normal?
- Is it necessary for athletes to take vitamin supplements?

The answers to these questions have varied through the years and the balance of opinion continues to change as new evidence appears (Clarkson 1991, 1995; van der Beek 1991; Fogelholm 1994; Armstrong & Maresh 1996). The focal points of the concerns for vitamin nutrition of athletes are the assumption that athletes need an increased vitamin intake, the optimum recommended dietary allowance (RDA) for athletes under different conditions, and the true effects of vitamin supplementation on physical performance.

It is accepted that the prevalence of vitamin deficiency diseases is low in the general population in industrialized societies. Theoretically, the athlete may have an increased requirement for dietary intake of vitamins induced by decreased absorption in the gastrointestinal tract, increased excretion in sweat, urine and faeces, increased turnover, as well as the adaptation for the initial stage of vigorous training and/or acute physical exercise which may enhance energy metabolism (van der Beek 1991, 1994). It is generally agreed that moderate physical activity *per se* does not adversely affect vitamin status when recommended amounts of vitamins are consumed in the diet (Clarkson 1991). Marginal vitamin deficiencies have been observed in athletes, but many of the published reports of vitamin deficiencies in athletes are invalid for methodological reasons: a shortfall in recommended intake relative to published recommended intakes is not indicative of a deficiency (van der Beek 1991, 1994; Chen & Wu 1996). Athletes with a balanced diet should receive the RDA provided energy intake is sufficient to balance expenditure (Shoorland 1988; Rokitzki *et al.* 1994a), although it must be recognized that not all athletes have a high energy intake, and not all eat a varied diet. Unfortunately, there are limited and conflicting data with regard to the micronutrient status of physically active individuals (van der Beek 1985; Belko 1987; Fogelholm 1992). Methods for the assessment of vitamin status are often inadequate, as outlined in the preceding chapter. Dietary surveys and food records have been used to assess the vitamin status of athletes, but tables of vitamin content are inherently unreliable, and the vitamin loss attributed to vitamin availability, processing, storage, and preparation of the foods is often not taken into account. Blood or other tissue levels of vitamins are affected by several factors including acute exercise and they may not be entirely accurate as measures of the nutritional status of athletes; caution should therefore be taken in interpreting the results (see Chapter 20). Furthermore, the RDAs are designed primarily to avoid nutritional deficiencies and do not focus on exercise or stressful environments. The RDA is determined by various professional bodies to designate the level of intake of a micronutrient that will meet the known nutritional needs of practically all healthy persons (Armstrong & Maresh 1996), and is based on an average-sized person with an average amount of physical activity and an average physiological requirement. This is then adjusted by a variable factor to compensate for incomplete utilization by the body, the variation in requirements among individuals and the bioavailability of the nutrients from different food sources (US National Research Council 1989). The definition of RDA is not identical for all nations and organizations (van der Beek 1991).

It is not clear that the RDA established for the general population may apply to athletes, labourers, or soldiers in heavy training (Shoorland 1988). There have been few reports on the setting of separate RDAs for athletes (Yakovlev 1957; Sports Science Committee of Japanese Association 1977; Grandjean 1989; Chen *et al.* 1992). The majority of dietary surveys conducted on athletic population clearly indicated that the vitamin intakes of all but a small minority of athletes exceed the RDA levels if a well-balanced diet is typically consumed (Sobal & Marquart 1994). Although vitamin intakes of less than the RDA do not indicate vitamin deficiencies *per se*, the further the intake falls below the RDA, the greater is the risk of developing a deficiency state.

Athletes have been targeted as a significant group for vitamin supplements, and dietary surveys and questionnaires of athletes confirm the widespread use of the vitamin supplements. Questionnaires completed by 2977 college and high school athletes have found that 44% of those surveyed took one or more vitamin supplements (Parr *et al.* 1984). In other, smaller surveys, 31% of 80 Australian athletes and 29% of 347 non-elite runners (Nieman *et al.* 1989) and 42–43% of football players, gymnasts and runners (Sobal & Marquart 1994) took vitamin supplements. Some studies have documented even higher percentages of athletes taking supplements, including 71% of female runners (Clark *et al.* 1988) and 100% of female bodybuilders (Lamar-Hildebrand *et al.* 1989). Supplementation is purported to enhance performance, delay fatigue, and speed up recovery by some ill-defined ergogenic mechanism. Despite the lack of evidence that large intakes of vitamin have positive effects on performance, many athletes are still taking vitamin supplements, because of a lack of nutritional knowledge and lack of familiarity with the dietary guidelines, and quite a number take very large doses. The concern is that not only the amounts of supplementation can be financially costly because of the large doses of up to 5000 times the recommended levels, but there is also the possibility that these excessive amounts may be harmful to health (see Chapter 20).

In the following sections, for each of the vitamin, there will be a brief description of exercise-induced changes in vitamin status and requirements, the effects of vitamin supplements, harmful effects of overdoses of vitamin intakes and the main food resources of vitamins (see Chapter 20). Vitamins are commonly classified into two groups, the fat soluble and the water soluble. Vitamins A, D, E and K are fat soluble. Vitamin C and members of the vitamin B complex are water soluble. Fat-soluble vitamins can be stored in appreciable amounts in the body, and their function is largely independent of energy metabolism. Water-soluble vitamins are not stored in large quantities in the body and must be ingested on a regular basis. Clinical symptoms can be developed in individuals with a diet deficient in B vitamins. Vitamin $B_{12}$ can be stored in the liver for a year or longer.

## Thiamin (vitamin $B_1$)

Vitamin $B_1$ as thiaminpyrophosphate (TPP, cocarboxylase), plays an important role in the oxidative decarboxylation of pyruvate to acetyl-coenzyme A (CoA) for entry into the Krebs cycle and subsequent oxidation to provide for adenosine triphosphate resynthesis. Thus, there is a possibility that the increased demand for acetyl-CoA during exercise would not be met in athletes with a thiamin deficiency. If this occurred, more pyruvate would be accumulated and converted to lactate, with the possibility that fatigue would develop more rapidly and aerobic performance could be impaired. Thiamin deficiency could also result in a reduced availability of succinate, a coingredient of haeme, leading to inadequate haemoglobin formation, another factor that could influence aerobic exercise capacity. However, little evidence has shown that ingestion of a vitamin $B_1$ supplement by athletes consuming a well-balanced diet has any effect on performance.

It has been noted that there is a good linear relationship between thiamin intake and energy intake (van der Beek 1994). It is generally accepted that the vitamin $B_1$ requirement is dependent on the total energy expenditure and is influenced by carbohydrate intake because vitamin $B_1$ is essential for the intermediary metabolism of carbohydrate. The vitamin $B_1$ necessary to meet the body's requirement intake may vary according to energy intake (Clarkson 1991), and 0.5 mg thiamin·4.2 MJ$^{-1}$ (1000 kcal$^{-1}$) is recommended for adults in most countries (US National Research Council 1989). Any increased requirement induced by exercise should be met by increased energy intake and well-balanced diet. However, reports from the Soviet Union in the early days indicated that the output of urinary vitamin $B_1$ of athletes decreased as the training load increased; it was reported that blood pyruvate levels increased by 30–40% as compared with sedentary individuals when vitamin $B_1$ intake was 2–3 mg·day$^{-1}$ (Yakovlev 1957). In order to keep pyruvate at normal levels, it was recommended that the vitamin $B_1$ intake should be 3–5 mg·day$^{-1}$ in the general population and 5–10 mg·day$^{-1}$ for athletes undergoing endurance training (Yakovlev 1957). Vytchikova (1958) indicated that the usual content of thiamin 1.5–2.0 mg·day$^{-1}$ in food rations of athletes is considered insufficient and that medical observation recommend approximately 10–20 mg daily supplementation.

Athletes do not have a lower intake of vitamin $B_1$ than the RDA and only very few have any signs of a biochemical deficiency (Fogelholm 1992), but athletes who are on energy-restricted diets for weight control are likely to have a less than adequate intake, and athletes who take a high percentage of their energy from low nutrient-density food such as candy, soda, etc. may be at risk (Clarkson 1991). Nutrition surveys in Chinese elite athletes indicated that about half of the athletes investigated had vitamin $B_1$ intakes that were lower than the RDA. The average dietary intakes of vitamin $B_1$ of the athletes undergoing vigorous training was 0.37–

**Table 21.1** Vitamin RDA for Chinese athletes. From Chen *et al.* (1992).

| Condition | Vitamin A (RE)* | Vitamin B$_1$ (mg) | Vitamin B$_2$ (mg) | Niacin (mg) | Vitamin C (mg) |
| --- | --- | --- | --- | --- | --- |
| Training | 1500 | 3–6 | 2.5 | 25 | 140 |
| Special condition† | 2400 | 5–10 | 2.5 | 25 | 200 |

*RE, retinol equivalent.
†Special condition refers to intensive vision for vitamin A, endurance training for vitamin B$_1$, competition period for vitamin C.

0.48 mg·4.2 MJ$^{-1}$ (1000 kcal$^{-1}$), and 25% of them have been found to be in a state of vitamin B$_1$ insufficiency as assessed by TPP method (blood transketolase coefficient) (Chen *et al.* 1989). In addition, systematic nutritional investigation showed that there has been a trend towards a decrease in vitamin B$_1$ intake because the consumption of cereal, especially whole grains, has decreased and the intake of animal foods has increased. The RDA of vitamin B$_1$ for Chinese athletes has been set at 3–6 mg·day$^{-1}$, which is about 1 mg·4.2 MJ$^{-1}$ (1000 kcal$^{-1}$) (Table 21.1) (Chen *et al.* 1989, 1992). The US National Research Council reported that the increased need of vitamin B$_1$ for athletes should be met by the larger quantities of food consumed. There has been no evidence for vitamin B$_1$ toxicity through oral ingestion. Good food sources of thiamin are identified in Chapter 20.

## Riboflavin (vitamin B$_2$)

Riboflavin functions as a coenzyme for a group of flavoproteins concerned with cellular oxidation: flavin adenine dinucleotide and flavin mononucleotide are the most common, and these act as hydrogen carriers in the mitochondrial electron transport system, being a component of oxidative enzymes, and are thus considered important for aerobic endurance activities. These coenzymes may also be important for the efficient functioning of glycolytic enzymes, and may have an effect on anaerobic type performance as well. The RDA of vitamin B$_2$ for adults is 1.5–1.7 mg·day$^{-1}$ for males and 1.2–1.3 mg·day$^{-1}$ for females (US National Research Council 1989;

Chinese Nutrition Society 1990). Since riboflavin is a component of several respiratory enzymes, the requirement is usually linked to energy intake, and the level of riboflavin intake recommended by the WHO is 0.5 mg·4.2 MJ$^{-1}$ (1000 kcal$^{-1}$). The RDA of vitamin B$_2$ for Chinese athletes has been set at 2.5 mg·day$^{-1}$ (Chen *et al.* 1992). Exercise training may increase the need of vitamin B$_2$. Using a RBC enzyme as an indicator of riboflavin status, it was noted that at an intake of 0.6 mg·4.2 MJ$^{-1}$ (1000 kcal$^{-1}$), young women who started a jogging programme developed a riboflavin deficiency (Belko *et al.* 1983), although riboflavin supplements have not been shown to have an effect on physical performance or aerobic capacity (Belko 1987). Most athletes have an adequate or greater than adequate intake of vitamin B$_2$ (Guilland *et al.* 1989; Burke & Read 1993), although biochemical insufficiencies were found for some athletes. The incidence of vitamin B$_2$ insufficiency has been reported to be relatively lower than that for thiamin (Haralambie 1976; Chen *et al.* 1989, 1992). Overdose problems have not been reported, and there is no evidence of toxicity. The possibility of riboflavin deficiency should be a concern for the vegetarian athlete if all dairy foods and other animal protein sources are omitted. Good sources include wheat germ, yeast, green leafy vegetables, and enriched cereals (see Chapter 20).

## Niacin (nicotinamide, nicotinic acid)

Niacin is a component of two important cofactors: nicotinamide adenine dinucleotide and nicotinamide adenine dinucleotide phosphate which serve as hydrogen acceptors and donors in glycolysis, fatty acid oxidation, and in the electron transport system. Niacin deficiency may possibly impair glycolysis and/or the oxidation processes of the citric acid cycle, so both anaerobic and aerobic type performances may be affected adversely. On the contrary, niacin supplementation in high doses may suppress free fatty acid release through decreased lipolysis which would result in a decreased availability of a major fuel source, forcing the muscle to rely more on its glycogen stores, and this may also adversely affect prolonged exercise performance (Williams 1985; Clarkson 1991).

The RDA for niacin is expressed as niacin equivalent because niacin may be synthesized in the body from tryptophan (1 mg of niacin is equivalent to 60 mg of dietary tryptophan). The requirement for niacin also usually is linked to energy intake which means that athletes who have a large energy intake need a proportionally higher niacin intake. The RDA for niacin in the general population has been set at $6.6 \, mg \cdot 4.2 \, MJ^{-1}$ ($1000 \, kcal^{-1}$) or about $14–19 \, mg \cdot day^{-1}$ for adults. The RDA for niacin for Chinese athletes has been set at 10 times that for riboflavin: $25 \, mg \cdot day^{-1}$. Since niacin is widely distributed in plant and animal food sources, most athletes show no evidence of niacin deficiency except those who have a chronically reduced dietary intake for weight control. Niacin deficiency symptoms may easily be solved by a well-balanced diet without recourse to specific supplementation. Good sources of niacin include poultry, meats, grain products, peanuts, yeast, fish, etc. (see Chapter 20).

## Pyridoxine (vitamin $B_6$)

Vitamin $B_6$ exists in five forms: pyridoxine, pyridoxal, pyridoxamine, pyridoxal phosphate (coenzyme form), and pyridoxamine phosphate (coenzyme form). The pyridines function in protein and amino acid metabolism, gluconeogenesis, and in formation of haemoglobin, myoglobin, and cytochromes, and are also a component of glycogen phosphorylase which plays a key role in glycogenolysis. Because exercise stresses metabolic pathways that use vitamin $B_6$, it has been suggested that the requirement for this vitamin is increased in athletes and active individuals (Manore 1994). Vitamin $B_6$ is essential in coenzymes related to nitrogen metabolism, and the requirement for vitamin $B_6$ is closely related to dietary protein intake. Currently the RDA for vitamin $B_6$ is $2.0 \, mg \cdot day^{-1}$ for men and $1.6 \, mg \cdot day^{-1}$ for women. If the dietary protein is more than $100 \, g \cdot day^{-1}$, then the intake of vitamin $B_6$ should be more than $2 \, mg \cdot day^{-1}$ (US National Research Council 1989; Manore 1994). Although the requirement for vitamin $B_6$ appears to increase when a high protein diet is consumed, vitamin $B_6$ is found in meats and other animal foods, and sufficient may be provided if these foods are the major source of protein in the diet. The incidence of acute toxicity of vitamin $B_6$ is low. Intakes of $117 \, mg$ of vitamin $B_6$ for more than 6 months can result in neurological impairment (US National Research Council 1989). Chronic ingestion of 2–6 g pyridoxine $\cdot day^{-1}$ has been shown to result in sensory neuropathy (Clarkson 1991). Some studies reported that athletes have low or marginal dietary intakes of vitamin $B_6$ (Hickson et al. 1987; Weight et al. 1988b; Guilland et al. 1989), whereas others reported mean intakes at or above the RDA (Faber et al. 1991; Singh et al. 1992a, 1992b, 1993). Young female athletes and those participating in sport training emphasizing low body weights need to be monitored regularly. Deficiencies should be corrected by a well-balanced diet, and if necessary, small amount of supplements within the RDA (Rokitzki et al. 1994a). There is no evidence suggesting that supplementation enhances athletic performance, so the use of vitamin $B_6$ as an ergogenic aid is contraindicated. Good food sources include meat, poultry, fish, whole grain, peanuts, soybeans, seeds, yeast and eggs (see Chapter 20).

## Cobalamin (vitamin $B_{12}$)

Vitamin $B_{12}$ is involved in a variety of metabolic

processes. It is an essential component in the formation and function of red blood cells. Because of this role, it is sometimes thought by athletes and their coaches that vitamin $B_{12}$ supplement should enhance the oxygen-carrying capacity of the blood and improve performance in those events where oxidative metabolism is important. In practice, however, vitamin $B_{12}$ supplementation will only help in cases of pernicious anaemia or macrocytic anaemia, and will not show benefits for the athlete with iron deficiency anaemia or for athletes whose iron stores are replete. In spite of this, vitamin $B_{12}$ injection is a common practice in sport, and it has been noted that some athletes have been receiving 1000 mg about 1 h before competition (Ryan 1977). The RDA for vitamin $B_{12}$ for the general adult population is $2 \mu g \cdot day^{-1}$, and the average diet contains about $5–15 \mu g \cdot day^{-1}$, so deficiency is rare. As for the general population, deficiency in athletes is rare, except for those who are complete vegetarians. This group may be susceptible to vitamin $B_{12}$ deficiency as the vitamin is found only in animal protein including meat, poultry, fish, egg, milk and milk products, and some fermented soybean products (see Chapter 20). Most vegetarians, however, are well aware of the need to ensure an adequate intake.

## Pantothenic acid

Pantothenic acid is a part of CoA, thus making it important in metabolism involving the Krebs cycle. The RDA for pantothenic acid is $4–7 mg \cdot day^{-1}$ (Williams 1985). Inadequate intakes of pantothenic acid are rare for the individual who has a normal diet, because it is widely distributed in foods including animal and plant foods such as eggs, yeast, whole grains, etc. It is not known if exercise increases the requirement for pantothenic acid. Results of studies on the effect of pantothenic acid supplementation on performance are equivocal (Nice *et al.* 1984; Litoff *et al.* 1985; Clarkson 1991). Nice *et al.* reported that supplementation with 1 g pantothenic acid · $day^{-1}$ (10 000% RDA) for 2 weeks had no effect on a treadmill run to exhaustion, pulse rate, blood

glucose levels, or several other blood measures in highly trained distance runners; it was concluded that pantothenic acid in pharmacological dosages has no significant effect on human exercise capacity (Nice *et al.* 1984).

## Folic acid (folate)

Folic acid acts as an coenzyme functioning in DNA synthesis for red blood cell formation, and is also important for nucleotide and amino acid metabolism. A deficiency state may cause anaemia, and at least in theory, a deficiency may affect aerobic endurance performance. The RDA has been set at $400 \mu g \cdot day^{-1}$ for non-trained adult males (US National Research Council 1989). The RDA set by the FAO/WHO is $200 \mu g \cdot day^{-1}$. No study is known to have been performed on the effects of folic acid supplements on physical performance. Since folate is present in large amounts in vegetables, fruits, and animal foods, a balanced diet would appear to provide adequate amounts of this vitamin (see Chapter 20).

## Vitamin B complex

Because of the close association of the vitamins in the B complex, the effects of deprivation of or supplementation with various combinations of the B vitamins have been studied. Results of some of the early studies showed that a deficiency of the B complex vitamins over a period of time, a few weeks at the most, could create a definite decrease in endurance capacity (Berryman *et al.* 1947). It is extremely unlikely that athletes on a well-balanced diet will encounter this level of deficiency. However, the effects of vitamin B complex supplements remain contradictory and further study is needed to determine the usefulness of vitamin B complex supplemention for athletes (Read & McGuffin 1983; Clarkson 1991).

## Ascorbic acid (vitamin C)

Vitamin C functions in the biosynthesis of collagen, catecholamines, serotonin and carnitine. It is also a powerful antioxidant which may aid intracellular oxidation-reduction reactions. Vitamin C also helps non-haem iron absorption, transport and storage. The deemed benefits of the effects of vitamin C supplements include stimulation of immune function and resistance to infection (Chen 1988) and a reduction in fatigue and muscle soreness, enhancing performance capacity and protecting cells from free radical damage (Kanter 1994), and thus it is perhaps the most widely used and studied of the vitamins.

The US RDA for vitamin C is $60\,mg \cdot day^{-1}$ (US National Research Council 1989), but recommended intakes vary widely between countries. In some countries, specific recommendations have been made for athletes, and the RDA for vitamin C has been set at $140\,mg \cdot day^{-1}$ during training and $200\,mg \cdot day^{-1}$ during competition periods for Chinese athletes on the basis of maintaining vitamin C in a saturation status as shown by urinary output (Chen et al. 1962, 1963, 1992). Most athlete groups studied have been reported to exceed the RDA for vitamin C, but a small percentage of athletes, particularly young gymnasts, have been found to have a less than adequate intake of vitamin C (Loosli et al. 1986; Chen et al. 1989). Megadoses of vitamin C can cause iron loading, may affect the availability of vitamin $B_{12}$ from food, and may also promote the formation of urinary stones, yet high intakes of vitamin C are relatively harmless (Clarkson 1991). A single bout of exercise may increase blood levels of ascorbic acid but decrease the ascorbic acid content of other tissues (Chen et al. 1965; Gleeson et al. 1987). Increases in plasma ascorbic acid levels correlate significantly with the increase in plasma cortisol, suggesting that exercise may cause ascorbic acid to be released from the adrenal gland or other organs into the circulation along with the release of cortisol. The effect of vitamin C supplementation on physical performance has been investigated intermittently over the past 50 years, but the results of these studies have been contradictory. The possible benefits of vitamin C supplementation on exercise-induced muscle damage remain doubtful and need further study.

Vitamin C is present in fresh fruits and vegetables, primarily the citrus fruits such as oranges, grapefruit, lemons and limes. Other good sources are broccoli, green peppers and greens. There is little doubt that a severe deficiency of vitamin C would have an adverse effect on work performance: the feelings of weakness and lassitude and the possibility of iron deficiency anaemia would certainly not be beneficial (Hodges 1980). Exercise may increase moderately the body's need for vitamin C, but to what extent exercise training will change an athlete's requirement for vitamin C is still not entirely clear. However, the inclusion of additional fruits and vegetables in the athletes' diet is advised.

## Vitamin A (retinol)

Vitamin A designates several compounds including retinol, retinaldehyde and retinoic acid. Vitamin A plays a major role in maintenance of proper vision and epithelial tissues, and is also involved in the development of bones and teeth as well as playing an important function in the body's immune response. β-carotene, the major carotenoid precursor of vitamin A, plays a role as an antioxidant. The need for vitamin A can be met by intake of carotenoid precursors commonly found in plants. The RDA for vitamin A is expressed in retinol equivalents (RE); one RE equals 1 μg retinol or 6 μg β-carotene. The RDA for vitamin A is 1000 RE (1000 μg retinol or 6000 μg β-carotene) for adult males and 800 RE (800 μg retinol or 4800 μg β-carotene) for adult females (US National Research Council 1989). Russian research suggested that extra vitamin A is needed in athletes requiring good visual acuity and alertness and during periods of stress (Williams 1985). The RDA for vitamin A for Chinese athletes was set at $1500\,RE \cdot day^{-1}$ (Chen et al. 1992).

The vitamin A intake of elite athletes has generally been found to be adequate, although it has been reported that 10–25% of the athletes investigated were ingesting less vitamin A than the RDA (Clarkson 1991). Studies that have assessed the vitamin A, C and E status of athletes have found that most had adequate blood levels of these vitamins (Weight *et al.* 1988b; Guilland *et al.* 1989; Fogelholm *et al.* 1992). Serum vitamin A levels of 5% of 182 athletes investigated had a value of less than $30 \mu g \cdot dl^{-1}$ (Chen *et al.* 1992). There has been no evidence of serious biochemical deficiencies of vitamin A existing in athletes. It is unlikely that vitamin A supplementation will enhance performance. Vitamin A supplementation is not necessary for athletes on an adequate diet (Williams 1985; Clarkson 1991). Whether the antioxidant role of β-carotene can reduce exercise damage due to free radical activity remains to be studied.

Vitamin A is one of the fat-soluble vitamins and hence may be stored in the body for considerable periods of time, unlike water-soluble vitamins. Overdosage over a period of time may cause a condition known as hypervitaminosis, characterized by anorexia, hair loss, hypercalcaemia, and kidney and liver damage (Aronson 1986). Sustained daily intakes exceeding 15 000 $\mu g \cdot day^{-1}$ of retinol can produce signs of toxicity (US National Research Council 1989). However, high doses of β-carotene are not generally considered to be toxic (US National Research Council 1989; Clarkson 1995). Bodily stores are available for short-term deficiency periods, and thus, no significant decrements would be revealed during short periods of reduced dietary intake of vitamin A. Good sources of vitamin A in the diet include liver, fish liver oils, butter, whole milk, cheese and egg yolk. Rich sources of the carotenoid are dark-green leafy vegetables, the yellow or orange fruits and vegetables (see Chapter 20).

## Vitamin D

Vitamin D represents any one of several sterol compounds in the body; vitamin $D_2$ (ergocalciferol) is the result of the irradiation of ergosterol. $D_3$ (cholecalciferol) is the naturally occurring compound in the skin, formed by exposure to the sunlight. The major function of vitamin D is its hormone-like action in the process of mineralization of bones and teeth and the regulation of calcium metabolism. It promotes absorption of calcium from the intestine and helps to prevent calcium deficiency. The RDA for vitamin D is $5 \mu g \cdot day^{-1}$ for adults (US National Research Council 1989), and no separate recommendations appear to have been made for athletes. Overdoses of vitamin D are potentially toxic and result in hypercalcaemia and hypercalciuria (US National Research Council 1989). Levels of five times the RDA are considered dangerous; intakes of $50 \mu g \cdot day^{-1}$ ($2000 IU \cdot day^{-1}$) for a prolonged time may pose considerable risk. Hypervitaminosis D leads to loss of weight, vomiting, nausea, lethargy and loss of muscle tone; calcium released from the bones may deposit in the soft tissues, in the walls of the blood vessels and in the kidneys.

Vitamin D deficiencies are rare in athletes with adequate intake of dairy products and exposure to sunlight, but those who have inadequate milk consumption and lack of sunshine may be at some risk for inadequate vitamin D nutriture. No known controlled research has been conducted on the role of vitamin D in physical performance (Van der Beek 1991). The role of vitamin D in providing calcium for newly forming muscle tissue is not clear and needs further investigation (Clarkson 1991). Vitamin D is present in fish liver oil and milk fortified with vitamin D (see Chapter 20).

## Vitamin E

Vitamin E is a fat-soluble vitamin. Its activity is derived from a number of tocopherols, the most active one of which is α-tocopherol. Vitamin E functions as an antioxidant of polyunsaturated fatty acids in cellular and subcellular membranes, and thus it serves as a free radical scavenger to protect cell membranes from lipid peroxidation. The RDA for vitamin E is 8–10 mg of α-tocopherol·$day^{-1}$. Vitamin E is relatively non-toxic up to $800 mg \cdot day^{-1}$ (US National Research Council 1989). Dietary records showed that between one third and one half of the athletes investigated consumed less than two thirds of the RDA (Loosli *et al.* 1986; Guilland *et al.* 1989). Guilland reported that the mean vitamin E intake of athletes was 77% of the RDA. However, vitamin E deficiencies are rare in athletes with a well-balanced diet. Although megadoses of vitamin E are relatively harmless, some individuals experience gastric disturbances and weakness when taking supplements ranging from 200 to 1000 IU (Clarkson 1991). Acute exercise has been shown to result in an increase of plasma levels of tocopherol, and the author suggested that tocopherol was mobilized from adipose tissue into the blood to be distributed to exercising muscles; however, this study did not correct for haemoconcentration and the small increase in plasma tocopherol was back to baseline after 10 min rest (Pincemail *et al.* 1988). This response to exercise has not been reported in another study (Duthie *et al.* 1990). It is not clear if the disparate findings are due to different exercise loads, different testing methods or to other factors.

Many studies have reported a significant effect of vitamin E supplementation on exercise performance, but the actual benefits are doubtful since many of these experiments were not well controlled. Those studies that have been well controlled have generally shown that vitamin E supplementation has no effect on performance (Shephard *et al.* 1974; Watt *et al.* 1974; Lawrence *et al.* 1975). On the contrary, supplements of vitamin E showed a beneficial effect on maximum oxygen uptake and a partially protective effect on cell membranes at high altitude; it was reported that mountain climbers with a vitamin E supplement working at an altitude of 5000 m exhaled lower levels of pentane, a marker of lipid peroxidation, and exhibited a higher anaerobic threshold than controls (Simon-Schnass & Pabst 1990). Another study also showed that the impairment of blood flow parameters was attenuated by vitamin E supplementation in mountaineers at altitude (Simon-Schnass & Korniszewski 1990). The positive effect may be due to the antioxidant properties of vitamin E. At high altitudes, vitamin E may counteract the effect of the increased lipid peroxidation of red blood cell membranes caused by the decreased availability of oxygen (Williams 1989). Vitamin E may also play a role in reducing muscle damage and oxidative stress, as shown by a reduction in muscle-specific enzyme levels in serum after strenuous exercise (Rokitzki *et al.* 1994b). However, results are equivocal as to whether muscle damage can be reduced by vitamin E supplementation (see Chapter 20).

In short, there has been much debate on the vitamin requirements of athletes, yet carefully controlled studies are limited.

## Conclusion

The following is a summary of the main viewpoints.

**1** Vitamin deficiencies may result in decreased exercise performance, and it has been demonstrated that vitamin supplements improve performance in persons with pre-existing vitamin deficiencies.

**2** Vitamin supplements are generally unnecessary in athletes consuming well-balanced diets.

**3** Athletes participating in strenuous training may need monitoring of vitamin status even if consuming the RDA levels of vitamins.

**4** Vitamin supplements should be suggested for athletes in special conditions including those who are on a weight loss diet, or have eating disorders, or low energy intakes. Supplementation is only warranted when there is reasonable evidence to suggest that a deficiency may be present.

**5** Excessive vitamin intake, especially of the fat-soluble vitamins, can be accumulated to a level that may be toxic. Prolonged excessive intake of water-soluble vitamins also may be harmful and cause nutritional imbalances. Attention to food choices, rather than specific supplementation, is the preferred option.

## References

Armstrong, L.E. & Maresh, C.M. (1996) Vitamin and mineral supplements as nutritional aids to exercise performance and health. *Nutrition Reviews* **54**, S149–S158.

Aroson, V. (1986) Vitamins and minerals as ergogenic aids. *Physician and Sports Medicine* **14**, 209–212.

Belko, A.Z. (1987) Vitamins and exercise: an update. *Medicine and Science in Sports and Exercise* **19**, S191–S196.

Belko, A.Z., Obarzenek, E., Karwalf, H.J. *et al.* (1983) Effect of exercise on riboflavin requirements of young women. *American Journal of Clinical Nutrition* **37**, 507–517.

Berryman, G., Henderson, C.R., Wheeler, N.C. *et al.* (1947) Effects in young men consuming restricted quantities of B-complex vitamines and proteins, and changes associated with supplementation. *American Journal of Physiology* **148**, 618–647.

Burke, L.M. & Read, R.S.D. (1993) Dietary supplements in sport. *Sports Medicine* **15**, 43–46.

Chen, J.D. (1988) Some sports nutrition researches in China. In *China's Sports Medicine* (ed. M.Y. Qu & C.L. Yu), pp. 94–113. Medicine and Sport Science, Vol. 28. Karger, Basel.

Chen, J.D. & Wu, L. (1996) Nutrition of vitamins and sports. In *Practical Sports Medicine* (ed. M.Y. Qu), pp. 244–246. Beijing Science and Technology Publishing House, Beijing.

Chen, J.D., Yu, X.X. & Nie, F.E. (1962) The study of vitamin C status and requirement of the gymnasts and middle-long distance runners. *Journal of Chinese Medicine* **7**, 454–457.

Chen, J.D., Liao, G.Z. & Yu, C.Y. (1963) Primary approach of the vitamin C requirement of athletes during competition period from the excretion of urinary vitamin C. *Journal of Chinese Medicine* **49**, 256–260.

Chen, J.D., Liao, G.Z. & Yu, C.Y. (1965) The vitamin C metabolism of organism in sports. *Journal of the Beijing Medical College* **1**, 1–72.

Chen, J.D., Wang, J.F., Li, K.J., Wang, S.W., Jiao, Y. & Hou, X.Y. (1989) Nutritional problems and measures in elite and amateur athletes. *American Journal of Clinical Nutrition* **49** (Suppl.), 1084–1089.

Chen, J.D., Wang, J.F., Wang, S.W., Li, K.J. & Chen, Z.M. (1992) Recommended dietary allowances for Chinese athletes. In *Integration of Medical and Sports Sciences* (ed. Y. Sato, J. Poortmans, I. Hashimoto & Y. Oshida), pp. 336–341. Medicine and Sport Science, Vol. 37. Basel, Karger.

Chinese Nutrition Society (1990) Document of the Chinese Nutrition Society: illustration of the recommended dietary allowances of the Chinese. *Acta Nutrimenta Sinica* **12**, 1–10.

Clark, N., Nelson, M. & Evans, W. (1988) Nutrition education for elite female runners. *Physician and Sports Medicine* **16**, 124–136.

Clarkson, P.M. (1991) Vitamins and trace element. In *Ergogenics*. Vol. 4. *Enhancement of Performance in Exercise and Sport* (ed. D.R. Lamb & M.H. Williams), pp. 123–182. W.C. Brown, USA.

Clarkson, P.M. (1995) Micronutrients and exercise: anti-oxidants and minerals. *Journal of Sports Sciences* **13**, S11–S24.

Daniel, L.J. (1991) Vitamins. In *The Encyclopedia Americana* (international edn). Vol. 30, pp. 183–191. Grolier, Danbury, CO.

Duthie, G.G., Robertson, J.D., Maughan, R.J. & Morrice, P.C. (1990) Blood antioxidant status and erythrocyte lipid peroxidation following distance running. *Archives of Biochemistry and Biophysics* **282**, 78–83.

Faber, M. & Spinnler Benade, A.-J. (1991) Mineral and vitamin intake in field athletes (discus-hammer, javelin-throwers and shot-putters). *International Journal of Sports Medicine* **12**, 324–327.

Fogelholm, M. (1992) Vitamin and mineral status in physically active people. In *Physical Activity and Nutritional Status: a Theoretical Basis for Balance in Vitamin and Mineral Status in Physically Active People* (ed. M. Fogelholm), pp. 3–19. Publications of the Social Insurance Institution, Turku, Finland.

Fogelholm, M. (1994) Vitamins, minerals and supplementation in soccer. *Journal of Sports Sciences* **12**, S23–S27.

Fogelholm, M., Rehunen, S., Gref, C.-G. *et al.* (1992) Dietary intake and thiamin, iron, and zinc status in elite nordic skiers during different training periods. *International Journal of Sport Nutrition* **2**, 351–365.

Gleeson, M., Robertson, J.D. & Maughan, R.J. (1987) Influence of exercise on ascorbic acid status in man. *Clinical Science* **73**, 501–505.

Grandjean, A.C. (1989) Macronutrient intake of US athletes compared with the general population and recommendation made for athletes. *American Journal of Clinical Nutrition* (Suppl.) **49**, 1070–1076.

Guilland, J.-C., Penaranda, T., Gallet, C., Boggio, V., Fuchs, F. & Klepping, J. (1989) Vitamin status of young athletes including the effects of supplementation. *Medicine and Science in Sports and Exercise* **21**, 441–449.

Haralambie, G. (1976) Vitamin B2 status in athletes and the influence of riboflavin administration on neuromuscular irritability. *Nutrition and Metabolism* **20**, 1–8.

Hickson, J.F., Duke, M.A., Risser, W.L., Johnson, C.W., Palmer, R. & Stockton, J.E. (1987) Nutritional intake from food sources of high school football athletes. *Journal of the American Dietetic Association* **87**, 1656–1659.

Hodges, R.E. (1980) Ascorbic acid. In *Modern Nutrition in Health and Disease* (ed. R.S. Goodhart & M.E. Shils), pp. 259–273. Lea and Febiger, Philadelphia, PA.

Kanter, M.M. (1994) Free radicals, exercise, and antioxidant supplementation. *International Journal of Sport and Nutrition* **4**, 205–220.

Lamar-Hilderbrand, N., Saldanha, L. & Endres, J. (1989) Dietary and exercise practices of college-aged female bodybuilders. *Journal of the American Dietetic Association* **89**, 1308–1310.

Lawrence, J.D., Bower, R.C., Riehl, W.P. & Smith, J.L. (1975) Effects of Alpha-tocopherol acetate on the swimming endurance of trained swimmers. *American Journal of Clinical Nutrition* **28**, 205–208.

Litoff, D., Scherzer, H. & Harrison, J. (1985) Effects of pantothenic acid supplementation on human exercise (abstract). *Medicine and Science in Sports and Exercise* **17**, 287.

Loosli, A.R., Benson, J., Gillien, D.M. & Bourdet, K. (1986) Nutrition habits and knowledge in competitive adolescent female gymnasts. *Physician and Sports Medicine* **14**, 118–130.

Manore, M.M. (1994) Vitamin B6 and exercise. *International Journal of Sport and Nutrition* **4**, 89–103.

Nice, C., Reeves, A.G., Brinck-Johnsen, T. & Noll, W. (1984) The effects of pantothenic acid on human exercise capacity. *Journal of Sports Medicine and Physical Fitness* **24**, 26–29.

Nieman, D.C., Gates, J.V., Butler, L.M., Pollett, S.J., Dietrich, S.J. & Lutz, R.D. (1989) Supplementation patterns in marathon runners. *Journal of the American Dietetic Association* **89**, 1615–1619.

Parr, R.B., Porter, M.A. & Hodgson, S.C. (1984) Nutrition knowledge and practices of coaches, trainers, and athletes. *Physician and Sports Medicine* **12**, 126–138.

Pincemail, J., Deby, C., Camus, G. *et al.* (1988) Tocopherol mobilization during intensive exercise. *European Journal of Applied Physiology* **57**, 189–191.

Read, M.H. & McGuffin, S.L. (1983) The effect of B-complex supplementation on endurance performance. *Journal of Sports Medicine and Physical Fitness* **23**, 178–184.

Rokitzki, L., Sagredos, A.N., Reub, F., Büchner, M. & Keul, J. (1994a) Acute changes in vitamin B6 status in endurance athletes before and after a marathon. *International Journal of Sport and Nutrition* **4**, 154–165.

Rokitzki, L., Logemann, E., Huber, G., Keck, E. & Keul, J. (1994b) Alpha-tocopherol supplementation in racing cyclists during extreme endurance training. *International Journal of Sport and Nutrition* **4**, 253–264.

Ryan, A. (1977) Nutritional practices in athletes abroad. *Physician and Sports Medicine* **5**, 33–41.

Shephard, R.J., Campbell, R., Pimm, P., Stuart, D. & Wright, G.R. (1974) Vitamin E, exercise, and the recovery from physical activity. *European Journal of Applied Physiology* **33**, 119–126.

Shoorland, F.B. (1988) Is our knowledge of human nutrition soundly based? *World Review of Nutrition and Diet* **57**, 126–213.

Simon-Schnass, I. & Pabst, H. (1988) Influence of vitamin E on physical performance. *International Journal of Vitamin and Nutrition Research* **58**, 49–54.

Simon-Schnass, I. & Korniszewski, L. (1990) The influ-

ence of vitamin E on rheological parameters in high altitude mountaineers. *International Journal of Vitamin and Nutrition Research* **60**, 26–34.

Singh, A., Moses, F.M. & Deuester, P.A. (1992a) Chronic multivitamin-mineral supplementation does not enhance physical performance. *Medicine and Science in Sports and Exercise* **24**, 726–732.

Singh, A., Moses, F.M. & Deuester, P.A. (1992b) Vitamin and mineral status in physically active men: effects of high-potency supplement. *American Journal of Clinical Nutrition* **55**, 1–7.

Singh, A., Evans, P., Gallagher, K.L. & Deuster, P.A. (1993) Dietary intakes and biochemical profiles of nutritional status of ultramarathoners. *Medicine and Science in Sports and Exercise* **25**, 328–334.

Sobal, J. & Marquart, L.F. (1994) Vitamin/mineral supplement use among athletes: a review of the literature. *International Journal of Sport and Nutrition* **4**, 320–334.

US National Research Council Food and Nutrition Board (1989) *Recommended Dietary Allowances*, 10th edn. National Academy Press, Washington, DC.

Van der Beek, E.J. (1985) Vitamins and endurance training. Food for running or faddish claims? *Sports Medicine* **2**, 175–197.

Van der Beek, E.J. (1991) Vitamin supplementation and physical exercise performance. *Journal of Sports Science* **9**, 79–89.

Van der Beek, E.J. (1994) Vitamin supplementation and physical exercise performance. In *Foods, Nutrition and Sports Performance* (ed. C. Williams & J.T. Delvin), pp. 95–107. E & FN Spon, London.

Vytchikova, M. (1958) Increasing the vitamin B1 content in the rations of athletes. *Chemistry Abstracts* **52**, 147–187.

Watt, T., Romet, T.T., McFarlane, I., McGuey, D., Allen, C. & Goode, R.C. (1974) Vitamin E and oxygen consumption (abstract). *Lancet* **2**, 354–355.

Weight, L.M., Myburgh, K.H. & Noakes, T.D. (1988a) Vitamin and mineral supplementation: effect on the running performance of trained athletes. *American Journal of Clinical Nutrition* **47**, 186–191.

Weight, L.M., Noakes, T.D., Labadarios, D., Graves, J., Jacobs, P. & Bermen, P.A. (1988b) Vitamin and mineral status of trained athletes including the effects of supplementation. *American Journal of Clinical Nutrition* **47**, 192–195.

Williams, M.H. (1985) The role of vitamins in physical activity. In *Nutrition Aspects of Human Physical and Athletic Performance*, 2nd edn (ed. M.H. Williams), pp. 147–185. Charles C. Thomas, Springfield, IL.

Williams, M.H. (1989) Vitamin supplementation and athletic performance, an overview. *International Journal of Vitamins and Nutrition Research* **30**, 161–191.

Yakovlev, N.N. (1957) Sports nutrition. *Nutrition Problems* (in Russian) **16**, 58–59.

# Chapter 22

# Exercise-induced Oxidative Stress and Antioxidant Nutrients

CHANDAN K. SEN, SASHWATI ROY AND LESTER PACKER

## Introduction

'Diradical' molecular oxygen has a strong affinity for four more electrons. Under normal resting conditions, approximately 95% of all oxygen consumed by the mammalian cells is reduced *via* the mitochondrial cytochrome oxidase to yield two molecules of water and energy. The remaining 3–5% of oxygen consumed at rest can be utilized in an alternative univalent pathway for the reduction of oxygen, and reactive oxygen species (ROS) are thus produced (Singal & Kirshenbaum 1990). Formation of superoxides and hydrogen peroxide can be regulated by either enzymatic or non-enzymatic mechanisms, whereas no enzymes are required for the formation of hydroxyl radical. Hydroxyl radical is highly reactive and may be formed either through a iron-catalysed Fenton reaction ($Fe^{2+} + H_2O_2 \rightarrow Fe^{3+} + OH^- + HO^\bullet$) or through the Haber–Weiss reaction ($O_2^{\bullet-} + H_2O_2 + Fe^{2+} \rightarrow O_2 + OH^- + HO^\bullet + Fe^{3+}$).

Partial reduction of oxygen, an event primarily underlying the generation of ROS, has been shown to be catalysed by a number of enzymes of rat liver. Some of the enzymes responsible for the generation of hydrogen peroxide or superoxide anion radical are listed in Table 22.1. Boveris *et al.* (1972) have shown that mitochondria, microsomes, peroxisomes and cytosolic enzymes are effective $H_2O_2$ generators, contributing in the rat liver, respectively, 15%, 45%, 35% and 5% to the cytosolic $H_2O_2$ at a $Po_2$ of 158 mmHg when fully supplemented by their substrates. Bio-

transformation of xenobiotics (e.g. pollutants and drugs), especially *via* cytochrome $P_{450}$-dependent mechanisms, may also contribute to the generation of reactive oxygen species (Archakov & Bachmanova 1990; Roy & Hanninen 1993).

Oxidative stress is now known to be implicated in the pathogenesis of a wide variety of health disorders, including coronary heart diseases, cerebrovascular diseases, emphysema, bronchitis, chronic obstructive lung disease, some forms of cancer, diabetes, skeletal muscular dystrophy, infertility, cataractogenesis, dermatitis, rheumatoid arthritis, AIDS-related dysfunctions, and Alzheimer's and Parkinson's diseases (Sen & Hanninen 1994; Davies & Ursini 1995). In addition, reactive oxygen species are thought to critically contribute to ageing and age-related disorders (Levine & Stadtman 1996). A late-breaking aspect of ROS action that has drawn the attention of current biomedical research is the ability of these reactive species to modulate a number of intracellular signal transduction processes that are critically linked to widespread pathologies such as cancer, human immuno-deficiency virus replication and atherosclerosis. ROS, at a concentration much below that required to cause oxidative damage to biological structures, can act on highly specific molecular loci inside the cell (Sen & Packer 1996).

## Exercise-induced oxidative stress

In exercise physiology, a common approach to

**Table 22.1** Rat liver enzymes that may contribute to the generation of reactive oxygen species. From Sies (1974).

| Enzyme | EC | Localization |
|---|---|---|
| Glycolate oxidase | 1.1.3.1 | Peroxisome |
| L-α-hydroxyacid oxidase | 1.1.3α | Peroxisome |
| L-gulonolactone oxidase | 1.1.3.8 | Cytosol |
| Aldehyde oxidase | 1.2.3.1 | Cytosol |
| Xanthine oxidase | 1.2.3.2 | Cytosol |
| D-amino-acid oxidase | 1.4.3.3 | Peroxisome |
| Monoamine oxidase | 1.4.3.4 | Mitochondrial outer membrane |
| Pyridoxamine oxidase | 1.4.3.5 | Endoplasmic reticulum |
| Diamine oxidase | 1.4.3.6 | Endoplasmic reticulum |
| NADPH-cytochrome $c$ reductase | 1.6.99.1 | Endoplasmic reticulum |
| NADPH-cytochrome $c$ reductase | 1.6.99.3 | Peroxisome core |
| Urate oxidase | 1.7.3.3 | Peroxisome core |
| Superoxide dismutase | 1.15.1.1 | Cytosol and mitochondrial matrix |

measure physical fitness is based on the ability of an individual to utilize atmospheric oxygen in a given interval of time per kilogram of body weight, i.e. the aerobic capacity. Therefore, athletes aim to boost their aerobic capacity to the highest possible limit. Supply of more and more oxygen to active tissues fuels oxidative metabolism that produces higher amounts, compared with anaerobic metabolism, of energy-rich phosphates and avoids the formation of lactate during the energy supply process. Physical exercise may be associated with a 10–20-fold increase in whole body oxygen uptake (Åstrand & Rodahl 1986). Oxygen flux in the active peripheral skeletal muscle fibres may increase by as much as 100–200-fold during exercise (Keul et al. 1972). Does this markedly enhanced consumption of oxygen by the tissue at exercise contribute to oxidative stress? This question was first addressed in 1978 when it was observed that strenuous physical exercise indeed induced oxidative damage to lipids in various tissues (Dillard et al. 1978). One of the early studies which kindled a strong motivation for further research in the area of exercise and oxygen toxicity was reported by Davies et al. (1982). Using the electron paramagnetic or spin resonance (EPR or ESR) spectroscopy for the direct detection of free radical species in tissues, it was shown that exhaustive exercise results in a two- to threefold increase in free radical concentrations of the muscle and liver of rats exercised on a treadmill. Since then, a considerable body of research has accumulated showing that strenuous physical exercise may be associated with oxidative stress (Sen et al. 1994c).

## Possible mechanisms

During exercise, several mechanisms may contribute to the generation of excess ROS. Some of the possibilities are listed below.

### Electron transport chain

Boveris et al. (1972) showed that mitochondria can generate $H_2O_2$. Exercise training increases electron flux capacity of skeletal muscle mitochondria, and this effect is known to be a mechanism by which aerobic capacity of trained muscles is increased (Robinson et al. 1994). It is likely that the exercise-associated increased electron flux in the mitochondria may result in enhanced 'leak' of partially reduced forms of oxygen centred radicals.

### Ischaemia reperfusion

During exercise, blood is shunted away from several organs and tissues (e.g. kidneys, splanchnic reserves) and fed to active working muscles. As a result, some of these organs or tissues may experience transient hypoxia. In addition, during exercise at or above $\dot{V}o_{2max}$, and perhaps at lower intensities, fibres within the working muscle may experience hypoxia. During the exercise recovery phase, these tissues, that were subject to transient hypoxia during exercise, are reoxygenated, resulting in the well-known burst of ROS production that is characteristic of ischaemia-reperfusion (Kellogg & Fridovich 1975; Wolbarsht & Fridovich 1989).

## Catecholamine auto-oxidation

During exercise, catecholamine levels in the circulation may increase severalfold (Singh 1992). Auto-oxidation of these catecholamines may represent a significant source of ROS during exercise.

## Xanthine oxidase activity

Mainly located in the vessel walls of most tissues, including cardiac and skeletal muscle, the enzyme xanthine dehydrogenase (XDH) catalyses the oxidation of hypoxanthine to xanthine, and xanthine to uric acid. While in its native form, XDH uses $NAD^+$ as an electron acceptor. Under certain conditions, e.g. ischaemia–reperfusion and extreme hypotension as in haemorrhagic shock, XDH may either reversibly or irreversibly be transformed to xanthine oxidase. In contrast to the native dehydrogenase form, xanthine oxidase utilizes $O_2$ as the electron acceptor and produces superoxides as a result while catalysing the oxidation of hypoxanthine to uric acid (Hellsten 1994).

## Neutrophil oxidative burst

As weapons for pathogen destruction and immunoprotection, ROS have been put to good use by phagocytes. Nicotinamide adenine dinucleotide phosphate (NADPH) oxidase located in the plasma membrane of neutrophils produces superoxides on purpose. Following spontaneous dismutation, superoxides generated in this way contribute to $H_2O_2$ formation. When activated by immune-challenge or such other stimuli, neutrophils release myeloperoxidase into the extracellular medium. Myeloperoxidase, released as such, complexes with $H_2O_2$ to form an enzyme–substrate complex with an oxidizing potential. The complex oxidizes chloride ($Cl^-$) to produce hypochlorous acid (HOCl). $O_2^{\bullet-}$, $H_2O_2$ and HOCl may be considered as broad spectrum physiological 'antibiotics' that eliminate pathogenic infection. Unfortunately, for this, the host cell has to pay a price in the form of inflammation (Edmonds & Blake 1994). Oxidative burst in leucocytes marginated to skeletal muscle during exercise may cause tissue damage (Weiss 1989; Ward 1991).

## Nitric oxide synthesis

Nitric oxide (NO) has one unpaired electron and is therefore a radical by definition. Cells like macrophages which are capable of producing both NO and superoxides are the likely host of a powerful ROS, the peroxynitrite anion ($ONOO^-$). Formed by the reaction of NO with superoxide, the peroxynitrite anion is a relatively long-lived ROS. In this way, NO may magnify superoxide toxicity. Human skeletal muscle expresses two different constitutive isoforms of NO synthase in different cellular compartments (Frandsen *et al.* 1996). Activity of skeletal muscle is known to be associated with a marked increase of NO production and release by the tissue (Balon & Nadler 1994). Increased end product of NO metabolism has been observed in the postexercise plasma of both athletes and non-athletes (Jungersten *et al.* 1997).

## Metal ions

Conditions, e.g. lowering of plasma pH to less than 6.0, haemolysis, ischaemia-reperfusion, that lead to the release of transition metal ions, e.g. iron and copper, may amplify ROS toxicity (Jenkins & Halliwell 1994).

Other conditions that may contribute to oxidative stress are cigarette smoking, alcoholism and high altitude (Moller *et al.* 1996). Each puff of a cigarette is estimated to contain approximately $10^{14}$ free radicals in the tar phase and approximately $10^{15}$ in the gas phase (Duthie & Arthur 1994). The metabolism of ethanol produces acetaldehyde that is known to consume the key physiological antioxidant, glutathione (GSH) (Videla & Valenzuela 1982). Ingestion of ethanol is associated with enhanced lipid peroxidation (Nadiger *et al.* 1988). Increased levels of lipid peroxidation by-products were observed in the alcohol-administered rat cerebral cortex, cerebellum and brain stem (Nadiger *et al.* 1986). Several factors, including hypoxia, altered mitochondrial respiration and exposure to UV radiation, are known contribute to oxidative stress at high altitude (Simon-Schnass 1994; Moller *et al.* 1996). It is also evident that exercise can induce changes in biochemical parameters that are indicative of oxidative stress in the fit horse and that this is exacerbated during exercise at high temperature and humidity (Mills *et al.* 1996).

## Evidence

Multiple unsaturation points in polyunsaturated fatty acids (PUFA) make them highly susceptible to ROS attack and oxidative damage. Uncontrolled and autocatalytic oxidative destruction of PUFA, commonly referred to as lipid peroxidation, is initiated when a ROS having sufficient energy to abstract a H-atom of a methylene ($-CH_2$) group (of the PUFA backbone) reacts with a PUFA (Alessio 1994). Peroxyl radicals thus formed are particularly dangerous because they are capable of propagating oxidative damage. These ROS are carried by the blood to distant targets where fresh oxidative damage may be initiated. Membrane lipid peroxidation may alter fluidity and permeability, and compromise the integrity of the barrier. Hence, the study of lipid peroxidation to estimate oxidative stress is a popular practice. In 1978, Dillard *et al.* first reported that in humans physical exercise at 75% $\dot{V}O_{2max.}$ increased the level of pentane, a possible by-product of oxidative lipid damage or lipid

peroxidation, by 1.8-fold in the expired air compared with resting subjects. Since then, considerable evidence has accumulated showing that physical exercise may trigger lipid peroxidation in several tissues including skeletal muscles, heart, liver, erythrocytes and plasma (Sen 1995). In a human study, serum lipid peroxidation was measured by three different methods during physical exercise of different duration with the aim of uncovering the significance of each method in measuring oxidative stress after physical exercise (Vasankari *et al.* 1995).

Oxidative protein damage is widespread within the body at rest. It has been estimated that, at rest, 0.9% of the total oxygen consumed by a cell contributes to protein oxidation (Floyd 1995). Most of this damage is irreparable, and by-products of such damage are either stored or degraded. Proteins that have been damaged by reactive oxygen are highly susceptible to proteolytic cleavage. The amount of oxidized protein in various tissues increases with age (Levine & Stadtman 1996). Certain components of protein such as tyrosine, methionine, tryptophan, histidine, and sulfhydryl residues are highly susceptible to oxidative damage. Following reactive oxygen attack, amino acid residues are converted to carbonyl derivatives. Alternatively, reducing sugars linked with the $\varepsilon$ amino group of Lys residues can be oxidized. As a result, protein carbonyl formation is widely used as an index of oxidative protein damage. Other specific markers of oxidative amino acid modification are dityrosine crosslinking and formation of disulphide bridges (-S-S-) and mixed disulphides in cysteine residues. For example, in dystrophic muscle the protein disulphide to sulphydryl (SS/SH) ratio has been observed to be increased, suggesting the possible involvement of oxidative damage (Kondo & Itokawa 1994). Oxidative modification of proteins may cause receptor modification, disturbance in intracellular ionic homeostasis, and altered signal transduction, and may also influence other fundamental cell-regulatory processes. Reznick *et al.* (1992) have reported that exhaustive exercise triggers skeletal muscle protein oxidation in rats. In another study where rats were subjected to exhaustive exercise, we (Sen *et al.* 1997a) observed consistent effects of physical exercise on tissue protein oxidation. Protein carbonyl levels in the red gastrocnemius muscle were roughly three time higher in exercised rats. In the vastus lateralis muscle, exercise increased the carbonyl content by 69%. Exhaustive exercise also increased protein oxidation in the liver, but the effect was much less pronounced than that in the muscles (Sen *et al.* 1997a). In another study, 10–15 min of swim exercise resulted in oxidation of rat erythrocyte membrane protein. Following exercise, skeletal muscle microsomes contained decreased sulphydryls and protein cross-linking was extensive (Rajguru *et al.* 1994). We observed that in skeletal muscle cells certain membrane $K^+$ transport proteins are highly sensitive to oxidant exposure (Sen *et al.* 1995).

In humans, the number of oxidative hits to the DNA per cell per day has been estimated to be as high as 10000 (Ames *et al.* 1993). Oxidative lesions of DNA accumulate with age. A 2-year-old rat is estimated to have two million oxidative DNA lesions per cell, which is about twice that in a young rat. In mammals, oxidative DNA damage appears to be roughly related to the metabolic rate (Ames *et al.* 1993). Such a trend, suggesting a relationship between metabolic rate and oxidative DNA damage, makes it important to study the effect of exercise on oxidative DNA modifications. Information regarding exercise-induced oxidative DNA damage is limited, however. Ten hours after marathon running, the ratio of urinary oxidized nucleosides per creatinine increased 1.3-fold above rest (Alessio & Cutler 1990). Neutrophils represent 50–60% of the total circulating leucocytes, and Smith *et al.* (1990) have shown that a single bout of exercise may remarkably increase ROS production by the neutrophils. We were therefore interested to see how different intensities of exercise may affect leucocyte DNA in humans. Results obtained in our study (Sen *et al.* 1994d) indicate the possibility that exercise-associated oxidative stress may initiate DNA damage in leucocytes. Out of the 36 measurements carried out with nine subjects

during four exercise tests, DNA damage was not detected in 11 cases, however. In another study, no significant increase in the urinary level of the oxidized RNA adduct 8-hydroxyguanosine following 90 min of bicycle exercise by young healthy men was observed (Viguie *et al.* 1993). In a later study, the single-cell gel test or COMET assay was employed to detect exercise-induced DNA damage in human white blood cells with increased sensitivity. Incremental exercise on a treadmill performed by healthy non-smoking men clearly caused DNA damage (Hartmann *et al.* 1995). Strenuous exercise for approximately $10 \text{ h} \cdot \text{day}^{-1}$ for 30 days also increased the rate of oxidative DNA modification by 33% (95% confidence limits, 3–67%; $P < 0.02$) in 20 men. It was suggested that oxidative DNA damage may increase the risk of the development of cancer and premature ageing in humans performing strenuous exercise on a regular basis (Poulsen *et al.* 1996).

Another line of evidence that supports the hypothesis that physical exercise may induce oxidative stress is the lowering of tissue levels of antioxidants during exercise. In view of the above-mentioned increases in tissue oxidative stress indices following exercise, such lowering of tissue antioxidant levels in response to physical exercise is thought to be a result of increased antioxidant consumption in oxidative stress challenged tissues. Several studies have shown that physical exercise decreases tissue levels of vitamin E (Goldfarb & Sen 1994). It is thought that exercise-induced mobilization of free fatty acids from the adipose tissues is accompanied by the loss of tocopherols from the tissue. As a result, tocopherol levels increased in human blood following intense cycling. This elevation of tocopherol levels in the circulation is transient and the level returns to normal in the early phase of recovery (Pincemail *et al.* 1988). Treadmill exercise-induced decrease in total antioxidant capacity of blood has also been evident in male claudication patients (Khaira *et al.* 1995).

It has been consistently reported from several laboratories (Gohil *et al.* 1988; Sen *et al.* 1994d; Tessier *et al.* 1995; Vina *et al.* 1995; Laaksonen *et al.*

1996) that physical exercise induces blood GSH oxidation even at submaximal intensities. This response is relatively rapid and can be observed after only a few minutes of exercise. Given the critical role of GSH in the antioxidant defence network and other physiological functions, this effect of exercise on blood GSH may be expected to have important implications (Sen & Packer 1999).

## Exercise training

In 1973, Caldarera *et al.* were the first to show that acute exercise increases catalase activity in rat liver, heart and skeletal muscle. Since then a relatively large number of studies have shown that endurance exercise training regimes may strengthen antioxidant defences in organs such as the skeletal muscle, heart and liver (Ji 1994; Ohno *et al.* 1994; Sen & Hanninen 1994; Powers & Criswell 1996). Results from needle biopsy samples collected from the vastus lateralis muscle of healthy men showed that individuals with high aerobic capacity had significantly greater activities of catalase and superoxide dismutase in their muscles. A strong positive correlation ($r=0.72$, $P<0.01$) between the subject's maximum oxygen uptake and muscle catalase was noted. A similar correlation was also observed between the subject's maximum oxygen uptake and muscle superoxide dismutase ($r=0.60$, $P<0.05$). The study also found that there was a rank order relationship between tissue oxygen consumption and antioxidant enzyme activity (Jenkins *et al.* 1984). In a study on exercise-induced oxidative stress in diabetic young men, we observed that levels of lipid peroxidation by-products in the resting plasma, and the exercise-induced increase in plasma lipid peroxidation by-products, strongly correlated ($r=-0.82$ and $0.81$, respectively) with the aerobic capacity of the individuals, suggesting a protective effect of physical fitness (Laaksonen *et al.* 1996). It has been observed that GSH-dependent antioxidant defence in the skeletal muscle is tightly regulated by the state of physical activity; endurance training enhances and chronic

inactivity diminishes such protection (Sen *et al.* 1992).

Compared with information on the effect of endurance training on tissue antioxidant defences, very limited information is currently available on the effect of sprint training. Criswell *et al.* (1993) studied the effect of 12-week interval training and observed favourable changes in the skeletal muscle of rat. It was proposed that 5-min interval high-intensity training was superior to moderate-intensity continuous exercise in upregulating muscle antioxidant defences. In another study, it was observed that sprint training of rats significantly increased the total GSH pool of skeletal muscles (Fig. 22.1) and GSH peroxidase activity of the heart and skeletal muscle. Skeletal muscle or heart superoxide dismutase activity was not influenced by sprint training (Atalay *et al.* 1997). Similar results were observed in a human study testing the effect of sprint cycle training on skeletal muscle antioxidant enzymes. After 7 weeks, sprint training significantly increased activities of GSH peroxidase and GSH reductase in muscle (Hellsten *et al.* 1996). Thus, habitual physical exercise is crucial to maintain and promote our natural capacity to defend against the ravages of reactive oxygen.

## Nutrition

The 1988 United States Surgeon General's report on Nutrition and Health state that 'for the two out of three adult Americans who do not smoke and do not drink excessively, one personal choice seems to influence long-term health prospect more than any other: what we eat'. As discussed above, in several conditions including physical exercise and cigarette smoking, generation of ROS in tissues may overwhelm endogenous antioxidant defence systems (Table 22.2). Epidemiological studies have emphasized the relevance of antioxidants in the prevention of health disorders that may have an oxidative stress-related aetiology (Sies 1997). It is not only what we eat but also how much we eat that may have marked implications in the management of oxidative stress. Dietary restriction is known

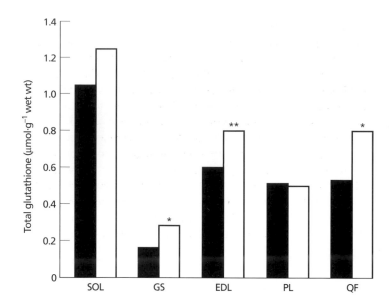

**Fig. 22.1** Sprint-training-dependent increase in skeletal muscle glutathione. Rats were either not trained (■) or treadmill trained 5 days per week for 6 weeks on a treadmill at speed close to the physiological limit of rats (□) (see Atalay *et al.* 1996). EDL, extensor digitorum longus; GS, gastrocnemius; PL, plantaris; QF, quadriceps femoris; SOL, soleus. Effect of sprint training: *, $P<0.001$; **, $P<0.01$.

**Table 22.2** Endogenous proteins with antioxidant properties.

| Protein | Function |
|---|---|
| Superoxide dismutases (Cu, Zn, Mn) | Dismutases superoxides to hydrogen peroxide |
| Catalase (Fe) | Hydroperoxide decomposition |
| Glutathione peroxidase (Se) | Hydroperoxide decomposition |
| Glutathione *S*-transferase | Hydroperoxide decomposition (secondary property) |
| Glutathione reductase | Glutathione recycling |
| Thioredoxin peroxidase | Hydroperoxide decomposition |
| Methionine sulphoxide reductase | Oxidized –SH repair in proteins |
| Thioredoxin | Reduces oxidized protein disulphides |
| Transferrin | Iron transport |
| Ferritin | Iron storage |
| Ceruloplasmin | Copper storage |
| 'Peroxiredoxin' (a 24 kD thiol-specific protein) | Hydroperoxide/ radical scavenging |

to effectively strengthen cellular antioxidant defences and protect against oxidative stress. Nutritional manipulations that have significant potential to circumvent exercise-induced oxidative stress are discussed below.

## Dietary restriction

Dietary restriction delays the loss of several cellular immune functions, retards age-related functional disorders and has been proven to significantly extend lifespan in laboratory animals (Sohal *et al.* 1994). Several studies suggest that dietary restriction may strengthen tissue antioxidant defence systems and alleviate oxidative stress-related damage including cataractogenesis (Taylor *et al.* 1995). Activities of certain components of the physiological antioxidant defence system are upregulated during the course of ageing, perhaps to cope with age-related increased oxidative stress. In the skeletal muscle, activities of catalase and GSH peroxidase increased progressively and markedly with ageing in rats fed *ad libitum*. Dietary restriction clearly suppressed such responses, suggesting that the ageing tissue may have been exposed to less oxidative stress challenge than that of rats fed *ad libitum* (Luhtala *et al.* 1994). In mice, ageing has been observed to be associated with marked oxidative protein damage in organs such as the brain, heart and kidney. This adverse effect could be considerably limited when mice were fed with a diet 40% lower in energy. Ageing increases the resting respiratory rate of mitochondria resulting in increased generation of mitochondrial superoxides and hydrogen peroxide. A protective effect of dietary restriction under such conditions has been also evident (Sohal *et al.* 1994). In rats, dietary restriction has been shown to suppress ROS generation in hepatic microsomes. Interestingly, a synergistic effect of dietary restriction and exercise was observed to protect mitochondrial membrane fluidity against oxidative damage (Kim *et al.* 1996a). Another study investigated the effect of dietary restriction and physically active lifestyle on lipid peroxidation and antioxidant defences of the rat heart. Diet restricted rats were fed 60% of the *ad libitum* level for 18.5 months. Both dietary restriction and a physically active lifestyle decreased lipid peroxidation damage in cardiac mitochondria. Dietary restriction significantly increased the activities of cytosolic antioxidant enzymes such as superoxide dismutase, selenium dependent GSH peroxidase and GSH S-transferase. It is thus evident that long-term dietary restriction and a physically active life style may alleviate the extent of free radical damage in the heart by strengthening endogenous antioxidant defences (Kim *et al.* 1996b).

Food deprivation, on the other hand, may adversely affect liver GSH reserves and wholebody GSH metabolism. Starvation is followed by lowered GSH levels in the plasma, lung and skeletal muscles (Cho *et al.* 1981; Lauterburg *et al.* 1984). The influences of food deprivation and refeeding on GSH status, antioxidant enzyme activity and lipid peroxidation in response to an acute bout of exercise have been investigated in the liver and skeletal muscles of male rats. Food deprivation depleted tissue GSH stores and caused increased lipid peroxidation in the liver and skeletal muscles. Leeuwenburgh and Ji (1996) showed that both food deprivation–refeeding and exhaustive exercise influence liver and skeletal muscle GSH status and that these changes may be controlled by hepatic GSH synthesis and release due to hormonal stimulation.

## Antioxidant nutrients

The chemical nature of any antioxidant determines its solubility, and thus its localization in biological tissues. For example, lipid-soluble antioxidants are localized in membranes and function to protect against oxidative damage of membranes. Water-soluble antioxidants, located, for example, in the cytosol, mitochondrial matrix or extracellular fluids, may not have access to ROS generated in membranes. Vitamins E and A, coenzyme Q, carotenoids, flavonoids, and polyphenols represent the most extensively studied naturally occurring fat-soluble antioxidants. Vitamin C, GSH, uric acid and lipoic acid are the most commonly known water-soluble antioxidants. The antioxidants that have been tested in exercise studies are briefly introduced in the following section.

### Vitamin E

Vitamin E refers to all tocol and tocotrienol derivatives which exhibit the biological activity of α-tocopherol (Sheppard *et al.* 1993). The form of vitamin E that has most biological activity is RRR-α-tocopherol, previously known as d-α-tocopherol. Vitamin supplements are marketed as mixed tocopherols, α-tocopherol or esterified derivatives, e.g. α-tocopheryl-acetate, -nicotinate or -succinate. Edible vegetable oils are the richest natural source of vitamin E. Unprocessed cereal grains and nuts are also good sources of vitamin E. Animal sources of vitamin E include meat, especially fat. One of the most significant properties of vitamin E is that it is an antioxidant. Vitamin E especially protects polyunsaturated fatty acids within phospholipids of biological membranes and in plasma lipoproteins (Burton *et al.* 1983). The phenolic moiety of tocopherol reacts with peroxyl (ROO•, where R=alkyl residue) radicals to form the corresponding organic hydroperoxide and the tocopheroxyl radical (Fig. 22.2). In this radical form, vitamin E is not an effective antioxidant, and when sufficiently accumulated may even have toxic prooxidant effects. The effect of vitamin E on the oxidation of various biological molecules, membranes and tissues have been extensively studied. Vitamin E suppresses the oxidative damage of biological membranes, lipoproteins and tissues. Tocopherols are unstable and are

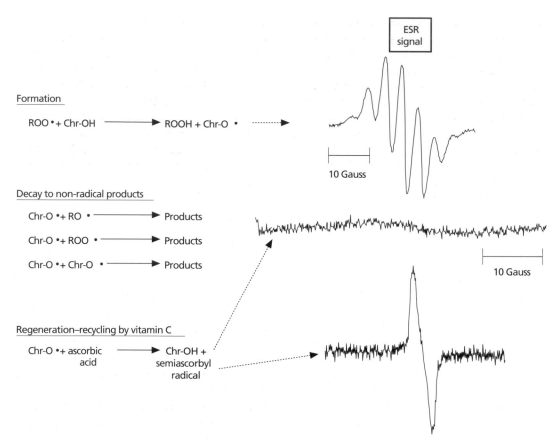

**Fig. 22.2** Interaction of vitamin E and C during the course of the lipid peroxidation chain reaction termination. During termination of the lipid peroxidation reaction, vitamin E may be oxidized to its corresponding radical configuration (Chr-O•) that has no antioxidant potency and may be even toxic. Vitamin C may regenerate Chr-O• to Chr-OH and itself be oxidized to the semiascorbyl radical. Spontaneous radical–radical recombination may lead to the decay of some radicals to non-reactive products. Chr-OH, chromanol head with the phenolic OH in tocopherol; ESR, electron spin resonance spectroscopy; ROO•, peroxyl radical; semiascorbyl radical, one electron oxidation product of vitamin C or ascorbic acid.

readily oxidized by air, especially in the presence of iron and other transition metal ions. The resulting tocopherylquinone has no biological activity. To prevent this loss of biological potency in nutritional supplements, vitamin E is presented in the esterified form. In the gastrointestinal tract, the ester is enzymatically hydrolysed and free tocopherol is absorbed (Traber & Sies 1996).

### Carotenoids

Carotenoid designates a long-chain molecule with 40 carbon atoms and an extensive conjugated system of double bonds. Plant and microorganism-derived carotenoids are efficient scavengers of several forms of ROS (Handelman 1996). The major forms of carotenoids that have been studied for their antioxidant properties include α-, β- and γ-carotene, lycopene, β-cryptoxanthin, lutein, zeaxanthin, astaxanthin, canthaxanthin, violaxanthin, and β-carotene-5,6-epoxide. Photosynthetic plant leaves are rich in carotenoids typical of the choloroplast, containing predominantly β-carotene, lutein, and epoxycarotenoids, e.g. violaxanthin. Storage bodies such as carrot, papaya or squash contain mostly β-carotene, α-carotene and β-cryptoxanthin. Tomatoes are rich in lycopene because the β-carotene biosynthetic pathway terminates prior to the formation of the terminal rings. Chemically, carotenoids are highly unstable and are susceptible to auto-oxidation (Handelman *et al.* 1991). Although most reports indicate that carotenoids do have effective antioxidant functions in biological systems, some studies show that carotenoids may also show toxic pro-oxidant effects (Burton & Ingold 1984; Andersen & Andersen 1993).

## Ubiquinone

Coenzyme $Q_{10}$, also called ubiquinone, is an integral component of the mitochondrial electron transport chain. Coenzyme $Q_{10}$ is found in the phospholipid bilayer of plasma membranes, all intracellular membranes and also in low-density lipoproteins. The actual mechanism of antioxidant action of ubiquinones is still conjectural. One possibility is that ubiquinols act independently as lipid peroxidation chain-breaking antioxidants. Alternatively, a redox interaction of ubiquinol with vitamin E has been suggested in which ubiquinol mainly acts by regenerating vitamin E from its oxidized form (Kagan *et al.* 1996).

## Vitamin C

Vitamin C or ascorbate is an excellent water-soluble antioxidant. Although in most higher organisms it is synthesized from abundant glucose precursors, other species, including humans, solely depend on nutritional supply. Because of its strong reducing properties, ascorbate readily reduces $Fe^{3+}$ and $Cu^{2+}$ to $Fe^{2+}$ and $Cu^+$, respectively. In this way, ascorbate can contribute to the redox cycling of these metals, generating transition metal ions that can stimulate free radical chemistry. Thus, ascorbate may have pro-oxidant effects in the presence of free metals (Aust *et al.* 1985; Buettner 1986). Apart from direct free radical scavenging activity, ascorbate

may also enhance the antioxidant action of vitamin E. The phenol group of tocopherol, which is the basis of its antioxidant action, appears to be located at the water–membrane interface of biological membranes. Such localization facilitates ascorbate–vitamin E interaction (see Fig. 22.2). Dehydroascorbate, the two-electron oxidation product of ascorbate, is reduced to ascorbate by reduced GSH. Thus, ascorbate plays a central role in the antioxidant network.

## Glutathione

Glutathione (L-γ-glutamyl-L-cysteinylglycine) is implicated in the circumvention of cellular oxidative stress and maintenance of intracellular thiol redox status (Meister 1992a, 1992b, 1995; Sen & Hanninen 1994). GSH peroxidase is specific for its hydrogen donor, reduced GSH, but may use a wide range of substrates extending from $H_2O_2$ to organic hydroperoxides. The cytosolic and membrane-bound monomer GSH phospholipid hydroperoxide-GSH peroxidase and the distinct tetramer plasma GSH peroxidase are able to reduce phospholipid hydroperoxides without the necessity of prior hydrolysis by phospholipase $A_2$. The protective action of phospholipid hydroperoxide-GSH peroxidase against membrane-damaging lipid peroxidation has been directly demonstrated (Thomas *et al.* 1990). Reduced GSH is a major cellular electrophile conjugator as well. GSH S-transferases catalyse the reaction between the -SH group of GSH and potential alkylating agents, thereby neutralizing their electrophilic sites and rendering them more water-soluble. GSH S-transferases represent a major group of phase II detoxification enzymes (Hayes & Pulford 1995).

Intracellular synthesis of GSH is a tightly regulated two-step process, both steps being adenosine triphosphate dependent. γ-Glutamylcysteine synthetase (also referred to as glutamate-cysteine ligase) catalyses the formation of the dipeptide γ-glutamylcysteine (DeLeve & Kaplowitz 1990) and subsequently the addi-

LIVERPOOL JOHN MOORES UNIVERSITY
LEARNING SERVICES

tion of glycine is catalysed by GSH synthetase. Substrates for such synthesis are provided both by direct amino acid transport and by γ-glutamyl transpeptidase (also known as glutamyl transferase) that couple the γ-glutamyl moiety to a suitable amino acid acceptor for transport into the cell. GSH is also generated intracellularly from its oxidized form GSH disulphide (GSSG) by GSSG reductase activity in the presence of NADPH. Under normal conditions, the rate-limiting factor in cellular GSH synthesis is the availability of the constituent amino acid cysteine. Thus, given that the GSH-synthesizing enzymes have normal activity, improving cysteine delivery to cells is effective in increasing cell GSH. Cysteine *per se* is highly unstable in its reduced form, and considerable research has been focused on alternative strategies for cysteine delivery (Sen & Packer 1999).

Administered GSH *per se* is not effectively transported into cells (Meister 1991) except in the small intestine (Vina *et al.* 1989; Hagen *et al.* 1990; Martensson *et al.* 1990; Aw *et al.* 1991); it is mostly degraded in the extracellular compartment. The degradation products, i.e. the constituent amino acids, may be used as substrates for GSH neosynthesis inside the cell. Two clinically relevant pro-GSH agents that have been extensively studied so far are N-acetyl-L-cysteine (NAC; 2-mercaptopropionyl glycine) and α-lipoate (Borgstrom *et al.* 1986; Issels *et al.* 1988; Aruoma *et al.* 1989; Holdiness 1991; Ferrari *et al.* 1995; Huupponen *et al.* 1995; Packer *et al.* 1995, 1997; van Zandwijk 1995; Akerlund *et al.* 1996; Atalay *et al.* 1996; Sen *et al.* 1997b, 1997c; Sen & Packer 1999). In addition to its reactive oxygen detoxifying properties (Aruoma *et al.* 1989; Sen *et al.* 1994d), NAC is thought to function as a cysteine delivery compound (Issels *et al.* 1988; Sjödin *et al.* 1989). After free NAC enters a cell, it is rapidly hydrolysed to release cysteine. NAC, but not N-acetyl-D-cysteine or the oxidized disulphide form of NAC, is deacetylated in several tissues to release cysteine. NAC is safe for human use and it has been used as a clinical mucolytic agent for many years.

## Lipoic acid

α-Lipoate is also known as thioctic acid, 1,2-dithiolane-3-pentanoic acid, 1,2-dithiolane-3-valeric acid or 6,8-thioctic acid. Biologically, lipoate exists as lipoamide in at least five proteins, where it is covalently linked to a lysyl residue (Packer *et al.* 1995, 1997; Sen *et al.* 1997b, 1997c; Sen & Packer 1999). Lipoic acid has been detected in the form of lipoyllysine in various natural sources. In the plant material studied, lipoyllysine content was highest in spinach ($3.15\,\mu g \cdot g^{-1}$ dry weight; $92.51\,\mu g \cdot mg$ protein). When expressed as weight per dry weight of lyophilized vegetables, the abundance of naturally existing lipoate in spinach was over three- and fivefold higher than that in broccoli and tomato, respectively. Lower concentrations of lipoyllysine were also detected in garden peas, brussel sprouts and rice bran. Lipoyllysine concentration was below detection limits in acetone powders of banana, orange peel, soybean and horseradish. In animal tissues, the abundance of lipoyllysine in bovine acetone powders can be represented in the following order: kidney > heart > liver > spleen > brain > pancreas > lung. The concentration of lipoyllysine in bovine kidney and heart was $2.64 \pm 1.23$ and $1.51 \pm 0.75\,\mu g \cdot g^{-1}$ dry weight, respectively (Lodge *et al.* 1997).

Studies with human Jurkat T-cells have shown that when added to the culture medium, lipoate readily enters the cell where it is reduced to its dithiol form, dihydrolipoate (DHLA). DHLA accumulated in the cell pellet, and when monitored over a 2-h interval, the dithiol was released to the culture medium (Handelman *et al.* 1994). As a result of lipoate treatment to the Jurkat T-cells and human neonatal fibroblasts, accumulation of DHLA in the culture medium was observed. The redox potential of the lipoate–DHLA couple is $-320\,mV$. Thus, DHLA is a strong reductant capable of chemically reducing GSSG to GSH. Following lipoate supplementation, extracellular DHLA reduces cystine outside the cell to cysteine. The cellular uptake mechanism for cysteine by the ASC system is approximately 10 times faster than that for cystine by the $x_c^-$ system (Watanabe & Bannai 1987). Thus, DHLA markedly improves cysteine availability within the cell resulting in accelerated GSH synthesis (Han *et al.* 1997; Sen *et al.* 1997b). Both lipoate and DHLA have remarkable reactive oxygen detoxifying properties (Packer *et al.* 1995, 1997).

## Selenium

Forty years ago, traces of dietary selenium were observed to prevent nutritional liver necrosis in vitamin E-deficient rats (Schwarz & Foltz 1957). At present, selenium is widely used in agriculture to prevent a variety of selenium- and vitamin E-sensitive conditions in livestock and poultry (Board on Agriculture 1983). In animal tissues, selenium is either present as selenocysteine in selenoproteins such as GSH peroxidase, selenoprotein P or thioredoxin reductase. Alternatively, selenium may present in animal tissues as selenomethionine, which is incorporated in place of methionine in a variety of proteins. Selenomethionine-containing proteins serve as a reservoir of selenium that provides selenium to the organism when the dietary supply of selenium is interrupted. Selenocysteine is the form of selenium that accounts for its biological activity. Perhaps the most prominent biological activity of selenium is that it is an essential cofactor for the critical hydroperoxide-metabolizing enzyme GSH peroxidase (Rotruck *et al.* 1973). It has been suggested that selenium may also have direct antioxidant effects in biological systems (Burk *et al.* 1980). The selenium content of food sources may markedly vary depending on the selenium content of the feed for animals, or selenium content in the agricultural soil. Organ meats, seafoods and muscle meat are considerable sources of selenium. Dairy products, cereal and grains may also provide significant amounts to meet the RDA value of 70 and $55 \mu g \cdot day^{-1}$ calculated for adult men and women, respectively (International Programme of Chemical Safety 1987).

## Antioxidant deficiency in exercise

The antioxidant deficiency model has been used to test the significance of various antioxidants in exercise-induced oxidative stress. Several studies have consistently indicated that vitamin E deficiency can lead to enhanced free radical formation resulting in compromised exercise performance and increased tissue lipid peroxidation (Dillard *et al.* 1978; Quintanilha *et al.* 1982; Quintanilha & Packer 1983; Salminen *et al.* 1984; Gohil *et al.* 1986; Jackson 1987; Amelink *et al.* 1991). These studies suggest that inadequate amounts of dietary vitamin E may decrease endurance performance by as much as 40% and lead to enhanced oxidative lipid damage of several tissues (Dillard *et al.* 1977; Davies *et al.* 1982; Gohil *et al.* 1984, 1986). Also, vitamin E deficiency was associated with increased fragility of lysosomal membranes and greater haemolysis of red blood cells (Davies *et al.* 1982; Gohil *et al.* 1986). Vitamin E deficiency also decreased oxidative phosphorylation (Quintanilha *et al.* 1982; Gohil *et al.* 1984) in skeletal muscle, liver and adipose tissues. In female rats, however, vitamin E deficiency does not appear to influence the ability to run nor does it enhance tissue lipid peroxidation (Tiidus *et al.* 1993). It has been suggested that female rats may be less susceptible to free radical damage compared to male rats because of higher levels of oestrogen, a potential antioxidant, in the circulation (Davies *et al.* 1982; Salminen *et al.* 1984; Bar & Amelink 1997). The effects of an ascorbate-depleting diet on run time were examined in guinea pigs, which do not synthesize vitamin C. Run time of ascorbate-depleted guinea pigs was significantly less than ascorbate-adequate animals (Packer *et al.* 1986).

Dietary selenium deficiency impairs tissue antioxidant defences by markedly downregulating GSH peroxidase activity in tissues such as the liver and muscle. This effect on the antioxidant enzyme did not influence endurance to treadmill run, however. This suggests that muscle GSH peroxidase activity is not a limiting factor in physical performance (Lang *et al.* 1987). Selenium deficiency has also been found to enhance lipid peroxidation in skeletal muscle mitochondria of rats that were exercised for 1 h (Ji et al. 1988). Activity of antioxidant enzymes in both liver and skeletal muscle have been observed to adapt in response to selenium deficiency, suggesting that the organs may have encountered and responded to an enhanced oxidative challenge. The role of endogenous GSH in the circumvention of exhaustive exercise-induced oxidative stress has been investigated using GSH-deficient rats. GSH synthesis was inhibited by intraperitoneally administered L-buthionine-sulphoxamine (BSO) to produce GSH deficiency. The BSO treatment resulted in (i) approximately 50% decrease in the total GSH pools of the liver, lung, blood and plasma, and (ii) 80–90% decrease in the total GSH pools of the skeletal muscle and heart. GSH-deficient rats had higher levels of tissue lipid peroxides than controls had, and they could run for only about half the interval when compared to the saline-injected controls. This observation underscores the critical role of tissue GSH in the circumvention of exercise-induced oxidative stress and as a determinant of exercise performance (Sen et al. 1994a). Increased susceptibility to oxidative stress was also observed in muscle-derived cells pretreated with BSO (Sen et al. 1993).

Leeuwenburgh and Ji (1995) studied the effect of chronic in vivo GSH depletion by BSO on intracellular and interorgan GSH homeostasis in mice both at rest and after an acute bout of exhaustive swim exercise. BSO treatment for 12 days decreased concentrations of GSH in the liver, kidney, quadriceps muscle, and plasma to 28%, 15%, 7% and 35%, respectively, compared with GSH-adequate mice. GSH depletion was associated with adaptive changes in the activities of several enzymes related to GSH metabolism. Exhaustive exercise in the GSH-adequate state severely depleted the GSH content of the liver (–55%) and kidney (–35%), whereas plasma and muscle GSH levels remained constant. However, exercise in the GSH-depleted state exacerbated the GSH deficit in the liver (–57%), kidney (–33%), plasma (–65%), and muscle (–25%) in the

absence of adequate reserves of liver GSH. Hepatic lipid peroxidation increased by 220% and 290%, respectively, after exhaustive exercise in the GSH-adequate and -depleted mice. It was concluded that GSH homeostasis is an essential component of the prooxidant-antioxidant balance during prolonged physical exercise.

## Antioxidant supplementation in exercise

Venditti and Di Meo (1996) observed that free radical-induced damage in muscle could be one of the factors terminating muscle effort. They suggested that greater antioxidant levels in the tissue should allow trained muscle to withstand oxidative processes more effectively, thus lengthening the time required so that the cell function is sufficiently damaged as to make further exercise impossible. Whether oxidative stress is the single most important factor determining muscle performance is certainly a debatable issue. The contention that strengthened antioxidant defence of the muscle may protect against exercise-induced oxidative-stress-dependent muscle damage is much more readily acceptable (Dekkers et al. 1996). Animal experiments studying the effect of vitamin E have shown mixed results on the prevention of lipid peroxidation (Sen 1995), with the general trend that such supplementation may diminish oxidative tissue damage. Brady and coworkers (Brady et al. 1979) examined the effects of vitamin E supplementation (50 IU · kg⁻¹ diet) on lipid peroxidation in liver and skeletal muscle at rest and following exhaustive swim exercise. Vitamin E effectively decreased lipid peroxidation in liver independent of selenium supplementation, whereas skeletal muscle lipid peroxidation response was unaffected by the supplementation. Goldfarb et al. (1994) observed that vitamin E supplementation can protect against run-induced lipid peroxidation in the skeletal muscle and blood. The effect in skeletal muscle was muscle fibre type dependent. The protective effect of vitamin E was more clearly evident when the animals were exposed to an additional stressor, dehydroepiandrosterone.

Jackson *et al.* (1983) examined the effect of both vitamin E deficiency and supplementation on the contractile activity of muscle. Male rats and female mice were given either a standard diet, a vitamin E-deficient diet with $500 \mu g \cdot kg^{-1}$ selenium or a diet supplemented with 240 mg $\alpha$-tocopherol acetate per kilogram of diet. The animals were given this diet for 42–45 days. Vitamin E deficiency, in both mice and rats, was associated with increased susceptibility to contractile damage. Vitamin E supplementation clearly protected against such damage. Despite the fact that vitamin E supplementation protected the muscles from damage, as indicated by creatine kinase and lactate dehydrogenase leakage, there was no apparent effect on muscle lipid peroxidation. Kumar *et al.* (1992) noted that vitamin E supplementation for 60 days in female adult albino rats completely abolished the increase in free radical-mediated lipid peroxidation in the myocardium as a result of exhaustive endurance exercise. They reported that exercise-induced lipid peroxidation in heart tissue increased in control rats but did not increase in the vitamin E-supplemented rats. Consistently, it has been also observed that vitamin E supplementation for 5 weeks attenuated exercise-induced increase in myocardial lipid peroxidation (Goldfarb *et al.* 1993, 1994, 1996).

Vitamin E-supplemented diet prevented dehydroepiandrosterone-induced increase of peroxisomal fatty acid oxidation and leakage of alanine aminotransferase and aspartate aminotransferase into the plasma (McIntosh *et al.* 1993a, 1993b). Exercised animals on a normal diet demonstrated similar peroxisomal fatty acid oxidation profile and plasma enzyme levels as the vitamin E-supplemented group. Novelli *et al.* (1990) examined the effects of intramuscular injections of three spin-trappers and vitamin E on endurance swimming to exhaustion in mice. Mice were injected on three successive days. It was observed that, compared to either the control or placebo saline-injected animals, the spin-trap- and vitamin E-injected groups had significantly increased swim endurance. In a study reported by Quintanilha and Packer (1983), rats were given one of the following three diets and compared for liver mitochondrial respiration and lipid peroxidation: a diet deficient in vitamin E, a diet with 40 IU vitamin $E \cdot kg^{-1}$, or a diet with 400 IU vitamin $E \cdot kg^{-1}$. Hepatic mitochondrial respiratory control ratios were highest in the group supplemented with 400 IU $\cdot kg^{-1}$. Additionally, liver lipid peroxidation in nuclei and microsomes was lowest in the vitamin E-supplemented group, especially when NADPH was present. Warren *et al.* (1992) studied the effects of vitamin E supplementation, 10 000 IU $\cdot kg^{-1}$ diet, for 5 weeks, on muscle damage and free radical damage to membranes as indicated by alterations in plasma enzymes. Susceptibility of the skeletal muscles to oxidative stress was markedly decreased in response to vitamin E supplementation but this did not attenuate muscle injury triggered by eccentric contractions. It was concluded that vitamin E supplementation may be beneficial in protecting against free radical damage, but that the injury caused by eccentric exercise may not be ROS-mediated. The effect of dietary vitamin E on exercise-induced oxidative protein damage has been investigated in the skeletal muscle of rats. For a period of 4 weeks, rats were fed with high vitamin E diet (10 000 IU $\cdot kg^{-1}$ diet), a $\alpha$-tocopherol- and tocotrienol (7000 mg tocotrienol $\cdot kg^{-1}$ diet)-rich palm oil diet or control diet with basal levels of $\alpha$-tocopherol (30 IU $\cdot kg^{-1}$ body weight). Uphill exhaustive treadmill exercise caused oxidative protein damage in skeletal muscles. A protective effect of vitamin E supplementation against exercise-induced protein oxidation in skeletal muscles was clearly evident (Reznick *et al.* 1992).

Fish oils have been shown to have a beneficial effect on cardiovascular mortality based on numerous epidemiological studies (Kromhout *et al.* 1985), presumably *via* effects on triglyceride levels, membrane fluidity and platelet and leucocyte function (Schmidt & Dyerberg 1994). Not all studies show beneficial effects, however (Ascherio *et al.* 1995). Because the *(n-3)* fatty acids making up fish oil are highly polyunsaturated, concerns have been raised regarding increased oxidative stress from fish oil intake (Hu *et al.* 1989; Nalbone *et al.* 1989; Leibovitz *et al.* 1990; Demoz *et al.* 1992, 1994). Furthermore, fish oils induce peroxisomal β-oxidation, in which fatty-acyl oxidation yields hydrogen peroxide ($H_2O_2$) as a normal by-product, and upregulate the activity of the $H_2O_2$ decomposing enzyme catalase (Aarsland *et al.* 1990; Demoz *et al.* 1992, 1994). Under normal conditions, up to 20% of cellular $O_2$ consumption has in fact been estimated to occur in the peroxisome (Chance *et al.* 1979). The beneficial effects of regular exercise on cardiovascular and overall mortality (Paffenbarger *et al.* 1984) may be decreased by uncontrolled exercise-induced oxidative stress. This may be particularly concerning in groups predisposed to oxidative stress, including that induced by fish oil (Hu *et al.* 1989; Nalbone *et al.* 1989; Leibovitz *et al.* 1990). Sen *et al.* (1997a) assessed the effect of fish oil and vitamin E supplementation compared to placebo soy oil and vitamin E supplementation on physiological antioxidant defences and resting and exercise-induced oxidative stress in rat liver, heart and skeletal muscle. The effects of 8-week vitamin E and fish oil supplementation on resting and exercise-induced oxidative stress was examined. Lipid peroxidation was 33% higher in fish oil fed rats than in the placebo group in the liver, but oxidative protein damage remained similar in both liver and red gastrocnemius muscle. Vitamin E supplementation markedly decreased liver and muscle lipid peroxidation induced by fish oil diet. Vitamin E supplementation also markedly decreased oxidative protein damage in the liver and muscle. Exhaustive treadmill exercise increased liver and muscle lipid peroxidation, and muscle oxidative protein damage. Vitamin E effectively decreased exercise-induced lipid peroxidation and protein oxidation (Sen *et al.* 1997a).

A limited number of studies have examined the effect of vitamin E supplementation in humans. Exercise performance and physical fitness have multifactorial determinants and may not serve as reasonable end points to test the efficacy of antioxidant supplementation. Vitamin E supplementation ($900\,IU \cdot day^{-1}$ for 6 months) in trained swimmers did not alter their swim performance nor their lactate response in plasma (Lawrence *et al.* 1975). Neither did vitamin E supplementation ($800\,IU \cdot day^{-1}$ for 4 weeks) alter the work load needed to run at 80% $\dot{V}o_{2max.}$ in trained and untrained males (Goldfarb *et al.* 1989). Volunteers given 400 IU vitamin E per day for 6 weeks showed no influence on cycle time, swim time, or step time (Sharman *et al.* 1976). Additionally no changes in $\dot{V}o_{2max.}$, a marker of physical fitness, was noted in humans following vitamin E supplementation (Watt *et al.* 1974; Goldfarb *et al.* 1989; Sumida *et al.* 1989). However, Cannon *et al.* (1990) reported that supplementation of 400 IU vitamin E daily for 48 days decreased the amount of creatine kinase leakage from muscles during recovery from a downhill run. Sumida *et al.* (1989) examined the effects of 4 weeks of vitamin E supplementation in 21 healthy college-aged males. The subjects ingested 300 mg of vitamin E daily and blood levels of several enzymes and lipid peroxides were determined before and for up to 3 h after cycling exercise to exhaustion. Exercise increased the level of lipid peroxidation by-products in plasma immediately after the cycling and returned to normal at 1 and 3 hours of recovery. Vitamin E supplementation significantly decreased the resting level of plasma lipid peroxides. Meydani *et al.* (1993) reported that urinary excretion of lipid peroxidation by-products tended to be lower in vitamin E-supplemented individuals (400-IU doses, twice daily, for 48 days) than in the corresponding placebo group, but this effect was only significant 12 days after downhill running. The subjects ran at 16% downhill inclination at 75% of their maximum heart rate for three 15-min periods. Muscle biopsies were obtained from the vastus lateralis of young subjects. It was observed that exercise increased the level of lipid peroxidation by-products in the muscle of the placebo group, whereas in the muscle of the vitamin E-supplemented group, no such oxidative lipid damage was evident. Another study examined the effect of vitamin E supplementation (800 IU daily for 4 weeks) and compared that with a placebo treatment in the same individuals at a specific exercise intensity (Goldfarb *et al.* 1989). Subjects were randomly assigned to either a placebo or vitamin E treatment group in a counterbalanced design. Subjects were exercised for 30 min at 80% $\dot{V}o_{2max.}$ and blood was collected before and after the run. Vitamin E treatment attenuated the level of resting plasma lipid peroxidation by-products and also protected against the exercise response. The effects of 5 months of α-tocopherol supplementation has been studied in 30 top-class cyclists. Although the supplementation did not improve physical performance, it was evident that exercise-induced muscle damage was less in response to antioxidant supplementation (Rokitzki *et al.* 1994a).

In 1980, the United States daily allowance for vitamin E was reduced from 30 IU (recommended in 1968) to 15 IU. In the same year it was estimated that in the United States, the amount of vitamin E supplied by a 'normal' diet is about 11 IU (7.4 mg). Packer and Reznick (1992) have discussed that such dosages are insufficient for active athletes and that dosages of up to 400 IU daily may be reasonable recommendation for active athletes engaged in moderate to heavy exercise. Vitamin E is proven to be safe at levels of intake up to approximately 3000 mg for prolonged periods of time (Bendich & Machlin 1988). However, individuals taking anticoagulants should refrain from taking very high doses (>4000 IU) of vitamin E because vitamin E can act synergistically with this class of drug (Corrigan 1979).

Vitamin C supplements (3 g · kg$^{-1}$ diet) given to rats who were placed on a vitamin E-deficient diet did not alter the run time to exhaustion in the vitamin E-deficient animals (Gohil *et al.* 1986). Vitamin C was unable to counter the deleterious effects of vitamin E deficiency. In a preliminary report, the effect of vitamin C supplementation in humans was documented. A mild protective effect of vitamin C supplementation, based on elevated total antioxidant capacity of the plasma, was observed (Alessio *et al.* 1993).

Other nutrients that have been ascribed to be beneficial as antioxidants, such as selenium and β-carotene, have not been examined individually but have been assessed in conjunction with either vitamin E deficiency or in combination with other antioxidants. The effects of selenium supplementation (0.5 ppm diet) or deprivation have been tested in liver, muscle and blood of swim-exercised rats (Brady *et al.* 1979). Some rats were additionally supplemented with vitamin E (50 IU · kg$^{-1}$). Selenium supplementation increased the activity of the hydroperoxide metabolizing enzyme GSH peroxidase in the liver. A tight regulation of tissue GSH peroxidase activity by dietary selenium was observed because a selenium-deficient diet markedly downregulated the activity of the enzyme. Muscle GSH peroxidase activity demonstrated similar responses to selenium intervention compared with the liver. Increased tissue lipid peroxidation was evident when both selenium and vitamin E were deficient. However, selenium deficiency had little effect when vitamin E was present. Selenium appeared to have minimal effects on swim-induced lipid peroxidation in the liver or muscle. Dietary selenium supplementation in horses (0.15 ppm daily for 4 weeks) had minimal effects on exercise-induced lipid peroxidation as indicated by blood level of lipid peroxidation by-products (Brady *et al.* 1978). In a double-blind human study, no effect of selenium supplementation on human physical performance was observed (Tessier *et al.* 1995). Selenium poisoning is rare in the United States, but the case of a man who was poisoned by selenium-containing vitamin tablets has been described (Clark *et al.* 1996).

A few studies have examined the effects of coenzyme $Q_{10}$ to determine if additional amounts of this factor in the electron transport chain would be beneficial in preventing free radical damage (Zuliani *et al.* 1989; Shimomura *et al.* 1991; Snider *et al.* 1992). Dietary coenzyme $Q_{10}$ supplementation protected against leakage of creatine kinase and lactate dehydrogenase from the muscles to serum following downhill run (Shimomura *et al.* 1991). In two human studies, however, this beneficial effect of coenzyme $Q_{10}$ could not be observed (Zuliani *et al.* 1989; Snider *et al.* 1992). The effects of ubiquinone supplementation ($120\,mg\cdot day^{-1}$ for 6 weeks) on aerobic capacity and lipid peroxidation during exercise has been investigated in 11 young (aged 22–38 years) and 8 older (aged 60–74 years), trained men. This cross-over study was double-blind and placebo-controlled. Ubiquinone supplementation effectively increased serum concentration of the element in both age groups but did not influence maximal aerobic capacity. Consistent with previous reports, oral ubiquinone supplementation was ineffective as an ergogenic aid in both the young and older, trained men (Laaksonen *et al.* 1995).

Two brief rodent studies have shown that exogenous GSH may remarkably increase endurance to physical exercise (Cazzulani *et al.* 1991; Novelli *et al.* 1991). Compared with placebo-treated controls, 0.5, 0.75 and $1\,g\cdot kg^{-1}$ intraperitoneal doses of GSH increased endurance to swimming by a marked 102.4%, 120% and 140.7%, respectively (Novelli *et al.* 1991). At a dose $0.25\,g\cdot kg^{-1}$, GSH did not affect endurance when injected once but such a dose could significantly increase endurance when injected once a day for 7 consecutive days. In another study, oral GSH at dosages of 0.25–$1\,g\cdot kg^{-1}$ caused a dose-dependent significant improvement in swim endurance (Cazzulani *et al.* 1991). Both above-mentioned studies employed brief bursts of swimming as the exercise challenge and did not report any biochemical data related to either GSH metabolism or other indices of oxidative stress. Sen *et al.* (1994a) sought to clarify the possible mechanism of such beneficial effect of GSH supplementation. An extensive biochemical investigation was necessary before any hypothesis regarding the role of exogenous GSH in endurance enhancement could be formulated. Almost all the evidence supporting the contention that a single bout of exercise may induce oxidative stress have been obtained from studies using exercise types that were long in duration, and mostly running or cycling in nature. Because we aimed to test the efficacy of exogenous GSH in controlling exercise-induced oxidative stress, an enduring ($\approx 2\,h$) treadmill run protocol was used. Intraperitoneal injection of GSH solution ($1\,g\cdot kg^{-1}$ body weight) resulted in a rapid appearance of GSH in the plasma and was followed by a rapid clearance of the thiol. Following the injection excess plasma GSH was rapidly oxidized. GSH injection did not influence GSH status of other tissues studied. Following the repeated administration of GSH, blood and kidney total GSH levels were increased. Plasma total GSH of GSH-supplemented animals was rapidly cleared during exhaustive exercise. The GSH administration protocol, as used in this study, did not influence the endurance to exhaustive physical exercise of rats. In a previous study, Sen *et al.* (1994b) observed that treadmill run to exhaustion is associated with a remarkable increase in immunoreactive manganese superoxide dismutase (Mn-SOD, a mitochondrial protein) in the plasma. GSH supplementation ($500\,mg\cdot kg^{-1}$ body weight) marginally suppressed such release of the mitochondrial protein to the plasma (Sen *et al.* 1994b). The inability of exogenous GSH to provide added antioxidant protection to tissues may be largely attributed to the poor availability of exogenous administered GSH to the tissues. In another part of this study, Atalay *et al.* (1996) tested the effect of GSH supplementation on exercise-induced leucocyte margination and neutrophil oxidative burst activity. Exercise-associated leucocyte margination was prevented by GSH supplementation. Peripheral blood neutrophil counts were significantly higher in GSH-supplemented groups than in the placebo control groups. Also, exercise-induced increase in peripheral blood neutrophil oxidative burst activity, as measured by luminol-enhanced chemiluminescence per volume of blood, tended to be higher in the GSH-supplemented group and lower in the GSH-deficient rats, suggesting high plasma GSH may have augmented exercise-dependent neutrophil priming. In these experiments, for the first time it was shown that GSH supplementation can induce neutrophil mobilization and decrease exercise-induced leucocyte margination, and that exogenous and endogenous GSH can regulate exercise-induced priming of neutrophil for oxidative burst response (Atalay *et al.* 1996).

In another human study, the effect of oral NAC on exercise-associated rapid blood GSH oxidation in healthy adult males who performed two identical maximal bicycle ergometer exercises 3 weeks apart was investigated. Before the second maximal exercise test, the men took effervescent NAC tablets ($4 \times 200 \, mg \cdot day^{-1}$) for 2 days, and an additional 800 mg on the morning of the test. The NAC supplementation protocol used in the study (i) increased the net peroxyl radical scavenging capacity of the plasma, and (ii) spared exercise-induced blood GSH oxidation (Fig. 22.3) (Sen *et al.* 1994d).

Reid and associates have shown that antioxidant enzymes are able to depress contractility of unfatigued diaphragm fibre bundles and inhibit development of acute fatigue. NAC has been tested for similar effects. Fibre bundles were removed from diaphragms and stimulated directly using supramaximal current intensity. Studies of unfatigued muscle showed that 10 mM NAC reduced peak twitch stress, shortened time

to peak twitch stress, and shifted the stress-frequency curve down and to the right. Fibre bundles incubated in 0.1–10 mM NAC exhibited a dose-dependent decrease in relative stresses developed during 30-Hz contraction with no change in maximal tetanic (200 Hz) stress. NAC (10 mM) also inhibited acute fatigue. In a later experiment, this effect of NAC was tested in humans. Healthy volunteers were studied on two occasions each. Subjects were pretreated with NAC 150 mg·kg⁻¹ or 5% dextrose in water by intravenous infusion. It was evident that NAC pretreatment can improve performance of human limb muscle during fatiguing exercise, suggesting that oxidative stress plays a causal role in the fatigue process and identifying antioxidant therapy as a novel intervention that may be useful clinically (Khawli & Reid 1994; Reid *et al.* 1994).

The first study testing the efficacy of α-lipoate supplementation in exercise-induced oxidative stress has been just reported. Khanna *et al.* (1997) studied the effect of intragastric lipoate supplementation ($150 \, mg \cdot kg^{-1}$ body weight for 8 weeks) on lipid peroxidation and GSH-dependent antioxidant defences in liver, heart,

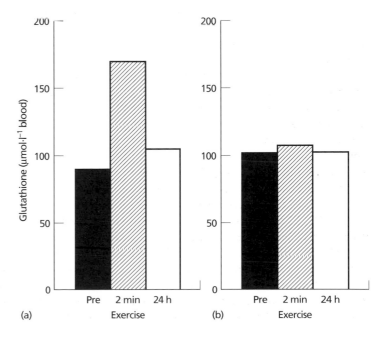

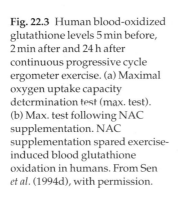

**Fig. 22.3** Human blood-oxidized glutathione levels 5 min before, 2 min after and 24 h after continuous progressive cycle ergometer exercise. (a) Maximal oxygen uptake capacity determination test (max. test). (b) Max. test following NAC supplementation. NAC supplementation spared exercise-induced blood glutathione oxidation in humans. From Sen *et al.* (1994d), with permission.

kidney and skeletal muscle of male Wistar rats. Lipoate supplementation significantly increased total GSH levels in liver and blood. These results are consistent with those from previously discussed cell experiments, and show that indeed lipoate supplementation may increase GSH levels of certain tissues *in vivo*. Lipoate supplementation, however, did not affect the total GSH content of organs such as the kidney, heart and skeletal muscles. Lipoate supplementation-dependent increase in hepatic GSH pool was associated with increased resistance to lipid peroxidation. This beneficial effect against oxidative lipid damage was also observed in the heart and red gastrocnemius skeletal muscle. Lower lipid peroxide levels in certain tissues of lipoate fed rats suggest strengthening of the antioxidant network defence in these tissues (Khanna *et al.* 1997).

From the biochemistry of antioxidant action it is evident that antioxidants function in a network and interaction between several major antioxidants have been clearly evident. As a result, some studies have attempted to investigate the efficacy of a combination of several antioxidants as supplements (Viguie *et al.* 1989; Kanter & Eddy 1992; Kanter *et al.* 1993). Supplementation of individuals with a vitamin mixture containing 37.5 mg β-carotene, 1250 mg vitamin C and 1000 IU of vitamin E for 5 weeks decreased the level of lipid peroxidation by-products in the serum and breath, both at rest and following exercise at both 60% and 90% $\dot{V}o_{2max.}$ (Kanter *et al.* 1993). In contrast, a previous study, which used a similar mixture of antioxidants and exercised the subjects at 65% of maximal heart rate in a downhill run, was unable to demonstrate any positive effects (Kanter & Eddy 1992). This inconsistency in observation was explained by differences in the nature and intensity of the exercise in the two studies. The effects of an antioxidant mixture (10 mg β-carotene, 1000 mg vitamin C and 800 IU of vitamin E) on human blood GSH system and muscle damage has been determined (Viguie *et al.* 1989). A protective effect on the blood GSH system and muscle damage was evident. A randomized and placebo-controlled study has been carried out on 24 trained long-distance runners who were substituted with α-tocopherol (400 IU · day⁻¹) and ascorbic acid (200 mg daily) for 4.5 weeks before a marathon race. Serum content of ascorbic acid as well as α-tocopherol were elevated in supplemented individuals. In this study the antioxidant supplementation protocol was observed to significantly protect against exercise-induced muscle damage as manifested by the loss of creatine kinase from the muscle to the serum (Rokitzki *et al.* 1994b).

## Perspectives

Several lines of evidence consistently show that physical exercise may induce oxidative stress. The relationship between physical activity, physical fitness and total radical trapping antioxidant potential was examined in the Northern Ireland Health and Activity Survey. This was a large cross-sectional population study ($n = 1600$) using a two-stage probability sample of the population. A necessity for antioxidant supplementation, especially in physically active and fit individuals, was indicated (Sharpe *et al.* 1996). Depending on nutritional habits and genetic disposition, susceptibility to oxidative stress may vary from person to person. Determination of tissue antioxidant status of individuals is thus recommended. Such information will be necessary to identify specific necessities and formulate effective antioxidant therapy strategies. Nutritional antioxidant supplements are known to be bioavailable to tissues and may strengthen defence systems against the ravages of reactive oxygen. Results from antioxidant supplementation studies considerably vary depending on the study design and measures of outcome. Physical performance is regulated by multifactorial processes and may not serve as a good indicator to test the effect of antioxidant supplementation. The general trend of results show no effect of antioxidant supplementation on physical performance. However, in a large number of studies it has been consistently evident that antioxidant supplementation protects against exercise-induced tissue damage. The diet of laboratory animals is often heavily enriched with antioxidant vitamins, particularly vitamin E. This may be one reason why antioxidant supplementation to animals fed regular diets do not influence several measures of outcome. At present there is a growing trend among people to cut out fat-containing diet. While this does markedly decrease caloric intake, in many cases this may also contribute to marked decrease in the intake of fat-soluble essential nutrients, including vitamins. From available information, we know that under regular circumstances antioxidants such as α-tocopherol, ascorbic acid and β-carotene are well tolerated and free from toxicity, even when consumed at doses several-fold higher than the recommended dietary allowances (Garewal & Diplock 1995). In view of this and the tremendous potential of antioxidant therapy, consumption of a diet rich in a mixture of different antioxidants may be expected to be a prudent course.

## References

Aarsland, A., Lundquist, M., Borretsen, B. & Berge, R.K. (1990) On the effect of peroxisomal beta-oxidation and carnitine palmitoyltransferase activity by eicosapentaenoic acid in liver and heart from rats. *Lipids* **25**, 546–548.

Akerlund, B., Jarstrand, C., Lindeke, B., Sonnerborg, A., Akerblad, A.C. & Rasool, O. (1996) Effect of N-acetylcysteine (NAC) treatment on HIV-1 infection: a double-blind placebo-controlled trial. *European Journal of Clinical Pharmacology* **50**, 457–461.

Alessio, H.M. (1994) Lipid peroxidation processes in healthy and diseased models. In *Exercise and Oxygen Toxicity* (ed. C.K. Sen, L. Packer & O. Hanninen), pp. 269–295. Elsevier Science, Amsterdam.

Alessio, H.M. & Cutler, R.G. (1990) Evidence that DNA damage and repair cycle activity increases following a marathon race. *Medicine and Science in Sports and Exercise* **25**, 218–224.

Alessio, H.M., Goldfarb, A.H., Cao, G. & Cutler, R.G. (1993) Short and long term vit C supplementation exercise and oxygen radical absorption capacity (Abstract). *Medicine and Science in Sports and Exercise* **25**, S79.

Amelink, G.J., van der Wal, W.A., Wokke, J.H., van Asbeck, B.S. & Bar, P.R. (1991) Exercise-induced muscle damage in the rat: the effect of vitamin E deficiency. *Pflugers Archives* **419**, 304–309.

Ames, B.N., Shigenaga, M.K. & Hagen, T.M. (1993) Oxidants, antioxidants, and the degenerative diseases of aging. *Proceedings of the National Academy of Science, USA* **90**, 7915–7922.

Andersen, H.R. & Andersen, O. (1993) Effects of dietary alpha-tocopherol and beta-carotene on lipid peroxidation induced by methyl mercuric chloride in mice. *Pharmacology and Toxicology* **73**, 192–201.

Archakov, A.I. & Bachmanova, G.I. (eds) (1990) *Cytochrome P-450 and Active Oxygen*. Taylor and Francis, London.

Aruoma, O.I., Halliwell, B., Hoey, B.M. & Butler, J. (1989) The antioxidant action of N-acetylcysteine: its reaction with hydrogen peroxide, hydroxyl radical, superoxide, and hypochlorous acid. *Free Radical Biology and Medicine* **6**, 593–597.

Ascherio, A., Rimm, E.B., Stampfer, M.J., Giovannucci, E.L. & Willett, W.C. (1995) Dietary intake of marine *n*-3 fatty acids, fish intake, and the risk of coronary disease among men [see comments]. *New England Journal of Medicine* **332**, 977–982.

Åstrand, P.-O. & Rodahl, K. (1986) *Textbook of Work Physiology*. McGraw Hill, New York.

Atalay, M., Marnila, P., Lilius, E.M., Hanninen, O. & Sen, C.K. (1996) Glutathione-dependent modulation of exhausting exercise-induced changes in neutrophil function of rats. *European Journal of Applied Physiology* **74**, 342–347.

Atalay, M., Laaksonen, D.E., Niskanen, L., Uusitupa, M., Hanninen, O. & Sen, C.K. (1997) Altered antioxidant enzyme defences in insulin-dependent diabetic men with increased resting and exercise induced oxidative stress. *Acta Physiologica Scandinavica* **161**, 195–201.

Aust, S.D., Morehouse, L.A. & Thomas, C.E. (1985) Role of metals in oxygen radical reactions. *Free Radical Biology and Medicine* **1**, 3–25.

Aw, T.Y., Wierzbicka, G. & Jones, D.P. (1991) Oral glutathione increases tissue glutathione *in vivo*. *Chemical and Biological Interactions* **80**, 89–97.

Balon, T.W. & Nadler, J.L. (1994) Nitric oxide release is present from incubated skeletal muscle preparations [see comments]. *Journal of Applied Physiology* **77**, 2519–2521.

Bar, P.R. & Amelink, G.J. (1997) Protection against muscle damage exerted by oestrogen: hormonal or antioxidant action. *Biochemical Society Transactions* **25**, 50–54.

Bendich, A. & Machlin, L.J. (1988) Safety of oral intake of vitamin E. *American Journal of Clinical Nutrition* **48**, 612–619.

Board on Agriculture, Committee on Animal Nutrition (1983) *Selenium in Nutrition*, revised edn. National Research Council, National Academy of Sciences, Washington, DC.

Borgstrom, L., Kagedal, B. & Paulsen, O. (1986) Pharmacokinetics of N-acetylcysteine in man. *European Journal of Clinical Pharmacology* **31**, 217–222.

Boveris, A., Oshino, N. & Chance, B. (1972) The cellular production of hydrogen peroxide. *Biochemical Journal* **128**, 617–630.

Brady, P.S., Ku, P.K. & Ullrey, D.E. (1978) Lack of effect of selenium supplementation on the response of the equine erythrocyte glutathione system and plasma enzymes to exercise. *Journal of Animal Science* **47**, 492–496.

Brady, P.S., Brady, L.J. & Ullrey, D.E. (1979) Selenium, vitamin E and the response to swimming stress in the rat. *Journal of Nutrition* **109**, 1103–1109.

Buettner, G.R. (1986) Ascorbate autoxidation in the presence of iron and copper chelates. *Free Radical Research Communications* **1**, 349–353.

Burk, R.F., Lawrence, R.A. & Lane, J.M. (1980) Liver necrosis and lipid peroxidation in the rat as the result of paraquat and diquat administration. Effect of selenium deficiency. *Journal of Clinical Investigation* **65**, 1024–1031.

Burton, G.W. & Ingold, K.U. (1984) Beta-carotene: an unusual type of lipid antioxidant. *Science* **224**, 569–573.

Burton, G.W., Joyce, A. & Ingold, K.U. (1983) Is vitamin E the only lipid-soluble, chain breaking antioxidant in human blood plasma and erythrocyte membranes? *Archives of Biochemistry and Biophysics* **221**, 281–290.

Cannon, J.G., Orencole, S.F., Fielding, R.A. *et al.* (1990) Acute phase response in exercise: interaction of age and vitamin E on neutrophils and muscle enzyme release. *American Journal of Physiology* **259**(6), R1214–1219.

Cazzulani, P., Cassin, M. & Ceserani, R. (1991) Increased endurance to physical exercise in mice given oral reduced glutathione GSH. *Medical Science Research* **19**, 543–544.

Chance, B., Sies, H. & Boveris, A. (1979) Hydroperoxide metabolism in mammalian organs. *Physiology Review* **59**, 527–605.

Cho, E.S., Sahyoun, N. & Steglink, L.D. (1981) Tissue glutathione as a cyst(e)ine reservoir during fasting and refeeding of rats. *Journal of Nutrition* **111**, 914–922.

Clark, R.F., Strukle, E., Williams, S.R. & Manoguerra, A.S. (1996) Selenium poisoning from a nutritional supplement [letter]. *Journal of the American Medical Association* **275**, 1087–1088.

Corrigan, J.J. Jr (1979) Coagulation problems relating to vitamin E. *American Journal of Pediatric Hematology and Oncology* **1**, 169–173.

Criswell, D., Powers, S., Dodd, S. *et al.* (1993) High intensity training-induced changes in skeletal muscle antioxidant enzyme activity. *Medicine and Science in Sports and Exercise* **25**, 1135–1140.

Davies, K.J.A. & Ursini, F. (eds) (1995) *The Oxygen Paradox*. CLEUP University Press, Padua.

Davies, K.J., Quintanilha, A.T., Brooks, G.A. & Packer, L. (1982) Free radicals and tissue damage produced by exercise. *Biochemical and Biophysical Research Communications* **107**, 1198–1205.

Dekkers, J.C., van Doornen, L.J. & Kemper, H.C. (1996) The role of antioxidant vitamins and enzymes in the prevention of exercise-induced muscle damage. *Sports Medicine* **21**, 213–238.

DeLeve, L.D. & Kaplowitz, N. (1990) Importance and regulation of hepatic glutathione. *Seminars in Liver Disease* **10**, 251–266.

Demoz, A., Willumsen, N. & Berge, R.K. (1992) Eicosapentaenoic acid at hypotriglyceridemic dose enhances the hepatic antioxidant defense in mice. *Lipids* **27**, 968–971.

Demoz, A., Asiedu, D.K., Lie, O. & Berge, R.K. (1994) Modulation of plasma and hepatic oxidative status and changes in plasma lipid profile by $n$-3 (EPA and DHA), $n$-6 (corn oil) and a 3-thia fatty acid in rats. *Biochimica Biophysica Acta* **1199**, 238–244.

Dillard, C.J., Dumelin, E.E. & Tappel, A.L. (1977) Effect of dietary vitamin E on expiration of pentane and ethane by the rat. *Lipids* **12**, 109–114.

Dillard, C.J., Litov, R.E., Savin, W.M., Dumelin, E.E. & Tappel, A.L. (1978) Effects of exercise, vitamin E, and ozone on pulmonary function and lipid peroxidation. *Journal of Applied Physiology* **45**, 927–932.

Duthie, G.G. & Arthur, J.R. (1994) Cigarette smoking as an inducer of oxidative stress. In *Exercise and Oxygen Toxicity* (eds C.K. Sen, L. Packer & O. Hanninen), pp. 297–317. Elsevier Science, Amsterdam.

Edmonds, S.E. & Blake, D.R. (1994) Hypoxia, oxidative stress, and exercise in rheumatoid arthritis. In *Exercise and Oxygen Toxicity* (eds C.K. Sen, L. Packer & O. Hanninen), pp. 398–422. Elsevier Science, Amsterdam.

Ferrari, G., Yan, C.Y. & Greene, L.A. (1995) N-acetylcysteine (D- and L-stereoisomers) prevents apoptotic death of neuronal cells. *Journal of Neuroscience* **15**, 2857–2866.

Floyd, R.A. (1995) Measurement of oxidative stress *in vivo*. In *The Oxygen Paradox* (ed. K.J.A. Davies & F. Ursini), pp. 89–103. CLEUP University Press, Padua.

Frandsen, U., Lopez-Figueroa, M. & Hellsten, Y. (1996) Localization of nitric oxide synthase in human skeletal muscle. *Biochemical and Biophysical Research Communications* **227**, 88–93.

Garewal, H.S. & Diplock, A.T. (1995) How 'safe' are antioxidant vitamins? *Drug Safety* **13**, 8–14.

Gohil, K., Henderson, S., Terblanche, S.E., Brooks, G.A. & Packer, L. (1984) Effects of training and exhaustive exercise on the mitochondrial oxidative capacity of brown adipose tissue. *Bioscience Reports* **4**, 987–993.

Gohil, K., Packer, L., de Lumen, B., Brooks, G.A. &

Terblanche, S.E. (1986) Vitamin E deficiency and vitamin C supplements: exercise and mitochondrial oxidation. *Journal of Applied Physiology* **60**, 1986–1991.

Gohil, K., Viguie, C., Stanley, W.C., Brooks, G.A. & Packer, L. (1988) Blood glutathione oxidation during human exercise. *Journal of Applied Physiology* **64**, 115–119.

Goldfarb, A. & Sen, C.K. (1994) Antioxidant supplementation and the control of oxygen toxicity during exercise. In *Exercise and Oxygen Toxicity* (ed. C.K. Sen, L. Packer & O. Hanninen), pp. 163–189. Elsevier Science, Amsterdam.

Goldfarb, A.H., Todd, M.K., Boyer, B.T., Alessio, H.M. & Cutler, R.G. (1989) Effect of vitamin E on lipid peroxidation to 80% maximum oxygen consumption (Abstract). *Medicine and Science in Sports and Exercise* **21**, S16.

Goldfarb, A.H., McIntosh, M.K. & Boyer, B.T. (1993) Effects of vitamin E DHEA and exercise on heart oxidative stress. *Medicine and Science in Sports and Exercise* **25**, S129.

Goldfarb, A.H., McIntosh, M.K., Boyer, B.T. & Fatouros, J. (1994) Vitamin E effects on indexes of lipid peroxidation in muscle from DHEA-treated and exercised rats. *Journal of Applied Physiology* **76**, 1630–1635.

Goldfarb, A.H., McIntosh, M.K. & Boyer, B.T. (1996) Vitamin E attenuates myocardial oxidative stress induced by DHEA in rested and exercised rats. *Journal of Applied Physiology* **80**, 486–490.

Hagen, T.M., Wierzbicka, G.T., Bowman, B.B., Aw, T.Y. & Jones, D.P. (1990) Fate of dietary glutathione: disposition in the gastrointestinal tract. *American Journal of Physiology* **259**, G530–535.

Han, D., Handelman, G., Marcocci, L. *et al.* (1997) Lipoic acid increases de novo synthesis of cellular glutathione by improving cysteine utilization. *Biofactors* **6**, 321–338.

Handelman, G.J. (1996) Carotenoids as scavengers of active oxygen species. In *Handbook of Antioxidants* (ed. E. Cadenas & L. Packer), pp. 259–314. Marcel Dekker, New York.

Handelman, G.J., van Kuijk, F.J., Chatterjee, A. & Krinsky, N.I. (1991) Characterization of products formed during the autoxidation of beta-carotene. *Free Radical Biology Medicine* **10**, 427–437.

Handelman, G.J., Han, D., Tritschler, H. & Packer, L. (1994) Alpha-lipoic acid reduction by mammalian cells to the dithiol form, and release into the culture medium. *Biochemical Pharmacology* **47**, 1725–1730.

Hartmann, A., Niess, A.M., Grunert-Fuchs, M., Poch, B. & Speit, G. (1995) Vitamin E prevents exercise-induced DNA damage. *Mutation Research* **346**, 195–202.

Hayes, J.D. & Pulford, D.J. (1995) The glutathione S-transferase supergene family: regulation of GST and the contribution of the isoenzymes to cancer chemo-protection and drug resistance. *Critical Reviews in Biochemical and Molecular Biology* **30**, 445–600.

Hellsten, Y. (1994) The role of xanthine oxidase in exercise. In *Exercise and Oxygen Toxicity* (ed. C.K. Sen, L. Packer & O. Hanninen), pp. 211–234. Elsevier Science, Amsterdam.

Hellsten, Y., Apple, F.S. & Sjodin, B. (1996) Effect of sprint cycle training on activities of antioxidant enzymes in human skeletal muscle. *Journal of Applied Physiology* **81**, 1484–1487.

Holdiness, M.R. (1991) Clinical pharmacokinetics of N-acetylcysteine. *Clinical Pharmacokinetics* **20**, 123–134.

Hu, M.L., Frankel, E.N., Leibovitz, B.E. & Tappel, A.L. (1989) Effect of dietary lipids and vitamin E on *in vitro* lipid peroxidation in rat liver and kidney homogenates. *Journal of Nutrition* **119**, 1574–1582.

Huupponen, M.R., Makinen, L.H., Hyvonen, P.M., Sen, C.K., Rankinen, T., Vaisanen, S. & Rauramaa, R. (1995) The effect of N-acetylcysteine on exercise-induced priming of human neutrophils: a chemiluminescence study. *International Journal of Sports Medicine* **16**, 399–403.

International Programme of Chemical Safety (1987) *Selenium*. World Health Organization, Geneva.

Issels, R.D., Nagele, A., Eckert, K.G. & Wilmanns, W. (1988) Promotion of cystine uptake and its utilization for glutathione biosynthesis induced by cysteamine and N-acetylcysteine. *Biochemical Pharmacology* **37**, 881–888.

Jackson, M.J. (1987) Muscle damage during exercise: possible role of free radicals and protective effect of vitamin E. *Proceedings of the Nutrition Society* **46**, 77–80.

Jackson, M.J., Jones, D.A. & Edwards, R.H.T. (1983) Biology of vitamin E. In *Biology of Vitamin E: Proceedings of a Ciba Foundation Symposium* (ed. R. Porter & J. Wheelan), pp. 224–239. Pitman Medical, London.

Jenkins, R.R. & Halliwell, B. (1994) Metal binding agents: possible role in exercise. In *Exercise and Oxygen Toxicity* (ed. C.K. Sen, L. Packer & O. Hanninen), pp. 59–76. Elsevier Science, Amsterdam.

Jenkins, R.R., Friedland, R. & Howald, H. (1984) The relationship of oxygen uptake to superoxide dismutase and catalase activity in human skeletal muscle. *International Journal of Sports Medicine* **5**, 11–14.

Ji, L.L. (1994) Exercise induced oxidative stress in heart. In *Exercise and Oxygen Toxicity* (ed. C.K. Sen, L. Packer & O. Hanninen), pp. 249–267. Elsevier Science, Amsterdam.

Ji, L.L., Stratman, F.W. & Lardy, H.A. (1988) Antioxidant enzyme systems in rat liver and skeletal muscle: influences of selenium deficiency, chronic training, and acute exercise. *Archives of Biochemistry and Biophysics* **263**, 150–160.

Jungersten, L., Ambring, A., Wall, B. & Wennmalm, A.

(1997) Both physical fitness and acute exercise regulate nitric oxide formation in healthy humans. *Journal of Applied Physiology* **82**, 760–764.

Kagan, V., Nohl, H. & Quinn, P.J. (1996) Coenzyme Q: its role in scavenging and generation of radicals in membranes. In *Handbook of Antioxidants* (ed. C. Cadenas & L. Packer), pp. 157–201. Marcel Dekker, New York.

Kanter, M.M. & Eddy, D.E. (1992) Effects of antioxidant supplementation on serum markers of lipid peroxidation and skeletal muscle damage following eccentric exercise. *Medicine and Science in Sports and Exercise* **24**, S17.

Kanter, M.M., Nolte, L.A. & Holloszy, J.O. (1993) Effects of an antioxidant vitamin mixture on lipid peroxidation at rest and postexercise. *Journal of Applied Physiology* **74**, 965–969.

Kellogg, E.W. III & Fridovich, I. (1975) Superoxide, hydrogen peroxide, and singlet oxygen in lipid peroxidation by a xanthine oxidase system. *Journal of Biological Chemistry* **250**, 8812–8817.

Keul, J., Doll, E. & Koppler, D. (1972) *Energy Metabolism and Human Muscle*. S. Karger, Basel.

Khaira, H.S., Maxwell, S.R. & Shearman, C.P. (1995) Antioxidant consumption during exercise in intermittent claudication. *British Journal of Surgery* **82**, 1660–1662.

Khanna, S., Atalay, M., Laaksonen, D.E. *et al.* (1997) Tissue glutathione homeostasis in response to lipoate supplementation and exercise. Paper presented at the Annual Meeting of the Oxygen Club of California, Santa Barbara, CA, 27 February–1 March.

Khawli, F.A. & Reid, M.B. (1994) N-acetylcysteine depresses contractile function and inhibits fatigue of diaphragm *in vitro*. *Journal of Applied Physiology* **77**, 317–324.

Kim, J.D., McCarter, R.J. & Yu, B.P. (1996a) Influence of age, exercise, and dietary restriction on oxidative stress in rats. *Aging (Milano)* **8**, 123–129.

Kim, J.D., Yu, B.P., McCarter, R.J., Lee, S.Y. & Herlihy, J.T. (1996b) Exercise and diet modulate cardiac lipid peroxidation and antioxidant defenses. *Free Radical Biological Medicine* **20**, 83–88.

Kondo, H. & Itokawa, Y. (1994) Oxidative stress in muscular atrophy. In *Exercise and Oxygen Toxicity* (ed. C.K. Sen, L. Packer & O. Hanninen), pp. 319–342. Elsevier Science, Amsterdam.

Kromhout, D., Bosschieter, E.B. & de Lezenne Coulander, C. (1985) The inverse relation between fish consumption and 20-year mortality from coronary heart disease. *New England Journal of Medicine* **312**, 1205–1209.

Kumar, C.T., Reddy, V.K., Prasad, M., Thyagaraju, K. & Reddanna, P. (1992) Dietary supplementation of vitamin E protects heart tissue from exercise-induced oxidant stress. *Molecular and Cellular Biochemistry* **111**, 109–115.

Laaksonen, D.E., Atalay, M., Niskanen, L., Uusitupa, M., Hanninen, O. & Sen, C.K. (1996) Increased resting and exercise-induced oxidative stress in young IDDM men. *Diabetes Care* **19**, 569–574.

Laaksonen, R., Fogelholm, M., Himberg, J.J., Laakso, J. & Salorinne, Y. (1995) Ubiquinone supplementation and exercise capacity in trained young and older men. *European Journal of Applied Physiology* **72**, 95–100.

Lauterburg, B.H., Adams, J.D. & Mitchell, J.R. (1984) Hepatic glutathione homeostasis in the rat: efflux accounts for glutathione turnover. *Hepatology* **4**, 586–590.

Lawrence, J.D., Bower, R.C., Riehl, W.P. & Smith, J.L. (1975) Effects of alpha-tocopherol acetate on the swimming endurance of trained swimmers. *American Journal of Clinical Nutrition* **28**, 205–208.

Leeuwenburgh, C. & Ji, L.L. (1995) Glutathione depletion in rested and exercised mice: biochemical consequence and adaptation. *Archives of Biochemistry and Biophysics* **316**, 941–949.

Leeuwenburgh, C. & Ji, L.L. (1996) Alteration of glutathione and antioxidant status with exercise in unfed and refed rats. *Journal of Nutrition* **126**, 1833–1843.

Leibovitz, B.E., Hu, M.L. & Tappel, A.L. (1990) Lipid peroxidation in rat tissue slices: effect of dietary vitamin E, corn oil-lard and menhaden oil. *Lipids* **25**, 125–129.

Levine, R.L. & Stadtman, E.R. (1996) Protein modifications with aging. In *Handbook of the Biology of Aging* (ed. E.L. Schneider & J.W. Rowe), pp. 184–197. Academic Press, San Diego.

Lodge, L., Handelman, G.J., Konishi, T., Matsugo, S., Mathur, V.V. & Packer, L. (1997) Natural sources of lipoic acid: determination of lipoyllysine released from protease-digested tissues by high performance liquid chromatography incorporating electrochemical detection. *Journal of Applied Nutrition* **49**, 3–11.

Luhtala, T.A., Roecker, E.B., Pugh, T., Feuers, R.J. & Weindruch, R. (1994) Dietary restriction attenuates age-related increases in rat skeletal muscle antioxidant enzyme activities. *Journal of Gerontology* **49**, B231–238.

McIntosh, M.K., Goldfarb, A.H., Cote, P.S. & Griffin, K. (1993a) Vitamin E reduces peroxisomal fatty acid oxidation and indicators of oxidative stress in untrained exercised rats treated with dehydroepiandrosterone DHEA. *Journal of Nutritional Biochemistry* **4**, 298–303.

McIntosh, M.K., Goldfarb, A.H., Curtis, L.N. & Cote, P.S. (1993b) Vitamin E alters hepatic antioxidant enzymes in rats treated with dehydroepiandrosterone (DHEA). *Journal of Nutrition* **123**, 216–224.

Martensson, J., Jain, A. & Meister, A. (1990) Glutathione is required for intestinal function. *Proceedings of the National Academy of Science, USA* **87**, 1715–1719.

Meister, A. (1991) Glutathione deficiency produced by inhibition of its synthesis, and its reversal: applications in research and therapy. *Pharmacology Therapy* **51**, 155–194.

Meister, A. (1992a) Biosynthesis and functions of glutathione, an essential biofactor. *Journal of Nutrition Science and Vitaminology (Tokyo)*, Special No., 1–6.

Meister, A. (1992b) On the antioxidant effects of ascorbic acid and glutathione. *Biochemical Pharmacology* **44**, 1905–1915.

Meister, A. (1995) Glutathione metabolism. *Methods in Enzymology* **251**, 3–7.

Meydani, M., Evans, W.J., Handelman, G. *et al.* (1993) Protective effect of vitamin E on exercise-induced oxidative damage in young and older adults. *American Journal of Physiology* **264**, R992–998.

Mills, P.C., Smith, N.C., Casas, I., Harris, P., Harris, R.C. & Marlin, D.J. (1996) Effects of exercise intensity and environmental stress on indices of oxidative stress and iron homeostasis during exercise in the horse. *European Journal of Applied Physiology* **74**, 60–66.

Moller, P., Wallin, H. & Knudsen, L.E. (1996) Oxidative stress associated with exercise, psychological stress and life-style factors. *Chemical and Biological Interactions* **102**, 17–36.

Nadiger, H.A., Marcus, S.R., Chandrakala, M.V. & Kulkarni, D.D. (1986) Malonyl dialdehyde levels in different organs of rats subjected to acute alcohol toxicity. *Indian Journal of Clinical Biochemistry* **1**, 133–136.

Nadiger, H.A., Marcus, S.R. & Chandrakala, M.V. (1988) Lipid peroxidation and ethanol toxicity in rat-brain: effect of viatmin E deficiency and supplementation. *Medical Science Research* **16**, 1273–1274.

Nalbone, G., Leonardi, J., Termine, E. *et al.* (1989) Effects of fish oil, corn oil and lard diets on lipid peroxidation status and glutathione peroxidase activities in rat heart. *Lipids* **24**, 179–186.

Novelli, G.P., Braccitiotti, G. & Falsini, S. (1990) Spin-trappers and vitamin E prolong endurance to muscle fatigue in mice. *Free Radical Biology and Medicine* **8**, 9–13.

Novelli, G.P., Falsini, S. & Bracciotti, G. (1991) Exogenous glutathione increases endurance to muscle effort in mice. *Pharmacological Research* **23**, 149–156.

Ohno, H., Suzuki, K., Fujii, J. *et al.* (1994) Superoxide dismutases in exercise and disease. In *Exercise and Oxygen Toxicity* (ed. C.K. Sen, L. Packer & O. Hanninen), pp. 127–161. Elsevier Science, Amsterdam.

Packer, L. & Reznick, A.Z. (1992) Significance of vitamin E for the athlete. In *Vitamin E in Health and Disease* (ed. J. Fuchs & L. Packer), pp. 465–471. Marcel Dekker, New York.

Packer, L., Gohil, K., deLumen, B. & Terblanche, S.E. (1986) A comparative study on the effects of ascorbic acid deficiency and supplementation on endurance and mitochondrial oxidative capacities in various tissues of the guinea pig. *Comparative Biochemistry and Physiology B* **83**, 235–240.

Packer, L., Witt, E.H. & Tritschler, H.J. (1995) alpha-Lipoic acid as a biological antioxidant. *Free Radical Biology and Medicine* **19**, 227–250.

Packer, L., Roy, S. & Sen, C.K. (1997) Alpha-lipoic acid: a metabolic antioxidant and potential redox modulator of transcription. *Advances in Pharmacology* **38**, 79–101.

Paffenbarger, R.S. Jr, Hyde, R.T., Wing, A.L. & Steinmetz, C.H. (1984) A natural history of athleticism and cardiovascular health. *Journal of the American Medical Association* **252**, 491–495.

Pincemail, J., Deby, C., Camus, G. *et al.* (1988) Tocopherol mobilization during intensive exercise. *European Journal of Applied Physiology* **57**, 189–191.

Poulsen, H.E., Loft, S. & Vistisen, K. (1996) Extreme exercise and oxidative DNA modification. *Journal of Sports Science* **14**, 343–346.

Powers, S.K. & Criswell, D. (1996) Adaptive strategies of respiratory muscles in response to endurance exercise. *Medicine and Science in Sports and Exercise* **28**, 1115–1122.

Quintanilha, A.T. & Packer, L. (1983) Vitamin E, physical exercise and tissue oxidative damage. *Ciba Foundation Symposia* **101**, 56–69.

Quintanilha, A.T., Packer, L., Davies, J.M., Racanelli, T.L. & Davies, K.J. (1982) Membrane effects of vitamin E deficiency: bioenergetic and surface charge density studies of skeletal muscle and liver mitochondria. *Annals of the NY Academy of Science* **393**, 32–47.

Rajguru, S.U., Yeargans, G.S. & Seidler, N.W. (1994) Exercise causes oxidative damage to rat skeletal muscle microsomes while increasing cellular sulfhydryls. *Life Sciences* **54**, 149–157.

Reid, M.B., Stokic, D.S., Koch, S.M., Khawli, F.A. & Leis, A.A. (1994) N-acetylcysteine inhibits muscle fatigue in humans. *Journal of Clinical Investigations* **94**, 2468–2474.

Reznick, A.Z., Witt, E., Matsumoto, M. & Packer, L. (1992) Vitamin E inhibits protein oxidation in skeletal muscle of resting and exercised rats. *Biochemical and Biophysical Research Communications* **189**, 801–806.

Robinson, D.M., Ogilvie, R.W., Tullson, P.C. & Terjung, R.L. (1994) Increased peak oxygen consumption of trained muscle requires increased electron flux capacity. *Journal of Applied Physiology* **77**, 1941–1952.

Rokitzki, L., Logemann, E., Huber, G., Keck, E. & Keul, J. (1994a) alpha-Tocopherol supplementation in racing cyclists during extreme endurance training [see comments]. *International Journal of Sport Nutrition* **4**, 253–264.

Rokitzki, L., Logemann, E., Sagredos, A.N., Murphy, M., Wetzel-Roth, W. & Keul, J. (1994b) Lipid peroxidation and antioxidative vitamins under extreme endurance stress. *Acta Physiologica Scandinavica* **151**, 149–158.

Rotruck, J.T., Pope, A.L., Ganther, H.E., Swanson, A.B., Hafeman, D.G. & Hoekstra, W.G. (1973) Selenium: biochemical role as a component of glutathione peroxidase. *Science* **179**, 588–590.

Roy, S. & Hanninen, O. (1993) Biochemical monitoring of the aquatic environment: possibilities and limitations. In *Ecotoxicology Monitoring* (ed. M. Richardson), pp. 119–135. VCH Publishers, London.

Salminen, A., Kainulainen, H., Arstila, A.U. & Vihko, V. (1984) Vitamin E deficiency and the susceptibility to lipid peroxidation of mouse cardiac and skeletal muscles. *Acta Physiologica Scandinavica* **122**, 565–570.

Schmidt, E.B. & Dyerberg, J. (1994) Omega-3 fatty acids: current status in cardiovascular medicine. *Drugs* **47**, 405–424.

Schwarz, K. & Foltz, C.M. (1957) Selenium as an integral part of factor 3 against dietary necrotic liver degeneration. *Journal of the American Chemical Society* **79**, 3292–3293.

Sen, C.K. (1995) Oxidants and antioxidants in exercise. *Journal of Applied Physiology* **79**, 675–686.

Sen, C.K. & Hanninen, O. (1994) Physiological antioxidants. In *Exercise and Oxygen Toxicity* (ed. C.K. Sen, L. Packer & O. Hanninen), pp. 89–126. Elsevier Science, Amsterdam.

Sen, C.K. & Packer, L. (1996) Antioxidant and redox regulation of gene transcription. *Faseb Journal* **10**, 709–720.

Sen, C.K. & Packer, L. (1999) Thiol homeostasis and supplementation in physical exercise. *American Journal of Clinical Nutrition*, in press.

Sen, C.K., Marin, E., Kretzschmar, M. & Hanninen, O. (1992) Skeletal muscle and liver glutathione homeostasis in response to training, exercise, and immobilization. *Journal of Applied Physiology* **73**, 1265–1272.

Sen, C.K., Rahkila, P. & Hanninen, O. (1993) Glutathione metabolism in skeletal muscle derived cells of the L6 line. *Acta Physiologica Scandinavica* **148**, 21–26.

Sen, C.K., Atalay, M. & Hanninen, O. (1994a) Exercise-induced oxidative stress: glutathione supplementation and deficiency. *Journal of Applied Physiology* **77**, 2177–2187.

Sen, C.K., Ookawara, T., Suzuki, K., Taniguchi, N., Hanninen, O. & Ohno, H. (1994b) Immunoreactivity and activity of mitochondrial superoxide dismutase following training and exercise. *Pathophysiology* **1**, 165–168.

Sen, C.K., Packer, L. & Hanninen, O. (eds) (1994c) *Exercise and Oxygen Toxicity*. Elsevier Science, Amsterdam.

Sen, C.K., Rankinen, T., Vaisanen, S. & Rauramaa, R. (1994d) Oxidative stress after human exercise: effect of N-acetylcysteine supplementation [published erratum appears in *Journal of Applied Physiology* 1994 Nov; **77** (5): following table of contents and 1994 Dec; **77** (6): following volume table of contents]. *Journal of Applied Physiology* **76**, 2570–2577.

Sen, C.K., Kolosova, I., Hanninen, O. & Orlov, S.N. (1995) Inward potassium transport systems in skeletal muscle derived cells are highly sensitive to oxidant exposure. *Free Radical Biology and Medicine* **18**, 795–800.

Sen, C.K., Atalay, M., Agren, J., Laaksonen, D.E., Roy, S. & Hanninen, O. (1997a) Fish oil and vitamin E supplementation in oxidative stress at rest and after physical exercise. *Journal of Applied Physiology* **83**, 189–195.

Sen, C.K., Roy, S., Han, D. & Packer, L. (1997b) Regulation of cellular thiols in human lymphocytes by alpha-lipoic acid: a flow cytometric analysis. *Free Radical Biology and Medicine* **22**, 1241–1257.

Sen, C.K., Roy, S. & Packer, L. (1997c) Therapeutic potential of the antioxidant and redox properties of alpha-lipoic acid. In *Oxidative Stress Cancer, AIDS and Neurodegenerative Diseases* (ed. L. Montagnier, R. Olivier & C. Pasquier), pp. 251–267. Marcel Dekker Inc., New York.

Sharman, I.M., Down, M.G. & Norgan, N.G. (1976) The effects of vitamin E on physiological function and athletic performance of trained swimmers. *Journal of Sports Medicine and Physical Fitness* **16**, 215–225.

Sharpe, P.C., Duly, E.B., MacAuley, D. *et al.* (1996) Total radical trapping antioxidant potential (TRAP) and exercise. *Quarterly Journal of Medicine* **89**, 223–228.

Sheppard, A.J., Pennington, J.A.T. & Weihrauch, J.L. (1993) Analysis and distribution of vitamin E in vegetable oils and foods. In *Vitamin E in Health and Disease* (ed. L. Packer & J. Fuchs), pp. 9–31. Marcel Dekker, New York.

Shimomura, Y., Suzuki, M., Sugiyama, S., Hanaki, Y. & Ozawa, T. (1991) Protective effect of coenzyme Q10 on exercise-induced muscular injury. *Biochemical and Biophysical Research Communications* **176**, 349–355.

Sies, H. (1974) Biochemistry of the peroxisome in liver cell. *Angewandte Chemie* (*International Edition*) **13**, 706–718.

Sies, H. (1997) *Antioxidants in Disease Mechanisms and Therapeutic Strategies*. Academic Press, San Diego, CA.

Simon-Schnass, I. (1994) Risk of oxidative stress during exercise at high altitude. In *Exercise and Oxygen Toxicity* (ed. C.K. Sen, L. Packer & O. Hanninen), pp. 191–210. Elsevier Science, Amsterdam.

Singal, P.K. & Kirshenbaum, L.A. (1990) A relative deficit in antioxidant reserve may contribute in cardiac failure. *Canadian Journal of Cardiology* **6**, 47–49.

Singh, V.N. (1992) A current perspective on nutrition and exercise. *Journal of Nutrition* **122**, 760–765.

Sjödin, K., Nilsson, E., Hallberg, A. & Tunek, A. (1989)

Metabolism of N-acetyl-L-cysteine: some structural requirements for the deacetylation and consequences for the oral bioavailability. *Biochemical Pharmacology* **38**, 3981–3985.

Smith, J.A., Telford, R.D., Mason, I.B. & Weidemann, M.J. (1990) Exercise training and neutrophil mcrobicidal activity. *International Journal of Sports Medicine* **11**, 179–187.

Snider, I.P., Bazzarre, T.L., Murdoch, S.D. & Goldfarb, A. (1992) Effects of coenzyme athletic performance system as an ergogenic aid on endurance performance to exhaustion. *International Journal of Sport Nutrition* **2**, 272–286.

Sohal, R.S., Ku, H.H., Agarwal, S., Forster, M.J. & Lal, H. (1994) Oxidative damage, mitochondrial oxidant generation and antioxidant defenses during aging and in response to food restriction in the mouse. *Mechanisms of Ageing and Development* **74**, 121–133.

Sumida, S., Tanaka, K., Kitao, H. & Nakadomo, F. (1989) Exercise-induced lipid peroxidation and leakage of enzymes before and after vitamin E supplementation. *International Journal of Biochemistry* **21**, 835–838.

Taylor, A., Jahngen-Hodge, J., Smith, D.E. *et al.* (1995) Dietary restriction delays cataract and reduces ascorbate levels in Emory mice. *Experiments in Eye Research* **61**, 55–62.

Tessier, F., Margaritis, I., Richard, M.J., Moynot, C. & Marconnet, P. (1995) Selenium and training effects on the glutathione system and aerobic performance. *Medicine and Science in Sports and Exercise* **27**, 390–396.

Thomas, J.P., Maiorino, M., Ursini, F. & Girotti, A.W. (1990) Protective action of phospholipid hydroperoxide glutathione peroxidase against membrane-damaging lipid peroxidation: in situ reduction of phospholipid and cholesterol hydroperoxides. *Journal of Biological Chemistry* **265**, 454–461.

Tiidus, P.M., Behrens, W.A., Madere, R., Kim, J.J. & Houston, M.E. (1993) Effect of vitamin E status and exercise training on tissue lipid peroxidation based on two methods of assessment. *Nutritional Research* **13**, 219–224.

Traber, M.G. & Sies, H. (1996) Vitamin E in humans: demand and delivery. *Annual Review of Nutrition* **16**, 321–347.

van Zandwijk, N. (1995) N-acetylcysteine (NAC) and glutathione (GSH): antioxidant and chemopreventive properties, with special reference to lung cancer. *Journal of Cell Biochemistry* **22** (Suppl.), 24–32.

Vasankari, T., Kujala, U., Heinonen, O., Kapanen, J. & Ahotupa, M. (1995) Measurement of serum lipid peroxidation during exercise using three different methods: diene conjugation, thiobarbituric acid reac-

tive material and fluorescent chromolipids. *Clinica Chimica Acta* **234**, 63–69.

Venditti, P. & Di Meo, S. (1996) Antioxidants, tissue damage, and endurance in trained and untrained young male rats. *Archives of Biochemical Biophysics* **331**, 63–68.

Videla, L.A. & Valenzuela, A. (1982) Alcohol ingestion, liver glutathione and lipoperoxidation: metabolic interrelations and pathological implications. *Life Science* **31**, 2395–2407.

Viguie, C.A., Packer, L. & Brooks, G.A. (1989) Antioxidant supplementation affects indices of muscle trauma and oxidant stress in human blood during exercise. *Medicine and Science in Sports and Exercise* **21**, S16.

Viguie, C.A., Frei, B., Shigenaga, M.K., Ames, B.N., Packer, L. & Brooks, G.A. (1993) Antioxidant status and indexes of oxidative stress during consecutive days of exercise. *Journal of Applied Physiology* **75**, 566–572.

Vina, J., Perez, C., Furukawa, T., Palacin, M. & Vina, J.R. (1989) Effect of oral glutathione on hepatic glutathione levels in rats and mice. *British Journal of Nutrition* **62**, 683–691.

Vina, J., Sastre, J., Asensi, M. & Packer, L. (1995) Assay of blood glutathione oxidation during physical exercise. *Methods in Enzymology* **251**, 237–243.

Ward, P.A. (1991) Mechanisms of endothelial cell killing by $H_2O_2$ or products of activated neutrophils. *American Journal of Medicine* **91**, 89S–94S.

Warren, J.A., Jenkins, R.R., Packer, L., Witt, E.H. & Armstrong, R.B. (1992) Elevated muscle vitamin E does not attenuate eccentric exercise-induced muscle injury. *Journal of Applied Physiology* **72**, 2168–2175.

Watanabe, H. & Bannai, S. (1987) Induction of cystine transport activity in mouse peritoneal macrophages. *Journal of Experimental Medicine* **165**, 628–640.

Watt, T., Romet, T.T., McFarlane, I., McGuey, D., Allen, C. & Goode, R.C. (1974) Vitamin E and oxygen consumption (Letter). *Lancet* **2**, 354–355.

Weiss, S.J. (1989) Tissue destruction by neutrophils [see comments]. *New England Journal of Medicine* **320**, 365–376.

Wolbarsht, M.L. & Fridovich, I. (1989) Hyperoxia during reperfusion is a factor in reperfusion injury [see comments]. *Free Radical Biology Medicine* **6**, 61–62.

Zuliani, U., Bonetti, A., Campana, M., Cerioli, G., Solito, F. & Novarini, A. (1989) The influence of ubiquinone (Co Q10) on the metabolic response to work. *Journal of Sports Medicine and Physical Fitness* **29**, 57–62.

# Chapter 23

# Minerals: Calcium

KARIN PIEHL AULIN

## Introduction

Calcium is a micronutrient with great importance to many cellular events in different tissues in the body, as well as forming the major structural component of bone. Athletes are often concerned that their normal diet will not provide sufficient micronutrients, and the need for an adequate dietary intake of calcium is as much a concern for athletes as it is for the general population. Augmentation of the diet with specific calcium supplements and with calcium-enriched foods is common practice among athletes and non-athletes alike, but there is limited information as to whether the need for calcium is increased by physical activity, and whether such supplementation is warranted.

The US Surgeon General's Report (1988) states that 'inadequate dietary calcium consumption in the first three to four decades of life may be associated with increased risk for osteoporosis in later life due to a low peak bone mass'. Osteoporosis is a chronic disease characterized by a progressive loss of bone mass: it affects women more than men, partly because of the role played by a falling oestrogen level after the menopause. Bone loss is widely accepted as a normal part of the ageing process, and occurs at a rate of about 0.5–1.0% per annum after the age of 40 (Cohn *et al.* 1976): by age 90, one third of women and one sixth of men will have suffered hip fractures as a consequence. However, a number of nutritional and lifestyle factors have a major impact on the rate of mineral loss from the skeleton:

these factors can be important in slowing this process, and thus in delaying the point at which the bone mineral density becomes so low that the fracture threshold is easily exceeded. Other important factors reported to be associated with the maintenance of bone health are an adequate level of physical activity and avoidance or cessation of cigarette smoking and excess alcohol intake. However, while there is a clear role for physical activity in maintaining bone mass, very high levels of exercise in women have been associated with some degree of bone loss (Drinkwater *et al.* 1990), so there are clearly a number of issues of importance for women, and perhaps also to a lesser extent for men, involved in sports where high training loads are involved.

## Roles of calcium in the body

Calcium is an essential nutrient and a major component of mineralized tissue and is the mineral found in the largest quantity in the body, representing about 1.5–2% of body mass in the average adult: for men, total body calcium content is about 1000–1100 g, and for women, about 800 g (Cohn *et al.* 1976). Approximately 99% of the total body calcium is located in the bones. The remaining 1% is accounted for by the calcium found in the blood, muscle and nervous tissue where calcium is necessary for blood coagulation, muscle contraction and nerve conduction: although the amounts are small, the role of calcium is crucial for normal functioning.

Bone matrix is a mixture of tough fibres (made of type I collagen), which resist pulling forces, and solid particles (calcium phosphate as hydroxyapatite crystals), which resist compression. Bone is by no means a permanent and immutable tissue. There is a continuous turnover and remodelling of the matrix with a concomitant release and uptake of calcium: the cells involved in bone breakdown are osteoclasts, while the osteoblasts are involved in bone formation. The regulators of calcium metabolism in bone tissue are two hormones, parathyroid hormone (PTH) and calcitonin. Excess PTH results in a rise in the blood calcium with a corresponding fall in the calcium content of the bones, and a loss of calcium from the body by increased excretion in the urine. PTH, and exposure to sunlight, also stimulates the formation of the active form of vitamin D, which governs the absorption of calcium from the small intestine. The ability to regulate the uptake of calcium is important, and differences in bone mineral density can be demonstrated in response to exercise, even between groups with the same dietary calcium intake. Calcitonin is released when plasma calcium increases and stimulates bone formation. Calcium is excreted by the large intestine and, to a lesser extent, by the kidney and by the dermis.

In the overall function of skeletal muscle, calcium plays two essential regulatory roles. First, calcium is the link between excitation and contraction. The concentration of free calcium in the cytosol is low (about $10^{-8}$ M) in resting muscle (Martonosi & Beeler 1983), whereas its concentration in the extracellular fluid and in the endoplasmic reticulum (ER) is high. Calcium is involved in a series of events which converts the electrical signal of the action potential arriving at the synaptic terminal into a chemical signal that travels across the synapse where it is converted back into an electrical signal in the postsynaptic cell. Release of calcium from the terminal cisternae of the sarcoplasmic reticulum in response to membrane depolarization upon the arrival of an action potential allows the actin and myosin filaments to interact. The plasma membrane and the ER membrane have mechanisms to regulate the calcium concentration gradient during resting conditions and to restore it after muscle and nerve cell stimulation (Alberts *et al.* 1994). The activation process involves the binding of calcium to troponin C, one of the regulatory proteins associated with the actin filaments, and the change in shape of these proteins allows interaction between actin and myosin to occur. Calcium is then pumped back into the terminal cisternae by an energy-dependent transporter in a process that consumes adenosine triphosphate (ATP), allowing relaxation of the muscle to occur. There is good evidence that fatigue during high-intensity exercise may involve a disruption of the cell's calcium-handling capability (Maughan *et al.* 1997). A number of substances, including caffeine, can alter the response of the muscle to a single action potential, and the effects of some of these compounds on exercise capacity may be mediated by effects on calcium transport. These processes are described in detail by Jones and Round (1990).

A second key process requiring calcium is the activation of numerous cellular enzymes involved in energy production, and calcium is important to both glycogenolysis and the glycolytic pathway in generating ATP (Tate *et al.* 1991; Clarkson & Haymes 1995). It seems sensible that the same process that allows the muscle to do work is involved in the regulation of ATP provision. The activity of phosphorylase, the key enzyme involved in glycogen breakdown, is stimulated by increasing cytosolic calcium concentration (Maughan *et al.* 1997) and this is important for the activation of the glycolytic pathway at the onset of exercise.

## Calcium intake

An adequate calcium intake is needed to achieve optimal peak bone mass in the first two or three decades of life, to maintain bone mass throughout the middle years of life, and to minimize bone loss in the later years (Andersson 1996). A daily calcium intake that is sufficient to meet the requirement may be achieved through diet alone, if some attention is paid to the composition of the diet. Alternatively, calcium-fortified food or calcium supplementation may be employed to meet the need. The amount of calcium available from the diet depends on the total dietary calcium intake, the bioavailability, which depends in turn on the amount of calcium in solution and on the presence of other dietary components, and on the activity of the intestinal calcium transport systems. The bioavailability is influenced by the presence of anions that form insoluble compounds that cannot be absorbed: these include oxalate (which is present in rhubarb and spinach) and polyphosphate. Vitamin D status will determine the activity of the calcium transporters in the intestine. All of these factors, in addition to the ongoing losses of calcium from the body, will influence the amount of calcium that the diet must supply to meet the individual's requirement.

When body mass is taken into account, growing children require as much as two to four times as much calcium as adults, and the United States recommended dietary allowance (RDA) for calcium is greatest during adolescence (11–18 years) and early adulthood (19–24 years), being in the order of 1200 mg · day$^{-1}$ (National Research Council 1989). Males and females of all ages have the same calcium requirement except when females are pregnant or lactating. The RDA for children (1–10 years) and adults 25 years and older is 800 mg · day$^{-1}$. The National Academy of Science Food and Nutrition Board recently suggested new guidelines for calcium intake. They recommend: during early childhood (1–3 years) 500 mg · day$^{-1}$, 800 mg · day$^{-1}$ between 4 and 8 years, 1300 mg · day$^{-1}$ during adolescence (9–18 years) and 1000 mg · day$^{-1}$ between the ages of 18 and 50 years.

In the general US population, it is estimated that the average dietary calcium intake of men is about 115% of the 1989 RDA, but for women the figure is only 78%: for children, it is estimated that the mean intake is about 105% of the RDA (US Surgeon General 1988). Corresponding figures for the UK indicate rather similar values, with a daily mean intake of 940 mg for men and 717 mg for women (Gregory et al. 1990). However, as the RDA for calcium in the UK is only 500 mg for men and for women, the average intake was well above the RDA. This discrepancy between countries in recommendations for dietary intake reflects the uncertainty as to requirements: the dietary intake necessary to maintain calcium balance has been reported to be anything between 200 mg · day$^{-1}$ and over 1000 mg · day$^{-1}$ (Irwin & Kienholz 1973). The high value recommended for the American population greatly exceeds the desirable intake recommended by the WHO/FAO, and reflects the high dietary content of protein and phosphate in that country: both protein and phosphate are reported to increase calcium loss.

Surveys of dietary habits in female adolescent athletes (gymnasts, ballet dancers and distance runners) show their average calcium intake to be well below RDA and often related to their low-energy intake in order to maintain a low body weight (Carroll et al. 1983). Low energy intake together with a high weekly training load will lead to a decreased percentage of body fat, and insufficient levels of circulating oestrogen, resulting in menstrual dysfunctions such as oligomenorrhea or amenorrhea (Drinkwater et al. 1984, 1990). Several cross-sectional studies have shown significant relationships between body mass and bone mineral density and between body mass and susceptibility to osteoporotic fracture (Sowers et al. 1991; Lindsay et al. 1992). Restriction of energy intake (which resulted in a 5% reduction in dietary calcium intake) for a period as short as 6 months has been shown to result in a significant reduction in bone mineral density in healthy young women, even though there was only a moderate (3.4 kg) loss of body mass in these subjects (Ramsdale & Bassey 1994). The combination of low body mass, low circulating oestrogen levels and low dietary calcium intake clearly creates a high risk situation for development of early osteoporosis, and the possibility of stress fractures due to overload of bone tissue will then increase. Resumption of menses by regain in body weight may restore some of the lost bone tissue but not all is likely to be regained, depending on the persistence of the amenor-rhoea (Drinkwater *et al.* 1986).

Foods rich in calcium include dairy products, some canned fish (especially if eaten with bones), some vegetables, including broccoli, spinach and collard greens, tofu, and some calcium-enriched grain products. UK data for the general population indicate that milk and milk products provided about one half of the total calcium intake, while cereal products provided about 25%: vegetables contributed only about 7%, and the use of supplements was negligible (Gregory *et al.* 1990). Where energy intake is a concern, as in weight category sports, or when energy intake is otherwise restricted, the use of reduced-fat dairy products should be encouraged: a wide range of low to moderate fat varieties can be used to add variety to the diet.

Calcium has been reported to inhibit the absorption of iron from the food and it is therefore suggested that these two nutrients should not be taken together in large amounts (Gleerup *et al.* 1995). When both iron status and calcium status are precarious, special attention must be paid to the initiation of any supplementation regimen. This may be particularly relevant to female athletes, who may suffer from anaemia due to both low energy intake and loss of iron through the menses.

## Calcium balance

Whole body net calcium balance reflects the relationship between the dietary calcium intake and all routes of calcium loss. Positive calcium balance occurs when calcium intake exceeds calcium loss, and is necessary for bone growth and peak bone mass to be achieved. Negative calcium balance will lead to a decrease in bone mass and density. Calcium loss is the sum of the faecal, urinary, and dermal calcium losses. Faecal calcium loss accounts for about 75–80% of the dietary calcium ingested (Schroeder *et al.* 1972), but about 20% of this is of endogenous origin (Melvin *et al.* 1970). As discussed further below, the urinary calcium loss may be influenced by a number of factors, and the acidity of the urine,

which may in turn be influenced by the composition of the diet, appears to be an important factor (Ball & Maughan 1997). The loss of calcium through the skin is often estimated at $60\,mg \cdot day^{-1}$, but this may substantially underestimate the actual calcium loss of individuals who engaged in strenuous training programmes (Matkovic 1991). Sweat calcium losses as high as $57\,mg \cdot h^{-1}$ have been reported during exercise (Krebs *et al.* 1988). Sweat calcium concentration is typically about $1\,mmol \cdot l^{-1}$ $(40\,mg \cdot l^{-1})$, so losses may be very much greater than this when sweat rates are high or when prolonged exercise is performed, especially in hot environments (Shirreffs & Maughan 1997).

Dietary factors other than calcium intake may be of importance, and the association between high protein diets and an increased urinary calcium loss is widely accepted (Lutz 1984; Kerstetter & Allen 1990); this effect appears to be a consequence of the acid load that results from protein metabolism. The effects of an acid load in increasing urinary calcium output are well established, and the US Surgeon General's Report on Nutrition and Health (1988) concluded that 'increased acidity induces calcium loss by increasing renal excretion directly as well as by increasing the dissolution of mineral from the skeleton and impairing mineral deposition.'

A recent comparison of the dietary intake of omnivorous women and a matched group of vegetarians showed that the vegetarians had a lower dietary protein intake and a lower 24-h total urinary acid excretion than the omnivorous women (Ball & Maughan 1997). Although there were no differences between these groups in the estimated (7-day weighed intake) dietary calcium intake, the daily urinary calcium excretion of the omnivores was significantly higher than that of the vegetarians. These results are consistent with the suggestion that the acid/alkaline characteristics of the habitual diet have implications for calcium balance, and that this may be amenable to manipulation by alteration of specific dietary components.

There have been numerous recent reviews of the current state of knowledge regarding nutri-

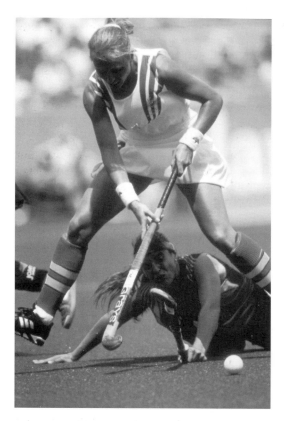

**Fig. 23.1** Most forms of exercise are good for bone health and should be encouraged in youngsters. Only a few athletes, most commonly young women in sports where low body mass confers an advantage, are likely to suffer accelerated bone mass. Photo © Allsport / M. Powell.

tion and bone metabolism and these have been summarized in the US Surgeon General's Report on Nutrition and Health (1988) (see Chapter 7).

## Exercise and calcium balance

Acute exercise results in a prompt increase in serum calcium, both in its ionized and non-ionized forms. This may be due in part to lactic acidosis rather than to changes in PTH and calcitonin concentrations, and haemoconcentration is also likely to be a significant factor (Vora *et al.* 1983; Cunningham *et al.* 1985). Marathon running was found to be accompanied by a transient decrease in urinary calcium and serum osteocalcin levels (Malm *et al.* 1992). Endurance

training has been reported to be associated with increased serum levels of the active form of vitamin D, leading to increased calcium absorption and a rise in total body calcium (Yeh & Aloia 1990). A few studies have demonstrated exercise-related elevations in PTH (Ljunghall *et al.* 1985, 1986; Salvesen *et al.* 1994), but this has not been confirmed in other studies (Aloia *et al.* 1985).

The influence of calcium intake and physical activity on peak bone mass has been the subject of much attention (Kanders *et al.* 1988; Mazess & Barden 1991; Recker *et al.* 1992). There are both cross-sectional and longitudinal studies that favour a beneficial effect of calcium on the adult skeleton and there are others that find no relationship between dietary calcium and bone mass and rate of bone loss. Peak bone mass is achieved during the third decade of life. Apart from calcium intake, heredity is also an important factor determining peak bone mass. A study on identical twins, where one twin in each pair received calcium supplementation and the other a placebo, suggested that extra calcium in the diet is beneficial to the achievement of peak bone mass prior to puberty (Johnston *et al.* 1992).

The role of physical activity in optimizing bone growth as well as maintaining bone mass is well established (Torgerson *et al.* 1995): acute reductions in weight-bearing activity are associated with a dramatic loss of calcium. Measurements of prolonged bed rest in healthy volunteers and in patients, as well as in astronauts subjected to microgravity, have all shown an increased calcium loss and a reduced skeletal mass (Anonymous 1983). Increased physical activity, and in particular running, has been shown to be associated with an increased bone density (Lane *et al.* 1986), and it seems clear that the physical stress imposed on the bone is an important factor (Lanyon 1992; Wolman 1994). This is supported by a recent study showing increases in bone area in adult male rats subjected to a resistance training programme (Westerlind *et al.* 1998). There is, however, little information on the type, frequency, duration and intensity of exercise that will optimize bone mass and minimize the age-related loss.

Apart from the implications for the development of osteoporosis in later life, a low bone density may be detrimental in athletes. Myburgh et al. (1990) found that athletes with lower extremity stress fractures had significantly lower femoral and lumbar mineral densities than matched athletic control subjects. Athletes with stress fractures had significantly lower calcium intakes and had lower intakes of dairy products. Injured female athletes were more likely to have irregular menstrual cycles and less likely to use oral contraceptives. This was not confirmed among female ballet dancers but a great number of dancers with stress fractures avoided dairy products (Frusztajer et al. 1990). A lifetime history of calcium intakes exceeding 800 mg· day$^{-1}$ appears to reduce the risk for hip fractures in older women compared with women with lower calcium intake (<450 mg·day$^{-1}$) and this also seems to hold for men (Matkovic et al. 1979). Milk consumption during childhood and adolescence and as an adult was associated with a greater bone mass in postmenopausal women, but total calcium intake was not associated with bone mass (Sandler et al. 1985; Bauer et al. 1993). Exercise appears to be more important in preventing trabecular bone loss while calcium intake may be a more important influence on cortical bone loss.

## Conclusion

Intake of sufficient amounts of energy to balance the expenditure, maintenance of circulating hormone levels, and regular participation in some form of weight-bearing exercise are of greatest importance to achieve and preserve skeletal health. This is important for the avoidance of stress fractures in young athletes and for the preservation of bone health in later life. An adequate dietary intake of calcium is also essential, and this can be achieved by consumption of dairy products (which may be reduced-fat varieties) and other foods rich in calcium. Exercise per se does not seem to lead to an increased requirement for calcium by the body and there is generally no need for calcium supplementation for athletes provided that the amount of energy consumed is sufficient. The RDA for calcium in both men and women is different in different countries, and is usually between 800 and 1200 mg·day$^{-1}$. The recommended intake is the same for males and females of all ages, except when females are pregnant or lactating. In postmenopausal women, adequate hormone supplementation, physical exercise and dietary calcium intake will prevent loss of bone tissue and delay the development of osteoporosis.

## References

Alberts, B., Bray, D., Lewis, J., Raff, M., Roberts, K. & Watson, J.D. (1994) Molecular Biology of the Cell. Garland Publishing, New York.

Aloia, J.F., Rasulo, P., Deftos, L., Vaswani, A. & Yeh, J.K. (1985) Exercise-induced hypercalcemia and the calciotropic hormones. Journal of Laboratory and Clinical Medicine 106, 229–232.

Anderson, J. (1996) Calcium, phosphorus and human bone development. Journal of Nutrition 126, 1153S–1158S.

Anonymous (1983) Osteoporosis and activity. Lancet i, 1365–1366.

Ball, D. & Maughan, R.J. (1997) Blood and urine acid-base status of pre menopausal omnivorous and vegetarian women. British Journal of Nutrition 78, 683–693.

Bauer, D.C., Browner, W.S. & Cauley, J.A. (1993) Factors associated with appendicular bone mass in older women. Annals of Internal Medicine 118, 657–665.

Carroll, M.D., Abraham, S. & Dresser, C.M. (1983) Dietary Source Intake Data: United States, 1976–1980 (Publication (PHS) no. 83-i 68). Hyattsville, MD, US Department of Human Services.

Clarkson, P.M. & Haymes, E.M. (1995) Exercise and mineral status of athletes: calcium, magnesium phosphorus, and iron. Medicine and Science in Sports and Exercise 6, 831–843.

Cohn, S.H., Vaswani, A., Zanzi, I., Aloia, F., Roginski, M.S. & Ellis K.J. (1976) Changes in body chemical composition with age measured by total-body neutron activation. Metabolism 25, 85–95.

Cunningham, J., Segre, G.V., Slatopolsky, E. & Aviobi, L.V. (1985) Effect of heavy exercise on mineral metabolism and calcium regulating hormones in humans. Calcified Tissue International 37, 598–601.

Drinkwater, B.L., Nilson, K. & Chesnut, C.H. (1984) Bone mineral content of amenorrheic and eumenorrheic athletes. New England Journal of Medicine 311, 277–281.

Drinkwater, B.L., Nilson, K. & Ott, S. (1986) Bone mineral density after resumption of menses in amenorrheic athletes. *Journal of the American Medical Association* **256**, 380–382.

Drinkwater, B.L., Bruemner, B. & Chesnut, C.H. (1990) Menstrual history as determinant of current bone density in young athletes. *Journal of the American Medical Association* **263**, 545–548.

Frusztajer, N.T., Dhuper, S., Warren, M.P., Brooks-Gunn, J. & Fox, R.P. (1990) Nutrition and the incidence of stress fractures in ballet dancers. *American Journal of Clinical Nutrition* **51**, 779–783.

Gleerup, A., Rossander-Hulten, L., Gramatkovski, E. & Hallberg, L. (1995) Iron absorption from the whole diet: comparison of the effect of two different distributions of daily calcium intake. *American Journal of Clinical Nutrition* **61**, 97–104.

Gregory, J., Foster, K., Tyler, H. & Wiseman, M. (1990) *The Dietary and Nutritional Survey of British Adults.* HMSO, London.

Irwin, M.I. & Kienholz, E.W. (1973) A conspectus of research on calcium requirements of man. *Journal of Nutrition* **103**, 1019–1025.

Johnstone, C.C., Miller, J.Z., Slemdna, C.W., Reister, T.K., Christian, J.C. & Peacock, M. (1992) Calcium supplementation and increase in bone mineral density in children. *New England Journal of Medicine* **327**, 82–87.

Jones, D.A. & Round, J.M. (1990) *Skeletal Muscle in Health and Disease.* Manchester University Press, Manchester.

Kanders, B., Dempster, D.W. & Lindsay, R. (1988) Interaction of calcium nutrition and physical activity on bone mass in young women. *Journal of Bone and Mineral Research* **3**, 145–149.

Kerstetter, J.E. & Allen, L.H. (1990) Dietary protein increases urinary calcium. *Journal of Nutrition* **120**, 134–135.

Krebs, J.V., Schneider, J., Smith, A., Leblanc, W., Thornton, J. & Leach, C. (1988) Sweat calcium loss during running. *FASEB J* **2**, A1099.

Lane, N.E., Bloch, D.A., Jones, H.H., Marshall, W.H., Wood, P.D. & Fries, J.F. (1986) Long-distance running, bone density and osteoarthritis. *Journal of the American Medical Association* **255**, 1147–1151.

Lanyon, L.E. (1992) Control of bone architecture by functional load bearing. *Journal of Bone and Mineral Research* **7** (Suppl. 2), S369–S375.

Lindsay, R., Cosman, F., Herrington, B.S. & Himmelstein, S. (1992) Bone mass and body composition in normal women. *Journal of Bone and Mineral Research* **7**, 55–63.

Ljunghall, S., Joborn, H., Lundin, I., Rastad, J., Wide, L. & Akerstrom, G. (1985) Regional and systemic effects of short-term intense muscular work on plasma concentrations and content of total and ionised calcium. *European Journal of Clinical Investigation* **15**, 248–252.

Ljunghall, S., Joborn, H., Roxin, L.E., Rostad, J., Wide, L. & Akerstrom, G. (1986) Prolonged low intensity exercise raises the serum parathyroid hormone levels. *Clinical Endocrinology* **25**, 535–542.

Lutz, J. (1984) Calcium balance and acid-base status of women as affected by increased protein intake and by sodium bicarbonate ingestion. *American Journal of Clinical Nutrition* **39**, 281–288.

Malm, H.T., Ronni-Sivula, H.M., Viinikka, L.U. & Ylikorkala, O.R. (1992) Marathon running accompanied by transient decreases in urinary calcium and serum osteocalcin levels. *Calcified Tissue International* **52**, 209–211.

Martonosi, A.N. & Beeler, T.J. (1983) Mechanisms of $Ca^{2+}$ uptake by sarcoplasmic reticulum. In *Handbook of Physiology.* Section 10. *Skeletal Muscle* (ed. L.D. Peachey, R.H. Adrian & S.R. Geiger), pp. 417–485. American Physiological Society, Bethesda, MD.

Matkovic, V. (1991) Calcium metabolism and calcium requirements during skeletal modeling and consolidation of bone mass. *American Journal of Clinical Nutrition* **54**, 245S–260S.

Matkovic, V., Kostial, K., Simonovic, I., Buzina, R., Brodarec, A. & Nordin, B.E.C. (1979) Bone status and fracture rates in two regions of Yugoslavia. *American Journal of Clinical Nutrition* **32**, 540–549.

Maughan, R.J., Gleeson, M. & Greenhaff, P.L. (1997) *Biochemistry of Exercise and Training.* Oxford University Press, Oxford.

Mazess, R.B. & Barden, H.S. (1991) Bone density in premenstrual women: effects of age, dietary intake, physical activity, smoking and birth-control pills. *American Journal of Clinical Nutrition* **53**, 132–142.

Melvin, K.E.W., Hepner, G.W., Bordier, P., Neale, G. & Joplin, G.F. (1970) Calcium metabolism and bone pathology in adult coeliac disease. *Quarterly Journal of Medicine* **39**, 83–112.

Myburg, K.H., Hutchins, J., Fataar, A.B., Hough, S.F. & Noakes, T.D. (1990) Low bone density is an etiological factor for stress fractures in athletes. *Annals of Internal Medicine* **113**, 754–759.

National Research Council (1989) *Recommended Dietary Allowances,* 10th edn. National Academy Press, Washington, DC.

Ramsdale, S. & Bassey, E.J. (1994) Changes in bone mineral density associated with dietary-induced loss of body mass in young women. *Clinical Science* **87**, 343–348.

Recker, R.R., Davies, K.M., Hinders, S.M., Heaney, R.P., Stegman, R.M. & Kimmel, D.B. (1992) Bone gain in young adult women. *Journal of the American Medical Association* **268**, 2403–2408.

Salvesen, H., Johansson, A., Foxdal, P., Wide, L., Piehl Aulin, K. & Ljunghall, S. (1994) Intact serum parathyroid hormone levels increase during running exercise in well-trained men. *Calcified Tissue International* **54**, 253–261.

Sandler, R.B., Slemenda, C.W. & Laporte, R.E. (1985) Postmenopausal bone density and milk consumption in childhood and adolescence. *American Journal of Clinical Nutrition* **42**, 270–274.

Schroeder, H.A., Tipton, I.H. & Nason, A.P. (1972) Trace metals in man: strontium and barium. *Journal of Chronic Disease* **25**, 491–517.

Shirreffs, S.M. & Maughan, R.J. (1997) Whole body sweat collection in man: an improved method with some preliminary data on electrolyte composition. *Journal of Applied Physiology* **82**, 336–341.

Sowers, M., Khirsagar, A., Crutchfield, M. & Updike, S. (1991) Body composition, age and femoral bone mass of young adult women. *Annals of Epidemiology* **1**, 245–254.

Tate, C.H., Michael, F., Hyek, G. & Taffet, E. (1991) The role of calcium in the energetics of contracting skeletal muscle. *Sports Medicine* **12**, 208–217.

Torgerson, D.J., Campbell, M.K. & Reid, D.M. (1995) Life-style, environmental and medical factors influencing peak bone mass in women. *British Journal of Rheumatology* **34**, 620–624.

US Surgeon General (1988) *Report on Nutrition and Health*. DHHS (PHS) Publication no. 88–50210. US Dept of Health and Human Services, Washington DC.

Vora, N.M., Kukreja, S.C., York, P.A.J., Bowser, E.N., Hargis, G.K. & Williams, G.A. (1983) Effect of exercise on serum calcium and parathyroid hormone. *Journal of Clinical and Endocrinology Metabolism* **57**, 1067–1069.

Westerlind, K.C., Fluckey, J.D., Gordon, S.E., Kraemer, W.J., Farrell, P.A. & Turner, R.T. (1998) Effect of resistance exercise training on cortival and cancellous bone in mature male rats. *Journal of Applied Physiology* **84**, 459–464.

Wolman, R. (1994) Osteoporosis and exercise. *British Medical Journal* **309**, 400–403.

Yeh, J.K. & Abia, J. (1990) Effect of physical activity on calciotropic hormones and calcium balance in rats. *American Journal of Physiology* **285** (Endocrinol. Metab. 21), E263–E268.

# Chapter 24

# Minerals: Iron

E. RANDY EICHNER

## Introduction

Nearly all living things need iron, the fourth most abundant element on Earth. In humans, the nutritional need for iron centres on its role in energy metabolism. Iron is necessary for the formation of haemoglobin and myoglobin, the oxygen carriers in red blood cells and muscles, respectively. Iron is also a constituent of several enzymes—including catalase, peroxidase, and succinate dehydrogenase—and of the cytochromes, which enable electron transport in cellular respiration (and foster drug metabolism in the liver). In other words, because it delivers oxygen *to* cells and facilitates the use of oxygen *by* cells, iron is essential for energy metabolism. Simply put, iron is as vital as oxygen in converting chemical energy from food into metabolic energy for life.

Because it is vital for energy metabolism, iron is critical in sports nutrition. Concerns include: (i) whether athletes need more iron than nonathletes; (ii) the prevalence of iron deficiency among athletes; (iii) the effect of iron deficiency anaemia on athletic performance; (iv) whether low ferritin level in the absence of anaemia impairs performance; (v) how to ensure that athletes—vegetarian or not—get the iron they need from their diet; and (vi) the pros and cons of iron supplementation for athletes.

Iron deficiency may be the most common nutritional deficiency in the world. When it leads to anaemia, the paramount problem for athletes is diminished exercise capacity. Iron deficiency

may also impair two other functions key to athletes—immunity and cognition (Dallman 1982; Cook & Lynch 1986; Bruner *et al.* 1996)—but because supporting evidence is limited and inconclusive, these areas will be omitted here.

The value of dietary iron has been known for centuries. It is said the Persian physician Melampus in 4000 BC gave iron supplements to sailors who bled in battle. Other accounts of iron as therapy date to ancient Egypt and Rome. In the 16th and 17th centuries, poets, painters and playwrights portrayed the 'green sickness', or chlorosis, and attributed it to unrequited passion, or 'lovesickness.' Shakespearean heroines and heroes, disappointed by love, were smitten by the green sickness (Farley & Foland 1990). It was Thomas Sydenham in 1681 who first cured the green sickness with iron; he prescribed a syrup made by steeping iron filings in cold Rhenish wine (London 1980).

The symptoms of the green sickness—dyspnoea, fatigue and palpitations—are recognized today as those of anaemia. But the grave olive pallor that gave the condition its name is no longer common because today anaemia is diagnosed early, especially in athletes. Indeed, today 'anaemia' is found so early among athletes—and vague 'fatigue' often ascribed to it—that iron deficiency is sometimes overdiagnosed and overtreated. Today, we have the Humpty-Dumpty problem.

Humpty Dumpty, when challenged by Alice on word usage, said, 'When I use a word, it means just what I choose it to mean, neither more

nor less. The question is, which is to be master?'
So it goes today with 'anaemia' and 'fatigue' and
'iron deficiency' in athletes. As I will cover, these
words mean different things to different people.
First, a description of normal iron balance is in
order.

## Normal iron balance

Because iron—as the core of the oxygen-
delivering haemoglobin molecule—is the most
precious metal in the body, it is recycled. Recycling ensures a constant *internal* supply of iron—
independent of *external* sources such as diet—to
maintain an optimal red cell mass. So the bulk of
the iron needed for the daily synthesis of haemoglobin (20–30 mg) comes from recycling the iron
in senile red cells.

Senile red cells are destroyed by macrophages
in the spleen, releasing iron that is taken up by
transferrin (the iron-transporting protein in
plasma), carried to the bone marrow, removed by
developing red cells (normoblasts), and incorporated into haemoglobin of new-born red cells
(reticulocytes).

Because of this avid recycling—a 'closed
system'—little iron is lost from the body. Indeed,
the body has no active mechanism to excrete
unneeded iron. The average man loses only 1 mg
iron·day$^{-1}$; the average woman (because of
menses), 2 mg. The small obligatory loss (other
than menses) is in sweat and in epithelial cells
shed largely from skin, intestine and genitouri-
nary tract.

Because obligatory loss of iron is small, only
small amounts must be absorbed. The normal
USA diet provides 10–20 mg of iron daily; each
1000 calories in food is usually associated with
5–6 mg of iron. To maintain iron balance, the
average man absorbs 1 mg·day$^{-1}$; the average
woman, 2 mg. During times of increased iron
need—growth, pregnancy, bleeding—the intestine increases its absorption of iron, up to 4 or
5 mg·day$^{-1}$. When the need declines, absorption
returns to baseline.

The average total body iron of an adult man is
4000 mg. Up to three quarters of this iron is in the
'functional compartment,' mainly haemoglobin
and myoglobin, and about one quarter, or
1000 mg, is in storage, a bountiful buffer against
deprivation of dietary iron. In contrast, iron
stores are typically lower in adult women
(300–500 mg), marginal to absent in college-aged
women, and absent in young children and many
adolescents. Unlike most adult male athletes,
then, female and adolescent athletes need a
steady dietary supply of iron to maintain iron
balance and avoid anaemia.

Body iron is stored in parenchymal cells of the
liver and macrophages of the liver, spleen and
bone marrow. The main storage protein is ferritin. Soluble ferritin is released from cells (into
plasma) in direct proportion to cellular ferritin
content. So in general, the level of ferritin in the
plasma parallels the level of storage iron in the
body (Finch & Huebers 1982; Baynes 1996).
Unfortunately, as will be covered below, the use
of serum ferritin level to gauge 'iron deficiency'
among athletes is fraught with problems, not the
least of which is that one can have low ferritin
level (low iron stores) yet still be absorbing
enough iron from the diet to avoid anaemia. Put
another way, iron deficiency evolves through
predictable stages of severity, in which depletion
of storage iron, the first stage, precedes anaemia.
The development of iron deficiency anaemia
goes through the following stages.

1 Absent marrow iron stores; serum ferritin less
than 12 µg·l$^{-1}$.
2 Low serum iron; high iron-binding capacity; increase in level of free erythrocyte
protoporphyrin.
3 Normocytic, normochromic anaemia with
abnormal red cell distribution width.
4 Microcytic, hypochromic anaemia.

## Effect of training and competition

Training, especially endurance training, and
competition, especially ultramarathons or events
spanning several days or weeks, affect haemoglobin concentration and iron profile in ways
both physiological and pathophysiological. Mis-
interpretations of these perturbations, notably

the training-induced declines in haemoglobin concentration and serum ferritin concentration, have created confusion and controversy about 'anaemia' and 'iron deficiency' in athletes.

### 'Sports anaemia'

A prime 'Humpty-Dumpty problem' has been the failure of some authors to understand or point out that a 'low' or 'subnormal' haematocrit or haemoglobin concentration in a given athlete—especially an endurance athlete—is not necessarily 'anaemia.' Anaemia is best defined as a *subnormal number or mass of red blood cells* for a given individual. In this sense, most endurance athletes (particularly male athletes) with 'subnormal' haematocrit or haemoglobin concentration have not anaemia, but *pseudoanaemia*.

It is true that athletes, notably endurance athletes, tend to have lower haemoglobin concentrations than non-athletes. This has been called 'sports anaemia'. Sports anaemia, however, is a Humpty-Dumpty misnomer because the most common cause of a low haemoglobin level in an endurance athlete is a false anaemia. This false anaemia accrues from regular aerobic exercise, which expands the baseline plasma volume, diluting the red blood cells and haemoglobin concentration. In other words, the naturally lower haemoglobin level of the endurance athlete is a *dilutional pseudoanaemia*.

The increase in baseline plasma volume that causes athlete's pseudoanaemia is an adaptation to the acute loss of plasma volume during each workout. Vigorous exercise acutely reduces plasma volume by up to 10–20% in three ways. First, the exercise-induced rise in systolic blood pressure and the muscular compression of venules increase capillary hydrostatic pressure. Second, the generation of lactic acid and other metabolites in working muscle increases tissue osmotic pressure. These two forces, in concert, drive an ultrafiltrate of plasma from blood to tissues. Third, some plasma volume is lost in sweat.

To compensate for these bouts of exercise-induced haemoconcentration, the body releases renin, aldosterone and vasopressin, which conserve water and salt. Also, more albumin is added to the blood. The net result is an increase in baseline plasma volume (Convertino 1991).

So baseline plasma volume waxes and wanes according to physical activity. For example, if non-athletic men begin cycling vigorously $2\,h\cdot day^{-1}$, in less than a week, baseline plasma volume will expand by 400–500 ml. If they then quit cycling, plasma volume will decline as fast as it once expanded. Baseline plasma volume can increase by 10% 1 day after a half-marathon (Robertson *et al.* 1990) and by 17% 1 day after a full marathon (Davidson *et al.* 1987). Even a single brief session of intense exercise can expand the baseline plasma volume by the next day. For example, when six athletic men performed eight brief bouts at 85% of $\dot{V}o_{2max.}$ on a cycle ergometer, baseline plasma volume decreased by 15% during the exercise session, but was expanded by 10% 1 day later (Gillen *et al.* 1991). In short, the endurance athletes who train the hardest have the highest plasma volumes and the lowest haemoglobin levels. This is pseudoanaemia, a facet of aerobic fitness (Eichner 1992).

### Training and iron profile

Training, especially endurance training, tends to decrease the serum ferritin level. For example, after pilot research found iron deficient profiles in adolescent female runners during seasons of cross-country running, Nickerson *et al.* (1985) reported the first controlled trial of iron supplements for such runners. Eight (40%) of 20 adolescent female runners given placebo (vs. only one of 20 given iron supplements) developed 'iron deficiency' (serum ferritin $<20\,\mu g\cdot l^{-1}$) after 5 or 10 weeks of the cross-country running season. No runner developed iron deficiency anaemia.

Adolescent *male* runners, with higher iron stores, are less apt to develop iron deficient profiles. Nickerson *et al.* (1989) found that 34% of female but only 8% of male runners 'developed iron deficiency' (ferritin $<12\,\mu g\cdot l^{-1}$ and transferrin saturation $<16\%$) during a season. Two girls but no boys developed iron deficiency anaemia. But at the outset, 29% of the female runners had ferritins of less than $12\mu g \cdot l^{-1}$, so this study, without non-athletic controls, exaggerates the contribution of training to the iron deficient profiles. Instead, it describes the typically low iron stores of adolescent females—athletic or not—with a small superimposed effect (fall in ferritin level) from training.

Rowland *et al.* (1987) found the same trend in adolescent runners. At the start of a season, eight of 20 females but only one of 30 males was iron deficient (ferritin $<12\mu g \cdot l^{-1}$). By the end of the season, one additional female and four additional males had become 'iron deficient' by the same definition. No runner developed iron deficiency anaemia.

Besides running, many other types of training have been shown to decrease ferritin level. When young men and women underwent a 7-week ($8 h \cdot day^{-1}$) military-type basic training programme, ferritin levels fell an average of 50% and haemoglobin levels fell more than 5% (Magazanik *et al.* 1988). When untrained men cycled $2 h \cdot day^{-1}$ four to five times a week for 11 weeks, mean serum ferritin fell 73%, from 67 to $18\mu g \cdot l^{-1}$ (Shoemaker *et al.* 1996). Rowland and Kelleher (1989) found no significant fall in serum ferritin during 10 weeks of swim training in adolescents, but nearly half of the female swimmers studied *began* with ferritin levels under $12\mu g \cdot l^{-1}$ (so there was little room to fall). In contrast, Roberts and Smith (1990) reported a decrease in ferritin over 2 years in female synchronized swimmers.

Even strength training decreases ferritin, as shown by the 35% fall in ferritin in 12 untrained men who underwent a 6-week strength-training programme (Schobersberger *et al.* 1990). A modest fall in ferritin was seen when young women underwent a 13-week programme of modest aerobic calisthenics (Blum *et al.* 1986). Training also can decrease ferritin level in cross-country skiers (Candau *et al.* 1992), female basketball players (Jacobsen *et al.* 1993) and in speed skaters and field hockey players (Cook 1994).

So athletic training can decrease the ferritin level. This decrease, however, is not necessarily pathophysiologic; it may reflect only a shift of iron from stores to functional compartment (haemoglobin and myoglobin). Also, any 'anaemia' that develops in the same athlete may be only pseudoanaemia, not necessarily iron deficiency anaemia.

## Competition and iron profile

In contrast to prudent training, all-out competition, especially a prolonged or muscle-damaging event, clouds interpretation of iron status by evoking the acute phase response (Eichner 1986). The acute phase response is an innate, generalized host defense against infection or inflammatory injury. In athletes, this may begin as damaged muscle activates complement, which recruits and activates neutrophils and monocytes (and fibroblasts), which release cytokines (e.g. interleukins 1 and 6, tumour necrosis factor). The cytokines trigger muscle proteolysis and the hepatic synthesis of proteins (e.g. C-reactive protein, ceruloplasmin, haptoglobin, fibrinogen and *ferritin*) that may contribute to host defense. The interleukins also activate lymphocytes, cause mild fever and sleepiness, and decrease serum iron level. So in the acute phase response, as during a US Army Ranger training programme (weeks of intense physical activity, stress and sleep deprivation) serum iron falls (and later rebounds), yet serum ferritin rises (Moore *et al.* 1993).

In light of recent research on bench-stepping exercise (Gleeson *et al.* 1995), it seems likely that any exercise bout that evokes delayed onset muscle soreness and damages muscle (sharply increases serum creatine kinase level) can spur an acute phase response that alters the markers of iron balance. Indeed, an integration of diverse field studies of athletes confirms this.

For example, during marathons and ultramarathons (Dickson *et al.* 1982; Strachan *et al.* 1984; Lampe *et al.* 1986a; Schmidt *et al.* 1989), multiday foot races (Dressendorfer *et al.* 1982; Seiler *et al.* 1989), triathlons (Rogers *et al.* 1986; Taylor *et al.* 1987) and distance ski races (Pattini *et al.* 1990), serial sampling and analysis of blood markers suggests the following sequence of events and mechanisms.

**1** An early (first day or two) decline in plasma haptoglobin level and *rise in serum iron* level, likely from exertional or 'footstrike' haemolysis; along with an increase in plasma volume and fall in haematocrit (i.e. dilutional pseudoanaemia) that can not be prevented by iron supplementation (Dressendorfer *et al.* 1991).

**2** A later (next few days) *fall in serum iron and increase in serum ferritin*, likely from the acute phase response.

**3** A late (e.g. later stages of a 20-day foot race) *return of serum iron and ferritin toward baseline*, as the body seems to adapt to the stress of racing and the acute phase response abates.

The above perturbations—some physiological, some pathophysiological—make it difficult to gauge iron balance in a given athlete who may be resting, training or racing. For example, an 'anaemia' may reflect dilution or iron deficiency; the serum iron may be normal, high, or low depending on the stage of the race; and serum ferritin falls with training yet rises if muscle damage evokes the acute phase response. Bearing these confounders in mind, practical issues of iron balance in athletes are covered next.

## Iron status of fit athletes

Because training decreases ferritin level (iron stores), one might expect highly trained athletes to be iron deficient compared with non-athletes. Indeed, beginning two decades ago, a spate of cross-sectional surveys suggested that certain athletes, especially distance runners, tended to be iron deficient. This area of inquiry began in part with concern that iron intake was insufficient in young Canadian women, and that haemoglobin levels of Canada's 1976 Olympic athletes were 'suboptimal' (meaning lower than those of the 1968 Australian Olympic Team). This led to a survey of 52 collegiate distance runners in Canada (Clement & Asmundson 1982), concluding that 29% of male and 82% of female runners were 'at risk for iron deficiency' (had serum ferritin of less than $25\,\mu g \cdot l^{-1}$).

Corroborating surveys followed. Low bone marrow iron stores were seen in competitive distance runners in Sweden and Israel (Ehn *et al.* 1980; Wishnitzer *et al.* 1983). In a second study from Sweden (Magnusson *et al.* 1984), 43 elite male distance runners had lower ferritin levels and marrow iron scores than 100 non-athletic controls. 'Systemic iron deficiency' (low saturation of transferrin) was found in 56% of 113 joggers and runners in Denmark (Hunding *et al.* 1981). Competitive distance runners in Germany had lower ferritin levels than elite rowers or professional cyclists (Dufaux *et al.* 1981). From South Africa came reports that 14% of male ultramarathoners (but just 2% of controls) had low ferritin levels, as did 16% of female marathon runners (Dickson *et al.* 1982; Matter *et al.* 1987). From the USA came a report that one third of women—and 7% of men—at a marathon fitness exposition had low ferritins (Lampe *et al.* 1986b). Other reports followed suit, as reviewed by Cook (1994).

These surveys are limited, however, by small sample size, no or few non-athletic controls, and widely different definitions of 'iron deficiency' (Humpty Dumpty redux). The most reliable studies are those based on ferritin assay, but these used different ferritin 'cut points' for diagnosing iron deficiency (e.g. 12, 20, 25 or $40\,\mu g \cdot l^{-1}$). The median ferritin value for young women in the USA is $25–30\,\mu g \cdot l^{-1}$ (Cook *et al.* 1986). A cut point of $40\,\mu g \cdot l^{-1}$ (Matter *et al.* 1987) classifies most young women—athletic or not—as iron deficient. Even $25\,\mu g \cdot l^{-1}$ (Clement & Asmundson 1982) is too high; experts say that less than $12\,\mu g \cdot l^{-1}$ is the proper ferritin cut point for diagnosing iron deficiency (Cook 1994).

Other surveys question whether athletes differ from non-athletes in iron balance, but these surveys too have problems. In one study, 19 top-level soccer players had ferritins similar to 20 controls (Resina *et al.* 1991). Likewise, ferritin was similar in 72 elite runners vs. 48 non-runners (Balaban *et al.* 1989). In this survey, however, one third of the male and two thirds of the female runners (but few controls) were taking iron supplements, and when those taking iron were excluded, sample sizes were small. When 100 female collegiate athletes were compared with 66 non-athletic controls, differences in iron balance were minor (Risser *et al.* 1988), but only 8% of the athletic women were distance runners.

Despite these problems, it seems likely that among athletes, distance runners at least have some reduction in iron stores compared to non-athletes. So concluded a comprehensive survey in South Carolina of 111 adult female runners vs. 65 inactive controls (Pate *et al.* 1993). The mean ferritin of the runners was lower than that of the controls ($25\,\mu g \cdot l^{-1}$ vs. $36\,\mu g \cdot l^{-1}$), and twice as many runners as nonrunners (50% vs. 22%) had ferritin levels of less than $20\,\mu g \cdot l^{-1}$. Anaemia, however, was rare (3%) in both groups.

So distance runners—especially female runners—tend to have lower iron stores than non-athletes and seem prone to iron deficiency anaemia. But frank iron deficiency (ferritin $<12\,\mu g \cdot l^{-1}$) among athletes, even among female runners, is not as common as once thought, and anaemia is not clearly more common in athletes than non-athletes. Then, too, most ultraendurance athletes studied—especially males—have adequate iron stores (Burke & Read 1987; Singh *et al.* 1993). Most iron studies are on runners; we need studies of women in 'low-bodyweight' sports such as ballet, gymnastics, diving and ice skating. But future studies of iron status are apt to be biased by the increasing use of iron supplements by athletes.

## Causes of low ferritin level in athletes

We have established that athletic training tends to decrease serum ferritin level (i.e. iron stores) and that some athletes, particularly female distance runners, may be prone to iron deficiency anaemia. Now the question becomes: *How* does training deplete iron stores? In theory, training can reduce serum ferritin level in at least eight ways, not all pathophysiological:

- haemodilution;
- increase in myoglobin mass;
- increase in red cell mass;
- inadequate iron intake;
- gastrointestinal bleeding;
- iron loss in sweat;
- iron loss in urine;
- shift of iron to liver.

### Haemodilution

As reviewed above, training—especially endurance training—can expand baseline plasma volume by as much as 10–20%, and if the training is regular, this expansion is maintained. This adaptation to exercise dilutes haemoglobin (pseudoanaemia). It seems likely, if not yet demonstrated, that the expansion of plasma volume in a highly fit athlete dilutes serum ferritin concentration by 10% or more.

### Increase in myoglobin mass

When adolescent boys undergo a growth spurt, stored iron is shifted into the increased mass of myoglobin, lowering ferritin. This must also occur in athletes who develop muscles by training, and surely accounts for much of the fall in ferritin with strength training (Schobersberger *et al.* 1990). This likely shifting of iron from stores to functional compartment (myoglobin) has not been quantified in athletes, but seems evident. To paraphrase Yogi Berra, you can observe a lot by just looking.

### Increase in red cell mass

Because cross-sectional studies show an expanded red cell mass in athletes—men and women—compared to non-athletes (Dill *et al.* 1974; Brotherhood *et al.* 1975; Weight *et al.* 1991), it seems likely that training can increase red cell mass. Yet longitudinal studies are inconclusive. Restricting it to studies that employ radiolabelled red cells, the best way to gauge red cell mass, two studies are positive and two 'negative'. Remes (1979) found that 6 months of military training increased red cell mass by 4%. Young *et al.* (1993) found a 4% increase after 8 weeks of regular cycling, but the unusual protocol (cycling immersed to the neck in water) prevented the expected increase in plasma volume. Ray *et al.* (1990) found that regular, upright cycling for 8 weeks increased red cell mass about 220 ml, but this increase was not significant. Shoemaker *et al.* (1996) found no increase in red cell mass when untrained men cycled regularly for 11 weeks, but it seems possible that blood-drawing for testing offset an increase in red cell mass.

If training does increase the red cell mass, a likely mechanism would be via erythropoietin. But whether training—or competing—increases serum erythropoietin level is also unclear; studies finding an exercise-induced increase are slightly exceeded by studies finding no change (Weight *et al.* 1991; Klausen *et al.* 1993; Shoemaker *et al.* 1996). All told, it seems likely that strenuous, long-term athletic training (at sea level) can increase red cell mass, but this is by no means proven, and the mechanism for any increase remains unclear. We need more research here.

### Inadequate iron intake

If dietary iron is inadequate for physiological needs, ferritin will decline. Insufficient dietary iron can be a problem for female athletes who are dieting, who have eating disorders, or who are vegetarians. It is rarely a problem in men. No good evidence exists for impaired absorption of iron in athletes; the one such report (in male distance runners) seems flawed by abnormally high iron-absorption in the non-athletic controls, blood donors who may have been iron deficient (Ehn *et al.* 1980).

### Gastrointestinal bleeding

Gastrointestinal bleeding in athletes has been widely studied and reviewed (Eichner 1989, 1996). It occurs most often in distance runners and ranges from occult and trivial to overt and grave. If all reports are lumped, about 2% of recreational marathoners and triathletes have seen blood in their stool after running and about 20% have occult faecal blood after distance races. In general, the longer the event and/or the greater the effort, the greater the likelihood of bleeding. In a recent study of 20 male triathletes who provided stool samples during training, taper and competition, 80% of the men had occult faecal blood on one or more of the tests (Rudzki *et al.* 1995).

The source of gastrointestinal bleeding varies. Anorectal disorders (e.g. fissures, haemorrhoids) can be the source. Gastro-oesophageal reflux commonly occurs in runners, but no reports have identified an oesophageal source of bleeding. In some athletes, no source is found depite endoscopies. The most common source is likely the stomach, as verified by endoscopy studies of runners after distance races (Schwartz *et al.* 1990). Usually, this is a mild gastritis with superficial erosions that heal quickly. Rarely, however, an athlete bleeds massively from a peptic ulcer during or just after running (Eichner 1996). Aspirin or other analgesics can increase the risk of gastrointestinal bleeding, as shown in a field study of marathoners (Robertson *et al.* 1987). In a recent study, aspirin sharply increased gastrointestinal permeability when volunteers ran 1 h on a treadmill (Ryan *et al.* 1996).

The second most common source seems to be the colon, usually from a segmental haemorrhagic colitis, presumably ischaemic. During strenuous exercise, splanchnic blood flow may decrease by as much as 80%, as blood diverts to working muscles. Normally, the gut tolerates this, but occasionally the colonic mucosa becomes ischaemic, in line with level of effort, unfitness, sympathetic response and dehydration. The result is superficial haemorrhage and erosions. Most cases are mild and soon reversible, but rare cases require subtotal colectomy (Eichner 1996).

Repeated bouts of ischaemic colitis in female runners could contribute to iron deficiency anaemia. In a recent German study, seven of 45 elite male distance runners had ferritins of less than $20\,\mu g \cdot l^{-1}$ (vs. only one of 112 controls). In eight of the runners, faecal iron (gastrointestinal blood) loss was gauged by radiolabelling haem iron and testing stool samples. When the runners were not training, average gastrointestinal blood loss was $1–2\,ml \cdot day^{-1}$. With training or racing, average loss increased to $5–6\,ml \cdot day^{-1}$. In general, gastrointestinal blood loss correlated with intensity of running, not distance (Nachtigall *et al.* 1996).

### Iron loss in sweat

Controversy continues on whether athletes can lose enough iron in sweat to cause iron deficiency (Haymes & LaManca 1989). The most meticulous study in resting subjects, one that minimized iron loss in desquamated cells and iron contamination of skin, found a very low sweat iron loss, averaging $23\,\mu g \cdot l^{-1}$, compared with much higher values in previous studies. The authors concluded that variations in sweating have only marginal effects on body iron loss (Brune *et al.* 1986).

The most recent study in athletes also suggests that sweat iron loss is modest (Waller & Haymes 1996). It shows that sweat iron level drops over time, at least during the first hour of exercise. It finds that exercising men have about twice the sweat iron loss as women, because of higher sweat rates in men and likely also because of greater iron stores in men. The authors estimate that 6–11% of the iron typically absorbed per day is lost in sweat during 1 h of exercise. They conclude that sweat iron losses would likely not deplete iron stores in men but might do so in female athletes whose diets are low in iron.

### Iron loss in urine

Some iron is lost in urine (Haymes & Lamanca 1989), but the amounts are negligible (Nachtigall *et al.* 1996). Athletes can develop haematuria from diverse causes, but not enough haematuria to drain iron stores (Eichner 1990a, 1990b). Exertional haemolytis rarely depletes haptoglobin and so does not increase urinary iron loss

(Eichner 1985; O'Toole *et al.* 1988). Urinary iron loss in athletes is negligible.

### Shift of iron to liver

The 'liver shift' hypothesis sought to explain why some runners had low ferritins (and low bone marrow iron scores) yet seemed *not* iron deficient by other criteria (Magnusson *et al.* 1984). The notion was that 'footstrike haemolysis' shifted iron from normal storage sites (macrophages) to hepatocytes, and that iron in hepatocytes was not readily available for reuse and not registered by the serum ferritin. This hypothesis lacked experimental support and should be put to rest by the finding in elite distance runners that when ferritin is low, hepatic iron is also low (Nachtigall *et al.* 1996).

## Iron status and athletic performance

### Anaemia and athleticism

It is well known that anaemia, even mild anaemia, impairs all-out athletic performance (Dallman 1982; Cook 1994); this needs no review. In my experience with runners, even a $1–2\,g \cdot dl^{-1}$ decrement in haemoglobin from baseline slows race performance. Coaches, trainers and sports medicine physicians, then, need to be alert for mild anaemia in athletes. When anaemia is mild and serum ferritin is marginal, it is difficult to distinguish pseudoanaemia from iron deficiency anaemia; indeed, they may coexist. When in doubt, a therapeutic trial of oral iron is wise; a rise in haemoglobin of $1–2\,g \cdot dl^{-1}$ is the 'gold standard' for diagnosing iron deficiency anaemia (Eichner 1990a).

### Low ferritin without anaemia

About two decades ago, a myth arose that low ferritin alone, without anaemia, impairs athletic performance. This led to monitoring ferritin as a marker of performance potential. When runners without anaemia were told that their ferritin was $30\,\mu g \cdot l^{-1}$ and 'should be much higher', they immediately felt tired. When, on iron pills, their serum ferritin rose to $90\,\mu g\cdot l^{-1}$, they felt three times stronger (despite no rise in haemoglobin). Alas, later, off iron pills, when their ferritin fell again to $30\,\mu g\cdot l^{-1}$, they felt weak again.

This myth is a Hydra; it keeps growing new heads. It stems from misinterpreting research on rodents—research probing the extent to which, in the face of iron deficiency, exercise capacity is limited by impaired oxygen *delivery* (anaemia) vs. impaired oxygen *use* (impaired oxidative metabolism in muscle). This model is not relevant to athletes because it first creates *severe iron deficiency anaemia* and muscle iron deficiency in weanling rats (deprived of dietary iron) and then, by blood transfusion, *reverses only the anaemia*. When this is done, the rats cannot run maximally because, although they are no longer anaemic, their muscles are still iron deficient (Dallman 1982).

This research was misread on two counts. One, it is a model of severe, 'lifelong,' bodywide iron deficiency with severe anaemia. As such, it is at the opposite end of the spectrum (of iron deficiency) from the athlete who has low ferritin but no anaemia yet. Two, as the rats grew ever more deficient in iron, there was a parallel decrease in all haem proteins measured (haemoglobin, cytochrome c, myoglobin). In other words, when haemoglobin was still normal, muscle myoglobin and iron-containing enzymes were also still normal. These rats developed 'iron deficient muscles' as they got anaemic. Rats—and athletes—with low ferritin but no anaemia have normal muscles.

Fortunately, accumulating studies may kill the Hydra. In one study (Celsing *et al.* 1986), mild iron deficiency anaemia was induced by venesection of nine healthy men. When the anaemia (but not the iron deficiency) was obviated by transfusion, the subjects' exercise capacity was unchanged from baseline. Also, the activity of iron-containing muscle enzymes remained normal. Three studies now show that when non-anaemic women with ferritin of less than $20\,\mu g\cdot l^{-1}$ or less than $25\,\mu g\cdot l^{-1}$ are randomized to iron therapy vs. placebo for 8 weeks, neither group

improves in work performance or endurance capacity (Newhouse *et al.* 1989; Fogelholm *et al.* 1992; Klingshirn *et al.* 1992). In two other studies in which mildly anaemic women were randomized to iron vs. placebo, performance improved only as anaemia was reversed (Schoene *et al.* 1983; LaManca & Haymes 1993). Finally, a recent study analyses the 10 most relevant articles in this field and concludes that low serum ferritin in the absence of frank anaemia is not associated with reduced endurance performance (Garza *et al.* 1997). It adds that ferritin can be used to detect 'prelatent anaemias,' but not as an independent marker for performance in athletes. Amen.

## Increasing iron supply

The pre-eminent cause of iron deficiency in women in sports (as in all women) is inadequate dietary iron. Athletic women, notably 'low-bodyweight' athletes, are notorious for consuming too few calories. The recommended dietary allowance (RDA) for iron is $10\,mg\cdot day^{-1}$ for children to age 10 and males 15 and above (some say 18 and above), $12\,mg\cdot day^{-1}$ for boys 11–15 years, and $15\,mg\cdot day^{-1}$ for females 11–50 years (Clarkson & Haymes 1995). Yet many elite female athletes consume no more than 8400 kJ (2000 kcal) daily, for a total of 12 mg of iron.

Also, because some female athletes are modified vegetarians, much of their dietary iron is not highly bioavailable. Meats are an excellent source of iron because they contain haem iron, which is easily absorbed. In contrast, cereals, legumes, whole grain or enriched breads and deep green leafy vegetables contain non-haem iron, which is not so easily absorbed. Four studies agree that some active or athletic women get too little iron. In one study, female recreational runners who were modified vegetarians had low ferritin levels, only one third those of counterparts who ate red meat (Snyder *et al.* 1989). In another study of distance runners, the men met the RDA for iron but the women did not (Weight *et al.* 1992b). In a study of active women in a university community, ferritins were highest in those who consumed red meat (Worthington-

Roberts *et al.* 1988). Finally, in the South Carolina study of female runners and non-runners, the runners (who had lower ferritins than the non-runners) consumed less meat, more carbohydrate, more fibre and more coffee or tea (Pate *et al.* 1993).

Iron supply can be increased by:
1 eating more lean red meat;
2 not consuming tea or coffee with meals
3 drinking orange juice with breakfast;
4 cooking in cast-iron cookware;
5 frequently eating mixed meals;
6 the wise use of iron supplements.

The best way is to consume some red meat — say, 80 g of lean beef three to four times a week. Poultry and fish also contain haem iron, but less than red meat. Meat, fish, poultry and ascorbic acid enhance non-haem iron absorption. Conversely, inhibitors include tea (tannins), coffee (polyphenols), eggs and cow's milk (calcium and phosphoproteins), wheat bran (phytate), soy products and fibre. The threat of inhibitors, however, seems overblown. For example, any inhibition of fibre on non-haem iron absorption is modest (Cook *et al.* 1983), and with a varied Western diet, the net effect of inhibitors (or enhancers) is small, because no given inhibitor (or enhancer) is contained within enough meals to shape iron balance (Cook *et al.* 1991a, 1991b).

Avoiding tea or coffee with breakfast (they can be drunk 1–2 h before or after) and taking a source of vitamin C (orange juice) can triple the amount of iron absorbed from the meal (Rossander *et al.* 1979). Cooking occasionally in cast-iron (vs. stainless steel) skillets and pots, especially when simmering acidic foods like vegetable soup or tomato sauce, can leach absorbable iron into the food. Eating mixed meals is key, because meat, fish and poultry contain enhancers, so when meat and vegetables are eaten together, more non-haem iron is absorbed from the vegetables than if the vegetables had been eaten alone.

It is preferable for female athletes to meet their iron need by consuming iron-rich foods, but for such women who repeatedly develop iron deficiency anaemia and are unable to follow dietary advice, one can prescribe supplementary iron (e.g. ferrous sulphate, 325 mg three times a week). As for other common supplements, women who take calcium supplements should avoid them with meals (because they inhibit non-haem iron absorption), whereas women who take vitamin C supplements should take them with meals to enhance iron absorption (Cook & Monsen 1977; Cook *et al.* 1991a, 1991b).

Vegetarians need to heed their supply of iron (and zinc) because plants are paltry providers. So vegetarians should eat iron-rich foods such as dried fruit (apricots, prunes, dates), beans, peas, tofu, kale, spinach (a recent report claims spinach has only one tenth the iron as formerly thought), collard greens, and blackstrap molasses. Vegetarians should also consider taking a multivitamin and mineral supplement that provides the RDA for iron (and zinc).

Finally, among male athletes especially, injudicious use of iron supplements is a potential hazard. In the USA at least, one person in 200 is genetically programmed to develop hereditary haemochromatosis; over the years, he or she becomes iron-overloaded because daily absorption of dietary iron is about twice normal. In men, who have no physiological means to excrete excess iron (i.e. no menses), problems from iron overload in hereditary haemochromatosis develop earlier in life (than in women). In such men, iron supplements accelerate haemochromatosis. As a concluding rule of thumb, if many female athletes need more iron than they get, many male athletes get more iron than they need.

## References

Balaban, E.P., Cox, J.V., Snell, P., Vaughan, R.H. & Frenkel, E.P. (1989) The frequency of anemia and iron deficiency in the runner. *Medicine and Science in Sports and Exercise* **21**, 643–648.

Baynes, R.D. (1996) Refining the assessment of body iron status. *American Journal of Clinical Nutrition* **64**, 793–794.

Blum, S.M., Sherman, A.R. & Boileau, R.A. (1986) The effects of fitness-type exercise on iron status in adult women. *American Journal of Clinical Nutrition* **43**, 456–463.

Brotherhood, J., Brozovic, B. & Pugh, L.G.C. (1975)

Haematological status of middle- and long-distance runners. *Clinical Science and Molecular Medicine* **48**, 139–145.

Brune, M., Magnusson, B., Persson, H. & Hallberg, L. (1986) Iron losses in sweat. *American Journal of Clinical Nutrition* **43**, 438–443.

Bruner, A.B., Joffe, A., Duggan, A.K., Casella, J.F. & Brandt, J. (1996) Randomized study of cognitive effects of iron supplementation in non-anaemic iron-deficient adolescent girls. *Lancet* **348**, 992–996.

Burke, L. & Read, R.S.D. (1987) Diet patterns of elite Australian male triathletes. *Physician and Sportsmedicine* **15**, 140–155.

Candau, R., Busson, T. & Lacour, J.R. (1992) Effects of training on iron status in cross-country skiers. *European Journal of Applied Physiology* **64**, 497–502.

Celsing, F., Blomstrand, E., Werner, B., Pihlstedt, P. & Ekblom, B. (1986) Effects of iron deficiency on endurance and muscle enyzme activity in man. *Medicine and Science in Sports and Exercise* **18**, 156–161.

Clarkson, P. & Haymes, E.M. (1995) Exercise and mineral status of athletes: calcium, magnesium, phosphorus, and iron. *Medicine and Science in Sports and Exercise* **27**, 831–843.

Clement, D.B. & Asmundson, R.C. (1982) Nutritional intake and hematological parameters in endurance runners. *Physician and Sportsmedicine* **10**, 37–43.

Convertino, V.A. (1991) Blood volume: its adaptation to endurance training. *Medicine and Science in Sports and Exercise* **23**, 1338–1348.

Cook, J.D. (1994) The effect of endurance training on iron metabolism. *Seminars in Hematology* **31**, 146–154.

Cook, J.D. & Lynch, S. (1986) The liabilities of iron deficiency. *Blood* **68**, 803–809.

Cook, J.D. & Monsen, E.R. (1977) Vitamin C, the common cold, and iron absorption. *American Journal of Clinical Nutrition* **30**, 235–241.

Cook, J.D., Noble, N.L., Morck, T.A., Lynch, S.R. & Petersium, S.J. (1983) Effect of fiber on nonheme iron absorption. *Gastroenterology* **85**, 1354–1358.

Cook, J.D., Skikne, B.S., Lynch, S.R. & Rausser, M.E. (1986) Estimates of iron sufficiency in the US population. *Blood* **68**, 726–731.

Cook, J.D., Dassenko, S.A. & Lynch, S.R. (1991a) Assessment of the role of nonheme-iron availability in iron balance. *American Journal of Clinical Nutrition* **54**, 717–722.

Cook, J.D., Dassenko, S.A. & Whittaker, P. (1991b) Calcium supplementation: effect on iron absorption. *American Journal of Clinical Nutrition* **53**, 106–111.

Dallman, P.R. (1982) Manifestations of iron deficiency. *Seminars in Hematology* **19**, 19–30.

Davidson, R.J.L., Robertson, J.D., Galea, G. & Maughan, R.J. (1987) Hematological changes associated with marathon running. *International Journal of Sports Medicine* **8**, 19–25.

Dickson, D.N., Wilkinson, R.L. & Noakes, T.D. (1982) Effects of ultra-marathon training and racing on hematologic parameters and serum ferritin levels in well-trained athletes. *International Journal of Sports Medicine* **3**, 111–117.

Dill, D.B., Braithwaite, K., Adams, W.C. & Beernauer, E.M. (1974) Blood volume of middle-distance runners: effect of 2,300-m altitude and comparison with non-athletes. *Medicine and Science in Sports and Exercise* **6**, 1–7.

Dressendorfer, R.H., Wade, C.E., Keen, C.L. & Scaff, J.H. (1982) Plasma mineral levels in marathon runners during a 20-day road race. *Physician and Sportsmedicine* **10**, 113–118.

Dressendorfer, R.H., Keen, C.L., Wade, C.E., Claybaugh, J.R. & Timmis, G.C. (1991) Development of runner's anemia during a 20-day road race: effect of iron supplements. *International Journal of Sports Medicine* **12**, 332–336.

Dufaux, B., Hoederath, A., Streitberger, I., Hollmann, W. & Assmann, G. (1981) Serum ferritin, transferrin, haptoglobin, and iron in middle- and long-distance runners, elite rowers, and professional racing cyclists. *International Journal of Sports Medicine* **2**, 43–46.

Ehn, L., Carlmark, B. & Hoglund, S. (1980) Iron status in athletes involved in intense physical activity. *Medicine and Science in Sports and Exercise* **12**, 61–64.

Eichner, E.R. (1985) Runner's macrocytosis: a clue to footstrike hemolysis. *American Journal of Medicine* **78**, 321–325.

Eichner, E.R. (1986) The marathon: is more less? *Physician and Sportsmedicine* **14**, 183–187.

Eichner, E.R. (1989) Gastrointestinal bleeding in athletes. *Physician and Sportsmedicine* **17**, 128–140.

Eichner, E.R. (1990a) Facts and myths about anemia in active women. *Your Patient and Fitness* **5**, 12–16.

Eichner, E.R. (1990b) Hematuria: a diagnostic challenge. *Physician and Sportsmedicine* **18**, 53–63.

Eichner, E.R. (1992) Sports anemia, iron supplements, and blood doping. *Medicine and Science in Sports and Exercise* **24**, S315–S318.

Eichner, E.R. (1996) Gastrointestinal disorders in active people. *Your Patient and Fitness* **10**, 13–19.

Farley, P.C. & Foland, J. (1990) Iron deficiency anemia. *Postgraduate Medicine* **87**, 89–101.

Finch, C.A. & Huebers, H. (1982) Perspectives in iron metabolism. *New England Journal of Medicine* **306**, 1520–1528.

Fogelholm, M., Jaakkola, L. & Lampisjarvi, T. (1992) Effects of iron supplementation in female athletes with low serum ferritin concentration. *International Journal of Sports Medicine* **13**, 158–162.

Garza, D., Shrier, I., Kohl, H.W., Ford, P., Brown, M. & Matheson, G.O. (1997) The clinical value of serum ferritin tests in endurance athletes. *Clinical Journal of Sport Medicine* **7**, 46–53.

Gillen, C.M., Lee, R., Mack, G.W., Tomaselli, C.M.,

Nishiyasu, T. & Nadel, E.R. (1991) Plasma volume expansion in humans after a single intense exercise protocol. *Journal of Applied Physiology* **71**, 1914–1920.

Gleeson, M., Almey, J., Brooks, S., Cave, R., Lewis, A. & Griffiths, H. (1995) Haematological and acute-phase responses associated with delayed-onset muscle soreness in humans. *European Journal of Applied Physiology* **71**, 137–142.

Haymes, E.M. & LaManca, J.J. (1989) Iron loss in runners during exercise. *Sports Medicine* **7**, 277–285.

Hunding, A., Jordal, R. & Paulev, P.E. (1981) Runner's anemia and iron deficiency. *Acta Medica Scandinavica* **209**, 315–318.

Jacobsen, D.J., Crouse, S.F., Rohack, J.J., Lowe, R.C. & Pronk, N.P. (1993) Hematological status of female basketball players. *Clinical Journal of Sports Medicine* **3**, 82–85.

Klausen, T., Breum, L., Fogh-Andersen, N., Bennett, P. & Hippe, H. (1993) The effect of short and long duration exercise on serum erythropoietin concentrations. *European Journal of Applied Physiology* **67**, 213–217.

Klingshirn, L.A., Pate, R.R., Bourque, S.P., Davis, J.M. & Sargent, R.G. (1992) Effect of iron supplements on endurance capacity in iron-depleted female runners. *Medicine and Science in Sports and Exercise* **24**, 819–824.

LaManca, J.J. & Haymes, E.M. (1993) Effects of iron repletion on VO2 max, endurance, and blood lactate in women. *Medicine and Science in Sports and Exercise* **12**, 1386–1392.

Lampe, J.W., Slavin, J.L. & Apple, F.S. (1986a) Elevated serum ferritin concentrations in master runners after a marathon race. *International Journal of Vitamin and Nutrition Research* **56**, 395–398.

Lampe, J.W., Slavin, J.L. & Apple, F.S. (1986b) Effects of moderate iron supplementation on the iron status of runners with low serum ferritin. *Nutrition Reports International* **34**, 959–966.

London, I.M. (1980) Iron and heme: crucial carriers and catalysts. In *Blood, Pure and Eloquent*. McGraw-Hill, New York.

Magazanik, A., Weinstein, Y., Dlin, R.A., Derin, M., Schwartzman, S. & Allalouf, D. (1988) Iron deficiency caused by 7 weeks of intensive physical exercise. *European Journal of Applied Physiology* **57**, 198–202.

Magnusson, B., Hallberg, L., Rossander, L. & Swolin, B. (1984) Iron metabolism and 'sports anemia.' *Acta Medica Scandinavica* **216**, 157–164.

Matter, M., Stittfall, T., Graves, J., Myburgh, K., Adams, B., Jacobs, P. & Noakes, T.D. (1987) The effect of iron and folate therapy on maximal exercise performance in female marathon runners with iron and folate deficiency. *Clinical Science* **72**, 415–422.

Moore, R.J., Friedl, K.E., Tulley, R.T. & Askew, E.W. (1993) Maintenance of iron status in healthy men during an extended period of stress and physical activity. *American Journal of Clinical Nutrition* **58**, 923–927.

Nachtigall, D., Nielsen, P., Fischer, R., Engelhardt, R. & Gabbe, E.E. (1996) Iron deficiency in distance runners: a reinvestigation using 59Fe-labelling and non-invasive liver iron quantification. *International Journal of Sports Medicine* **17**, 473–479.

Newhouse, I.J., Clement, D.B., Taunton, J.E. & McKensie, D.C. (1989) The effects of prelatent/latent iron deficiency on physical work capacity. *Medicine and Science in Sports and Exercise* **21**, 263–268.

Nickerson, H.J., Holubets, M., Tripp, A.D. & Pierce, W.E. (1985) Decreased iron stores in high school female runners. *American Journal of the Diseases of Childhood* **139**, 1115–1119.

Nickerson, H.J., Holubets, M.C., Weiler, B.R., Haas, R.G., Schwartz, S. & Ellefson, M.E. (1989) Causes of iron deficiency in adolescent athletes. *Journal of Pediatrics* **114**, 657–663.

O'Toole, M.L., Hiller, W.D.B., Roalstad, M.S. & Douglas, P.S. (1988) Hemolysis during triathlon races: its relation to race distance. *Medicine and Science in Sports and Exercise* **20**, 272–275.

Pate, R.R., Miller, B.J., Davis, J.M., Slentz, C.A. & Klingshirn, L.A. (1993) Iron status of female runners. *International Journal of Sport Nutrition* **3**, 222–231.

Pattini, A., Schena, F. & Guidi, G.C. (1990) Serum ferritin and serum iron changes after cross-country and roler ski endurance races. *European Journal of Applied Physiology* **61**, 55–60.

Ray, C.A., Cureton, K.J. & Ouzts, H.G. (1990) Postural specificity of cardiovascular adaptations to exercise training. *Journal of Applied Physiology* **69**, 2202–2208.

Remes, K. (1979) Effect of long-term physical training on total red cell volume. *Scandinavian Journal of Clinical and Laboratory Investigation* **39**, 311–319.

Resina, A., Gatteschi, L., Giamgerardino, M.A., Imreh, F., Rubenni, M.G. & Vecchiet, L. (1991) Hematological comparison of iron status in trained top-level soccer players and control subjects. *International Journal of Sports Medicine* **12**, 453–456.

Risser, W.L., Lee, E.J., Poindexter, H.B.W., West, M.S., Pivarnik, J.M., Risser, J.M.H. & Hickson, J.F. (1988) Iron deficiency in female athletes: its prevalence and impact on performance. *Medicine and Science in Sports and Exercise* **20**, 116–121.

Roberts, D. & Smith, D. (1990) Serum ferritin values in elite speed and synchronized swimmers and speed skaters. *Journal of Laboratory and Clinical Medicine* **116**, 661–665.

Robertson, J.D., Maughan, R.J. & Davidson, R.J.L. (1987) Faecal blood loss in response to exercise. *British Medical Journal* **295**, 303–305.

Robertson, J.D., Maughan, R.J., Walker, K.A. & Davidson, R.J.L. (1990) Plasma viscosity and the haemodilution following distance running. *Clinical Hemorheology* **10**, 51–57.

Rogers, G., Goodman, C., Mitchell, D. & Hattingh, J. (1986) The response of runners to arduous triathlon competition. *European Journal of Applied Physiology* **55**, 405–409.

Rossander, L., Halberg, L. & Bjorn-Rasmussen, E. (1979) Absorption of iron from breakfast meals. *American Journal of Clinical Nutrition* **32**, 2484–2489.

Rowland, T.W. & Kelleher, J.F. (1989) Iron deficiency in athletes. *American Journal of the Diseases of Childhood* **143**, 197–200.

Rowland, T.W., Black, S.A. & Kelleher, J.F. (1987) Iron deficiency in adolescent endurance athletes. *Journal of Adolescent Health Care* **8**, 322–326.

Rudzki, S.J., Hazard, H. & Collinson, D. (1995) Gastrointestinal blood loss in triathletes: its etiology and relationship to sports anaemia. *Australian Journal of Science and Medicine* **27**, 3–8.

Ryan, A.J., Chang, R.T. & Gisolfi, C.V. (1996) Gastrointestinal permeability following aspirin intake and prolonged running. *Medicine and Science in Sports and Exercise* **28**, 698–705.

Schmidt, W., Maassen, N., Tegtbur, U. & Braumann, K.M. (1989) Changes in plasma volume and red cell formation after a marathon competition. *European Journal of Applied Physiology* **58**, 453–458.

Schobersberger, W., Tschann, M., Hasibeder, W. *et al.* (1990) *European Journal of Applied Physiology* **60**, 163–168.

Schoene, R.B., Escourrou, P., Robertson, H.T., Nilson, K.L., Parsons, J.R. & Smith, N.J. (1983) Iron repletion decreases maximal exercise lactate concentrations in female athletes with minimal iron-deficiency anemia. *Journal of Laboratory and Clinical Medicine* **102**, 306–312.

Schwartz, A.V., Vanagunas, A. & Kamel, P.L. (1990) Endoscopy to evaluate gastrointestinal bleeding in marathon runners. *Annals of Internal Medicine* **113**, 632–633.

Seiler, D., Nagel, D., Franz, H., Hellstern, P., Leitzmann, C. & Jung, K. (1989) Effects of long-distance running on iron metabolism and hematological parameters. *International Journal of Sports Medicine* **10**, 357–362.

Shoemaker, J.K., Green, H.J., Coates, J., Ali, M. & Grant, S. (1996) Failure of prolonged exercise training to increase red cell mass in humans. *American Journal of Physiology* **270**, H121–H126.

Singh, A., Evans, P., Gallagher, K.L. & Deuster, P.A. (1993) Dietary intakes and biochemical profiles of nutritional status of ultramarathoners. *Medicine and Science in Sports and Exercise* **25**, 328–334.

Synder, A.C., Dvorak, L.L. & Roepke, J.B. (1989) Influence of dietary iron source on measures of iron status among female runners. *Medicine and Science in Sports and Exercise* **21**, 7–10.

Strachan, A.F., Noakes, T.D., Kotzenberg, G., Nel, A.E. & DeBeer, F.C. (1984) C reactive protein concentrations during long distance running. *British Medical Journal* **289**, 1249–1251.

Taylor, C., Rogers, G., Goodman, C., Baynes, R.D., Bothwell, T.H., Bezwoda, W.R., Kramer, F. & Hattingh, J. (1987) Hematolotic, iron-related, and acute-phase protein responses to sustained strenuous exercise. *Journal of Applied Physiology* **62**, 464–469.

Waller, M.F. & Haymes, E.M. (1996) The effects of heat and exercise on sweat iron loss. *Medicine and Science in Sports and Exercise* **28**, 197–203.

Weight, L.M., Darge, B.L. & Jacobs, P. (1991) Athletes' pseudoanaemia. *European Journal of Applied Physiology* **62**, 358–362.

Weight, L.M., Alexander, D., Elliot, T. & Jacobs, P. (1992a) Erythropoietic adaptations to endurance training. *European Journal of Applied Physiology* **64**, 444–448.

Weight, L.M., Jacobs, P. & Noakes, T.D. (1992b) Dietary iron deficiency and sports anaemia. *British Journal of Nutrition* **68**, 253–260.

Wishnitzer, R., Vorst, E. & Berrebi, A. (1983) Bone marrow iron depression in competitive distance runners. *International Journal of Sports Medicine* **4**, 27–30.

Worthington-Roberts, B.S., Breskin, M.W. & Monsen, E.R. (1988) Iron status of premenopausal women in a university community and its relationship to habitual dietary sources of protein. *American Journal of Clinical Nutrition* **47**, 275–279.

Young, A.J., Sawka, M.N., Quigley, M.D. *et al.* (1993) Role of thermal factors on aerobic capacity improvements with endurance training. *Journal of Applied Physiology* **75**, 49–54.

# Chapter 25

# Trace Minerals

PRISCILLA M. CLARKSON

## Introduction

Trace minerals are required by the body in very small quantities, generally less than $20\,mg \cdot day^{-1}$ for healthy adults. Fourteen essential trace minerals have been identified, but only six are related to exercise, and these are iron, zinc, copper, selenium, chromium and vanadium. Vanadium is known to be essential for animals and is likely essential for humans, although not enough information exists to establish a requirement. Boron has been associated with bone health and exercise, but it is not yet considered an essential trace element.

The reason these minerals have received attention in the sports medicine arena is that some, like zinc, serve as components of enzymes involved in energy production, and others, like selenium and copper, work with enzymes and proteins that function as antioxidants. Chromium and vanadium have been purported to increase muscle mass because they are involved in either amino acid uptake or growth. Moreover, there is concern that many athletes may not ingest sufficient quantities of certain trace minerals to meet possible losses in sweat and urine induced by exercise.

This paper will discuss physiological function, dietary intake and status of athletes, changes induced by exercise and training, and effects of supplementation for each trace mineral mentioned above (except iron, which is discussed in Chapter 24).

## Zinc

Zinc functions as a component of more than 200 enzymes which affect many processes of life (Hunt & Groff 1990; Lukaski 1997). The recommended dietary allowance (RDA) is set at $15\,mg \cdot day^{-1}$ and $12\,mg \cdot day^{-1}$ for males and females, respectively, 11 years and older (Food and Nutrition Board 1989). Diets containing meat generally provide sufficient amounts of zinc to meet the RDA. Animal products, such as meat, fish, poultry and especially oysters, contain the most zinc.

Most, but not all, male athletes and some female athletes ingest sufficient amounts of zinc (Lukaski et al. 1983, 1990; Peters et al. 1986; Singh et al. 1989; Fogelholm et al. 1991, 1992a, 1992b), but many female athletes do not (Deuster et al. 1986, 1989; Nieman et al. 1989; Steen et al. 1995). Lower zinc intakes have been reported for female compared with male swimmers (Lukaski et al. 1990, 1996b). Those athletes maintaining low body weights, such as wrestlers, dancers and gymnasts, do not appear to meet their requirement for zinc (Benson et al. 1985; Loosli et al. 1986; Steen & McKinney 1986).

### Zinc status and effects of exercise

Zinc status is most commonly assessed in serum or plasma samples, although this measurement can be affected by stress, infection and oral contraceptives (Hunt & Groff 1990). Several studies reported that male athletes and some female athletes have adequate blood zinc levels (Weight *et al.* 1988; Fogelholm & Lahtinen 1991; Fogelholm *et al.* 1991, 1992a; Bazzarre *et al.* 1993; Lukaski 1997). However, many endurance athletes were found to have relatively low resting blood levels of zinc (Dressendorfer & Sockolov 1980; Haralambie 1981; Dressendorfer *et al.* 1982; Deuster *et al.* 1986; Couzy *et al.* 1990; Marrella *et al.* 1990; Singh *et al.* 1990), and Singh *et al.* (1989) reported low blood zinc levels in a significant number of Navy Seals.

Deuster *et al.* (1986) did not find a strong correlation between dietary zinc intake and serum zinc, although they did find a relationship between zinc intake and red blood cell zinc. Relying on plasma or serum zinc as a measure of status will probably not show impaired zinc status when indeed it may occur. In a study of induced zinc deficiency, Prasad (1991) found that 5 mg zinc·day$^{-1}$ did not result in a decrease in plasma zinc until 4–5 months. However, zinc concentration in lymphocytes, granulocytes and platelets decreased within 8–12 weeks and may be a more sensitive indicator of mild zinc deficiency.

Exercise can result in a loss of zinc in the sweat as well as the urine (Anderson *et al.* 1984; Van Rij *et al.* 1986; Anderson & Guttman 1988). Couzy *et al.* (1990) found that serum zinc was significantly decreased after 5 months of intensive training. Because the lower zinc values could not be explained by changes in dietary habits, plasma protein concentration, hormonal changes, or infection, they were considered to result from the stress of exercise. However, Manore *et al.* (1993) reported that after 6 weeks of an aerobic training programme, there was a significant decrease in plasma zinc but at 12 weeks the values were back to baseline, suggesting only a transient change. Also, subjects who were on a combination of anaerobic and aerobic exercise programmes did not show a change in plasma zinc. Hübner-Woźniak *et al.* (1996) found that plasma zinc increased after 10 weeks of weight training, and Ohno *et al.* (1990) reported that 10 weeks of training resulted in an increase in erythrocyte levels of zinc, but no change in plasma zinc. Fogelholm (1992) suggested that the increase

in erythrocyte zinc may reflect a high concentration of zinc-dependent enzymes as a result of training.

Examination of changes in blood levels of zinc after an acute bout of exercise may prove helpful in understanding the chronic effects of exercise. However, the results of these studies are equivocal (Dressendorfer *et al.* 1982; Anderson *et al.* 1984; Ohno *et al.* 1985; Marrella *et al.* 1993). High-intensity exercise appears to produce an increase in plasma zinc while endurance activity either showed no change or a decrease (Bordin *et al.* 1993; Lukaski 1997). Increases may be due to a redistribution of zinc. For example, zinc may be released from erythrocytes in response to exercise or may be released from muscle (Lukaski 1997). Aruoma *et al.* (1988) suggested that a decrease in plasma zinc immediately after exercise may reflect an acute phase response to exercise stress. Postexercise changes in plasma zinc levels were found to be sensitive to the zinc status of the individual, and this may affect the variability in response (Lukaski *et al.* 1984). The changes that occur are temporary, returning to baseline within a few hours to a day. Dressendorfer *et al.* (1982) found that over a 20-day road race, plasma zinc increased on the first exercise day but thereafter returned to near baseline values.

From the above studies it appears that an acute bout of exercise induces an alteration in zinc distribution in the blood. Because zinc is an integral part of carbonic anhydrase in erythrocytes, erythrocytes may serve as a readily exchangeable store zinc (Ohno *et al.* 1995). Further study of the process of redistribution of zinc among body compartments is needed to understand how exercise can exert an effect on zinc status. When examining chronic changes in zinc status due to training, the activity level of the subjects must be carefully controlled prior to taking samples because of the variable responses to an acute exercise bout.

### Performance and supplementation

Few studies examined the relationship between zinc status and performance or the effects of zinc supplementation. Lukaski *et al.* (1983) reported no correlation between blood zinc levels and $\dot{V}o_{2max.}$. In a later report, however, Lukaski (1995) presented evidence that zinc intake was significantly related to swim times in collegiate swimmers. Another study reported that $50\,mg\cdot day^{-1}$ of zinc had no effect on physiological changes or time to exhaustion during a run at 70–75% $\dot{V}o_{2max.}$ (Singh *et al.* 1994). Krotkiewski *et al.* (1982) examined the effect of $135\,mg\,zinc\cdot day^{-1}$ for 2 weeks on measures of knee extension strength. The supplement resulted in a significant increase in isokinetic strength at fast angular velocities ($180\,s^{-1}$) only and in isometric endurance, but no change in dynamic endurance or isokinetic strength at 60 or $120\,s^{-1}$. However, no studies have substantiated these findings regarding strength improvement.

The popularity of zinc supplements arises from their purported effect of increasing muscle mass. The reason for this belief may partially stem from the Krotkiewski *et al.* (1982) study, since the increase in strength could be due to increased muscle mass, although this was not assessed. Animal and human studies have found that zinc deficiency results in a stunting of growth that can be reversed by zinc supplements (Prasad 1991). Also, a relationship between zinc deficiency and lower testosterone in patients who were ill has been reported (Prasad *et al.* 1981). However, zinc supplementation has not been found to have any positive effect on testosterone or muscle growth in individuals with adequate or near adequate status.

Nishiyama *et al.* (1996) examined haematological factors in two groups of female endurance runners, one with impaired zinc status and one with normal status. The zinc-deficient group had a lower number of red blood cells, serum haemoglobin and iron. They were then given an iron or an iron-plus-zinc supplement. The subjects who received the iron-plus-zinc showed a greater increase in haemoglobin and red blood cells. The authors suggested that zinc plays a role in haematopoiesis and can prevent anaemia.

The effect of zinc supplementation for 6 days on exercise-induced changes in immune function in male runners has been assessed (Singh *et al.* 1994). By examining the respiratory burst activity of neutrophils after exercise, it was found that the supplement compared to a placebo blocked the increase in reactive oxygen species which cause an increase in free radical damage. Free radicals have an unpaired electron, making them highly reactive and damaging to the cell. These data suggest that supplemental zinc may serve as an antioxidant, but because the supplement suppressed T-lymphocyte activity, it may also increase susceptibility to infection.

### Summary

Many athletes are not ingesting the recommended quantities of zinc, and zinc status may be compromised. However, accurate assessment of zinc status or balance in athletes is lacking. Studies that examined the effects of acute and chronic exercise on blood zinc levels are equivocal, and the disparate results are unexplained. Well-controlled studies are needed to examine the changes in blood levels of zinc induced by various types of exercise and redistribution pathways. Even though exercise may result in some loss of zinc in sweat and urine, it is not known whether the body will adapt to this loss by increasing retention.

Zinc supplementation at levels in excess of the RDA may have negative consequences (Lukaski 1997). Excessive zinc can inhibit copper absorption, reduce high-density lipoprotein levels, and prevent an exercise-induced increase in high-density lipoproteins (Lukaski 1997). Female athletes and many male athletes, especially vegetarians and those maintaining low body weights, should be concerned that they ingest foods rich in zinc, or take a multivitamin-mineral supplement with micronutrient concentrations equal or less than the RDA.

## Copper

Copper is a component of many metalloenzymes in several key reactions (Hunt & Groff 1990). The copper-containing protein, ceruloplasmin, serves as a multifaceted oxidative enzyme playing a role as a scavenger of free radicals and a modulator of the inflammatory response as an acute phase protein. Copper is also part of superoxide dismutase, the enzyme that converts the harmful superoxide radical into the less harmful hydrogen peroxide. As part of cytochrome c oxidase, copper functions in the electron transport chain of the mitochondria. Copper is also needed for haemoglobin formation. A complete review of copper containing enzymes and proteins can be found elsewhere (Linder 1996).

There is not sufficient information to establish an RDA, so the Food and Nutrition Board recommended an estimated safe and adequate daily dietary intake (ESADDI) of between 1.5 and $3.0 \, mg \cdot day^{-1}$. Copper is found in organ meats (especially liver), seafoods (especially oysters), nuts and seeds (Food and Nutrition Board 1989). Many diets in the general population contain less than $1.6 \, mg \cdot day^{-1}$ but this value may underestimate intake (Food and Nutrition Board 1989). Most studies reported that athletes ingest adequate amounts of copper (Deuster et al. 1986; Worme et al. 1990; Bazzarre et al. 1993; Singh et al. 1993). However, in many of these studies, there was a small fraction of athletes ingesting less than two thirds of the ESADDI for copper. For example, about 5% of Navy Seals did not ingest two thirds the ESADDI (Singh et al. 1989).

**Copper status and effects of exercise**

Blood levels of copper are most commonly used to assess status. Several studies have found that athletes had similar or higher levels than controls (Dressendorfer & Sockolov 1980; Olha et al. 1982; Lukaski et al. 1983, 1990; Weight et al. 1988; Singh et al. 1989; Bazzarre et al. 1993; Wang et al. 1995; Tuya et al. 1996). One study reported that male distance runners had lower plasma copper levels than controls (Resina et al. 1990). However, the weight of the data suggests that copper deficiency, as assessed by blood copper levels, is rare in trained athletes.

Wang et al. (1995) reported that female orienteers had higher serum copper concentrations than male orienteers, which they suggested may

be due to the use of oestrogen-containing oral contraceptives. Newhouse et al. (1993) found that the mean copper values for females on oral contraceptives was $30.1 \, \mu mol \cdot l^{-1}$ vs. $18.8 \, \mu mol \cdot l^{-1}$ for women not on oral contraceptives. The reason for high circulating copper in women on oral contraceptives is not known but could be due to higher plasma ceruloplasmin levels from altered liver function and/or increased absorption of dietary copper with no change in urine loss (Newhouse et al. 1993). This effect is related to oestrogen use because oestrogen replacement therapy by postmenopausal women also significantly increased serum copper levels.

Results of training on blood copper levels are equivocal. Dressendorfer et al. (1982) reported an increase in plasma copper over the first 8 days of a 20-day road race which remained elevated throughout the duration of the race. These authors suggested that the elevation in plasma copper may be due to an increase in the liver's production of ceruloplasmin in response to exercise stress. In contrast, Hübner-Woźniak et al. (1996) found that bodybuilders who began a strength training programme for 10 weeks showed no pre- to posttraining change in blood copper levels. Anderson et al. (1995) reported that an acute bout of strenuous exercise increased blood copper levels in both moderately trained runners and untrained men, demonstrating that the release of copper into the circulation was independent of the degree of training. However, Olha et al. (1982) found that trained runners had a significantly greater increase in serum copper after exercise than untrained subjects.

Several studies reported that an acute bout of exercise results in an increase in plasma copper levels immediately after exercise which returned to baseline within a couple of hours (Olha et al. 1982; Ohno et al. 1984). In contrast, Anderson et al. (1984) found no increase in serum copper immediately or 2 h after a 9.6-km run, Marrella et al. (1990) found a slight but significant decrease in plasma copper after a 1-h cycling test, and Bordin et al. (1993) found a decrease in plasma copper after approximately 30 min of a run-to-exhaustion test. The reason for these discrepant findings is unclear. Because most of plasma copper is bound to ceruloplasmin, an increase in copper may be required for increased antioxidant capacity in response to muscle damage (Dressendorfer *et al.* 1982; Anderson & Guttman 1988; Aruoma *et al.* 1988). Apparently, exercise results in a redistribution of copper, but how this occurs is not known, nor is how this might affect adaptation to training.

### Copper status and performance

Little data exist regarding the effects of copper status and performance. Lukaski *et al.* (1996) reported that nutritional status and dietary intake of several micronutrients including copper were useful predictors of 100-yard (91-m) freestyle swimming performance in collegiate male swimmers. However, no significant correlation between $\dot{V}o_{2max.}$ and plasma copper levels in trained athletes or untrained subjects was found (Lukaski *et al.* 1983). No studies have examined the effect of copper supplementation on performance. Although copper can be lost in sweat (Gutteridge *et al.* 1985), it is not likely that exercise and training will lead to a deficiency.

### Summary

Most athletes appear to have adequate copper status. There is concern that some athletes, especially females, are not ingesting sufficient amounts of copper in their diet, but whether the body adapts to slightly smaller dietary amounts than the ESADDI needs to be determined. Results from studies examining changes in blood copper levels after acute and chronic exercise are equivocal. After acute exercise, there appears to be a transient redistribution of copper among body compartments leading to copper changes in the blood, but how this occurs is not known and requires further study (Marrella *et al.* 1993). Studies are needed to assess how copper status, the type of exercise and training, and the duration and intensity of exercise affect acute and chronic changes in blood copper levels. There is no basis to recommend copper supplementation

for athletes, rather athletes should ingest foods rich in copper. It should be noted that high amounts of vitamin C and high levels of dietary zinc can reduce the absorption of copper and may lead to reduced copper status (Reeves 1997). On the other hand, iron supplements do not affect blood copper levels (Newhouse *et al.* 1993).

## Selenium

Selenium has received recent attention in the media because of an interesting randomized controlled trial where it was found that 200 µg selenium·day$^{-1}$ for about 4 years resulted in a significant reduction in total cancer mortality and incidence of lung, colorectal and prostate cancers (Clark *et al.* 1996). Before selenium supplements are recommended, further studies are needed to confirm these findings and evaluate circumstances where selenium may have adverse effects (Colditz 1996). The reason that selenium may exert this positive effect on cancer occurrence is likely due to its role as an antioxidant.

Selenium functions as an antioxidant by serving as a cofactor for the enzyme glutathione peroxidase (Levander & Burk 1996). This enzyme catalyses the reduction of organic peroxides, including the tissue damaging hydrogen peroxide ($H_2O_2$) (Hunt & Groff 1990). The reduction of peroxides renders them harmless. Glutathione (GSH) reacts with $H_2O_2$, thereby 'inactivating' it to produce glutathione disulphide (GSSG; the oxidized form of glutathione). Also, glutathione reacts with organic peroxides formed by an increase in the hydroxyl radical.

Exercise increases oxygen consumption which can lead to an increase in free radicals, such as superoxide, by the incomplete reduction of oxygen in the electron transport system. Superoxide is converted to hydrogen peroxide by the enzyme superoxide dismutase (SOD) or can form the hydroxy radical. Thus, the increased hydroxy radicals and hydrogen peroxide levels can be rendered harmless by glutathione peroxidase and its essential cofactor selenium.

Because selenium serves as an antioxidant, adequate levels may reduce oxidative stress during exercise and aid in recovery, thereby allowing athletes to train harder. For more information on selenium, oxidative stress and exercise, see Aruoma (1994), Clarkson (1995) and Halliwell (1996).

## Selenium intake and status in athletes

The content of selenium in foods, especially plants, is highly variable because of the variation in the soil content of selenium. Blood selenium values vary among countries; for example, they are relatively high for adults in the USA and Canada, but low for adults in Sweden and New Zealand, where soil content of selenium is low (Hunt & Groff 1990). Food sources of selenium are seafoods, liver, organ meats, muscle meats, cereals and grain (Levander & Burk 1996).

The RDA for selenium is 70 and 55 μg for males and females, respectively, 19 years and older (Food and Nutrition Board 1989). There is no completely acceptable measure of selenium status (Gibson 1990). Whole blood or erythrocyte measures are somewhat more accurate than plasma or serum values that fluctuate from day to day (Gibson 1990). However, published means of serum selenium in adults are fairly consistent varying from 0.53 to 2.4 $\mu mol \cdot l^{-1}$ (Malvy et al. 1993). The activity of glutathione peroxidase has been used to assess selenium status, but normal values have not been well standardized (Gibson 1990).

Little data exist on selenium intake or status of athletes. Wrestlers were found to have intakes of selenium below 90% of the RDA in about half of those competing while only one in eight of non-competing wrestlers had lower intakes than the RDA (Snook et al. 1995). Despite the lower selenium intake, selenium status assessed by plasma and erythrocyte glutathione peroxidase activity indicated that all wrestlers had adequate status (Snook et al. 1995). Robertson et al. (1991) reported that sedentary subjects had lower blood glutathione peroxidase activity and concentra-tion of selenium than trained runners. And, of the trained runners, those who trained 80–147 $km \cdot week^{-1}$ had higher levels than those who trained only 16–43 $km \cdot week^{-1}$ for at least 2 years. Athletes in countries where the food content of selenium is adequate generally have adequate status (Fogelholm & Lahtinen 1991; Wang et al. 1995). Wang et al. (1995) found that Swedish orienteers had lower serum selenium values than Finnish orienteers. Since 1984, Finland has been enriching fertilizer with selenium to increase the selenium content of cereal crops, which is not the case in Sweden.

## Changes due to exercise

Few studies have examined either exercise changes in blood selenium or glutathione peroxidase. Duthie et al. (1990) reported no significant change in erythrocyte glutathione peroxidase, catalase or SOD activity after a half marathon and up to 120 h postrace in trained subjects. In contrast, sedentary subjects who exercised on a cycle ergometer at 70% of maximal heart rate for 1 h showed decreases in erythrocyte enzyme activities of superoxide dismutase, catalase and glutathione peroxidase at 5 min after exercise and remained low for up to 48 h (Toskulkao & Glinsukon 1996). This change was accompanied by an increase in plasma malondialdehyde, an indirect indicator of increased lipid peroxidation. Thus, the large production of free radicals may result in a decrease in activity of the enzymes. In the Duthie et al. study (1990), trained subjects may be better able to handle the increase in free radicals such that changes in these enzyme activities were not apparent.

Toskulkao and Glinsukon (1996) also examined the changes in antioxidant enzyme activity in trained athletes but the results were inconsistent. Rokitzki et al. (1994) found that trained athletes did not show an increase in activity of glutathione peroxidase in erythrocytes after a marathon. However, these authors suggested that the lack of change may be due to the inappropriate use of erythrocytes rather than muscle where the greater stress is taking place.

Selenium intake and plasma levels were examined before and after a week of sustained physical activity, psychological stress and lack of sleep in Navy Seals during 'Hell Week' (Singh *et al.* 1991). Physical activity stress included simulated combat exercise and obstacle course trials; psychological stress included performance anxiety, verbal confrontation and uncertainty of events. Selenium intake was substantially higher during Hell Week, but plasma selenium values at the end of the week were lower. Lower serum selenium values may reflect a redistribution of selenium to other tissues requiring antioxidant protection (Singh *et al.* 1991). The authors suggested that the decrease in selenium and other accompanying changes, such as a decrease in plasma zinc, iron and albumin, and an increase in ferritin, ceruloplasmin, white blood cell count and creatine kinase, were indicative of an acute-phase response to tissue damage and the inflammatory effect of prolonged physical activity.

Fogelholm *et al.* (1991) examined serum micronutrient levels in a sailing crew during a transatlantic race and compared these values to those of a control group. While there was no pre- to postrace difference in serum selenium values, the values for the sailors were lower than the control values. Whether this indicates a slight lowering of serum selenium values with training is not known. It should be noted that the values for the sailors were within the reference range. However, if exercise results in an increase in oxidative stress, the body may require greater than reference levels of selenium (and other antioxidants) to keep pace (Duthie 1996). This does not necessarily mean that more selenium should be ingested, because the body may become more efficient in retention or action in trained individuals.

## Selenium supplementation and lipid peroxidation

Two of the first studies to examine the effects of selenium supplementation used a crossover design, where the length of time of the washout may not have been adequate. Drăgan *et al.* (1990) examined the effect of an acute dose of 140 µg of selenium or placebo in trained Romanian swimmers, where subjects repeated the treatment after 1 week. In a second experiment, 100 µg of selenium (or placebo) were administered for 14 days and then the treatments were crossed for another 14 days with no washout period in between. Before and after the treatments, subjects performed a 2-h endurance swimming exercise. The acute dose resulted in no significant change in the exercise-induced increase in lipid peroxides. However, after 14 days of supplementation, the group who received the selenium supplement on the second bout showed a decrease in lipid peroxides in response to the exercise. This was not true for the group who received the selenium first.

A second study by the same laboratory (Drăgan *et al.* 1991) found that 3 weeks of supplementing with a mixture containing selenium, vitamin E, glutathione and cysteine (concentrations were unspecified) in trained Romanian cyclists resulted in a smaller change in lipid peroxidation compared with the group ingesting a placebo. After 1 week, the groups crossed over, but the group taking the placebo showed less of an increase in lipid peroxides. It appeared the first leg of the crossover may have affected the response to the second leg of the crossover.

Tessier *et al.* (1995a, 1995b) administered 180 µg·day$^{-1}$ of selenium or a placebo for 10 weeks during an endurance training programme after a 4-week deconditioning period. The selenium supplement resulted in an increase in the resting plasma levels of glutathione peroxidase activity. A moderate correlation between erythrocyte glutathione peroxidase activity and $\dot{V}o_{2max.}$ was found in the supplemented group only (Tessier *et al.* 1995a), but the supplement did not affect $\dot{V}o_{2max.}$. In another report from the same study (Tessier *et al.* 1995b), there was an increase in muscle glutathione peroxidase activity in response to an acute exercise bout in the supplemented group only (Tessier *et al.* 1995b). These results lend support for selenium supplements enhancing antioxidant capacity.

## Summary

Little is known about selenium intake and status of athletes or changes in selenium status with training. A few studies suggested a benefit of selenium supplementation in improving antioxidant capacity, but these studies require corroboration. It is possible that selenium may be most effective in athletes who are ingesting insufficient amounts, yet it is not known if marginally insufficient intake will compromise status or antioxidant capacity. Excessive amounts of selenium ($>200\,\mu g \cdot day^{-1}$) could have toxic effects (Levander & Burk 1996; Boylan & Spallholz 1997).

## Chromium

Chromium's primary function is to potentiate the effects of insulin in stimulating the uptake of glucose, amino acids and triglycerides by cells (Hunt & Groff 1990; Stoecker 1996; Anding et al. 1997). How chromium affects insulin action is not fully known but chromium is thought to help bind insulin to its receptor (Trent & Thieding-Cancel 1995). Release of insulin may stimulate the release of chromium from body stores (Hunt & Groff 1990). The physiological role of chromium was first identified when it was shown that a substance containing chromium was necessary for maintaining normal glucose tolerance (Stoecker 1996; Anding et al. 1997). This organic compound, referred to as the glucose tolerance factor, was found to be a complex of chromium, nicotinic acid and glutathione (Hunt & Groff 1990).

In addition to insulin's role in transport of nutrients into muscle cells, it may act as a physiological antagonist to bone resorption and promote collagen production by osetoblasts (McCarty 1995). At present there have been no trials to assess chromium's effectiveness on bone health, but this may prove a fruitful area for research, especially in amenorrhoeic athletes. McCarty (1995) suggests that rather than relying on mononutrient therapy with calcium, a micronutrient cocktail of several nutrients that affect bone, such as calcium, chromium, zinc, boron, copper and manganese and vitamins D and K, be studied in the maintenance of bone mineral density.

The US Food and Nutrition Board was unable to establish an RDA for chromium due to insufficient data. Instead, the ESADDI is set at 50–$200\,\mu g \cdot day^{-1}$ (Food and Nutrition Board 1989). Many people may not be ingesting the minimum ESADDI (Anderson et al. 1991; Stoecker 1996). A diet that would appear adequate for most nutrients can have less than $16\,\mu g$ of chromium per $4.2\,kJ$ (1000 cal), and high-fat diets may have less chromium than isocaloric low-fat diets (Stoecker 1996). Anderson and Kozlovsky (1985) analysed the chromium content of 7-day self-selected diets for 10 men and 22 women and found that the mean (and range) chromium content of the food was $33\,\mu g \cdot day^{-1}$ (range, 22–48) for the men and $25\,\mu g \cdot day^{-1}$ (range, 13–36) for the women. Even individuals with the largest content of chromium in the diet had less than the minimum ESADDI. However, there is some concern that the ESADDI may be set too high because earlier studies used less sophisticated equipment so that the requirement determination may have been inaccurately high (Stoecker 1996).

Chromium ingestion has been related to several health benefits. Studies have found that subjects with impaired glucose tolerance who were supplemented with chromium demonstrated improved glucose tolerance (Anderson 1992). Chronic insufficient chromium ingestion could predispose an individual to developing glucose intolerance and maturity-onset diabetes (Anderson 1992). Chromium supplements resulted in a lowering of blood lipids in subjects with high values (Hermann et al. 1994), and one study found that blood lipids were lowered in bodybuilders taking chromium supplements (Lefavi et al. 1993).

Food sources rich in chromium are Brewer's yeast, mushrooms, prunes, nuts, asparagus, wine, beer and whole grains (Hunt & Groff 1990). Absorption of chromium is enhanced when given in conjunction with vitamin C, and foods prepared in stainless steel cookware can increase the amount of chromium available due to the leaching of chromium from the pans by the action of acidic foods (Stoecker 1996). Chromium supplements are available in three forms: chromium picolinate, chromium nicotinate and chromium chloride.

### Chromium status and effects of exercise and diet

Because many national nutrient databases do not include chromium, there is little information on chromium intake of athletes. Athletes who ingest high-calorie diets to meet their energy needs may have diets adequate in chromium. There may be concern that athletes who restrict calories to maintain low body weights do not ingest sufficient chromium. Kleiner et al. (1994) examined nutrient intake of male and female elite bodybuilders during 8–10 days prior to competition. The mean chromium intake for the males was $143 \mu g \cdot day^{-1}$ and for the females was only $21 \mu g \cdot day^{-1}$. The low value for the females was related to low caloric intake and food choices low in chromium. Of interest, nine of the 11 females were amenorrhoeic at contest time.

Exercise produces an increase of chromium in the blood followed by an increase in the urine (Anderson et al. 1982, 1984; Gatteschi et al. 1995). Apparently there is a release of chromium from the body stores that cannot be re-uptaken by tissues or the kidney and is therefore lost into the urine (Anderson et al. 1984; Anding et al. 1997). Several studies from the same laboratory showed urinary chromium excretion is increased by exercise such that 24-h chromium losses were twice as high on the exercise day as on the rest day (Anderson et al. 1982, 1984, 1991). Whether this loss can result in a negative chromium balance is not known. Resting urinary excretion of chromium was lower in trained athletes than untrained individuals (Anderson et al. 1988), which suggests that the body may be able adapt to the increased loss by retaining more of the

ingested chromium. For more detailed reviews of chromium and exercise, see Anding et al. (1997), Clarkson (1991), Clarkson and Haymes (1994) and Lefavi et al. (1992).

CHO content of the diet also influences chromium loss. Although a high-CHO diet did not produce an increased chromium excretion (Anderson et al. 1991), ingestion of glucose/fructose (simple sugar) drinks did (Anderson et al. 1990). Anderson et al. (1990) found that beverages resulting in the greatest increase in circulating insulin caused the most change in urinary excretion of chromium in subjects with a normal insulin response. Those who ingest high amounts of simple sugars may have an enhanced loss of chromium.

### Chromium supplementation and lean body mass

Chromium has been marketed as a supplement to increase lean body mass and decrease fat. The increase in lean body mass was thought to occur due to chromium's facilitation of amino acid transport into muscle cells. In 1989, Evans reported data from two studies showing that $200 \mu g \cdot day^{-1}$ of chromium increased lean body weight in untrained subjects and trained athletes during 40 days of weight training. Supplemental chromium was then touted as the healthy alternative to anabolic steroids. The Evans studies (1989) estimated lean body mass from skinfold measurements which may not provide an accurate indication of fat or muscle mass.

Four studies then attempted to confirm the above results but, for the most part, could not. Hasten et al. (1992) examined the effect of $200 \mu g \cdot day^{-1}$ of chromium picolinate (or placebo) for 12 weeks in male and female college students enrolled in a weight training class. Over the 12 weeks there was only a slight increase in body weight for the males (placebo and supplemented groups) and for the female placebo group, with no difference among the groups (range, 0.9–2.0% increase). However, the females taking the supplement demonstrated a 4.3% increase in body weight. The chromium supplement did not affect the change in skinfolds, circumferences or strength. The authors suggested that the chromium supplement may affect the females to a greater extent because the dose per body weight was higher for the females or that females produce more insulin than males and would therefore be more sensitive to chromium. The greater effect for the females also could be due to the fact that females may ingest less chromium than males and have insufficient status. However, this study did not assess chromium ingestion. The authors also suggested that the relatively large gains in muscle mass for untrained subjects may have masked the effect of the supplement for the males.

Clancy et al. (1994) examined the effects of chromium picolinate in football players who ingested 200 μg·day$^{-1}$ or a placebo for 9 weeks during spring training that included a weight-lifting programme. This study improved upon the prior studies in that hydrostatic weighing was used to assess body composition and urinary chromium excretion was assessed. The results showed no significant difference in lean body mass or strength between groups. However, the subjects who ingested the supplement had an increased level of chromium in the urine at 4 and then 9 weeks of training. Whether some of the chromium was retained is not known, but the results suggest that a large portion of the supplement was excreted, which may indicate that the body stores were close to optimal prior to supplementation. A near duplicate study (Hallmark et al. 1996) to the Clancy et al. study also reported no effects of 200 μg chromium picolinate on strength or lean body mass after 12 weeks of resistance training, and chromium excretion was increased in the supplemented group.

In the most well-controlled study of chromium supplementation, Lukaski et al. (1996a) matched subjects for specific physical and nutritional characteristics and placed them into one of three groups: placebo, chromium picolinate and chromium chloride. The groups were studied for 8 weeks while on a weight training pro-gramme. The two supplements similarly increased serum chromium levels and urinary chromium excretion. There was no difference among the groups in body composition assessed by dual X-ray absortiometry or in strength gain, suggesting that the chromium supplement was ineffective.

## Chromium supplementation and weight loss

Although chromium supplements received initial attention as a means to gain muscle mass, more recently they have been marketed as a weight loss product. Two studies investigated the effectiveness of chromium picolinate supplements on fat loss. Trent and Thieding-Cancel (1995) examined the effect of 16 weeks of 400 μg chromium picolinate or a placebo in Navy personnel who exceeded the Navy percentage body fat standards of 22% for men and 30% for women. During the 16 weeks, subjects participated in a physical conditioning programme. Body fat was determined only from body circumference measures and height. No significant difference in total exercise time or dietary habits (a ratio of good to bad food choices) was observed between the placebo and chromium groups. The supplement was found to be ineffective as a weight loss agent. The authors stated that chromium picolinate was 'not a quick cure for obesity and perhaps not a remedy at all'.

Kaats et al. (1996) had subjects ingest a placebo, 200 μg or 400 μg chromium picolinate·day$^{-1}$ for 72 days. Subjects were free living. Body composition was assessed by hydrostatic weighing and a body composition index (BCI) was calculated by adding the loss of body fat and gain in nonfat mass and subtracting fat gained and lean lost. At the end of the 72 days, both supplemented groups had demonstrated high positive changes in BCIs compared to the placebo, with no difference between groups taking the 200 or the 400 μg. These authors concluded that chromium supplementation did improve body composition. However, further studies are needed to confirm these results.

### Negative effects of chromium supplementation

Because chromium has a low absorption rate, it is not considered to be toxic (Anding *et al.* 1997). However, Stearns *et al.* (1995a) reported that chromium picolinate produced chromosome damage in isolated cells *in vitro*. This study received criticism due to its use of supraphysiological doses in cell cultures rather than oral doses in animals or humans (McCarty 1996). In a second report, Stearns *et al.* (1995b) employed a pharmacokinetic model to predict how ingested chromium could accumulate and be retained in human tissue. These authors cautioned against taking supplements with concentrations greater than the ESADDI and concluded that the normal dietary intake of chromium may be adequate to maintain a positive chromium balance in most people, even at levels of ingestion somewhat below the 50–200 μg range.

Other anecdotal accounts, case histories and studies suggest that chromium supplements may cause headaches, sleep disturbances, mood changes, increased excretion of trace minerals, altered iron metabolism and changes in perceptual processes (Lefavi *et al.* 1992; Trent & Thieding-Cancel 1995). Lukaski *et al.* (1996a) found that chromium supplementation for 8 weeks resulted in a small decrease in transferrin saturation which was greater for the chromium picolinate supplement than the chromium chloride supplement. This may be due to the fact that chromium competes with iron for binding on transferrin. Lukaski *et al.* (1996a) speculated that chromium supplementation may predispose an individual to iron deficiency. However, it should be noted that the change in transferrin saturation was not statistically significant, thus further studies are needed to confirm this finding.

### Summary

Exercise can increase urinary excretion, as can ingestion of simple sugars; however, whether this will induce a chromium deficiency or whether athletes are able to increase efficiency or retention of chromium is not known. Because the long-term safety of chromium is a concern (Anding *et al.* 1997), athletes should ingest foods rich in chromium. For added assurance, a multivitamin-mineral supplement containing between 50 and 200 μg of chromium would not be harmful. Studies of the effects of chromium supplementation on lean body mass in athletes show that it is not effective. Results of the two studies to assess chromium's efficacy as a weight loss agent are equivocal. Chromium may only be effective in individuals with impaired status, but this has not been assessed.

## Vanadium

Vanadium, like chromium, is purported to have an insulin-like effect and promote the transport of amino acids into cells. Because this effect is thought to be anabolic, vanadium, in the form of vanadyl sulphate, is widely marketed to bodybuilders. There is not sufficient information to state that vanadium is an essential element for humans (Food and Nutrition Board 1989). Data suggesting that vanadium may be anabolic come from *in vitro* study of cells and pharmacological studies of animals (Nielsen 1996). For example, growth rate is reduced in vanadium deficient rats (Nielsen 1996). The Food and Nutrition Board (1989) came to the conclusion that if nutritional requirements exist they are low and easily met by levels naturally occurring in foods.

Fawcett *et al.* (1996) cite anecdotal evidence that athletes are taking up to 60 mg·day$^{-1}$ for 2–3 months to increase muscle mass. In the only study to evaluate vanadium supplements, Fawcett *et al.* (1996) had subjects ingest 0.5 mg·kg$^{-1}$·day$^{-1}$ of vanadyl sulphate or placebo for 12 weeks during a weight training programme. The results showed no beneficial effect of the supplement on body composition as assessed by anthropometric measures or DEXA scans. Vanadium supplements could have detrimental effects when taken for a long period of time, but this has not been adequately studied (Moore & Friedl 1992). There is no basis at this time to suggest that vanadyl sulphate will have any beneficial effects for athletes.

## Boron

Boron has been found to be an essential element for plant growth, and it may be an essential nutrient for animals (Food and Nutrition Board 1989; Nielsen 1996). Boron affects calcium and magnesium metabolism and can influence membrane function (Chrisley 1997). Nielsen *et al.* (1987) found that boron supplementation of $3\,mg\cdot day^{-1}$ lowered urinary calcium loss in a low-magnesium diet and increased serum oestrogen and testosterone in postmenopausal women. These data suggested that boron may play a role in the prevention of bone loss (Volpe *et al.* 1993a, 1993b). Also, boron supplements have been purported to increase testosterone and muscle mass in athletes (Green & Ferrando 1994).

There is a paucity of information on boron requirements in general (there is no RDA or ESADDI set) and no information on dietary intake or status in athletes. A national database for boron content of foods does not yet exist so it is impossible to evaluate boron intake. However, the average daily intake of boron is estimated to range between 0.5 and 3.1 mg (Nielsen 1996). Rich food sources of boron are leafy vegetables, nuts, legumes and non-citrus fruits (Nielsen 1996).

A few studies of boron supplementation in athletes exist. Meacham *et al.* (1994, 1995) and Volpe *et al.* (1993a, 1993b) examined the effect of $3\,mg\cdot day^{-1}$ of boron (or placebo) for 10 months in four groups of subjects: athletes taking boron, athletes taking placebo, sedentary taking boron, and sedentary taking placebo. Serum phosphorus concentrations were lower and serum magnesium higher in the subjects taking the boron supplement. The sedentary subjects taking boron had the lowest serum phosphorus levels and the highest serum magnesium levels. Urinary boron increased in the subjects supplemented with boron. Bone mineral density was not affected by boron supplementation, nor were circulating levels of 1,25-dihydroxyvitamin $D_3$, 17-β oestradiol, progesterone or testosterone. Thus, it appeared that boron supplementation did not affect bone mineral density or hormonal status, but had some effect on mineral levels in the blood. Whether these changes in serum phosphate and magnesium are meaningful remains to be determined.

Green and Ferrando (1994) examined the effect of 2.5 mg boron or placebo for 7 weeks in male bodybuilders. Of the 10 subjects receiving the boron supplement, six demonstrated an increase in plasma boron levels. Both groups showed an increase in lean body mass, total testosterone level and strength over the course of the 7 weeks but there was no difference between the group taking the boron and the group taking the placebo. At present there is not sufficient information to suggest that boron supplements will have any beneficial effects for athletes.

## Conclusion

Although athletes may not be ingesting sufficient amounts of some trace minerals, in all cases, an improved diet is recommended, or a multi-vitamin–mineral supplement containing no more than the RDA or ESADDI level. Despite a lower dietary intake, often blood indicators of status are normal, which may suggest that dietary analyses are in error perhaps due to under-reporting of certain foods or that databases are inadequate. Futhermore, there may be a long-term homeostatic adaptation to low mineral intake. Exercise promotes a loss of some trace minerals in sweat and urine, but it is not known whether athletes can counteract this loss by increasing absorption, retention, or efficiency of the micronutrient. Thus, mineral balance studies of athletes are needed. Also, exercise produces acute changes in trace minerals in the blood but how this occurs has not been adequately explained.

Supplementation of various micronutrients on performance or body composition has not proven very effective. There are no data to show that zinc will enhance muscle growth or testosterone levels. Unconfirmed results show that zinc supplements produced some strength gains but the data are inconclusive. A few studies have reported benefits of selenium supplements on antioxidant defense. The purported benefit of chromium supplementation on increasing lean body mass has not been proven. Limited data on chromium as a weight loss agent are equivocal. The only published study of vanadyl sulphate did not show a change in body composition. The few studies on boron supplementation did not find any beneficial effect on bone mass, muscle mass, or testosterone levels. It is unlikely that micronutrient supplements will enhance performance or body composition in athletes who have sufficient status. Athletes should maintain adequate status by ingesting a variety of foods rich in trace minerals.

## References

Anderson, R.A. (1992) Chromium, glucose tolerance, and diabetes. *Biological Trace Element Research* **32**, 19–24.

Anderson, R.A. & Guttman, H.N. (1988) Trace minerals and exercise. In *Exercise, Nutrition, and Energy Metabolism* (ed. E.S. Horton & R.L. Terjung), pp. 180–195. Macmillan, New York.

Anderson, R.A. & Kozlovsky, A.S. (1985) Chromium intake, absorption and excretion of subjects consuming self-selected diets. *American Journal of Clinical Nutrition* **41**, 1177–1183.

Anderson, R.A., Polansky, M.M., Bryden, N.A., Roginski, E.E., Patterson, K.Y. & Reamer, D.C. (1982) Effect of exercise (running) on serum glucose, insulin, glucagon, and chromium excretion. *Diabetes* **31**, 212–216.

Anderson, R.A., Polansky, M.M. & Bryden, N.A. (1984) Strenuous running: acute effects on chromium, copper, zinc, and selected clinical variables in urine and serum of male runners. *Biological Trace Element Research* **6**, 327–336.

Anderson, R.A., Bryden, N.A., Polansky, M.M. & Deuster, P.A. (1988) Exercise effects on chromium excretion of trained and untrained men consuming a constant diet. *Journal of Applied Physiology* **64**, 249–252.

Anderson, R.A., Bryden, N.A., Polansky, M.M. & Reiser, S. (1990) Urinary chromium excretion and insulinogenic properties of carbohydrates. *American Journal of Clinical Nutrition* **51**, 864–868.

Anderson, R.A., Bryden, N.A., Polansky, M.M. & Thorp, J.W. (1991) Effects of carbohydrate loading and underwater exercise on circulating cortisol, insulin and urinary losses of chromium and zinc. *European Journal of Applied Physiology* **63**, 146–150.

Anderson, R.A., Bryden, N.A., Polansky, M.M. & Deuster, P.A. (1995) Acute exercise effects on urinary losses and serum concentrations of copper and zinc of moderately trained and untrained men consuming a controlled diet. *Analyst* **120**, 867–870.

Anding, J.D., Wolinsky, I. & Klimis-Tavantzis, D.J. (1997) Chromium. In *Sports Nutrition: Vitamin and Trace Elements* (ed. I. Wolinsky & J.A. Driskell), pp. 189–194. CRC Press, Boca Raton.

Aruoma, O.I. (1994) Free radicals and antioxidant strategies in sports. *Journal of Nutritional Biochemistry* **5**, 370–381.

Aruoma, O.I., Reilly, T., MacLaren, D. & Halliwell, B. (1988) Iron, copper and zinc concentrations in human sweat and plasma: the effect of exercise. *Clinica Chimica Acta* **177**, 81–88.

Bazzarre, T.L., Scarpino, A., Sigmon, R., Marquart, L.F., Wu, S.L. & Izurieta, M. (1993) Vitamin-mineral supplement use and nutritional status of athletes. *Journal of the American College of Nutrition* **12**, 162–169.

Benson, J., Gillien, D.M., Bourdet, K. & Loosli, A.R. (1985) Inadequate nutrition and chronic calorie restriction in adolescent ballerinas. *Physician and Sportsmedicine* **13**, 79–90.

Bordin, D., Sartorelli, L., Bonanni, G., Mastrogiacomo, I. & Scalco, E. (1993) High intensity physical exercise induced effects on plasma levels of copper and zinc. *Biological Trace Element Research* **36**, 129–134.

Boylan, M & Spallholz, J.E. (1997) Selenium. In *Sports Nutrition: Vitamin and Trace Elements* (ed. I. Wolinsky & J.A. Driskell), pp. 195–204. CRC Press, Boca Raton.

Chrisley, B.Mc. (1997) Other substances in foods. In *Sports Nutrition: Vitamin and Trace Elements* (ed. I. Wolinsky & J.A. Driskell), pp. 205–220. CRC Press, Boca Raton.

Clancy, S.P., Clarkson, P.M., DeCheke, M.E. *et al.* (1994) Effects of chromium picolinate supplementation on body composition, strength, and urinary chromium loss in football players. *International Journal of Sport Nutrition* **4**, 142–153.

Clark, L.C., Combs, G.F., Turnbull, B.W. *et al.* for the Nutritional Prevention of Cancer Study Group (1996) Effects of selenium supplementation for cancer prevention in patients with carcinoma of the skin: a randomized controlled trial. *Journal of the American Medical Association* **276**, 1957–1963.

Clarkson, P.M. (1991) Nutritional ergogenic aids: chromium, exercise, and muscle mass. *International Journal of Sport Nutrition* **3**, 289–293.

Clarkson, P.M. (1995) Antioxidants and physical performance. *Critical Reviews in Food Science and Nutrition* **35**, 131–141.

Clarkson, P.M. & Haymes, E.M. (1994) Trace mineral

requirements for athletes. *International Journal of Sport Nutrition* **4**, 104–119.

Colditz, G.A. (1996) Selenium and cancer protection: promising results indicate further trials required. *Journal of the American Medical Association* **276**, 1984–1985.

Couzy, F., Lafargue, P. & Guezennec, C.Y. (1990) Zinc metabolism in the athlete: influence of training, nutrition and other factors. *International Journal of Sports Medicine* **11**, 263–266.

Deuster, P.A., Kyle, S.B., Moser, P.B., Vigersky, R.A., Singh, A. & Schoomaker, E.B. (1986) Nutritional survey of highly trained women runners. *American Journal of Clinical Nutrition* **45**, 954–962.

Deuster, P.A., Day, B.A., Singh, A., Douglass, L. & Moser-Veillon, P.B. (1989) Zinc status of highly trained women runners and untrained women. *American Journal of Clinical Nutrition* **49**, 1295–1301.

Drăgan, I., Dinu, V., Mohora, M., Cristea, E., Ploesteanu, E. & Stroescu, V. (1990) Studies regarding the antioxidant effects of selenium on top swimmers. *Revue Roumaine de Physiologie* **27**, 15–20.

Drăgan, I., Dinu, V., Cristea, E., Mohora, M., Ploesteanu, E. & Stroescu, V. (1991) Studies regarding the effects of an antioxidant compound in top athletes. *Revue Roumaine de Physiologie* **28**, 105–108.

Dressendorfer, R.H. & Sockolov, R. (1980) Hypozincemia in runners. *Physician and Sportsmedicine* **8**, 97–100.

Dressendorfer, R.H., Wade, C.E., Keen, C.L. & Scaff, J.H. (1982) Plasma mineral levels in marathon runners during a 20-day road race. *Physician and Sportsmedicine* **10**, 113–118.

Duthie, G.G. (1996) Adaptations of the antioxidant defence systems to chronic exercises. In *Human Muscular Function during Dynamic Exercise*. Vol. 41. *Medicine and Sport Science* (ed. P. Marconnet, B. Saltin, P. Komi & J. Poortmans), pp. 95–101. Karger, Basel.

Duthie, G.G., Robertson, J.D., Maughan, R.J. & Morrice, P.C. (1990) Blood antioxidant status and erythrocyte lipid peroxidation following distance running. *Archive of Biochemistry and Biophysics* **282**, 78–83.

Evans, G.W. (1989) The effect of chromium picolinate on insulin controlled parameters in humans. *International Journal of Biosocial and Medical Research* **11**, 163–180.

Fawcett, J.P., Farquhar, S.J., Walker, R.J., Thou, T., Lowe, G. & Goulding, A. (1996) The effect of oral vanadyl sulfate on body composition and performance in weight-training athletes. *International Journal of Sport Nutrition* **6**, 382–390.

Fogelholm, M. (1992) Micronutrient status in females during a 24-week fitness-type exercise programme. *Annals of Nutrition and Metabolism* **36**, 209–218.

Fogelholm, G.M. & Lahtinen, P.K. (1991) Nutritional evaluation of a sailing crew during a transatlantic race. *Scandinavian Journal of Medicine and Science in Sports* **1**, 99–103.

Fogelholm, M., Laakso, J., Lehto, J. & Ruokonen, I. (1991) Dietary intake and indicators of magnesium and zinc status in male athletes. *Nutrition Research* **11**, 1111–1118.

Fogelholm, G.M., Himberg, J., Alopaeus, K., Gref, C., Laakso, J.T. & Mussalo-Rauhamaa, H. (1992a) Dietary and biochemical indices of nutritional status in male athletes and controls. *Journal of the American College of Nutrition* **11**, 181–191.

Fogelholm, M., Rehunen, S., Gref, C.-G., Laasko, J.T., Lehto, J.J., Ruokonen, I. & Himberg, J.-J. (1992b) Dietary intake and thiamin, iron and zinc status in elite skiers during different training periods. *International Journal of Sports Nutrition* **2**, 351–365.

Food and Nutrition Board (1989) *Recommended Dietary Allowances,* 10th edn, pp. 205–213, 217–224, 224–230, 241–243, 267. National Academy Press, Washington, DC.

Gatteschi, L., Castellani, W., Galvan, P., Parise, G., Resina, A. & Rubenni, M.G. (1995) Effects of aerobic exercise on plasma chromium concentrations. In *Sports Nutrition: Minerals and Electrolytes* (ed. C.V. Kies & J.A. Driskell), pp. 199–204. CRC Press, Boca Raton.

Gibson, R.S. (1990) *Principles of Nutritional Assessment,* pp. 532–541. Oxford Press, New York.

Green, N.R. & Ferrando, A.A. (1994) Plasma boron and the effects of boron supplementation in males. *Environmental Health Perspectives* **102**, 73–77.

Gutteridge, J.M.C., Rowley, D.A., Halliwell, B., Cooper, D.F. & Heeley, D.M. (1985) Copper and iron complexes catalytic for oxygen radical reactions in sweat from human athletes. *Clinica Chimica Acta* **145**, 267–273.

Halliwell, B. (1996) Antioxidants. In *Present Knowledge in Nutrition*, 7th edn (ed. E.E. Ziegler & L.J. Filer), pp. 596–603. International Life Sciences Institute, Washington, DC.

Hallmark, M.A., Reynolds, T.H., DeSouza, C.A., Dotson, C.O., Anderson, R.A. & Roger, M.A. (1996) Effects of chromium and resistive training on muscle strength and body composition. *Medicine and Science in Sports and Exercise* **28**, 139–144.

Haralambie, G. (1981) Serum zinc in athletes in training. *International Journal of Sports Medicine* **2**, 135–138.

Hasten, D.L., Rome, E.P., Franks, B.D. & Hegsted, M. (1992) Effects of chromium picolinate on beginning weight training students. *International Journal of Sport Nutrition* **2**, 343–350.

Hermann, J., Arquitt, A. & Stoecker, B.J. (1994) Effect of chromium supplementation on plasma lipids, apoproteins, and glucose in elderly subjects. *Nutrition Research* **14**, 671–674.

Hübner-Woźniak, E., Lutoslawska, G., Sendecki, W.,

Dentkowski, A., Sawicka, T. & Drozd, J. (1996) Effects of a 10 week-training on biochemical and hematological variables in recreational bodybuilders. *Biology of Sport* **13**, 105–112.

Hunt, S.M. & Groff, J.L. (1990) *Advanced Nutrition and Human Metabolism*, pp. 286–348. West Publishing, St Paul, MN.

Kaats, G.R., Blum, K., Fisher, J.A. & Adelman, J.A. (1996) Effects of chromium picolinate supplementation on body composition: a randomized, double-masked, placebo-controlled study. *Current Therapeutic Research: Clinical and Experimental* **57**, 747–756.

Kleiner, S.M., Bazzarre, T.L. & Ainsworth, B.E. (1994) Nutritional status of nationally ranked elite bodybuilders. *International Journal of Sport Nutrition* **4**, 54–69.

Krotkiewski, M., Gudmundsson, M., Backstrom, P. & Mandroukas, K. (1982) Zinc and muscle strength and endurance. *Acta Physiologica Scandinavica* **116**, 309–311.

Lefavi, R.G., Anderson, R.A., Keith, R.E., Wilson, G.D., McMillan, J.L. & Stone, M.H. (1992) Efficacy of chromium supplementation in athletes: emphasis of anabolism. *International Journal of Sport Nutrition* **2**, 111–122.

Lefavi, R.G., Wilson, G.D., Keith, R.E., Anderson, R.A., Blessing, D.L., Hames, C.G. & McMillan, J.L. (1993) Lipid-lowering effect of a dietary chromium (III)–nicotinic acid complex in male athletes. *Nutrition Research* **13**, 239–249.

Levander, O.A. & Burk, R.F. (1996) Selenium. In *Present Knowledge in Nutrition*, 7th edn (ed. E.E. Ziegler & L.J. Filer Jr), pp. 320–328. International Life Sciences Institute, Washington, DC.

Linder, M.C. (1996) Copper. In *Present Knowledge in Nutrition*, 7th edn (ed. E.E. Ziegler & L.J. Filer Jr), pp. 307–319. International Life Sciences Institute, Washington, DC.

Loosli, A.R., Benson, J., Gillien, D.M. & Bourdet, K. (1986) Nutrition habits and knowledge in competitive adolescent female gymnasts. *Physician and Sportsmedicine* **14**, 118–130.

Lukaski, H.C. (1995) Interactions among indices of mineral element nutriture and physical performance of swimmers. In *Sports Nutrition: Minerals and Electrolytes* (ed. C.V. Kies & J.A. Driskell), pp. 267–279. CRC Press, Boca Raton.

Lukaski, H.C. (1997) Zinc. In *Sports Nutrition: Vitamin and Trace Elements* (ed. I. Wolinsky & J.A. Driskell), pp. 157–175. CRC Press, Boca Raton.

Lukaski, H.C., Bolonchuk, W.W., Klevay, L.M., Milne, D.B. & Sandstead, H.H. (1983) Maximum oxygen consumption as related to magnesium, copper, and zinc nutriture. *American Journal of Clinical Nutrition* **37**, 407–415.

Lukaski, H.C., Bolonchuk, W.W., Klevay, L.M., Milne, D.B. & Sandstead, H.H. (1984) Changes in plasma zinc content after exercise in men fed a low-zinc diet. *American Journal of Physiology* **247**, E88–E93.

Lukaski, H.C., Hoverson, B.S., Gallagher, S.K. & Bolonchuk, W.W. (1990) Physical training and copper, iron and zinc status of swimmers. *American Journal of Clinical Nutrition* **51**, 1093–1099.

Lukaski, H.C., Bolonchuk, W.W., Siders, W.A. & Milne, D.B. (1996a) Chromium supplementation and resistance training: effects of body composition, strength, and trace element status of men. *American Journal of Clinical Nutrition* **63**, 954–965.

Lukaski, H.C., Siders, W.A., Hoverson, B.S. & Gallagher, S.K. (1996b) Iron, copper, magnesium, and zinc status as predictors of swimming performance. *International Journal of Sports Medicine* **17**, 535–540.

McCarty, M.F. (1995) Anabolic effects of insulin on bone suggest a role for chromium picolinate in preservation of bone density. *Medical Hypotheses* **45**, 241–246.

McCarty, M.F. (1996) Chromium (III) picolinate (Letter). *FASEB Journal* **10**, 365–367.

Malvy, D.J.-M., Arnaud, J., Burtschy, B., Richard, M.-J., Favier, A., Houot, O. & Amédée-Manesme, O. (1993) Reference values for serum zinc and selenium of French healthy children. *European Journal of Epidemiology* **9**, 155–161.

Manore, M.M., Helleksen, J.M., Merkel, J. & Skinner, J.S. (1993) Longitudinal changes in zinc status in untrained men: effect of two different 12 week exercise training programs and zinc supplementation. *Journal of the American Dietetic Association* **93**, 1165–1168.

Marrella, M., Guerrini, F., Tregnaghi, P.L., Nocini, S., Velo, G.P. & Milanino, R. (1990) Effect on exercise on copper, zinc and ceruloplasmin levels in blood of athletes. *Metal Ions in Biology and Medicine: Proceedings of the 1st International Symposium, 16–19 May*, pp. 111–113.

Marrella, M., Guerrini, F., Solero, P.L., Tregnaghi, P.L., Schena, F. & Velo, G.P. (1993) Blood copper and zinc changes in runners after a marathon. *Journal of Trace Elements Electrolytes and Health Disorders* **7**, 248–250.

Meacham, S.L., Taper, L.J. & Volpe, S.L. (1994) Effects of boron supplementation on bone mineral density and dietary, blood, and urinary calcium, phosphorus, magnesium, and boron in female athletes. *Environmental Health Perspectives* **102**, 79–82.

Meacham, S.L., Taper, L.J. & Volpe, S.L. (1995) Effect of boron supplementation on blood and urinary calcium, magnesium, and phosphorus, and urinary boron in athletic and sedentary women. *American Journal of Clinical Nutrition* **61**, 341–345.

Moore, R.J. & Friedl, K.E. (1992) Physiology of nutritional supplements: chromium picolinate and vanadyl sulfate. *National Strength and Conditioning Association Journal* **14**, 47–51.

Newhouse, I.J., Clement, D.B. & Lai, C. (1993) Effects of iron supplementation and discontinuation on serum copper, zinc, calcium, and magnesium levels in women. *Medicine and Science in Sports and Exercise* **25**, 562–571.

Nielsen, F.H. (1996) Other trace elements. In *Present Knowledge in Nutrition*, 7th edn (ed. E.E. Ziegler & L.J. Filer Jr), pp. 353–377. International Life Sciences Institute, Washington, DC.

Nielsen, F.H., Hunt, C.D., Mullen, L.M. & Hunt, J.R. (1987) Effect of dietary boron on mineral, estrogen, and testosterone metabolism in postmenopausal women. *FASEB Journal* **1**, 394–397.

Nieman, D.C., Butler, J.V., Pollett, L.M., Dietrich, S.J. & Lutz, R.D. (1989) Nutrient intake of marathon runners. *Journal of the American Dietetic Association* **89**, 1273–1278.

Nishiyama, S., Inomoto, T., Nakamura, T., Higashi, A. & Matsuda, I. (1996) Zinc status related to hematological deficits in women endurance runners. *American College of Nutrition* **4**, 359–363.

Ohno, H., Yahata, T., Hirata, F. *et al.* (1984) Changes in dopamine-Beta-hydroxylase, and copper, and catecholamine concentrations in human plasma with physical exercise. *Journal of Sports Medicine* **24**, 315–320.

Ohno, H., Yamashita, K., Doi, R., Yamamura, K., Kondo, T. & Taniguchi, N. (1985) Exercise-induced changes in blood zinc and related proteins in humans. *Journal of Applied Physiology* **58**, 1453–1458.

Ohno, H., Sato, Y., Ishikawa, M. *et al.* (1990) Training effects on blood zinc levels in humans. *Journal of Sports Medicine and Physical Fitness* **30**, 247–253.

Ohno, H., Sato, Y., Kizaki, T., Yarnashita, H., Ookawara, T. & Ohira, Y. (1995) Physical exercise and zinc metabolism. In *Sports Nutrition: Minerals and Electrolytes* (ed. C.V. Kies & J.A. Driskell), pp. 129–138. CRC Press, Boca Raton.

Olha, A.E., Klissouras, V., Sullivan, J.D. & Skoryna, S.C. (1982) Effect of exercise on concentration of elements in the serum. *International Journal of Sports Medicine* **22**, 414–425.

Peters, A.J., Dressendorfer, R.H., Rimar, J. & Keen, C.L. (1986) Diet of endurance runners competing in a 20-day road race. *Physician and Sportsmedicine* **14**, 63–70.

Prasad, A.S. (1991) Discovery of human zinc deficiency and studies in an experimental human model. *American Journal of Clinical Nutrition* **53**, 403–412.

Prasad, A.S., Abbasi, A.A., Rabbani, P. & DuMouchelle, E. (1981) Effect of zinc supplementation on serum testosterone level in adult male sickle cell anemia subjects. *American Journal of Hematology* **19**, 119–127.

Reeves, P.G. (1997) Copper. In *Sports Nutrition: Vitamins and Trace Elements* (ed. I. Wolinsky & J.A. Driskell), pp. 175–187. CRC Press, Boca Raton.

Resina, A., Fedi, S., Gatteschi, L. *et al.* (1990) Comparison of some serum copper parameters in trained runners and control subjects. *International Journal of Sports Medicine* **11**, 58–60.

Robertson, J.D., Maughan, R.J., Duthie, G.G. & Morrice, P.C. (1991) Increased blood antioxidant systems of runners in response to training load. *Clinical Science* **80**, 611–618.

Rokitzki, L., Logemann, E., Sagredos, A.N., Murphy, M., Wetzel-Roth, W. & Keul, J. (1994) Lipid peroxidation and antioxidative vitamins under extreme endurance stress. *Acta Physiologica Scandinavica* **151**, 149–158.

Singh, A., Day, B.A., Debolt, J.E., Trostmann, U.H., Bernier, L.L. & Deuster, P.A. (1989) Magnesium, zinc, and copper status of US Navy SEAL trainees. *American Journal of Clinical Nutrition* **49**, 695–700.

Singh, A., Deuster, P.A. & Moser, P.B. (1990) Zinc and copper status in women by physical activity and menstrual status. *Journal of Sports Medicine and Physical Fitness* **30**, 29–36.

Singh, A., Smoak, B.L., Patterson, K.Y., LeMay, L.G., Veillon, C. & Deuster, P.A. (1991) Biochemical indices of selected trace minerals in men: effect of stress. *American Journal of Clinical Nutrition* **53**, 126–131.

Singh, A., Evans, P., Gallagher, K.L. & Deuster, P.A. (1993) Dietary intakes and biochemical profiles of nutritional status of ultramarathoners. *Medicine and Science in Sports and Exercise* **25**, 328–334.

Singh, A., Failla, M.I. & Deuster, P.A. (1994) Exercise-induced changes in immune function: effects of zinc supplementation. *Journal of Applied Physiology* **76**, 2298–2303.

Snook, J.T., Cummin, D., Good, P.R. & Grayzar, J. (1995) Mineral and energy status of groups of male and female athletes participating in events believed to result in adverse nutritional status. In *Sports Nutrition: Minerals and Electrolytes* (ed. C.V. Kies & J.A. Driskell), pp. 293–304. CRC Press, Boca Raton.

Stearns, D.M., Belbruno, J.J. & Wetterhahn, K.E. (1995a) A prediction of chromium (III) accumulation in humans from chromium dietary supplements. *FASEB Journal* **9**, 1650–1657.

Stearns, D.M., Wise, J.P. Sr, Patierno, S.R. & Wetterhahn, K.E. (1995b) Chromium (III) picolinate produces chromosome damage in Chinese hamster ovary cells. *FASEB Journal* **9**, 1643–1649.

Steen, S.N. & McKinney, S. (1986) Nutritional assessment of college wrestlers. *Physician and Sportsmedicine* **14**, 101–116.

Steen, S.N., Mayer, K., Brownell, K.D. & Wadden, T.A. (1995) Dietary intake of female collegiate heavyweight rowers. *International Journal of Sport Nutrition* **5**, 225–231.

Stoecker, B.J. (1996) Chromium. In *Present Knowledge in Nutrition*, 7th edn (ed. E.E. Ziegler & L.J. Filer Jr), pp. 344–353. International Life Sciences Institute, Washington, DC.

Tessier, F., Hida, H., Favier, A. & Marconnet, P. (1995a) Muscle GSH-Px activity after prolonged exercise training and selenium supplementation. *Biological Trace Element Research* **47**, 279–285.

Tessier, F., Margaritis, I., Richard, M., Moynot, C. & Marconnet, P. (1995b) Selenium and training effects of the glutathione system and aerobic performance. *Medicine and Science in Sports and Exercise* **27**, 390–396.

Toskulkao, C. & Glinsukon, T. (1996) Endurance exercise and muscle damage: relationship to lipid peroxidation and scavenging enzymes in short and long distance runners. *Japanese Journal of Physical Fitness and Sports Medicine* **45**, 63–70.

Trent, L.K. & Thieding-Cancel, D. (1995) Effects of chromium picolinate on body composition. *Journal of Sports Medicine and Physical Fitness* **35**, 273–280.

Tuya, I.R., Gil, E.P., Marino, M.M., Carra, R.M.G. & Misiego, A.S. (1996) Evaluation of the influence of physical activity on the plasma concentrations of several trace metals. *European Journal of Applied Physiology* **73**, 299–303.

Van Rij, A.M., Hall, M.T., Dohm, G.L., Bray, J. & Pories, W.J. (1986) Changes in zinc metabolism following exercise in human subjects. *Biological Trace Element Research* **10**, 99–106.

Volpe, S.L., Taper, L.J. & Meacham, S. (1993a) The relationship between boron and magnesium status and bone mineral density in the human: a review. *Magnesium Research* **6**, 291–296.

Volpe, S.L., Taper, L.J. & Meacham, S. (1993b) The effect of boron supplementation on bone mineral density and hormonal status in college female athletes. *Medicine, Exercise, Nutrition, and Health* **2**, 323–330.

Wang, W., Heinonen, O., Mäkelä, A., Mäkelä, P. & Näntö, V. (1995) Serum selenium, zinc and copper in Swedish and Finnish orienteers: a comparative study. *Analyst* **120**, 837–840.

Weight, L.M., Noakes, T.D., Labadarios, D., Graves, J., Jacobs, P. & Berman, P.A. (1988) Vitamin and mineral status of trained athletes including the effects of supplementation. *American Journal of Clinical Nutrition* **47**, 186–191.

Worme, J.D., Doubt, T.J., Singh, A., Ryan, C.J., Moses, F.M. & Deuster, P.A. (1990) Dietary patterns, gastrointestinal complaints, and nutrition knowledge of recreational triathletes. *American Journal of Clinical Nutrition* **51**, 690–697.

# Chapter 26

# Nutritional Ergogenic Aids*

MELVIN H. WILLIAMS AND BRIAN C. LEUTHOLTZ

## Introduction

The optimal production, control and efficiency of human energy is the key composite determinant of all muscular power for movement in sport. In general, as noted in previous chapters, sport scientists recognize three major human muscle energy systems important for the generation of adenosine triphosphate (ATP) for muscle contraction and subsequent power production. The ATP–phosphocreatine (ATP–PCr) energy system, which uses adenosine triphosphate and creatine phosphate as its fuel sources, generates maximal anaerobic power for very short periods of time, such as 10 s for a 100-m dash. The lactic acid energy system, which utilizes carbohydrate via anaerobic glycolysis, is capable of sustaining high anaerobic power production, such as 45 s for a 400-m run. The oxidative energy system, which uses carbohydrates via aerobic glycolysis and fats via β-oxidation, can sustain aerobic power for prolonged endurance events, such as 130 min for a 42.2-km marathon.

The three human muscle energy systems depend on various dietary nutrients for optimal functioning. Dietary carbohydrates and fats, two of the macronutrients, provide the main sources of energy. Protein, another macronutrient, may also serve as an energy source, but as the amino

acids released by protein degradation are either reutilized or oxidized, the amount of protein oxidized per day must be replenished by dietary intake. Protein is utilized primarily to synthesize muscle tissue that serves as the structural basis for energy production, and to synthesize enzymes, hormones, and other physiological substances that, along with vitamins and minerals (micronutrients), help regulate the myriad of neural, hormonal and metabolic processes involved in the release of energy from carbohydrates and fats for use during sport-related exercise tasks.

Most sport nutritionists recommend that athletes consume a balanced diet of macronutrients and micronutrients to provide adequate energy, regulate metabolic processes properly, and maintain an optimal body mass specific to their sport. In general, dietary guidelines for healthy eating developed for the average population are also applicable to athletes. However, considerable research effort has been expended to determine whether or not dietary manipulation may be able to enhance sport performance, and much of this research has focused on the identification and development of specific nutritional ergogenic aids.

Nutritional ergogenic aids are purported to enhance sport performance beyond that associated with the typical balanced diet. The major categories targeted to physically active individuals include: megadoses of essential nutrients, such as 1000 mg of vitamin C; engineered metabolic byproducts of essential nutrients, such as β-

---

*Small segments of this chapter have been extracted from Melvin H. Williams, *The Ergogenics Edge: Pushing the Limits of Sports Performance*, Human Kinetics Publishers, Champaign, IL, 1998.

hydroxy-β-methylbutyrate (HMB) from leucine; nutraceuticals or phytochemicals, non-drug substances found in plants that are purported to affect metabolism, such as ginseng; non-essential nutrients, such as creatine; and drug nutrients, legal drugs found naturally in foods or beverages consumed by humans, such as alcohol and caffeine. Examples of these nutritional ergogenic aids can be categorized as follows.

1 Megadoses of essential nutrients:
   (a) amino acids: arginine, ornithine, lysine and tryptophan;
   (b) vitamins: vitamin $B_{12}$, vitamin C and vitamin E;
   (c) minerals: boron, chromium and phosphates.
2 Engineered metabolic by-products of essential nutrients:
   (a) HMB (β-hydroxy-β-methylbutyrate);
   (b) DHAP (dihydroxyacetone plus pyruvate);
   (c) FDP (fructose diphosphate).
3 Non-essential nutrients:
   (a) carnitine;
   (b) choline;
   (c) glycerol;
   (d) inosine.
4 Plant extracts (phytochemicals):
   (a) gamma oryzanol;
   (b) ginseng;
   (c) wheat germ oil;
   (d) yohimbine.
5 Drug nutrients:
   (a) alcohol;
   (b) caffeine.

Nutritional ergogenic aids may be used in attempts to increase sport performance in various ways, such as: increased energy supply in the muscle (e.g. creatine supplements); increased energy-releasing metabolic processes in the muscle (e.g. L-carnitine supplements); enhanced oxygen delivery to the muscle (e.g. iron supplements); increased oxygen utilization in the muscle (e.g. coenzyme $Q_{10}$ supplements); decreased production or accumulation of fatigue-causing metabolites in the muscle (e.g. sodium bicarbonate supplements); and improved neural control of muscle contraction

(e.g. choline supplements). Because all nutrients may be involved in energy production or control in one way or another, every nutrient may be potentially ergogenic for specific sport tasks. The potential capacity of many specific essential and non-essential nutrients to enhance the three human energy systems is detailed in other chapters of this volume, including the role of creatine supplementation to enhance the ATP–PCr energy system, the ingestion of sodium bicarbonate to improve performance in sport events associated with the lactic acid energy system, and dietary carbohydrate regimens to increase aerobic endurance capacity associated with the oxygen energy system.

This brief review will focus on several nutritional ergogenics commonly marketed to athletes as dietary supplements with alleged ergogenic properties to improve performance in (i) strength/power sport tasks, and (ii) aerobic endurance sport tasks.

## Strength/power sport tasks

### Arginine, ornithine and lysine

THEORY

Human growth hormone (hGH), a polypeptide, is released from the pituitary gland into the bloodstream and affects all body tissues. Supplementation with various amino acids, particularly arginine, ornithine and lysine, has been used in attempts to stimulate the release of hGH. Increased serum levels of hGH in turn may stimulate production and release of insulin-like growth factor-1 that may lead to increases in muscle mass and strength. Additionally, amino acid supplementation is theorized to stimulate the release of insulin, another anabolic hormone.

EFFICACY

In early research, Elam (1989) reported that in conjunction with a weight-training programme, supplementation with arginine ($1\,g \cdot day^{-1}$) and ornithine ($1\,g \cdot day^{-1}$) reduced body fat, increased

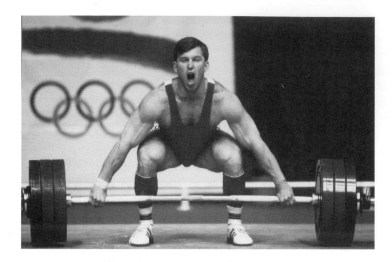

**Fig. 26.1** Some athletes consume nutritional ergogenic aids in attempts to increase serum levels of anabolic hormones, with resultant expected benefits of increased muscle mass, strength and power. Photo © Allsport / Botterill.

lean body mass, and increased strength over a 5-week period. However, this study has been criticized on the grounds of poor experimental design and statistical analysis. More recent well-controlled studies (Fogelholm *et al.* 1993; Lambert *et al.* 1993; Mitchell *et al.* 1993) with experienced weightlifters or bodybuilders do not support any ergogenic effect of various combinations of arginine, ornithine and lysine on hGH secretion, increased muscle mass, strength or power.

Moreover, two well-controlled studies revealed that hGH supplementation itself did not increase muscle protein synthesis, muscle size or strength in untrained males undergoing a 12-week resistance-training programme (Yarasheski *et al.* 1992) or muscle protein synthesis or whole body protein breakdown in trained weightlifters over a 2-week period (Yarasheski *et al.* 1993).

Although moderate doses of amino acid supplements may be safe, larger doses, e.g. 170mg ornithine·kg$^{-1}$ body weight, may lead to gastrointestinal distress (osmotic diarrhoea). Moreover, the potential adverse health effects of hGH administration are substantial, and most researchers caution that the long-term health risks of hGH administration, either genetically

engineered or produced by amino acid supplementation, are unknown (Bucci 1993).

## β-Hydroxy-β-methylbutyrate

### THEORY

β-Hydroxy-β-methylbutyrate is a metabolite of the essential amino acid leucine, and is currently being marketed as a dietary supplement, calcium-HMB-monohydrate. Although its metabolic role in humans is uncertain, HMB supplementation is proposed to help exercisers maximize muscle gains during resistance training by counteracting the catabolic effects of exercise-induced stress on protein metabolism. Investigators hypothesize that HMB may be an essential component of the cell membrane that is jeopardized during exercise stress or that it may regulate enzymes important to muscle growth.

### EFFICACY

Animal studies involving poultry, cattle and pigs have indicated that HMB supplementation may increase lean muscle mass and decrease body fat. (Nissen *et al.* 1994; Van Koevering *et al.* 1994).

However, HMB research with humans is very limited and has emanated from a single laboratory. Collectively, three studies provide some evidence supportive of an anabolic, or an anticatabolic, effect of HMB supplementation. In one study, HMB supplementation (1.5 or 3.0 g·day$^{-1}$), in a dose–response manner, induced significant improvements in lean body mass and muscle strength in untrained men over a 3-week period (Nissen *et al.* 1996b). In two other studies, HMB supplementation (3 g·day$^{-1}$) increased strength in physically active males in the 1-repetition maximal bench press (Nissen *et al.* 1996b) and decreased body fat and increased lean body mass and bench press strength in both trained and untrained subjects over a 4-week period of resistance training (Nissen *et al.* 1996a).

Although these preliminary findings are impressive, replication from other laboratories is needed. Additionally, each study included several threats to internal validity, including the use of unorthodox measures of muscle strength or absence of a true placebo, and in tests of multiple dependent variables, such as multiple measures of strength, HMB benefited performance in some tests, but not all.

### SAFETY

Studies in humans at doses of 1.5–3.0 g·day$^{-1}$ for several weeks have reported no acute adverse effects. Chronic supplementation has not evidenced adverse effects in animals, but no data appear to be available for humans.

## Herbal products

### THEORY

Numerous herbal products have been marketed as potential ergogenics for physically active individuals. Three such products have been marketed as bodybuilding supplements as a means to enhance muscle size and strength: γ-oryzanol, a ferulic acid ester derived from rice bran oil; yohimbine (yohimbe), a nitrogen-containing alkaloid from the bark of the yohimbe tree; and smilax, an extract of phytosterols from the dried roots of *Smilax officinalis* or various forms of sarsaparilla. Advertisers theorize that these herbal products contain the male hormone testosterone

or stimulate its endogenous production, thus inducing increases in muscle size and strength.

### EFFICACY

A scientific literature review revealed no research to validate the claims made by the manufacturers that γ-oryzanol, smilax or yohimbine either raise serum testosterone levels or induce gains in muscle size or strength, confirming the findings of previous scientific reviews (Wheeler & Garleb 1991; Grunewald & Bailey 1993). Wheeler and Garleb (1991) speculated that γ-oryzanol might actually decrease serum testosterone. Well-controlled research with these herbal products, and other plant-derived purported ergogenics such as dehydroepiandrosterone (DHEA), is limited, but that which is available does not substantiate advertising claims. For example, Fry and others (1997) recently reported that γ-oryzanol supplementation (500 mg·day$^{-1}$ for 9 weeks), in comparison to a placebo condition, did not increase circulating concentrations of testosterone or improve 1-repetition maximum muscular strength in the bench press or squat exercise.

### SAFETY

Although herbal dietary supplements may be safe, most lack appropriate safety data. Some preparations have been reported to cause various health problems, including anaphylactic reactions.

## Aerobic endurance sport tasks

### Phosphorus (phosphates)

### THEORY

Dietary phosphates, the source of the essential nutrient phosphorus, are incorporated into many compounds in the body that are involved in energy metabolism, such as ATP as an energy substrate, thiamin pyrophosphate as a vitamin cofactor, sodium phosphate as a buffer, and 2,3-diphosphoglycerate (2,3-DPG) for red blood cell function. All of these roles could provide ergogenic potential, but the most researched theory involves the effect of phosphate salt supplementation on 2,3-DPG levels. Increased levels of 2,3-DPG could facilitate release of oxygen from haemoglobin in the red blood cell and possibly enhance aerobic endurance exercise performance.

### EFFICACY

Current research is equivocal as to whether or not phosphate loading may improve physiological functions important to endurance performance. About a dozen studies have been conducted. No study has reported decreases in performance, and four well-controlled studies (Cade *et al.* 1984; Kreider *et al.* 1990, 1992; Stewart *et al.* 1990) have reported that phosphate supplementation may enhance exercise performance. However, the underlying mechanism has not been clarified. For example, 2,3-DPG did not increase in all studies. Increased maximal oxygen uptake and improved performance on cycle ergometer exercise tests are the most consistent findings. Although these results are impressive, a number of confounding variables in previous research have been identified and more controlled research has been recommended (Tremblay *et al.* 1994).

### SAFETY

Phosphate supplements may cause gastrointestinal distress unless consumed with ample fluids or food. Chronic consumption, particularly with limited calcium intake, can lead to a decreased calcium to phosphate ratio, which may increase parathyroid hormone secretion and impair calcium balance.

## L-Carnitine

### THEORY

Carnitine, a non-essential short-chain carboxylic acid, is a vitamin-like compound found naturally in animal foods but may also be synthesized in the liver and kidney. L-Carnitine is the physiologically active form in the body and has been the form most commonly used as a dietary supplement.

L-Carnitine may affect various physiological functions important to exercise; most of the effects are ergogenic in nature but some may possibly impair performance, i.e. be ergolytic (Wagenmakers 1991; Williams 1995). A primary function of L-carnitine is to facilitate transfer of free fatty acids (FFA) into the mitochondria to help promote oxidation of the FFA for energy. Theoretically, L-carnitine supplementation could enhance FFA oxidation and help to spare the use of muscle glycogen, which might be theorized to

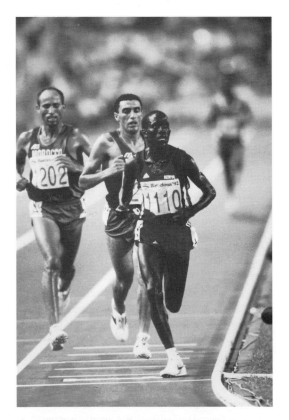

**Fig. 26.2** Theoretically, nutritional ergogenic aids may enhance physiological or metabolic processes deemed important for aerobic energy production. Photo © Allsport / Martin.

improve prolonged aerobic endurance capacity. Additionally, by decreasing the ratio of acetyl-coenzyme A (CoA) to CoA and hence stimulating the activity of pyruvate dehydrogenase, L-carnitine supplementation may be theorized to facilitate the oxidation of pyruvate. Such an effect could reduce lactic acid accumulation and improve anaerobic endurance exercise performance (Wagenmakers 1991). On the other hand, the increased oxidation of glucose could lead to an earlier depletion of muscle glycogen and impair performance, an ergolytic effect (Wagenmakers 1991).

### EFFICACY

Although L-carnitine supplementation will increase plasma levels of carnitine, it has not been shown to consistently increase muscle carnitine levels, the site of its action relative to the use of FFA for energy production during exercise (Wagenmakers 1991; Williams 1995). The data are equivocal relative to the effects of L-carnitine supplementation on the use of FFA during exercise and $\dot{V}o_{2max}$, with some studies providing evidence of enhanced FFA utilization and increased $\dot{V}o_{2max}$ and other studies showing no effect on energy metabolism (Kanter & Williams 1995; Williams 1995; Heinonen 1996). On the other hand, research data clearly indicate that L-carnitine supplementation does not affect lactic acid accumulation in a fashion that may be considered to be ergogenic (Kanter & Williams 1995; Williams 1995). Also, in general, in those studies that included physical performance measures, L-carnitine supplementation has not been shown to enhance either aerobic or anaerobic exercise performance (Kanter & Williams 1995; Williams 1995). However, research is needed to investigate the potential ergogenic effects of chronic L-carnitine supplementation on prolonged aerobic endurance exercise tasks, such as marathon running, to test the possibility of muscle glycogen sparing and subsequent improved performance. Colambani and others (1996) found that acute supplementation of L-carnitine ($2g \cdot 2h^{-1}$ before the events) had no significant effect on performance in either a marathon or a 20-km run, but this dose may have been insufficient compared to chronic supplementation protocols.

### SAFETY

L-Carnitine appears to be safe in dosages utilized in these studies, although large doses may cause diarrhoea. Individuals should not use supplements containing D-carnitine. The D-carnitine isomer may impair the synthesis of L-carnitine in the body leading to symptoms of L-carnitine deficiency, including myopathy and muscular weakness.

## Coenzyme Q$_{10}$

### THEORY

Coenzyme Q$_{10}$ (CoQ$_{10}$), a non-essential nutrient, is a lipid with characteristics common to vitamins. It is located primarily in the mitochondria of the cells, such as heart and muscle cells, and is involved in the processing of oxygen for the production of cellular energy. Increased processing of oxygen could increase sport performance in aerobic endurance events. CoQ$_{10}$ is also an antioxidant. CoQ$_{10}$ is also referred to as ubiquinone, or ubiquinone-10.

### EFFICACY

Bucci (1993) cites six studies showing beneficial effects of CoQ$_{10}$ supplementation to various subject populations, but these studies appeared in the proceedings of a conference and do not appear to have been published in peer-reviewed journals. Moreover, each study suffered one or more experimental design flaws, e.g. no control group (Williams 1999).

A recent review of six well-controlled scientific studies involving CoQ$_{10}$ supplementation ($\approx$ 70–150 mg $\cdot$ day$^{-1}$ for 4–8 weeks) either administered separately or in combination with other putative ergogenic nutrients, indicated that although blood levels of CoQ$_{10}$ may be increased, there was no effect on lipid peroxidation, substrate utilization, serum lactate levels, oxygen uptake, cardiac function or anaerobic threshold during submaximal exercise or serum lactate levels and oxygen uptake during maximal exercise. Additionally, there was no effect on time to exhaustion on a cycle ergometer in two studies (Williams 1999).

## SAFETY

Bucci (1993) indicates that the long-term safety of $CoQ_{10}$ has been thoroughly documented, although others indicate that it may actually serve as a pro-oxidant and generate free radicals (Demopoulous *et al.* 1986). In a recent study, Malm and others (1996) reported evidence of muscle tissue damage in exercising subjects who were supplemented with 120 mg $CoQ_{10} \cdot day^{-1}$ for 20 days.

## Choline

### THEORY

Choline, a non-essential nutrient, is an amine widely distributed in foods and may also be synthesized in the body. Its primary metabolic role in humans is to serve as a precursor for the formation of phosphatidylcholine (lecithin) and other essential components of cell membranes and for the formation of acetylcholine, the neurotransmitter at the myoneural junction that initiates electrical events in muscle contraction. Conlay *et al.* (1992) reported significantly lower plasma choline levels following a 42.2-km marathon, suggestive as an aetiologic factor in the development of fatigue because of the possibility of decreased acetylcholine production and resultant impaired muscular contractility. Theoretically, choline supplementation will enhance acetylcholine synthesis and prevent acetylcholine depletion and subsequent fatigue in endurance events.

### EFFICACY

Von Allwörden *et al.* (1993) noted that lecithin supplementation helped prevent a decrease in serum choline in triathletes and adolescent runners following long-term hard physical stress, but they did not evaluate the effects on performance. No studies of choline supplementation and physical performance were presented in a recent review (Kanter & Williams 1995). Subsequent to this review, a double-blind, placebo-controlled, crossover study with trained male cyclists, using a single dosage of 2.43 g choline bitartrate, reported that although there was a significant increase in serum choline, compared with the placebo there were no significant effects on time to exhaustion in either a high intensity (150% $\dot{V}o_{2max.}$) or a prolonged (70% $\dot{V}o_{2max.}$) cycle exercise test (Spector *et al.* 1995). At the present time, there are no data to support choline supplementation as an effective ergogenic, but confirming research is desirable.

## SAFETY

Choline is a natural dietary component and small supplemental doses are not considered unsafe.

## Inosine

### THEORY

Inosine, a non-essential nutrient, is a nucleoside. Some *in vitro* research has led to the theory that inosine supplementation increases the amount of 2,3-DPG in the red blood cell. Theoretically, increased levels of 2,3-DPG may facilitate the release of oxygen from the red blood cells to the muscle and enhance aerobic endurance exercise.

### EFFICACY

Only two well-controlled studies have evaluated the purported ergogenic effect of inosine supplementation. Two days of inosine supplementation (6000 mg $\cdot$ day$^{-1}$) exerted no significant effect on heart rate, ventilation, oxygen consumption, or lactic acid production in highly trained runners during both submaximal and maximal exercise, nor was there any effect on performance in a 4.8-km treadmill run for time (Williams *et al.* 1990). Five days of inosine supplementation (5000 mg·day⁻¹) did not influence peak power, end power, a fatigue index, total work, or post-test lactate in competitive male cyclists undertaking several cycle ergometer exercise tasks (Starling *et al.* 1996). In both studies, inosine supplementation actually impaired performance in some of the tests, including run time to exhaustion in a peak oxygen uptake test (Williams *et al.* 1990) and time to fatigue in a supramaximal cycling sprint (Starling *et al.* 1996).

### SAFETY

Inosine supplementation appears to be relatively safe, but may increase production of uric acid which could lead to complications in those afflicted with gout.

## Glycerol

### THEORY

Glycerol is an alcohol derived from triglycerides. Investigators theorize that a combination of glycerol-water supplementation may be a more effective hyperhydration technique than water hyperhydration alone. Increasing body water stores may be theorized to enhance aerobic endurance performance, either by increasing blood volume or by increasing resistance to dehydration while exercising under heat-stress environmental conditions.

### EFFICACY

Glycerol-induced hyperhydration (≈1 g glycerol·kg⁻¹ body weight with 20–25 ml water·g⁻¹ glycerol), when compared with water hyperhydration alone, has been shown to increase total body water, including blood volume, to a greater extent (DeLuca *et al.* 1993; Freund *et al.* 1993; Sawka *et al.* 1993). Several studies have shown that glycerol-induced hyperhydration improves cardiovascular responses, temperature regula-tion, and cycling exercise performance under warm/hot environmental conditions (Lyons *et al.* 1990; Montner *et al.* 1992). However, Lamb and others (1997) reported that glycerol-induced hyperhydration exerted no significant effect on temperature regulation, physiological or meta-bolic responses to exercise, or prolonged cycling performance. Additional research is needed to help resolve these contradictory findings, particularly so in sports in which the extra body mass needs to be moved, such as distance running.

### SAFETY

Although the dosages used in these studies appear to be safe, larger doses may lead to abnor-mal pressures in tissue spaces.

## Ginseng

### THEORY

Ginseng, a plant extract, is a generic term encom-passing a wide variety of compounds derived from the family Araliaceae. The ergogenic effect of ginseng is attributed to specific glycosides, also referred to as ginseng saponins or gin-senosides. The specific physiological effects of ginseng extracts depend on the plant species, the various forms including Chinese or Korean ginseng (*Panax ginseng*), American ginseng (*P. quinquefolium*), Japanese ginseng (*P. japonicum*) and Russian/Siberian ginseng (*Eleutherococcus senticosus*). Although the mechanism underlying the alleged ergogenicity of ginseng on physical performance has not been defined, theories include stimulation of the hypothalamic–pituitary-adrenal cortex axis and increased resistance to the stress of exercise, enhanced myocardial metabolism, increased haemoglobin levels, vasodilation, increased oxygen extraction by muscles, and improved mitochondrial metab-olism in the muscle, all of which theoretically could enhance aerobic exercise performance (Dowling *et al.* 1996).

EFFICACY

There are very few well-controlled studies supporting an ergogenic effect of ginseng supplementation. In their major recent review of the ergogenic properties of ginseng, Bahrke and Morgan (1994) indicated that because of methodological and statistical shortcomings, there is no compelling evidence to indicate ginseng supplementation consistently enhances human physical performance and there remains a need for well-designed research to address this issue. One recent well-designed study (Pieralisi *et al.* 1991) did find an ergogenic effect of Geriatric Pharmaton (a preparation including ginseng G115 and other elements, including dimethylaminoethanol) on various physiologic variables, including $\dot{V}o_{2max}$, and performance during the Bruce treadmill protocol. However, the investigators noted that the ergogenic effect is attributed to the total preparation used, i.e. Geriatric Pharmaton, and not to the standardized ginseng G115, because some research has supported a beneficial effect of dimethylaminoethanol bitartrate, possibly by affecting favourably the choline–acetylcholine complex. However, several recent studies with appropriate designs have not reported any benefits to endurance performance. For example, no significant ergogenic effects were associated with 6 weeks of *Eleutherococcus senticosus* Maxim L (ESML) supplementation in highly trained runners on any metabolic, psychological or performance parameters measured in both a submaximal and maximal aerobic exercise task, including heart rate, $\dot{V}o_2$, $\dot{V}_E$, $\dot{V}_E/\dot{V}o_2$, and respiratory exchange ratio during both exercise and recovery, ratings of perceived exertion during exercise, serum (lactate) following exercise, and run time to exhaustion in a maximal test (Dowling *et al.* 1996). Additionally, Morris and others (1996), in a double-blind, placebo-controlled study, reported no effect of a standardized ginseng extract (8 or 16 mg·kg$^{-1}$ body mass for 7 days) on ratings of perceived exertion or time to exhaustion on a cycle ergometer test.

Nevertheless, quality research evidence

regarding the effect of ginseng supplementation on exercise performance is limited and more controlled research is needed with varying types, dosages, and physical performance parameters.

SAFETY

Animal studies indicate that extracts of ginseng have a low acute or chronic toxicity and the doses normally used with humans are regarded as safe. However, Beltz and Doring (1993) noted a ginseng-abuse syndrome has been reported, with such symptoms as hypertension, nervousness, sleeplessness and oedema.

## Conclusion

Nutritional ergogenics have been used since time immemorial, and will continue to be used as long as athletes believe they may gain a competitive advantage. However, before using such supplements for their purported ergogenic effects, one should address the following questions.

Is it effective? If the supplement has not been shown to be effective, either by appropriately designed research or repeated personal experiences, there is no reason to buy it.

Is it safe? Most nutrient and dietary supplements are presumed to be safe if consumed in recommended dosages. However, athletes often believe that if one is good, 10 is better, and may take amounts in excess of normal needs (Burke & Read 1993). Excess amounts of various nutrients and dietary supplements may pose health risks to some individuals.

Is it legal? Most nutritional ergogenics are considered legal because they are regulated as food or dietary supplements, not drugs. However, the same dietary supplements may contain drugs, such as caffeine and ephedrine, which may lead to a positive doping test.

Athletes should be allowed to utilize any effective, safe and legal nutritional supplement in attempts to enhance sport performance, just as they should be able to use the most effective and legal equipment specific to their sport which may provide a mechanical edge.

# References

Bahrke, M. & Morgan, W. (1994) Evaluation of the ergogenic properties of ginseng. *Sports Medicine* **18**, 229–248.

Beltz, S. & Doering, P. (1993) Efficacy of nutritional supplements used by athletes. *Clinical Pharmacy* **12**, 900–908.

Bucci, L. (1993) *Nutrients as Ergogenic Aids for Sports and Exercise*. CRC Press, Boca Raton, FL.

Burke, L. & Read, R. (1993) Dietary supplements in sport. *Sports Medicine* **15**, 43–65.

Cade, R., Conte, M., Zauner, C. *et al.* (1984) Effects of phosphate loading on 2,3-diphosphoglycerate and maximal oxygen uptake. *Medicine and Science in Sports and Exercise* **16**, 263–68.

Colombani, P., Wenk, C., Kunz, I. *et al.* (1996) Effects of L-carnitine supplementation on physical performance and energy metabolism of endurance-trained athletes: a double-blind crossover field study. *European Journal of Applied Physiology* **73**, 434–439.

Conlay, L., Sabounjian, L. & Wurtman, R. (1992) Exercise and neuromodulators: choline and acetylcholine in marathon runners. *International Journal of Sports Medicine* **13**, S141–42.

DeLuca, J., Freund, B., Montain, S., Latzka, W. & Sawka, M. (1993) Hormonal responses to hyperhydration with glycerol vs. water alone (Abstract). *Medicine and Science in Sports and Exercise* **25**, S36.

Demopoulous, H., Santomier, J., Seligman, M., Hogan, P. & Pietronigro, D. (1986) Free radical pathology: rationale and toxicology of antioxidants and other supplements in sports medicine and exercise science. In *Sport, Health and Nutrition* (ed. F. Katch), pp. 139–189. Human Kinetics, Champaign, IL.

Dowling, E., Redondo, D., Branch, J., Jones, S., McNabb, G. & Williams, M. (1996) Effect of *Eleutherococcus senticosus* on submaximal and maximal exercise performance. *Medicine and Science in Sports and Exercise* **28**, 482–489.

Elam, R. (1989) Effects of arginine and ornithine on strength, lean body mass and urinary hydroxyproline in adult males. *Journal of Sports Medicine and Physical Fitness* **29**, 52–56.

Fogelholm, M., Nagueri, H., Kiilavuori, K. & Haarkaonen, M. (1993) No effects on serum human growth hormone and insulin in male weightlifters. *International Journal of Sport Nutrition* **3**, 290–297.

Freund, B., Montain, S., McKay, J., Laird, J., Young, A. & Sawka, M. (1993) Renal responses to hyperhydration using aqueous glycerol vs. water alone provide insight to the mechanism for glycerol's effectiveness (Abstract). *Medicine and Science in Sports and Exercise* **25**, S35.

Fry, A., Bonner, E., Lewis, D., Johnson, R., Stone, M. &

Kraemer, W. (1997) The effects of gamma-oryzanol supplementation during resistance exercise training. *International Journal of Sport Nutrition* **7**, 318–329.

Grunewald, K. & Bailey, R. (1993) Commercially marketed supplements for bodybuilding athletes. *Sports Medicine* **15**, 90–103.

Heinonen, O. (1996) Carnitine and physical exercise. *Sports Medicine* **22**, 109–132.

Kanter, M. & Williams, M. (1995) Antioxidants, carnitine and choline as putative ergogenic aids. *International Journal of Sport Nutrition* **5**, S120–131.

Kreider, R., Miller, G., Williams, M., Somma, C. & Nassar, T. (1990) Effects of phosphate loading on oxygen uptake, ventilatory anaerobic threshold, and run performance. *Medicine and Science in Sports and Exercise* **22**, 250–56.

Kreider, R., Miller, G., Schenck, D. *et al.* (1992) Effects of phosphate loading on metabolic and myocardial responses to maximal and endurance exercise. *International Journal of Sport Nutrition* **2**, 20–47.

Lamb, D., Lightfoot, W. & Myhal, M. (1997) Prehydration with glycerol does not improve cycling performance vs. 6% CHO-electrolyte drink (Abstract). *Medicine and Science in Sports and Exercise* **29**, S249.

Lambert, M., Hefer, J., Millar, R. & Macfarlane, P. (1993) Failure of commercial oral amino acid supplements to increase serum growth hormone concentrations in male bodybuilders. *International Journal of Sport Nutrition* **3**, 298–305.

Lyons, T., Riedesel, M., Meuli, L. & Chick, T. (1990) Effects of glycerol-induced hyperhydration prior to exercise in the heat on sweating and core temperature. *Medicine and Science in Sports and Exercise* **22**, 477–483.

Malm, C., Svensson, M., Sjoberg, B., Ekblom, B. & Sjodin, B. (1996) Supplementation with ubiquinone-10 causes cellular damage during intense exercise. *Acta Physiologica Scandinavica* **157**, 511–512.

Mitchell, M., Dimeff, R. & Burns, B. (1993) Effects of supplementation with arginine and lysine on body composition, strength and growth hormone levels in weightlifters (Abstract). *Medicine and Science in Sports and Exercise* **25**, S25.

Montner, P., Chick, T., Riedesel, M., Timms, M., Stark, D. & Murata, G. (1992) Glycerol hyperhydration and endurance exercise (Abstract). *Medicine and Science in Sports and Exercise* **24**, S157.

Morris, A., Jacobs, I., McLellan, T., Klugerman, A., Wang, L. & Zamecnik, J. (1996) No ergogenic effect of ginseng ingestion. *International Journal of Sport Nutrition* **6**, 263–271.

Nissen, S., Faidley, T., Zimmerman, D., Izard, R. & Fisher, C. (1994) Colostral milk fat percentage and pig performance are enhanced by feeding the leucine metabolite β-hydroxy-β-methyl butyrate to sows. *Journal of Animal Science* **72**, 2331–2337.

Nissen, S., Panton, L., Wilhelm, R. & Fuller, J. (1996a) Effect of β-hydroxy-β-methylbutyrate (HMB) supplementation on strength and body composition of trained and untrained males undergoing intense resistance training (Abstract). *FASEB Journal* (Suppl.), A287.

Nissen, S., Sharp, R., Ray, M. *et al.* (1996b) Effect of leucine metabolite β-hydroxy-β-methylbutyrate on muscle metabolism during resistance-exercise training. *Journal of Applied Physiology* **81**, 2095–2104.

Pieralisi, G., Ripari, P. & Vecchiet, L. (1991) Effects of a standardized ginseng extract combined with dimethylaminoethanol bitartrate, vitamins, minerals, and trace elements on physical performance during exercise. *Clinical Therapeutics* **13**, 373–382.

Sawka, M., Freund, B., Roberts, D., O'Brien, C., Dennis, R. & Valen, C. (1993) Total body water (TBW), extracellular fluid (ECF) and plasma responses to hyperhydration with aqueous glycerol (Abstract). *Medicine and Science in Sports and Exercise* **25**, S35.

Spector, S., Jackman, M., Sabounjian, L., Sakkas, C., Landers, D. & Willis, W. (1995) Effect of choline supplementation on fatigue in trained cyclists. *Medicine and Science in Sport and Exercise* **27**, 668–673.

Starling, R., Trappe, T., Short, K. *et al.* (1996) The effect of inosine supplementation on aerobic and anaerobic cycling performance. *Medicine and Science in Sports and Exercise* **28**, 1193–1198.

Stewart, I., McNaughton, L., Davies, P. & Tristram, S. (1990) Phosphate loading and the effects on VO$_{2max}$ in trained cyclists. *Research Quarterly for Exercise and Sport* **61**, 80–84.

Tremblay, M., Galloway, S. & Sexsmith, J. (1994) Ergogenic effects of phosphate loading: physiological fact or methodological fiction? *Canadian Journal of Applied Physiology* **19**, 1–11.

Van Koevering, M., Dolezal, H., Gill, D. *et al.* (1994) Effects of β-hydroxy-β-methyl butyrate on performance and carcass quality of feedlot steers. *Journal of Animal Science* **72**, 1927–1935.

von Allwörden, H., Horn, S., Kahl, J. & Feldheim, W. (1993) The influence of lecithin on plasma choline concentrations in triathletes and adolescent runners during exercise. *European Journal of Applied Physiology* **67**, 87–91.

Wagenmakers, A. (1991) L-carnitine supplementation and performance in man. *Medicine and Sport Science* **32**, 110–127.

Wheeler, K. & Garleb, K. (1991) Gamma oryzanol-plant sterol supplementation: metabolic, endocrine, and physiologic effects. *International Journal of Sport Nutrition* **1**, 170–77.

Williams, M. (1995) Nutritional ergogenics in athletics. *Journal of Sports Sciences* **13**, S63-S74.

Williams, M. (1999) *Nutrition for Health, Fitness and Sport*. WCB/McGraw-Hill, Boston.

Williams, M., Kreider, R., Hunter, D. *et al.* (1990) Effect of inosine supplementation on 3-mile treadmill performance and VO$_{2peak}$. *Medicine and Science in Sports and Exercise* **22**, 517–22.

Yarasheski, K., Campbell, J., Smith, K., Rennie, M., Holloszy, J. & Bier, D. (1992) Effect of growth hormone and resistance exercise on muscle growth in young men. *American Journal of Physiology* **262**, E261–E267.

Yarasheski, K., Zachwieja, J., Angelopoulos, T. & Bier, D. (1993) Short-term growth hormone treatment does not increase muscle protein synthesis in experienced weight lifters. *Journal of Applied Physiology* **74**, 3073–3076.

# Chapter 27

# Creatine

PAUL L. GREENHAFF

## Distribution and biosynthesis

Creatine, or methyl guanidine-acetic acid, is a naturally occurring compound found in abundance in skeletal muscle. It is also found in small quantities in brain, liver, kidney and testes. In a 70-kg man, the total body creatine pool amounts to approximately 120 g, of which 95% is situated in muscle (Myers & Fine 1915; Hunter 1922).

In the early part of this century there was already literature pointing to an important function for creatine in muscle contraction. The knowledge of its fairly specific distribution and its absence from normal urine led to the realization that it is not merely a waste product of metabolism. This realization was confirmed when Chanutin (1926) observed that creatine administration resulted in a major portion of the compound being retained by the body.

Creatine synthesis has been shown to proceed via two successive reactions involving two enzymes (Fig. 27.1). The first reaction is catalysed by glycine transamidinase, and results in an amidine group being reversibly transferred from arginine to glycine, forming guanidino-acetic acid. The second reaction involves irreversible transfer of a methyl group from S-adenosylmethionine catalysed by guanidino-acetate methyltransferase, resulting in the methylation of guanidinoacetate and the formation of creatine (Fitch 1977; Walker 1979). The distribution of the two enzymes differs between tissues across mammalian species. In the case of humans, however, it is generally accepted that

the majority of *de novo* creatine synthesis occurs in the liver. As little creatine is found in the major sites of synthesis, it is logical to assume that transport of creatine from sites of synthesis to storage must occur, thus allowing a separation of biosynthesis from utilization.

Two mechanisms have been proposed to explain the very high creatine concentration within skeletal muscle. The first involves the transport of creatine into muscle by a specific saturable entry process, and the second entails the trapping of creatine within muscle (Fitch & Shields 1966; Fitch *et al.* 1968; Fitch 1977). Early studies demonstrated that creatine entry into muscle occurs actively against a concentration gradient, possibly involving creatine interacting with a specific membrane site which recognizes the amidine group (Fitch & Shields 1966; Fitch *et al.* 1968; Fitch 1977). Recently, a specific sodium-dependent creatine transporter has been identified in skeletal muscle, heart and brain (Schloss *et al.* 1994). It has been suggested that some skeletal muscles do not demonstrate a saturable uptake process, thereby supporting the idea of intracellular entrapment of creatine (Fitch 1977). About 60% of muscle total creatine exists in the form of phosphocreatine, which is therefore unable to pass through membranes because of its polarity, thus trapping creatine. This entrapment will result in the generation of a concentration gradient, but phosphorylation alone cannot be the sole mechanism of cellular retention of creatine. Other mechanisms that have been proposed include binding to intracellular components and

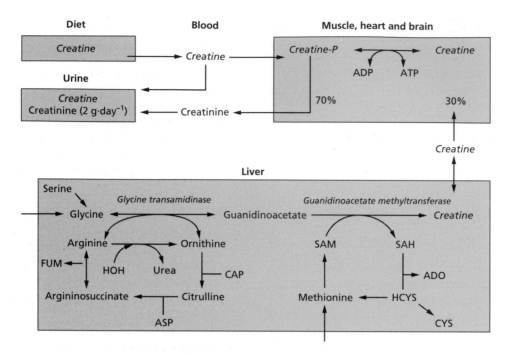

**Fig. 27.1** The biosynthesis of creatine. Italics indicate enzymes. Adapted from Walker (1979).

the existence of restrictive cellular membranes (Fitch 1977).

Creatinine has been established as the sole end-product of creatine degradation being formed non-enzymatically in an irreversible reaction (Fitch & Sinton 1964; Fitch et al. 1968). As skeletal muscle is the major store of the body creatine pool, this is the major site of creatinine production. Daily renal creatinine excretion is relatively constant in an individual, but can vary between individuals (Fitch 1977), being dependent on the total muscle mass in healthy individuals (Heymsfield et al. 1983). Once generated, creatinine enters circulation by simple diffusion and is filtered in a non-energy-dependent process by the glomerulus and excreted in urine.

## Effect of dietary creatine supplementation on muscle creatine concentration

In normal healthy individuals, muscle creatine is replenished at a rate of approximately

$2 \text{g} \cdot \text{day}^{-1}$ by endogenous creatine synthesis and/or dietary creatine intake (Walker 1979). Oral ingestion of creatine has also been demonstrated to suppress biosynthesis, an effect which has been shown to be removed upon cessation of supplementation (Walker 1979). Conversely, the absence of creatine from the diet has been shown to result in low rates of urinary creatine and creatinine appearance (Delanghe et al. 1989). Augmented creatine retention occurs during subsequent dietary creatine supplementation in vegetarians, suggesting that endogenous synthesis may not match creatine requirements in these individuals (Green et al. 1997). In this respect, creatine could be viewed as an essential constituent of a 'normal' diet.

Early studies demonstrated that creatine ingestion resulted in a small increase in urinary creatinine excretion. In general, urinary creatinine excretion rose slowly during prolonged creatine administration and, upon cessation, around 5 weeks elapsed before a significant fall in creatinine excretion was observed (Benedict &

Osterberg 1923; Chanutin 1926). From these early studies, creatine retention in the body pool was thought to be much greater during the initial stages of administration. These early studies also demonstrated that there was no increase in creatinine excretion until a significant amount of the administered creatine had been retained (Benedict & Osterberg 1923; Chanutin 1926).

These early studies invariably involved chronic periods of creatine ingestion. With the application of the muscle biopsy technique, however, it has now become clear that the ingestion of 20g of creatine each day for 5 days by healthy volunteers can lead to, on average, more than a 20% increase in muscle total creatine concentration, of which approximately 20% is in the form of phosphocreatine (PCr) (Fig. 27.2) (Harris *et al.* 1992). It is important to note that most studies to date have involved 5g of creatine being ingested in a warm solution on four equally spaced occasions per day. This procedure was adopted principally because it results in a rapid (within 20min), marked ($\approx 1000\,\mu$mol$\cdot$l$^{-1}$ increase) and sustained ($\approx 3$h) increase in plasma creatine (Harris *et al.* 1992), to a concentration above the $K_m$ reported for creatine transport in isolated rat skeletal muscle (Fitch *et al.* 1968). A warm liquid was used because this has been

shown to facilitate the dissolving of creatine. In agreement with earlier work, it has also been demonstrated that the majority of tissue creatine uptake occurs during the initial days of supplementation, with close to 30% of the administered dose being retained during the initial 2 days of supplementation, compared with 15% from days 2–4 (Harris *et al.* 1992). It was also shown by Harris *et al.* (1992) that the initial presupplementation muscle total creatine concentration is an important determinant of creatine accumulation during supplementation in healthy volunteers (Fig. 27.2). Furthermore, when submaximal exercise was performed by healthy subjects during the period of supplementation, muscle uptake was increased by a further 10% (Harris *et al.* 1992). With the exception of vegetarians and some disease states, it is not yet clear what determines whether a person has a high or low muscle creatine store. Interestingly, normal healthy females, for reasons as yet unknown, appear to have a slightly higher muscle creatine concentration than males (Forsberg *et al.* 1991). This may be a consequence of their muscle mass, and therefore their creatine distribution space, being smaller.

Based on more recently published experimental findings (Hultman *et al.* 1996), it would

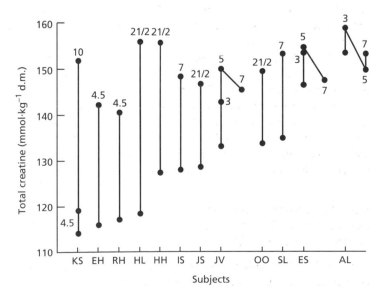

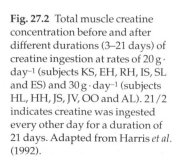

**Fig. 27.2** Total muscle creatine concentration before and after different durations (3–21 days) of creatine ingestion at rates of 20 g · day$^{-1}$ (subjects KS, EH, RH, IS, SL and ES) and 30 g · day$^{-1}$ (subjects HL, HH, JS, JV, OO and AL). 21/2 indicates creatine was ingested every other day for a duration of 21 days. Adapted from Harris *et al.* (1992).

appear that, as might be expected, a 2–3-week period of lower dose creatine supplementation ($3 g \cdot day^{-1}$) increases tissue creatine content at a slower rate than a 6-day regimen of $20 g \cdot day^{-1}$. However, following 4 weeks of supplementation, no difference in muscle creatine stores is evident when comparing the two dosage regimens. The same study clearly demonstrated that muscle creatine stores can be maintained at an elevated concentration when the 6-day supplementation dose of $20 g \cdot day^{-1}$ is immediately followed by a lower dose of $2 g \cdot day^{-1}$ (Fig. 27.3). This lower dose was aimed at sustaining dietary creatine intake at a slightly higher level than degradation of muscle creatine to creatinine. The natural time-course of muscle creatine decline following supplementation was also investigated by Hultman *et al.* (1996), where it was found to take at least 4 weeks for muscle creatine 'wash-out' to occur following 6 days of creatine ingestion at the rate of $20 g \cdot day^{-1}$. This fits with earlier studies which investigated the time-course of creatinine excretion following creatine ingestion (Benedict & Osterberg 1923; Chanutin 1926), and with the suggestion of Fitch (1977) that creatine is 'trapped' within skeletal muscle once taken up. Thus, it would appear that a rapid

way to 'load' and then maintain muscle creatine stores is to ingest $20 g \cdot day^{-1}$ for 5–6 days followed by $2 g \cdot day^{-1}$ thereafter.

It is also clear from the literature that there is considerable variation between subjects in the extent of muscle creatine accumulation during supplementation (Harris *et al.* 1992; Greenhaff *et al.* 1994). A concentration of $160 mmol \cdot kg^{-1}$ dry muscle (d.m.) appears to be the maximal total creatine concentration achievable as a result of creatine supplementation, and occurs in about 20% of subjects. Conversely, about 20–30% of subjects do not respond to creatine ingestion, i.e. they demonstrate less than $10 mmol \cdot kg^{-1}$ d.m. increase in muscle total creatine as a result of supplementation. Of particular importance, recent work has revealed that muscle total creatine accumulation can be increased by a further 60% when creatine is ingested in solution (5 days of creatine at $20 g \cdot day^{-1}$) in combination with simple carbohydrates ($370 g$ carbohydrate $\cdot day^{-1}$; Green *et al.* 1996a, 1996b), elevating muscle creatine concentration in all subjects closer to the upper limit of $160 mmol \cdot kg^{-1}$ d.m. As might be expected, urinary creatine excretion and plasma creatine concentration were reduced in parallel with the increase in muscle total creatine (Green *et al.* 1996a, 1996b).

The mean and individual increases in muscle total creatine concentration from the study of Green *et al.* (1996b) are shown in Fig. 27.4. This figure highlights the major difference between ingesting creatine in combination with carbohydrate compared with ingesting creatine alone. As can be seen, 50% of the subjects who ingested creatine alone ($4 \times 5 g \cdot day^{-1}$ for 5 days) experienced an increase in muscle total creatine concentration of less than $20 mmol \cdot kg^{-1}$ d.m. (Fig. 27.4a). This contrasts with the subjects who ingested creatine in combination with carbohydrate, all of whom experienced an increase of more than $20 mmol \cdot kg^{-1}$ d.m. (Fig. 27.4b). In agreement with the work of Harris *et al.* (1992), there was a significant inverse relationship between the initial muscle total creatine concentration and the magnitude of accumulation seen following creatine supplementation alone ($r = -0.579$, $n = 12$; $P <$

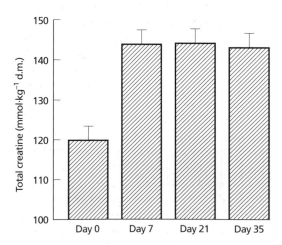

**Fig. 27.3** Total muscle creatine concentration before and after 34 days of creatine ingestion. Creatine was ingested at a rate of $20 g \cdot day^{-1}$ for the initial 6 days and at a rate of $2 g \cdot day^{-1}$ thereafter.

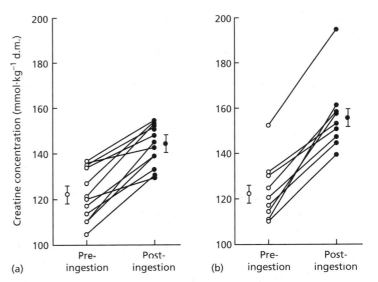

**Fig. 27.4** Mean and individual values for total muscle creatine concentration before (○) and following (●) 5 days of: (a) creatine (20 g · day⁻¹) ingestion, and (b) creatine (20 g · day⁻¹) and carbohydrate (370 g · day⁻¹) ingestion.

0.05). However, this was not the case for those subjects who ingested creatine in combination with carbohydrate ($r=0.058$, $n=9$; $P>0.05$), where the initial muscle creatine concentration was found to have little association with the extent of muscle creatine accumulation when creatine was ingested in combination with carbohydrate. Evidence was also presented in the studies of Green *et al.* (1996a, 1996b) to indicate that the augmentation of muscle creatine accumulation following carbohydrate ingestion occurred as a result of a stimulatory effect of insulin on muscle creatine transport, and that this effect outweighed the positive effect that exercise has on muscle creatine accumulation. The exact mechanisms by which muscle contraction and insulin stimulate muscle creatine transport are currently under investigation. As muscle creatine is elevated to above the $K_m$ concentration reported for muscle creatine transport when creatine alone is ingested, it is possible that insulin operates by increasing the $\dot{V}_{max}$ of creatine transport. This could perhaps be achieved by insulin stimulating sodium–potassium, adenosine triphosphatase (ATP)-dependent, pump activity, and thereby sodium-dependent creatine transport. Interestingly, other hormones have also been shown to stimulate muscle creatine transport (Odoom *et al.* 1996).

## Health risks associated with dietary creatine supplementation

There have been anecdotal reports of creatine supplementation being linked with kidney damage and muscle cramps. At the time of writing this author is unaware of any definitive data to support these conclusions. Creatine supplementation does cause an increase in urinary creatinine excretion, which is often used as an indicator of kidney function, but this increase correlates well with the increase in muscle creatine observed during supplementation and reflects the increased rate of muscle creatine degradation to creatinine rather than any abnormality of renal function (Hultman *et al.* 1996). Furthermore, chronic high-dose creatine supplementation (20 g · day⁻¹ for 5 days followed by 10 g · day⁻¹ for 51 days) has been reported to have no effect on serum markers of hepatorenal function and routine clinical chemistry (Almada *et al.* 1996; Earnest *et al.* 1996). It should be stressed, nevertheless, that the long-term health risks of chronic creatine ingestion are presently unknown. Equally, however, the regimen of ingesting 20 g · day⁻¹ for 5–6 days has been reported to have no known side-effects, providing the creatine is dissolved prior to ingestion (undissolved creatine may cause slight gastrointestinal discomfort). Furthermore, the $2g \cdot day^{-1}$ 'maintenance dose' of creatine ingestion currently advocated to maintain muscle creatine concentration during chronic periods of creatine supplementation (Hultman *et al.* 1996) is only slightly greater than the quantity of creatine found in a meat eater's diet.

## Effect of dietary creatine supplementation on exercise performance

In human skeletal muscle, creatine is present at a concentration of about $125 mmol \cdot kg^{-1}$ d.m., of which approximately 60% is in the form of PCr at rest. A reversible equilibrium exists between creatine and PCr:

$$(PCr + ADP + H^+ \leftrightarrow ATP + creatine)$$

and together they function to maintain intracellular ATP availability, modulate metabolism and buffer hydrogen ion accumulation during contraction. The availability of PCr is generally accepted to be one of the most likely limitations to muscle performance during intense, fatiguing, short-lasting contractions, its depletion resulting in an increase in cellular adenosine diphosphate (ADP) concentration and, thereby, the development of fatigue via an inhibition of muscle cross-bridge formation. This conclusion has been drawn from human studies involving short bouts of maximal electrically evoked contraction (Hultman *et al.* 1991) and voluntary exercise (Katz *et al.* 1986), and from animal studies in which the muscle creatine store has been depleted, prior to maximal electrical stimulation, using the creatine analogue β-guanidinopropionate (Fitch *et al.* 1975; Meyer *et al.* 1986). Recent studies from this laboratory (Casey *et al.* 1996a) and from others (Bogdanis *et al.* 1996) have demonstrated that the extent of PCr resynthesis during recovery following a single bout of maximal exercise is positively correlated with exercise performance during a subsequent bout of exercise. For example, in the study of Casey *et al.* (1996a), eight subjects performed two bouts of maximal exercise, each

lasting 30s, which were separated by 4min of recovery. Rapid PCr resynthesis occurred during this recovery period, but was incomplete, reaching on average 88% of the pre-exercise concentration. However, the extent of PCr resynthesis during recovery was positively correlated with performance during the second bout of exercise ($r=0.80$, $P<0.05$). More detailed analysis also revealed that whilst the magnitude of PCr degradation in the second bout of exercise was less than that in the first, this fall in PCr utilization was restricted solely to the fast twitch muscle fibres (Fig. 27.5), and was probably attributable to incomplete PCr resynthesis in this fibre type during recovery following the initial bout of exercise (Casey *et al.* 1996a). Creatine in its free and phosphorylated forms appears therefore to occupy a pivotal role in the regulation and homeostasis of skeletal muscle energy metabolism and fatigue. This being the case, it is pertinent to suggest that any mechanism capable of increasing muscle creatine availability might be expected to delay PCr depletion and the rate of ADP accumulation during maximal exercise and/or stimulate PCr resynthesis during recovery.

In 1934, Boothby (see Chaikelis 1940) reported that the development of fatigue in humans could be delayed by the addition of large amounts of

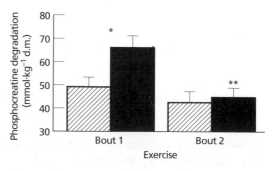

**Fig. 27.5** Changes in phosphocreatine in slow (type I, ▨) and fast (type II, ■) muscle fibres during two bouts of 30 s maximal intensity, isokinetic cycling exercise in humans. Each bout of exercise was performed at 80 pedal rev·min$^{-1}$ and separated by 4 min of passive recovery. *, $P<0.05$ between fibre types; **, $P<0.01$ from exercise bout 1 in type II fibres.

the creatine precursor glycine to the diet, which he attributed to an effect on muscle creatine concentration. Later, Ray and co-workers (Ray *et al.* 1939) concluded that the ingestion of 60 g gelatin·day⁻¹ for several weeks could also postpone the development of fatigue in humans. The authors reasoned that because glycine constitutes 25% of gelatin by weight, the increased ingestion of gelatin would result in an increased muscle creatine concentration and thereby an increase in muscle function. Maison (1940), however, could not reproduce these findings and concluded that gelatin, and therefore glycine, had no effect on work capacity during repeated bouts of fatiguing muscle contractions. Shortly after this, however, Chaikelis (1940) reported that the ingestion of 6 g glycine·day⁻¹ in tablet form for 10 weeks markedly improved performance (≈20%) in a number of different muscle groups and reduced creatinine excretion by 30%. In the discussion of results, the author implicated a change in the muscle creatine pool as being responsible for the observations made.

Other than these initial reports, which do not relate to creatine ingestion *per se*, little has been published concerning creatine ingestion and exercise performance until recently. Sipila *et al.* (1981) reported that in a group of patients receiving 1 g creatine·day⁻¹ as a treatment for gyrate atrophy (a condition in which creatine biosynthesis is impaired), there was a comment from some of a sensation of strength gain following a 1-year period of supplementation. Indeed, creatine ingestion was shown to reverse the type II muscle fibre atrophy associated with this disease and one athlete in the group of patients improved his personal best record for the 100 m by 2 s. Muscle creatine availability has been implicated in the control of muscle protein synthesis (Bessman & Savabi 1990), and the pathology of muscle-wasting diseases (Fitch & Sinton 1964; Fitch 1977) and in-born errors of metabolism (Stockler *et al.* 1994) have been related to abnormalities of creatine metabolism.

Based on published results from placebo-controlled laboratory experiments, it would appear that the ingestion of 4×5 g creatine·day⁻¹

for 5 days can significantly increase the amount of work which can be performed by healthy normal volunteers during repeated bouts of maximal knee-extensor exercise (Greenhaff *et al.* 1993), maximal dynamic exercise (Balsom *et al.* 1993a) and maximal isokinetic cycling exercise (Birch *et al.* 1994). In addition, it has been demonstrated that creatine supplementation can facilitate muscle PCr resynthesis during recovery from maximal intensity exercise in individuals who demonstrate an increase of 20 mmol·kg⁻¹ d.m. or more in muscle creatine as a consequence of supplementation (Greenhaff *et al.* 1994). The author is also aware of published work demonstrating that creatine ingestion has no effect on maximal exercise performance (Cooke *et al.* 1995). Undoubtedly, one reason for the lack of agreement between studies will be the large variation between subjects in the extent of creatine retention during supplementation with creatine, which will be discussed in more detail later. However, the most prevalent finding from published performance studies seems to be that creatine ingestion can significantly increase exercise performance by sustaining force or work output during exercise. For example, in the study of Greenhaff *et al.* (1993), two groups of subjects (*n* = 6) performed five bouts of 30 maximal voluntary unilateral knee extensions at a constant angular velocity of 180°·s⁻¹ before and after placebo or creatine ingestion (4×5 g creatine·day⁻¹ for 5 days). No difference was seen when comparing muscle torque production during exercise before and after placebo ingestion. However, following creatine ingestion, torque production was increased by 5–7% in all subjects during the final 10 contractions of exercise bout 1 and throughout the whole of exercise bouts 2–4. In the study of Birch *et al.* (1994), two groups of seven healthy male subjects performed three bouts of maximal isokinetic cycling exercise at 80 rev·min⁻¹ before and after creatine or placebo ingestion (4×5 g creatine·day⁻¹ for 5 days). Each exercise bout lasted for 30 s and was interspersed by 4 min rest. The total amount of work performed during bouts 1–3 were similar when comparing values obtained before and after placebo ingestion (<2%

change). After creatine ingestion, work output was increased in all seven subjects during exercise bouts 1 ($P<0.05$) and 2 ($P<0.05$), but no difference was observed during exercise bout 3. It should be noted, however, that results also suggest that creatine ingestion has no effect on performance or metabolism during submaximal exercise (Balsom *et al.* 1993b; Stroud *et al.* 1994), which is perhaps not surprising, given that PCr availability is not thought to limit energy production during this type of exercise.

More recently, data have been published to indicate that creatine supplementation mediates its performance-enhancing effect during maximal-intensity exercise by increasing PCr availability principally in fast-twitch muscle fibres (Casey *et al.* 1996b). This finding is in agreement with previous suggestions of a specific depletion of PCr in fast muscle fibres limiting exercise performance under these conditions (Hultman *et al.* 1991; Casey *et al.* 1996a), and with the hypothesis that PCr acts as a temporal buffer of cytosolic ADP accumulation in this fibre type during exercise (Walliman *et al.* 1992).

As mentioned previously, it is important to note that the extent of muscle creatine retention during supplementation is highly variable between subjects. This finding is of special interest because it has recently been shown that this will have important implications to individuals wishing to gain exercise performance benefits from creatine supplementation. For example, work has revealed that the extent of improvement in exercise performance (Casey *et al.* 1996b) and the magnitude of postexercise PCr resynthesis following creatine supplementation (Greenhaff *et al.* 1994) are closely related to the extent of muscle creatine accumulation during supplementation. Figure 27.6a demonstrates the muscle total creatine concentration of eight subjects before and after 5 days of dietary creatine supplementation ($4\times5\,g\cdot day^{-1}$) from the study of Casey *et al.* (1996b). Each subject has been assigned a number based on their initial muscle total creatine concentration (1 being the lowest and 8 being the highest). Figure 27.6b shows the change in cumulative work production achieved

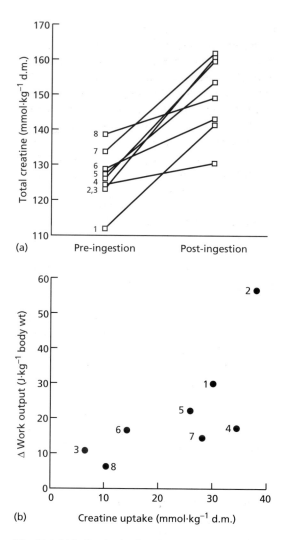

**Fig. 27.6** (a) Individual values for total muscle creatine concentration before and after 5 days of creatine ingestion ($20\,g\cdot day^{-1}$). Subjects have been numbered 1–8 based on the initial total muscle creatine concentration. (b) Individual increases in muscle total creatine for the same group of subjects, plotted against the cumulative change in work production during $2\times 30\,s$ bouts of maximal isokinetic cycling after creatine ingestion. Values on the $y$ axis were calculated by subtracting total work output during exercise before creatine ingestion from the corresponding value after creatine ingestion.

during two bouts of maximal exercise (each lasting 30 s) following creatine ingestion plotted against the increase in muscle total creatine as a result of supplementation in the same eight subjects. The positive relationship found ($r=0.71$, $P<0.05$) led to the conclusion that it may be necessary to increase muscle total creatine concentration by close to or more than $20 \text{ mmol} \cdot \text{kg}^{-1}$ d.m. to obtain substantial improvements in exercise performance as a result of creatine supplementation. These findings may provide some insight to those studies which have reported no improvement in exercise performance following creatine supplementation. In this context, the combination of results from several recent studies undertaken in the author's laboratory has revealed that approximately 20–30% of individuals 'do not respond' to creatine supplementation, i.e. they demonstrate an increase of less than $10 \text{ mmol} \cdot \text{kg}^{-1}$ d.m. (8%) in muscle total creatine following 5 days of $20 \text{ g} \cdot \text{day}^{-1}$ oral creatine supplementation ($4 \times 5 \text{ g}$ doses dissolved in $\approx 250 \text{ ml}$). Thus, as suggested previously, to gain 'optimal' functional and metabolic benefits from creatine supplementation, recent data indicate that it is important to consume creatine in combination with a carbohydrate solution (Green et al. 1996a, 1996b).

## Mechanism of action of dietary creatine supplementation on exercise performance

As previously stated, the literature indicates that if the muscle creatine concentration can be increased by close to or more than $20 \text{ mmol} \cdot \text{kg}^{-1}$ d.m. as a result of acute creatine ingestion, then performance during single and repeated bouts of maximal short-duration exercise will be significantly improved. However, the exact mechanism by which this improvement in exercise performance is achieved is not yet clear. The available data indicate that it may be related to the stimulatory effect that creatine ingestion has upon pre-exercise PCr availability, particularly in fast-twitch muscle fibres (Casey et al. 1996b). For example, in the study of Casey et al. (1996b), the

increase in resting type II muscle fibre PCr concentration as a consequence of creatine supplementation in a group of eight male subjects was positively correlated with the increase in PCr degradation measured during exercise in this fibre type ($r=0.78$, $P<0.01$) and with the increase in total work production observed during exercise following supplementation ($r=0.66$, $P<0.05$). No such associations were found in the type I fibres ($r=0.22$ and $r=0.32$, respectively). Given that PCr availability in type II fibres is generally accepted to limit exercise capacity during maximal exercise (Hultman et al. 1991; Casey et al. 1996a), the increase in type II muscle fibre PCr concentration as a consequence of creatine supplementation may have improved contractile function during exercise by maintaining ATP turnover in this fibre type. This suggestion is supported by reports showing that the accumulation of plasma ammonia and hypoxanthine are reduced during maximal exercise following creatine ingestion (both metabolites are accepted plasma markers of the disruption of muscle ATP resynthesis), despite a higher work output being achieved (Balsom et al. 1993a; Greenhaff et al. 1993). Furthermore, more direct supportive evidence comes from a recent study showing that creatine supplementation reduced the decline in muscle ATP by approximately 30% during maximal isokinetic cycling exercise, while, at the same time, increasing work output (Casey et al. 1996b).

It should be recognized, however, that the positive effects of creatine supplementation on muscle energy metabolism and function are also likely to be the result of the stimulatory effect that an increase in cytoplasmic free creatine will have on mitochondrial mediated PCr resynthesis (Greenhaff et al. 1994), which will be particularly important during repeated bouts of maximal exercise. This suggestion is supported by in vitro studies showing that an increase in the creatine concentration of an incubation medium can accelerate the rate of respiration in isolated skeletal muscle mitochondria (Bessman & Fonyo 1966) and skinned cardiac fibres (Field et al. 1994), and by in vivo human studies showing that the increase in muscle total creatine concentration following creatine supplementation is principally in the form of free creatine (Harris *et al.* 1992; Greenhaff *et al.* 1994).

Of further interest, it has recently been demonstrated that caffeine (5 mg·kg⁻¹ body mass·day⁻¹, single dose) ingested in combination with creatine (0.5 g·kg⁻¹ body mass·day⁻¹, eight equal doses per day) can counteract the positive effect of creatine supplementation on performance during repeated bouts of high intensity exercise (Vandenberghe *et al.* 1996). The authors hypothesized that caffeine ingestion would augment muscle creatine accumulation via a direct and indirect (catacholamine-mediated) stimulation of sodium-dependent muscle creatine transport and thereby may enhance exercise performance further. However, caffeine appeared to have no stimulatory effect on muscle creatine accumulation as the authors demonstrated a 4–6% increase in resting muscle PCr concentration, irrespective of whether caffeine was ingested or not (muscle total creatine was not assessed directly but PCr was determined using phosphorous magnetic resonance spectroscopy). Surprisingly, therefore, the ergolytic effect of caffeine ingestion was not attributable to caffeine inhibiting muscle creatine accumulation during supplementation. The authors offered no clear alternative explanation for their performance findings, but did point out that it was unlikely to be attributable to an effect of caffeine on 'muscle energetics' as the final caffeine dose preceded the postsupplementation exercise test by at least 20 h, which is easily sufficient time for caffeine elimination to have occurred.

In conclusion, information relating to the effects of dietary creatine ingestion on muscle function and metabolism during exercise in healthy normal individuals and in disease states is relatively limited. Based on recent findings, it would appear that it is important to optimize tissue creatine uptake in order to maximize performance benefits, and therefore further work is required to elucidate the principal factors regulating tissue creatine uptake in humans. More information is needed about the exact mecha-

nisms by which creatine achieves its ergogenic effect and on the long term effects of creatine supplementation. With respect to this last point, it should be made clear that the health risks associated with prolonged periods of high-dose creatine supplementation are unknown; equally, however, research to date clearly shows it is not necessary to consume large amounts of creatine to load skeletal muscle. Creatine supplementation may be viewed as a method for producing immediate improvements to athletes involved in explosive sports. In the long run, creatine may also allow athletes to benefit from being able to train without fatigue at an intensity higher than that to which they are normally accustomed. For these reasons alone, creatine supplementation could be viewed as a significant development in sports related nutrition.

## Acknowledgements

The author wishes to acknowledge the Wellcome Trust, Smithkline Beecham and the Defence Research Agency for their support of the experiments described in this chapter and his past and present collaborators for their greatly valued contributions.

## References

Almada, A., Mitchell, T. & Earnest, C. (1996) Impact of chronic creatine supplementation on serum enzyme concentrations. *FASEB Journal* **10**, 4567.

Balsom, P.D., Ekblom, B., Soderlund, K., Sjodin, B. & Hultman, E. (1993a) Creatine supplementation and dynamic high-intensity intermittent exercise. *Scandinavian Journal of Medicine in Science and Sports* **3**, 143–149.

Balsom, P.D., Harridge, S.D.R., Soderlund, K., Sjodin, B. & Ekblom, B. (1993b) Creatine supplementation *per se* does not enhance endurance exercise performance. *Acta Physiologica Scandinavica* **149**, 521–523.

Benedict, S.R. & Osterberg, E. (1923) The metabolism of creatine. *Journal of Biological Chemistry* **56**, 229–230.

Bessman, S.P. & Fonyo, A. (1966) The possible role of mitochondrial bound creatine kinase in regulation of mitochondrial respiration. *Biochemistry and Biophysics Research Communications* **22**, 597–602.

Bessman, S.P. & Savabi, F. (1990) The role of the phosphocreatine energy shuttle in exercise and muscle hypertrophy. In *Biochemistry of Exercise VII* (ed. A.W. Taylor, P.D. Gollnick, H.J. Green, C.D. Ianuzzo, E.G. Noble, G. Metivier & J.R. Sutton), pp. 167–178. Human Kinetics Publishers, Champaign, IL.

Birch, R., Noble, D. & Greenhaff, P.L. (1994) The influence of dietary creatine supplementation on performance during repeated bouts of maximal isokinetic cycling in man. *European Journal of Applied Physiology* **69**, 268–270.

Bogdanis, G.C., Nevill, M.E., Boobis, L.H. & Lakomy, H.K.A. (1996) Contribution of phosphocreatine and aerobic metabolism to energy supply during repeated sprint exercise. *Journal of Applied Physiology* **80**, 876–884.

Casey, A., Constantin-Teodosiu, D., Howell, S., Hultman, E. & Greenhaff, P.L. (1996a) The metabolic response of type I and II muscle fibres during repeated bouts of maximal exercise in humans. *American Journal of Physiology* **271**, E38–E43.

Casey, A., Constantin-Teodosiu, D., Howell, S., Hultman, E. & Greenhaff, P.L. (1996b) Creatine supplementation favourably affects performance and muscle metabolism during maximal intensity exercise in humans. *American Journal of Physiology* **271**, E31–E37.

Chaikelis, A.S. (1940) The effect of glycocoll (glycine) ingestion upon the growth, strength and creatinine-creatine excretion in man. *American Journal of Physiology* **133**, 578–587.

Chanutin, A. (1926) The fate of creatine when administered to man. *Journal of Biological Chemistry* **67**, 29–37.

Cooke, W.H., Grandjean, P.W. & Barnes, W.S. (1995) Effect of oral creatine supplementation on power output and fatigue during bicycle ergometry. *Journal of Applied Physiology* **78**, 670–673.

Delanghe, J., De Slypere, J.-P., Debuyzere, M., Robbrecht, J., Wieme, R. & Vermeulen, A. (1989) Normal reference values for creatine, creatinine and carnitine are lower in vegetarians. *Cinical Chemistry* **35**, 1802–1803.

Earnest, C., Almada, A. & Mitchell, T. (1996) Influence of chronic creatine supplementation on hepatorenal function. *FASEB Journal* **10**, 4588.

Field, M.L., Clark, J.F., Henderson, C., Seymour, A.M.-L. & Radda, G. (1994) Alterations in the myocardial creatine kinase system during chronic anaemic hypoxia. *Cardiovascular Research* **28**, 86–91.

Fitch, C.D. (1977) Significance of abnormalities of creatine metabolism. In *Pathogenesis of Human Muscular Dystrophies* (ed. L.P. Rowland), pp. 328–340. Excerpta Medica, Amsterdam.

Fitch, C.D. & Shields, R.P. (1966) Creatine metabolism in skeletal muscle. I. Creatine movement across muscle membranes. *Journal of Biological Chemistry* **241**, 3610–3614.

Fitch, C.D. & Sinton, D.W. (1964) A study of creatine metabolism in diseases causing muscle wasting. *Journal of Clinical Investigation* **43**, 444–452.

Fitch, C.D., Lucy, D.D., Bornhofen, J.H. & Dalrymple, M. (1968) Creatine metabolism in skeletal muscle. *Neurology* **18**, 32–39.

Fitch, C.D., Jellinek, M., Fitts, R.H., Baldwin, K.M. & Holloszy, J.O. (1975) Phosphorylated β-guanidinopropionate as a substitute for phosphocreatine in rat muscle. *American Journal of Physiology* **288**, 1123–1125.

Forsberg, A.M., Nilsson, E., Werneman, J., Bergstrom, J. & Hultman, E. (1991) Muscle composition in relation to age and sex. *Clinical Science* **81**, 249–256.

Green, A.L., Hultman, E., Macdonald, I.A., Sewell, D.A. & Greenhaff, P.L. (1996a) Carbohydrate ingestion augments skeletal muscle creatine accumulation during creatine supplementation in man. *American Journal of Physiology* **271**, E812–E826.

Green, A.L., Simpson, E.J., Littlewood, J.J., Macdonald, I.A. & Greenhaff, P.L. (1996b) Carbohydrate ingestion augments creatine retention during creatine feeding in man. *Acta Physiologica Scandinavica* **158**, 195–202.

Green, A.L., Macdonald, I.A. & Greenhaff, P.L. (1997) The effects of creatine and carbohydrate on whole-body creatine retention in vegetarians. *Proceedings of the Nutrition Society* **56**, 81A.

Greenhaff, P.L., Casey, A., Short, A.H., Harris, R.C., Soderlund, K. & Hultman, E. (1993) Influence of oral creatine supplementation on muscle torque during repeated bouts of maximal voluntary exercise in man. *Clinical Science* **84**, 565–571.

Greenhaff, P.L., Bodin, K., Soderlund, K. & Hultman, E. (1994) The effect of oral creatine supplementation on skeletal muscle phosphocreatine resynthesis. *American Journal of Physiology* **266**, E725–E730.

Harris, R.C., Soderlund, K. & Hultman, E. (1992) Elevation of creatine in resting and exercised muscle of normal subjects by creatine supplementation. *Clinical Science* **83**, 367–374.

Heymsfield, S.B., Arteaga, C., McManus, C., Smith, J. & Moffitt, S. (1983) Measurement of muscle mass in humans: validity of the 24-hour urinary creatinine method. *American Journal of Clinical Nutrition* **36**, 478–494.

Hultman, E., Greenhaff, P.L., Ren, J.-M. & Soderlund, K. (1991) Energy metabolism and fatigue during intense muscle contraction. *Biochemical Society Transactions* **19**, 347–353.

Hultman, E., Soderlund, K., Timmons, J., Cederblad, G. & Greenhaff, P.L. (1996) Muscle creatine loading in man. *Journal of Applied Physiology* **81**, 232–237.

Hunter, A. (1922) The physiology of creatine and creatinine. *Physiological Reviews* **2**, 586–599.

Katz, A., Sahlin, K. & Henriksson, J. (1986) Muscle ATP

turnover rate during isometric contractions in humans. *Journal of Applied Physiology* **60**, 1839–1842.

Maison, G.L. (1940) Failure of gelatin or amino-acetic acid to increase the work ability. *Journal of the American Medical Association* **115**, 1439–1441.

Meyer, R.A., Brown, T.R., Krilowicz, B.L. & Kushmerick, M.J. (1986) Phosphagen and intracellular pH changes during contraction of creatine-depleted rat muscle. *American Journal of Physiology* **250**, C264–C274.

Myers, V.C. & Fine, M.S. (1915) The metabolism of creatine and creatinine. VII. The fate of creatine when administered to man. *Journal of Biological Chemistry* **21**, 377–383.

Odoom, J.E., Kemp, G.J. & Radda, G.K. (1996) The regulation of total creatine content in a myoblast cell line. *Molecular and Cellular Biochemistry* **158**, 179–188.

Ray, G.B., Johnson, J.R. & Taylor, M.M. (1939) Effect of gelatin on muscular fatigue. *Proceedings of the Society for Experimental Biology and Medicine* **40**, 157–161.

Schloss, P., Mayser, W. & Betz, H. (1994) The putative rat choline transporter chot1 transports creatine and is highly expressed in neural and muscle-rich tissues. *Biochemistry and Biophysics Research Communications* **198**, 637–645.

Sipila, I., Rapola, J., Simell, O. & Vannas, A. (1981) Supplementary creatine as a treatment for gyrate atrophy of the choroid and retina. *New England Journal of Medicine* **304**, 867–870.

Stockler, S., Holzbach, U., Hanefeld, F. *et al.* (1994) Creatine deficiency in the brain: a new, treatable inborn error of metabolism. *Pediatric Research* **36**, 409–413.

Stroud, M.A., Holliman, D., Bell, D., Green, A., Macdonald, I.A. & Greenhaff, P.L. (1994) Effect of oral creatine supplementation on respiratory gas exchange and blood lactate accumulation during steady-state incremental treadmill exercise and recovery. *Clinical Science* **87**, 707–710.

Vandenberghe, K., Gills, N., Van Leemputte, M., Van Hecke, P., Vanstapel, F. & Hespel, P. (1996) Caffeine counteracts the ergogenic action of muscle creatine loading. *Journal of Applied Physiology* **80**, 452–457.

Walker, J.B. (1979) Creatine: biosynthesis, regulation and function. *Advances in Enzymology and Related Areas of Molecular Medicine* **50**, 177–242.

Walliman, T., Wyss, M., Brdiczka, D., Nicolay, K. & Eppenberger, H.M. (1992) Intracellular compartmentation, structure and function of creatine kinase isoenzymes in tissues with high and fluctuating energy demands: the 'phosphocreatine circuit' for cellular energy homeostasis. *Biochemical Journal* **281**, 21–40.

# Chapter 28

# Caffeine

LAWRENCE L. SPRIET AND RICHARD A. HOWLETT

## Introduction

Caffeine is a socially acceptable drug that is widely consumed throughout the world. It is also commonly used by athletes in their daily lives and in preparation for athletic training and competitions. Caffeine is a 'controlled or restricted drug' in the athletic world. Urinary caffeine levels greater than $12\,\mu g \cdot ml^{-1}$ following competitions are considered illegal by the International Olympic Committee (IOC). However, most athletes who consume caffeine beverages prior to exercise would not approach the illegal limit following a competition. Therefore, if caffeine ingestion enhances sports performance, it occupies a unique position in the sports world. It is an accepted component of the diet of many athletes, although it has no nutritional value and would be a 'legal' drug and ergogenic aid in these situations.

Review articles in the early 1990s concluded that the effects of caffeine ingestion on exercise performance and metabolism were inconsistent (Wilcox 1990; Conlee 1991). The authors stated that many experiments had not been well controlled and Conlee (1991) summarized the factors which appeared to confound the caffeine results: the exercise modality, exercise power output, caffeine dose used in the experimental design; the nutritional status, training status, previous caffeine use of the subjects; and individual variation. An additional factor is the ability to reliably measure exercise performance, which improves with increased training frequency and intensity.

Recent research has attempted to control these factors and has demonstrated an ergogenic effect of caffeine during prolonged endurance exercise (>40 min). Investigations examining the effects of caffeine on exercise performance during intense exercise lasting approximately 20 min and shorter durations ($\approx$4–7 min) and sprinting (<90 s) have also appeared. At this point it is difficult to conclude whether caffeine is ergogenic during exercise lasting less than 20 min (for review, see Spriet 1997).

Caffeine appears to be taken up by all tissues of the body, making it difficult to independently study its effects on the central nervous system (CNS) and the peripheral tissues (skeletal muscle, liver and adipose tissue) in the exercising human. It is also likely that multiple and/or different mechanisms may be responsible for performance enhancement in different types of exercise.

This chapter provides a brief but comprehensive review of the issues surrounding caffeine's ability to enhance exercise performance in humans and the mechanisms which may explain the ergogenic effects. The chapter does not contain a complete list of citations but highlights current thinking in the caffeine area and indicates where information is lacking.

# Caffeine and endurance exercise performance

### Early studies

The interest in caffeine as an ergogenic aid during endurance exercise was initially stimulated by work from Costill's laboratory in the late 1970s. Trained cyclists improved their cycle time to exhaustion at 80% of maximal oxygen consumption ($\dot{V}o_{2max.}$) from 75 min in the placebo condition to 96 min following caffeine (330 mg) ingestion (Costill *et al.* 1978). A second study demonstrated a 20% increase in the amount of work performed in 2 h following 250 mg caffeine (Ivy *et al.* 1979). These studies reported increased venous free fatty acid (FFA) concentrations, decreased respiratory exchange ratios (RER) and increased fat oxidation ($\approx$30%) in the caffeine trials. A third study reported that ingestion of 5 mg caffeine·kg$^{-1}$ body mass spared muscle glycogen and increased muscle triacylglycerol (TG) use (Essig *et al.* 1980). In the 1980s, most investigators examined only the effects of caffeine on metabolism and not on endurance performance. Furthermore, conclusions regarding the metabolic effects of caffeine were equivocal and based on changes in plasma FFA and RER. This work has been extensively reviewed (Wilcox 1990; Graham *et al.* 1994; Tarnopolsky 1994; Spriet 1995).

### Recent endurance performance and metabolic studies

Several well-controlled studies in the 1990s examined the performance and metabolism effects of caffeine in well-trained athletes, accustomed to exhaustive exercise and race conditions. These experiments examined the effects of 9 mg caffeine·kg$^{-1}$ body mass (in capsule form) on running and cycling time to exhaustion at 80–85% $\dot{V}o_{2max}$ (Graham & Spriet 1991; Spriet *et al.* 1992), the effects of varying doses (3–13 mg·kg$^{-1}$) of caffeine on cycling performance (Graham & Spriet 1995; Pasman *et al.* 1995) and the effects of a moderate caffeine dose

(5 mg·kg$^{-1}$) on performance of repeated 30-min bouts of cycling (5 min rest between bouts) at 85–90% $\dot{V}o_{2max.}$ (Trice & Haymes 1995).

Collectively, this work produced or confirmed several important findings. Endurance performance was improved by approximately 20–50% compared with the placebo trial (40–77 min) following ingestion of varying caffeine doses (3–13 mg·kg$^{-1}$) in elite and recreationally trained athletes while running or cycling at approximately 80–90% $\dot{V}o_{2max.}$ (Figs 28.1, 28.2). Without exception, the 3, 5 and 6 mg·kg$^{-1}$ doses produced an ergogenic effect with urinary caffeine levels below the IOC acceptable limit (Fig. 28.3). Three of four experiments using a 9 mg·kg$^{-1}$ dose reported performance increases, while 6/22 athletes tested in these studies had urinary caffeine at or above 12 µg·ml$^{-1}$. Performance was enhanced with a 13 mg·kg$^{-1}$ dose, but 6/9 athletes had urinary caffeine well above 12 µg·ml$^{-1}$ (Fig. 28.3). The side-effects of caffeine ingestion (dizziness, headache, insomnia and gastrointestinal distress) were rare with doses at or below 6 mg·kg$^{-1}$, but prevalent at higher doses (9–13 mg·kg$^{-1}$) and associated with decreased perfor-

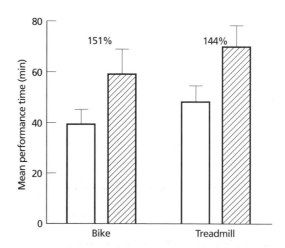

**Fig. 28.1** Performance times for subjects running and cycling to exhaustion at approximately 85% $\dot{V}o_{2max.}$ after placebo (□) or caffeine (▨) ingestion. Performance was significantly improved by 51% during running and 44% while cycling. From Graham and Spriet (1991), with permission.

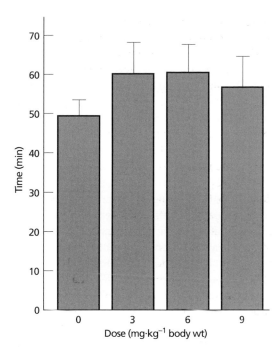

Fig. 28.2 Performance times during running to exhaustion at 85% $\dot{V}o_{2max.}$ following placebo or caffeine ingestion (3, 6 or 9 mg · kg⁻¹ body weight) 1 h prior to exercise. All caffeine conditions were significantly different from placebo. From Graham and Spriet (1995), with permission.

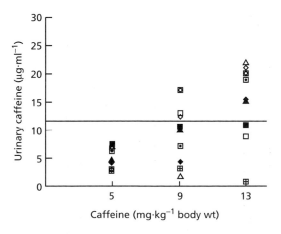

Fig. 28.3 Individual urine caffeine concentrations in 15 men following exhaustive cycling at approximately 80% $\dot{V}o_{2max.}$ and the ingestion of 5, 9 or 13 mg caffeine · kg⁻¹ body weight. The horizontal line depicts the acceptable level of less than 12 µg caffeine · ml⁻¹ urine, as outlined by the International Olympic Committee. From Pasman *et al.* (1995), with permission.

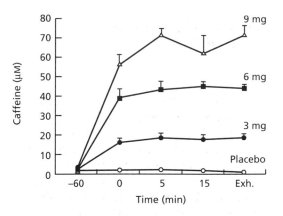

Fig. 28.4 Plasma caffeine concentrations during exhaustive (Exh.) cycling at 80% $\dot{V}o_{2max.}$ following the ingestion of placebo or 3, 6 and 9 mg caffeine · kg⁻¹ body mass 1 h prior to exercise. Exhaustion occurred between 50 and 62 min in all trials. From Graham and Spriet (1995), with permission.

mance in some athletes at 9 mg · kg⁻¹ (Graham & Spriet 1995).

Caffeine generally produced no change in venous plasma noradrenaline (norepinephrine) concentration at rest or exercise, a twofold increase in plasma adrenaline (epinephrine) concentration at rest and exercise and increased plasma FFA concentration at rest. The elevated FFA concentration at the onset of exercise with caffeine was no longer present after 15–20 min of exercise. At the lowest caffeine dose (3 mg · kg⁻¹), performance was increased without a significant increase in plasma venous adrenaline and FFA. Muscle glycogen utilization was reduced following caffeine ingestion, but the 'sparing' was limited to the initial 15 min of exercise at approximately 80% $\dot{V}o_{2max.}$.

## Caffeine and short-term exercise performance

There has been recent interest in the effects of caffeine ingestion on performance of short-term exercise lasting between 30 s and 20–40 min. If caffeine has an ergogenic effect during short-term exercise, the mechanism will not be related to increased fat oxidation and decreased carbohydrate (CHO) oxidation, as CHO availability does not limit performance in this type of exercise.

### Graded exercise tests: 8–20 min

Several studies reported no effect of moderate doses of caffeine on time to exhaustion and $\dot{V}o_{2max.}$ during graded exercise protocols lasting 8–20 min (Dodd *et al.* 1993). However, two studies reported prolonged exercise times when doses of 10–15 mg caffeine·$kg^{-1}$ were given (McNaughton 1987; Flinn *et al.* 1990). Unfortunately, no mechanistic information presently exists to explain how these high caffeine doses prolong exercise time during a graded test, although it might be predicted that central effects would be the most likely cause.

### Intense aerobic exercise: ≈ 20–40 min

Competitive races lasting approximately 20–40 min require athletes to exercise at power outputs of approximately 80–95% $\dot{V}o_{2max.}$. Caffeine (6 mg·$kg^{-1}$) significantly reduced 1500-m swim trial time, from 21:22 ($\pm$38 s) to 20:59 ($\pm$36 s) (min:s), in trained distance swimmers (MacIntosh & Wright 1995). The authors reported lower pre-exercise venous plasma [$K^+$] and higher post-exercise venous blood glucose concentration with caffeine and suggested that electrolyte balance and exogenous glucose availability may be related to caffeine's ergogenic effect. A second study reported no ergogenic effect of caffeine in mildly trained military recruits when cycling to exhaustion (26–27 min) at approximately 80% $\dot{V}o_{2max.}$ at sea level (Fulco *et al.* 1994). However, cycle time was improved upon acute (35 vs. 23 min) and chronic (39 vs. 31 min) exposure to altitude.

### Intense aerobic exercise: ≈ 4–7 min

Exercise events at high power outputs (≈100–110% $\dot{V}o_{2max.}$) that last for approximately 4–7 min require near-maximal or maximal rates of energy provision from both aerobic and anaerobic sources.

Collomp *et al.* (1991) reported that moderate caffeine doses increased cycle time to exhaustion at 100% $\dot{V}o_{2max.}$, from 5:20 with placebo to 5:49 in one group and 5:40 in a second group, although the increases were not statistically significant. Wiles *et al.* (1992) reported that coffee ingestion (≈ 150–200 mg caffeine) improved 1500-m race time on a treadmill by 4.2 s over placebo (4:46.0 vs. 4:50.2). The runners in this study were well-trained, but clearly not elite. In a second experiment, subjects consumed coffee or placebo and then ran for 1100 m at a predetermined pace, followed by a final 400 m where they ran as fast as possible. The time to complete the final 400 m was 61.25 s with coffee and 62.88 s without. Following coffee, all subjects ran faster and the mean $\dot{V}o_{2max.}$ during the final 400 m was higher. To document such small changes, the average response to three trials in the caffeine and placebo conditions was determined in both experiments.

Jackman *et al.* (1996) examined the effects of caffeine ingestion (6 mg·$kg^{-1}$) on the performance and metabolic responses to three bouts of cycling at 100% $\dot{V}o_{2max.}$. Bouts 1 and 2 lasted 2 min and bout 3 was to exhaustion, with rest periods of 6 min between bouts. Time to exhaustion in bout 3 was improved with caffeine (4.93 $\pm$ 0.60 min vs. placebo, 4.12 $\pm$ 0.36 min; $n$=14). Muscle and blood lactate measurements suggested a higher production of lactate in the caffeine trial, even in bouts 1 and 2, when power output was fixed. The glycogenolytic rate was not different during bouts 1 and 2 and less than 50% of the muscle glycogen store was used in either trial during the protocol. The authors concluded that the ergogenic effect of caffeine during short-term intense exercise was not associated with glycogen sparing and may be caused by either a direct action on the muscle or altered CNS function.

### Sprint exercise

Sprinting is defined as exercise or sporting

events at power outputs corresponding to 150–300% $\dot{V}o_{2max.}$ lasting less than 90s. The amount of energy derived from anaerobic processes would be approximately 75–80% of the total in the first 30s, approximately 65–70% over 60s and approximately 55–60% of the total energy over 90s.

Williams *et al.* (1988) reported that caffeine ingestion had no effect on maximal power output or muscular endurance during short, maximal bouts of cycling. Collomp *et al.* (1992) reported that 5 mg caffeine·kg⁻¹ did not increase peak power or total work during a 30-s Wingate test, but the same group later reported that 250 mg caffeine produced a 7% improvement in the maximal power output generated during a series of 6-s sprints at varying force–velocity relationships (Anselme *et al.* 1992). The authors also examined the effects of 4.3 mg caffeine·kg⁻¹ on two 100-m freestyle swims, separated by 20 min (Collomp *et al.* 1990). In well-trained swimmers, caffeine increased swim velocity by 2% and 4% in the two sprints, but performance times were not reported. Caffeine had no effect on sprint performance in untrained swimmers.

Therefore, given the present information, it is not possible to conclude whether caffeine has an ergogenic effect on sprint performance. The brief and intense nature of sprint exercise makes it difficult to study and demonstrate significant differences.

## Field studies

Exercise performance in most laboratory studies is measured as the time taken to reach exhaustion at a given power output or the amount of work that can be performed in a given amount of time. However, in the field, performance is usually measured as the time taken to complete a certain distance. Consequently, extrapolations from the laboratory to field settings may not be valid. Occasionally, laboratory studies simulate race conditions and other studies measure performance in the field (track, swimming pool) in time trial settings without actual race conditions. However, these studies still do not simulate real

competitions. In field studies that do simulate race conditions, it is often impossible to employ the controls required to generate conclusive results. For example, Berglund and Hemmingsson (1982) reported that caffeine increased cross-country ski performance by 1–2.5 min with a control race lasting 1–1.5 h. This improvement occurred at altitude but not at sea level. Unfortunately, the weather and snow conditions were variable in both locations, requiring normalization of the performance times in order to compare results. A recent field study reported that ingesting 0, 5 or 9 mg caffeine·kg⁻¹ had no effect on 21-km road-race performance in hot and humid environments (Cohen *et al.* 1996). While subjects acted as their own controls, no subjects received the placebo treatment in all three races to assess whether between race environmental differences affected race performance, independent of caffeine.

The problems associated with field trials raise questions about the validity of the results and indicate how difficult it is to perform well-controlled and meaningful field trials. However, there is clearly a need for more field studies.

## Theories of ergogenicity

The mechanisms that may contribute to the ergogenic effects of caffeine are categorized into three general theories. The first theory is the classic or 'metabolic' explanation for the ergogenic effects of caffeine during endurance exercise involving an increase in fat oxidation and reduction in CHO oxidation. The metabolic category also includes factors which may affect muscle metabolism and performance in a direct manner, including inhibition of phosphodiesterase, leading to an elevated cyclic adenosine monophosphate (AMP) concentration, and direct effects on key enzymes such as glycogen phosphorylase (PHOS). The second theory proposes a direct effect of caffeine on skeletal muscle performance via ion handling, including $Na^+$–$K^+$-ATPase activity and $Ca^{2+}$ kinetics. The third theory suggests that caffeine exerts a direct effect on portions of the CNS that alter the perception of effort and/or motor unit recruitment.

## Metabolic mechanisms for improved exercise performance

Presently, it seems that metabolic mechanisms are part of the explanation for the improvement in endurance performance following caffeine ingestion ($5$–$13\,mg \cdot kg^{-1}$), except at low caffeine doses ($2$–$4\,mg \cdot kg^{-1}$) where this has not been fully examined. The increased plasma FFA concentration at the onset of exercise, the glycogen sparing in the initial 15 min of exercise and increased intramuscular TG use during the first 30 min of exercise suggest a greater role for fat metabolism early in exercise following caffeine doses of at least $5\,mg \cdot kg^{-1}$. However, there are currently no definitive measurements of increased plasma FFA use following caffeine ingestion. Also, these metabolic findings do not preclude other factors contributing to enhanced endurance performance as discussed below.

It has been suggested that the increased fat oxidation and decreased glycogen use in muscle following caffeine ingestion could be explained by the classic glucose–fatty acid cycle proposed by Randle and colleagues (Spriet & Dyck 1996). In this scheme, elevated FFA availability to the muscle produced increases in muscle citrate and acetyl-coenzyme A, which were believed to inhibit the enzymes phosphofructokinase and pyruvate dehydrogenase. The subsequent decrease in glycolytic activity increased glucose 6-phosphate content, leading to inhibition of hexokinase and ultimately decreased muscle glucose uptake and oxidation. However, these mechanisms were not involved in the CHO sparing during exercise at 85% $\dot{V}o_{2max.}$ with caffeine ingestion or increased fat availability (Spriet et al. 1992; Dyck et al. 1993). Instead, the mechanism for muscle glycogen sparing following caffeine ingestion appeared related to the regulation of glycogen PHOS activity via the energy status of the cell (Chesley et al. 1998). Subjects who spared muscle glycogen had smaller decreases in muscle phosphocreatine and smaller increases in free AMP during exercise in the caffeine vs. placebo trials. The resultant lower free inorganic phosphate and AMP concentrations decreased the flux through the more active $a$ form of PHOS. There were no differences in these metabolites between trials in subjects who did not spare muscle glycogen. It is not presently clear how caffeine defends the energy state of the cell at the onset of intense exercise, but it may be related to the availability of fat (Chesley et al. 1998).

It also appears that adrenaline does not contribute to the metabolic changes which lead to enhanced endurance performance following caffeine ingestion. First, performance was enhanced with $3\,mg\ caffeine \cdot kg^{-1}$ without significant increases in plasma adrenaline and FFA, although FFA were increased twofold at rest (Graham & Spriet 1995). Second, an infusion of adrenaline, designed to produce resting and exercise adrenaline concentrations similar to those induced by caffeine had no effect on plasma FFA concentration or muscle glycogenolysis during exercise (Chesley et al. 1995). Third, Van Soeren et al. (1996) gave caffeine to spinal-cord injured subjects and reported an increased plasma FFA concentration without changes in adrenaline concentration. These findings suggest that caffeine ingestion affects the mobilization of fat by antagonizing the adenosine receptors in adipose tissue.

Therefore, while it is clear that metabolic changes contribute to the ergogenic effect of caffeine during endurance exercise, aspects of the metabolic contribution have not been adequately examined in all situations. Measurements of muscle glycogen and TG use and plasma FFA turnover are required to determine the magnitude of the metabolic link to improved performance at all caffeine doses and endurance exercise situations.

There is some evidence that caffeine has an ergogenic effect on short-term intense exercise. The mechanism will not be related to increased fat oxidation and decreased CHO oxidation, as CHO availability does not limit performance in this situation. It is possible that increased anaerobic energy provision from glycogen breakdown and the glycolytic pathway may contribute to the improvement in performance during repeated bouts of intense exercise (100% $\dot{V}o_{2max}$) lasting 2–5 min (Jackman *et al.* 1996). If this occurred, it would likely be the result of a direct effect of caffeine or a caffeine metabolite.

A few additional metabolic mechanisms have been suggested to contribute to the ergogenic effects of caffeine. It is commonly stated that caffeine inhibits phosphodiesterase, leading to an increase in cyclic AMP concentration and muscle glycogen PHOS activation. However, the support for these conclusions is from *in vitro* or 'test tube' studies that used pharmacological caffeine levels and it is now generally accepted that these effects would not be present at physiological caffeine concentrations (for review, see Tarnopolsky 1994; Spriet 1995). Vergauwen *et al.* (1994) recently reported that adenosine receptors mediate the stimulation of glucose uptake and transport by insulin and contractions in rat skeletal muscle. Caffeine, as an adenosine receptor antagonist and at a physiological level (77 μM), decreased glucose uptake during contractions. This may be an additional mechanism whereby CHO use is spared following caffeine ingestion and replaced by increased fat oxidation. However, there have been no definitive reports demonstrating that adenosine receptors exist in human skeletal muscle.

### Ion handling in skeletal muscle

Caffeine may alter the handling of ions in skeletal muscle and contribute to an ergogenic effect during exercise. Most of the supporting evidence has come from *in vitro* experiments using pharmacological doses of methylxanthines. The candidates that have been suggested to contribute to an ergogenic effect in a physiological environment are increased $Ca^{2+}$ release during the latter stages of exercise and increased $Na^+$–$K^+$-ATPase activity, which may help maintain the membrane potential during exercise. These are the most likely candidates since the lowest methylxanthine concentration used to show these effects in the *in vitro* experiments approached the actual methylxanthine concentrations that have been shown to be ergogenic *in vivo* (Lindinger *et al.* 1993; Tarnopolsky 1994).

It has been demonstrated *in vitro* that pharmacological levels of methylxanthine affect several steps in skeletal muscle excitation–contraction coupling:

**1** increasing the release of $Ca^{2+}$ from the sarcoplasmic reticulum;

**2** enhancing troponin/myosin $Ca^{2+}$ sensitivity; and

**3** decreasing the reuptake of $Ca^{2+}$ by the sarcoplasmic reticulum (Tarnopolsky 1994).

Methylxanthines also stimulate $Na^+$–$K^+$-ATPase activity in inactive skeletal muscle leading to increased rates of $K^+$ uptake and $Na^+$ efflux. This attenuates the rise in plasma [$K^+$] with exercise, which may help maintain the membrane potential in contracting muscle and contribute to caffeine's ergogenic effect during exercise (Lindinger *et al.* 1993, 1996). Any of these changes could produce increases in skeletal muscle force production. However, at the present time, it is not clear if these potential ion-handling effects of caffeine contribute to an ergogenic effect, given the physiological or *in vivo* methylxanthine concentration normally found in humans.

### Central effects of caffeine

While it is almost universally accepted that some of the ergogenic effects of caffeine are manifested through effects on the CNS, it is almost impossible to quantify how much of caffeine's ability to delay fatigue is due to central or peripheral effects. Complicating the problem is the fact that it is not clear how caffeine exerts its actions on the CNS. Caffeine is certainly a CNS stimulant, causing increased wakefulness and vigilance (Van Handel 1983; Nehlig *et al.* 1992; Daly 1993). Some have attributed the increased performance derived from caffeine simply to this increased alertness or improved mood (Nehlig & Debry 1994). However, the ability of caffeine to delay fatigue points to more complex mechanisms than simply heightened arousal. Because they are also related to peripheral metabolic effects, the following topics are of special interest in a discussion of caffeine's central effects: adenosine receptor antagonism, lowered perceived exertion and the central fatigue hypothesis.

## Adenosine receptor antagonism

Since caffeine can freely pass through the blood–brain barrier (Nehlig *et al.* 1992), its concentration in the brain and CNS increases rapidly following ingestion, in concert with changes in other body tissues (Daly 1993). Caffeine increases brain neurotransmitter concentration, causing increases in spontaneous locomotor activity and neuronal firing in animals (Nehlig *et al.* 1992). It is generally accepted that the mechanism for neurotransmitter increases is adenosine receptor antagonism and high adenosine receptor levels in the brain support this hypothesis (Fernstrom & Fernstrom 1984; Snyder 1984; Daly 1993; Fredholm 1995).

Adenosine is both a neurotransmitter and neuromodulator, capable of affecting the release of other neurotransmitters (Fernstrom & Fernstrom 1984). Adenosine and adenosine analogues generally cause lowered motor activity, decreased wakefulness and vigilance, and decreases in other neurotransmitter concentrations. Caffeine and adenosine receptor antagonists have the opposite effect by blocking the adenosine receptors. It is generally believed that the inhibition (adenosine) or stimulation (caffeine) of neurotransmitter release is presynaptic (Snyder 1984; Fredholm 1995). It has been demonstrated that caffeine increases the concentration, synthesis and/or turnover of all major neurotransmitters, including serotonin, dopamine, acetylcholine, noradrenaline and glutamate. These neurotransmitters are all inhibited by adenosine. The exact consequences of these changes in neurotransmitters with regards to performance is currently not known. Both dopamine and serotonin levels have been implicated in the central effects of caffeine on fatigue and behaviour (Fernstrom & Fernstrom 1984; Daly 1993), and in the development of central fatigue exclusive of caffeine ingestion (Davis & Bailey 1997). It has been suggested that an increase in excitatory neurotransmitters could lead to decreases in motorneurone threshold, resulting in greater motor unit recruitment (Waldeck 1973) and subsequently lower perceived exertion for a given power output (Nehlig & Debry 1994; Cole *et al.* 1996). However, this theory has not been demonstrated during exercise, although it continues to be cited as a potential mechanism (Nehlig & Debry 1994; Cole *et al.* 1996).

Complicating the effects of caffeine on adenosine antagonism is the existence of two main classes of adenosine receptors, $A_1$ and $A_2$ (Snyder 1984; Graham *et al.* 1994), each having differing affinities for endogenous adenosine and xanthines, and affecting the release of different neurotransmitters (Daly 1993) Likewise, antagonism of these receptors is dependent on the caffeine concentration, which will either inhibit ($A_1$) or stimulate ($A_2$) adenylate cyclase, leading to differential effects and possibly explaining the biphasic response to caffeine. Increasing caffeine doses are stimulatory, but very high physiological doses are depressant (Snyder 1984). As well, some adenosine antagonists display the same affinity as xanthines for adenosine receptors, but do not cause the same effects (Snyder 1984; Daly 1993). Finally, the binding of caffeine to benzodiazepine receptors and the relationship to gamma-aminobutyric acid (GABA) and excitatory amino acids is currently being explored (Nehlig *et al.* 1992; Daly 1993). Some authors assert that adenosine receptor antagonism, while likely the primary mechanism, cannot account for all of caffeine's actions on the CNS (Graham *et al.* 1994).

## Ratings of perceived exertion

One quantifiable aspect of caffeine's central effects is a lower rating of perceived exertion (RPE) during exercise. Several studies have demonstrated that (i) RPE at a standard power output was lower in subjects following caffeine ingestion than in controls (Costill *et al.* 1978), and

(ii) subjects accomplished a greater amount of work following caffeine ingestion than controls when RPE was held constant (Ivy *et al.* 1979; Cole *et al.* 1996). This significant decline in experimental RPE is certainly supported by anecdotal evidence. It has been speculated that the lowered RPE with caffeine is due to a decrease in the firing threshold of motorneurones (Nehlig & Debry 1994; Cole *et al.* 1996) or changes in muscle contraction force (Tarnopolsky 1994). Both mechanisms would result in lowered afferent feedback from the working muscle and a lowered RPE, the first mechanism because more motor units would be recruited for a given task and the second because the force for a given stimulus would be greater. However, the ability of physiological caffeine concentration to alter contractile function is equivocal as discussed earlier (Graham *et al.* 1994; Tarnopolsky 1994). Another hypothesis is that caffeine directly affects the release of β-endorphins and other hormones that modulate the feelings of discomfort and pain associated with exhaustive exercise (Nehlig *et al.* 1992). A final explanation for the reduced RPE may involve the central fatigue hypothesis (Tarnopolsky 1994).

### CENTRAL FATIGUE HYPOTHESIS

Given that caffeine affects the CNS, it is appealing to link it to one proposed mechanism of fatigue currently being investigated, the central fatigue hypothesis (see Chapter 12). Briefly, this hypothesis argues that the central component of fatigue caused by exhaustive exercise is mediated by elevated levels of serotonin (5-HT) in the brain, caused by an increase in its precursor, tryptophan (TRP) (Blomstrand & Newsholme 1996). Tryptophan is the only amino acid that is transported in plasma bound to albumin and it competes for transport into the brain with branched-chain amino acids (BCAA). Evidence for the central fatigue theory includes increased levels of brain 5-HT at fatigue, increased plasma free TRP at fatigue caused by high FFAs, and decreased fatigue with BCAA supplementation (Blomstrand & Newsholme 1996). If caffeine delayed the onset of CNS fatigue via serotonin levels, then it must lower 5-HT levels or inhibit the rise in 5-HT. However, the effects of caffeine on the CNS and peripheral metabolism appear to counter this process for two reasons. First, acute caffeine ingestion has been shown to significantly increase brain 5-HT levels, most likely due to increases in brain free TRP levels (Fernstrom & Fernstrom 1984; Nehlig *et al.* 1992). Second, caffeine ingestion prior to exercise elevates plasma FFA concentration at the onset of exercise, which should increase free TRP, due to competition for albumin binding, and hasten fatigue. It is possible that the rise in 5-HT at the onset of exercise is overridden by other factors, such as increased sympathetic drive, or favourable metabolic factors. Similarly, since it has been postulated that the ratio of 5-HT to dopamine is a larger determinant in fatigue than the [5-HT] alone (Davis & Bailey 1997), the caffeine-induced rise in both neurotransmitters could offset each other.

In summary, the caffeine-induced mechanism(s) that may delay central fatigue are still undiscovered, but the link between caffeine and the central fatigue hypothesis remains intriguing.

## Complications of studying caffeine, exercise performance and metabolism

It is important to note in a discussion of the performance, metabolic and central effects of caffeine ingestion that the mechanism(s) of action may not be entirely due to the primary effects of caffeine. Caffeine is a trimethylxanthine compound, which is rapidly metabolized in the liver to three dimethylxanthines, paraxanthine, theophylline and theobromine. These are released into the plasma as the caffeine concentration declines and remain in the circulation longer. While the plasma dimethylxanthine concentrations are not large, paraxanthine and theophylline are potential adenosine antagonists and metabolic stimuli. Therefore, as caffeine and its metabolites are often present at the same time, it is difficult to resolve which tissues are directly or indirectly affected by which compound (Fig. 28.5). Due to this uncertainty, the reader should note that when the term 'caffeine' is used in this chapter, it could be any of the methylxanthines.

Another complication of studying caffeine ingestion is the variability of individual responses, affecting central, metabolic and exercise performance responses to caffeine. This problem affects all categories of subjects, but is a larger problem with less aerobically fit individuals. Chesley *et al.* (1998) reported a variable glycogen sparing response to a high caffeine dose (9 mg·kg$^{-1}$) in untrained men. Only 6/12 subjects demonstrated glycogen sparing during 15 min of cycling at approximately 85% $\dot{V}o_{2max.}$, whereas the sparing response was more uniform in a group of trained men (Spriet *et al.* 1992). Variability is also present in all groups of caffeine users, including mild and heavy users, users withdrawn from caffeine and non-users. Therefore, while mean results in groups of subjects and athletes predict improved athletic performance, predictions that a given person will improve are less certain.

There has been a recent report comparing the effects of 4.5 mg caffeine·kg$^{-1}$, given in 'pure'

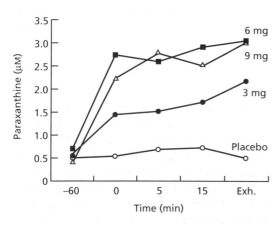

**Fig. 28.5** Plasma paraxanthine concentrations during exhaustive (Exh.) cycling at 80% $\dot{V}o_{2max.}$ following the ingestion of placebo or 3, 6 and 9 mg caffeine·kg$^{-1}$ body mass 1 h prior to exercise. Exhaustion occurred between 50 and 62 min in all trials. From Graham and Spriet (1995), with permission.

capsule form or in two mugs of strong coffee (Graham *et al.* 1998). Caffeine in capsule form resulted in the usual metabolic and performance effects, but the ingested coffee produced less of a response in plasma adrenaline concentration and little or no effect on performance, even though the plasma caffeine concentrations were identical. It appears that the hundreds of additional chemicals in coffee negated the usual ergogenic benefit. On the other hand, there have been reports where caffeine administration in coffee produced strong ergogenic performance effects (Wiles *et al.* 1992). Therefore, while it is common to equate caffeine with coffee, it should be noted that rarely is coffee the method of administration in research studies and it may be misleading to equate the two.

The study of caffeine ingestion and exercise performance has been generally limited to male subjects. There has been little systematic study of the response of females to caffeine ingestion at rest and during exercise. It will be important to control for menstrual status in future studies, as oestrogen may affect the half-life of caffeine.

## Other considerations of ingesting caffeine

### Caffeine dose

Caffeine is a 'controlled or restricted substance' with respect to the IOC. Athletes are permitted up to 12 µg caffeine·ml$^{-1}$ urine before it is considered illegal. This allows athletes who normally consume caffeine in their diet to continue this practice prior to competition. An athlete can consume a very large amount of caffeine before reaching the 'illegal limit'. A 70-kg person could drink three or four mugs or six regular-size cups of drip-percolated coffee approximately 1 h before exercise, exercise for 1–1.5 h, and a subsequent urine sample would only approach the urinary caffeine limit. A caffeine level above 12 µg·ml$^{-1}$ suggests that a person has deliberately taken caffeine in capsule or tablet form or as suppositories, in an attempt to improve performance. Not surprisingly, only a few athletes have been caught with illegal levels during competitions, although formal reports of the frequency of caffeine abuse are rare. One study reported that 26/775 cyclists had illegal urinary caffeine levels when tested following competition (Delbecke & Debachere 1984).

## Urinary caffeine and doping

The use of urinary caffeine levels to determine caffeine abuse in sport has been criticized (Duthel *et al.* 1991). Only 0.5–3% of orally ingested caffeine actually reaches the urine as the majority is metabolized in the liver. The excreted caffeine by-products are not measured in doping tests. Other factors also affect the amount of caffeine that reaches the urine, including body weight, gender and hydration status of the athlete. The time elapsed between caffeine ingestion and urine collection is also important and affected by the exercise duration and environmental conditions. Sport governing bodies may not regard these concerns as problems since most people caught with illegal levels of caffeine will have used the drug in a doping manner. However, it is possible that someone who metabolizes caffeine slowly or who excretes 3% of the ingested dose rather than 0.5% could have illegal urine levels following a moderate dose.

## Habitual caffeine consumption

An athlete's normal caffeine intake habits may affect whether acute caffeine ingestion improves performance. Many investigators ask users to refrain from caffeine consumption for 2–3 days prior to experiments. Caffeine metabolism is not increased by use, but the effects of caffeine may be altered by habitual use via alterations in adenosine receptor populations. As reviewed by Graham *et al.* (1994), several studies suggest that chronic caffeine use dampens the adrenaline response to exercise and caffeine, but does not affect plasma FFA concentration or exercise RER (Bangsbo *et al.* 1992; Van Soeren *et al.* 1993). However, these changes do not appear to dampen the ergogenic effect of 9 mg caffeine·

kg$^{-1}$. Endurance performance increased in all subjects when both caffeine users and non-users were examined and users abstained from caffeine for 48–72 h prior to experiments (Graham & Spriet 1991; Spriet *et al.* 1992). However, the performance results were more variable in a subsequent study with more non-users (Graham & Spriet 1995). In addition, Van Soeren and Graham (1998) reported no effect of up to 4 days of caffeine withdrawal on exercise hormonal and metabolic responses to doses of 6 or 9 mg caffeine·kg$^{-1}$ in recreational cyclists. Time to exhaustion at 80–85% $\dot{V}o_{2max.}$ improved with caffeine and was unaffected by 0–4 days of withdrawal.

## Caffeine and high carbohydrate diets

An early investigation suggested that a high CHO diet and a prerace CHO meal negated the expected increase in plasma FFA concentration following caffeine ingestion during 2 h of exercise at approximately 75% $\dot{V}o_{2max.}$ (Weir *et al.* 1987). These results implied that high CHO diets negated the ergogenic effects of caffeine, although performance was not measured. However, a high CHO diet and a pretrial CHO meal did not prevent caffeine-induced increases in performance in a number of recent studies using well-trained/recreational runners and cyclists (Spriet 1995).

## Diuretic effect of caffeine

Because caffeine is a diuretic, it has been suggested that caffeine ingestion may lead to poor hydration status prior to and during exercise. However, no changes in core temperature, sweat loss or plasma volume were reported during exercise following caffeine ingestion (Gordon *et al.* 1982; Falk *et al.* 1990). It has also been demonstrated that urine flow rate, decreases in plasma volume, sweat rate and heart rate were unaffected by caffeine ($\approx$600 mg), ingested in a CHO electrolyte drink ($\approx$2.5 l) during 1 h at rest and 3 h of cycling at 60% $\dot{V}o_{2max.}$ (Wemple *et al.* 1997).

# Conclusion

Caffeine ingestion ($3–13 \, mg \cdot kg^{-1}$ body mass) prior to exercise increases performance during prolonged endurance cycling and running in the laboratory. Caffeine doses below $9 \, mg \cdot kg^{-1}$ generally produce urine caffeine levels below the IOC allowable limit of $12 \, \mu g \cdot ml^{-1}$. Moderate caffeine doses ($5–6 \, mg \cdot kg^{-1}$) may also increase short-term intense cycling performance ($\approx 4–7$ min) in the laboratory and decrease 1500-m swim time ($\approx 20 \, min$). These results are generally reported in well-trained or recreational athletes, but field studies are lacking to confirm the ergogenic effects of caffeine in the athletic world. The mechanisms for the improved endurance have not been clearly established. Caffeine ingestion generally increases resting venous plasma FFA concentration and reduces muscle glycogen use and increases muscle TG use early during endurance exercise, suggesting greater fat oxidation and reduced CHO oxidation in the working muscles. However, a single metabolic explanation for the ergogenic effect of caffeine is unlikely, especially at low caffeine doses that do not cause major metabolic changes. All human performance studies have been unable to separate the central effects of caffeine from peripheral effects. Therefore, a central contribution to the enhancement of endurance exercise performance following caffeine ingestion is a strong possibility. Potential mechanisms for improved performance during short-term intense exercise include direct caffeine effects on the CNS and/or ion handling in skeletal muscle and increased anaerobic energy provision in muscle. Definitive research into the mechanisms of the ergogenic effects of caffeine in exercising humans is hampered by the ability of this drug and its byproducts to affect both central and peripheral processes.

# References

Anselme, F., Collomp, K., Mercier, B., Ahmaidi, S. & Prefaut, C. (1992) Caffeine increases maximal anaerobic power and blood lactate concentration. *European Journal of Applied Physiology* **65**, 188–191.

Bangsbo, J., Jacobsen, K., Nordberg, N., Christensen, N.J. & Graham, T. (1992) Acute and habitual caffeine ingestion and metabolic responses to steady-state exercise. *Journal of Applied Physiology* **72**, 1297–1303.

Berglund, B. & Hemmingsson, P. (1982) Effects of caffeine ingestion on exercise performance at low and high altitudes in cross country skiers. *International Journal of Sports Medicine* **3**, 234–236.

Blomstrand, E.E. & Newsholme, E.A. (1996) Glucose-fatty acid cycle and fatigue involving 5-hydroxytryptamine. In *Biochemistry of Exercise IX* (ed. R.J. Maughan & S.M. Shirreffs), pp. 185–195. Human Kinetics, Champaign, IL.

Chesley, A., Hultman, E. & Spriet, L.L. (1995) Effects of epinephrine infusion on muscle glycogenolysis during intense aerobic exercise. *American Journal of Physiology* **268** (Endocrinology Metabolism), E127–E134.

Chesley, A., Howlett, R.A., Heigenhauser, G.J.F., Hultman, E. & Spriet, L.L. (1998) Regulation of muscle glycogenolytic flux during intense aerobic exercise after caffeine ingestion. *American Journal of Physiology* **275**, R596–603.

Cohen, B.S., Nelson, A.G., Prevost, M.C., Thompson, G.D., Marx, B.D. & Morris, G.S. (1996) Effects of caffeine ingestion on endurance racing in heat and humidity. *European Journal of Applied Physiology* **73**, 358–363.

Cole, K.J., Costill, D.L., Starling, R.D., Goodpaster, B.H., Trappe, S.W. & Fink, W.J. (1996) Effect of caffeine ingestion on perception of effort and subsequent work production. *International Journal of Sport Nutrition* **6**, 14–23.

Collomp, K., Caillaud, C., Audran, M., Chanal, J.-L. & Prefaut, C. (1990) Influence of acute and chronic bouts of caffeine on performance and catecholamines in the course of maximal exercise. *Comptes Rendues des Seances de la Societe de Biologie* **184**, 87–92.

Collomp., K., Ahmaidi, S., Audran, M., Chanal, J.-L. & Prefaut, C. (1991) Effects of caffeine ingestion on performance and anaerobic metabolism during the Wingate test. *International Journal of Sports Medicine* **12**, 439–443.

Collomp, K., Ahmaidi, S., Chatard, J.C., Audran, M. & Prefaut, C. (1992) Benefits of caffeine ingestion on sprint performance in trained and untrained swimmers. *European Journal of Applied Physiology* **64**, 377–380.

Conlee, R.K. (1991) Amphetamine, caffeine and cocaine. In *Ergogenics: Enhancement of Performance in Exercise and Sport* (ed. D.R. Lamb & M.H. Williams), pp. 285–330. Brown and Benchmark, Indianapolis, IN.

Costill, D.L., Dalsky, G.P. & Fink, W.J. (1978) Effects of caffeine on metabolism and exercise performance. *Medicine and Science in Sports* **10**, 155–158.

Daly, J.W. (1993) Mechanism of action of caffeine. In *Caffeine, Coffee, and Health* (ed. S. Garatttini), pp. 97–150. Raven Press, New York.

Davis, J.M. & Bailey, S.P. (1997) Possible mechanisms of central nervous system fatigue during exercise. *Medicine and Science in Sports and Exercise* 29, 45–57.

Delbecke, F.T. & Debachere, M. (1984) Caffeine: use and abuse in sports. *International Journal of Sports Medicine* 5, 179–182.

Dodd, S.L., Herb, R.A. & Powers, S.K. (1993) Caffeine and exercise performance: an update. *Sports Medicine* 15, 14–23.

Duthel, J.M., Vallon, J.J., Martin, G., Ferret, J.M., Mathieu, R. & Videman, R. (1991) Caffeine and sport: role of physical exercise upon elimination. *Medicine and Science in Sports and Exercise* 23, 980–985.

Dyck, D.J., Putman, C.T., Heigenhauser, G.J.F., Hultman, E. & Spriet, L.L. (1993) Regulation of fat–carbohydrate interaction in skeletal muscle during intense aerobic cycling. *American Journal of Physiology* 265, E852–859.

Essig, D., Costill, D.L. & VanHandel, P.J. (1980) Effects of caffeine ingestion on utilization of muscle glycogen and lipid during leg ergometer cycling. *International Journal of Sports Medicine* 1, 86–90.

Falk, B., Burstein, R., Rosenblum, J., Shapiro, Y., Zylber-Katz, E. & Bashan, N. (1990) Effects of caffeine ingestion on body fluid balance and thermoregulation during exercise. *Canadian Journal of Physiology and Pharmacology* 68, 889–892.

Fernstrom, J.D. & Fernstrom, M.H. (1984) Effects of caffeine on monamine neurotransmitters in the central and peripheral nervous system. In *Caffeine* (ed. P.B. Dews), pp. 107–118. Springer-Verlag, Berlin.

Flinn, S., Gregory, J., McNaughton, L.R., Tristram, S. & Davies, P. (1990) Caffeine ingestion prior to incremental cycling to exhaustion in recreational cyclists. *International Journal of Sports Medicine* 11, 188–193.

Fredholm, B.B. (1995) Adenosine, adenosine receptors and the actions of caffeine. *Pharmacology and Toxicology* 76, 93–101.

Fulco, C.S., Rock, P.B., Trad, L.A. *et al.* (1994) Effect of caffeine on submaximal exercise performance at altitude. *Aviation Space and Environmental Medicine* 65, 539–545.

Gordon, N.F., Myburgh, J.L., Kruger, P.E. *et al.* (1982) Effects of caffeine on thermoregulatory and myocardial function during endurance performance. *South African Medical Journal* 62, 644–647.

Graham, T.E. & Spriet, L.L. (1991) Performance and metabolic responses to a high caffeine dose during prolonged exercise. *Journal of Applied Physiology* 71, 2292–2298.

Graham, T.E. & Spriet, L.L. (1995) Metabolic, catecholamine and exercise performance responses to varying doses of caffeine. *Journal of Applied Physiology* 78, 867–874.

Graham, T.E., Rush, J.W.E. & van Soeren, M.H. (1994) Caffeine and exercise: metabolism and performance. *Canadian Journal of Applied Physiology* 19, 111–138.

Graham, T.E., Hibbert, E. & Sathasivam, P. (1998) Metabolic and exercise endurance effects of coffee and caffeine ingestion. *Journal of Applied Physiology* 85, 883–889.

Ivy, J.L., Costill, D.L., Fink, W.J. & Lower, R.W. (1979) Influence of caffeine and carbohydrate feedings on endurance performance. *Medicine and Science in Sports* 11, 6–11.

Jackman, M., Wendling, P., Friars, D. & Graham, T.E. (1996) Metabolic, catecholamine and endurance responses to caffeine during intense exercise. *Journal of Applied Physiology* 81, 1658–1663.

Lindinger, M.I., Graham, T.E. & Spriet, L.L. (1993) Caffeine attenuates the exercise-induced increase in plasma [K+] in humans. *Journal of Applied Physiology* 74, 1149–1155.

Lindinger, M.I., Willmets, R.G. & Hawke, T.J. (1996) Stimulation of Na+, K+-pump activity in skeletal muscle by methylxanthines: evidence and proposed mechanisms. *Acta Physiologica Scandinavica* 156, 347–353.

MacIntosh, B.R. & Wright, B.M. (1995) Caffeine ingestion and performance of a 1500-metre swim. *Canadian Journal of Applied Physiology* 20, 168–177.

McNaughton, L. (1987) Two levels of caffeine ingestion on blood lactate and free fatty acid responses during incremental exercise. *Research Quarterly of Exercise and Sport* 58, 255–259.

Nehlig, A. & Debry, G. (1994) Caffeine and sports activity: a review. *International Journal of Sports Medicine* 15, 215–223.

Nehlig, A., Daval, J.-L. & Debry, G. (1992) Caffeine and the central nervous system: mechanisms of action, biochemical, metabolic, and psychostimulant effects. *Brain Research Reviews* 17, 139–170.

Pasman, W.J., VanBaak, M.A., Jeukendrup, A.E. & DeHaan, A. (1995) The effect of different dosages of caffeine on endurance performance time. *International Journal of Sports Medicine* 16, 225–230.

Snyder, S.H. (1984) Adenosine as a mediator of the behavioral effects of xanthines. In *Caffeine* (ed. P.B. Dews), pp. 129–141. Springer-Verlag, Berlin.

Spriet, L.L. (1995) Caffeine and performance. *International Journal of Sports Nutrition* 5, S84–S99.

Spriet, L.L. (1997) Ergogenic aids: recent advances and retreats. In *Recent Advances in the Science and Medicine of Sport*, Vol. 10 (ed. D.R. Lamb & R. Murray), pp. 186–238. Cooper Publishing, Carmel.

Spriet, L.L. & Dyck, D.J. (1996) The glucose-fatty acid cycle in skeletal muscle at rest and during exercise. In *Biochemistry of Exercise IX* (ed. R.J. Maughan & S.M. Shirreffs), pp. 127–155. Human Kinetics, Champaign, IL.

Spriet, L.L., MacLean, D.A., Dyck, D.J., Hultman, E.,

Cederblad, G. & Graham, T.E. (1992) Caffeine ingestion and muscle metabolism during prolonged exercise in humans. *American Journal of Physiology* **262** (Endocrinology Metabolism), E891–E898.

Tarnopolsky, M.A. (1994) Caffeine and endurance performance. *Sports Medicine* **18**, 109–125.

Trice, I. & Haymes, E.M. (1995) Effects of caffeine ingestion on exercise-induced changes during high-intensity, intermittent exercise. *International Journal of Sports Nutrition* **5**, 37–44.

Van Handel, P. (1983) Caffeine. In *Ergogenic Aids in Sport* (ed. M.H. Williams), pp. 128–163. Human Kinetics, Champaign, IL.

Van Soeren, M.H. & Graham, T.E. (1998) Effect of caffeine on metabolism, exercise endurance, and catecholamine responses after withdrawal. *Journal of Applied Physiology* **85**, 1493–1501.

Van Soeren, M.H., Sathasivam, P., Spriet, L.L. & Graham, T.E. (1993) Caffeine metabolism and epinephrine responses during exercise in users and non-users. *Journal of Applied Physiology* **75**, 805–812.

Van Soeren, M.H., Mohr, T., Kjaer, M. & Graham, T.E. (1996) Acute effects of caffeine ingestion at rest in humans with impaired epinephrine responses. *Journal of Applied Physiology* **80**, 999–1005.

Vergauwen, L., Hespel, P. & Richter, E.A. (1994) Adenosine receptors mediate synergistic stimulation of glucose uptake and transport by insulin and by contractions in rat skeletal muscle. *Journal of Clinical Investigation* **93**, 974–981.

Waldeck, B. (1973) Sensitization by caffeine of central catecholamine receptors. *Journal of Neural Transmission* **34**, 61–72.

Weir, J., Noakes, T.D., Myburgh, K. & Adams, B. (1987) A high carbohydrate diet negates the metabolic effect of caffeine during exercise. *Medicine and Science in Sports Exercise* **19**, 100–105.

Wemple, R.D., Lamb, D.R. & McKeever, K.H. (1997) Caffeine vs. caffeine-free sports drinks: effects on urine production at rest and during prolonged exercise. *International Journal of Sports Medicine* **18**, 40–46.

Wilcox, A.R. (1990) Caffeine and endurance performance. In *Sports Science Exchange*, pp. 1–5. Gatorade Sports Science Institute, Barrington, IL.

Wiles, J.D., Bird, S.R., Hopkins, J. & Riley, M. (1992) Effect of caffeinated coffee on running speed, respiratory factors, blood lactate and perceived exertion during 1500-m treadmill running. *British Journal of Sports Medicine* **26**, 116–120.

Williams, J.H., Signoille, J.F., Barnes, W.S. & Henrich, T.W. (1988) Caffeine, maximal power output and fatigue. *British Journal of Sports Medicine* **229**, 132–134.

# Chapter 29

# Bicarbonate and Citrate

LARS R. MCNAUGHTON

## Introduction

The ability to resist fatigue is an important aspect of many types of sporting activity, whether it be short-term, high-intensity anaerobic type work, or longer, high-intensity endurance activity. Athletes who fatigue early do not perform as well as those who fatigue more slowly, so, in order to maximize performance, it is important that fatigue is minimized wherever possible.

Fatigue is generally defined as the failure to maintain an expected or required force or power output (Edwards 1981). The causes of fatigue are multifaceted (see Green 1990 and Hultman *et al.* 1990 for reviews) and can be roughly divided into either physiological or psychological. In the physiological realm, fatigue can be described as either central or peripheral (Green *et al.* 1987). In the latter case, there is a myriad of factors which can interact to decrease power output and hinder performance. During high-intensity work of short duration, potential contributors to fatigue could be related to muscle energy production (for example, a decline in muscle adenosine triphosphate, ATP) or they could be related to impaired electrochemical events of muscle contraction/relaxation production. Alternatively, fatigue could be related to the accumulation of metabolites — for example lactate, hydrogen ions and ammonia. During prolonged submaximal effort, energy substrate depletion is generally regarded as the major cause of fatigue, but a number of other factors such as hyperthermia, dehydration and oxygen transport problems may also contribute in differing amounts.

Athletes and their coaches have always sought ways to improve performance and overcome the fatigue process. In doing so, they have targeted a number of different areas, including training methodology, nutritional practices, medical interventions and the use of both legal and illegal drugs — for a review of ergogenic aids, see Chapter 26. With a 'win at all costs' mentality, many athletes have ingested substances which are claimed to have an ergogenic effect by overcoming the fatigue process. Over the last decade or so, the use of sodium bicarbonate and sodium citrate have become popular to offset fatigue during short-term, high-intensity exercise. It is claimed that these substances improve performance by buffering the acids which are produced during exercise.

The aim of this chapter is to discuss the current knowledge with respect to metabolic acidosis during both short-term, high-intensity and endurance exercise and the effects of sodium bicarbonate and sodium citrate ingestion on these types of performance.

## Basics of acid–base balance

Substances that release $H^+$ when they dissociate in solution are called *acids*, whereas substances that accept $H^+$ ions and form hydroxide ions ($OH^-$) are called *bases*. In the body there must be a balance between the formation of hydrogen ions and the removal of hydrogen ions for homeosta-

**Table 29.1** Approximate relationship between [H+] and pH.

| [H+] (nmol·l⁻¹) | pH |
|---|---|
| 20 | 7.7 |
| 30 | 7.5 |
| 40 | 7.4 |
| 50 | 7.3 |
| 60 | 7.2 |
| 70 | 7.15 |

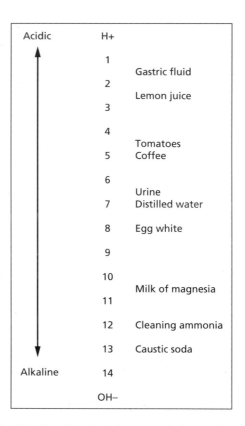

**Fig. 29.1** The pH scale with some typical examples.

sis to be maintained. When this is not the case, and the number of H+ ions increases, the pH of the blood (which is normally around 7.4) decreases to lower levels (7.0 or lower) (Table 29.1). Muscle pH is normally at 7.0 and decreases to 6.8 or lower (Robergs & Roberts 1997). The pH of a given substance is the negative logarithm of the hydrogen ion concentration ($-\log$ [H+]). Since it is logarithmic, a unit increase of 1.0 means a tenfold increase in the number of H+ ions. Basic solutions have few H+ ions and acids have plentiful amounts of H+ ions. Distilled water is considered a neutral substance at a pH of 7.0 (25°C). The pH scale is shown in Fig. 29.1 and was initially devised by the Danish chemist Soren Sorensen. Body fluids differ in their pH level, with gastric fluids being an acidic 1.0 and arterial and venous blood being slightly basic at *c.* 7.45.

During normal activity, the blood and extracellular fluid remain at a pH of approximately 7.4, a slightly alkalotic state. When the number of H+ ions increases, such as during intense exercise, the blood pH drops to below 7.0 (muscle pH is even lower), and a state of acidosis exists. As metabolism is highly H+ ion sensitive, the regulation of alkalosis and acidosis is extremely important. Figure 29.2 shows the relationship between pH and [H+] with the extreme physiological realms.

The body has three basic mechanisms for adjusting and regulating acid–base balance and which minimize changes within the body. First, there are the chemical buffers which adjust [H+] within seconds. Secondly, pulmonary ventilation excretes H+ through the reaction

$$H+ + HCO_3^- \leftrightarrow H_2CO_3 \leftrightarrow H_2O + CO_2$$

adjusting [H+] within minutes. Finally, the kidneys excrete [H+] as fixed acid and work on a long-term basis to maintain acid–base balance. We are concerned with the bicarbonate buffer system (Vick 1984).

The body's chemical buffer, and more specifically the bicarbonate buffer, consists of a weak acid (carbonic acid) and the salt of that acid (sodium bicarbonate), often termed a conjugate acid–base pair. Discussion of blood pH regulation has generally focused on the role of bicarbonate, since it can accept a proton to form carbonic acid in the following equation:

$$HCO_3^- + H+ \leftrightarrow H_2CO_3$$

When metabolism produces an acid such as lactic acid, which is much stronger than carbonic acid, a proton is liberated, binds with bicarbonate and

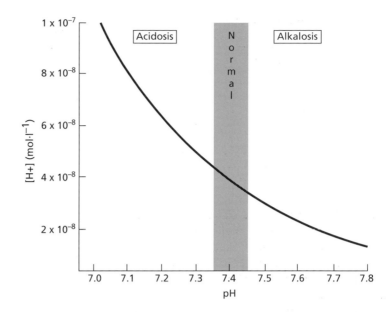

**Fig. 29.2** The relationship between [H+] and pH within the extreme physiological range.

forms sodium lactate and carbonic acid. Eventually this forms added carbon dioxide and water.

## Effects of sodium bicarbonate and citrate on performance

High-intensity exercise can be maintained for only short periods of time (Parry-Billings & MacLaren 1986). Energy for this type of activity comes predominantly from the anaerobic glycolysis system. In this process, energy is provided in the absence of oxygen as shown in the following equation:

$$Glycogen + 3\,ADP + 3\,P_i \leftrightarrow 3\,ATP + 2\,lactic\ acid + 2H_2O$$

The energy for the muscle contractions then comes from the ATP molecules which are produced. The above equation indicates that the breakdown of glucose anaerobically results in the formation of lactic acid, which dissociates almost immediately at a normal physiological pH to a lactate anion and a proton [H+] (Brooks 1985), which in turn would decrease intramuscular pH (Fletcher & Hopkins 1907; Hermansen & Osnes 1972; Osnes & Hermansen 1972; Sahlin et al. 1978) if the H+ was not buffered. High rates of glycolysis decreases pH even further, which eventually shuts down the contractile process (Fuchs et al. 1970; Donaldson & Hermansen 1978; Bryant-Chase & Kushmerick 1988). Force generation in isolated muscle (Mainwood & Cechetto 1980) has also been shown to be pH sensitive. More specifically, the myofibrillar protein troponin does not bind as efficiently to calcium when pH decreases, and this impairs the formation of the actomyosin complex (Fuchs et al. 1970). This reaction is reversible, so that when pH is reversed, bringing it towards a normal level, recovery of force generation takes place (Bryant-Chase & Kushmerick 1988). Changes in pH have also been shown to have an effect on energy production (Hill & Lupton 1923; Hill 1955; Krebs 1964). When muscle intracellular pH reaches 6.3, the process of glycolysis is inhibited by an impairment of the activity of the glycolytic enzyme phosphofructokinase (Trivedi & Danforth 1966). In order to reduce or delay these fatigue-producing processes, the ingestion of sodium bicarbonate has been used both experimentally and practically.

Research into acid–base balance during exercise commenced many decades ago. Dennig et al. (1931) used acid salts to make runners more

LIVERPOOL JOHN MOORES UNIVERSITY
LEARNING SERVICES

acidic and established that this regimen made them less able to use oxygen efficiently. In turn, this led the researchers to infer that induced alkalosis could have an opposite effect. Dill *et al.* (1932) demonstrated that runners could have a 1% decrease in running times when alkalotic. While it has been shown previously the muscle cell membranes are impervious to $HCO_3^-$ (Katz *et al.* 1984; Costill *et al.* 1988), an increase in extracellular $HCO_3^-$ increases the pH gradient between the intracellular and extracellular environment. The effect of this increased pH gradient is to facilitate the efflux of intracellular lactate and $H^+$, thus reducing the fall in intracellular pH (Katz *et al.* 1984; Costill *et al.* 1988). Both lactate and $H^+$ have been shown to follow a favourable pH gradient (Roth & Brooks 1990). The time course for the production of lactate has been shown to vary from 5s (Pernow & Wahren 1968; Saltin *et al.* 1971; Jacobs *et al.* 1983) to several minutes (Wilkes *et al.* 1983). In an early, well-conducted study, Osnes and Hermansen (1972) measured postexercise blood lactate levels in subjects who ran distances from 100 to 5000 m. Lactate concentrations increased with increasing distance up to 1500 m, after which there was no further increase: pH and blood bicarbonate concentrations were lowest after the 1500-m run. This would seem to suggest that acid–base balance shifts occur most dramatically after exercise lasting 4–5 min. It is reasonable to assume, therefore, that if sodium bicarbonate were to be effective as an ergogenic aid, it would be so over a similar time span, since these time periods are dependent upon high rates of energy production from anaerobic glycolysis.

There has been some suggestion that the mechanisms whereby sodium bicabonate loading is effective lie not with the bicarbonate ion but are possibly due to the sodium load (Saltin 1964; Kozak-Collins *et al.* 1994). Sodium could change intravascular volume, which in turn could alter performance. Kozak-Collins *et al.* (1994) tested this hypothesis with the ingestion of either $NaHCO_3$ or NaCl, which both provided equimolar amounts of sodium given prior to repeated bouts of 1-min exercise. Performance was not enhanced in either condition but haematocrit measures suggested that intravascular fluid status remained similar. pH was significantly raised in the bicarbonate trial when compared with that in the NaCl trial. Further studies are required to determine whether intravascular volume is responsible for the increased performance.

A greater understanding of acid–base balance during rest and exercise can be gained by reading Jackson (1990), Jones (1990), Lindinger and Heigenhauser (1990) and Heigenhauser *et al.* (1990).

The work of Jervell (1928), Dennig *et al.* (1931) and Dill *et al.* (1932) was, by and large, forgotten by the coaching and scientific communities. The modern era of the study of acid–base balance during exercise performance essentially began in the 1970s, with publication of the work of Jones *et al.* (1977). These workers studied five men who acted as their own controls, through treatments consisting of either a placebo (calcium carbonate), 0.3 g ammonium chloride (acidic) per kilogram of body mass, or sodium bicarbonate in the same dosage. All doses were taken after an overnight fast and over a 3-h time period. The exercise consisted of cycle ergometry utilizing three different protocols: 20 min at both 33% and 66% of previously determined maximum oxygen uptake ($\dot{V}o_{2max.}$), followed by exercise to exhaustion at 95% $\dot{V}o_{2max.}$, without rest in between. Time to exhaustion at the 95% $\dot{V}o_{2max.}$ power output level was approximately 4 min for the control condition. In the bicarbonate treatment, exhaustion time was approximately twice that of the control, whilst in the acidic condition, it was about half the control time. Blood lactate concentration in the bicarbonate treatment was significantly greater ($P < 0.01$) than the control at both the 66% power output level and at exhaustion. In the ammonium chloride condition, blood lactate levels were significantly lower in these two work periods. Blood pH was consistently higher in the bicarbonate treatment group and lower in the ammonium chloride treatment than in the control during the dosing phase and throughout the exercise. At the start of the final exercise phase, pH in the bicarbonate treatment group was about 7.41, while the control was 7.34 and the acidic treatment was 7.19. At exhaustion, the pH was 7.34, 7.26 and 7.14, respectively.

A number of studies in the early 1980s suggested that ingestion of sodium bicarbonate could be effective in performance enhancement. Wilkes *et al.* (1983), conducting a field type study, examined six well-trained competitive 800-m runners and compared the effects of sodium bicarbonate, placebo (calcium carbonate) and control treatments. The substances were both given over a 2-h period in a dose of $300\,mg \cdot kg^{-1}$ body mass and water was taken *ad libitum* (average intake was 504 ml). Each subject completed their normal 30-min warm-up prior to the race. Each runner completed all three protocols, thus acting as his own control. In the bicarbonate condition, runners were 2.9 s faster, on average, than in the control condition ($P < 0.05$), while the control and placebo results were not significantly different. Control, placebo and bicarbonate mean times (min : s) were, respectively, 2 : 05.8, 2 : 05.1 and 2 : 02.9. While not particularly fast, the difference between control and bicarbonate (2.9 s) might mean the difference between first and last place within a race.

In work from our own laboratory, Goldfinch *et al.* (1988) saw improvements in 400-m race performance due to ingestion of sodium bicarbonate in six competitive, trained runners. The experimental design was similar to that of Wilkes *et al.* (1983), but with a major difference: the bicarbonate dose was $400\,mg \cdot kg^{-1}$ body mass. This was done deliberately in order to eliminate ambiguities around dose size. The control, the calcium carbonate placebo or the experimental treatment were given over a 1-h period in a low-energy drink to try to disguise the taste. Each of the subjects ran as part of a two-man competitive race to simulate, as closely as possible, real competition. The mean time of the bicarbonate ingestion group was 56.94 s, and was significantly better by 1.25 s ($P < 0.005$) than the control and placebo,

which were not different from each other. The time difference was equivalent to approximately a 10-m distance at the finish, again enough to warrant a first or last place finish.

A number of studies have also shown $NaHCO_3$ loading to be ineffective in delaying fatigue or improving performance. Katz *et al.* (1984) exercised eight trained men at 125% of their predetermined $\dot{V}o_{2max.}$ in either a bicarbonate or control condition. Bicarbonate was given in a dose of $200\,mg \cdot kg^{-1}$ body mass, while the placebo consisted of NaCl. No significant difference between the two conditions was noticed. In the bicarbonate condition, subjects cycled for 100.6 s, while with the placebo, the time to exhaustion was 98.6 s. These results are of interest, since even though pH and base excess (which is the measure of extra base above normal, principally bicarbonate ions) after correction for haemoglobin content (Guyton & Hall 1981) were significantly elevated following ingestion of sodium bicarbonate, no improvement in performance was seen. In other words, the bicarbonate increased the amount of buffer available to the body, but this was not used. The pH values seen after exercise in this experiment were lower in the control condition, possibly suggesting the subjects could have worked harder in the experimental condition, thus utilizing the extra buffer available. In another study from the same laboratory, Horswill and colleagues (1988) found no difference in performance when subjects performed four bouts of intense, 2-min sprint exercise. Again, the levels of blood bicarbonate were significantly elevated in two of the conditions tested prior to the performance tests, as was pH, but again this increased buffering capacity did not result in improved performance by the subjects.

A number of practical problems have arisen in the study of sodium bicarbonate loading due to the nature of the experimental paradigms used. That is, there is no single method employed by researchers in order to detect any benefit. While this is a natural process in research, from a practical sporting point of view it is a hindrance, as athletes are unable to make concrete choices about, for example, how much sodium bicarbonate/citrate should be used or over what time periods it is effective.

Several authors (Wijnen *et al.* 1984; McKenzie *et al.* 1986; Parry-Billings & MacLaren 1986) have used a research paradigm involving multiple exercise bouts interspersed with rest/recovery. The exercise periods have varied, but have been between 30 and 60 s with rest/recovery periods from 60 s (Wijnen *et al.* 1984; McKenzie *et al.* 1986) to 6 min (Parry-Billings & MacLaren 1986). The results of this work have generally been inconclusive. Wijnen *et al.* (1984) infused bicarbonate intravenously in one of two doses (180 or 360 mg·kg$^{-1}$ body mass) while subjects rode a cycle ergometer for 60 s with a rest period of 60 s, and repeated this a further three times. Both dosages of NaHCO$_3$ significantly raised pH ($P < 0.01$) above the control condition in a manner which was dependent upon the dosage. However, as has been shown in some studies previously, the increased pH did not lead to an increase in performance in all subjects. McKenzie *et al.* (1986) used a protocol similar to that of Wijnen *et al.* (1984), but used dosages of either 150 or 300 mg·kg$^{-1}$ body mass. Blood pH and blood bicarbonate levels increased in both experimental conditions when compared with the control treatment. When time to fatigue and the amount of work done were compared, the two experimental conditions both increased these parameters but with no difference between the two dose levels. In another interval type paradigm, Parry-Billings and MacLaren (1986) again found that a dose of 300 mg·kg$^{-1}$ body mass had no effect on 30 s of exercise when interspersed with 6-min recovery periods. Again, this was despite an increase in blood bicarbonate levels of approximately 8 mmol·l$^{-1}$ above control levels.

## Bicarbonate dose and exercise

Various studies have suggested, either directly or indirectly, that there is a minimum level of sodium bicarbonate ingestion needed to improve performance. Katz *et al.* (1984) found no differ-

ences in performance time on a cycle ergometer test at 125% $\dot{V}o_{2max.}$ after subjects ingested 200 mg NaHCO$_3$·kg$^{-1}$ body mass despite significant ($P < 0.001$) rises in pH prior to exercise. Blood bicarbonate and base excess also significantly increased and the hydrogen ion to lactate ratio (nmol/mmol) was significantly lower in the experimental trial than in the control trial, all of which suggest that buffering was available but for some reason was not effective. Horswill *et al.* (1988) also found no improvement in exercise performance with dosages between 100 and 200 mg·kg$^{-1}$. In this interesting experiment, the authors (Horswill *et al.* 1988) had subjects undertake four 2-min sprint tests after they had consumed either a placebo or one of three doses of sodium bicarbonate (100, 150 or 200 mg·kg$^{-1}$). Pretest plasma bicarbonate levels were not different, nor were they different between the placebo and 100 mg·kg$^{-1}$ groups 1 h after the test, but they were significantly increased in the 150 and 200 mg·kg$^{-1}$ conditions. Even though plasma bicarbonate levels increased with the latter dosages, subjects were still unable to use the increased buffer capacity given by the NaHCO$_3$.

In a study from our laboratory (McNaughton 1992a), we attempted to extend the work of Horswill *et al.* (1988) to determine which dosage was most efficacious. We also decided to use an exercise bout of 60 s, since previous experience had led us to believe this would elicit high blood lactate levels and low levels of blood pH. Each of the subjects undertook a total of seven tests: one control, one placebo and one of five doses of NaHCO$_3$ (100, 200, 300, 400 and 500 mg·kg$^{-1}$) (Fig. 29.3). These were undertaken in a random fashion, after the control test, which was always first. The ingestion of sodium bicarbonate as a dose of 100 mg·kg$^{-1}$ did not increase blood bicarbonate levels, in agreement with the work of Horswill *et al.* (1988). Larger doses had the effect of significantly increasing the levels of blood bicarbonate.

Unlike Horswill *et al.* (1988), this author found a significant increase in performance with a dose of 200 mg·kg$^{-1}$ and this improvement increased

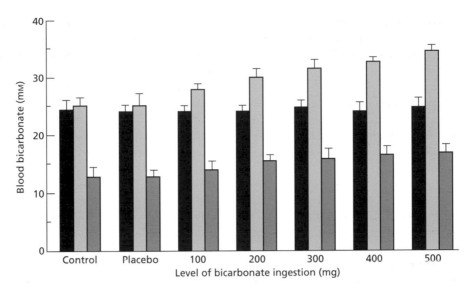

**Fig. 29.3** Bicarbonate levels in the blood after the ingestion of different levels of sodium bicarbonate, before and after exercise. ■, before exercise, ▢, after ingestion; ▨, after exercise. From McNaughton (1992a).

in a linear fashion with increasing dosage. Improvements in performance, however, did not follow the increasing levels of blood bicarbonate, with the highest amount of work being performed after a dosage of $300\,mg \cdot kg^{-1}$, although there were no significant differences between 300, 400 or $500\,mg \cdot kg^{-1}$.

In another approach to answering the question of sodium bicarbonate and performance, Kindermann *et al.* (1977) intravenously induced metabolic alkalosis by infusing an 8.4% sodium bicarbonate solution until the arterial pH reached 7.5. They then had subjects exercise by running 400 m, but found no difference in performance when they compared them with performance in a control run. Similarly, Wijnen *et al.* (1984) found no differences in the fifth bout of an interval exercise regimen on a bicycle ergometer when $NaHCO_3$ was administered intravenously in a dosage of $180\,mg \cdot kg^{-1}$. Again, this was despite finding a significant increase in pH in the 30 min prior to the exercise test. In a second stage of this study (Wijnen *et al.* 1984), the authors used a higher dosage and found that a greater number (80%) of their subjects performed significantly better than in the control trial.

### Exercise time

A further question to be asked is, 'Over what time period is sodium bicarbonate effective?' The plethora of research papers examining the ergogenic benefits of $NaHCO_3$ have used time periods ranging from 30 s (McCartney *et al.* 1983) to 6 min (McNaughton & Cedaro 1991a).

McCartney and colleagues (1983) had six subjects perform 30 cycle ergometer tests in a control, an alkalosis and two acidotic trials, one caused by ammonium chloride ingestion and a respiratory acidosis trial caused by inhalation of a 5% $CO_2$ mixture. There were small, but not significant, differences in the amount of work accomplished by the subjects. In the alkalotic trial, the work accomplished was 101% of control, suggesting a difference of 0.3 s (over a 30-s trial), not statistically different, but certainly practically so!

We (McNaughton *et al.* 1991) investigated the effects of bicarbonate loading on anaerobic work and maximal power output during exercise of 60 s duration. The dosage of $NaHCO_3$ used was $400\,mg \cdot kg^{-1}$ body mass with a control and placebo trial which were randomly assigned to each of the eight subjects. The work output increased significantly ($P < 0.01$) in the experimental condition when compared with the control or placebo condition (9940, 9263 and 9288 J, respectively). In the $NaHCO_3$ trial, pretest blood bicarbonate levels increased significantly above either the resting or control/placebo pretest levels. An interesting finding in this study was that the peak power, as measured in watts, achieved by the subjects, also increased significantly ($P < 0.05$) in the experimental condition when compared with that in the control or placebo conditions.

In order to examine more closely the time periods over which sodium bicarbonate can be used as an ergogenic aid, McNaughton (1992b) studied four different time periods (10, 30, 120 and 240 s) with a dosage of $300 \, mg \cdot kg^{-1}$ body mass. Subjects ingested sodium bicarbonate or a placebo and undertook a control test. There were eight male subjects in each time group, and each subject undertook three test sessions. As is usual with a dosage of this size ($300 \, mg \cdot kg^{-1}$), the blood bicarbonate levels were increased in the experimental trial when compared with those in either the control or placebo trials. This was also true for the base excess and pH measurements. However, the work and power data collected during the cycle ergometer tests over the four time periods were only significantly different in the latter two time periods (120 and 240 s), even though the blood lactate levels in both the 10- and 30-s trial were significantly higher after exercise than the pre-exercise levels.

This work is in agreement with several other studies suggesting that $NaHCO_3$ loading is not effective for short-term anaerobic work (McCartney *et al.* 1983; Katz *et al.* 1984) but that it is effective for longer-term work (Wilkes *et al.* 1983; McKenzie *et al.* 1986; Goldfinch *et al.* 1988). McNaughton and Cedaro (1991) found the same dosage of sodium bicarbonate to be effective in rowing performance of 6 min duration using elite rowers.

## Sodium citrate

A number of authors (Simmons & Hardt 1973; Parry-Billings & MacLaren 1986; McNaughton 1990; McNaughton & Cedaro 1991b) have used sodium citrate as an alkalizing agent rather than sodium bicarbonate. The results of work from our laboratory (McNaughton 1990) would suggest that sodium citrate is an effective ergogenic substance when given in dosages between 300 and $500 \, mg \cdot kg^{-1}$ body mass, with anaerobic capacity increasing in a linear fashion in relation to these doses (McNaughton 1990). In relation to duration of exercise, the high dosage of sodium citrate appears to be effective in time periods of between 2 and 4 min (McNaughton & Cedaro 1991b). Sodium citrate does not appear to be an effective ergogen when used with short-term (30 s) maximal exercise (Parry-Billings & MacLaren 1986; McNaughton & Cedaro 1991b). A recent article (Potteiger *et al.* 1996) has also suggested that large doses ($500 \, mg \cdot kg^{-1}$ body mass) of sodium citrate may improve 30-km cycling performance. These competitive cyclists completed the placebo 30-km trial in $3562.3 \pm 108.5$ s, while in the citrate trial they completed the same distance in $3459.6 \pm 97.4$ s. More work needs to be undertaken to determine if this regimen can be applied to other endurance activities.

Some subjects have reported short-term gastrointestinal distress as a side-effect of sodium bicarbonate/citrate use (Wilkes *et al.* 1983; Goldfinch *et al.* 1988; McNaughton & Cedaro 1991b). Other possible side-effects have been noted including gastric rupture (Downs & Stonebridge 1989; Reynolds 1989), muscle spasms and cardiac arrhythmias (Reynolds 1989; Heigenhauser & Jones 1991).

Although detection of sodium bicarbonate and citrate is difficult, several authors (Wilkes *et al.* 1983; Gledhill 1984; McKenzie 1988) have suggested it is possible to detect, and therefore control, using existing procedures (urine sample, post-exercise). The work of McKenzie (1988) is most detailed, with subjects providing a post-exercise urine sample. Of the 65 subjects, no subjects who had ingested $NaHCO_3$ had a urinary pH of less than 6.8, whereas in the placebo group, none was greater than a pH of 7.0. McKenzie (1988) suggested using a pH of 7.0 as a baseline, which would have captured 92% of the subjects using NaHCO$_3$ in his study. Even though this was the case in the McKenzie (1988) study, other factors, such as vomiting, a high-carbohydrate diet (results in metabolic alkalosis) (Greenhaff *et al.* 1987a, 1987b, 1988a, 1988b), a high-protein diet (results in metabolic acidosis; Maughan & Greenhaff 1991), a vegetarian diet and a low glomerular filtration rate (Kiil 1990), can change the alkalinity of the urine which normally ranges from 4.5 to 8.2, thus giving a false positive result (for a review, see Charney & Feldman 1989). It would be virtually impossible to detect confidently those who had used a buffering agent to improve performance.

## Conclusion

Several reviews on the use of substances to induce metabolic alkalosis in order to improve short-term maximal performance have been written (Gledhill 1984; Heigenhauser & Jones 1991; Linderman & Fahey 1991; Maughan & Greenhaff 1991; Williams 1992; McNaughton *et al.* 1993; Linderman & Gosselink 1994). Although no firm conclusions can be drawn from the plethora of research conducted, there does appear to be some general agreement on a number of factors. Firstly, both sodium bicarbonate and sodium citrate are effective buffering agents. Second, there is a minimum level of NaHCO$_3$ or sodium citrate ingestion below which no improvement in performance takes place and this is approximately 200 mg·kg$^{-1}$ body mass; the optimum dosage would appear to be only slightly higher, at 300 mg·kg$^{-1}$ body mass. Dosages higher than 300 mg·kg body mass do not appear to have any greater benefit to performance. Higher dosages of sodium citrate may be more effective than sodium bicarbonate, but this has not yet been confirmed. Thirdly, these buffering agents have no effect on performance of less than 30 s but do enhance performance between 1 and 10 min. Finally, these substances

may be effective in enhancing high-intensity endurance performance but more work needs to be conducted.

## Practical implications

Many substances used by athletes to improve performance have been banned by such bodies as the International Olympic Committee (IOC). Presently, no ban exists for the use of sodium bicarbonate or sodium citrate and they are hard to detect. However, their use may be considered a violation of the IOC Doping Rule which states, at least in part, that athletes shall not use any physiological substance taken in an attempt to artificially enhance performance. An athlete may attempt to legitimize the use of these substances, however, by likening it to the use of carbohydrate loading. If athletes decide to use these buffering agents, then they should do so for short-term, high-intensity exercise only and should use dosages of approximately 300 mg·kg$^{-1}$ body mass dose. The substances should be taken in or with fluid, preferably water, and in large quantities (0.5 l or greater). Subjects should be made familiar with possible side-effects prior to usage.

## References

Brooks, G.A. (1985) Anaerobic threshold: review of the concept and directions for future research. *Medicine and Science in Sports and Exercise* **17**, 22–31.

Bryant-Chase, P. & Kushmerick, M.J. (1988) Effects of pH on contraction of rabbit fast and slow skeletal muscle fibres. *Biophysics Journal* **53**, 935–946.

Charney, A.N. & Feldman, F. (1989) Internal exchanges of hydrogen ions: gastrointestinal tract. In *The Regulation of Acid-Base Balance* (ed. D.W. Seldin & G. Giebisch), pp. 89–105. Raven Press, New York.

Costill, D.L., Flynn, M.G. & Kirwan, J.P. (1988) Effects of repeated days of intensified training on muscle glycogen and swimming performance. *Medicine and Science in Sports and Exercise* **20**, 249–254.

Dennig, H., Talbot, J.H., Edwards, H.T. & Dill, B. (1931) Effects of acidosis and alkalosis upon the capacity for work. *Journal of Clinical Investigation* **9**, 601–613.

Dill, D.B., Edwards, H.T. & Talbot, J.H. (1932) Alkalosis and the capacity for work. *Journal of Biological Chemistry* **97**, 58–59.

Donaldson, S.K.B. & Hermansen, L. (1978) Differential direct effects of H+ and Ca2+-activated force of skinned fibres from the soleus, cardiac, adductor magnus muscle of rabbits. *Pflügers Archive* **376**, 55–65.

Downs, N. & Stonebridge, P. (1989) Gastric rupture due to excessive sodium bicarbonate ingestion. *Scottish Medical Journal* **34**, 534–535.

Edwards, R.H.T. (1981) Human muscle function and fatigue. In *Human Muscle Fatigue: Physiological Mechanisms* (ed. R. Porter & J. Whelan), Ciba Foundation Symposium No. 82, pp. 1–18. Pitman Medical, London.

Fletcher, W.W. & Hopkins, F.G. (1907) Lactic acid in mammalian muscle. *Journal of Physiology* **35**, 247–303.

Fuchs, F., Reddy, Y. & Briggs, F.N. (1970) The interaction of cations with the calcium binding site of troponin. *Biochimica Biophysica Acta* **221**, 407–409.

Gledhill, N. (1984) Bicarbonate ingestion and anaerobic performance. *Sports Medicine* **1**, 177–180.

Goldfinch, J., McNaughton, L.R. & Davies, P. (1988) Bicarbonate ingestion and its effects upon 400-m racing time. *European Journal of Applied Physiology* **57**, 45–48.

Green, H.J. (1990) Manifestations and sites of neuromuscular fatigue. In *Biochemistry of Exercise*. Vol. 7 (ed. A.W. Taylor, P.D. Gollnick, H.J. Green *et al.*), pp. 13–35. Human Kinetics, Champaign, IL.

Green, H.J., Jones, S. & Mills, D. (1987) Interactive effects of post-tetanic potentiation on low frequency fatigue in human muscle. *Federation Proceedings* **46**, 640–644.

Greenhaff, P.L., Gleeson, M. & Maughan, R.J. (1987a) The effects of dietary manipulation on blood acid base status and performance of high intensity exercise. *European Journal of Applied Physiology* **56**, 331–337.

Greenhaff, P.L., Gleeson, M., Whiting, P.H. & Maughan, R.J. (1987b) Dietary composition and acid-base status: limiting factors in performance of maximal exercise in man? *European Journal of Applied Physiology* **56**, 444–450.

Greenhaff, P.L., Gleeson, M. & Maughan, R.J. (1988a) Diet induced metabolic acidosis and the performance of high intensity exercise in man. *European Journal of Applied Physiology* **57**, 583–590.

Greenhaff, P.L., Gleeson, M. & Maughan, R.J. (1988b) The effect of a glycogen-loading regimen on acid base status and blood lactate concentrations before and after a fixed period of high intensity exercise in man. *European Journal of Applied Physiology* **57**, 254–259.

Guyton, A.C. & Hall, J.E. (1996) *Textbook of Medical Physiology*, 9th edn. W.B. Saunders, Philadelphia, PA.

Heigenhauser, G.J.F. & Jones, N.L. (1991) Bicarbonate loading. In *Perspectives in Exercise Science and Sports Medicine*. Vol. 4. *Ergogenics Enhancement of Performance in Exercise and Sport* (ed. D.R. Lamb & M.H. Williams), pp. 183–212. Wm C. Brown, Dubuque, IA.

Heigenhauser, G.J.F., Jones, N.L., Kowalchuk, J.M. & Lindinger, M.I. (1990) The role of the physiochemical systems in plasma in acid base control in exercise. In *Biochemistry of Exercise*. Vol. 7 (ed. A.W. Taylor, P.D. Gollnick, H.J. Green *et al.*), pp. 359–374. Human Kinetics, Champaign, IL.

Hermansen, L. & Osnes, J. (1972) Blood and muscle pH after maximal exercise in man. *Journal of Applied Physiology* **32**, 304–308.

Hill, A.V. (1955) The influence of the external medium on the internal pH of the muscle. *Proceedings of the Royal Society of London* **144**, 1–22.

Hill, A.V. & Lupton, H. (1923) Muscular exercise, lactic acid and the supply and utilization of oxygen. *Quarterly Journal of Medicine* **16**, 135–171.

Horswill, C.A., Costill, D.L., Fink, W.J. *et al.* (1988) Influence of sodium bicarbonate on sprint performance, relationship to dosage. *Medicine and Science in Sports and Exercise* **20**, 566–569.

Hultman, E., Bergstrom, M., Spriet, L.L. & Soderlund, K. (1990) Energy metabolism and fatigue. In *Biochemistry of Exercise*. Vol. 7 (ed. A.W. Taylor, P.D. Gollnick, H.J. Green *et al.*), pp. 73–92. Human Kinetics, Champaign, IL.

Jackson, D.C. (1990) Ion regulation in exercise: lessons from comparative physiology. In *Biochemistry of Exercise*. Vol. 7. (ed. A.W. Taylor, P.D. Gollnick, H.J. Green *et al.*), pp. 375–386. Human Kinetics, Champaign, IL.

Jacobs, I., Tesch, P.A., Bar-Or, O., Karlsson, J. & Dotan, R. (1983) Lactate in human skeletal muscle after 10 and 30s of supramaximal exercise. *Journal of Applied Physiology* **55**, 365–367.

Jervell, O. (1928) Investigation of the concentration of lactic acid in blood and urine. *Acta Medica Scandinavica* **24** (Suppl.), 1–135.

Jones, N.L. (1990) [H+] control in exercise: concepts and controversies. In *Biochemistry of Exercise*. Vol. 7 (ed. A.W. Taylor, P.D. Gollnick, H.J. Green *et al.*), pp. 333–339. Human Kinetics, Champaign, IL.

Jones, N., Sutton, J.R., Taylor, R. & Toews, C.J. (1977) Effect of pH on cardiorespiratory and metabolic responses to exercise. *Journal of Applied Physiology* **43**, 959–964.

Katz, A., Costill, D.L., King, D.S., Hargreaves, M. & Fink, W.J. (1984) Maximal exercise tolerance after induced alkalosis. *International Journal of Sports Medicine* **5**, 107–110.

Kiil, F. (1990) The paradox of renal bicarbonate reabsorption. *News in Physiology and Science* **5**, 13–17.

Kindermann, W., Keul, J. & Huber, G. (1977) Physical exercise after induced alkalosis (bicarbonate and tris-buffer). *European Journal of Applied Physiology* **37**, 197–204.

Kozak-Collins, K., Burke, E. & Schoene, R.B. (1994) Sodium bicarbonate ingestion does not improve cycling performance in women cyclists. *Medicine and Science in Sports and Exercise* **26**, 1510–1515.

Krebs, H. (1964) Gluconeogenesis. *Proceedings of the Royal Society of London* (Series B) **159**, 545–564.

Linderman, J. & Fahey, T.D. (1991) Sodium bicabonate ingestion and exercise performance: an update. *Sports Medicine* **11**, 71–77.

Linderman, J.K. & Gosselink, K.L. (1994) The effects of sodium bicarbonate ingestion on exercise perfor-mance. *Sports Medicine* **18**, 75–80.

Lindinger, M.I. & Heigenhauser, G.J.F. (1990) Acid base systems in skeletal muscle and their response to exercise. In *Biochemistry of Exercise*. Vol. 7 (ed. A.W. Taylor, P.D. Gollnick, H.J. Green *et al.*), pp. 341–357. Human Kinetics, Champaign, IL.

McCartney, N., Heigenhauser, G.F.C. & Jones, N.L. (1983) Effects of pH on maximal power output and fatigue during short term dynamic exercise. *Journal of Applied Physiology* **55**, 225–229.

McKenzie, D.C. (1988) Changes in urinary pH follow-ing bicarbonate loading. *Canadian Journal of Sports Science* **13**, 254–256.

McKenzie, D.C., Coutts, K.D., Stirling, D.R., Hoeben, H.H. & Kuzara, G. (1986) Maximal work production following two levels of artificially induced metabolic alkalosis. *Journal of Sports Science* **4**, 35–38.

McNaughton, L.R. (1990) Sodium citrate and anaerobic performance: implications of dosage. *European Journal of Applied Physiology* **61**, 392–397.

McNaughton, L.R. (1992a) Bicarbonate ingestion: effects of dosage on 60s cycle ergometry. *Journal of Sports Science* **10**, 415–423.

McNaughton, L.R. (1992b) Sodium bicarbonate inges-tion and its effects on anaerobic exercise of differing durations. *Journal of Sports Science* **10**, 425–435.

McNaughton, L.R. & Cedaro, R. (1991a) The effect of sodium bicarbonate on rowing ergometer perfor-mance in elite rowers. *Australian Journal of Science and Medicine in Sport* **23**, 66–69.

McNaughton, L.R. & Cedaro, R. (1991b) Sodium citrate ingestion and its effects on maximal anaerobic exer-cise of different durations. *European Journal of Applied Physiology* **64**, 36–41.

McNaughton, L.R., Curtin, R., Goodman, G., Perry, D., Turner, B. & Showell, C. (1991) Anaerobic work and power output during cycle ergometer exercise: Effects of bicarbonate loading. *Journal of Sports Science* **9**, 151–160.

Mainwood, G.W. & Cechetto, D. (1980) The effect of

bicarbonate concentration on fatigue and recovery in isolated rat diaphragm. *Canadian Journal of Physiology and Pharmacology* **58**, 624–632.

Maughan, R.J. & Greenhaff, P.L. (1991) High intesnity exercise performance and acid-base balance: the influence of diet and induced metabolic alkalosis. In *Advances in Nutrition and Top Sport* (ed. F. Brouns), pp. 147–165. Karger, Basel.

Osnes, J.B. & Hermansen, L. (1972) Acid-base balance after maximal exercise of short duration. *Journal of Applied Physiology* **32**, 59–63.

Parry-Billings, M. & MacLaren, D.P.M. (1986) The effect of sodium bicarbonate and sodium citrate ingestion on anaerobic power during intermittent exercise. *European Journal of Applied Physiology* **55**, 224–229.

Pernow, B. & Wahren, J. (1968) Lactate and pyruvate formation and oxygen utilization in the human forearm muscle during work of high intensity and varying duration. *Acta Physiologica Scandinavica* **56**, 267–285.

Potteiger, J.A., Nickel, G.L., Webster, M.J., Haub, M.D. & Palmer, R.J. (1996) Sodium citrate ingestion enhances 30 km cycling performance. *International Journal of Sports Medicine* **17**, 7–11.

Reynolds, J. (1989) *The Extra Pharmacopoeia*. Pharma-ceutical Press, London.

Robergs, R.A. & Roberts, S.O. (1997) *Exercise Physiology Exercise, Performance and Clinical Applications*. Mosby, St Louis, MO.

Roth, D.A. & Brooks, G.A. (1990) Lactate and pyruvate transport is dominated by a pH gradient-sensitive carrier in rat skeletal muscle sarcolemmal vesicles. *Archives in Biochemistry and Biophysics* **279**, 386–394.

Sahlin, K., Alvestrand, A., Brandt, R. & Hultman, E. (1978) Acid-base balance in blood during exhaustive bicycle exercise and the following recovery period, *Acta Physiologica Scandinavica* **104**, 370–372.

Saltin, B., Gollnick, P.D., Eriksson, B.O. & Piehl, K. (1971) Metabolic and circulatory adjustments at onset of maximal work. In *Onset of Exercise* (ed. A. Gilbert & P. Guile), pp. 63–76. University of Toulouse Press, Toulouse.

Saltin, G. (1964) Aerobic and anaerobic work capacity after dehydration. *Journal of Applied Physiology* **19**, 114–118.

Simmons, R.W.F. & Hardt, A.B. (1973) The effect of alkali ingestion on the performance of trained swim-mers. *Journal of Sports Medicine* **13**, 159–163.

Trivedi, B. & Danforth, W.H. (1966) Effect of pH on the kinetics of frog muscle phosphofructokinase. *Journal of Biological Chemistry* **241**, 4110–4114.

Vick, R.L. (1984) *Contemporary Medical Physiology*. Addison Wesley, Menlo Park, CA.

Wijnen, S., Verstappen, F. & Kuipers, H. (1984) The

influence of intravenous $NaHCO_3^-$ administration on interval exercise: acid-base balance and endurance. *International Journal of Sports Medicine* **5**, 130–132.

Wilkes, D., Gledhill, N. & Smyth, R. (1983) Effect of acute induced metabolic alkalosis on 800-m racing time. *Medicine and Science in Sports and Exercise* **15**, 277–280.

Williams, M.H. (1992) Bicarbonate loading. *Gatorade Sports Science Exchange* **4**(36), 1–6.

# Chapter 30

# Alcohol in Sport

LOUISE M. BURKE AND RONALD J. MAUGHAN

## Introduction

Ancient civilizations dating back to thousands of years BC recorded the intake of drinks containing alcohol (or, more correctly, ethanol) as part of social rituals. One practice which has persisted, even throughout the last decades, is the intake of alcohol before or during sport in the belief that it might improve performance (for review, see Williams 1991). Today, the major strong link between sport and alcohol is through sponsorship and advertising, with many sporting organizations, leagues, teams and events being financed by beer and liquor brewing companies. While a small number of athletes may still consume alcohol specifically to attempt to improve their sports performance, the overwhelming majority of athletes who drink alcohol, do so for social reasons. However, this is often in the context of rituals that are part of the culture of their sport. The aim of this chapter is to overview the effect of alcohol on sports performance, particularly related to the typical patterns of consumption by athletes, and to provide some guidelines for sensible use of alcohol by sports people.

## Alcohol use by athletes

Typically, alcohol intake provides less than 5% of the total energy intake of adults, although recent UK data suggest that alcohol accounted on average for 6.9% of the total energy intake of men aged between 18 and 64 years (Gregory et al.

1990); the corresponding value for women was 2.8%. Since the contribution to total energy intake is regarded as minor, it is often excluded from the results of dietary surveys of athletes. Furthermore, while the general limitations of dietary survey methodology are acknowledged, it is likely that self-reported data on alcohol intake are particularly flawed. For example, people are unlikely to report accurately and reliably about their consumption of a nutrient or food that is regarded so emotively; there is potential for both significant under-reporting and over-reporting. These factors help to explain the lack of reliable data on the alcohol intakes and drinking practices of athletes. It is also important to note that, because many people abstain completely from alcohol, the data are skewed, and mean values may be misleading: in the survey of Gregory et al. (1990) quoted above, for example, men and women who were alcohol drinkers obtained an average of 8.7% and 4.3%, respectively, of total energy from alcohol.

There are clearly gender-related differences in consumption patterns, but age, socio-economic background, and geographical location also influence drinking habits. It is not clear whether the consumption patterns of athletes are greatly different from those of the non athletic population. In general, though, dietary surveys of athletes which include alcohol suggest that it contributes 0–5% of total energy intake in the everyday diet. However, there is evidence that this provides a misleading view of the alcohol intakes of athletes. For example, in a dietary survey of 45 professional football players from the leading team in the national Australian Rules Football League, mean daily alcohol intake was estimated to be 20 g, accounting for 3.5% of total energy intake (Burke & Read 1988). However, these players rarely drank alcohol during the training week, in accordance with the club policy, and instead confined their intake to weekends, particularly after the weekly football match. Closer examination of the football data revealed that the mean intake of alcohol immediately after the match was 120 g (range, 27–368 g), with alcohol providing a mean contribution of 19% of total energy intake on match day (range, 3–43% of total energy intake).

Such 'binge' drinking practices were confirmed in a separate study in these same subjects. Blood samples were taken from 41 players who attended a 9.00 a.m. training session on the morning following a weekend match. Fourteen of these players still registered a positive blood alcohol content (BAC) from their previous evening's intake, with levels ranging from 0.001 to 0.113 g · 100 ml⁻¹. Blood alcohol content in four players exceeded the legal limit for driving a motor vehicle (0.05 g · 100 ml⁻¹). The lay press provides ample anecdotal evidence of binge drinking patterns of some athletes, particularly in the immediate celebration or commiseration of their competition performances, or in the off-season. In some cases these episodes are romanticized and the drinking prowess of the athletes is admired.

Whether total alcohol intake, or the prevalence of episodes of heavy alcohol intake, by athletes is different from that of the general population remains unclear. Surveys which have examined this issue report conflicting results. Various hypotheses have been proposed to explain likely associations between sport and alcohol use. It has been suggested that athletes might have a lower intake due to increased self-esteem, a more rigid lifestyle and greater interest in their health and performance. Equally, alcohol has been associated with the rituals of relaxation and celebration in sport, and it has been suggested that athletes might be socialized into certain behav-

iours and attitudes to drinking as a result of their sports participation.

Several dietary surveys comparing different groups of athletes have reported that the mean daily alcohol intakes of team sport athletes are significantly greater than those of athletes involved in endurance and strength sports (van Erp-Baart *et al.* 1989; Burke *et al.* 1991). While these studies were not specifically designed to collect data on alcohol intake, the findings are supported by data collected in some population surveys on alcohol use. Watten (1995), in a national survey of Norwegian adults, reported that men and women involved in team sports reported a higher intake of alcohol, particularly beer and liquor, than those involved in individual sports or those with no sports involvement. However, some of these differences were explained by the age and educational backgrounds of subjects. O'Brien (1993) reported difference between sports in alcohol use by elite Irish athletes, but the overall intake of this group was exceptionally low, at an average of 0.5% of total energy intake.

Clearly, while there is anecdotal evidence to suggest that some athletes may consume alcohol in excessive amounts, on at least some occasions, further studies are needed to fully determine the alcohol intake and patterns of use by athletes. Information on the attitudes and beliefs of athletes about alcohol is also desirable, since it would allow education about current drinking practices which are detrimental to the athlete's performance or health to be specifically targeted.

## Metabolism of alcohol

The metabolism of ethanol occurs primarily in the liver, where it is oxidized, first to acetaldehyde, and then to acetate. The first step is catalysed by a number of hepatic enzymes, the most important of which is the nicotinamide adenine dinucleotide (NAD)-dependent alcohol dehydrogenase:

$$CH_3CH_2OH + NAD^+ \rightarrow CH_3CHO + NADH + H^+$$

Aldehyde dehydrogenase catalyses the further oxidation of acetaldehyde to acetate:

$$CH_3CHO + NADH^+ + H_2O \rightarrow CH_3COO^- + NADH + 2H^+$$

The NADH which is formed in these reactions must be reoxidized within the mitochondria, but transfer of the hydrogen atoms into the mitochondria might be a limiting process leading to an alteration in the redox potential of the cell. This can interfere with the conversion of lactate to pyruvate, and explains the increased blood lactate concentration that may be observed after high alcohol intakes.

Acetaldehyde is metabolized within the liver, and the acetaldehyde concentration in the blood remains low, but it is acetaldehyde that is thought to be responsible for many of the adverse effects of ethanol. The rate of hepatic gluconeogenesis is markedly suppressed by the metabolism of ethanol as a result of the altered NAD/NADH ratio and the reduced availability of pyruvate (Krebs *et al.* 1969). If the liver glycogen stores are low because of a combination of exercise and a low carbohydrate intake, the liver will be unable to maintain the circulating glucose concentration, leading to hypoglycaemia. The rate at which ethanol is cleared by the liver varies widely between individuals, and the response of the individual will depend on the amount of ethanol consumed in relation to the habitual intake. It is not altogether clear whether the rate of metabolism of alcohol is increased by exercise, and there are conflicting data in the literature (Januszewski & Klimek 1974). Table 30.1 indicates the amount of alcohol contained in some standard measures.

## Effects of acute alcohol ingestion on exercise

The variety of effects of alcohol on different body tissues, and the variability of subject responses to alcohol, make it difficult to study the direct effects on sports performance. Generally, the ergogenic benefits of alcohol intake immediately before and during exercise are psychologically

**Table 30.1** A standard drink contains approximately 10 g of alcohol.

| Drink | Amount (ml) |
| --- | --- |
| Standard beer (4% alcohol) | 250 |
| Low alcohol beer (2% alcohol) | 500 |
| Cider, wine coolers, alcoholic soft drinks | 250 |
| Wine | 100 |
| Champagne | 100 |
| Fortified wines, sherry, port | 60 |
| Spirits | 30 |

driven. Alcohol has been used to decrease sensitivity to pain, improve confidence, and to remove other psychological barriers to performance. However, it may also be used to stimulate the cardiovascular system, or to lessen the tremor and stress-induced emotional arousal in fine motor control sports. Although it is no longer on the general doping list of the IOC, it is still considered a banned substance in some sports, such as shooting and fencing. In some sports, such as darts and billiards, it is still popularly used as a (proposed) performance aid, but it remains to be seen whether this simply reflects the culture of sports that are widely played in a hotel environment (for review, see Williams 1991).

### Exercise metabolism and performance

The American College of Sports Medicine (1982), and a more recent review by Williams (1991), have summarized the acute effects of alcohol ingestion on metabolism and performance of exercise. Alcohol does not contribute significantly to energy stores used for exercise, but in situations of prolonged exercise it may increase the risk of hypoglycaemia due to a suppression of hepatic gluconeogenesis. Increased heat loss may be associated with this hypoglycaemia as well as the cutaneous vasodilation caused by exercise, causing an impairment of temperature regulation in cold environments. Studies of the effects of alcohol on cardiovascular, respiratory and muscular function have provided conflicting results, but ingestion of small amounts of alcohol has been reported not to significantly alter the cardiorespiratory and metabolic responses to submaximal exercise (Bond *et al.* 1983; Mangum *et al.* 1986). Dose–response relationships, inter- and intrasubject variability, and difficulty with providing a suitable placebo may all help to explain the difficulty of conducting and interpreting alcohol studies. In general it has been concluded that the acute ingestion of alcohol has no beneficial effects on aspects of muscle function and performance tasks: because it may actually produce detrimental responses, it is best avoided.

The few studies of acute alcohol ingestion and actual sports performance show variability in results and responses. For example, Houmard and others (1987) reported that the ingestion of small amounts of alcohol (keeping BAC below $0.05\,g\cdot100\,ml^{-1}$) did not have a significant effect on the performance of a 8-km treadmill time trial, although there was a trend towards performance deterioration at higher blood alcohol levels. Meanwhile, McNaughton and Preece (1986) tested the performance of runners over various distances ranging from 100 to 1500 m, at four different levels of alcohol consumption (BAC estimated at $0–0.1\,g\cdot100\,ml^{-1}$). Alcohol intake did not affect performance of 100-m times in sprinters, but reduced performance over 200 and 400 m as alcohol intake increased. Middle-distance runners showed impaired performance in 800 and 1500 m run times, with these effects also being dose-related. An earlier study by Hebbelinck (1963) showed no effect of alcohol ($0.6\,ml$ of 94% ethanol $\cdot\,kg^{-1}$ body mass) on isometric strength, but a 6% reduction in vertical jump height and a 10% decrease in performance in an 80-m sprint.

### Motor control and skill performance

There is a limited amount of information available on the effects of acute ingestion of alcohol on motor control and the performance of skilled tasks. It is, however, clear from the controlled studies that have been conducted that alcohol has an adverse effect on tasks where concen-

tration, visual perception, reaction time, and co-ordination are involved (Williams 1995). In many of the earlier studies that showed a detrimental effect of even small doses of alcohol on components of athletic performance, the performance measures were not well standardized and the results are difficult to interpret. Hebbelinck (1963), however, showed that posture control deteriorated after alcohol ingestion, with both the extent and frequency of sway being markedly increased: this represents a mild version of the unsteadiness and ataxia that is apparent after higher levels of alcohol intake.

In 1982, the American College of Sports Medicine published a Position Statement on the use of alcohol in sports, and this included a review of the research to date on the effects of alcohol on performance: this literature was also reviewed by Williams (1985). The available evidence showed a detrimental effect of small to moderate amounts of alcohol on reaction time, hand–eye co-ordination, accuracy, balance and complex skilled tasks, with no evidence cited to support the purported beneficial effects of reduced tremor. It has, however, been proposed that the ingestion of small amounts of alcohol may result in a greater feeling of self-confidence in athletes (Shephard 1972), and this may, in turn, improve performance in some situations. The interference of alcohol with the judgement and skill involved in the fine motor skills required for driving accounts for the legislation to prevent individuals who have been drinking from driving automobiles.

### Effects of acute alcohol ingestion on postexercise recovery

There is evidence that the postcompetition situation is often associated with alcohol intake and binge drinking, and it is likely that social rituals after training or practice sessions in some sports (particularly in lower level competitions) may also involve moderate to heavy intake of alcohol. Given that athletes may be dehydrated and have eaten little on the day of competition, it is likely that alcohol consumed after exercise is more quickly absorbed and has increased effects. Therefore it is important to examine the effects of alcohol on processes that are important in the recovery from prolonged exercise, and on the performance of subsequent exercise bouts. Unfortunately, postexercise drinking is subject to many rationalizations and justifications by athletes, including 'everyone is doing it', 'I only drink once a week' and 'I can run/sauna it off the next morning'.

## Rehydration

The restoration of the body fluid deficit incurred during exercise is a balance between the amount of fluid that athletes can be induced to drink after exercise, and their ongoing fluid losses. The palatability of postexercise fluids is an important factor in determining total fluid intake, while replacement of sodium losses is a major determinant of the success in retaining this fluid (see Chapter 19). It has been suggested that beer is a valuable postexercise beverage since large volumes can be voluntarily consumed by some athletes! However, the absence of an appreciable sodium content (unless it is accompanied by the intake of salty foods), and the diuretic action of alcohol are factors that are likely to promote increased urine losses. A recent study (Shirreffs & Maughan 1997) examined the effect

of alcohol on postexercise rehydration from an exercise task which dehydrated subjects by 2% of body mass. Subjects replaced 150% of the volume of their fluid deficits with drinks containing 0%, 1%, 2% or 4% alcohol within 90 min of finishing the exercise. The total volume of urine produced during the 6 h of recovery was positively related to the alcohol content of the fluid. However, only in the 4% alcohol drink trial did the difference in total urine approach significance, with a net retention of 40% of ingested fluid compared with 59% in the no-alcohol trial, equating to a difference of about 500 ml in urine losses. Subjects were still dehydrated at the end of the recovery period with the 4% alcohol drink, despite having consumed 1.5 times the volume of their fluid deficit (Fig. 30.1). Although individual variability must be taken into account, this study suggests that the intake of significant amounts of alcohol will impede rehydration. It also indicated that beer is not a suitable rehydration drink, even in the low alcohol forms that are available, because of the low content of electrolytes, particularly sodium (Maughan & Shirreffs 1997).

In practical terms, low alcohol beers (<2% alcohol) or beer 'shandies' (beer mixed in equal proportions with lemonade, thus diluting the alcohol content and providing some carbohydrate) may not be detrimental to rehydration.

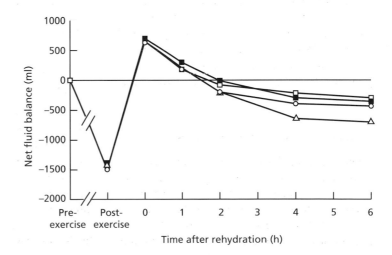

**Fig. 30.1** Whole-body water balance after exercise- induced dehydration followed by ingestion of a volume equal to 1.5 times the sweat loss of fluids containing alcohol at concentrations of 0% (□), 1% (■), 2% (○) and 4% (△). There is clearly an increasing urine output in the postingestion period as the alcohol concentration increases. Adapted from Shirreffs and Maughan (1997).

Furthermore, notwithstanding other effects of small to moderate amounts of alcohol, these drinks might be useful in encouraging large fluid intakes in dehydrated athletes. However, drinks with more a concentrated alcohol content are not advised, since the combination of a smaller fluid volume and a greater alcohol intake will reduce the rate of effective fluid replacement. Nevertheless, when aggressive rehydration is required, the planned intake of fluids containing sodium, or fluid intake in conjunction with sodium-rich foods, provides a more reliable strategy to replace fluid losses (see Chapter 19).

### Glycogen storage

Since alcohol has a number of effects on the intermediary metabolism of carbohydrate, it is possible that postexercise intake might impair the restoration of depleted glycogen stores. In the absence of carbohydrate intake, alcohol intake is known to impair the carbohydrate status of the liver by inhibiting hepatic gluconeogenesis and increasing liver glycogenolysis. Alcohol intake has been reported to impair muscle glycogen storage in rats following depletion by fasting or exercise (for review, see Palmer *et al.* 1991). The effect of alcohol intake on muscle glycogen storage in humans was recently studied by Burke and co-workers (in press), who undertook two separate studies to examine refuelling over 8 h and 24 h of recovery from a prolonged cycling bout.

In these studies, athletes undertook three different diets following their glycogen-deleting exercise: a control (high carbohydrate) diet, an alcohol displacement diet (kept isoenergetic with the control diet by reducing the carbohydrate intake) and an alcohol + carbohydrate diet (alcohol added to the control diet). In the two diets containing alcohol, the athletes were required to consume 1.5 g alcohol·kg$^{-1}$ body mass of alcohol in the 3 h immediately after exercise (e.g. ≈100 g alcohol or 10 standard drinks). Muscle glycogen storage was significantly reduced on the alcohol displacement diets in both the 8 h and 24 h study compared with the

high carbohydrate diets. There was a trend towards a reduction in glycogen storage over 8 h of recovery with alcohol + carbohydrate diet; however, glycogen storage on the alcohol + carbohydrate diet on the 24-h study was identical to the control diet. Therefore, there was no clear evidence of a direct impairment of muscle glycogen storage by alcohol when adequate substrate was provided to the muscle; however, this may have been masked by intersubject variability.

The results of these studies suggest that the major effect of alcohol intake on postexercise refuelling is indirect, that high intakes of alcohol are likely to prevent the athlete from consuming adequate carbohydrate intake to optimize muscle glycogen storage. In general, athletes who participate in alcoholic binges are unlikely to eat adequate food or make suitable high-carbohydrate food choices. Furthermore, food intake over the next day may also be affected as the athletes 'sleep off their hangover'. Further studies are needed to determine the direct effect of alcohol on muscle glycogen storage.

### Other effects

Alcohol is known to exert other effects which may impede postexercise recovery. Many sporting activities are associated with muscle damage and soft tissue injuries, either as a direct consequence of the exercise, as a result of accidents, or due to the tackling and collisions involved in contact sports. Standard medical practice is to treat soft tissue injuries with vasoconstrictive techniques (e.g. rest, ice, compression, elevation). Since alcohol is a potent vasodilator of cutaneous blood vessels, it has been suggested that the intake of large amounts of alcohol might cause or increase undesirable swelling around damaged sites, and might impede repair processes. Although this effect has not been systematically studied, there are case histories that report these findings. Until such studies are undertaken, it seems prudent that players who have suffered considerable muscle damage and soft tissue injuries should avoid alcohol in the immediate recovery phase (e.g. for 24 h after the event).

Another likely effect of cutaneous vasodilation following alcohol intake is an increase in heat loss from the skin. This may be exacerbated by hypoglycaemia, which results from the combined effects of carbohydrate depletion and impaired liver gluconeogenesis. Therefore, athletes who consume large quantities of alcohol in cold environments may incur problems with thermoregulation. An increased risk of hypothermia may be found in sports or recreational activities undertaken in cold weather, particularly hiking or skiing, where alcohol intake is an integral part of *après-ski* activities.

As in the case of postexercise refuelling, it is likely that the major effect of excessive alcohol intake comes from the athlete's failure to follow guidelines for optimal recovery. The intoxicated athlete may fail to undertake sensible injury management practices or to report for treatment; they may fail to seek suitable clothing or shelter in cold conditions or to notice early signs of hypothermia. While studies which measure the direct effect of alcohol on thermoregulation and soft tissue damage are encouraged, these effects are likely to be minor or at least additive to the failure to undertake recommended recovery practices.

## Accidents and high-risk behaviour

The most important effect of alcohol is the impairment of judgement. Coupled with a reduced inhibition, it is easy to see how intoxicated athletes might undertake high-risk behaviour and suffer an increased risk of accidents. Alcohol consumption is highly correlated with accidents of drowning, spinal injury and other problems in recreational water activities (see O'Brien 1993), and is a major factor in road accidents. The lay press frequently contains reports of well-known athletes being caught driving while severely intoxicated, or being involved in brawls or other situations of domestic or public violence. There have been a disturbing number of deaths of elite athletes in motor car accidents following excess alcohol intake. Clearly, athletes are not immune to the social and behavioural problems following excess alcohol intake; there is some discussion that certain athletes may be more predisposed (see O'Brien 1993). Further studies are required before it can be determined whether athletes, or some groups of athletes, are more likely to drink excessively or suffer a greater risk of alcohol-related problems. However, it appears that athletes should at least be included in population education programmes related to drink-driving and other high-risk behaviour.

## Effect of previous day's intake (i.e. 'hangover') on performance

Some athletes will be required to train (or even compete again) on the day after a competition and its postevent drinking binge. In some cases, athletes may choose to drink heavily the night before a competition, as a general part of their social activities, or in the belief that this will help to 'relax' them prior to the event. The effect of an 'alcohol hangover' on performance is widely discussed by athletes, but has not been well studied. Karvinen and coworkers (1962) used a crossover design to examine 'next day' performance following the consumption of large amounts of alcohol (approximately eight standard drinks), and reported that a hangover did not impair power or strength, but impaired the ability to undertake a bout of high-intensity cycling. O'Brien (1993) undertook 'aerobic' and 'anaerobic' testing of a team of Rugby Union players on a Friday night, and then requested them to return for repeat testing the next day after consuming their 'typical Friday night's alcohol intake'. A standardized sleep time and breakfast were followed. He reported that $\dot{V}O_{2max.}$ was significantly reduced the following day, and that any level of alcohol intake appeared to impair this measure of aerobic capacity. However, since no control trial was undertaken, it is hard to dissociate the effects of alcohol from the effects and variability of repeated testing. Meanwhile it is interesting to note that the mean alcohol intake reported by players as typical of their prematch activities was approximately 130 g (range, 1–38 units).

Research in other areas of industrial work (e.g. machine handling and flying) suggests that impairment of psychomotor skills may continue during the hangover phase. Clearly this will be of detriment in team sports and court sports which demand tactical play and a high skill level.

## Effects of chronic alcohol intake on issues of sports performance

Athletes who chronically consume large amounts of alcohol are liable to the large number of health and social problems associated with problem drinking. Early problems to have impact on sports performance include inadequate nutrition and generally poor lifestyle (e.g. inadequate rest). Since alcohol is an energy-dense nutrient (providing 27 kJ·g$^{-1}$), frequent episodes of heavy alcohol intake are generally accompanied by weight gain. Weekend binge drinkers tend to maintain their food consumption, since alcohol does not seem to regulate total energy intake in the short term. However, erratic eating patterns and choice of high fat foods can lead to excess energy consumption. A common issue, particularly in team sports, is the significant gain in body fat during the off-season due to increased alcohol intake coupled with reduced exercise expenditure. Many players need to devote a significant part of their pre-season (and even early season) conditioning to reversing the effects of their off-season activities. Clearly this is a disadvantage to performance and to the longevity of a sports career.

## Guidelines for sensible use of alcohol by athletes

The following guidelines are suggested to promote sensible use of alcohol by athletes.

1 Alcohol is not an essential component of a diet. It is a personal choice of the athlete whether to consume alcohol at all. However, there is no evidence of impairments to health and performance when alcohol is used sensibly.

2 The athlete should be guided by community guidelines which suggest general intakes of alcohol that are 'safe and healthy'. This varies from country to country, but in general, it is suggested that mean daily alcohol intake should be less than 40–50 g (perhaps 20–30 g·day$^{-1}$ for females), and that 'binge' drinking is discouraged. Since individual tolerance to alcohol is variable, it is difficult to set a precise definition of 'heavy' intake or an alcohol 'binge'. However, intakes of about 80–100 g at a single sitting are likely to constitute a heavy intake for most people.

3 Alcohol is a high-energy (and nutrient-poor) food and should be restricted when the athlete is attempting to reduce body fat.

4 The athlete should avoid heavy intake of alcohol on the night before competition. It appears unlikely that the intake of one or two standard drinks will have negative effects in most people.

5 The intake of alcohol immediately before or during exercise does not enhance performance and in fact may impair performance in many people. Psychomotor performance and judgement are most affected. Therefore the athlete should not consume alcohol deliberately to aid performance, and should be wary of exercise that is conducted in conjunction with the social intake of alcohol.

6 Heavy alcohol intake is likely to have a major impact on postexercise recovery. It may have direct physiological effects on rehydration, glycogen recovery and repair of soft tissue damage. More importantly, the athlete is unlikely to remember or undertake strategies for optimal recovery when they are intoxicated. Therefore, the athlete should attend to these strategies first before any alcohol is consumed. No alcohol should be consumed for 24 h in the case of an athlete who has suffered a major soft-tissue injury.

7 The athlete should rehydrate with appropriate fluids in volumes that are greater than their existing fluid deficit. Suitable fluid choices include sports drinks, fruit juices, soft drinks (all containing carbohydrate) and water (when refuelling is not a major issue). However, sodium replacement via sports drinks, oral rehydration

solutions or salt-containing foods is also important to encourage the retention of these rehydration fluids. Low alcohol beers and beer–soft drink mixes may be suitable and seem to encourage large volume intakes. However, drinks containing greater than 2% alcohol are not recommended as ideal rehydration drinks.

8 Before consuming any alcohol after exercise, the athlete should consume a high carbohydrate meal or snack to aid muscle glycogen recovery. Food intake will also help to reduce the rate of alcohol absorption and thus reduce the rate of intoxication.

9 Once postexercise recovery priorities have been addressed, the athlete who chooses to drink is encouraged to do so 'in moderation'. Drink-driving education messages in various countries may provide a guide to sensible and well-paced drinking.

10 Athletes who drink heavily after competition, or at other times, should take care to avoid driving and other hazardous activities.

11 It appears likely that it will be difficult to change the attitudes and behaviours of athletes with regard to alcohol. However, coaches, managers and sports medicine staff can encourage guidelines such as these, and specifically target the old wives tales and rationalizations that support binge drinking practices. Importantly, they should reinforce these guidelines with an infrastructure which promotes sensible drinking practices. For example, alcohol might be banned from locker rooms and fluids and foods appropriate to postexercise recovery provided instead. In many cases, athletes drink in a peer-group situation and it may be easier to change the environment in which this occurs than the immediate attitudes of the athletes.

## Conclusion

Alcohol is strongly linked with modern sport. The alcohol intakes and drinking patterns of athletes are not well studied; however, it appears that some athletes undertake binge drinking practices, often associated with postcompetition socializing. There is no evidence that alcohol improves sports performance; in fact there is evidence that intake during or immediately before exercise, or that large amounts consumed the night before exercise may actually impair performance. There are considerable differences in the individual responses to alcohol intake. It is likely that recovery after exercise is also impaired; but particularly by the failure of the intoxicated athlete to follow guidelines for optimum recovery. Athletes are not immune to alcohol-related problems, including the greatly increased risk of motor vehicle accidents following excess alcohol intake. Not only should athletes be targeted for education about sensible drinking practices, but they might be used as spokespeople for community education messages. Athletes are admired in the community and may be effective educators in this area. Alcohol is consumed by the vast majority of adults around the world, and merits education messages about how it might be used to enhance lifestyle rather than detract from health and performance.

## References

American College of Sports Medicine (1982) Position statement on the use of alcohol in sports. *Medicine and Science in Sports and Exercise* 14, ix–x.

Bond, V., Franks, B.D. & Howley, E.T. (1983) Effects of small and moderate doses of alcohol on submaximal cardiorespiratory function, perceived exertion and endurance performance in abstainers and moderate drinkers. *Journal of Sports Medicine* 23, 221–228.

Burke, L.M. & Read, R.S.D. (1988) A study of dietary patterns of elite Australian football players. *Canadian Journal of Sports Science* 13, 15–19.

Burke, L.M., Gollan, R.A. & Read, R.S.D. (1991) Dietary intakes and food use of groups of elite Australian male athletes. *International Journal of Sport Nutrition* 1, 378–394.

Burke, L.M., Collier, G.R., Broad, E.M. *et al.* (submitted for publication) The effect of alcohol intake on muscle glycogen storage following prolonged exercise.

Gregory, J., Foster, K., Tyler, H. & Wiseman, M. (1990) *The Dietary and Nutritional Survey of British Adults.* HMSO, London.

Hebbelinck, M. (1963) The effects of a small dose of ethyl alcohol on certain basic components of human physical performance. *Archives in Pharmacodynamics* 143, 247–257.

Houmard, J.A., Langenfeld, M.E., Wiley, R.L. & Siefert, J. (1987) Effects of the acute ingestion of small amounts of alcohol upon 5-mile run times. *Journal of Sports Medicine* **27**, 253–257.

Januszewski, J. & Klimek, A. (1974) The effect of physical exercise at varying loads on the elimination of blood alcohol. *Acta Physiologica Polonica* **25**, 541–545.

Karvinin, E.A., Miettinen, A. & Ahlman, K. (1962) Physical performance during hangover. *Quarterly Journal of Studies of Alcohol* **23**, 208–215.

Krebs, H.A., Freedland, R.A., Hems, R. & Stubbs, M.(1969) Inhibition of hepatic gluconeogenesis by ethanol. *Biochemistry Journal* **112**, 117–124.

McNaughton, L. & Preece, D. (1986) Alcohol and its effects on sprint and middle distance running. *British Journal of Sports Medicine* **20**, 56–59.

Mangum, M., Gatch, W., Cocke, T.B. & Brooks, E. (1986) The effects of beer consumption on the physiological responses to submaximal exercise. *Journal of Sports Medicine* **26**, 301–305.

Maughan, R.J. & Shirreffs, S.M. (1997) Recovery from prolonged exercise, restoration of water and electrolyte balance. *Journal of Sports Science* **15**, 297–303.

O'Brien, C.P. (1993) Alcohol and sport: impact of social drinking on recreational and competitive sports performance. *Sports Medicine* **15**, 71–77.

Palmer, T.N., Cook, E.B. & Drake, P.G. (1991) Alcohol abuse and fuel homeostasis. In *Alcoholism: A Molecular Perspective* (ed. T.N. Palmer), pp. 223–235. Plenum Press, New York.

Shephard, R. (1972) *Alive Man: The Physiology of Physical Activity*. CC Thomas, Springfield, IL.

Shirreffs, S.M. & Maughan, R.J. (1997) Restoration of fluid balance after exercise-induced dehydration, effects of alcohol consumption. *Journal of Applied Physiology* **83**, 1152–1158.

Van Erp-Baart, A.M.J., Saris, W.H.M., Binkhorst, R.A., Vos, J.A. & Elvers, J.W.H. (1989) Nationwide survey on nutritional habits in elite athletes. Part 1. Energy, carbohydrate, protein and fat intake. *International Journal of Sports Medicine* **10** (Suppl.), S3–S10.

Watten, R.G. (1995) Sports, physical exercise and use of alcohol. *Scandinavian Journal of Sports Medicine* **5**, 364–368.

Williams, M.H. (1985) *Nutritional Aspects of Human Physical and Athletic Performance*. CC Thomas, Springfield, IL.

Williams, M.H. (1991) Alcohol, marijuana and beta blockers. In: *Perspectives in Exercise Science and Sports Medicine. Vol. 4. Erogenics: Enhancement of Performance in Exercise and Sport* (ed. D.R. Lamb & M.H. Williams), pp. 331–372. Cooper Publishing Group, Carmel, CA.

Williams, M.H. (1995) *Nutrition for Fitness and Sport*. Brown & Benchmark, Madison.

# PART 2

## SPECIAL CONSIDERATIONS

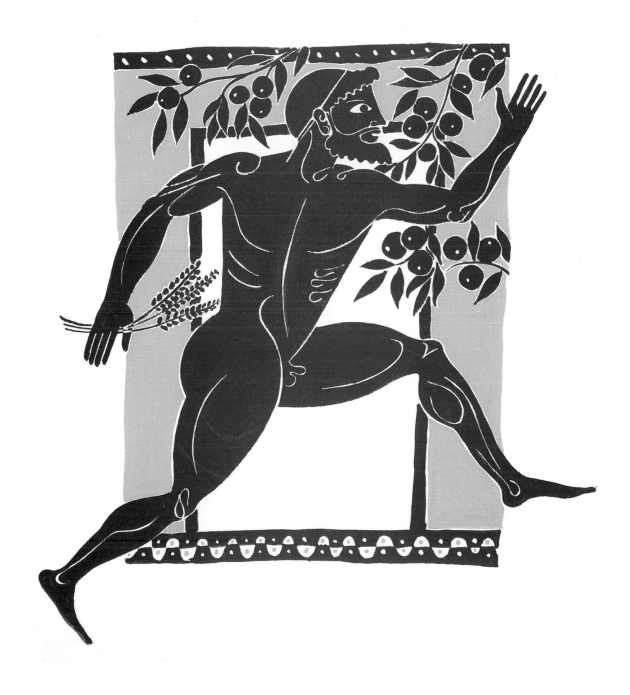

# Chapter 31

# The Female Athlete

KATHE A. GABEL

## Introduction

As increasing numbers of women participate in sport and exercise, recommendations for their dietary intake to enhance general health and performance become important. Unfortunately, physical and metabolic differences between men and women generally have not been considered in the development of current dietary guidelines, except for calcium and iron. However, gender differences exist that could potentially affect a woman's energy and nutrient needs: upper body muscle mass and strength (Miller *et al.* 1993), endurance capacity in isometric and dynamic exercise at relatively low intensities (Maughan *et al.* 1986), resting metabolic rate (Arciero *et al.* 1993) and heart rate measured during different exercise modalities (Kravitz *et al.* 1997). Rather than deriving recommendations from research involving mixed-gender or female populations, dietary guidelines for protein (Lemon 1995) and carbohydrate (CHO) (Williams 1989) intakes have been developed from studies using male subjects. In consideration of dietary guidelines for the female athlete, this chapter will address limitations of the use of current recommendations for athletes, present evidence for gender differences related to lipid and substrate metabolism and provide discussion regarding macro- and micronutrient recommendations. A brief clarification of terms used to define nutrient needs and recommendations for intake to meet these needs in populations and in individuals will precede these topics of discussion.

## Clarification of dietary guideline nomenclature

Terms that reflect estimates of nutrient requirements vary among countries. In the United Kingdom, nomenclature consists of *dietary reference values* (DRV), *estimated average requirement* (EAR), *lower reference nutrient intake* (LRNI) and *reference nutrient intake* (RNI) (Department of Health 1991). The term *recommended dietary allowance* (RDA) (National Research Council 1989) has traditionally been used in the United States, but is expected to change in the next edition of guidelines to terminology similar to that currently used in the UK. In Canada, recommended intakes of energy and certain nutrients are called *recommended nutrient intakes* (RNI) (Health and Welfare Canada 1983). To simplify reading, *dietary guideline* will be used in this chapter when referring to RNI, RDA or terms used by other countries.

## Limitations of the use of current dietary guidelines for athletes

Dietary guidelines used in the US are expressed as quantities of a nutrient for a reference individual *per day*, a term that should be interpreted as an average intake over time (National Research Council 1989). For dietary assessments of athletes, food intake should be recorded for a

417

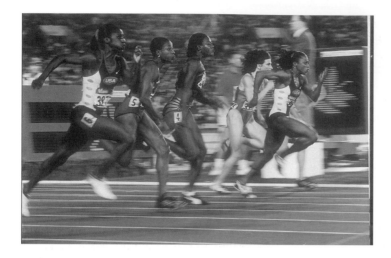

**Fig. 31.1** Performances of elite female athletes have improved rapidly with increased opportunities for participation and increased training loads. Photo © Allsport / John Gichigi.

minimum of 3 days. Dietary guidelines of most nutrients are intended to be intakes averaged over at least 3 days and over several months for those nutrients stored by the body, e.g. vitamin A.

Physical activity levels, climate and other factors can change dietary requirements. Anyone who exercises and/or is exposed to cold or hot environments may require different levels of some nutrients as compared to levels listed in current guidelines. As the reader evaluates dietary assessments of physically active populations, these limitations of the dietary guidelines should be considered.

## Requirement for energy

Energy needs are related to body mass. In the UK, median weights and heights of the population, recorded in 1980, are used to calculate energy needs ($MJ \cdot day^{-1}$). Total energy expenditure (TEE) is expressed as a multiple of the basal metabolic rate (BMR) and is affected by the physical activity level. Examples of TEE calculations for men and women can be found in the *UK Report on Dietary Reference Values* (Department of Health 1991). Current US energy calculations are based on median heights and weights found in the second National Health and Nutrition Examination Survey with empirically derived

equations developed by the World Health Organization (WHO 1985) specifically used to estimate resting energy expenditure (REE). To estimate total energy expenditure (TEE), REE is multiplied by a factor that represents an activity level which needs to be recorded over a sufficiently long time accounting for weekdays and weekends to increase validity of the estimate of energy expenditure. Examples of this calculation can be found in the US reference (National Research Council 1989).

Agreement regarding which equation to use for TEE estimation does not exist. As published in the WHO's *Report on Energy and Protein Requirements*, BMR forms the basis of the factorial method to estimate TEE (WHO 1985). However, examination of the calculations indicates that the equations overestimate BMR of some population groups (Piers *et al*. 1997). Carpenter *et al*. (1995), in a meta-analysis of 13 studies that utilized doubly labelled water technique as the method to measure TEE in free-living humans, concluded that there are insufficient published data to permit development of practical models to predict TEE in adults.

Acknowledgement of potential limitations of TEE calculations and of the derivation of energy recommendations is necessary to prevent inappropriate energy-related conclusions made in sports nutrition research or recommendations given to athletes. It is also expected that most female athletes will have a different weight/height ratio as compared to the women in the UK or US surveys. This difference is illustrated by comparing estimates of body fat and weights for national-level competitive female rhythmic gymnasts to controls of the same age and height. Female gymnasts averaged 10% body fat (range, 6–17%) as compared to controls, whose mean percentage body fat was 19% (range, 14–27%). An average weight of the gymnasts was reported to be 42 kg as opposed to 54 kg average weight for the controls (Sundgot-Borgen 1996).

Depending upon desired level for accuracy of energy estimates and in spite of the identified limitations, TEE equations may still be useful to calculate an estimate of energy expenditure for the female athlete. Additional research is needed to better predict TEE for athletic populations and understand the influence of exercise on TEE, particularly in relation to the female athlete. Gender differences in substrate metabolism as discussed in the next section also support this need.

## Substrate metabolism

Levels of triacylglycerol, total cholesterol (TC), high-density lipoprotein cholesterol (HDL-C) and low-density lipoprotein (LDL-C) can be affected by the presence of oestrogen. Major proteins for HDL and LDL are apo $A_{-1}$ and apo B, respectively, and were investigated in 25 female runners and 36 age-matched non-exercising women (controls) (Lamon-Fava et al. 1989). Lower concentrations of TC, apo B, triacylglycerol and higher apo $A_{-1}$ to apo B ratios were observed in the eumenorrhoeic female runners ($n=16$) as compared with nonexercising controls. All blood parameters in the amenorrhoeic runners ($n=9$) were similar to levels in the controls, except that apo B-values were 20% lower. Except for the effect on apo B levels, the positive effects of exercise on serum lipids were negated in those females with decreased oestrogen, i.e. amenorrhoeic runners.

In considering oestrogen's effect on lipid metabolism, one may ask whether there is a difference between men and women in the substrates used for energy during exercise. Tarnopolsky et al. (1990) matched subjects for maximal oxygen consumption, training status, and competition histories; tested females during the midfollicular phase of their menstrual cycles; and controlled the macronutrient content of the diet to prevent confounding effects of these factors on results. Subjects ran 15.5 km on a treadmill at a velocity requiring oxygen consumption of about 65% of maximal. Glycogen utilization was estimated from muscle biopsies, with respiratory exchange ratio (RER) used to determine substrate utilization during the exercise. Females demonstrated greater lipid utilization based on RER values, less muscle glycogen use and less urea nitrogen excretion than males during moderate-intensity, long-duration exercise. Given that a female athlete could oxidize greater fat stores while preserving CHO and protein, females would have an advantage in endurance and ultra-endurance events in which fat oxidation becomes metabolically more important. However, one may also argue that controlling for training level and substrate availability between genders is unlikely. This presents researchers with a challenging task in answering the question of gender-related substrate use.

Hormonal status of the female may need consideration by the researcher and sport nutritionist when evaluating energy intake of the female athlete. Barr et al. (1995) provide evidence that energy intakes of normally ovulating women are higher during the luteal phase of their menstrual cycles. While it is possible to ignore differences when conducting cross-sectional studies, it would be necessary to consider these energy intake differences in longitudinal studies. Whether a dietary assessment is taken over time or for 1 day, inquiry about the athlete's menstrual cycle may provide useful information related to energy intake, as well as nutritional and health status.

## Carbohydrate recommendations

Recommended percentages of energy from CHO

in the total diet have been listed as 55–70% for those engaged in exercise and training (Williams 1995). The percentage of energy (E%) derived from CHO may be helpful in comparison of dietary intakes, but has limited value for counselling athletes and, if used alone, can be misleading. For example, an endurance cyclist could consume a diet of 63% energy from CHO which would normally be considered less than the recommended level of 70% for the intake of an athlete engaged in endurance-type exercise. Yet, when the actual daily intake of approximately 18 g CHO·kg$^{-1}$ body weight (BW) is considered (Gabel et al. 1995), intake of the athlete cycling 14–16 h·day$^{-1}$ is greater than current recommendations. To obtain a greater understanding of an athlete's food intake, the optimal analysis would include values for g CHO·kg$^{-1}$ BW, E% from CHO and total amount of CHO.

Reports of dietary intakes for female athletes illustrate a lower than expected energy and CHO intake in relation to current dietary recommendations for those engaged in exercise and training. Review of CHO and energy intake in female athletes (Walberg-Rankin 1995) revealed consumption of 3.2–5.4 g CHO·kg$^{-1}$ BW·day$^{-1}$ and energy intakes of 6.4–9.6 MJ·day$^{-1}$ (1540–2300 kcal·day$^{-1}$) for female athletes involved in anaerobic sports (bodybuilding, gymnastics, basketball). Ranges of 4.4–6.2 g CHO·kg$^{-1}$ BW·day$^{-1}$ and 7–10 MJ·day$^{-1}$ (1660–2400 kcal) were reported for those participating in aerobic sports (running, cycling, triathlons). In preparation for a 90-km ultramarathon, 23 South African female runners consumed an average of 49.5% of their energy intake (7.5 MJ) from CHO or 4 g CHO·kg$^{-1}$ BW·day$^{-1}$ as part of their training diet (Peters & Goetzsche 1997). The female athletes reported running an average of 73.4 (±12.1) km·week$^{-1}$. Dietary assessments included two 24-h food records obtained 4 weeks prior to the race and no associations were found among energy, macro- and micronutrient intake and performance in the event. The use of 24-h records limits interpretation of these results.

Steen et al. (1995) reported average energy and CHO intakes of female heavyweight collegiate rowers below those expected for athletes engaged in training for 12 h and 2 h of weight training per week. Average intakes of 11 MJ (2630 kcal; range, 2025–3858 kcal) and 51% of energy from CHO (4.9 g·kg$^{-1}$ BW) were estimated from 5-day food records (3 weekdays and 2 weekend days). Simonsen et al. (1991) investigated energy needs of 24 collegiate rowers during 4 weeks of twice daily training 6 days per week. A high-CHO diet providing 10 g CHO·kg$^{-1}$ BW promoted greater muscle glycogen content and greater power output than a diet containing 5 g CHO·kg$^{-1}$ BW. However, the moderate-CHO diet provided a constant level of muscle glycogen (119 mmol·kg$^{-1}$) and did not lead to glycogen depletion or performance impairment.

Dietary recommendations for CHO intake do not differentiate for gender nor are the current CHO dietary recommendations derived from female athletic populations. Current recommendations include a minimum CHO intake of 5 g·kg$^{-1}$·day$^{-1}$ that has been suggested for a recreational athlete (Clark 1990) and increased levels for a more competitive athlete. For counselling women who participate in endurance and ultra-endurance events, sports nutritionists are encouraged to use recommendations of more than 6 g CHO·kg$^{-1}$ BW currently suggested to athletes involved in endurance sports and a minimum of 5 g CHO·kg$^{-1}$ BW for other female athletes. Researchers are encouraged to pursue the question of macro-nutrient needs of female athletes at all levels of exercise intensity and related performance.

It is worth repeating the advice for analysing the female athlete's food intake using values of g CHO·kg$^{-1}$ BW, E% from CHO and total amount of CHO. The findings from Simonsen et al. (1991) suggested that 10 g CHO·kg$^{-1}$ BW will promote greater muscle glycogen content and power output. If this CHO recommendation was used for a female rower who weighed 60 kg, consider the ramifications.

10 g CHO/kg BW × 60 kg BW = 600 g CHO
× 16.7 kJ (or 4 kcal)/g CHO
= 10 MJ (or 2400 kcal)

If perchance the athlete consumed a total of $10.9 \, \text{MJ} \cdot \text{day}^{-1}$ $(2600 \, \text{kcal} \cdot \text{day}^{-1})$ (Steen *et al.* 1995), only 840 kJ (200 kcal) would remain for protein and fat needs. This yields an impossible task not only in providing adequate levels of protein and fat, but in a practical sense as well. Another CHO recommendation comes in the form of total amount of CHO per day. The currently used $500–600 \, \text{g CHO} \cdot \text{day}^{-1}$ recommendation was derived from four trained male runners whose average weight was 80 kg (Costill *et al.* 1981). As illustrated and reflected in current intakes of females, these higher recommended levels of CHO are not practical for the typically lower weight female athlete.

## Protein recommendations

When compared with CHO and fat, protein is a nutrient with greater biological diversity in the body, greater methodological challenges in its study and with corresponding controversy in the findings. The reader can find in-depth reviews of amino acid metabolism in Chapter 9 and of protein requirements in Chapter 10.

Recognized as important for the athlete, protein is an energy nutrient that has a dietary guideline of about $0.75 \, \text{g} \cdot \text{kg}^{-1} \cdot \text{day}^{-1}$ in the UK (Department of Health 1991) and US (National Research Council 1989). As previously mentioned, these recommendations are not set with consideration for the effects of physical activity or climate. Rationale for using the recommended level of protein for both sexes stems from limited evidence found during a nitrogen balance study of six young women that requirement values, when expressed per kilogram of body weight, are not substantially different from those for young adult men. Calloway and Kurzer (1982) also noted in their study the importance of hormonal influences on the gain and loss of nitrogen and cautioned others that failure to consider the effect of the menstrual cycle could lead to inaccurate estimates of nitrogen/protein requirements.

Endurance athletes have greater protein requirements than those of sedentary persons (Tarnopolsky *et al.* 1988; Meredith *et al.* 1989). Phillips *et al.* (1993) considered protein needs for individuals engaged in habitual physical exercise and concluded that $0.86 \, \text{g} \cdot \text{kg}^{-1} \cdot \text{day}^{-1}$ was inadequate for endurance athletes. Females in the study were eumenorrhoeic, not taking oral contraceptives and matched to training levels of males with the use of training and performance histories. Male athletes exhibited higher absolute leucine oxidation than females, yet an increase in oxidation with exercise was proportionally greater in the females. This was not explained by the authors. In respect to methodology, a [15]N-glycine isotope revealed a higher protein turnover in elderly women ($n=6$) after they consumed 20% of their total energy as protein than after a 10% protein diet and no difference was observed when a [1-[13]C] leucine method was used (Pannemans *et al.* 1997). Care must therefore be taken in choosing the stable isotope tracer to measure protein turnover. The age of these subjects and small sample size limit the application of this research to female athletes, yet may pose questions for researchers who investigate protein utilizing leucine as a tracer.

While investigations of the most appropriate isotope tracer may redirect protein research, the more traditional nitrogen balance studies still support increased protein needs for active individuals. Without support for a specific protein requirement for the female athlete, reliance on a thorough dietary assessment of protein quality and energy intake followed with the provision of current recommendations for protein is suggested. Lemon (1995) suggests that endurance athletes consume protein levels of $1.2–1.4 \, \text{g} \cdot \text{kg}^{-1} \cdot \text{day}^{-1}$ and increased amounts for the strength athlete, $1.4–1.8 \, \text{g protein} \cdot \text{kg}^{-1} \cdot \text{day}^{-1}$. Unfortunately, these recommendations are based on data derived from male subjects aged 20–40 years. In consideration of recent data suggesting gender differences in substrate utilization, the protein levels may be excessive for the female; however, Lemon (1995) suggests that any adverse effect of excessive protein intake is minimal for individuals with normal kidney function.

Concern regarding protein intake for the female athlete stems from whether or not the individual consumes a low-energy intake or a strict vegetarian diet. Negative nitrogen balance can result in situations when energy intake is insufficient or consumed protein is of lesser biological quality. In these situations, heightened attention to the protein quality and adequate energy levels is warranted in the dietary assessment.

## Fat

Dietary fat guidelines promoted by different countries and agencies (James *et al.* 1988; Committee on Diet and Health 1989) vary from 20 to 35 E%. Developed for the general public, these levels stem from research that associates high fat intake with a variety of chronic diseases. Some have proposed the use of high-fat diets or *fat loading* to improve endurance capability of athletes. In their review of studies testing the fat-loading hypothesis, Sherman and Leenders (1995) concluded that the use of high-fat diets to improve endurance is not supported by a sufficient number of valid, credible and replicated studies. See Chapter 14 for more support of this conclusion.

Concern for a lower weight and percentage of body fat, as indicated by a score on the Eating Attitudes Test, motivates amenorrhoeic female athletes to consume less fat (11 E%) than eumenorrhoeic athletes (17 E%) (Perry *et al.* 1996), while other female athletes could benefit from counselling to reduce fat content in their diets (Steen *et al.* 1995). Consideration for the female athlete's weight history, appropriate goals for body composition and weight, current eating habits and serum lipid chemistries, family history of disease, and factors that influence energy and fat intake is important in the development of appropriate recommendations for fat intake. For the sport nutritionist, a thorough dietary and health

assessment will provide the best basis for any recommendation that can be made for fat intake by female athletes.

## Vitamins

It is generally supported that vitamin supplementation is not needed for those athletes consuming a variety of foods and that vitamin supplementation in athletes with an adequate vitamin status has no effect on performance (van der Beek 1991). For further discussion of vitamins, see Chapters 20 and 21. For the female athlete, research on vitamin $B_6$ and the antioxidant vitamins requires further discussion in this chapter.

### Vitamin $B_6$

Energy metabolism during exercise relies on several biological functions of vitamin $B_6$. The six biologically active forms of vitamin $B_6$ may function as a cofactor for enzymes used in metabolic transformation of amino acids, in gluconeogenesis and glycogenolysis. Other functions related to exercise include serotonin formation and synthesis of haemoglobin and carnitine. With the possibility of an increased need for this vitamin in young women, it may be beneficial to consider vitamin $B_6$ intake of the female athlete.

Female athletes tend to report vitamin $B_6$ intakes that are less than two thirds of the dietary guideline. However, it is important to note the possible influences of underreporting, low energy intakes or inadequate vitamin $B_6$ data in dietary computer software programs as possible contributors to the reported lower than expected intakes of vitamin $B_6$.

Manore (1994) summarized post-1985 studies reporting average dietary intakes of vitamin $B_6$ for female athletes. With the majority of researchers using a 3-day record to record intakes, 10–60% of the subjects reported consumption of less than two thirds of the dietary guideline for vitamin $B_6$. However, levels of the vitamin expressed as milligrams of vitamin $B_6$ per gram of protein were not below the currently recommended level of 0.016. The results of a study by Huang *et al.* (1998) provide recent evidence that the level of 0.016 mg vitamin $B_6 \cdot g^{-1}$ protein is inadequate for young women. Their study of eight women residing in a metabolic unit for 92 days suggests that 0.019 mg vitamin $B_6 \cdot g^{-1}$ protein is needed to normalize vitamin $B_6$ measures to controlled baseline values. If vitamin $B_6$ needs are indeed higher than current guidelines for young women, more attention to an adequate intake of this vitamin is needed for female athletes.

It is advisable for those working with athletes who typically report low energy intakes, i.e. gymnasts, figure skaters, and runners, to appropriately assess food intakes while noting completeness of the nutrient data bank used to estimate vitamin $B_6$ intake. Based on a thorough assessment, one may potentially proceed to recommend consumption of additional vitamin $B_6$-rich foods.

### Antioxidant vitamins

Exercise-induced oxidative stress may be a concern for an athlete. Oxidative stress occurs at submaximal levels of exercise (Leaf *et al.* 1997), and at peak $\dot{V}o_{2max.}$ (Viguie *et al.* 1990). The human body constantly forms free radicals and other oxygen-derived species that can damage DNA, lipids and proteins. When exposed to mild oxidative stress, the body can respond by increasing its defensive antioxidant enzymes and proteins; however, severe damage may lead to cell transformation and the increased oxidative damage has been associated with human disease, specifically cardiovascular disease and cancer (Halliwell 1994).

To diminish the effect of naturally occurring oxidative damage, it has been suggested that antioxidant nutrients should be added to the diet (Jacob & Burri 1996). Carotenoids, ascorbic acid, α-tocopherol, flavonoids, and other plant phenolics are a few of those suggested as important in protecting against oxidative damage. In other words, inclusion of fruits and vegetables in the athlete's diet can partially provide a solution to the concern for increased oxidative stress from exercise.

Some reports suggest that supplementation with antioxidant nutrients, such as vitamin E, can attenuate the exercise-induced lipid peroxidation (Sumida *et al.* 1989). A daily combination of 294 mg vitamin E, 1000 mg ascorbic acid and 60 mg ubiquinone was found to be effective in preventing LDL oxidation in male endurance athletes; however, 4 weeks' supplementation with the antioxidant nutrients did not reduce LDL oxidation products, i.e. conjugated dienes (Vasankari *et al.* 1997). Limited data specifically on female athletes are again noted in the area of antioxidant research.

For possible increased antioxidant vitamin requirements for those who exercise, the recommendation for an increased fruit and vegetable intake is worthy of emphasis. Dietary guidelines from several US organizations recommend five or more daily servings of fruits and vegetables to help reduce the risk of heart disease and certain kinds of cancer (Jacob & Burri 1996). For the female athlete, increased intake of fruits and vegetables can provide additional CHO and several essential nutrients. For those athletes limiting energy intake to reduce body fat, these foods will provide a higher nutrient to calorie ratio known to be beneficial for consuming a more nutrient adequate food intake.

## Minerals

### Macrominerals: calcium

A nutrient worthy of consideration for supplementation to the female athlete's diet is calcium. For detailed discussion of this mineral's roles in the body, calcium intake and its relationship to exercise, refer to Chapter 23. Discussion supporting the concern for adequate intake of this mineral and of practical ways to increase calcium intake in female athletes follows.

Peak bone mass development depends upon adequate calcium intake during skeletal growth (Matkovic 1991; Johnston *et al.* 1992) as well as for gain in bone mass until the third decade of life

(Recker *et al.* 1992). The combination of suboptimal calcium intakes by female athletes (Chen *et al.* 1989; Steen *et al.* 1995; Peters & Goetzsche 1997) and differences of opinion regarding recommended dietary guidelines for this mineral (Health and Welfare Canada 1983; National Research Council 1989; Department of Health 1991) prompts some concern and questions among those who care for, work with or feed female athletes.

Why should one have concern? Since physical activity, particularly high impact, is associated with greater bone density (Dook *et al.* 1997), one might expect that female athletes need not worry about the possibility of bone loss. However, identification of a syndrome of disordered eating, amenorrhoea and reduced bone density (Loucks 1987) overshadows this positive aspect of physical activity and may contribute to a greater consideration for adequate calcium intakes in female athletes.

The important questions regarding calcium are:

**1** What is an optimal calcium intake to promote and support adequate bone density in a female athlete?

**2** How can suboptimal calcium intakes be improved?

The answer to the first question is currently unknown. Differences of opinion regarding optimal calcium intakes for adults exist among countries, agencies and researchers. Even though physical activity has been identified as a positive factor in promoting greater bone density, no one has identified either the optimal level of exercise or calcium intake to support adequate bone density in the female athlete. To recommend an appropriate level of calcium intake, one needs to rely on a thorough nutritional, exercise and medical history of the athlete. Answers to questions about the following will provide added perspective on whether to recommend the dietary guideline for calcium or potentially a higher level.

• Family history of osteoporosis

• Typical intake of calcium, fluoride, other bone-related minerals, protein and energy

• Training intensity and type of sport

• Menstrual history and current status

• Supplement and/or drug use and any malabsorption conditions

For the athlete who avoids calcium-rich foods or is restricting energy intake to lose weight, discussion of low-fat calcium-rich foods, food choices not normally recognized as calcium-rich or those that are fortified with calcium, e.g. calcium-fortified orange juice, is recommended. Consumption of a mineral water that has a high calcium content may also be appropriate for a possible source of dietary calcium (Couzy *et al.* 1995).

The second choice would be that for supplementation of the female athlete's diet with calcium tablets. Determination of the typical calcium intake from food will help determine the appropriate level of supplement to recommend. However, supplementation with minerals is not without potential adverse effects. Wood and Zheng (1997) report that high dietary calcium intakes during a 36-day study reduced zinc absorption in healthy postmenopausal women. Limitations of the study include that activity level was not reported for the subjects and that differences will exist in nutrient absorption between a postmenopausal female and a young female. Cook *et al.* (1991) reported calcium supplements could inhibit the absorption of ferrous sulphate when consumed with food, although Reddy and Cook (1997) found no significant influence of calcium intake on non-haem iron absorption when varying levels of calcium ($280–1281\,mg \cdot day^{-1}$) were consumed as part of the diet.

In general, most experts agree that a calcium-rich diet is the most appropriate dietary prescription to promote and support optimal bone density. If this is not possible, consideration for low to moderate levels of a calcium supplement in addition to the dietary calcium intake to meet optimal levels is reserved for an alternative action.

The relationship between the macrominerals and microminerals warrants more attention as athletes look to supplementation as solutions to their possible dietary inadequacies. Lukaski (1995) has expressed concern for the adverse effects of trace mineral supplementation, particularly magnesium, zinc, and copper; while Clarkson and Haymes (1994) recommend a multivitamin/mineral supplement containing no more than the dietary guideline to athletes whose diets may be less than optimal.

### Microminerals: iron

Iron is another mineral worthy of consideration for supplementation. Deficiency of this mineral has the distinction of being common in female athletes and is frequently reported in physically active populations. In a comparison of 111 adult female habitual runners with 65 inactive females of comparable age, Pate *et al.* (1993) found serum ferritin levels, indicative of iron status, 28% lower in the runners than controls. However, frank iron deficiency indicated by suboptimal haemoglobin levels was rare in both groups. Dr Eichner provides insight into the reasons for iron depletion and expanded discussion of the effect of exercise on this mineral (see Chapter 24).

Challenges in maintaining adequate iron stores in the female athlete include the complexity of the mineral's absorption, lower intakes of energy by females, low levels of iron in food, avoidance of meat products, and monthly menstrual losses. More challenge is added to understanding this issue when one needs to decide which haematological assessment to use for iron status determination. Lack of standardization of the blood parameters and values used to classify the stages of iron depletion lends to the variability reported for the incidence of iron depletion in athletic populations.

However, most agree that iron supplements are appropriately given to those athletes who are diagnosed with iron deficiency anaemia (Haymes 1987). This is related to reports by some researchers that aerobic capacity in female athletes with mild anaemia can be improved with iron supplementation (Fogelholm 1995).

### Supplement use by athletes

Sobal and Marquart (1994) reviewed 51 studies in which 10274 athletes were investigated regarding the prevalence, patterns and explanations for their vitamin/mineral supplement use. Mean percentage of supplement use among female athletes was 57% (33 study groups). Several reasons were noted by the athletes for their supplement use: performance enhancement, prevention of illness, substitute for inadequate diet, provision of additional energy, and the meeting of specific nutrient demands for exercise. It was also noted that vitamin and mineral supplements were more frequently used by female athletes consuming low energy diets. Small sample sizes (<50 athletes) of most of the reviewed studies (56%) and the minor focus on supplements in the studies limits our understanding of supplement use by athletes. The authors recommended that those who study dietary intake of athletes consider vitamin/mineral supplement use as an important part of their study designs and sport nutritionists include a vitamin/mineral supplement history as part of their dietary assessment.

If the female athlete consumes adequate amounts of a variety of foods, she does not require vitamin/mineral supplementation to her food intake. However, for those athletes who consistently restrict energy intake, a one-a-day multiple vitamin/mineral supplement can provide some insurance in meeting nutrient needs for overall good health and exercise.

## Fluid intake and recommendations

Due to the wide variation in individual fluid losses during exercise, it is not reasonable to differentiate hydration recommendations for the female athlete. In spite of the physical, physiological and hormonal differences between males and females, individual variations in fluid balance surpass any gender differences (R.J. Maughan, personal communication).

## Conclusion

Dietary guidelines based on data from sedentary or male populations pose challenges, as well as opportunities, for the sports nutritionist and researcher who are interested in the nutritional needs of the female athlete. Since macronutrient dietary guidelines for athletes have been based on male subjects and micronutrient needs derived from non-athletic populations, the researcher has the opportunity to explore these needs of the female athlete, while faced with the challenge of understanding and controlling for the hormonal influences on metabolism. The sports nutritionist is presented with opportunities to systematically collect food intakes and supplementation information from female athletes, yet challenged with the lack of dietary guidelines specifically designed for the female athlete.

Presently, information obtained from a thorough diet, supplement and health history, 3–5-day food record, and training schedule; estimation of energy expenditure during exercise; plus anthropometric and biochemical data can provide a good basis for providing appropriate nutritional advice. Observation of the female athlete while training and competing, as well as during meal times, can also help to understand better the energy and nutrient requirements of the individual.

# References

Arciero, P.J., Goran, M.I. & Poehlman, E.T. (1993) Resting metabolic rate is lower in women than in men. *Journal of Applied Physiology* **75**, 2514–2520.

Barr, S.I., Janelle, K.C. & Prior, J.C. (1995) Energy intakes are higher during the luteal phase of ovulatory menstrual cycles. *American Journal of Clinical Nutrition* **61**, 39–43.

Calloway, D.H. & Kurzer, M.S. (1982) Menstrual cycle and protein requirements of women. *Journal of Nutrition* **112**, 356–366.

Carpenter, W.H., Poehlman, E.T., O'Connell, M. & Goran, M.I. (1995) Influence of body composition and resting metabolic rate on variation in total energy expenditure: a meta-analysis. *American Journal of Clinical Nutrition* **61**, 4–10.

Chen, J.D., Wang, J.F., Li, K.J. *et al.* (1989) Nutritional problems and measures in elite and amateur athletes. *American Journal of Clinical Nutrition* **49**, 1084–1089.

Clark, N. (1990) *Sport Nutrition Guide: Eating to Fuel Your Lifestyle.* Leisure Press, Champaign, IL.

Clarkson, P.M. & Haymes, E.M. (1994) Trace mineral requirements for athletes. *International Journal of Sport Nutrition* **4**, 104–119.

Committee on Diet and Health, National Research Council (1989) *Diet and Health: Implications for Reducing Chronic Disease Risk.* National Academy Press, Washington, DC.

Cook, J.D., Dassenko, S.A. & Whittaker, P. (1991) Calcium supplementation: effect on iron absorption. *American Journal of Clinical Nutrition* **53**, 106–111.

Costill, D.L., Sherman, W.M., Fink, W.J., Maresh, C., Witten, M. & Miller, J.M. (1981) The role of dietary carbohydrates in muscle glycogen resynthesis after strenuous running. *American Journal of Clinical Nutrition* **34**, 1831–1836.

Couzy, F., Kastenmayer, P., Vigo, M., Clough, J., Munoz-Box, R. & Barclay, D.V. (1995) Calcium bioavailability from a calcium- and sulfate-rich mineral water, compared with milk, in young adult women. *American Journal of Clinical Nutrition* **62**, 1239–1244.

Department of Health (1991) *Dietary Reference Values for Food Energy and Nutrients for the United Kingdom.* HMSO, London.

Dook, J.E., James, C., Henderson, N.K. & Price, R.I. (1997) Exercise and bone mineral density in mature female athletes. *Medicine and Science in Sports and Exercise* **29**, 291–296.

Fogelholm, M. (1995) Indicators of vitamin and mineral status in athletes' blood: a review. *International Journal of Sport Nutrition* **5**, 267–284.

Gabel, K., Aldous, A. & Edgington, C. (1995) Dietary intake of two elite male cyclists during 10-day, 2,050-mile ride. *International Journal of Sport Nutrition* **5**, 56–61.

Halliwell, B. (1994) Free radicals, antioxidants, and human disease: curiosity, cause, or consequence? *Lancet* **334**, 721–724.

Haymes, E.M. (1987) Nutritional concerns: need for iron. *Medicine and Science in Sports and Exercise* **19**, S197–S200.

Health and Welfare Canada (1983) *Recommended Nutrient Intakes for Canadians.* Bureau of Nutritional Sciences, Health Protection Branch, Health and Welfare, Ottawa.

Huang, Y.-C., Chen, W., Evans, M.A., Mitchell, M.E. & Shultz, T.D. (1998) Vitamin B-6 requirement and status assessment of young women fed a high-protein diet with various levels of vitamin B-6. *American Journal of Clinical Nutrition* **67**, 208–220.

Jacob, R.A. & Burri, B.J. (1996) Oxidative damage and defense. *American Journal of Clinical Nutrition* **63**, 985S–990S.

James, W.P.T., Ferro-Luzzi, A., Isaksson, B. & Szostak, W.B. (1988) *Healthy Nutrition: Preventing Nutrition-*

*Related Diseases in Europe*. WHO Regular Publication, European Series, no. 24, WHO, Copenhagen.

Johnston, C.C., Miller, J.Z., Slemenda, C.W. *et al.* (1992) Calcium supplementation and increases in bone mineral density in children. *New England Journal of Medicine* **327**, 82–87.

Kravitz, L., Robergs, R.A., Heyward, V.H., Wagner, D.R. & Powers, K. (1997) Exercise mode and gender comparisons of energy expenditure at self-selected intensities. *Medicine and Science in Sports and Exercise* **29**, 1028–1035.

Lamon-Fava, S., Fisher, E.C., Nelson, M.E., Evans, W.J., Millar, J.S., Ordovas, J.M. & Schaefer, E.J. (1989) Effect of exercise and menstrual cycle status on plasma lipids, low density lipoprotein particle size, and apolipoproteins. *Journal of Clinical Endocrinology and Metabolism* **68**, 17–21.

Leaf, D.A., Kleinman, M.T., Hamilton, M. & Barstow, T.J. (1997) The effect of exercise intensity on lipid peroxidation. *Medicine and Science in Sports and Exercise* **29**, 1036–1039.

Lemon, P.W.R. (1995) Do athletes need more dietary protein and amino acids? *International Journal of Sport Nutrition* **5**, S39–S61.

Loucks, A.B. (1987) Skeletal demineralisation in the amenorrheic athlete. In *Exercise: Benefits, Limits and Adaptations* (ed. D. Macleod, R. Maughan, M. Nimmo, T. Reilly & C. Williams), pp. 255–269. E. & F.M. Spon, London.

Lukaski, H.C. (1995) Micronutrients (magnesium, zinc, and copper): are mineral supplements needed for athletes? *International Journal of Sport Nutrition* **5**, S74–S83.

Manore, M.M. (1994) Vitamin $B_6$ and exercise. *International Journal of Sport Nutrition* **4**, 89–103.

Matkovic, V. (1991) Calcium metabolism, and calcium requirements during skeletal modeling and consolidation of bone mass. *American Journal of Clinical Nutrition* **54**, 245S–260S.

Maughan, R.J., Harmon, M., Leiper, J.B., Sale, D. & Delman, A. (1986) Endurance capacity of untrained males and females in isometric and dynamic muscular contractions. *European Journal of Applied Physiology* **55**, 395–400.

Meredith, C.N., Zackin, M.J., Frontera, W.R. & Evans, W.J. (1989) Dietary protein requirements and body protein metabolism in endurance-trained men. *Journal of Applied Physiology* **66**, 2850–2856.

Miller, A.E.J., MacDougall, J.D., Tarnopolsky, M.A. & Sale, D.G. (1993) Gender differences in strength and muscle fiber characteristics. *European Journal of Applied Physiology* **66**, 254–262.

National Research Council (1989) *Recommended Dietary Allowances*, 10th edn. National Academy of Science, Washington, DC.

Pannemans, D.L.E., Wagenmakers, A.J.M., Westerterp, K.R., Schaafsma, G. & Halliday, D. (1997) The effect of an increase of protein intake on whole-body protein turnover in elderly women is tracer dependent. *Journal of Nutrition* **127**, 1788–1794.

Pate, R.R., Miller, B.J., Davis, J.M., Slentz, C.A. & Klingshirn, L.A. (1993) Iron status of female runners. *International Journal of Sport Nutrition* **3**, 222–231.

Perry, A.C., Crane, L.S., Applegate, B., Marquez-Sterling, S., Signorile, J.F. & Miller, P.C. (1996) Nutrient intake and psychological and physiological assessment in eumenorrheic and amenorrheic female athletes: a preliminary study. *International Journal of Sport Nutrition* **6**, 3–13.

Peters, E.M. & Goetzsche, J.M. (1997) Dietary practices of South African ultradistance runners. *International Journal of Sport Nutrition* **7**, 90–103.

Phillips, S.M., Atkinson, S.A., Tarnopolsky, M.A. & MacDougall, J.D. (1993) Gender differences in leucine kinetics and nitrogen balance in endurance athletes. *Journal of Applied Physiology* **75**, 2134–2141.

Piers, L.S., Diffey, B., Soares, M.J., Frandsen, S.L., McCormack, L.M., Lutschini, M.J. & O'Dea, K. (1997) The validity of predicting the basal metabolic rate of young Australian men and women. *European Journal of Clinical Nutrition* **51**, 333–337.

Recker, R.R., Davies, K.M., Hinders, S.M., Heaney, R.P., Stegman, M.R. & Kimmel, D.B. (1992) Bone gain in young adult women. *Journal of the American Medical Association* **268**, 2403–2408.

Reddy, M.B. & Cook, J.D. (1997) Effect of calcium intake on nonheme-iron absorption from a complete diet. *American Journal of Clinical Nutrition* **65**, 1820–1825.

Sherman, W.M. & Leenders, N. (1995) Fat loading: the next magic bullet? *International Journal of Sport Nutrition* **5**, S1–S12.

Simonsen, J.C., Sherman, W.M., Lamb, D.R., Dernbach, A.R., Doyle, J.A. & Strauss, R. (1991) Dietary carbohydrate, muscle glycogen, and power output during rowing training. *Journal of Applied Physiology* **70**, 1500–1505.

Sobal, J. & Marquart, L.F. (1994) Vitamin/mineral supplement use among athletes: a review of the literature. *International Journal of Sport Nutrition* **4**, 320–334.

Steen, S.N., Mayer, K., Brownell, K.D. & Wadden, T.A. (1995) Dietary intake of female collegiate heavyweight rowers. *International Journal of Sport Nutrition* **5**, 225–231.

Sumida, S., Tanaka, K., Kitao, H. & Nakadomo, F. (1989) Exercise-induced lipid peroxidation and leakage of enzymes, before and after vitamin E supplementation. *International Journal of Biochemistry* **21**, 835–838.

Sundgot-Borgen, J. (1996) Eating disorders, energy intake, training volume, and menstrual function in high-level modern rhythmic gymnasts. *International Journal of Sport Nutrition* **6**, 100–109.

Tarnopolsky, L.J., MacDougall, J.D., Atkinson, S.A., Tarnopolsky, M.A. & Sutton, J.R. (1990) Gender differences in substrate for endurance exercise. *Journal of Applied Physiology* **68**, 302–308.

Tarnopolsky, M.A., MacDougall, J.D. & Atkinson, S.A. (1988) Influence of protein intake and training status on nitrogen balance and lean body mass. *Journal of Applied Physiology* **64**, 187–193.

van der Beek, E.J. (1991) Vitamin supplementation and physical exercise performance. *Journal of Sports Science* **9**, 77–89.

Vasankari, T.J., Kujala, U.M., Vasankari, T.M., Vuorimaa, T. & Ahotupa, M. (1997) Increased serum and low-density lipoprotein antioxidant potential after antioxidant supplementation in endurance athletes. *American Journal of Clinical Nutrition* **65**, 1052–1056.

Viguie, C.A., Frei, B., Shigenanga, M.K., Ames, B.N., Packer, L. & Brooks, G.A. (1990) Oxidant stress in human beings during consecutive days of exercise (Abstract). *Medicine and Science in Sports and Exercise* **22**, 86S.

Walberg-Rankin, J. (1995) Dietary carbohydrate as an ergogenic aid for prolonged and brief competitions in sport. *International Journal of Sport Nutrition* **5**, S13–S28.

WHO (1985) *Energy and Protein Requirements: Report of a Joint FAO/WHO/UNU Expert Consultation.* Technical Report Series 724, World Health Organization, Geneva.

Williams, C. (1989) Diet and endurance fitness. *American Journal of Clinical Nutrition* **49**, 1077–1083.

Williams, M. (1995) *Nutrition Related to Fitness and Sport.* Brown and Benchmark, Dubuque, IA.

Wood, R.J. & Zheng, J.J. (1997) High dietary calcium intakes reduce zinc absorption and balance in humans. *American Journal of Clinical Nutrition* **65**, 1803–1809.

# Chapter 32

# The Young Athlete

VISWANATH B. UNNITHAN AND ADAM D.G. BAXTER-JONES

## Introduction

Unlike most adults, children naturally engage in spontaneous, vigorous physical activity. It is postulated that this phenomenon represents more than mere play; rather, it is an essential biological process that likely plays a key role in the child's growth and development (Cooper 1995). Adequate food intake is essential for a growing child, perhaps more so for one engaged in physical training for several hours a day. Research into the nutritional needs of the young athlete therefore needs to be addressed in the wider context of not just the effects diet may have on performance, but also the interactions between nutritional intake, exercise and physiological growth. In the past, there was a preoccupation with meeting a child's nutrient needs, but, there is now a significant shift in thinking to address concerns with regard to nutritional behaviour during childhood and its impact on health outcomes in later life (Lucas 1997).

Although the nutritional requirements and nutritional habits of top-level adult sport performers have been extensively researched (Burke & Deakin 1994), there is little information with regard to the young athlete. This limitation is not just in the area of youth sport; our knowledge of the dietary requirements of normal healthy children is also still very limited. As is the case for the nutritional needs of the young athlete, recommendations for a child's nutritional intake are based mainly on adult requirements. The nutritional preparation of the elite young athlete, however, raises special problems for the nutritionist and dietician. These physically gifted youngsters are often highly motivated, and undergo prolonged strenuous exercise in training on a daily basis. This period of exercise stress often coincides with a period of rapid growth, so there are some real difficulties in making simple extrapolations from adult data.

Organized sport for youth is characterized today by increasing rates of participation, at ever-decreasing initial ages. In Western societies, youngsters (particularly girls) in their early teens are likely to have undergone intensive training and high-level international competition for several years and this highlights the 'catch them young' philosophy (Rowley 1987). There is a widely held, although unsubstantiated, belief that in order to achieve performance success at senior level, training and competition should begin before puberty.

As already outlined, the issue of adequate nutrition with regard to sports performance must be viewed in light of the physiological changes occurring during childhood which require increased amounts of energy for growth (Tanner 1989). The challenge for those working with young athletes is to integrate sports nutrition into the child's training regimen and to ensure that the nutritional needs for growth and development are met (Nelson Steen 1996). As well as being highly motivated, young athletes are often easily impressed by their heroes and will seek to emulate not only their training programmes but also their dietary habits. This can lead to extreme behaviour. A recent study of American adolescent athletes found that over a third were taking vitamin/mineral supplements and that over two thirds believed that such supplementation was improving their athletic performance (Sobal & Marquart 1994). This is despite the consensus in the nutrition literature that supplements do not help performance (Haymes 1991). Such findings suggest that improved education and dietary counselling are necessary to clarify such issues.

The first part of this review discusses the interactions between nutrition and a child's normal growth and the effects that training may have on growth. The second part concentrates on nutritional requirements for performance.

## Nutritional requirements of the growing child

From birth to approximately 10 years of age, children are highly dependent on their elders for their nutritional requirements and dietary habits. Studies of the nutritional requirements for this age group have been relatively neglected, apart from infant nutrition. Healthy boys and girls are expected to gain around 30 cm in height and 12 kg in weight between 5 and 10 years of age (Tanner 1989). Whilst percentage body fat remains fairly constant in boys during this period, it usually increases slowly in girls (Forbes 1987). At this age there is a considerable need for energy and essential nutrients for growth. In girls, sexual maturation begins around 8 years of age and this also affects nutritional requirements. For most essential nutrients, requirements for schoolchildren have been estimated by interpolating between infant and adult data, which raises concerns with regard to the validity of these estimated requirements.

The next stage of childhood growth is adolescence (10–19 years). Adolescence includes puberty, which consists of characteristic development of biological age, which differs in boys and girls, and leads to 'final' adult height, shape, body composition, and physical and sexual function. This hormonally driven development involves a linear growth spurt which commences about 2 years earlier in girls (around 12 years of age) than boys, acceleration of growth of muscle in boys and adipose tissue in girls, the emergence of secondary sexual characteristics and finally, in girls, menarche, or the onset of periods (Tanner 1989). Once menarche is attained, girls lose blood (on average 44 ml) approximately every 4 weeks. This loss of blood is equivalent to a loss of 12.5 μmol iron·day$^{-1}$. However, there is wide variation in blood loss among girls, with the 95th centile estimated at 118 ml·period$^{-1}$, or 34 μmol iron·day$^{-1}$ (Hallberg et al. 1966). Consequently, the iron requirement for postmenarcheal girls is higher than for boys, and much higher than the prepubertal requirement.

In boys, the linear growth spurt is greater than in girls and is accompanied by accelerated muscle growth. Boys' nutritional requirements therefore rapidly diverge from those of girls. During this time, bone density increases quickly by the incorporation of calcium and phosphate. It is estimated that 25% of peak bone mass is acquired during adolescence. Studies have shown positive effects of increasing the intake of dairy products on bone-density development (Lee et al. 1996). Although there is clear evidence that calcium intake during growth influences bone mineral density (Barr 1995), debate still exists as to the levels of calcium intake required. It also appears that physical activity is at least as important an influence on the increase in bone density in adolescence (Welten et al. 1994).

## Adolescent dieting behaviour

Adolescence is the peak period for dietary change, from self-imposed dietary restraint to veganism and beyond. In girls, dieting to reduce weight, whether needed or not, is common, particularly in some sporting events. While adolescent boys tend to exercise as much or more than previously and eat as dictated by appetite, girls today tend to eat towards a thin body ideal, and exercise less than previously.

The complex and ill-understood illnesses, anorexia nervosa and bulimia nervosa, almost always commence with 'simple' dieting. In a comprehensive review of eating disorders in young athletes, Wilmore (1995) concluded that athletes are at an increased risk of eating disorders, particularly female athletes in endurance sports or appearance sports. Dieting is also likely to contribute to suboptimal peak bone mass in early adulthood and early osteoporosis in the long term (Bailey *et al.* 1996). Dieting and vegetarian diets nearly always contribute to iron deficiency. Iron deficiency is a major problem in adolescence, occurring in boys as well as girls (Kurz 1996). This is likely to contribute to reduced physical activity and hence reduced peak bone mass, reduced immunity and, though not proven, reduced cognitive function.

Although, in contrast to their non-athletic peers, adolescent athletes are concerned with regard to their nutrition, studies have shown that their dietary intake may be less than adequate (Perron & Endres 1985; Lindholm *et al.* 1995). Martinez *et al.* (1993) found in a group of male high school American football players that the majority consumed inadequate food energy, iron and calcium, when compared to recommended dietary allowances (RDA), and consumed too much salt. However, as no measures of body mass were recorded, it was not possible to determine whether this shortfall in RDAs resulted in progressive weight loss. What is suggested is that these male athletes did not have any better or worse dietary habits than other male teenagers (Martinez *et al.* 1993). Studies of adolescent female athletes have also found that energy intakes are significantly lower than estimated energy needs (Perron & Endres 1985; Lindholm *et al.* 1995). A Swedish study compared the nutritional intake of 22 elite female gymnasts (age range, 13.5–16.6 years) and 22 healthy girls (age range, 14.1–15.9 years). This study found that both groups had energy intakes below their estimated energy needs, but this did not seem to influence their health status (Lindholm *et al.* 1995). One criticism of this type of study relates to the interpretation of recommended RDAs. How valid are RDAs for children? Can standard recommendations for a child of average weight at a given chronological age be used for comparison with an elite young gymnast, especially given the fact that elite gymnasts are known to be small for their chronological age, due in part to their late sexual development (Baxter-Jones & Helms 1996)? It is therefore suggested that a gymnast's recommended RDA would be lower than the average child's.

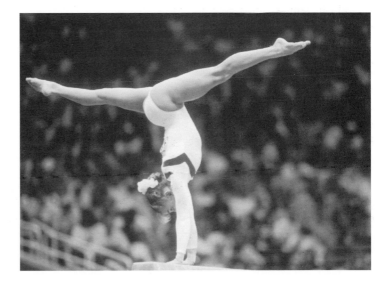

**Fig. 32.1** Adolescents excel in some sports: gymnastics, especially women's gymnastics, has traditionally been dominated by young performers. Small stature and low body fat content are also characteristic of elite performers. Photo © Allsport.

## Influence of exercise and diet on a child's growth and development

Some authors (Martinez *et al.* 1993; Lindholm *et al.* 1995) suggest that, in the long term, if children's energy intake is insufficient in relation to their energy needs, this could affect their growth and sexual development. It is well recognized that young female gymnasts are shorter and lighter than sedentary girls of the same age: they also show signs of late maturation, as evidenced by late menarche (Baxter-Jones *et al.* 1994; Lindholm *et al.* 1994; Malina 1994). Hence, although there is clear evidence of an effect of intensive training on the hormones of the hypothalamic–pituitary axis, it is not clear whether this effect accounts for what appears to be a loss of growth potential in some elite young athletes (Theintz *et al.* 1993). What is known is that malnutrition delays growth. Children subjected to episodes of acute starvation recover more or less completely, provided the adverse conditions are not too severe and do not last too long, and will reach their predicted adult height. Chronic malnutrition, on the other hand, causes individuals to grow to be smaller adults than they should (Tanner 1989), but there is no evidence to suggest that young athletes are malnourished.

## The elite young athlete

It has been demonstrated that, although restricted energy intake can delay maturation and sexual development, the late development which is observed in some sports is more related to inherited characteristics than to the effects of intensive training and/or nutritional inadequacy. Several studies have compared the physical characteristics of elite junior performers in different sports with those of non-elite competitors and non-athletic children (McMiken 1975; Buckler & Brodie 1977; Bloomfield *et al.* 1990). Data from a longitudinal study of young female British athletes indicated differences in stature between three sporting groups and UK growth standards (Fig. 32.2). At all ages, swimmers and tennis players were above average height on British growth standard charts (Tanner 1989). In contrast, gymnasts were below average height, particularly from 12 to 16 years of age. However, at 17 years of age, the gymnasts' height was again similar to the average height seen on the standard charts, indicating that what was being observed was a late attainment of the adolescent growth spurt. The parents of these gymnasts were also of less than average height (Baxter-Jones 1995), in accord with other data (Theintz

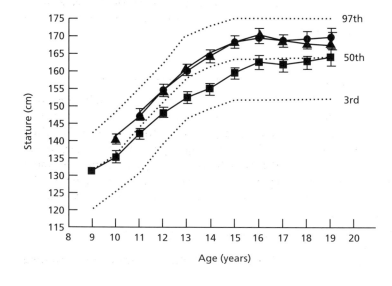

**Fig. 32.2** Development of stature in British female athletes compared with standard growth percentiles (dotted lines). Means and standard errors are shown at each age. Standard growth data are taken from height percentiles of British children (Tanner 1989). ●, swimming; ▲, tennis; ■, gymnastics. From Baxter-Jones and Helms (1996), with permission (based on data from Tanner 1989).

*et al.* 1989), suggesting that the short stature of the elite gymnast is determined largely by genetic rather than training and nutritional factors. Although Theintz *et al.* (1989) found no evidence that the predicted adult height for a group of elite young female gymnasts, who had already been training intensively for a period of 5 years, was less than the target height, their subsequent work suggested otherwise (Theintz *et al.* 1993). However, for this question to be resolved, both groups of athletes (Theintz *et al.* 1993; Baxter-Jones 1995) need to be reassessed to ascertain their actual adult height.

The biological maturity status of athletes has also been studied extensively, especially age at menarche (Malina 1994; Beunen & Malina 1996). When considering the influence of nutrition on the biological development of the elite young athlete, it is important to remember that this analysis is beset with a number of difficulties. Firstly, the definition of what constitutes an elite young athlete is vague, and secondly, as already discussed, it is likely that young athletes self-selected themselves for their sport due to their appropriate size and physique (Baxter-Jones & Helms 1996). A girl's menarcheal age is closely related to her mother's menarcheal age and this appears to be due mainly to a genetic influence on hormonal changes (Tanner 1989). Potential environmental influences include physical activity and nutrition (Malina 1983). In abnormal circumstances, nutrition may play an important role in the attainment of menarche, although this clearly relates to the malnourished child. It has been hypothesized that young athletes undertaking intensive training have delayed menarche due to the effects of training at an early age. In the British longitudinal study (Baxter-Jones & Helms 1996), all the sports (gymnastics, swimming and tennis) had later mean ages of menarche (14.3, 13.3 and 13.2 years, respectively) than the previously reported UK reference value of 13.0 years (Fig. 32.3). A positive correlation was found between menarcheal age in mothers and daughters ($n=201$, $r=0.27$, $P<0.01$; Baxter-Jones *et al.* 1994). Analysis of covariance, using maternal menarcheal age, socio-economic group, duration

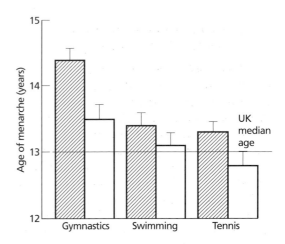

**Fig. 32.3** Mean age of menarche and associated standard errors for British mothers (□) and daughter athletes (▨) in different sports, with reference to the UK median age (Tanner 1989). Significant differences were found between mothers' and daughters' age of menarche in gymnastics and tennis ($P<0.05$). From Baxter-Jones *et al.* (1994), with permission of Taylor & Francis.

of training and type of sport confirmed that maternal menarcheal age and type of sport have a significant influence on the subject's age of menarche. As maternal menarcheal age and sport were the best predictors of menarcheal age in the athletes studied, it would appear that menarche was intrinsically late rather than delayed (Baxter-Jones *et al.* 1994); this suggests that some form of sport-specific selection had occurred.

## Nutrition and performance

The remainder of this review will be limited to nutritional factors that could affect performance in the young athlete. Performance will be delimited to three major sporting areas: strength and flexibility-based sports (gymnastics), endurance sports (running/cycling) and high-intensity intermittent sports (soccer, rugby, basketball).

### Carbohydrate and fat

The major substrates used by the muscles during

exercise are carbohydrate derived from muscle glycogen or blood glucose from hepatic glycogen stores, and fatty acids which may come from the adipose triglyceride via plasma free fatty acids (FFA) or from the intramuscular triglyceride stores. The relative contributions of these fuels during exercise is intensity dependent, with the contribution of carbohydrate increasing as exercise intensity increases. As documented by Rowland (1985), effective aerobic training for the child athlete requires a relatively high volume of exercise at high intensity, thus placing large demands on the body's limited carbohydrate stores (Coyle 1992).

In order to appreciate the nutritional consequences of carbohydrate and fat manipulation in the diet of the young athlete, it is necessary to understand the underpinning physiological bases of the child athlete. Erikksson *et al.* (1973), Keul (1982) and Kindermann *et al.* (1978) have all demonstrated lower levels of muscle phosphofructokinase activity and a reduced glycolytic potential in children aged 11–13 years than in adults. Conversely, Haralambie (1979) demonstrated higher tricarboxylic-acid cycle enzyme activity and increased lactate dehydrogenase activity in 11–14-year-old girls than in adult women and men.

Children performing prolonged exercise indicate a preference for fat rather than carbohydrate metabolism (Bar-Or & Unnithan 1994). Berg *et al.* (1980) and Macek and Vavra (1981) demonstrated significant increases in glycerol levels in blood with prolonged (30–120 min) activity in children. In addition, Martinez and Haymes (1992) concluded that prepubertal girls relied more on fat than on carbohydrate utilization during exercise of moderate to heavy intensity. Not only have higher glycerol (0.425 vs. 0.407 mmol·l$^{-1}$) and FFA levels (1.97 vs. 1.82 mmol·l$^{-1}$) been noted in young children (10–12 years) vs. adolescents (15–17 years) during exercise, but the increase in glycerol (five times resting values) occurred at an earlier time than seen in adults (Berg *et al.* 1980). FFA uptake expressed per minute per litre of $O_2$ uptake has been found to be greater in children than in adults during pro-

longed submaximal exercise. It is theorized that a large immediate increase in noradrenaline and a greater utilization of FFA is used by children to offset hypoglycaemia during prolonged exercise at the same relative exercise intensity (Delamarche *et al.* 1992). A confounding factor in the interpretation of the above observations is the fact that it is assumed that a true maximal oxygen uptake has been achieved by the individuals under investigation. However, it has been shown that only a minority of children and adolescents attain a true maximal oxygen uptake (Armstrong & Welsman 1994).

Respiratory exchange ratio (RER) data also suggest a preference for fat utilization in children. Asano and Hirakoba (1984), Macek and Vavra (1981) and Martinez and Haymes (1992) demonstrated lower RER values for children than for adults during prolonged exercise. Again, interpretation of these results is confounded by the fact that a failure to achieve a true maximal oxygen uptake will result in overestimated submaximal work loads in children. Therefore, comparisons between children's and adults' data may not be appropriate. Macek and Vavra (1981) demonstrated significant reductions in RER over 60 min of submaximal exercise, in conjunction with increases in glycerol levels in blood. Magnetic resonance spectroscopy work by Zanconato *et al.* (1993) also demonstrated that children were less able than adults to effect adenosine triphosphate rephosphorylation by anaerobic metabolic pathways during high-intensity exercise. In conclusion, muscle enzyme, RER and magnetic resonance spectroscopy data suggest that children, as compared with adults, seem better suited for aerobic than anaerobic energy metabolism (Bar-Or & Unnithan 1994).

While it is acknowledged that children may use fat rather than carbohydrate as the major fuel during exercise, the ability to sustain this exercise over a number of months and in high-intensity exercise bouts would still depend upon adequate carbohydrate stores being present. Hence, appropriate knowledge and guidance regarding carbohydrate intake are critical. Loosli and Benson (1990) showed that in the absence of directed eating from the child's parent or guardian, inherent nutritional knowledge with respect to carbohydrate was poor. In a survey of 97 competitive female gymnasts (11–17 years), 77% rated protein as their favourite energy source; 53% were unaware of what a complex carbohydrate was and 36% chose nutrient-poor foods such as doughnuts and soft drinks as their favourite energy food (Loosli & Benson 1990).

Whilst the lower levels of glycolytic and higher levels of citrate-cycle enzyme activity of the child would imply that increased dietary fat would produce the best responses during prolonged exercise, it is clear that certain reservations apply to this procedure. Firstly, it would be medically unsound, as the risk of developing coronary heart disease, stroke and certain cancers has been associated with eating a chronic high fat diet; and secondly, following the hypothesis of central fatigue, increased FFA levels may promote fatigue by enhancing free tryptophan levels, leading to raised levels of serotonin in the brain (Davis *et al.* 1992). However, it has also been shown that increased FFA in the presence of heprin increases endurance (see Chapter 13). Serotonin (5-hydroxytrytamine or 5-HT) is responsible for causing a state of tiredness in both man and experimental animals (Young 1991). Hence, an elevation of serotonin may exacerbate the sensation of fatigue.

## Protein intake

There is no evidence that protein metabolism differs between adults and children (Lemon 1992). Hence, the increased need for protein intake by active adolescents is purely the product of the extra demand imposed by exercise and growth, and not the result of any inadequacies of the child's metabolism of protein. The RDA values for the adult population vary widely between countries ($0.8–1.2\,g\cdot kg^{-1}\cdot day^{-1}$): where separate values are established for adolescents, they are generally in the region of $1\,g\cdot kg^{-1}\cdot day^{-1}$ (Lemon 1992). Bar-Or and Unnithan (1994) suggest an increase, in non-athletic children, from the adult value of $0.8\,g\cdot kg^{-1}\cdot day^{-1}$ to $1.2\,g\cdot$ $kg^{-1}\cdot day^{-1}$ for boys and girls between 7 and 10 years, and a value of $1.0\,g\cdot kg^{-1}\cdot day^{-1}$ for 11–14 years. These figures are based upon tables generated by the American Academy of Paediatrics (1991): after this age, recommendations are in line with adult figures.

O'Connor (1994) demonstrated that young people (age range, 7–19 years) achieve a mean dietary intake of $1.6\,g\cdot kg^{-1}\cdot day^{-1}$, even in those sports where energy intake is restricted (e.g. gymnastics). In contrast, Martinez *et al.* (1993), assessing the diet of adolescent American footballers, via the use of dietary recall, found that in 87 subjects 95% consumed less than the RDA ($16.8\,MJ\cdot day^{-1}$ or $4000\,kcal\cdot day^{-1}$) (Pipes 1989) for the adolescent male athlete. These results parallel the findings for adolescents not engaged in sports training and therefore it would appear that those engaged in sports do not practice any better nutritional habits than those who are not. Concern was noted with regard to protein intake: the mean protein intake was almost twice the RDA and accounted for 16% of total energy consumed (Martinez *et al.* 1993). Even taking into account the validity of the RDAs, the resultant excess protein in the blood could be harmful to liver function. Although, the sports practitioner (coach) and parent should be made aware of a possible increased protein requirement during periods of rapid growth and intensive training, protein supplementation, as seen in adults, should also be discouraged. Finally, it still has to be ascertained whether protein requirements differ depending upon the sport selected and the level of competition undertaken.

## Fluid intake and composition

In order to understand the significance of fluid intake and drink composition for the child athlete, it is necessary to review briefly the underpinning thermoregulatory physiology of the child compared to that of the adult.

Primarily as a result of their greater surface area to body mass ratio, children and adolescents absorb heat quicker at high ambient temperatures and lose heat faster at low ambient temperatures during activities such as walking and running (MacDougall *et al.* 1983). In an attempt to control for differences in stature between adults and children, sweating rate is normalized to body surface area, but, even after this adjustment, children demonstrate a lower sweating rate than adults (Bar-Or 1980; Falk *et al.* 1992). This decrease exists in spite of the fact that children have a greater number of heat-activated sweat glands per unit skin area (Falk *et al.* 1992). The sweating threshold is considerably higher in children than in adults (Araki *et al.* 1979). Meyer *et al.* (1992) demonstrated that adults have elevated sodium (Na) and chloride (Cl) concentrations in sweat. It has also been shown that body core temperature increases at a higher rate for any given level of hypohydration in children than in adults (Bar-Or *et al.* 1980). Despite the multitude of differences in the physiological responses of the child, the critical question is whether these characteristics will limit performance in children. There is no definite answer, but it is clear that in a hot environment, children are at a disadvantage compared with adults. In adult studies, it has been found that there is a clear effect of temperature on exercise capacity which appears to follow an inverted-U relationship. Galloway and Maughan (1997) found under their study conditions that exercise duration was longest at 11°C: below this temperature (at 4°C) and above this temperature (at 21° and 31°C), a reduction in exercise capacity was observed.

Bar-Or *et al.* (1992) identified that children, like adults, do not drink enough when offered fluids *ad libitum* during exercise in the heat, a condition known as voluntary dehydration. The physiological consequences for the child athlete are serious; at any given level of hypohydration, children's core temperature rises faster than that of adults, and it is therefore critically important to reduce voluntary dehydration (Bar-Or *et al.* 1992). The general guidelines that should be issued to children exercising in the heat are to drink until the child does not feel thirsty, and then to drink an additional half a glass (100–125 ml); for adolescents, a full glass extra is recom-

mended. However, in order to implement these guidelines for sporting competitions under climatic heat stress conditions, competition regulations need to be altered for the child athlete. Suggestions include allowing the child to leave the field of play periodically, or, as in the 1994 soccer World Cup, the positioning of drinking bottles on the perimeter of the field to allow for fluid intake during natural stoppages in play.

In order to encourage the child to take on board sufficient fluid to offset voluntary dehydration, the fluid of choice has to be palatable and should stimulate further thirst. Thirst perception is influenced by drink flavour and drink composition. Meyer *et al.* (1994) demonstrated in prepubertal children, at rest after a maximal aerobic test and for rehydration purposes after prolonged exercise in the heat, that grape flavouring was preferred to apple, orange and unflavoured water. Wilk and Bar-Or (1996) attempted to determine which of the two factors played the more important role. Trials were undertaken using flavoured water and an identically flavoured carbohydrate (6%)–electrolyte (NaCl) drink. It was shown that the flavoured water (grape) maintained euhydration over a 90-min exercise period under heat stress conditions. The carbohydrate–electrolyte drink produced a slight overhydration over the same time period. These studies suggest that voluntary dehydration could be reduced by drinking flavoured water and prevented by drinking a carbohydrate–electrolyte drink (Fig. 32.4).

The concentration of sodium ions in the extracellular fluid is critical to the rate of replenishment of body fluids. Nose *et al.* (1988) demonstrated that the ingestion of 0.45 g NaCl in capsule form per 100 ml of water enhanced volume restoration after dehydration relative to water alone. Wilk and Bar-Or (1996) demonstrated that there was a 45% increase in drinking volume in favour of the grape flavoured water, and an additional 47% increase in voluntary drinking on the addition of carbohydrate and NaCl (Fig. 32.5). Their study design did not allow the partitioning out of the carbohydrate and NaCl effects, but previous studies (Nose *et al.*

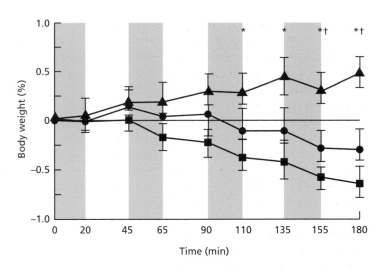

**Fig. 32.4** Net body weight changes throughout chamber sessions in unflavoured water (W), flavoured water (FW) and carbohydrate–electrolyte (CNa) trials. Vertical lines denote SE values; tinted areas show exercise periods. ●, swimming; ▲, tennis; ■, gymnastics; $n = 12$; *, $P < 0.05$ (CNa–W); †, $P < 0.05$ (CNa–FW). From Wilk and Bar-Or (1996), with permission.

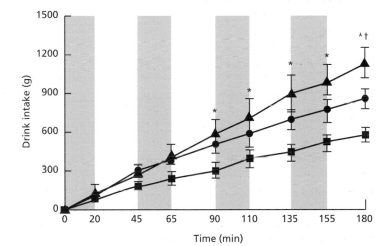

**Fig. 32.5** Cumulative drink intake throughout chamber sessions in unflavoured water (W; ■), flavoured water (FW; ●), and carbohydrate–electrolyte (CNa; ▲) trials. Vertical lines denote SE values; tinted areas show exercise periods. $n = 12$ subjects. *, $P < 0.05$ (CNa–W); †, $P < 0.05$ (CNa–FW). From Wilk and Bar-Or (1996), with permission.

1988; Bar-Or *et al.* 1992) suggest that most of the benefit was obtained through the addition of NaCl. A limitation to these findings is that the population was pre- and early pubertal only; further research is necessary in older children and adolescents.

## Micronutrients

In recent times there has been much concern over the adequacy of specific micronutrients in the diets of young athletes. Vitamins, iron and calcium are most commonly considered, although zinc, sodium, potassium and magnesium have also received attention (Shephard 1982). Supplementation of the diet with vitamins or minerals is not generally warranted in athletes, irrespective of age: additional demand for these nutrients imposed by training should be met if the energy intake is sufficient to meet the additional energy expenditure incurred in training and competition, and if a varied diet is consumed. One of the major sources of inadequate (defined as less than the required RDA) micronutrient intake is the actual methodology used to collect the information. Dietary recall procedures are susceptible to under-reporting of nutritional information and for the absence of selected micronutrients from the food tables. Hence, the reported intake may not be true.

Few studies have been published on the vitamin status of young athletes. Those studies that are available suggest inadequate vitamin consumption resulting from diets of excessive consumption of confectionery, soft drinks and other low nutrient-density foods (O'Connor 1994). This is contrary to the American Dietetic Association's (1980) stance that athletes who consume adequate amounts of energy do not present with vitamin deficiencies and therefore do not require supplements. It is therefore suggested that while indiscriminate use of vitamin supplements in young athletes should be discouraged, their use may be appropriate in athletes who restrict their food intake (O'Connor 1994).

Iron deficiency in the absence of anaemia is common in adolescent distance runners. However, whether non-anaemic iron deficiency affects athletic performance is unclear (Rowland & Kelleher 1989). The effect of iron deficiency is associated with incorporation of iron into haemoglobin and other processes requiring iron such as enzyme cofactors. However, evidence of such deficiencies is limited; Pate *et al.* (1979), Rowland *et al.* (1987) and Rowland and Kelleher (1989) all demonstrated limited evidence of anaemia in athletic children and adolescents. In addition, Nickerson *et al.* (1989) demonstrated limited evidence of gastrointestinal bleeding in cross-country runners with iron deficiency. It is unlikely that non-anaemic iron deficiency will have a significant effect upon athletic performance. Performance may possibly be impaired in females (see Chapter 24) with low ferritin levels and borderline haemoglobin ($12 \, g \cdot dl^{-1}$). If decrements in performance are noted, then serum ferritin and haemoglobin are worth assessing. General guidelines for the child athlete would be to encourage eating poultry, lean red meat, iron-enriched breakfast cereals and green vegetables.

Calcium requirements are highest during childhood and adolescence, aside from during pregnancy and lactation. Concern has centred on those athletic populations whose total food, and hence calcium, intake is likely to be low—for example, gymnasts and dancers (O'Connor 1994). A combination of inadequate calcium intake and amenorrhoea in these athletes has raised serious concerns because of its association with osteoporosis (Bailey *et al.* 1996). Although the effectiveness of calcium supplementation in childhood is still unclear (Welten *et al.* 1994), every effort should be made to educate young athletes about the importance of adequate dietary calcium.

## Nutritional knowledge

As already discussed, one of the major factors that influences the nutrition of the young athlete is a sound basis of nutritional knowledge. Work by Richbell (1996) demonstrated in élite junior swimmers, track and field athletes and soccer players that whilst the three groups followed the recommended ratio of 55:30:15 for carbohydrate, fat and protein intake, the nutritional knowledge in all three disciplines was poor. This type of pattern was also demonstrated by Perron and Endres (1985), who assessed the dietary intake of female volleyball players (13–17 years) and showed that no significant correlation existed between nutritional knowledge and attitudes and dietary intake. These findings seemed to indicate that at this age other factors such as weight concerns and dependence on others for food selection are significant. As previously mentioned by Loosli and Benson (1990), competitive female gymnasts had poor nutritional knowledge. Swedish gymnasts have been shown to have energy intakes insufficient in relation to their high energy needs; it is suggested that, if left unchecked, this could affect their pubertal development and menstrual patterns (Lindholm *et al.* 1995). However, although the gymnasts in this study (Lindholm *et al.* 1995) had body weights at least 1 SD below the normal weight for Swedish children of similar chronological age, they also had late sexual development. Therefore, interpretation of the data with normal growth charts is confounded by the effects of biological age (BA): you would expect individuals with the same chronological age but lower BA to have lower body weights. The above observations do, however, suggest that young athletes need supervision of their diet not only as an aid to performance but, more importantly, for their general health.

## Challenges for future research

1 Longitudinal studies of non-athletic and athletic children are required to elucidate the relationship between nutritional intake, growth and development and intensive training during childhood and adolescence. It is recommended that a mixed-longitudinal study design is chosen so that information can be collected over a shorter period (Baxter-Jones & Helms 1996).

2 Care is advised in the interpretation of data, especially when comparing athletic and non-athletic groups; they must be matched for both chronological and biological age. When comparing submaximal exercise data from adults and children, it is essential that the failure of children to reach a true maximal oxygen uptake be taken into account.

3 Further work is needed to identify the relationship between the intensity of exercise and appropriate dietary intervention. In one of the few studies that investigated the role of exercise intensity, Rankinen et al. (1993) established that micronutrient intake of 12–13-year-old Finnish ice-hockey players increased with an increase in training intensity.

4 There is a need to understand more about the muscle metabolism of children, possibly through magnetic resonance spectroscopy, thereby allowing us to understand more fully whether dietary deficiencies impinge upon the functioning of the cellular functioning of the muscle.

5 Optimization of pre- and postcompetition diet is an area that warrants further investigation in the child athlete.

6 Sport specificity (contact vs. non-contact, strength/power vs. endurance) and the level of competition that the child undertakes may well determine the level of protein requirement. Further research is needed in this area.

7 The results for dietary intake are usually compared with RDA, but the validity of the current age-related RDAs is questioned. Further work is necessary to find out if these standards, developed for the average child, are relevant for the young athlete of the same age.

## References

American Academy of Paediatrics (1991) Nutrition and the athlete. In Sport Medicine: Health Care for Young Athletes, pp. 99–109, American Academy of Paediatrics, Evanston, IL.

American Dietetic Association (1980) Nutrition and physical fitness. Journal of the American Dietetic Association 76, 437–443.

Araki, T., Toda, Y., Matsushita, K. & Tsujino, A. (1979) Age differences in sweating during muscular exercise. Japanese Journal of Physical Fitness and Sports Medicine 28, 239–248.

Armstong, N. & Welsman, J.R. (1994) Assessment and interpretation of aerobic fitness in children and adolescents. Exercise and Sports Sciences Reviews 22, 435–476.

Asano, K. & Hirakoba, K. (1984) Respiratory and circulatory adaptation during prolonged exercise in 10–12-year-old children and in adults. In Children and Sport (eds J. Ilmarinen & I. Valimaki), pp. 119–28. Springer-Verlag, Berlin.

Bailey, D.A., Faulkner, R.A. & McKay, H.A. (1996) Growth, physical activity, and bone mineral acquisition. Exercise and Sport Sciences Reviews 24, 233–266.

Bar-Or, O. (1980) Climate and the exercising child. International Journal of Sports Medicine 1, 53–65.

Bar-Or, O. & Unnithan, V.B. (1994) Nutritional requirements of young soccer players. Journal of Sports Sciences 12, S39–42.

Bar-Or, O., Blimkie, C.J.R., Hay, J.A., MacDougall, J.D., Ward, D.S. & Wilson, W.M. (1992) Voluntary dehydration and heat intolerance in patients with cystic fibrosis. Lancet 339, 696–699.

Barr, S.I. (1995) Nutritional factors in bone growth and development. In New Horizons in Pediatric Exercise Science (eds C.J.R. Blimkie & O. Bar-Or), pp. 109–20. Human Kinetics, Champaign, IL.

Baxter-Jones, A.D.G. (1995) Physical effects of training during puberty and adolescence. PhD thesis, University of Aberdeen, Aberdeen, UK.

Baxter-Jones, A.D.G. & Helms, P.J. (1996) Effects of training at a young age: a review of the training of young athletes (TOYA) study. *Pediatric Exercise Science* **8**, 310–327.

Baxter-Jones, A.D.G., Helms, P., Baines Preece, J. & Preece, M. (1994) Menarche in intensively trained gymnasts, swimmers and tennis players. *Annals of Human Biology* **21**, 407–415.

Berg, A., Keul, J. & Huber, G. (1980) Biochemische aktuveranderungen bei ausdauerbelastungen im kindesund jugendalter. *Monatsschrift Kinderheilk* **128**, 590–595.

Beunen, G. & Malina, R.M. (1996) Growth and maturation: relevance to athletic performance. In *The Child and Adolescent Athlete* (ed. O. Bar-Or), pp. 3–24. Blackwell Science, Oxford.

Bloomfield, J., Blanksby, B.A. & Ackland, T.R. (1990) Morphological and physiological growth of competitive swimmers and non-competitors through adolescence. *Australian Journal of Science and Medicine in Sport* **22**, 4–12.

Buckler, J.M.H. & Brodie, D.A. (1977) Growth and maturity characteristics of schoolboy gymnastics. *Annals of Human Biology* **4**, 455–463.

Burke, L.M. & Deakin, V. (1994) *Clinical Sports Nutrition*. McGraw-Hill, Sydney.

Cooper, D.M. (1995) New horizons in pediatric exercise research. In *New Horizons in Pediatric Exercise Science* (ed. C.J.R Blimkie & O. Bar-Or), pp. 1–24. Human Kinetics, Champaign, IL.

Coyle, E.F. (1992) Timing and method of increasing carbohydrate intake to cope with heavy training, competition and recovery. *Journal of Sports Sciences* **9** (Special Issue), 29–52.

Davis, J.M., Bailey, S.P., Galiano, F.J., Deacon, W.S., Merril, T.L., Bynoe, R.P. & Pettigrew, C. (1992) Increased free fatty acid and glucose availability and fatigue during prolonged exercise in man. *Medicine and Science in Sports and Exercise* **24** (Supplement), S71.

Delamarche, P., Monnier, M., Gratas-Delamarche, A., Koubi, H.E., Mayet, M.H. & Favier, R. (1992) Glucose and free fatty acid utilisation during prolonged exercise in pre-pubertal boys in relation to catecholamine responses. *European Journal of Applied Physiology* **65**, 66–72.

Erikkson, B.O., Gollnick, P.D. & Saltin, B. (1973) Muscle metabolism and enzyme activities after training in boys 11–13 years old. *Acta Physiologica Scandinavica* **87**, 485–497.

Falk, B., Bar-Or, O. & MacDougall, J.D. (1992) Thermoregulatory responses of pre-, mid- and late-pubertal boys. *Medicine and Science in Sports and Exercise* **24**, 688–694.

Forbes, G.B. (1987) Body composition in infancy, childhood and adolescence. In *Human Body Composition* (ed. G.B. Forbes), pp. 125–68. Springer Verlag, New York.

Galloway, S.D.R. & Maughan, R.J. (1997) Effects of ambient temperature on the capacity to perform prolonged cycle exercise in man. *Medicine and Science in Sports and Exercise* **29**, 1240–1249.

Hallberg, L., Hogdahl, A.M., Nilsson, L. & Rybo, G. (1966) Menstrual blood loss: a population study. Variation at different ages and attempts to define normality. *Acta Obstetrica et Gynecologica Scandinavica* **45**, 320–351.

Haralambie, G. (1979) Skeletal muscle enzyme activities in female subjects of various ages. *Bulletin of European Physiopathology and Respiration* **15**, 259–267.

Haymes, E.M. (1991) Vitamin and mineral supplementation to athletes. *International Journal of Sport Nutrition* **1**(2), 146–169.

Keul, J. (1982) Zur belastbarkeit des kinlichen organismus aus biochemischer sicht. In *Kinder im Leistungsport* (ed. H. Howald & E. Hatin), pp. 31–49. Birkhauser Verlag, Basel.

Kindermann, W., Keul, J., Simon, G. & Reindell, H. (1978) Anpassungerscheinungen durch Schul-und Leistungssport im Kindesalter. *Sportwissenschaft* **8**, 222–234.

Kurz, K.M. (1996) Adolescent nutritional status in developing countries. *Proceedings of the Nutrition Society* **55**, 321–331.

Lee, W.T.K., Leung, S.S.F., Leung, D.M.Y. & Cheng, J.C.Y. (1996) A follow-up study on the effects of calcium-supplement withdrawal and puberty on bone acquisition of children. *American Journal of Clinical Nutrition* **64**, 71–77.

Lemon, P. (1992) Effect of exercise on protein requirements. *Journal of Sports Sciences* **9** (Special Issue), 53–70.

Lindholm, C., Hagenfeldt, K. & Ringertz, B.M. (1994) Pubertal development in elite juvenile gymnasts: effects of physical training. *Acta Obstetrica Gynecologica Scandinavica* **73**, 269–273.

Lindholm, C., Hagenfeldt, K. & Hagman, U. (1995) A nutrition study in juvenile elite gymnasts. *Acta Paediatrica* **84**, 273–277.

Loosli, A.R. & Benson, J. (1990) Nutritional intake of adolescent athletes. *Pediatric Clinics of North America* **37**, 1143–1152.

Lucas, A. (1997) Paediatric nutrition as a new subspecialty: is the time right? *Archives of Disease in Childhood* **76**, 3–5.

MacDougall, J.D., Roche, P.D., Bar-Or, O. & Moroz, J.R. (1983) Maximal aerobic capacity of Canadian school children: predicted based on age-related oxygen cost of running. *International Journal of Sports Medicine* **4**, 194–198.

Macek, M. & Vavra, J. (1981) Prolonged exercise in 14-year-old girls. *International Journal of Sports Medicine* **2**, 228–30.

McMiken, D.F. (1975) Maximum aerobic power and

physical dimensions of children. *Annals of Human Biology* **3**, 141–147.

Malina, R.M. (1983) Menarche in athletes: a synthesis and hypothesis. *Annals of Human Biology* **10**, 1–24.

Malina, R. (1994) Physical growth and biological maturation of young athletes. *Exercise and Sports Science Reviews* **22**, 389–434.

Martinez, J., Lowenstein, M.K., Montague, A. & Munios, W. (1993) Nutrition and substance use in the adolescent male football player. *International Paediatrics* **8**, 435–439.

Martinez, L.R. & Haymes, E.M. (1992) Substrate utilisation during treadmill running in prepubertal girls and women. *Medicine and Science in Sports and Exercise* **24**, 975–83.

Meyer, F., Bar-Or, O., MacDougall, J.D. & Heigenhauser, J.F. (1992) Sweat electrolyte loss during exercise in the heat: effects of gender and maturation. *Medicine and Science in Sports and Exercise* **24**, 776–81.

Meyer, F., Bar-Or, O., Salsberg, A. & Passe, D. (1994) Hypohydration during exercise in children: effect of thirst, drink preferences and rehydration. *International Journal of Sports Nutrition* **4**, 22–35.

Nelson Steen, S. (1996) Nutrition for the school-aged child athlete. In *The Child and Adolescent Athlete* (ed. O. Bar-Or), pp. 260–273. Blackwell Science, Oxford.

Nickerson, H.J., Holubets, M.C., Weiler, B.R., Haas, R.G., Schwartz, S. & Ellerfson, M.E. (1989) Causes of iron deficiency in adolescent athletes. *Journal of Paediatrics* **114**, 657–663.

Nose, H., Mack, G.W., Shi, X. & Nadel, E.R. (1988) Role of plasma osmolality and plasma volume during rehydration in humans. *Journal of Applied Physiology* **65**, 325–231.

O'Connor, H. (1994) Special needs: children and adolescents in sport. In *Clinical Sports Nutrition* (ed. L.M. Burke & V. Deakin), pp. 390–414. McGraw Hill, Sydney.

Pate, R.R., Maguire, M. & Van Wyke, J. (1979) Dietary iron supplementation in women athletes. *Physician and Sportsmedicine* **7**, 81–89.

Perron, M. & Endres, J. (1985) Knowledge, attitudes, and dietary practices of female athletes. *Journal of the American Dietetic Association* **85**, 573–576.

Pipes, P.L. (1989) *Nutrition in Infancy and Childhood*, 4th edn. Mosby, St Louis, MO.

Rankinen, T., Fogelholm, M., Isokaanta, M. & Hartikka, K. (1993) Nutritional status of exercising and control children. *International Journal of Sports Medicine* **14**, 293–297.

Richbell, M. (1996) *Nutritional habits of junior elite athletes*. Dissertation, University of Liverpool.

Rowland, T.W. (1985) Aerobic response to endurance training in pre-pubescent children: a critical analysis. *Medicine and Science in Sports and Exercise* **17**, 493–497.

Rowland, T.W. & Kelleher, J.F. (1989) Iron deficiency in athletes: insights from high school swimmers. *American Journal of Diseases in Childhood* **143**, 197–200.

Rowland, T.W., Black, S.A. & Kelleher, J.F. (1987) Iron deficiency in adolescent endurance athletes. *Journal of Adolescent Health Care* **8**, 322–326.

Rowley, S. (1987) Psychological effects of intensive training in young athletes. *Journal of Childhood Psychology and Psychiatry* **28**, 371–377.

Shephard, R.J. (1982) *Physiology and Biochemistry of Exercise*. Praeger, New York.

Sobal, J. & Marquart, L.M. (1994) Vitamin/mineral supplement use among high school athletes. *Adolescent* **29**, 835–843.

Tanner, J.M. (1989) *Foetus into Man: Physical Growth from Conception to Maturity*, 2nd edn. Castlemead Publications, Ware, UK.

Theintz, G., Howald, H., Allemann, Y. & Sizonenko, P.C. (1989) Growth and pubertal development of young female gymnasts and swimmers: a correlation with parental data. *International Journal of Sports Medicine* **10**, 87–91.

Theintz, G.E., Howald, H., Weiss, U. & Sizonenko, P.C. (1993) Evidence for a reduction of growth potential in adolescent female gymnasts. *Journal of Pediatrics* **122**, 306–313.

Welten, D., Kemper, H.C.G., Post, G.B. et al. (1994) Weight-bearing activity during youth is a more important factor for peak bone mass than calcium intake. *Journal of Bone Mineral Research* **9**, 1089–1096.

Wilk, B. & Bar-Or, O. (1996) Effect of drink flavour and NaCl on voluntary drinking and hydration in boys exercising in the heat. *Journal of Applied Physiology* **80**, 1112–1117.

Wilmore, J.H. (1995) Disordered eating in the young athlete. In *New Horizons in Pediatric Exercise Science* (ed. C.J.R. Blimkie & O. Bar-Or), pp. 161–178. Human Kinetics, Champaign, IL.

Young, S.J. (1991) The clinical psychopharmacology of tryptophan. In *Nutrition and the Brain* (ed. R.J. Wurtman & J.J. Wurtman), pp. 49–88. Raven Press, NY.

Zanconato, S., Buchtal, S., Barstow, T.J. & Cooper, D.M. (1993) $^{31}$P-magnetic resonance spectroscopy of leg muscle metabolism during exercise in children and adults. *Journal of Applied Physiology* **74**, 2214–2218.

# Chapter 33

# The Vegetarian Athlete

JACQUELINE R. BERNING

## Introduction

All athletes at some time in their career look at alternative ways of eating to reach their athletic potential. While some athletes take pills, powders or potions in the belief that these will enhance their performance, others have changed their eating styles to a vegetarian diet to gain advantages in training and performance. Unfortunately, after many years of research, the effects of elimination of animal products from the diet on athletic performance are still unclear. Some data do exist on elite athletes who consume a vegetarian diet, but studies that include Olympic-calibre athletes are limited. In addition, most of the research on vegetarianism in the past decade has been focused on the health aspects of a vegetarian diet, rather than on human performance issues. There is certainly a lack of information regarding vegetarianism and its relationship to athletic performance. However, an athlete who consumes a poorly planned vegetarian diet may be at risk of multiple nutritional deficiencies as well as poor physical performance.

## Early meat eaters

It well known that ancient Greek athletes consumed large amounts of meats and many of them believed that their performances were dependent upon animal protein. As an example, Milo of Croton, the legendary Greek wrestler, consumed huge amounts of animal protein and trained by carrying animals across his shoulders.

As the animals grew, so did his strength. While Milo's diet would be viewed today as containing excessive amounts of protein, he was never brought to his knees in the course of the five Olympiads in which he competed (Ryan 1981; Whorton 1982). This concept of the need for large amounts of animal protein was promoted in the early 1800s by Liebig, the pre-eminent physiological chemist of the time (Whorton 1982). He believed that protein was the main substrate for the exercising muscle. While Liebig's hypothesis was disproved by Atwater in the mid-1800s, his philosophy of consuming large amounts of protein continues to have influence even into the modern day. Today, many athletes still believe that, by consuming large amounts of protein, they will become stronger and gain lean body mass (Berning *et al.* 1991).

## Early vegetarians

While many ancient Greeks were consuming large amounts of animal protein for athletic prowess, the founder of the philosophical vegetarian movement was also Greek. Pythagoras, the Greek mathematician, is the father of vegetarianism, and until the middle of the 19th century, vegetarians referred to themselves as 'Pythagoreans' (Dombrowski 1984).

Many of the vegetarians in the mid- to late 1800s were determined to prove that their diet was superior to that of meat eaters. As a result, the London Vegetarian Society formed an athletic and cycling club in the late 1800s to compete against their carnivorous counterparts and in most cases outperformed them in athletic competition (Nieman 1988). Due to their success, many other vegetarian athletes joined the movement. One such competition was the 1893 race from Berlin to Vienna, a 599-km course in which the first two competitors to finish were vegetarian (Whorton 1982). Over the next 10–20 years many other vegetarian athletes performed well in endurance performances around Europe.

Because of the success of vegetarian athletes, a few researchers in the early part of the 20th century were interested in measuring their physical capabilities, and Fischer (1907) conducted experiments on Yale student athletes. The subjects were exposed to a wide variety of foods including meat and meatless choices and performed a variety of endurance tests. Those athletes who gravitated toward the meatless diet were classified as vegetarians and were compared with athletes who ate meat. Each subject was tested to determine the maximum length of time that they could hold their arms out horizontally and the number of maximum deep knee bends and leg raises they could perform. Fischer noted that the vegetarians scored better than their meat-eating counterparts.

Wishart (1934) reported on a 48-year-old Olympic cyclist who had been a vegetarian for 23 years. The subject was submitted to four different meatless meals with different levels of protein during the 4-week experimental period. The exercise protocol involved riding a cycle ergometer for 8.5 h on four occasions after stabilizing on a different level of dietary protein. During the ride, measurements were made of external work and total energy expenditure. Higher speeds were recorded on the cycle ergometer after consuming the diets with a higher protein content, especially after 4 h of riding. The improved performance was attributed to an increased supply of energy coming from the meatless protein foods. While the energy content of each of the four different meatless meals varied by about 840 kJ (200 kcal), the amount of carbohydrate was not calculated and the increase in protein content for each of the

four experimental diets came from dairy products which contain a significant amount of carbohydrates.

## Modern-day vegetarian athletes

The recent literature contains few publications dealing with vegetarianism and athletic performance. However, Cotes et al. (1970) studied the effect of a vegan diet on physiological responses to submaximal exercise in 14 females who had consumed a vegetarian diet for an average of more than 11 years. They compared the vegetarians with two different controls, one that included 66 females of comparable social background and a second group of 20 office cleaners who had a comparable level of activity to that of the vegetarians. All subjects performed a submaximal test on a cycle ergometer in which they cycled for 3 min at 30 and 60 W. Ventilation and cardiac frequency were obtained as well as width of the muscles in the thigh. Their results showed that the sedentary controls had a significantly higher cardiac frequency while having a significantly lower grade of activity ($P > 0.02$). No statistical differences exist between the groups for thigh circumference or anterior skinfold thickness. The authors concluded that the data do not support the hypothesis that a low dietary intake of animal protein impairs the physiological response to submaximal exercise.

Few data exist on the relationship between athleticism and vegetarian diets even today, in spite of the popular belief that a vegetarian diet may be beneficial to some athletes. However, anecdotal reports abound. The Tarahumara, a Ute-Aztecan tribe inhabiting the Sierra Madre Occidental Mountains in the north central state of Chihuahua, Mexico, have been reported to be capable of extraordinary physical fitness and endurance as long-distance runners (Balke & Snow 1965), while consuming a vegetarian diet. Their diet contains very little food from animal sources and they have reportedly run distances up to 320 km in 'kickball' races which often last several days (Balka & Snow 1965). Cerqueira and associates (1979) investigated the Tarahumaras' food intake and nutrient composition and reported that most of their daily energy and nutrients come from corn, beans and squash. About 94% of their daily protein intake is from vegetable sources and only 6% from animal sources. Since most of the fat in their diet (9–12%) was derived from corn, beans and squash, their diets are rich in linoleic acid and plant sterols. The Tarahumara diet is extremely low in cholesterol (71 mg·day$^{-1}$) since their primary source of cholesterol is eggs, of which they consume about two or three per week. Other sources of fat and cholesterol in the Tarahumara diet come from small, infrequent servings of meat, fish, poultry and dairy products and lard. Even though the diet of the Tarahumara Indians is a simple one consisting mainly of plant foods, it is of high nutritional quality and is nutritionally sound, resulting in little chronic deficiencies and no widespread undernutrition (Cerqueira *et al.* 1979).

Hanne *et al.* (1986) investigated various fitness parameters of vegetarian athletes and compared them with non-vegetarians. Forty-nine athletes (29 men and 20 women) who had been either lacto-ovo- or lactovegetarian for at least 2 years were compared with 49 controls (29 men and 20 women). Subject ages ranged from 17 to 60 years of age, with the majority of the subjects in the age range of 17–35 years. Fitness parameters included anthropometric measurements, pulmonary function, aerobic and anaerobic capacity and blood chemistries. The authors found no significant differences in body mass between the two groups, although the female vegetarians had a significantly ($P>0.01$) high percentage body fat than their non-vegetarian counterparts. No differences were found in pulmonary function, heart rate, blood pressure or in the electrocardiogram. No differences were found between the two groups of subjects in aerobic capacity or anaerobic capacity as determined from a submaximal test and a Wingate test, respectively. Results from the blood examination found that non-vegetarian controls had lower uric acid levels than the vegetarian males, but the non-vegetarian group were within the normal range.

Vegetarian women had lower haematocrit values than controls, but haemoglobin, total protein, and glucose were similar in both groups. While no differences were found between the two groups, it is always difficult to find significant differences, because vegetarianism does not embrace a single, well-defined diet, and the influence of other lifestyle factors, including habitual physical activity levels, may obscure possible effects of the diet itself. Herein may lie part of the problem, as past research on vegetarianism and athletic performance did not clearly define the type of diet being followed by groups of individuals studied. Many athletes may call themselves vegetarian when in fact they simply eliminate from their diet a food group or a certain class of foods. Information on the diet of vegetarian athletes would be helpful in defining limiting or beneficial factors.

## Classifications of vegetarian diets

Vegetarian diets range from the vegan diet, which excludes all animal proteins, to the semi-vegetarian diet, which may include some animal proteins (Table 33.1).

Whatever the term an individual uses, it appears that vegetarianism is a continuum of eating styles, which range from the sole consumption of plant foods to a diet restricting certain kinds of animal proteins or limiting the frequency of animal protein consumption (Ratzin 1995). Because of the variety of vegetarian eating styles among practitioners, it is difficult to define the variables that will influence human performance, but relationships have been found between vegetarianism and a reduction in specific health risks.

## Health implications of vegetarian diets

There is increasing tendency among researchers to conclude that the reduced disease risk observed among vegetarians is not explained so much by the absence of meat from the diet, but by the fact that they eat more plant foods. Results

**Table 33.1** Classifications of various types of vegetarian diets. From Rudd (1989), with permission.

| Diet | Description |
|---|---|
| Semivegetarian | Some but not all groups of animal-derived products, such as meat, poultry, fish, seafood, eggs, milk and milk products may be included in this diet |
| New vegetarian | Plant-food diet supplemented with some groups of animal products, but emphasis is placed on foods that are 'organic, natural and unprocessed or unrefined' |
| Pescovegetarian | Excludes red meats, but consumes fish as well as plant foods |
| Lacto-ovovegetarian | Milk and milk products and eggs included in this diet, but meat, poultry, fish, seafood and eggs excluded |
| Ovovegetarians | Eggs are included in this diet, but milk and milk products, meat, poultry, fish and seafood are excluded |
| Strict vegetarian/vegan | All animal-derived foods, including meat, poultry, fish, seafood, eggs, milk and milk products are excluded from this diet |
| Macrobiotic | Avoids all animal foods. Uses only unprocessed, unrefined, natural and organic foods. In some types there is fluid restriction. Tamari, miso and various seaweeds are used |
| Fruitarian | This diet consists of raw or dried fruits, nuts, seeds, honey and vegetable oil |

of epidemiological research are traditionally expressed in terms of relative risk, a difficult concept for the athletic and consumer population to grasp. In a recent re-examination of data from the Adventist Health Study (Fraser *et al.* 1995), novel statistical calculations show how certain effects may delay or advance the first expression of disease. The Adventist Health Study is a cohort investigation of approximately 34 000 Californian, non-Hispanic, white subjects living in Seventh Day Adventist households who were followed for 6 years. Some of the findings from this study are as follows.

**1** Non-vegetarians develop coronary disease 1.77 years earlier than vegetarians.

**2** Among males, non-vegetarians have a remaining lifetime risk of developing coronary disease that is 11.9% higher (*P*<0.05) than that of vegetarians.

**3** Non-vegetarian females have a remaining lifetime risk of developing coronary disease that is 0.26 percentage points lower than that of female vegetarians.

**4** Those who rarely consume nuts develop coronary disease 2.6 years earlier and have a remaining lifetime risk 11.9 percentage points greater

(*P*<0.05) than persons who eat nuts at least five times per week.

While Seventh Day Adventists show a reduced risk of several chronic diseases, many of them also abstain from smoking and alcohol, and they are more physically active than non-vegetarians, which also affects the prevalence of chronic diseases. To date, no one has followed a vegetarian athletic population to see if they show the same health benefits.

## Nutritional adequacy of vegetarian diets

### Protein quality

A nutritionally sound vegetarian diet is possible if adequate amounts of a wide variety of foods are consumed (Grandjean 1989; Harding *et al.* 1996), but there are certain nutrients that vegetarians must be aware of and plan for to ensure the presence of adequate amounts in their diets. The most obvious nutrient of concern is protein. Lacto-ovovegetarians and ovovegetarians receive high-quality complete proteins and are unlikely to incur protein deficiencies. Vegetarians who consume only plant proteins could become protein deficient unless they balance their amino acids. Plant proteins are incomplete and lack one or more essential amino acid. While it was once thought that all the amino acids must be consumed in one meal, it is now agreed that timing of the amino acid intake is less critical and that amino acid intake must be balanced over days rather than hours. Research now shows that the liver monitors the amino acid composition of proteins consumed in a meal: if the meal is low in an essential amino acid, the liver can break down its own proteins to supply it. When the amino acid is once again plentiful, the liver will replenish its protein source.

Because individual plant foods do not contain all the essential amino acids, it is recommended that vegetarians complement their proteins. For example, cereals are very low in the essential amino acid lysine, while legumes are slightly deficient in the sulphur-containing amino acids. By combining these two groups of foods (i.e. refried beans and corn tortillas), a vegetarian could provide a mixture of amino acids similar to that of a complete or high-quality protein food. Figure 33.1 illustrates different combinations of incomplete proteins to make a complete protein as well as demonstrating the fact that when an animal protein is combined with an incomplete

protein, the result is a complete, high-quality protein.

## Protein requirements for vegetarian athletes

A major concern for vegetarian athletes is to make sure that they have consumed enough food so that their protein requirement will be met. The total protein intake of athletes consuming a vegetarian diet may have to be increased slightly to take account of the lower digestibility, lower energy density and lower protein quality of plant foods consumed. This may lead to problems with the volume of food to be consumed, because athletes with high energy requirements may find it difficult to consume sufficient volume of foods to maintain energy balance on a purely vegetarian diet. Generally, if vegetarian athletes consume between 0.8 and 1.7 g protein·kg$^{-1}$ body mass·day$^{-1}$ and maintain energy balance, they should meet their protein requirement for exercise and health.

## Vitamin B$_{12}$

Another nutrient that may be low in a vegetarian diet is vitamin B$_{12}$, especially for those individuals on a strict plant-based diet (vegans). Rauma *et al.* (1995) studied the vitamin B$_{12}$ status of long-

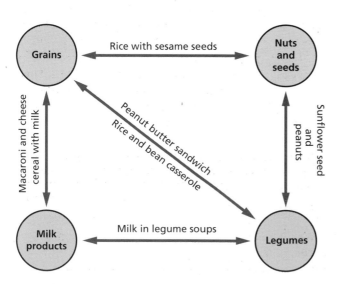

**Fig. 33.1** The concept of mutual supplementation, which is the strategy of combining two incomplete sources of protein so that the amino acids in each food make up for those lacking in other foods. Such protein combinations are sometimes called complementary proteins.

term adherents to a strict uncooked vegan diet called the 'living food diet' (LFD). Most food items in this diet are fermented or sprouted. Serum $B_{12}$ concentrations and the dietary intakes of 21 long-term adherents of the LFD were compared with those of 21 omnivorous controls. In a longitudinal study, the LFD diet resulted in a decrease in serum vitamin $B_{12}$ in six of nine subjects. The cross-sectional study revealed significantly lower serum vitamin $B_{12}$ in the LFD adherents than in their matched omnivorous controls. Those following the LFD who consumed nori or chinerilla seaweeds had somewhat better $B_{12}$ status than those who did not, but $B_{12}$ levels fell over time in all but one subject. While lower levels of vitamin $B_{12}$ have been found in strict vegans, few cases of clinical deficiency have been found. Helman and Darnton-Hill (1987) found the mean serum vitamin $B_{12}$ levels of vegetarians to be significantly lower ($350 \, pg \cdot ml^{-1}$) than those of omnivores ($490 \, pg \cdot ml^{-1}$), while 16% of the vegetarians had values less than $200 \, pg \cdot ml^{-1}$. Vitamin $B_{12}$ deficiency is rare among lacto-ovovegetarians because milk and eggs contain sufficient quantities of this nutrient. Vegans should be encouraged to use soybean milk fortified with vitamin $B_{12}$ or a vitamin $B_{12}$ supplement. Analogues of the vitamin found in algae, spirulina, nori or fermented soy products do not have vitamin activity for humans.

Individuals with low serum $B_{12}$ may manifest paraesthesia (numbness and tingling in the hands and legs), weakness, fatigue, loss of vibration and position sense, and a range of psychiatric disorders including disorientation, depression and memory loss. The use of alcohol, tobacco and drugs such as antacids, neomycin, colchicine and aminosalicylic acid may contribute to the problem by causing $B_{12}$ malabsorption in both omnivores and vegetarians.

### Iron availability in vegetarian diets

While both vegetarian and non-vegetarians may have difficulty in meeting the dietary requirements for iron, athletes who eat red meat are at less risk of iron deficiency anaemia. In absolute amounts, red meat contains only an average amount of iron, but the bioavailabilty of iron from red meat is superior to that derived from plant sources. There are two forms of iron in the diet: haem iron and non-haem iron. Haem iron found in meats, fish and poultry is better absorbed than non-haem iron, which is found in grains, vegetables and fruits. The fractional absorption of haem and non-haem iron varies between 3% and 35%, depending on the presence of dietary enhancing factors such as ascorbic acid, consumption of sources of haem iron and on the body stores of iron. Table 33.2 lists the ranges of intestinal absorption of iron from haem and non-haem food sources which is dependent upon body stores of iron.

Iron is classified as an essential nutrient and is required for the formation of haemoglobin and myoglobin, as well as the cytochromes, which are components of the electron transport chain in the mitochondria. Iron is also a cofactor for a number of enzymatic reactions, including those involved in the synthesis of collagen and of various neurotransmitters. In addition, iron is needed for proper immune function and plays a role in the drug detoxification pathways (Wardlaw & Insel 1995).

Since iron plays a critical role in oxidative energy metabolism, it is essential for athletes to have adequate iron stores. There are some differences of opinion about the prevalence of iron deficiency among athletes. A number of studies have used serum ferritin as a measure of iron deficiency anaemia, while other studies have used haemoglobin and haematocrit as determinants of iron deficiency anaemia. The number

**Table 33.2** Absorption rate (as % of intake) of haem and non-haem iron in relation to body stores of iron.

|  | Haem (%) | Non-haem (%) |
| --- | --- | --- |
| Low stores of iron | 35 | 20 |
| Normal stores of iron | 15 | 2–3 |

of athletes suffering from true iron deficiency anaemia is therefore difficult to establish (Eichner 1988). Further debates have been sparked by the fact that many athletes with low iron stores eat little haem iron and yet have no performance decrements (Dallongeville *et al.* 1989; Snyder *et al.* 1989; Lyle *et al.* 1992; Pate *et al.* 1993; Williford *et al.* 1993). It is, however, important to monitor iron status among athletes, especially female athletes. The Sports Medicine and Science Division of the United States Olympic Committee recommend screening for haemoglobin and haematocrit twice yearly. Other tests of iron stores are recommended based on menstruation records.

Snyder *et al.* (1989) investigated the iron intake and iron stores in female athletes who either were consuming a mixed diet or were classified as a modified vegetarian. The subjects were matched for age, body mass, aerobic capacity, training load and number of pregnancies. The modified vegetarians ($n = 9$) consumed less than 100 g of red meat per week while the subjects on the mixed diet ($n = 9$) included red meat in their diet. Both groups consumed the same amount of iron (14 mg·day$^{-1}$), but serum ferritin and total iron-binding capacity were significantly lower in the modified vegetarian group ($P < 0.05$). The authors also found that the bioavailability of the iron consumed by the two groups was different. Iron consumed by the modified vegetarian group was significantly less available than the iron consumed by the mixed-diet group. These data suggest that in female runners non-haem iron may not be as readily available as haem iron. These findings have also been confirmed in the non-athletic population. In 1995 Shaw *et al.* (1995) investigated the iron status of young Chinese Buddhist vegetarians (23 men and 32 women) and compared them with non-vegetarian students (20 men and 39 women). Dietary assessment of iron intake and haematological measurements of biochemical indices, including haemoglobin, plasma iron, transferrin saturation and plasma ferritin, were made. A characteristic of the vegetarian diets was that most of the protein was coming from soybean products, which have limited bioavailable iron. Daily iron intake was similar in both vegetarian and non-vegetarian men, but iron intake was significantly higher in female vegetarians than non-vegetarians. Results from the haematological measurements showed that for both sexes, the median plasma ferritin concentration of the vegetarians was about half that of the non-vegetarians. There was also a greater prevalence of low ferritin levels and anaemia in the vegetarian group, especially among the vegetarian women.

FOOD STRATEGIES FOR INCREASING
IRON IN A VEGETARIAN DIET

Because animal foods are the best and most absorbable source of iron, this presents a potential problem to the vegetarian who eats no red meat. Lacto-ovovegetarians also have a problem consuming enough iron, as milk and dairy products are poor sources of iron. Vegetarians can incorporate leafy green vegetables such as spinach and legumes as well as fortified and enriched whole grains into their diets. Dried fruit can also provide iron in the vegetarian diet. Dietary iron may also be derived from iron cooking utensils. When acidic foods are cooked in iron cookware, some of the iron is taken up with the food.

## Zinc status among athletes

Since the best food sources of zinc are meats, dairy products and seafood (especially oysters), zinc nutriture is of concern for vegetarians. Whole-grain cereals and cereal products are the primary sources of zinc in many vegetarian diets, but the phytate and fibre content of these products reduces the bioavailability of zinc (Reinhold *et al.* 1976). Zinc is found in almost every tissue in the body and is a cofactor for over 100 enzymes, of which several are important in the pathways for energy metabolism. Zinc is also needed for protein synthesis and is a part of the insulin molecule.

Several studies have demonstrated that

exercise increases zinc loss from the body (Dressendorfer & Socklov 1980; Haralambie 1981; Singh *et al.* 1990; Clarkson & Haymes 1994) and that levels may be low in athletes. Possible explanations for the reduced level of zinc stores include inadequate intake of zinc, low bioavailability, increased zinc loss during exercise, dilution of zinc by expansion of plasma volume, and redistribution of zinc in the body.

Contrary to these reports, Lukaski (1989; Lukaski *et al.* 1990) has found that zinc status is not affected by physical training as long as dietary intakes of zinc are adequate. Lukaski *et al.* (1990) studied 16 female and 13 male swimmers and 13 female and 15 male non-swimming controls. Plasma zinc values were within the normal range for all subjects and did not change throughout the swimming season. In addition to Lukaski's studies, Duester *et al.* (1989) investigated the effects of endurance training on zinc status in 13 highly trained women and compared them with 10 untrained controls. Three-day dietary records were evaluated for zinc intake while blood and 24 h urine samples were taken before and after a 25-mg oral zinc load. Mean daily zinc intakes did not differ and were below the recommended dietary allowance set for zinc for both groups. The authors reported no differences between fasting concentrations of plasma zinc, serum albumin, α-2-macroglobulin, and erythrocyte zinc content among the two groups. However, the trained women had significantly ($P<0.05$) higher urinary zinc excretion and reduced responses to the oral zinc load than did the untrained women. The authors concluded that the increase in zinc excretion in the highly trained women may reflect higher rates of skeletal muscle turnover.

## ZINC AND THE VEGETARIAN

In addition to these studies of athletes, several studies confirm lower zinc status among vegetarians (Freeland-Graves *et al.* 1980; Gibson 1994; Kadrabova *et al.* 1995).

Janelle and Barr (1995) recently reported a study comparing nutrient intakes between female vegetarians and non-vegetarians with similar health practices and found that vegans and lactovegetarians had lower zinc intakes (8.5 and 8.2 mg·day⁻¹, respectively) than the recommended dietary allowance of 15 mg·day⁻¹. Similar results were found in a study conducted by Donovan and Gibson (1995), who found that 33% of semivegetarians, 24% of lacto-ovovegetarians and 18% of omnivores had serum zinc levels below 10.7 nmol·l⁻¹. They also reported that the phytate to zinc ratio in the diet was negatively associated with the serum zinc concentration ($P<0.05$). The authors concluded that the suboptimal zinc status was the result of low intakes of poorly available zinc in all dietary groups.

## FOOD STRATEGIES FOR INCREASING ZINC IN A VEGETARIAN DIET

Foods for the vegetarian that have the highest zinc content are oysters, crab, shrimp, wheat germ and legumes. Incorporating other good sources of zinc into a vegetarian diet will also help meet the dietary recommendations: nuts, beans and whole grains can all contribute. Zinc is not part of the enrichment process, so refined flours are not a good source.

## Calcium requirements of vegetarians

The diets of strict vegetarians or vegans tend to be low in calcium unless adequate amounts of milk and dairy products or dark leafy greens are consumed daily. As with iron and zinc, the absorption of calcium may be reduced by phytates, oxalates, fibre and tannins (James *et al.* 1978; Weaver *et al.* 1996). Phytic acid is found in oatmeal and other whole-grain cereals, while oxalates are commonly found in beets, spinach and leafy greens. These binders seem to depress absorption of calcium present in some calcium-containing foods but not in others. That is why strict vegans who obtain most of their dietary calcium from leafy greens and whole-grain products are at a greater risk of an inadequate calcium availability than milk-drinking vegetarians. A purely vegan diet may also be low in vitamin D, which will further impair calcium absorption and utilization.

In an interesting anthropological study of prehispanic burials from the Canary Islands, Gonzalez-Reimers and Arnay-de-la-Rosa (1992) found a high prevalance of osteoporosis among the 117 skeletons analysed for trace elements. Bone trace element analysis showed that low concentrations of iron, zinc and copper were found in skeletons with a reduced trabecular bone mass. The authors state that during this prehispanic period many of the residents of the Canary Islands existed in a relative protein-energy malnutrition state which consisted mainly of a vegetarian diet which may have predisposed these individuals to osteoporosis.

It has been suggested that vegetarians who restrict their intake of dairy products should provide calcium-rich foods or supplements by consuming calcium-fortified soy products as well as consuming dark leafy green vegetables on a daily basis.

FOOD STRATEGIES FOR INCREASING
CALCIUM IN A VEGETARIAN DIET

Foods with the highest nutrient density for calcium are leafy greens, such as spinach and broccoli, non-fat milk, romano cheese, swiss cheese, sardines and canned salmon. The calcium found in some leafy greens is not well absorbed because of the presence of oxalic acid, but this effect is not as strong for kale, collard, turnip, and mustard greens. Overall, non-fat milk is the most nutrient-dense source of calcium because of its high bioavailability and low energy value. The new calcium-fortified orange juices and other beverages offer an alternative to the individual who is a strict vegetarian; other calcium-fortified foods include bread, breakfast cereal, breakfast bars, and snacks. Another good source for the vegetarian is soybean curd (tofu) if it is made with calcium carbonate (check the food label).

While there are concerns about the potential lack of some nutrients in a vegetarian diet, many of these concerns can be overcome by using a wide variety of foods and planning meals so that they complement proteins and include nutrient-dense foods. Table 33.3 summarizes the nutrients that may be lacking in a vegetarian diet and gives some examples of foods that could be included in a vegetarian diet to overcome these inadequacies.

## Hormonal alterations as a result of a vegetarian diet

There is evidence that nutritional status and diet can affect the reproductive system. Hill *et al.* (1984) found that Caucasian women ($n = 16$), who normally ate meat had a significantly ($P < 0.01$) shorter follicular phase of their second menstrual cycle when they ate a vegetarian diet for two cycles. The vegetarian diet decreased ($P < 0.01$) the pituitary response to releasing luteinizing hormone and decreased ($P < 0.05$) the episodic release of luteinizing hormone. The experiment also included supplementing nine vegetarian Black South African women with daily meat product: an increased length of the follicular phase was observed ($P < 0.01$). The authors concluded that a lower episodic release of gonadotrophins and a shorter duration of the follicular phase, when omnivorous women ate no animal protein, implies that a vegetarian diet plays a role in the control of ovulation through the hypothalamic axis of the central nervous system. In a similar study, Pirke *et al.* (1986) investigated the influence of a vegetarian diet on the menstrual cycles of 18 healthy normal weight women aged 17–27 years. Plasma levels of oestradiol, progesterone and luteinizing hormone were measured on Monday, Wednesday and Friday throughout the 6-week diet period. Nine women followed a vegetarian diet while nine followed an omnivorous diet. Both groups lost weight during the experimental period (1 kg body weight·week$^{-1}$). Seven of the nine vegetarian women became anovulatory and had significantly decreased luteinizing hormone during the mid-cycle and luteal phase. Oestrogen and progesterone levels were also signifi-

**Table 33.3** Nutrients that are of concern in a vegetarian diet and strategies to lower nutritional deficiencies. From Rudd (1990).

| Nutrient | RDA | Physiological function | Vegetarian food sources |
|---|---|---|---|
| Protein | $0.8\,g \cdot kg^{-1}\,BW$ | Build and repair tissues; major component of antibodies, enzymes, hormones; responsible for transport of nutrients and fluid balance | Eggs, fish, legumes, peanut butter, milk, brown rice, peanuts, soybeans |
| Vitamin $B_{12}$ | $2.0\,\mu g \cdot day^{-1}$ | Promotes growth; cofactor for several enzymes; maintains the sheath around nerve fibres; helps folate in preventing anaemia | Eggs, dairy products, clams, oysters, some seafood |
| Iron | Males, $10\,mg \cdot day^{-1}$; females, $15\,mg \cdot day^{-1}$ | Constituent of haemoglobin and myoglobin; carrier of $O_2$ and $CO_2$ | Clams, whole grains, enriched cereals, green leafy vegetables, dried fruits, tofu, legumes |
| Calcium | Teens, $1200\,mg \cdot day^{-1}$; adults, $800\,mg \cdot day^{-1}$ | Major component of hydroxyapatite for bones and teeth; regulation of muscle contraction, heart beat, clotting of blood, and transmission of nerve impulses; blood pressure | Dairy products, leafy green vegetables, fish and shellfish, tofu, legumes |
| Zinc | Males, $15\,mg \cdot day^{-1}$; females, $12\,mg \cdot day^{-1}$ | Part of over 100 enzymes; associated with insulin; involved in making DNA and RNA; involved with the immune system; transport of vitamin A; wound healing and normal development of the fetus | Fish, oysters, dairy products, black beans, kidney beans, tofu, beets, peas, whole-grain breads, bran flakes |
| Vitamin D | $400\,IU \cdot day^{-1}$ | Promotes normal bone and teeth formation, aids body's absorption, transportation and deposition of calcium and phosphorus | Fortified dairy products, egg yolk, shrimp, sunlight |

cantly decreased in the vegetarian group. In comparison, seven of nine women in the omnivorous group maintained ovulatory cycles and had no change in cycle length or in the length of the follicular phase. In both of these studies a vegetarian diet appears to be involved in the incidence of menstrual irregularities, but the underlying pathophysiology remains unclear.

### Vegetarian diets and oestrogen levels

Adlercreutz *et al.* (1986a, 1986b, 1995) have provided some possible reasons why a vegetarian diet may play a role in menstrual-cycle regularity. Dietary constituents such as fibre and a vegetarian eating pattern have been shown to alter oestrogen levels in humans by influencing oestrogen synthesis, availability, excretion metabolism and action. Currently there is a great deal of interest in plant-derived lignans and isoflavonic phyto-oestrogens, as they have been found in human urine and appear to exhibit, both *in vitro* and *in vivo*, weak oestrogenic and sometimes anti-oestrogenic activities. Plant lignans and isoflavonoids, glycosides from soybean products as well as whole grains, seeds and nuts are converted by intestinal microflora to hormone-like compounds. These compounds bind, with low affinity, to oestrogen receptors, and preliminary results suggest that they may induce production of sex hormone-binding globulin in the liver and in this way influence sex hormone metabolism and biological effects. Indeed, Gorbach and Goldin (1987) measured urinary, faecal and plasma levels of oestrogens in pre- and postmenopausal women eating different diets. Premenopausal US women consuming a 'Western' diet composed of 40% fat and low fibre were compared with age-matched vegetarians eating 30% of their energy intake as fat and a high-fibre diet. The researchers found that the vegetarian women excreted threefold more oestrogen in their faeces, had lower urinary oestrogen excretion, and had 15–20% lower plasma oestrogen than the omnivorous women. When pre- and postmenopausal women eating a Western diet were compared with Asian immigrants eating a very low fat diet (20–25% of total energy from fat), similar results were found, except that the plasma oestrogen levels were 30% lower among the Orientals than in the Western omnivore group. Correlation analysis of dietary components and plasma oestrogen showed that plasma oestrogen was positively associated with fat intake and negatively associated with dietary fibre. The authors concluded that diets high in fibre, like a vegetarian diet, can alter the route of excretion of oestrogen by influencing the enterohepatic circulation and thus influence plasma levels of oestrogen. In a similar study, Pedersen *et al.* (1991) examined the effect of different nutritional patterns on menstrual regularity in premenopausal women. Forty-one non-vegetarian and 34 vegetarian women were recruited and completed a questionnaire regarding menstrual history and a 3-day dietary record. The reported incidence of menstrual irregularity was 4.9% among the non-vegetarians and 26.5% among the vegetarians. The vegetarian group consumed significantly more polyunsaturated fatty acids, carbohydrates, vitamin $B_6$ and dietary fibre, whereas the non-vegetarians consumed significantly more caffeine, cholesterol, saturated fatty acids and alcohol. Logistic regression analysis showed that the probability of menstrual regularity among all subjects was positively correlated with increasing protein and cholesterol

intakes. The probability of developing menstrual irregularities was negatively correlated with increasing dietary fibre and increasing amounts of magnesium in the diet. This study is consistent with the notion that premenopausal vegetarian women as a group have decreased circulating oestrogen concentrations.

Additional data from Adlercreutz *et al.* (1986a) have also found that vegetarians may be excreting more oestrogen than omnivores: they investigated the possible effects of variations in dietary fibre intake on oestrogen metabolism in young Finnish women through one winter and one summer. Eleven of the subjects were lactovegetarians, while 12 were omnivorous. Within the groups there was a seasonal variation in fibre intake. The vegetarian group consumed more fibre ($P<0.02$), more grains ($P<0.02$) and more vegetables ($P<0.02$) during the winter than during the summer. The excretion of oestrogens was remarkably constant in the omnivorous group, while the vegetarian group had a significant seasonal variation of total and individual catecho-oestrogens and estrone ($P<0.05$–$0.005$). There were no differences between the groups in excretion of total or individual urinary oestrogens in any season or between mean values for both seasons, but a significant negative correlation was found between dietary intake of total grain fibre per kilogram of body weight and the excretion of individual oestrogens were found. These studies are consistent with the notion that menstrual regularity can be influenced by specific dietary nutrients that may have a direct effect on oestrogen.

## Hormonal responses of a vegetarian lifestyle on males

Most of the data collected on diet and hormone relationships among vegetarians is on women, and information on males is sparse. Howie and Shultz (1985) studied the relationship between dietary nutrients and plama testosterone, 5-α-dihydrotestosterone, oestradiol-17-β, luteinizing hormone, and prolactin levels in 12 Seventh Day Adventist vegetarian, 10 Seventh Day Adventist non-vegetarian and 8 non-Seventh Day Adventist, non-vegetarian males. Fasting blood samples and 3-day dietary intakes were obtained from all subjects. The Seventh Day Adventist vegetarians consumed significantly more crude and dietary fibre than the other non-vegetarian subjects. Plasma levels of testosterone and oestradiol-17-β were significantly lower in the Seventh Day Adventist vegetarians than in the ominvores. Additionally, plasma levels of testosterone and oestradiol-17-β of all subjects were negatively correlated with dietary fibre intake. The authors concluded that a vegetarian eating style may lead to decreased plasma concentrations of androgens and oestrogens in men. In contrast, Naik and Snyder (1997) examined the independent effects of diet and endurance training on basal serum testosterone concentration by comparing endurance-trained cyclists with vegetarian individuals who had abstained from eating red meat and poultry for 1 year. The aerobic ability of the endurance athletes was significantly greater than that of the sedentary vegetarians. Nutrient intake, however, was similar in both groups, except for dietary fibre intake, which was higher in the vegetarian group. Serum total and free testosterone concentrations were not different for either main effect (i.e. diet and exercise). Perhaps the lack of difference in sex hormones could be attributed to the fact that the diets were very similar in both groups.

## Implications of vegetarian diets for athletes

Vegetarian diets have been associated with a low incidence of cancers of the breast, endometrium and prostate. However, lowered plasma levels and increased urinary excretion of oestrogen can lead to menstrual abnormalities which may in turn lead to irregular menstrual cycles and compromised bone health in vegetarians. Brooks et al. (1984) noted that most female athletes with amenorrhoea were vegetarian. They compared the diets of amenorrhoeic runners (82% vegetarian) with regularly menstruating runners (13% vegetarian) and found that the runners with regular menstrual cycles ate five times more meat and significantly ($P < 0.05$) more fat than amenorrhoeic runners. Kaiserauer et al. (1989) also found that amenorrhoeic runners consumed significantly less fat, red meat and total energy than did regularly menstruating runners. Slavin et al. (1984) found that there was a high incidence of vegetarianism among amenorrhoeic athletes and speculated that trace elements or plant hormones may affect menstruation. While it appears that vegetarianism may influence menstrual function, the real importance of menstrual irregularities in female athletes is related to bone health.

In a landmark study on bone health and athletic amenorrhoea, Drinkwater et al. (1984) studied 28 female athletes, 14 of whom were amenorrhoeic. When compared with the regularly menstruating runners, the amenorrhoeic runners had significantly lower lumbar vertebral bone mineral densities. The mean age of the amenorrhoeic athletes was 25 years, but their average bone mineral density was equivalent to that of a 51-year-old. While there is a clear relationship between athletic amenorrhoea and bone health, there is a limited amount of information on the possible effects of a vegetarian lifestyle. Hunt et al. (1989) investigated the relationship of bone mineral content/bone width in elderly, independently living Methodist omnivores and Seventh Day Adventist vegetarians. Bone mass was measured by single photon absorptiometry and dietary intakes were assessed by 24-h dietary recall and food frequency methods. Bone mineral/bone width was not different in omnivores compared to vegetarians and no significant relationships were found to exist between current or early dietary intakes and bone mineral/bone width. Lloyd et al. (1991) also found no significant differences in bone density between vegetarian and non-vegetarian women despite a significantly higher prevalence of menstrual irregularities among the vegetarian subjects. These studies support the concept that, despite the differences in dietary practices, vegetarian and non-vegetarian women do not appear to differ in bone health. Caution must be taken, however, when dealing with an athlete who is a vegetarian. Bone mineral densitiy should be measured and adequate amounts of calcium should be consumed to ward off the potential harmful effects of low oestrogen on bone.

While vegetarianism is not a risk factor for the Female Athlete Triad, it may become a factor if an athlete is amenorrhoeic due to her vegetarian eating pattern.

## Conclusions and recommendations

Currently most information on vegetarianism relates to nutritional adequacy and the implications for lifestyle diseases such as heart disease and cancer. Little is known about the relationship between vegetarianism and athletic performance. What is clearly understood is that the vegetarian athlete must plan his or her diet carefully to avoid the risk of nutritional deficiencies and an adverse effect on performance. There are advantages to the athlete of consuming a vegetarian diet. Vegetarian athletes usually consume a higher proportion of energy in the form of carbohydrates. It is well documented that athletes, especially endurance athletes, should be consuming a higher proportion of carbohydrates in their diets to maximize muscle glycogen concentration. Prolonged strenuous exercise can deplete most of the glycogen stored in the muscles and the athlete can become chronically fatigued. Increasing dietary carbohydrates will be beneficial to the athlete involved in heavy training. More research is needed to answer some of the current concerns of vegetarian athletes, especially with regard to hormonal alterations and their impact on bone health as well as the questions on protein-energy requirements for strict vegetarians who consume no animal protein.

If athletes adopt a vegetarian lifestyle, they must become aware of the limitations of the diet and make sure that their nutritional requirements are met so as not to influence performance. Vegan diets should not be attempted by any athlete without previous experience or without consultation with a dietitian or health care provider. Young growing athletes should be discouraged from such a strict diet due to its possible limitations on growth and performance. Vegan diets should only be considered if an athlete is willing to devote time and effort to understanding the proper combinations and amounts of foods necessary to achieve a nutritionally balanced diet.

In planning vegetarian diets of any type, athletes should choose a wide variety of foods and ensure that the energy intake is adequate to meet their needs. Additionally, the American Dietetic Association (1993) gives the following recommendations for individuals who are vegetarian or thinking of becoming vegetarian.
• Keep the intake of foods with a low nutrient density, such as sweets and fatty foods, to a minimum.
• Choose whole or unrefined grain products, instead of refined products, whenever possible, or use fortified or enriched cereal products.
• Use a variety of fruits and vegetables, including a good food source of vitamin C.
• If milk or dairy products are consumed, use low-fat or non-fat varieties.
• Limit egg intake to three or four per week.
• Vegans should have a reliable source of vitamin $B_{12}$, such as some fortified commercial breakfast cereals, fortified soy beverage or a cyanocobalamin supplement. As long as the athlete is outdoors in the sun for part of the day, supplemental vitamin D may not be needed.
• Vegetarian and non-vegetarian infants who are solely breastfed beyond 4–6 months of age should receive supplements of iron and vitamin D if exposure to the sun is limited.

These recommendations, of course, were formulated for the non-athlete, and may need to be modified. When energy intake is very high, for example, there is room in the diet for foods with low nutrient density without compromising nutritional status.

## References

Adlercreutz, H., Fotsis, T., Bannwart, C., Hamalainen, E., Bloigu, S. & Ollus, A. (1986a) Urinary estrogen profile determination in young Finnish vegetarian and omnivorous women. *Journal of Steroid Biochemistry* **24**, 289–296.

Adlercreutz, H., Fotsis, T., Bannwart, C. *et al.* (1986b) Determination of urinary lignans and phytoestrogen metabolites, potential antiestrogens and anticarcinogens, in urine of women on various habitual diets. *Journal of Steroid Biochemistry* **25**, 791–797.

Adlercreutz, H., Goldin, B.R., Gorbach, S.L. *et al.* (1995) Soybean phytoestrogen intake and cancer risk. *Journal of Nutrition* **125** (Suppl.), S757–770.

American Dietetic Association (1993) Position of the American dietetic association: vegetarian diets. *Journal of the American Dietetic Association* **93**, 1317–1319.

Balke, B. & Snow, C. (1965) Anthropological and physiological observations on Tarahumara endurance runners. *American Journal of Physical Anthropology* **23**, 293–302.

Berning, J.R., Troup, J.P., VanHandel, P.J., Daniels, J. & Daniels, N. (1991). The nutritional habits of young adolescent swimmers. *International Journal of Sport Nutrition* **1**, 240–248.

Brooks, S.M., Sanborn, C.F., Albrecht, B.H. & Wagner, W.W. (1984) Diet in athletic amenorrhoea (letter). *Lancet* i, 559–660.

Cerqueira, M.T., Fry, M.M. & Connor, W.E. (1979) The food and nutrient intakes of the Tarahumara Indians of Mexico. *American Journal of Clinical Nutrition* **32**, 905–915.

Clarkson, P.M. & Haymes, E.M. (1994) Trace mineral requirements for athletes. *International Journal of Sport Nutrition* **4**, 104–119.

Cotes, J.E., Dabbs, J.M., Hall, A.M. *et al.* (1970) Possible effect of a vegan diet upon lung function and the cardiorespiratory response to submaximal exercise in healthy women. *Journal of Physiology* **209**, 30P–32P.

Dallongeville, J., Ledoux, M. & Brisson, G. (1989) Iron deficiency among active men. *Journal of the American College of Nutrition* **8**, 195–202.

Dombrowski, D.A. (1984) *The Philosophy of Vegetarianism*. University of Massachusetts Press, Amherst, MA.

Donovan, U.M. & Gibson, R.S. (1995) Iron and zinc status of young women aged 14–19 years consuming vegetarian and omnivore diets. *Journal of the American College of Nutrition* **14**, 463–472.

Dressendorfer, R.H. & Sockolov, R. (1980) Hypozincemia in runners. *Physician and Sports Medicine* **8**, 97–100.

Drinkwater, B.L., Nilson, K., Chesnut, C.H. *et al.* (1984) Bone mineral content of amenorrheic and eumenorrheic athletes. *New England Journal of Medicine* **311**, 277–281.

Duester, P.A., Day, G.A., Singh, A., Douglass, L. & Moser-Vellon, P.B. (1989) Zinc status of highly

trained women runners and untrained women. *American Journal of Clinical Nutrition* **49**, 1295–1301.

Eichner, R.E. (1988) Sports anemia: poor terminology for a real phenomenon. *Sports Science Exchange* **1** (6), 1–6.

Fisher, I. (1907) The effect of diet on endurance: based on an experiment, in thorough mastication, with nine healthy students at Yale University, January to June 1906. *Transactions of the Connecticut Academy of Arts and Science* **13**, 1–46.

Fraser, G.E., Lindsted, K.D. & Beeson, W.L. (1995) Effect of risk factor values on lifetime risk of and age at first coronary event: The Adventist Health Study. *American Journal of Epidemiology* **142**, 746–758.

Freeland-Graves, J.H., Ebangit, M.L. & Hendrikson, P.J. (1980) Alterations in zinc absorption and salivary sediment zinc after a lacto-ovo-vegetarian diet. *American Journal of Clinical Nutrition* **33**, 1757–1766.

Gibson, R.S. (1994) Content and bioavailability of trace elements in vegetarian diets. *American Journal of Clinical Nutrition* **59** (Suppl.), 1223s–1232s.

Gonzalez-Reimers, E. & Arnay-de-la-Rosa, M. (1992) Ancient skeletal remains of the Canary Islands: bone histology and chemical analysis. *Anthropologischer Anzeiger* **50**, 201–215.

Gorbach, S. & Goldin, B.R. (1987) Diet and the excretion of enterohepatic cycling of estrogens. *Preventive Medicine* **16**, 525–531.

Grandjean, A.C. (1989) Macronutrient intake of U.S. athletes compared with the general population and recommendations made for athletes. *American Journal of Clinical Nutrition* **49**, 1070–1076.

Hanne, N., Dlin, R. & Rotstein, A. (1986) Physical fitness, anthropometric and metabolic parameters in vegetarian athletes. *Journal of Sports Medicine* **26**, 180–185.

Haralambie, G. (1981) Serum zinc in athletes in training. *International Journal of Sports Medicine* **2**, 136–138.

Harding, M.G., Crooks, H. & Stare, F.J. (1996) Nutritional studies of vegetarians. *Journal of the American Dietetic Association* **48**, 25–28.

Helman, A.D. & Darnton-Hill, I. (1987) Vitamin and iron status in new vegetarians. *American Journal of Clinical Nutrition* **45**, 785–789.

Hill, P., Garbaczewski, L., Haley, L. & Wynder, E.L. (1984) Diet and follicular development. *American Journal of Clinical Nutrition* **39**, 771–777.

Howie, B.J. & Shultz, T.D. (1985) Dietary and hormonal interrelationships among vegetarian Seventh-Day Adventists and nonvegetarian men. *American Journal of Clinical Nutrition* **42**, 127–134.

Hunt, I.F., Murphy, N.J., Henderson, C. *et al.* (1989) Bone mineral content in postmenopausal women; comparison of omnivores and vegetarians. *American Journal of Clinical Nutrition* **50**, 517–523.

James, W.P.T., Branch, W.J. & Southgate, D.A.T. (1978) Calcium binding by dietary fibre. *Lancet* i, 638.

Janelle, K.C. & Barr, S.I. (1995) Nutrient intakes and eating behavior scores of vegetarian and nonvegetarian women. *Journal of the American Dietetic Association* 2, 180–186.

Kadrabova, J., Madaric, A., Kovacikova, Z. & Ginter, E. (1995) Selenium status, plasma zinc, copper and magnesium in vegetarians. *Biological Trace Element Research Journal* 50, 13–24.

Kaiserauer, S., Snyder, A.C., Sleeper, M. & Zierath, J. (1989) Nutritional, physiological, and menstrual status of distance runners. *Medicine and Science in Sports and Exercise* 21, 120–125.

Lloyd, T., Shaeffer, J.M., Walker, M.A. & Demers, L.M. (1991) Urinary hormonal concentrations and spinal bone densities of premenopausal vegetarian and nonvegetarian women. *American Journal of Clinical Nutrition* 54, 1005–1010.

Lukaski, H.C. (1989) Effects of exercise training on human copper and zinc nutrition. *Advances in Experimental Medicine and Biology* 258 (2), 163–170.

Lukaski, H.C., Hoverson, B.S., Gallagher, S.K. & Bolonchuk, W.W. (1990) Physical training and copper, iron, and zinc status of swimmers. *American Journal of Clinical Nutrition* 51, 1093–1099.

Lyle, R.M., Weaver, C.M., Sedlock, D.A., Rajaram, S., Martin, B. & Melby, C.L. (1992) Iron status in exercising women: the effect of oral iron therapy vs increased consumption of muscle foods. *American Journal of Clinical Nutrition* 56, 1049–1055.

Naik, J. & Snyder, A.C. (1997) The inter-relationship among endurance training, consumption of a vegetarian diet and serum testosterone concentration. *Medicine and Science in Sports and Exercise* 29, S295.

Nieman, D.C. (1988) Vegetarian dietary practices and endurance performance. *American Journal of Clinical Nutrition* 48, 754–761.

Pate, R.R., Miller, B.J., Davis, J.M., Slentz, C.A. & Klingshirn, L.A. (1993) Iron status of female athletes. *International Journal of Sport Nutrition* 3, 222–231.

Pedersen, A.B., Bartholomew, M.J., Dolence, L.A., Aljadir, L.P., Netteburg, K.L. & Lloyd, T. (1991) Menstrual differences due to vegetarian and nonvegetarian diets. *American Journal of Clinical Nutrition* 53, 879–885.

Pirke, K.M., Schweiger, U., Laessle, R., Dickhaut, B., Schweiger, M. & Waechtler, N. (1986) Dieting influences the menstrual cycle: vegetarian versus nonvegetarian diet. *Fertility Sterility* 46, 1083–1088.

Ratzin, R.A. (1995) Nutritional concerns for the vegetarian recreational athlete. In *Nutrition for the Recreational Athlete* (ed. C.G.R. Jackson). CRC Press, Boca Raton, FL.

Rauma, A.L., Torronen, R., Hanninen, O. & Mykkanen, H. (1995) Vitamin B-12 status of long-term adherents of a strict uncooked vegan diet ('living food diet') is compromised [see comments]. *Journal of Nutrition* 125, 2511–2515.

Reinhold, J.G., Faradji, B., Abadi, P. & Ismail-Beigi, F. (1976) Decreased absorption of calcium, magnesium, zinc and phosphorus by humans due to increased fiber and phsophorus consumption as wheat bread. *Journal of Nutrition* 106, 493–503.

Rudd, J. (1989) *Vegetarianism: Implications for Athletes.* US Olympic Committee, Sports Medicine and Science Division and International Center for Sports Nutrition, Omaha, NB.

Ryan, A.J. (1981) Anabolic steroids are fool's gold. *Federation Proceedings* 40, 2682–2685.

Shaw, N.S., Chin, C.J. & Pan, W.H. (1995) A vegetarian diet rich in soybean products compromises iron status in young students. *Journal of Nutrition* 125, 212–219.

Singh, A., Deuster, P.A. & Moser, P.B. (1990) Zinc and copper status in women by physical activity and menstrual status. *Journal of Sports Medicine and Physical Fitness* 30, 29–36.

Slavin, J., Lutter, J. & Cushman, S. (1984) Amenorrhoea in vegetarian athletes (Letter). *Lancet* 1, 1474–1475.

Snyder, A.C., Dvorak, L.L. & Roepke, J.B. (1989) Influence of dietary iron source on measures of iron status among female runners. *Medicine and Science in Sports and Exercise* 21, 7–10.

Wardlaw, G.M. & Insel, P.M. (1995) *Perspectives in Nutrition*, 3rd edn. Mosby Year Book, St Louis, MO.

Weaver, C.M., Heaney, R.P., Teegarden, D. & Hinders, S.M. (1996) Wheat bran abolishes the inverse relationship between calcium load size and absorption fraction in women. *Journal of Nutrition* 126, 303–307.

Whorton, J.C. (1982) *Crusaders for Fitness.* Princeton University Press, Princeton, NJ.

Williford, H.N., Olson, M.S., Keith, R.E. *et al.* (1993) Iron status in women aerobic dance instructors. *International Journal of Sport Nutrition* 3, 387–397.

Wishart, G.M. (1934) The efficiency and performance of a vegetarian racing cyclist under different dietary conditions. *Journal of Physiology* 82, 189–199.

# Chapter 34

# The Diabetic Athlete

JØRGEN JENSEN AND BRENDAN LEIGHTON

## Introduction

Diabetes mellitus is a disease of abnormal regulation of glucose metabolism, resulting in an elevated blood glucose concentration which may arise for different reasons. Consequently, the treatments of the disease are varied. Exercise training for people with diabetes mellitus must also be viewed in the light of the aetiology of the disease, as the physiological response to exercise can differ. In one form of diabetes mellitus, training is regarded as a cornerstone in the treatment of the disease, whereas training is a challenge in the other form of diabetes.

Diabetes mellitus is classified into two distinct types:

1 Insulin-dependent diabetes mellitus (IDDM, or type I or juvenile diabetes), which requires insulin replacement on a daily basis because insulin secretion is almost totally lacking.

2 Non-insulin-dependent diabetes mellitus (NIDDM, or type II), in which the early pathological lesion is a decreased sensitivity of skeletal muscle and liver to insulin (insulin resistance). The initial period of insulin resistance is associated with increased circulating concentrations of insulin, but the blood glucose concentration remains normal. NIDDM develops when the pancreatic β-cell is no longer able to secrete the appropriate amount of insulin to maintain adequate blood glucose concentrations and hyperglycaemia is the direct consequence.

The incidence of diabetes mellitus has increased during recent decades. In particular, the incidence of NIDDM has increased dramatically and up to 10–20% of people over 65 years old suffer from NIDDM in many countries. NIDDM is associated with an increased risk for many diseases such as coronary heart disease, neuropathy, renal failure, and blindness (Kahn 1998). In NIDDM, the management of blood glucose concentration with prescribed pharmaceutical drugs is poor and diet and regular physical exercise are important therapeutic treatments for the disease.

Only a small portion of diabetics (about 10%) are IDDM, but this group requires particularly close monitoring because IDDM develops early in life. Exercise training and physical activity are natural things for children to do and the opportunity to participate in sports is important for social development. IDDM is treated with insulin and the combination of exercise training and insulin injection may cause too high a stimulation of peripheral glucose uptake, resulting in hypoglycaemia. The requirement of insulin is influenced by exercise and the dose of insulin must therefore be varied with the intensity and duration of exercise. Thus, in people with IDDM physical exercise must be regarded as a challenge, but, with education and management, people with IDDM can participate in exercise training together with non-diabetics, and can achieve the same health benefits.

## Regulation of carbohydrate and fat metabolism during exercise

In working skeletal muscle, the demand for formation of adenosine triphosphate, which fuels muscle contraction, increases enormously (Newsholme & Leech 1983). The formation of adenosine triphosphate is driven by increased flux through glycolysis and the tricarboxylic cycle. Exercise mobilizes intramuscular fuels in the form of glycogen and triacylglycerol to supply glucose moieties and fatty acids, respectively. Exogenous fuels, in the form of glucose and non-esterified fatty acids (NEFA), are also taken up from the blood and oxidized together with intramuscular fuels.

The glucose concentration in the blood, however, remains relatively stable because the rate of peripheral glucose uptake is matched by the rate of release of glucose into the circulation. Regulation of blood glucose concentration is complex and, in addition to exercise, several hormones participate in this regulation. Insulin is the major hormone regulating the removal of glucose from the blood. Glucose entering the circulation may be absorbed from the intestine (from food or glucose drinks) but most of the time glucose is released from the liver as a result of glycogen breakdown or glucose synthesized via gluconeogenesis. During exercise, the concentrations of glucagon, catecholamines, cortisol and growth hormone all increase and these hormones stimulate glucose release from the liver and ensure that blood glucose concentration remains relatively constant (Cryer & Gerich 1985). The hormones that stimulate glucose release into the blood (and inhibit glucose uptake) are often called *counter-regulatory hormones*.

The rate of glucose uptake is elevated in skeletal muscle during exercise, although the insulin concentration decreases during exercise. Several studies have shown that glucose uptake is stimulated by exercise, even in the absence of insulin (Richter 1996) and the reduction of insulin concentration during exercise may be important for avoiding hypoglycaemia (Cryer & Gerich 1985). Insulin is a strong inhibitor of lipolysis in fat cells and of glucose release from the liver. A fall in the insulin concentration is important to optimize the supply of NEFA to the contracting muscles.

The decrease in basal insulin concentration aids the release of NEFA from adipose tissue and glucose from the liver.

During prolonged exercise, the concentration of glycogen in skeletal muscles decreases and glucose uptake from the blood becomes gradually more important. When skeletal muscles are depleted of glycogen, glucose uptake may account for nearly all carbohydrate oxidation (Wahren et al. 1971). When the liver is depleted of glycogen, glucose is released at much lower rates and the blood glucose concentration decreases. A decrease in blood glucose concentration is well recognized as a major factor in the fatigue that accompanies endurance exercise, and the reduced supply of carbohydrate to the central nervous system and to the muscle may both be factors in the fatigue process (Costill & Hargreaves 1992).

The intensity of exercise is also an important determinant of the rate of carbohydrate utilization. During exercise of an intensity of about 50% of $\dot{V}o_{2max.}$, the energy comes equally from fat and carbohydrate metabolism and, as the intensity of the exercise increases, the percentage contribution from carbohydrates rises. At intensities of exercise above 80% $\dot{V}o_{2max.}$, carbohydrates become the major metabolic fuel. At this intensity of exercise, glucose uptake is also much higher, and depletion of liver glycogen will occur in 1–2 h followed by a decrease in concentration of blood glucose. During exercise of short duration and high intensity, on the other hand, the hepatic glucose output can exceed the rate of glucose uptake and lead to hyperglycaemia.

## Regulation of carbohydrate and fat metabolism after exercise

The ability to convert chemical energy to fuel skeletal muscle contraction is essential for human movement. Skeletal muscles have, however, also an important role for regulation of the blood glucose concentration, as most of the glucose disposal stimulated by insulin occurs in skeletal muscle (Shulman et al. 1990).

After a carbohydrate-rich meal, the increased

concentration of glucose in the blood causes a release of insulin from the β-cells in the pancreas. Insulin binds to its receptor and stimulates glucose transport and metabolism, particularly in heart, skeletal muscle and adipose tissue. The signalling pathway for insulin has been studied extensively and during the last decade the mechanism of action of insulin has become much clearer (Kahn 1998).

Glucose is transported into cells by proteins called glucose transporters. There are different isoforms of the glucose transporters and their expression is tissue specific (Holman & Kasuga 1997). GLUT-4 is expressed in tissue where insulin stimulates glucose uptake (skeletal muscle, heart and adipose tissue) and GLUT-4 is named the insulin-regulated glucose transporter. Insulin stimulates glucose uptake by recruitment of GLUT-4 from intracellular sites to the sarcolemmal membrane (Fig. 34.1). GLUT-4 is normally located in vesicles in the cells, but during insulin stimulation, GLUT-4 is translocated to the cell membrane by exocytosis (Holman & Kasuga 1997). When GLUT-4 transporter proteins are in the sarcolemmal membrane, they will transport glucose into the cells, and the amount of GLUT-4 in the sarcolemmal membrane is regarded as the regulatory step for glucose uptake. GLUT-4 will be internalized when the insulin stimulation is removed and glucose transport will decrease to basal level again.

Skeletal muscle makes up 30–40% of the body weight and the 70–90% of the insulin-stimulated glucose uptake occurs in this tissue (Shulman et al. 1990). Therefore, it is evident that skeletal muscles play a central role in regulation of glucose metabolism. Glucose taken up in skeletal muscle during insulin stimulation is incorporated into glycogen (Shulman et al. 1990), but skeletal muscles are unable to release glucose into the bloodstream to maintain blood glucose concentration. Skeletal muscle glycogen can, however, be broken down to lactate and released from skeletal muscle for conversion to glucose in the liver via gluconeogenesis. Skeletal muscle glycogen is therefore indirectly a carbohydrate source for maintaining blood glucose.

Exercise recruits GLUT-4 to the sarcolemmal membrane in a manner similar to the effects of insulin. Although both exercise and insulin stimulate glucose uptake by translocation of GLUT-4 to the sarcolemmal membrane, this process seems to occur via different signalling pathways (Richter 1996) and exercise stimulates glucose uptake even in insulin resistant muscles (Etgen et al. 1996). Another effect of exercise is that insulin sensitivity increases in skeletal muscle after exercise (Richter 1996). This means that lower insulin

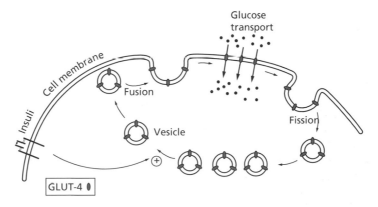

**Fig. 34.1** Schematic illustration showing regulation of glucose transport in skeletal muscle. When insulin binds to the insulin receptor, GLUT-4-containing vesicles are translocated to the sarcolemmal membrane. GLUT-4 transports glucose into the cell when they are located in the sarcolemmal membrane. In insulin-resistant muscles, translocation is reduced in response to insulin.

concentrations are required to remove glucose, and in line with this, highly trained people have lower circulating insulin levels and a reduced insulin response to a glucose challenge. However, the increased insulin sensitivity during and after exercise increases the risk for hypoglycaemia in insulin-treated diabetics.

## Insulin-dependent diabetes mellitus

In people with IDDM, insulin secretion is lacking or insufficient because of an almost total destruction of the insulin secreting β-cells in the pancreas. The β-cells are destroyed by the diabetic's own immune system (autoimmune destruction). IDDM is treated with life-long insulin therapy by insulin injection several times each day. Insulin is produced as long-acting (elevates blood insulin concentration for many hours) and rapid-acting (elevates blood insulin for a much shorter period of time) forms and most patients take a mixture of both forms. In the evening (and some times morning), long-acting insulin is injected to maintain the basal insulin concentration. Before each meal, rapid-acting insulin is injected to stimulate removal of the absorbed glucose. The insulin dose required depends on the individual and it is important to measure glucose concentration often to establish the correct dose.

### Exercise training for IDDM

IDDM normally develops at a young age and exercise is a natural activity for children. It is particularly important for their social development that they get the opportunity to participate in group exercises with other children. Although some children with IDDM develop fear of participation in sports, exercise is regarded as safe if children with IDDM are educated to adjust their dose of insulin to the intensity of exercise. Many people with IDDM participate in sport and there are several examples of athletes at the top of their sports.

These athletes clearly show that it is possible for diabetic athletes to achieve a high performance level. In non-diabetics, exercise training causes adaptations in skeletal muscle and circulatory system which is the background to the increased performance (Holloszy & Booth 1976). People with IDDM seem, however, to respond to training in a similar way and there are therefore no physiological reasons for not participating in sport (Wallberg-Henriksson 1992).

Exercise training for people with IDDM is, however, not without problems. The insulin concentration is important for control of the glucose concentration and too high a concentration of insulin in combination with exercise may cause hypoglycaemia. Too low a concentration of insulin, on the other hand, may cause elevation in blood glucose and ketoacidosis. The greatest problem is the development of hypoglycaemia because of the inability to regulate prevailing blood insulin concentrations. In people with IDDM the insulin concentration in blood will depend on the amount of insulin administered and the rate of release of insulin from the site of injection. The normal decrease in insulin level during exercise will therefore not occur in people with IDDM and, as exercise increases insulin sensitivity, glucose uptake in skeletal muscles may be too high. To mimic the reduction in concentration of insulin that occurs in normal subjects during exercise, insulin injections have to be avoided immediately prior to exercise in people with IDDM.

Before exercise, it is important that the glucose and insulin concentrations are neither too high nor too low (Horton 1988). The concentration of glucose should be measured to give information about the insulin level. If the blood glucose concentration is below 5 mM, it may be a result of too high a concentration of insulin and there is a high risk for hypoglycaemia if exercise is performed. It is therefore not advised to participate in exercise, and glucose should be taken to raise the blood glucose concentration before exercise is performed. Furthermore, it is important that athletes with IDDM should be able to recognize the symptoms of hypoglycaemia and respond accordingly.

Exercise is not recommended when the blood glucose concentration is above 16 mM (Wallberg-

Henriksson 1992). Too high a glucose concentration may be a result of a low concentration of insulin. Exercise in under-insulinated diabetics may result in a further increase in blood glucose concentration as the normal inhibition of glucose release from the liver is lacking (Wallberg-Henriksson 1992). Low insulin concentration will also cause elevated lipolysis and the high concentration of NEFA may increase production of ketone bodies, resulting in ketoacidosis (Wallberg-Henriksson 1992). In case of high glucose concentration, it is recommended that ketone body levels should be checked in urine (Horton 1988). However, if a large meal has been eaten shortly before exercise and minimal rapid-acting insulin is taken, exercise will decrease glucose concentration to a normal level (Sane *et al.* 1988).

Although exercise decreases blood glucose concentration and increases insulin sensitivity in skeletal muscle, exercise may not be regarded as a treatment for IDDM (Kemmer & Berger 1986; Horton 1988; Wallberg-Henriksson 1992). In contrast to NIDDM, training does not seem to improve glycaemic control in IDDM (Wallberg-Henriksson *et al.* 1984; Wallberg-Henriksson 1992; Ebeling *et al.* 1995). Elite athletes require a higher amount of carbohydrates in the diet, which makes the regulation of blood glucose more difficult. Furthermore, participation in elite sport is often accompanied with travelling and other changes in their daily routine which also make administration of insulin more difficult. For elite athletes it is therefore important that the blood glucose is monitored carefully and athletes must learn to correct the insulin requirements to the exercise performed. In learning this, it is recommended that the athletes write down the blood glucose concentration before and after exercise of different type, intensity, and duration and relate it to ingestion of carbohydrates and injection of insulin.

### Dietary considerations

An important part of treatment of IDDM is education. Today it is normal to have a small blood glucose analyser at home to monitor glucose concentration on a regular basis. The dose of insulin needed differs between individuals and the requirement for insulin to handle a meal varies even within the same individual since, for example, exercise increases insulin sensitivity and decreases the requirement for insulin. Ideally, IDDM subjects will want to achieve a normal pattern of food consumption. However, some foods with a high glycaemic index will be absorbed rapidly (e.g. glucose in a soft drink) and this may cause some metabolic problems. Importantly, the amount of insulin taken before a meal should be matched with the anticipated dietary glucose uptake. This means that if the blood glucose concentration is high after a meal, the insulin dose is increased and *vice versa*.

If postprandial exercise is planned, precautions can be taken to improve glucose regulation. To avoid hypoglycaemia, Horton (1988) suggests eating a large meal 1–3 h before planned exercise and to reduce insulin injection before this meal. Although it is difficult to give a standard recommendation, a reduction of 30–50% in rapid-acting insulin may be a starting point for adjustment of the dose to endurance exercise. Reduction of the insulin dose before strength training and ball games may be smaller. However, it is important to measure blood glucose concentration frequently, particularly when a new type of exercise is performed or when intensity or duration is changed. The dose of insulin before meals must be optimized to the new and unfamiliar exercises.

If the duration of the exercise is more than 30 min, extra glucose should be supplied. This glucose ingestion has two effects in IDDM; avoiding dangerous hypoglycaemia and improvement of performance. As in non-diabetics, glucose ingestion increases performance in prolonged endurance sport. In IDDM, glucose ingestion should also prevent hypoglycaemia. Severe hypoglycaemia causes coma and hypoglycaemic coma is potentially fatal for the diabetic (Cryer & Gerich 1985). The only energy substrate for the brain is glucose and severe brain damage will occur within minutes at very low glucose concentrations (Cryer & Gerich 1985). It is therefore required that glucose, which can be rapidly absorbed, is available when IDDM athletes perform exercise training, to prevent hypoglycaemia and to reduce the risk of coma if hypoglycaemia occurs. This is particularly important when running or cycling is performed in conditions where it will be difficult to obtain carbohydrates.

It seems that ingestion of 40 g carbohydrate·h⁻¹ is sufficient to avoid hypoglycaemia (Sane *et al.* 1988). Athletes with IDDM performed a 75-km ski race and ingested glucose at an average rate of 40 g·h⁻¹ (more in the later part of the exercise); ingestion of glucose at this rate prevented hypoglycaemia when insulin injection also was reduced (Fig. 34.2). The glucose concentration was, however, in the lower range for many of the IDDM athletes at the end and more glucose may have improved performance. Horton (1988) suggested that glucose should be ingested at a rate of

70–80 g·h⁻¹ during prolonged exercise. In normal subjects, glucose ingestion at a rate of 60 g·h⁻¹ is recommended (Costill & Hargreaves 1992) and glucose should be ingested at the same rate in athletes with IDDM. Furthermore, in addition to supply of carbohydrates, athletes with IDDM must always be aware of the risk of hypoglycaemia and ingest glucose when symptoms of hypoglycaemia come.

Exercise *per se* stimulates glycogen synthesis after the training session when glucose is available. In diabetics, regulation of blood glucose concentration is normally the focused subject and glycogen synthesis in skeletal muscles is regarded prerequisite for regulation of blood glucose. In sport, on the other hand, the replenishment of muscle glycogen stores is normally viewed from a performance perspective. Muscle glycogen is the most important energy substrate in most types of sport and for optimal performance, it is important that the glycogen stores are replenished after each bout of exercise (Ivy 1991). Glycogen can be synthesized in people with IDDM even in the absence of insulin injection after exercise (Mæhlum *et al.* 1978). In the absence of insulin, however, only half of the glycogen store seems to be replenished (Fig. 34.3). Injection of insulin is therefore necessary for optimal glycogen synthesis, even though the administration of insulin after exercise increases the risk for hypoglycaemia.

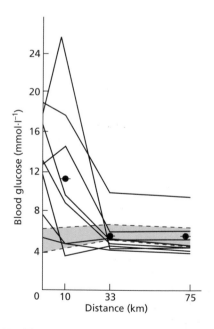

**Fig. 34.2** Blood glucose concentration (individual and mean) in athletes with IDDM during a 75-km ski race. The shaded area shows healthy controls. The athletes with IDDM reduced their daily insulin dose by about 35% and ingested about 270 g of carbohydrate during the exercise (36 g·h⁻¹). Adapted from Sane *et al.* (1988).

## Conclusion

The nature and intensity of any exercise training programme combined with the personal requirements of a person with IDDM make it difficult to generalize about factors, such as dose of insulin administered before exercise and amount of dietary intake. Monitoring the concentration of glucose prior to any exercise ensures that the performance is not undertaken in conditions which may be adverse for the IDDM subject. If the blood glucose level is low then the intensity of exercise should be decreased or delayed until ingested carbohydrate has time to boost the blood glucose concentration. High blood glucose

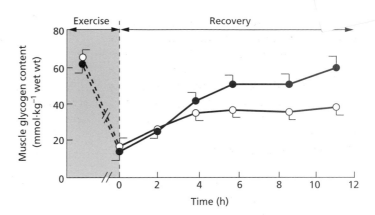

**Fig. 34.3** Glycogen synthesis in IDDM subjects after exercise in the presence (●) or absence (○) of insulin. Subjects exercised at 75% of $\dot{V}_{O_{2max}}$ until exhaustion and received a carbohydrate-rich diet and their normal insulin injection in the control experiment. On the other experimental day, insulin was not injected. Adapted from Mæhlum *et al.* (1978).

concentration should lead to the postponement of exercise for the reasons given above. The dose of insulin administered before any exercise should be scaled down to reflect the degree of intensity and duration of exercise. However, individual IDDM subjects may have to reach the optimum pre-exercise insulin dose by monitoring post-exercise glucose levels.

## Non-insulin-dependent diabetes mellitus

NIDDM is a world health problem and the disease is often regarded as a disease of abnormal lifestyle. About 90% of all diabetics are NIDDM and the disease develops gradually and is normally associated with obesity and hypertension. Initially, the skeletal muscles and liver becomes insulin resistant, but the body responds by producing more insulin and glucose concentration remains normal. However, as the insulin resistance increases, the pancreas becomes unable to produce enough insulin to regulate the metabolism of blood glucose concentration and hyperglycaemia occurs.

The pharmacological treatment of NIDDM is poor. As the muscles are insulin resistant, insulin therapy is not a satisfactory treatment of the disease. There are some other drugs prescribed, such as sulphonylureas and metformin. NIDDM is in most case initially treated with dietary manipulation and exercise. This treatment is sufficient for many people with NIDDM if the disease has not progressed too far. Exercise of moderate intensity in people with NIDDM is usually associated with a decrease in blood glucose towards the normal range. A further benefit of regular exercise is that it increases the sensitivity of skeletal muscle to insulin, which will have the beneficial effect of lowering the requirement for circulating insulin concentration. It is important to recognize that exercise also lowers the risk factors for cardiovascular disease in people with NIDDM.

### Exercise training for NIDDM

NIDDM is normally associated with obesity and a low exercise capacity. NIDDM develops later in life than IDDM and the majority of patients are over 50 years old. The aims of exercise training for people with NIDDM are therefore often different from those of young people with IDDM. People with NIDDM are often untrained and an improved level of physical fitness is normally the main goal. As for untrained people in general, there are large opportunities for improvement and training studies have shown that endurance training increases maximum oxygen uptake and oxidative capacity in skeletal muscle (Wallberg-Henriksson 1992).

Obesity may hinder training and a high body mass increases the risk of injury to joints and tendons. In people with NIDDM, it is also important to be aware of the risk for foot problems, particularly in diabetics with peripheral neuropathy, and good shoes and attention to hygiene must be stressed. In previously untrained NIDDM, the training must start slowly, as with all sedentary individuals who embark on an exercise programme. However, although a larger percentage of energy comes from fat at lower intensity endurance training, it is important to achieve a progressive increase in intensity to obtain the largest improvement in glucose tolerance. Endurance training at higher intensities is probably the most effective way to reduce body weight and increase insulin sensitivity (Koivisto et al. 1986; Kang et al. 1996).

In people with NIDDM, insulin-stimulated glucose uptake is reduced in skeletal muscles (Shulman et al. 1990). Much research is directed at finding the reason for this reduced insulin sensitivity. The amount of GLUT-4 is normal in insulin-resistant muscle but insulin is unable to translocate GLUT-4 to the cell membrane (Etgen et al. 1996). Exercise training, however, stimulates glucose uptake in skeletal muscle and increases insulin sensitivity in insulin-resistant muscles (Koivisto et al. 1986; Etgen et al. 1997). Insulin resistance in skeletal muscle develops prior to NIDDM and endurance training seems to prevent the development of insulin resistance. Furthermore, endurance training increases insulin sensitivity in people with NIDDM and improves the regulation of blood glucose concentration.

Strength training is normally not regarded to be as effective as endurance training in increasing insulin sensitivity (Koivisto et al. 1986). However, most people with NIDDM are older, untrained people and with increasing age the skeletal muscle atrophies. Reduction in the mass of muscle available to remove glucose from the blood during insulin stimulation decreases glucose tolerance. Strength training which increases muscle mass in older, untrained people with NIDDM may be more effective than endurance training to increase glucose tolerance. Strength training may, however, cause vascular side-effects and precautions should be taken (Wallberg-Henriksson 1992).

### Dietary considerations for NIDDM

NIDDM is often associated with obesity, hypertension and hyperlipidaemia (Koivisto et al. 1986). Obesity is a risk factor for NIDDM and weight reduction improves insulin sensitivity in skeletal muscles. Weight reduction is therefore, together with training, central in the treatment of most people with NIDDM. For the reduction of body mass, energy intake must be lower than energy utilization and food intake must normally be reduced. Furthermore, a high-fat diet causes insulin resistance in skeletal muscles. People with NIDDM are therefore recommended to reduce their fat intake. Furthermore, in contrast to IDDM, insulin treatment is unable to stimulate glucose disposal after a large meal in NIDDM. Large meals will therefore cause an elevation in blood glucose. It is therefore advised that people with NIDDM eat smaller meals and that the content of complex carbohydrates is high.

Hypoglycaemia during and after exercise is not a major problem in NIDDM when the therapy is changed diet and increased exercise training. Pharmacological treatments of NIDDM with insulin, sulphonylureas or metformin may increase the risk of hypoglycaemia. However, the risk for development of hypoglycaemia in pharmacologically treated diabetics with NIDDM is still much lower than in people with IDDM. During exercise, carbohydrate supply is normally not necessary in people with NIDDM and water should be drunk to replace fluid.

Replenishment of glycogen stores is important for performance (Ivy 1991). However, in most people with NIDDM, improved regulation of the blood glucose concentration is more important than improved performance. Most of the glucose taken up during insulin stimulation is incorporated into glycogen and a high glycogen concentration in skeletal muscle reduces insulin-stimulated glucose uptake (Jensen et al. 1997). Normal regulation of blood glucose metabolism requires that glucose can be incorporated into glycogen in skeletal muscles and a high glycogen content impedes this. The reduced glycogen concentration after exercise in people with NIDDM is important for improved glucose metabolism and reduced glycogen stores will aid the disposal of blood glucose.

### Conclusion

NIDDM is often associated with obesity and reduction of body mass is important to improve glucose metabolism. Exercise increases energy consumption and has an important role is any weight-loss programme. Exercise increases also insulin sensitivity in skeletal muscle, leading to an improved regulation of the blood glucose concentration. Exercise therefore has a central position in the management of most people with NIDDM. However, as most of the people with NIDDM are overweight, it is important to find types of exercise that can be performed. Endurance training such as running may cause joint and tendon problems because of the high body mass. Cycling or swimming may be good alternatives. Furthermore, strength training may be effective to increase glucose tolerance in older people. Most of the glucose is taken up by skeletal muscles during insulin stimulation and an increased muscle mass will improve removal of glucose from the blood.

## References

Costill, D.L. & Hargreaves, M. (1992) Carbohydrate nutrition and fatigue. *Sports Medicine* **13**, 86–92.

Cryer, P.E. & Gerich, J.E. (1985) Glucose counterregulation, hypoglycemia, and intensive insulin therapy in diabetes mellitus. *New England Journal of Medicine* **313**, 232–241.

Ebeling, P., Tuominen, J.A., Bourey, R., Koranyi, L. & Koivisto, V.A. (1995) Athletes with IDDM exhibit impaired metabolic control and increased lipid utilization with no increase in insulin sensitivity. *Diabetes* **44**, 471–477.

Etgen, G.J., Wilson, C.M., Jensen, J., Cushman, S.W. & Ivy, J.L. (1996) Glucose transport and cell surface GLUT-4 protein in skeletal muscle of the obese Zucker rat. *American Journal of Physiology* **271**, E294–E301.

Etgen, G.J., Jensen, J., Wilson, C.M., Hunt, D.G., Cushman, S.W. & Ivy, J.L. (1997) Exercise training reverses insulin resistance in muscle by enhanced recruitment of GLUT-4 to the cell surface. *American Journal of Physiology* **272**, E864–E869.

Holloszy, J.O. & Booth, F.W. (1976) Biochemical adaptations to endurance exercise in muscle. *Annual Review of Physiology* **38**, 273–291.

Holman, G.D. & Kasuga, M. (1997) From receptor to transporter: insulin signalling to glucose transport. *Diabetologia* **40**, 991–1003.

Horton, E.D. (1988) Role and management of exercise in diabetes mellitus. *Diabetes Care* **11**, 201–211.

Ivy, J.L. (1991) Muscle glycogen synthesis before and after exercise. *Sports Medicine* **11**, 6–19.

Jensen, J., Aslesen, R., Ivy, J.L. & Brørs, O. (1997) Role of glycogen concentration and epinephrine on glucose uptake in rat epitrochlearis muscle. *American Journal of Physiology* **272**, E649–E655.

Kahn, B.B. (1998) Type 2 diabetes: when insulin secretion fails to compensate for insulin resistance. *Cell* **92**, 593–596.

Kang, J., Robertson, R.J., Hagberg, J.M. *et al.* (1996) Effect of exercise intensity on glucose and insulin metabolism in obese individuals and obese NIDDM patients. *Diabetes Care* **19**, 341–349.

Kemmer, F.W. & Berger, M. (1986) Therapy and better quality of life: the dichotomous role of exercise in diabetes mellitus. *Diabetes/Metabolism Reviews* **2**, 53–68.

Koivisto, V.A., Yki-Järvinen, H. & DeFronzo, R.A. (1986) Physical training and insulin sensitivity. *Diabetes/Metabolism Reviews* **1**, 445–481.

Mæhlum, S., Høstmark, A.T. & Hermansen, L. (1978) Synthesis of muscle glycogen during recovery after prolonged severe exercise in diabetic subjects. Effect of insulin deprivation. *Scandinavian Journal of Clinical and Laboratory Investigations* **38**, 35–39.

Newsholme, E.A. & Leech, A.R. (1983) *Biochemistry for the Medical Sciences*. John Wiley & Sons, Chichester.

Richter, E.A. (1996) Glucose utilization. In *Handbook of Physiology*. Section 12. *Exercise: Regulation and Integration of Multiple Systems* (ed. L.B. Rowell & J.T. Shepherd), pp. 912–951. Oxford University Press, Oxford.

Sane, T., Helve, E., Pelkonen, R. & Koivisto, V.A. (1988) The adjustment of diet and insulin dose during long-term endurance exercise in type 1 (insulin-dependent) diabetic men. *Diabetologia* **31**, 35–40.

Shulman, G.I., Rothman, D.L., Jue, T., Stein, P., DeFronzo, R.A. & Shulman, R.G. (1990) Quantification of muscle glycogen synthesis in normal subjects and subjects with non-insulin-dependent diabetes by $^{13}C$ nuclear magnetic resonance spectroscopy. *New England Journal of Medicine* **322**, 223–228.

Wahren, J., Felig, P., Ahlborg, G. & Jorfeldt, L. (1971) Glucose metabolism during leg exercise in man. *Journal of Clinical Investigation* **50**, 2715–2725.

Wallberg-Henriksson, H. (1992)) Exercise and diabetes mellitus. *Exercise and Sport Sciences Reviews* **20**, 339–368.

Wallberg-Henriksson, H., Gunnarsson, R., Henriksson, J., Östman, J. & Wahren, J. (1984) Influence of physical training on formation of muscle capillaries in type I diabetes. *Diabetes* **33**, 351–357.

# PART 3

## PRACTICAL ISSUES

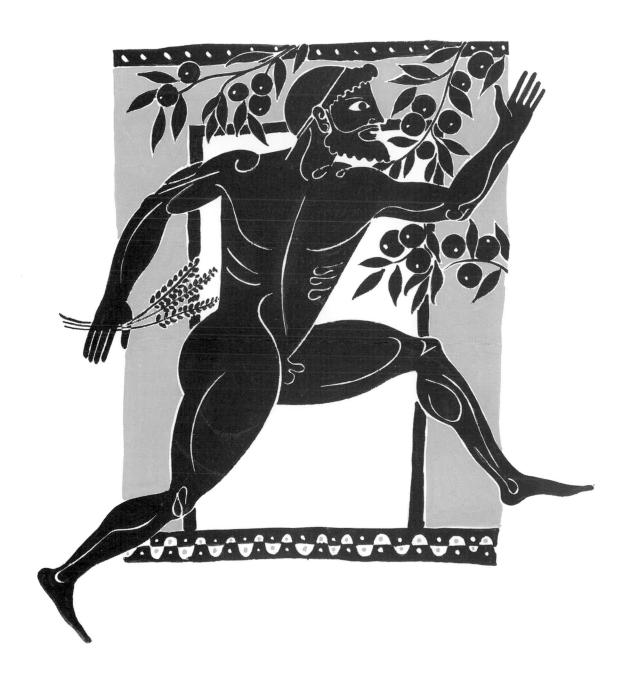

# Chapter 35

# The Overweight Athlete

MELINDA M. MANORE

## Introduction

For the sport medicine team, the overweight athlete can present numerous challenges. First, the type of athlete who wants or needs to lose weight can vary dramatically, from a small female participating in a lean build sport (gymnastics, track and field, figure skating) to a large male participating in a strength or power sport (weightlifting, heavy weight wrestling). Some of these athletes may also participate in sports that require 'making weight,' which adds a unique challenge to any health professional guiding them through the weight-loss process. These athletes may not be 'overfat or overweight' according to normal criteria, but may be considered heavy for their sport or for the weight category in which they must compete. To further complicate the weight-loss process, some athletes participate in sports in which they are judged on both performance and appearance. This can add pressure to reduce body weight lower than optimal for good health and performance. Second, the weight-loss programme needs to provide adequate energy so that exercise training can still occur. The diet cannot be too restrictive in energy without the athlete running the risk of injury, loss of fat-free mass (FFM), poor performance, feelings of deprivation, and eventual failure. Thus, adequate time needs to be allotted for weight loss to occur. Aerobic and strength training may also need to be added if they are not already a part of the athlete's normal training programme. Finally, the weight-loss programme needs to provide a strong educational component. The athlete needs to be taught good nutritional, exercise and behavioural techniques for long-term weight maintenance. Without an educational component, the athlete is susceptible to the many fad diets, diet products, and weight-loss drugs that frequently hit the consumer market. With the emphasis placed on physical appearance in Western society, dieting can become obsessive. The athlete is not immune to this pressure. In fact, they are pressured on two fronts: their sport and society. This pressure can lead to desperate means of weight loss and an eventual eating disorder.

This review will briefly outline the principles and components of energy balance that need to be considered before placing an athlete on a weight-loss programme. Specific methods for determining energy balance in an athlete will also be reviewed. Finally, practical applications and guidelines for determining the weight-loss goal and approaches to gradual weight loss will be given. For individuals working with athletes in weight-category sports, the effects of rapid weight loss on health and performance has been addressed elsewhere (Steen & Brownell 1990; Horswill 1992, 1993; Fogelholm 1994). Other excellent reviews are available on the effect of weight loss on sport performance (Wilmore 1992a), the techniques used in different sports (Fogelholm 1994; Burke 1995), the effect of weight loss on health and metabolism (Brownell *et al.* 1987), and the role of dieting in eating disorders (Wilmore 1991; Sundgot-Borgen 1993, 1994;

469

Beals & Manore 1994) and menstrual dysfunction (Dueck *et al.* 1996). Part 4 of this book gives more specific information about the weight and nutrition concerns of different sports, particularly weight-category sports.

## Energy and nutrient balance

The classic energy balance equation states that if energy intake equals energy expenditure then weight is maintained; however, this equation does not allow for changes in body composition and energy stores (Ravussin & Swinburn 1993). The maintenance of body weight and composition over time requires that energy intake equals energy expenditure, and that dietary intakes of protein, carbohydrate, fat and alcohol equal their oxidation rates (Flatt 1992; Swinburn & Ravussin 1993). If this occurs, an individual is considered to be in energy balance and body weight and composition will be maintained.

This approach to energy balance is dynamic and allows for the effect of changing energy stores on energy expenditure over time. For example, after a short period of positive energy balance, the extra energy would cause weight gain (of both fat and lean tissues). However, the larger body size would cause an increase in energy expenditure that would eventually balance the extra energy consumed. Thus, weight gain can be the consequence of an initial positive energy balance, but can also be a mechanism whereby energy balance is eventually restored. Conversely, weight loss must reverse this process. If body fat is to be lost, energy intake must be less than expenditure, and fat oxidation must exceed fat intake (Westerterp 1993).

## Nutrient balance

The alteration of energy intake and expenditure is just one part of the energy balance picture. Changes in the type and amount of nutrients consumed (i.e. protein, fat, carbohydrate and alcohol) and the oxidation of these nutrients within the body must also be considered. Under normal physiological conditions, carbohydrate,

protein and alcohol are not easily converted to body fat (Abbott *et al.* 1988; Swinburn & Ravussin 1993). Thus, increases in the intake of non-fat nutrients stimulate their oxidation rates proportionally. Conversely, an increase in fat intake does not immediately stimulate fat oxidation, hence increasing the probability that dietary fat will be stored as adipose tissue (Abbott *et al.* 1988; Westerterp 1993). Therefore, the type of food consumed plays a role in the amount of energy consumed and expended each day (Acheson *et al.* 1984; Swinburn & Ravussin 1993). Successful weight loss requires that an energy deficit be produced (either through increased energy expenditure and/or decreased energy intake) and diet composition and oxidation be altered (decreased fat intake and/or increased fat oxidation through exercise) (Hill *et al.* 1993).

### Carbohydrate balance

Carbohydrate balance is proposed to be precisely regulated (Flatt 1992), with the ingestion of carbohydrate stimulating both glycogen storage and glucose oxidation, and inhibiting fat oxidation (Fig. 35.1). Glucose not stored as glycogen is thought to be oxidized directly in almost equal balance to that consumed (Schutz *et al.* 1989; Thomas *et al.* 1992). Thus, the conversion of excess dietary carbohydrate to triglycerides does not appear to occur to any large extent in humans under normal physiological conditions (Acheson *et al.* 1988; Hellerstein *et al.* 1991).

### Protein balance

Like carbohydrate, the body alters protein oxidation rates to match protein intakes (Thomas *et al.* 1992). Once anabolic needs are met, the carbon skeletons of excess amino acids can be used for energy. The adequacy of both energy and carbohydrate intake dramatically affects this process. Inadequate energy or carbohydrate intakes will result in negative protein balance, while excess intake of energy or carbohydrate will spare protein (Krempf *et al.* 1993). Any excess dietary protein or that made available through protein

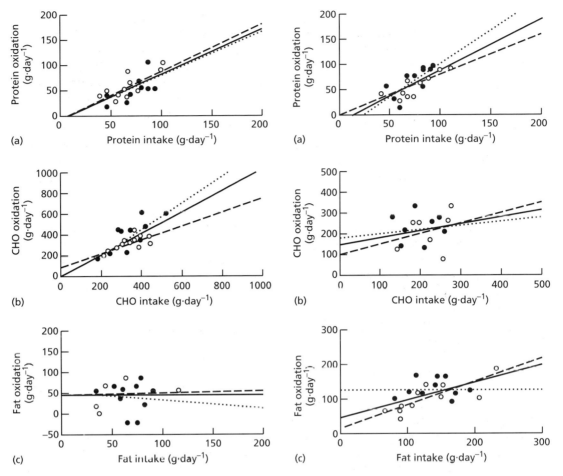

**Fig. 35.1** High-carbohydrate diet: the relationship between intake and oxidation of (a) protein, (b) carbohydrate (CHO), and (c) fat for all subjects on day 7 of a high carbohydrate feeding period. —, regression line for all 21 subjects; - - -, regression line for lean subjects (○); ····, regression line for obese subjects (●). (a) Lean subjects: $r = 0.79$, $P < 0.01$; obese subjects: $r = 0.59$, n.s. (b) Lean subjects: $r = 0.74$, $P < 0.01$; obese subjects: $r = 0.79$, $P < 0.01$. (c) Lean subjects: $r = 0.06$, n.s.; obese subjects: $r = -0.08$, n.s. From Thomas *et al.* (1992), with permission.

**Fig. 35.2** High-fat diet: the relationship between intake and oxidation of (a) protein, (b) carbohydrate (CHO), and (c) fat for all subjects on day 7 of a high fat feeding period. —, regression line for all 21 subjects; - - -, regression line for lean subjects (○); ····, regression line for obese subjects (●). (a) Lean subjects: $r = 0.78$, $P < 0.01$; obese subjects: $r = 0.74$, $P < 0.02$. (b) Lean subjects: $r = 0.32$, n.s.; obese subjects: $r = 0.14$, n.s. (c) Lean subjects: $r = 0.78$, $P < 0.01$; obese subjects: $r = 0.02$, n.s. From Thomas *et al.* (1992), with permission.

sparing may contribute indirectly to fat storage by sparing dietary fat.

### Fat balance

Fat balance is not as precisely regulated as either protein or carbohydrate balance (Flatt 1992).

Figure 35.2 shows that as fat intake increases, the oxidation of fat does not increase proportionately (Thomas *et al.* 1992). Thus, acute increases in fat intake have little influence on fat oxidation. For example, Jebb *et al.* (1996) overfed three lean men by 33% of energy requirements for 12 days. They found that carbohydrate and protein intake (grams per day) matched their oxidation rates, while fat oxidation rates did not change significantly even though fat intake increased (fat intake was 150 g·day[-1] while fat oxidation was only 59 g·day[-1]). The result was a 2.9-kg weight gain in 12 days. Thus, excess energy eaten as dietary fat is stored as triglycerides in adipose tissue with little loss of energy (Acheson et al. 1984; Swinburn & Ravussin 1993).

### Alcohol balance

When athletes ingest alcohol, it becomes a priority fuel, with a rapid rise in alcohol oxidation occurring until all the alcohol is cleared from the body. Alcohol also suppresses the oxidation of fat and, to a lesser degree, that of protein and carbohydrate (Shelmet et al. 1988). Alcohol is not stored as fat nor can it contribute to the formation of muscle or liver glycogen. It may, however, indirectly divert fat to storage by providing an alternative and preferred energy source for the body (Sonko et al. 1994). Thus, alcohol, at 29.4 kJ·g[-1] (7 kcal·g[-1]), can contribute significantly to total energy intake. Athletes who consume alcohol must reduce their intake of energy from other sources to maintain energy balance.

## Energy balance

Determination of energy balance requires the measurement or estimation of both energy intake and energy expenditure. Energy balance is then estimated by subtracting energy expenditure from energy intake. This section will briefly review the various components of energy intake and expenditure, how these components are measured, and the many factors that may influence them.

### Components of energy expenditure

The components of total daily energy expenditure (TDEE) are generally divided into three main categories: (i) resting metabolic rate (RMR), (ii) the thermic effect of food (TEF), and (iii) the thermic effect of activity (TEA) (Fig. 35.3). RMR is the energy required to maintain the systems of the body and to regulate body temperature at rest. In most sedentary healthy adults, RMR accounts for approximately 60–80% of TDEE (Bogardus et al. 1986; Ravussin et al. 1986). However, in an active individual this percentage can vary greatly. It is not unusual for some athletes to expend 4.2–8.4 MJ (1000–2000 kcal) per day in sport-related activities. For example, Thompson et al. (1993) determined energy balance in 24 elite male endurance athletes over a 3–7-day period and found that RMR represented only 38–47% of TDEE. Similar results are reported in female runners (Beidleman et al. 1995).

The TEF is the increase in energy expenditure above RMR that results from the consumption of food throughout the day. It includes the energy cost of food digestion, absorption, transport, metabolism and storage within the body, and the energy expended due to sympathetic nervous system activity brought about by seeing, smelling and eating food. TEF is usually expressed as a percentage of the energy content of the foods consumed and accounts for 6–10% of TDEE, with women usually having a lower value (approximately 6–7%) (Poehlman 1989). However, this value will vary depending on the energy density and size of the meal and types of foods consumed. In addition, if the absolute amount of energy intake is decreased, then it follows that the absolute amount of energy expended in TEF will decrease.

TEA is the most variable component of energy expenditure in humans. It includes the energy cost of daily activities above RMR and TEF, such as purposeful activities of daily living (making dinner, dressing, cleaning house) and planned exercise (running, weight training, cycling). It also includes the energy cost of involuntary muscular activity such as shivering and fidgeting. This type of movement is called *spontaneous physical activity*. TEA may be only 10–15% of TDEE in sedentary individuals, but may be as high as 50% in active individuals. The addition of RMR, TEF and TEA should account for 100% of

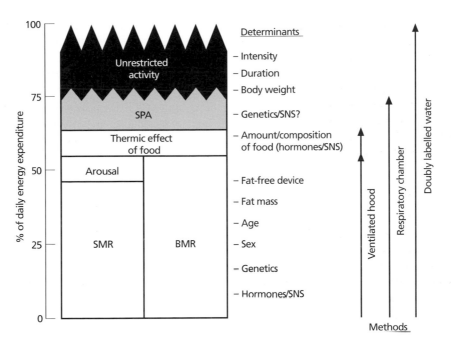

**Fig. 35.3** Components of daily energy expenditure in humans. Daily energy expenditure can be divided into three major components: (i) the basal metabolic rate (BMR) (the sum of the sleeping metabolic rate (SMR) and the energy cost of arousal), which represents 50–70% of daily energy expenditure; (ii) the thermic effect of food, which represents approximately 10% of daily energy expenditure; and (iii) the energy cost of physical activity (the sum of spontaneous physical activity (SPA) and unrestricted/voluntary physical activity), which represents 20–40% of daily energy expenditure. The major determinants of the different components of daily energy expenditure, as well as the methods to measure them, are presented. SNS, sympathetic nervous system. From Ravussin and Swinburn (1993).

TDEE. However, there are a variety of factors that may increase energy expenditure above normal, such as cold, fear, stress, and various medications or drugs. These factors are referred to as *adaptive thermogenesis* and represent a temporary increase in thermogenesis that may last for hours or days, depending on the duration and magnitude of the stimulus. For example, a serious injury, the stress associated with competition, going to high altitudes, or the use of certain drugs may all increase RMR.

### Factors that influence RMR

It is well documented that RMR is influenced by gender, age and body size, including the amount of FFM and fat mass. These four variables generally explain about 80% of the variability in RMR

(Bogardus *et al.* 1986). Since FFM has a high rate of metabolic activity, any change in FFM would dramatically influence RMR. In general, males have higher RMRs than females because they usually weigh more and have more FFM. However, Ferraro *et al.* (1992) found that females have a lower RMR than males (approximately 100 kcal less per day) even after differences in FFM, fat mass and age are controlled. Age is another variable known to influence RMR. It is estimated that the decline in RMR is less than 1–2% per decade from the second to the seventh decade of life (Keys *et al.* 1983).

It is now known that RMR also has a genetic component. This means that within a family members may have similar RMRs. Two studies illustrate this phenomenon. Bogardus *et al.* (1986) found that family membership could explain

11% of the variability in RMR ($P<0.0001$) in American Indians from 54 families. Similarly, Bouchard et al. (1989) found that in twins and parent–child pairs, heritability explained approximately 40% of the variability in RMR after adjusting for age, gender and FFM.

Research now indicates that RMR may fluctuate over the phases of the menstrual cycle, with RMR values lowest during the follicular phase and highest during the luteal phase (Solomon et al. 1982; Bisdee et al. 1989). The difference in RMR between these two phases is approximately 420–1260 kJ·day$^{-1}$ (100–300 kcal·day$^{-1}$). It also appears that adaptations in energy intake mimic the changes in RMR. Barr et al. (1995) found that females consume approximately 1260 kJ·day$^{-1}$ (300 kcal·day$^{-1}$) more during the luteal phase of the menstrual cycle than during the follicular phase. Thus, the increased energy expenditure, due to a higher RMR during the luteal phase, is compensated by an increase in energy intake during this period. However, if an athlete is amenorrhoeic, these changes in RMR will not occur. Data are not available for anovulatory females who may be menstruating but have depressed hormonal profiles. Although there is substantial research to suggest that RMR changes over the menstrual cycle, not all research is supportive of these findings. Weststrate (1993) showed no effect of menstrual cycle on RMR, and Piers et al. (1995) showed no effect of menstrual cycle phase on RMR or energy intake.

EFFECT OF EXERCISE ON RMR

For the athlete participating in an intense training programme, exercise may affect RMR both directly and indirectly. First, exercise can directly increase RMR if it increases FFM (Bogardus et al. 1986). Second, intense exercise training can temporarily increase resting energy expenditure above the typical RMR long after the exercise bout has ended. This short-term increase in energy expenditure is termed excess postexercise oxygen consumption (EPOC) and is the amount of energy expended above the typical RMR. The extent of EPOC after an exercise bout and the effect it has on TDEE appears to depend on the exercise intensity and/or the duration (Bahr 1992). For example, Bahr et al. (1987) found that aerobic exercise (70% $\dot{V}O_{2max.}$) lasting 80 min produced a 15% increase in EPOC lasting for 12 h after exercise. Similarly, 2 min of exercise at 108% $\dot{V}O_{2max.}$, repeated three times, produced a significant increase in EPOC for 4 h after exercise (Bahr et al. 1992). Although most research has examined the effect of aerobic exercise on EPOC, Melby et al. (1993) found a significant increase in EPOC after 90 min of weightlifting. Oxygen consumption was elevated by 5–10% over baseline the following morning.

Finally, it appears that energy flux can also alter RMR. Energy flux is defined as the amount of energy expended in exercise compared with the amount of energy consumed each day. An athlete who is exercising intensely and eating adequate energy would be in high energy flux, while an athlete who is exercising intensely, but restricting energy intake would be in negative energy flux. Bullough et al. (1995) examined the effect of energy flux on RMR in trained male athletes. They measured RMR after 3 days of high-intensity exercise (90 min of cycling at 75% $\dot{V}O_{2max.}$, while eating adequate energy) and after 3 days of exercise when energy intake was reduced (energy intake matching that required on a no-exercise day). They found that RMR was significantly higher during high energy than during negative energy flux. Thus, two athletes may be doing similar workouts, but have dramatically different energy expenditures if one is restricting energy intake and the other is not.

## Factors that influence TEF

A number of factors can influence how athletes' bodies respond metabolically to the food they consume. Some of these factors are associated with the physiological characteristics of an individual such as genetic background, age, level of physical fitness, sensitivity to insulin, or level of body fat. Other factors are associated with the meal, such as meal size, composition, palatability and timing.

## EFFECT OF FOOD COMPOSITION, MEAL SIZE AND EXERCISE

The TEF can last for several hours after a meal and will depend on the amount of energy consumed and the composition of the meal. In general, the thermic effect of a mixed meal is estimated to be 6–10% of total daily energy intake; however, the total TEF will also depend on the macronutrient composition of the diet. For example, the thermogenic effect of glucose is 5–10%, fat is 3–5% and protein is 20–30% (Flatt 1992). Carbohydrate and fat have a lower thermic effect than protein because less energy is required to process, transport and convert carbohydrate and fat into their respective storage forms. Conversely, protein synthesis and metabolism are more energy demanding. Thus, diets higher in fat will have a lower TEF than diets that contain more carbohydrate or protein. In addition, a diet high in energy will have a higher TEF than a diet lower in energy because there is more food to be digested, transported and stored. For example, the TEF of an individual who consumes 12.6 MJ (3000 kcal) daily would be approximately 756–1260 kJ · day$^{-1}$ (180–300 kcal · day$^{-1}$), while an individual consuming only 6.3 MJ (1500 kcal) daily would have a TEF of 378–630 kJ · day$^{-1}$ (90–150 kcal · day$^{-1}$). The total TEF for a day does not appear to be influenced by meal size or number, as long as the same amount of energy is consumed throughout the day (Belko & Barbieri 1987). Thus, the TEF will depend both on the amount of energy consumed each day and the composition of this energy.

Although exercise may influence the TEF, there are few data available on the effect of exercise before and after a meal in trained athletes. One study in trained swimmers reported that 45 min of swimming significantly increased the metabolic response to a meal when the meal preceded the exercise (104.2 kJ · h$^{-1}$, 24.8 kcal · h$^{-1}$) compared with no exercise (84.8 kJ · h$^{-1}$, 20.2 kcal · h$^{-1}$) (Nichols *et al.* 1988). However, this difference is so small that its long-term significance on energy regulation is negligible, especially considering the high variability in the termic effect of a meal (TEM) measurement between individuals. Similar results are reported by Bahr (1992), who exercised physically active males for 80 min at 75% $\dot{V}o_{2max.}$ and measured oxygen consumption after exercise. In the treatment condition subjects were fed a meal 2 h after exercise, while subjects fasted in the control condition. They found only a 42-kJ (10-kcal) difference between the two conditions over a 5-h postexercise period.

## Measurement of energy expenditure

Energy expenditure can be measured in the laboratory or estimated using prediction equations. Since access to a laboratory for the measurement of energy expenditure (calorimetry or doubly labelled water) may be limited, this review will focus on the prediction methods used to estimate energy expenditure.

### PREDICTING ENERGY EXPENDITURE

One of the most commonly used methods for estimating TDEE is to predict RMR using a prediction equation and then multiply RMR by an appropriate activity factor (Food and Nutrition Board 1989; Montoye *et al.* 1996). A number of prediction equations have been developed to estimate RMR, but most have been developed using sedentary populations. To date, no equation has been developed to predict the RMR of athletes who may spend hours in training each week. Some of the commonly used RMR prediction equations and the population from which these equations were derived are discussed below. To determine which of these equations work best for athletes, Thompson and Manore (1996) compared the measured RMR values from indirect calorimetry with predicted RMR values using the following equations. In all these equations, weight (wt) was measured in kilograms, height (ht) in centimetres and age in years; LBM stands for lean body mass.

• Harris and Benedict (1919); based on 239 subjects, 136 men (mean age, 27±9 years; mean weight, 64±10 kg) and 103 women (mean age,

33±14 years; mean weight, 56.5±11.5 kg), including trained male athletes. Harris and Benedict derived different equations for both men and women:

Males: RMR = 66.47 + 13.75 (wt) − 5 (ht)
       − 6.76 (age)

Females: RMR = 655.1 9.56 (wt) + 1.85 (ht)
         − 4.68 (age)

• Owen *et al.* (1986); based on 44 lean and obese women, eight of whom were trained athletes (age range, 18–65 years; weight range, 48–143 kg), none of whom were menstruating during the study, and all of whom were weight stable for at least 1 month:

Active females: RMR = 50.4 + 21.1 (wt)

Inactive females: RMR = 795 + 7.18 (wt)

• Owen *et al.* (1987); based on 60 lean and obese men (age range, 18–82 years; weight range, 60–171 kg), none of whom were athletes, and all of whom were weight stable for at least 1 month:

Males: RMR = 290 + 22.3 (LBM)

Males: RMR = 879 + 10.2 (wt)

• Mifflin *et al.* (1990); based on 498 healthy lean and obese subjects, 247 females and 251 males (age range, 18–78 years; weight range, 46–120 kg for women and 58–143 kg for men); no mention was made of physical activity level:

RMR = 9.99 (wt) + 6.25 (ht) − 4.92 (age)
      + 166 (sex; male = 1, female = 0) − 161

• Cunningham (1980); based on 223 subjects, 120 males and 103 females, from the Harris and Benedict data base. Cunningham eliminated 16 males who were identified as trained athletes. In this study, LBM accounted for 70% of the variability of RMR. LBM was not calculated in the Harris–Benedict equation, so Cunningham estimated LBM based on body mass and age:

RMR = 500 + 22 (LBM)

Thompson and Manore (1996) found that for both male and female athletes the Cunning-ham equation best predicted RMR, with the Harris–Benedict equation being the next best predictor. Because the Cunningham equation requires the measurement of FFM, the Harris–Benedict equation will be easier to use in settings where FFM cannot be measured.

Once RMR has been estimated, TDEE can then be estimated by a variety of different factorial methods. These methods vary in how labour intensive they are to use and the level of respondent burden. A detailed description of these methods is given elsewhere (Food and Nutrition Board 1989; Schutz & Jequier 1994; Montoye *et al.* 1996). The easiest method multiplies RMR by an appropriate activity factor, with the resulting value representing TDEE (Food and Nutrition Board 1989). Another method estimates a general activity factor (GAF) and a specific activity factor (SAF). The GAF represents the energy expended in doing everyday activities such as walking, standing, driving, and watching television. The SAF is the amount of activity expended in specific exercises (e.g. running, swimming or weight training) for a designated intensity and amount of time. The SAF is calculated by multiplying the amount of time spent in an activity by its energy requirement (Berning & Steen 1991; Montoye *et al.* 1996). The GAF and SAF are then added together to get the total amount of energy expended per day in activity. This value is added to the estimated RMR value, then an additional 6–10% is added to represent the TEF. The final number then represents the TDEE. This method is relatively easy to use with athletes who have specific training or exercise programmes and who already keep training logs. TDEE can also be estimated by recording all activities over a 24-h period and then calculating the energy expended in each of these activities ($kJ \cdot kg^{-1} \cdot min^{-1}$). The amount of energy expended in each activity is then added and represents TDEE. Many computer programs calculate energy expenditure in this way. Regardless of the method used, keep in mind that all values are estimates. The accuracy of these values will depend on a number of factors: the accuracy of the activity records, the accuracy of the data base used, and the accuracy with which the calculations are done.

### Energy intake

Since energy intake is one part of the energy balance equation, knowing total energy intake will give some indication of TDEE if body weight is stable. The assessment of dietary records is one of the most frequently used procedures for monitoring the energy and nutrient intakes of athletes. The goal of assessing dietary intake is to achieve the most accurate description of the athlete's typical food intake. This information is then used to assess mean energy intake and composition of the diet, make recommendations for improving food habits and adjusting energy intake, and determine the need for micronutrient supplements while dieting.

#### METHODS FOR COLLECTING ENERGY AND NUTRIENT INTAKE DATA

For the athlete with limited time and skills for recording food intake, retrospective methods, such as 24-h diet recalls, food frequency questionnaires or diet histories, can be used. If more specific energy or nutrient intake data are needed, food records or weighed food records should be used. Deciding which method to use will depend on the capabilities and dedication of the athlete, and the detail and specificity of the data required by the sports medicine team (Dwyer 1999).

The diet record is probably the most frequently used method for assessing the energy and nutrient intake of athletes. A diet record is a list of all food consumed over a specified time, such as 3–7 days. To more accurately predict energy and nutrient intakes, it is best if foods consumed can be weighed or measured, labels of convenience foods saved, and all supplements recorded from the label. This method also allows for the gathering of more in-depth information such as the time, place, feelings, and behaviours associated with eating. The dietitian working with the athlete can review the diet record to ensure its accuracy. A primary drawback of this method is the tendency for individuals to change their 'typical eating habits' on days they record food intake. This method is also more time consuming than a 24-h recall; thus, the accuracy of the diet record depends on the individual's cooperation and skill in recording foods properly.

How many days must be recorded to give an accurate picture of an athlete's diet? Diet records lasting from 3 to 14 days will provide good estimates of energy and nutrient intakes (Schlundt 1988). Within this range, reliability and accuracy appear to increase with each additional day up to 7 days. Thus, a 7-day diet record can give accurate data for energy and most nutrients. One advantage of the 7-day diet record is that it encompasses all the days of the week, including the dietary changes that frequently occur on weekends and the athlete's weekly training routine. The disadvantage of this method is that as the number of days increases, so does the respondent burden. If only 3–4-day diet records are used, care should be taken in choosing which days will be recorded.

## Practical guidelines for achieving a competitive body weight

For the overweight athlete, any weight loss attempt should be aimed at achieving a competitive body weight and composition that is optimal for performance and health. What is an optimal body weight for performance? How is this number determined? Who determines this goal? These are difficult questions that need to be addressed by the athlete in consultation with the sports medicine team before a weight loss programme can begin. If the athlete is young and still growing, these questions are even harder. Table 35.1 gives ranges of relative body fat levels for elite athletes in various sports; Berning and Steen (1998) also give body fat and $\dot{V}o_{2max.}$ data for athletes of varying ages. These ranges, however, do not take into account individual variability regarding body fat and performance. In addition, some athletes will perform at their best outside of these ranges. Remember that a certain amount of body fat is essential for good health. Finally, the inherent error of body composition assessment, 1–3% under ideal conditions, must be considered (Wilmore 1992a).

### Weight loss goals

The following outline offers some criteria and questions that may be helpful in determining an athlete's optimal body weight.

**1** Put emphasis on personal health and well being, and fitness and performance goals—not only weight.

 • Set realistic weight goals. (What is your current weight goal? Is body weight reduction necessary? Is there any indication that weight loss will improve performance? Have you ever maintained your goal weight without dieting? When was the last time you were at your goal weight? At what weight or body-fat level do you perform well, do you feel good and are you injury free? What was the last weight you could maintain without constantly dieting?)

 • Place less focus on the scale and more on changes in body composition and lifestyle, such as stress management and making good food choices.

 • Pick the appropriate weight loss technique that works with your training schedule. Weight loss should be gradual, at approximately 0.5–1.0 kg·week$^{-1}$.

 • Mark progress by measuring changes in fitness level and performance levels (personal record times, level of fatigue at the end of a workout, level of energy at the end of the day, strength and power changes), and general overall well-being.

**2** Make changes in diet and eating behaviour.

 • Do not starve yourself or restrict energy too severely. Do not go below 5–6.4 MJ (1200–1500 kcal) daily for women and 6.4–7.6 MJ (1500–1800 kcal) daily for men.

 • Do not constantly deprive yourself of favourite foods or set unrealistic dietary rules.

 • Make basic dietary changes that moderately reduce energy intake, that fit into your lifestyle, and that you know you can achieve.

 • Reduce fat intake but remember, a lower fat diet will not guarantee weight loss if a negative energy balance is not achieved.

 • Eat more whole grains, cereals, fruits, and vegetables, and get adequate fibre (>25 g·day$^{-1}$).

 • Do not skip meals and do not let yourself get too hungry. Eat something for breakfast. This will prevent you from being too hungry and overeating later in the day.

 • Reduce or eliminate late night eating.

 • Plan ahead and be prepared for when you might get hungry. Carry healthy snacks with you. Always eat high carbohydrate foods immediately after strenuous exercise.

 • Identify your dietary weaknesses; plan a strategy for dealing with these difficult times. Are you eating when you are bored, depressed, upset? Do you overeat when you are around food or eat out?

 • Do not go into a training session or competition without eating adequately. Be sure you are well fed both before and after you exercise.

**3** Make changes in exercise behaviour.

 • If you do not already do aerobic exercise and strength training, start and maintain an exercise programme that includes both of these components. This is an absolute requirement for burning fat and the maintenance of a healthy competitive body weight. Strength training will help maintain FFM while you are working to lose body fat.

 • Plan regular exercise into your day (outside your training sessions) and add additional exercise by walking instead of driving, or using the stairs instead of the elevator.

(Adapted from Burke 1995; Manore 1996.)

Optimal body weight should be a weight that promotes both good health and performance, and is 'reasonable' to achieve and maintain. If an athlete has never been able to achieve or maintain his or her goal weight, then this may be an unrealistic weight that places them under unnecessary psychological stress. Determination of an athlete's optimal weight must also consider the genetic background, age, gender, sport, health and past weight history. For the female athlete, knowing menstrual history will also be important in setting weight loss and dietary goals (Dueck *et al.* 1996).

Body composition should be measured and weight loss goals centred on the loss of body fat instead of just weight. This way the goal is shifted to changes in body composition instead of weight (Table 35.1). Knowing body composition also helps prevent the athlete from losing too much weight or setting an unachievable goal. This information can then be used to determine an optimal body weight and to set fat loss goals. For the athlete who is already lean, yet wants to diet, this process can help convince him or her

that weight loss is not necessary. Weight loss in a lean athlete is not possible without seriously compromising performance because of the inevitable loss of FFM. These athletes will benefit more from establishing good dietary practices than from weight loss. These guidelines can also be used with the young athlete who does not want to gain weight even though growth and weight gain should be occurring.

### Role of diet

If the athlete does need to lose weight (body fat), a weight loss plan needs to be developed early in the athlete's training programme to avoid potentially harmful dieting practices and weight cycling. Weight loss is not recommended during periods of intense endurance training; athletes cannot be expected to train intensely and improve performance on low energy intakes. Thus, weight loss goals should be set at approximately $0.5–1 \, kg \cdot week^{-1}$, depending on body size and gender, and focus on decreases in body fat, while maintaining or increasing FFM (Wilmore 1992b; Fogelholm 1994). The degree of energy restriction will depend on body size, typical energy intake and expenditure, and the period allotted for weight loss. In general, reducing energy intake by 10–25% (approximately 1680–3360 kJ or 400–800 kcal daily) may be all that is necessary. If the weight loss is occurring in the off season, then both the restriction of energy intake and increased energy expenditure need to occur.

Severe energy restriction or fasting should not be used with athletes. This approach to weight loss only decreases carbohydrate and protein intake and, thus, the ability to replace muscle glycogen (Bogardus *et al.* 1981) and repair and build muscle tissue after exercise. These types of diets also increase the risk of injury and the feelings of fatigue after routine workouts, which in turn can dramatically undermine self-confidence and performance. Finally, these diets increase FFM losses and decrease RMR (Donnelly *et al.* 1994; Thompson *et al.* 1996). These factors, combined with the feelings of deprivation that

**Table 35.1** Ranges of relative body fat for men and women athletes in various sports. From Wilmore (1992b), with permission.

| Sport | Men | Women |
| --- | --- | --- |
| Baseball, softball | 8–14 | 12–18 |
| Basketball | 6–12 | 10–16 |
| Body building | 5–8 | 6–12 |
| Canoeing and kayaking | 6–12 | 10–16 |
| Cycling | 5–11 | 8–15 |
| Fencing | 8–12 | 10–16 |
| Football | 6–18 | — |
| Golf | 10–16 | 12–20 |
| Gymnastics | 5–12 | 8–16 |
| Horse racing | 6–12 | 10–16 |
| Ice and field hockey | 8–16 | 12–18 |
| Orienteering | 5–12 | 8–16 |
| Pentathlon | — | 8–15 |
| Racketball | 6–14 | 10–18 |
| Rowing | 6–14 | 8–16 |
| Rugby | 6–16 | — |
| Skating | 5–12 | 8–16 |
| Ski jumping | 7–15 | 10–18 |
| Skiing | 7–15 | 10–18 |
| Soccer | 6–14 | 10–18 |
| Swimming | 6–12 | 10–18 |
| Synchronized swimming | — | 10–18 |
| Tennis | 6–14 | 10–20 |
| Track and field | | |
|   Field events | 8–18 | 12–20 |
|   Running events | 5–12 | 8–15 |
| Triathlon | 5–12 | 8–15 |
| Volleyball | 7–15 | 10–18 |
| Weightlifting | 5–12 | 10–18 |
| Wrestling | 5–16 | — |

accompany severe dieting, usually result in diet failure or relapse.

If energy intake decreases below 7.6–8 MJ· day⁻¹ (1800–1900 kcal·day⁻¹), nutrient intakes can be severely compromised (Beals & Manore 1994, 1998; Manore 1996). This level of energy intake is not adequate to replace muscle glycogen and fuel the athlete during intense training periods. Athletes have higher protein and carbohydrate requirements than their sedentary counterparts (Coyle 1995; Lemon 1995). When dieting, carbohydrate intake should remain as high as possible (60–70% of energy) and protein intake at 1.2–1.8 g·kg⁻¹ body weight (Lemon 1995), while fat intake is reduced to 15–25% of energy. Prolonged energy restriction also places that athlete at risk for low dietary intakes of calcium, iron, magnesium, zinc and B complex vitamins (Manore 1996; Beals & Manore, 1998). Thus, it may be necessary for athletes to use vitamin and mineral supplements during long periods of energy restriction (>3–4 weeks). This may be especially true if the athlete makes poor food choices, eats primarily processed or convenience foods, or eliminates various food groups from the diet.

Any weight loss plan for an athlete should moderately reduce energy intake while teaching good food choices. It is much easier to teach athletes how to eliminate or reduce high fat and energy dense foods from their diet than to count kilocalories. They also need to become aware of the situations and emotions that trigger overeating or binge eating. Athletes need to learn the nutrient composition of the foods they eat and why they eat them. This knowledge is useful in developing a diet plan around better food choices, training schedules, budgets and periods when overeating is most likely to occur.

### Role of exercise

Exercise is necessary for both weight loss and weight maintenance. Unlike the general population, most athletes participate in hard physical activity. However, which activities are best for fat loss? It is well documented that aerobic activity oxidizes fat; however, recent evidence indicates that high-intensity anaerobic activity added to an aerobic exercise programme may be better at reducing body fat than aerobic-only exercise (Trembly et al. 1994). Weight training can also help preserve FFM and strength while dieting if energy restriction is not too severe (Donnelly et al. 1994). Thus, the type of exercise added to a weight-loss programme will depend on the current training practices of the athlete.

### Behaviour modification and weight maintenance

In order for weight loss to be maintained, changes in diet and exercise habits need to become part of the athlete's lifestyle. Foreyt and Goodrick (1993) and Klem et al. (1996) found that individuals who are successful at losing and maintaining weight loss have the following characteristics in common: they modify diet, especially energy intake from fat; they exercise regularly and monitor their weight; and they have high levels of social support from family and friends. These changes can be achieved by first identifying the eating or exercise behaviour that needs to be changed, then setting specific and realistic goals for changing this behaviour. Changes in behaviour should be made slowly and modified as necessary. Finally, successful behaviour is rewarded. This approach to weight loss and maintenance will take time and may require continuous social and professional support (Foreyt & Goodrick 1991).

## Conclusion

Successfully guiding the overweight athlete through the weight loss process is a challenge for both the athlete and the sports medicine team. Identifying the appropriate weight loss goal and method is imperative for a successful outcome. These basic considerations need to be remembered before beginning any weight loss programme:
• Both energy intake and expenditure are important. If energy intake is less than energy expendi-

ture, weight will be lost. Increases in energy expenditure and moderate decreases in energy intake may help preserve FFM and muscle strength while dieting.

• Rate of weight loss is important. Do not use severe energy restriction or fasting as a means of weight loss. For most athletes, a weight loss of $0.5–1 \, \text{kg} \cdot \text{week}^{-1}$ is the maximum recommended.

• Composition of the diet is important, especially for weight maintenance. Carbohydrate, protein and alcohol oxidation appear to match their energy intake, while fat oxidation does not.

• The protein/energy intake ratio is important. When energy intake is low, a higher protein/energy ratio is required. In addition, athletes have higher protein requirement than sedentary individuals.

• Micronutrients are important. If dieting is longer than 3–4 weeks, micronutrient supplementation may be required to meet the recommended intakes.

## References

Abbott, W.G.H., Howard, B.V., Christin, L. *et al.* (1988) Short-term energy balance: relationship with protein, carbohydrate, and fat balances. *American Journal of Physiology* **255**, E332–E337.

Acheson, K.J., Schutz, Y., Bessard, T., Ravussin, E., Jequier, E. & Flatt, J.P. (1984) Nutritional influences on lipogenesis and thermogenesis after a carbohydrate meal. *American Journal of Physiology* **246**, E62–70.

Acheson, K.J., Schutz, Y., Bessard, T., Anantharaman, K., Flatt, J.P. & Jequier, E. (1988) Glycogen storage capacity and de novo lipogenesis during massive carbohydrate overfeeding in man. *American Journal of Clinical Nutrition* **48**, 240–247.

Bahr, R. (1992) Excess postexercise oxygen consumption: magnitude, mechanisms and practical implications. *Acta Physiologica Scandinavica* **144** (Suppl.), 1–70.

Bahr, R., Ingnes, I., Vaage, O., Sejersted, O.M. & Newsholme, E.A. (1987) Effect of duration of exercise on excess postexercise $O_2$ consumption. *Journal of Applied Physiology* **62**, 485–490.

Bahr, R., Gronnerod, O. & Sejersted, O.M. (1992) Effect of supramaximal exercise on excess postexercise $O_2$ consumption *Medicine and Science in Sports and Exercise* **24**, 66–71.

Barr, S.I., Janelle, K.C. & Prior, J.C. (1995) Energy intakes are higher during the luteal phase of ovulatory menstrual cycles. *American Journal of Clinical Nutrition* **61**, 39–43.

Beals, K.A. & Manore, M.M. (1994) The prevalence and consequences of subclinical eating disorders in female athletes. *International Journal of Sport Nutrition* **4**, 175–195.

Beals, K.A. & Manore, M.M. (1998) Nutritional status of female athletes with subclinical eating disorders. *Journal of the American Dietetic Association* **98**, 419–425.

Beidleman, B.A., Pahl, J.L. & De Souza, M.J. (1995) Energy balance in female distance runners. *American Journal of Clinical Nutrition* **61**, 303–311.

Belko, A.Z. & Barbieri, T.F. (1987) Effect of meal size and frequency on the thermic effect of food. *Nutrition Research* **7**, 237–242.

Berning, J.R. & Steen, S.N. (1998) *Nutrition for Sport and Exercise*, 2nd edn. Aspen Publishers, Gaithersburg, MD.

Bisdee, J.T., James, W.P.T. & Shaw, M.A. (1989) Changes in energy expenditure during the menstrual cycle. *British Journal of Nutrition* **61**, 187–199.

Bogardus, C., LaGrange, B.M., Horton, E.S. & Sims, E.A.H. (1981) Comparison of carbohydrate-containing and carbohydrate restricted hypocaloric diets in the treatment of obesity. *Journal of Clinical Investigation* **68**, 399–404.

Bogardus, C., Lillioja, S. & Ravussin, E. *et al.* (1986) Familial dependence of the resting metabolic rate. *New England Journal of Medicine* **315**, 96–100.

Bouchard, C., Tremblay, A., Nadeau, A. *et al.* (1989) Genetic effect in resting and exercise metabolic rates. *Metabolism* **38**, 364–370.

Brownell, K.D., Steen, S.N. & Wilmore, J.H. (1987) Weight regulation practices in athletes: analysis of metabolic and health effects. *Medicine and Science in Sports and Exercise* **19**, 546–556.

Bullough, R.C., Gillette, C.A., Harris, M.A. & Melby, C.L. (1995) Interaction of acute changes in exercise energy expenditure and energy intake on resting metabolic rate. *American Journal of Clinical Nutrition* **61**, 473–481.

Burke, L. (1995) *The Complete Guide to Food for Sports Performance: Peak Nutrition for Your Sport*, 2nd edn. Allen & Unwin, St Leonards, NSW.

Coyle, E.F. (1995) Substrate utilization during exercise in active people. *American Journal of Clinical Nutrition* **61** (Suppl.), 968S–979S.

Cunningham, J.J. (1980) A reanalysis of the factors influencing basal metabolic rate in normal adults. *American Journal of Clinical Nutrition* **33**, 2372–2374.

Donnelly, J.E., Jacobsen, D.J., Jakieic, J.M. & Whately, J.E. (1994) Very low calorie diet with concurrent vs. delayed and sequential exercise. *International Journal of Obesity* **18**, 469–475.

Dueck, C.A., Manore, M.M. & Matt, K.S. (1996) Role of

energy balance in athletic menstrual dysfunction. *International Journal of Sport Nutrition* **6**, 165–190.

Dwyer, J.T. (1999) Dietary assessment. In *Modern Nutrition in Health and Disease*, 9th edn (ed. M.E. Shils, J.A. Olson, M. Shike & A.C. Ross), pp. 937–959. Lea & Febiger, Baltimore, MD.

Ferraro, R., Lillioja, S., Fontvieille, A.M., Rising, R., Bodgarus, C. & Ravussin, E. (1992) Lower sedentary metabolic rate in women compared to men. *Journal of Clinical Investigation* **90**, 780–784.

Flatt, J.P. (1992) The biochemistry of energy expenditure. In *Obesity* (ed. P. Bjorntrop & B.N. Brodoff), pp. 100–116. J.B. Lippincott, New York.

Fogelholm, M. (1994) Effects of bodyweight reduction on sports performance. *Sports Medicine* **18**, 249–267.

Food and Nutrition Board (1989) *Recommended Dietary Allowances*, 10th edn. National Research Council, National Academy Press, Washington, DC.

Foreyt, J.P. & Goodrick, G.K. (1991) Factors common to successful therapy for the obese patient. *Medicine and Science in Sports and Exercise* **23**, 292–297.

Foreyt, J.P. & Goodrick, G.K. (1993) Weight management without dieting. *Nutrition Today* March/April, 4–9.

Harris, J.A. & Benedict, F.G. (1919) *A Biometric Study of Basal Metabolism in Man* (Carnegie Institute, Washington publication no. 279). F.B. Lippincott, Philadelphia, PA.

Hellerstein, M.K., Christiansen, M., Kaempfer, S. *et al.* (1991) Measurement of de novo hepatic lipogenesis in humans using stable isotopes. *Journal of Clinical Investigation* **87**, 1841–1852.

Hill, J.O., Drougas, H. & Peters, J.C. (1993) Obesity treatment: can diet composition play a role? *Annals of Internal Medicine* **119** (7 part 2), 694–697.

Horswill, C.A. (1992) Applied physiology of amateur wrestling. *Sports Medicine* **14**, 114–143.

Horswill, C.A. (1993) Weight loss and weight cycling in amateur wrestlers: implications for performance and resting metabolic rate. *International Journal of Sport Nutrition* **3**, 245–260.

Jebb, S.A., Prentice, A.M., Goldberg, G.R., Murgatroyd, P.R., Black, A.E. & Coward, W.A. (1996) Changes in macronutrient balance during over- and under-feeding assessed by 12-d continuous whole-body calorimetry. *American Journal of Clinical Nutrition* **64**, 259–266.

Keys, A., Taylor, H.L. & Grande, F. (1983) Basal metabolism and age of adult man. *Metabolism* **22**, 579–587.

Klem, M.L., McGuire, T.M., Wing, R.R., Seagle, H. & Hill, J.O. (1996) The national weight control registry: the diet and exercise behaviors of individuals highly successful at long-term maintenance of weight loss. *International Journal of Obesity* **4** (Suppl. 1), 7S.

Krempf, M., Hoerr, R.A., Pelletier, V.A., Marks, L.A., Gleason, R. & Young, V.R. (1993) An isotopic study of the effect of dietary carbohydrate on the metabolic fate of dietary leucine and phenylalanine. *American Journal of Clinical Nutrition* **57**, 161–169.

Lemon, P.R.W. (1995) Do athletes need more protein and amino acids? *International Journal of Sport Nutrition* **5**, S39–S61.

Manore, M.M. (1996) Chronic dieting in active women: what are the health consequences? *Women's Health Issues* **6**, 332–341.

Melby, C., Scholl, C., Edwards, G. & Bullough, R. (1993) Effect of acute resistance exercise on post-exercise energy expenditure and resting metabolic rate. *Journal of Applied Physiology* **75**, 1847–1853.

Mifflin, M.D., St Jeor, S., Hill, L.A., Scott, B.J., Daugherty, S.A. & Koh, Y.O. (1990) A new predictive equation for resting energy expenditure in healthy individuals. *American Journal of Clinical Nutrition* **51**, 241–247.

Montoye, H.J., Kemper, H.C.G., Saris, W.H.M. & Washburn, R.A. (1996) *Measuring Physical Activity and Energy Expenditure*. Human Kinetics, Champaign, IL.

Nichols, J., Ross, S. & Patterson, P. (1988) Thermic effect of food at rest and following swim exercise in trained college men and women. *Annals of Nutrition and Metabolism* **32**, 215–219.

Owen, O.E., Kavle, E., Owen, R.S. *et al.* (1986) A reappraisal of caloric requirements in healthy women. *American Journal of Clinical Nutrition* **44**, 1–19.

Owen, O.E., Holup, J.L., D'Alessio, D.A. *et al.* (1987) A reappraisal of the caloric requirements of men. *American Journal of Clinical Nutrition* **46**, 875–885.

Piers, L.S., Diggavi, S.N., Rijskamp, J., van Raaij, J.M.A., Shetty, P.S., & Hautvast, J.G.A.J. (1995) Resting metabolic rate and thermic effect of a meal in the follicular and luteal phases of the menstrual cycle in well-nourished Indian women. *American Journal of Clinical Nutrition* **61**, 296–302.

Poehlman, E.T. (1989) A review: exercise and its influence on resting energy metabolism in man. *Medicine and Science in Sports and Exercise* **21**, 515–525.

Ravussin, E. & Swinburn, B.A. (1993) Energy Metabolism. In *Obesity: Theory and Therapy*, 2nd edn (ed. A.J. Stunkard & T.A. Wadden), pp. 97–123. Raven Press, New York.

Ravussin, E., Lillioja, S., Anderson, T.E., Christin, L. & Bogardus, C. (1986) Determinants of 24-hour energy expenditure in man: methods and results using a respiratory chamber. *Journal of Clinical Investigation* **78**, 1568–1578.

Schlundt, D.G. (1988) Accuracy and reliability of nutrient intake estimates. *Journal of Nutrition* **118**, 1432–1435.

Schutz, Y. & Jequier, E. (1994) Energy needs: assessment and requirements. In *Modern Nutrition in Health and Disease*, 8th edn (ed. M.E. Shils, J.A. Olson & M. Shike), pp. 101–111. Lea & Febiger, Baltimore, MD.

Schutz, Y., Flatt, J.P. & Jequier, E. (1989) Failure of dietary fat intake to promote fat oxidation: a factor favoring the development of obesity. *American Journal of Clinical Nutrition* **50**, 307–314.

Shelmet, J.J., Reichard, G.A., Skutches, C.L., Hoeldtke, R.D., Owen, O.E. & Boden, G. (1988) Ethanol causes acute inhibition of carbohydrate, fat, and protein oxidation and insulin resistance. *Journal of Clinical Investigation* **81**, 1137–1145.

Solomon, S.J., Kurzer, M.S. & Calloway, D.H. (1982) Menstrual cycle and basal metabolic rate in women. *American Journal of Clinical Nutrition* **36**, 611–616.

Sonko, B.J., Prentice, A.M., Murgatroyd, P.R., Goldberg, G.R., van de Ven, M.L.H.M. & Coward, W.A. (1994) Effect of alcohol on postmeal fat storage. *American Journal of Clinical Nutrition* **59**, 619–625.

Steen, S.N. & Brownell, K.D. (1990) Patterns of weight loss and regain in wrestlers: has the tradition changed? *Medicine and Science in Sports and Exercise* **22**, 762–768.

Sundgot-Borgen, J. (1993) Prevalence of eating disorders in elite female athletes. *International Journal of Sport Nutrition* **3**, 29–40.

Sundgot-Borgen, J. (1994) Risk and trigger factors for the development of eating disorders in female elite athletes. *Medicine and Science in Sports and Exercise*. **26**, 414–419.

Swinburn, B. & Ravussin, E. (1993) Energy balance or fat balance? *American Journal of Clinical Nutrition* **57** (Suppl.), 766S–771S.

Thomas, C.D., Peters, J.C., Reed, W.G., Abumrad, N.N., Sun, M. & Hill, J.O. (1992) Nutrient balance and energy expenditure during ad libitum feeding of high-fat and high-carbohydrate diets in humans. *American Journal of Clinical Nutrition* **55**, 934–942.

Thompson, J.L. & Manore, M.M. (1996) Predicted and measured resting metabolic rate of male and female endurance athletes. *Journal of the American Dietetic Association* **96**, 30–34.

Thompson, J., Manore, M.M. & Skinner, J.S. (1993) Resting metabolic rate and thermic effect of a meal in low- and adequate-energy intake male endurance athletes. *International Journal of Sport Nutrition* **3**, 194–206.

Thompson, J.L., Manore, M.M. & Thomas, J.R. (1996) Effects of diet and diet-plus-exercise programs on resting metabolic rate: a meta-analysis. *International Journal of Sport Nutrition* **6**, 41–61.

Trembly, A., Simoneau, J. & Bouchard, C. (1994) Impact of exercise intensity on body fatness and skeletal muscle metabolism. *Metabolism* **43**, 814–818.

Westerterp, K.R. (1993) Food quotient, respiratory quotient, and energy balance. *American Journal of Clinical Nutrition* **57** (Suppl.), 759S–765S.

Weststrate, J.A. (1993) Resting metabolic rate and diet-induced thermogenesis: a methodological reappraisal. *American Journal of Clinical Nutrition* **58**, 592–601.

Wilmore, J.H. (1991) Eating and weight disorders in the female athlete. *International Journal of Sport Nutrition* **1**, 104–117.

Wilmore, J.H. (1992a) Body weight and body composition. In *Eating, Body Weight and Performance in Athletes: Disorders of Modern Society* (ed. K.D. Brownell, J. Robin & J. H. Wilmore), pp. 77–93. Lea & Febiger, Philadelphia, PA.

Wilmore, J.H. (1992b) Body weight standards and athletic performance. In *Eating, Body Weight and Performance in Athletes: Disorders of Modern Society* (ed. K.D. Brownell, J. Robin & J. H. Wilmore), pp. 315–329. Lea & Febiger, Philadelphia, PA.

# Chapter 36

# The Travelling Athlete

ANN C. GRANDJEAN AND JAIME S. RUUD

## Introduction

Spectators perceive the life of the international athlete as glamorous and exciting, but the travel involved in training and competition can have a devastating effect on performance. Many professional and elite athletes travel long distances on a regular basis to train and compete. Top American basketball players are away from home for a large part of the year, and travel is so much part of the routine that it has become a way of life. In many sports, travel must be accommodated in a rigorous training and competition schedule: jet lag and travel fatigue are not accepted as excuses when there is a high expectation of success. A good example is the US Women's Olympic basketball team, who travelled more than 161 000 km in 14 months prior to the games to promote women's basketball and to win the gold medal in Atlanta (Wolff 1996).

Whether flying for 12h or longer to another continent or jumping on a bus to compete in a neighbouring town, travel can cause a major disruption to an athlete's training programme. Major events may require extended periods of travel: the Sydney Olympics, for example, will require competitors from Europe to travel for at least 24h to reach their accommodation or pre-Games holding camps. Successful athletes should have an established training programme that includes a workout schedule, proper nutrition, adequate sleep and stress management, although in reality this is often not the case. When something happens to interfere with this

schedule, the break in routine can be physiologically and psychologically damaging. Diet is one of the major factors that may lead to disruption of an athlete's training programme away from home. Food intake often depends on local restaurant facilities, concession stands, or vendors, which means access to familiar foods may be limited. Consumption of unfamiliar foods and beverages, especially in large amounts, can result in severe gastrointestinal symptoms: even minor discomfort from gas, diarrhoea, or constipation may be enough to adversely affect performance. Potentially more serious, and even fatal, illness contracted from eating contaminated foodstuffs is as great a risk for the athlete as it is for all international travellers. Even where familiar foods are available, interrupting the athlete's normal eating and training schedule can negatively affect performance.

There seems to have been no serious attempt to quantify the effect of eating disturbances resulting from travel on sports performance, and there is little published information in this area. Much of the information in this chapter is based on the authors' professional experience and on experiences reported by athletes, coaches and team physicians. Inevitably, most of these reports are anecdotal, and even individual case reports are seldom available. To broaden the range of experiences, we surveyed sports nutritionists from each of the continents to glean information from their experiences and to provide the reader with practical suggestions. Interestingly, two problems were reported by all respondents: food availability and food safety. Jet-lag, risk of dehydration, body mass changes and food allergies were also identified as challenges for the travelling athlete.

## Food availability

Without hesitation, athletes, coaches, trainers and sports nutritionists list 'not having the food we need available' as the number one nutritional problem when travelling to a training camp or competition. While this can be a hurdle for all athletes, it is particularly difficult for those whose nutritional plan involves frequent small meals throughout the day: some athletes, especially those engaged in hard training, eat seven to eight meals or snacks each day. Local and regional events present fewer problems, as athletes can bring their own food, either on an individual or team basis, or can ensure that local restaurants or hotels have the appropriate food available. However, the greater the distance to be travelled and the longer the time to be spent away from home, the more important it is to plan well in advance if athletes are to be able to follow their nutritional plan. On long trips or training camps, it is not possible to be self-sufficient. One problem in such situations is the short menu cycle in many training camps: restaurant or hotel dining may be even worse, with no change of menu. A menu or self-service buffet that appears varied for the first day can become extremely monotonous after only a few days.

For high-altitude training, Finnish athletes train in countries such as Switzerland or Austria and often stay in small villages: the accommodation is usually in private hotels run by families where the food is plentiful but not always the high-carbohydrate foods that many athletes prefer, and again with little variety. At these locations, travel to training venues is usually by bus, and low-carbohydrate, high-fat foods purchased at fuel stations may be the only food available. Similar situations are reported from athletes in many other countries. Here, as in all situations, athletes require some nutritional knowledge to allow them to make the best food choices. Some-

times special arrangements can be made with hotel owners to ensure a menu that will meet the athletes' needs, and to provide meals that can be taken to the training venue, but such arrangements may not be possible. Many athletes use sports drinks and high-carbohydrate snacks to maintain carbohydrate intake, but this can lead to an unbalanced diet: while this may not be important in the short term, athletes may spend weeks or even months at some training camps. Chinese athletes, when travelling in the West, prefer to bring their own foods such as noodles, canned porridge, salted vegetables (such as hot pickled mustard tuber) and chocolate. While there is no single solution to all travel problems, as all athletes, coaches, team physicians and nutritionists know, planning ahead is essential if the athletes' needs are to be met.

Athletes or teams preferring to take food for the trip need to consider not only the perishability of food, but also airline restrictions on the weight and number of pieces of luggage. A US boxing team travelling abroad for a month of training and competition augmented their diet by taking canned tuna, peanut butter, crackers and chocolate bars. These items provided a significant amount of energy and nutrients while not adding significantly to the weight of the luggage. International travel is likely to impose limitations on the type of foods that can be taken. Many countries, including the US, have customs laws that prohibit the importation of fresh fruit, vegetables and meat products: such restrictions almost invariably apply to intercontinental travel. The penalties for contravening import regulations may be severe, apart from the confiscation of the team's food supply, and all team members must be aware of the restrictions that apply. Advance planning should prevent this situation from arising.

Some travelling athletes choose to take only enough food to serve as a backup, and expect to rely on local food sources for the majority of their needs. Common 'travel food' for US athletes include dried pasta, canned or powered sauces, cookies, canned meat and fish, peanut butter, soups, nuts, chocolate bars, crackers and sports bars. Other athletes travel with sufficient food to meet all of their needs and with cooking equipment which makes it possible to prepare food under a variety of travel and living conditions. Electrical current and plug adapters are an essential, but sometimes forgotten, part of this equipment. Distributing supplies and equipment throughout the baggage will help to ensure that it will reach the desired destination, and reduce the possibility of the entire supply being lost.

## Body mass changes

Another common concern related to travel and diet is body mass (weight) change. Athletes report that prevention of unwanted body mass loss or gain may be a major challenge while travelling. Body mass loss is likely to occur if athletes do not have access to an adequate supply of appropriate food and beverages, but it may also occur in the midst of dietary abundance. It is not uncommon, especially for athletes travelling abroad for the first time, for local foods to be avoided, perhaps because of a dislike of the unfamiliar, an uncertainty over the content or a fear of an adverse reaction. This is likely to lead to a reduction in energy intake and a loss of body mass. Athletes experienced at travelling will usually learn to eat in spite of taste preference or will ensure their own supply of food because they recognize that an inadequate intake leads to less than optimal performance. Even for the experienced traveller, however, some disruption is likely until a new routine is established. This involves identifying the location of dining facilities, restaurants, etc., as well as recovering for the effects of jet lag and travel fatigue, and it is during this period that a supply of snacks brought from home may be particularly valuable.

On the other hand, there are times when the local cuisine is so appetizing, that the athlete will overeat. This is typical in a dining hall setting where there is a variety of food choices and portion sizes are generous or where there is a self-service facility. Boredom, increased eating opportunities and the provision of food free of charge in a training camp are also factors that will lead some athletes to eat more than they would at home. This may be particularly the case at major championship events: the dining facilities at the Olympic Village, for example, provide a wide range of high-quality food free of charge $24 \, h \cdot day^{-1}$. For the athlete in a weight-category event whose first competition is not until near the end of the programme, 2 or 3 weeks spent in the Village, with a reduced training load and little to occupy the time, provides a severe challenge to self-restraint. This is a particular challenge for athletes from countries or from social backgrounds where such food is seldom available.

In both of these extreme situations, there may be advantages in regular monitoring of body mass as a guide to the adequacy of the dietary intake. This is not, however, as straightforward as might at first appear. A fall in body mass may be the result of an inadequate energy intake, but may also reflect some degree of hypohydration, particularly in warm weather. Athletes may experience some loss of body mass during a training camp if the training load is increased above the normal level, and this may be desirable or not, depending on whether there is a need for the athlete to reduce the body fat content and whether the mass loss does indeed reflect a loss of body fat. Ekblom and Bergh (Chapter 51) have reported that the daily energy requirement of elite cross-country skiers during normal training is about 20–25 MJ (4780–5970 kcal) and that this may increase by 4–8 MJ (950–1910 kcal) during training camps. An increased body mass may indicate overeating, but is also a normal response to a reduced training load in the days prior to competition. Changes in the diet may induce constipation, leading to a small increase in body mass.

## Dehydration

Travel increases the athlete's risk of dehydration. An adequate intake of fluids is essential, especially on long-range flights as the low water vapour pressure in aircraft cabins leads to an

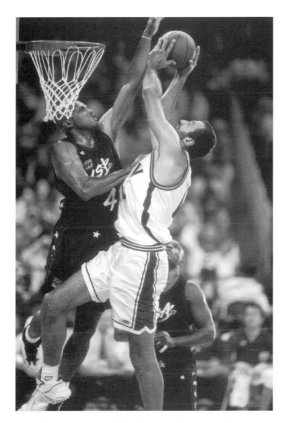

**Fig. 36.1** In many sports, elite performers travel long distances on a regular basis. This adds many problems when there is little time for recovery between competitions. Photo © Allsport / A. Bello.

increased loss of water from the respiratory tract and through skin. Drinking fluids before, during and after travel is essential. Carrying bottled water can provide fluid, while sport drinks, juice packs and soft drinks provide both carbohydrate and fluid. On transcontinental flights, most airlines are aware of the risks of dehydration and frequently offer water, juice or soft drinks. If this service is not sufficient, ring the flight attendant call button and request fluids on a routine (e.g. hourly) basis. Ask for a whole bottle or can, or even two, rather than a small glass. When a large team is travelling together, the airline might be warned in advance that demand for fluids is likely to be high and an extra provision requested. In any case, it is unwise to rely on

an adequate amount being available and each athlete should be self-sufficient for the duration of the flight. Particularly when travelling to hot climates, sufficient fluid should be taken to allow for delays at immigration and customs upon arrival.

## Jet lag

Jet lag is a common problem for athletes who travel through different time zones (Reilly *et al.* 1997a). It results from a disruption of the body's rhythms and sleep–wake cycle. Fatigue, disturbances of sleeping patterns, poor concentration, digestive problems and irritability are usual symptoms of jet lag. Studies have shown that the 'competitive edge' can be lost after crossing as few as one or two time zones (US Olympic Committee 1988). Symptoms of jet lag are generally more severe when travelling from west to east rather than in the opposite direction (Reilly *et al.* 1997b). Although athletes generally suffer less than sedentary individuals, in terms of general symptoms (Reilly *et al.* 1997a), the implications for performance are perhaps more serious for the athlete who may have to recover quickly and compete soon after arrival. A rough rule of thumb is that one day is required at the new destination for each time zone crossed, but it is clear that there is a large variability between individuals in the speed of adjustment.

Both the type of food consumed and timing of meals are important considerations in helping the body adapt to time zone shifts. Although the light–dark cycle is perhaps the most important signal involved in setting the body's internal clock, the timing of meals and of exercise are also important signals. The composition of meals and the amount of food eaten may also have some impact. High-protein foods (meats, cheese, fish, poultry and tofu) are reported to stimulate the adrenaline pathway and increase alertness. High-carbohydrate foods (pasta, rice, bread, fruit) increase insulin secretion, which facilitates the uptake of tryptophan, an essential amino acid which is then converted to serotonin, and ingestion of meals with a high carbohydrate content may be followed by a feeling of drowsiness. Thus, what and when an athlete eats may influence the severity and duration of jet-lag symptoms, and it has been suggested that high-protein foods should be eaten at breakfast time and high-carbohydrate meals taken at night (Reilly *et al.* 1997b). Central nervous system stimulants, such as the caffeine in tea and coffee, may be beneficial when taken in the mornings on arrival at the new destination, but are best avoided in the later part of the day. Drinking an adequate amount of fluids is also recommended, as dehydration can aggravate the symptoms of fatigue and jet lag. This implies a need for care in the use of caffeine-containing beverages and alcohol because of the possible diuretic effects.

Where a single major event involving long-distance travel is scheduled, there may be advantages for some individuals in preparing before departure. If this is to be attempted, it might be suggested that, 3 days before travel, athletes should begin training, sleeping, eating and drinking according to the time of their destination. It should be recognized, however, that attempts at preadjustment by changes in lifestyle have generally been found to be ineffective because of the difficulty in controlling all the factors involved.

In recent years, melatonin has been used by some athletes to avoid jet lag (Grafius 1996). Melatonin is a hormone derived from the pineal gland that affects the body's sleep–wake cycle. Research has shown that low doses of melatonin taken in the evening can help induce sleep (Zhdanova *et al.* 1995). Oral doses of melatonin (0.5–3 mg) taken 1 h before bedtime appears to be safe and effective (Grafius 1996). However, as with any substance, melatonin may be tolerated differently by each athlete. Morning grogginess and vivid dreams have been reported with use of melatonin. For the athlete who wants to try melatonin, experimenting with it prior to travel or competition is recommended. Melatonin is not included on the list of prohibited substances. The purity of commercial preparations is uncertain, and melatonin content of some preparations may be less than the stated dose.

## Traveller's diarrhoea and other infections

Once an athlete arrives in a new country, one of the greatest fears is becoming ill just prior to or during competition. Although there is little recent information, one report suggests that up to 60% of athletes travelling abroad may be affected by some form of gastroenteritis (Grantham 1983). Food-borne illnesses and gastrointestinal distresses of other aetiology can prohibit participation or diminish performance. Traveller's diarrhoea is a concern to athletes irrespective of the country of origin or destination.

Traveller's diarrhoea can be caused by food or water that contains bacteria, viruses or parasites. It is estimated that bacterial enteropathogens cause at least 80% of traveller's diarrhoea with *Escherichia coli* and *Shigella* being the two most common agents (DuPont & Ericsson 1993). Clinical features of traveller's diarrhoea include frequent loose stools and abdominal cramps, sometimes accompanied by nausea, vomiting or the passage of bloody stools. Since contaminated food and water can cause traveller's diarrhoea, athletes need to be cautious of what they eat and drink and to apply stringent food hygiene rules. Prevention of the problem involves selecting eating establishments that are well known or recommended by coaches or other individuals who have been to the area before and who are aware of the food safety issues. Contacting your country's embassy in the country of your destination to identify in advance potential problems can also be of value. Information on immunization requirements and recommended prophylactic precautions should also be established well in advance of travel, and this advice is readily available from travel agents, airlines and embassies.

Foods such as fruits that can be peeled and vegetables that have been thoroughly washed with boiling water are generally safe food choices. For the most part, athletes should drink only bottled water, juices or soft drinks from sealed containers. The following list provides guidance for foods and beverages generally considered safe. However, when in doubt, remember the phrase, 'Boil it, cook it, peel it or forget it' (Mayo Clinic Health Letter 1997).

Table 36.1 lists foods and beverages generally considered to be safe and those which are potentially dangerous.

Foods and beverages are not the only source of pathogens. If the level of water purity is unknown, athletes should use bottled water to brush their teeth and should not swallow water when bathing. Athletes participating in water sports, such as rowing or canoeing, need to avoid swallowing lake or river water.

Oral prophylactic drugs that have been used to prevent traveller's diarrhoea in adults include doxycycline, trimethoprim-sulfamethoxazole, norfloxacin, ciprofloxacin and bismuth subsalicylate. These drugs are generally taken on the first day of arrival and continued for one or two days after departure (DuPont & Ericsson 1993). However, the disadvantages of prophylaxis may outweigh the benefits. When used for an extended period of time, potential side-effects can occur, depending on the oral agent selected, such as blackening of the tongue and faeces, skin rashes and reactions to the sun. Prophylactic drugs may also give a false sense of security to an athlete who would otherwise exercise caution

when choosing food and beverages. Certain probiotic organisms, such as lactobacillus GG, have been shown to be effective in stimulating antibody production against rotavirus (Kaila *et al.* 1992, 1995), and to reduce the duration of diarrhoea (Isolauri *et al.* 1991). It would, however, be unwise to rely on these.

If diarrhoea develops, the athlete should seek medical attention as soon as possible. Because dehydration is likely to result, it is important to consume plenty of fluids: bottled beverages, broth, soup and tea made from bottled water. Sports drinks, which have a composition similar to that of oral rehydration solutions recommended for the treatment of childhood diarrhoea, are an effective remedy in this situation (Maughan 1994). If diarrhoea is a possible outcome, a supply of one of the commercially available oral rehydration solutions must be available: this may not be easily available locally and should be brought from home. These drinks contain higher electrolyte levels than sports drinks and will help maintain fluid balance and speed recovery: if a powdered or tablet formulation is used, bottled water must be used in the preparation. If a large fluid loss is incurred and the athlete has difficulty in taking oral fluids, intravenous rehydration may be warranted.

A variety of other medical problems, including upper respiratory infection, abscessed tooth and general infections, are known to impair performance and may even prevent an athlete from competing. Adequate sleep and rest, maintenance of hydration status and a nutritionally adequate diet can help ward off infections. A daily multiple vitamin/mineral supplement can also help ensure adequate vitamin and mineral intakes. In addition, the importance of frequent and careful hand washing with soap cannot be overemphasized.

## Food allergies and food intolerance

The athlete with food allergies has an additional challenge when travelling. A food allergy is any adverse reaction to an otherwise harmless food or food component that involves the body's

**Table 36.1** Foods and beverages generally considered to be safe or potentially unsafe.

| Safe | Unsafe |
| --- | --- |
| Steaming hot food | Moist foods at room |
| Dry food (e.g. breads) | temperature (e.g. |
| High sugar-content | sauces, salads and |
| foods (e.g. jellies and | buffet dishes) |
| syrups) | Raw or undercooked |
| Fruit which can be | meats, fish and |
| peeled (e.g. bananas, | shellfish |
| oranges and melons) | Unpeelable raw |
| Bottled drinks in their | vegetables and |
| original containers (e.g. | fruit (e.g. grapes |
| carbonated water, soda | and berries) |
| and sports drinks) | All dairy products |
| Coffee and tea, if | Tap water |
| steaming hot | Ice cubes |

immune system. A food allergen is the part of the food that stimulates the immune system of a food-allergic individual and a single food can contain multiple food allergens. Proteins in foods are most commonly the cause of an allergic response. It is estimated that less than 2% of the population has a true allergy to food.

Travel guides and books for people with allergies are available. Foreign sources of information have been published by the Food Allergy Network and the Information Centre for Food Hypersensitivity (LIVO). Translation of commonly used allergy terms, food labelling laws, emergency medical services, travel tips and a list of non-profit organizations working with food allergies can be obtained.*

A food intolerance is different from a food allergy: it occurs when people react adversely to food but without the involvement of the immune system. Food intolerances can occur for a number of reasons. The most common of these involve enzyme deficiencies, such as lactose intolerance, which results from a lactase deficiency.

## Developing an eating strategy

It is important that the nutritional needs of the travelling athlete are not left to chance. A clearly identified strategy is an essential part of the preparation process. For team sports, there should be an overall team plan, but an individualized programme should also be developed for each team member to take account of individual needs and preferences. The key elements of the strategy are as follows.

Recommendations for a nutritional survival plan include:
• think through your nutritional needs;

*These can be obtained from: The Food Allergy Network, 10400 Eaton Place, Fairfax, VA 22030–220, USA; Tel.: 703-691-3179; Fax: 703-691-2713; or The Information Centre for Food Hypersensitivity (LIVO), PO Box 84185, 2508 AD, The Hague, The Netherlands; Tel.: 703510893; Fax: 703547343.

• have a plan and a back-up plan;
• contact hotels and restaurants at your travel destination and make appropriate arrangements;
• be assertive in making plans and when ordering in restaurants;
• before flights, order special airplane meals if necessary;
• request extra potatotes, bread, rice, pasta or other carbohydrate-rich foods;
• take food and drink with you.
  Food appropriate for short trips includes:
• breads, biscuits, bagels;
• muffins, cookies, pretzels;
• canned vegetables;
• bottled, canned or boxed fruit juices;
• canned fruit, dried fruits;
• bottled water;
• sports drinks;
• canned meal replacement;
• nuts, trail mix.

Where there are special nutritional requirements, particular care in planning ahead is necessary. Favourite foods or drinks that are used in training or that make up the pregame meal may not be available. Vegetarian athletes may experience difficulty in some countries where their needs may not be catered for.

## Conclusion

Athletes are often expected to produce their best performance in unfamiliar surroundings far from home. Long-distance travel brings with it a multitude of challenges and opportunities. In ideal situations, a member of the sports staff assumes responsibility for travel arrangements, visa requirements, accommodation, equipment, money, itinerary and nutritional needs. It is important, however, that nutritional issues are not left to chance. While veteran travellers most often think of nutrition, the novice traveller may be more likely to forget. A clear eating strategy, well rehearsed in minor competitions closer to home, should be developed. The input of appropriately qualified and experienced staff to the development of this strategy is essential.

## Acknowledgements

The authors would like to thank Drs Louis Burke, JiDi Chen, Mikael Fogelholm, Michael Hamm, Jon Vanderhoof, Robert Voy and Ron Maughan for content contributions and Dr Kathy Kolasa for valuable editorial assistance.

## References

DuPont, H.L. & Ericsson, C.D. (1993) Prevention and treatment of traveler's diarrhea. *New England Journal of Medicine* **328**, 1821–1827.

Grafuis, S. (1996) Melatonin: a trusty travel companion? *Physician and Sportsmedicine* **24**, 19–20.

Grantham, P. (1983) Traveller's diarrhea in athletes. *Physician and Sportsmedicine* **11**, 65–70.

Isolauri, E., Juntunen, M., Rautanen, T., Sillanaukee, P. & Koivula, T. (1991) A human Lactobacillus strain (*Lactobacillus casei* sp. strain GG) promotes recovery from acute diarrhea in children. *Pediatrics* **88**, 90–97.

Kaila, M., Isolauri, E., Soppi, E., Virtanen, E., Laine, S. & Arvilommi, H. (1992) Enhancement of the circulating antibody secreting cell response in human diarrhea by a human Lactobacillus strain. *Pediatric Research* **32**, 141–144.

Kaila, M., Isolauri, E., Saxelin, M., Arvilommi, H. & Vesikari, T. (1995) Viable vs. inactivated Lactobacillus strain GG in acute rotavirus diarrhea. *Archives of Disease in Childhood* **72**, 51–53.

Maughan, R.J. (1994) Fluid and electrolyte loss and replacement in exercise. In *Oxford Textbook of Sports Medicine* (ed. M. Harries, C. Williams, W.D. Stanish & L.L. Micheli), pp. 82–93. Oxford University Press, New York.

Mayo Clinic Health Letter (1997) Traveler's diarrhea. *Mayo Clinic Health Letter* 6 January.

Reilly, T., Atkinson, G. & Waterhouse, J. (1997a) *Biological Rhythms and Exercise*. Oxford University Press, Oxford.

Reilly, T., Atkinson, G. & Waterhouse, J. (1997b) Travel fatigue and jet-lag. *Journal of Sports Science* **15**, 365–369.

United States Olympic Committee (1988) *From the US to Seoul: How to Beat Jet Lag*. USOC, Colorado Springs.

Wolff, A. (1996) Road show. *Sports Illustrated*, 94–97, 22 July.

Zhdanova, I.V., Wurtman, R.J., Lynch, H.J. *et al.* (1995) Sleep-inducing effects of low doses of melatonin ingested in the evening. *Clinical and Pharmacological Therapy* **57**, 552–558.

# Chapter 37

# Overtraining: Nutritional Intervention

HARM KUIPERS

## Introduction

The primary goal of athletic training is to enhance performance and to peak at the right moment. To push the performance capacity to its upper limit, relatively high amounts of intensive exercise are assumed to be necessary. Consequently, athletes are often balancing on the edge between training and overtraining. One of the most difficult parts of the training process is to find the optimal balance between training and recovery. A correct balance between training and recovery is of utmost importance, since the difference between winning and losing is small. Snyder and Foster (1994) reported that in the 1988 Olympic speedskating event in Calgary, the difference in average velocity between all gold and silver medal performances was 0.3%, while the mean difference between all the gold medalists and the fourth places was 1.3%. Similar differences can be found in other sports.

Unfortunately, few scientific data exist about the optimal amount of training for peak performance. The relatively scarce data available indicates that there appears to be an inverted U-shaped relationship between training volume and increase in performance. It is assumed that there is an optimal amount of training which will yield optimal performances (Fig. 37.1). However, this optimal amount of training is poorly defined, and passing this 'gray' area may lead to overtraining. Proper nutrition, consisting of adequate carbohydrate intake, may enhance recovery, and consequently may play a significant role

to optimize the training process by increasing the training loads that can be sustained.

The actual adaptation concludes the recovery phase and, therefore, recovery is one of the most important components of the training process. Too many athletes and coaches lay too much emphasis on the training but pay too little attention to recovery. Although little is known about recovery, it appears that the time required for the recovery phase is not always the same and depends among other things on several factors, such as: the volume of training, individual factors, and nutrition. It has been shown that after exercise, glycogen synthesis can be optimized by starting to consume easily absorbable carbohydrates immediately after exercise in an amount of $1-2\,g\cdot kg^{-1}$ body weight. Although direct evidence is still lacking, carbohydrate intake may indirectly also enhance other components of the recovery process. Carbohydrate ingestion stimulates insulin secretion, which is a powerful stimulator of protein synthesis, one of the key processes for recovery and adaptation.

When exercise and the concomitant disturbance in homeostasis are not matched by adequate recovery, an athlete is actually overdoing or overtraining, and may become overloaded or overtrained. In order to obtain optimal results in sports, it is important to detect too much training or incomplete recovery as soon as possible. Although overtraining is a general term, it may include different entities. Based on the pathogenesis and affected organ systems, three different types of overtraining can be distinguished:

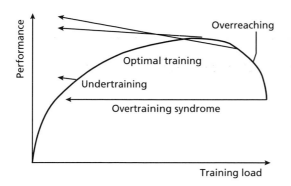

**Fig. 37.1** The relationship between training volume and increase in performance capacity. Courtesy of C. Foster.

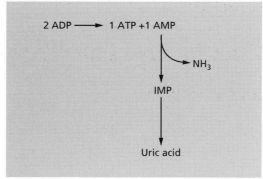

**Fig. 37.2** Metabolic pathway indicating the breakdown of ADP to uric acid, under the formation of ammonia. IMP, inosine monophosphate.

1 Mechanical overtraining.
2 Metabolic overtraining or overreaching.
3 Overtraining syndrome or staleness.

### Mechanical overtraining

Mechanical overload involves the locomotor system. An imbalance between exercise and recovery is usually local and is generally expressed as an overuse injury. Although little information is available about the role of nutrition in these injuries, there is some indication that a low calcium intake increases the risk for stress injuries to the skeleton. Another type of mechanical overtraining is exercise-induced muscle damage. Muscle damage is associated with inflammatory changes, which are followed by regeneration. There is some evidence that a deficit in vitamin E intake may increase the susceptibility to this type of mechanical damage. However, athletes who consume a normal mixed diet are unlikely to have a vitamin E deficiency. Therefore, supplementation of vitamin E in these athletes does not provide any protection against exercise-induced muscle soreness.

### Metabolic overtraining or overreaching

Nowadays athletic training includes a high volume of intensive exercise. Intensive exercise relies on carbohydrate supply, resulting in a rapid depletion of glycogen stores. When high-intensity exercise is done in association with low glycogen levels, this may lead to an imbalance between the rates of adenosine triphosphate (ATP) splitting and ATP generation. This in turn will lead to an accumulation of adenosine diphosphate (ADP). In order to restore the ADP/ATP ratio, 2 ADP form 1 ATP and 1 adenosine monophosphate (AMP), which is further broken down to inosine monophosphate and eventually to uric acid (Fig. 37.2), while ammonia is also formed (Sahlin & Katz 1993). When insufficient time for recovery is allowed, this may lead to a decline of the energy-rich phosphate pool. The metabolic type of overtraining is probably associated with overreaching.

Data suggest that insufficient carbohydrate intake may enhance the susceptibility for developing overreaching. Therefore, adequate carbohydrate intake and quick restoration of glycogen stores may decrease the risk of developing metabolic overtraining. Studies have shown that a high carbohydrate intake, starting immediately after exercise, may restore glycogen stores within 24 h. However, although insufficient carbohydrate intake may increase the susceptibility for metabolic overtraining, a high intake of carbohydrate may decrease the risk, but cannot prevent metabolic overtraining. Therefore, in addition to proper nutrition, adequate rest and recovery are of paramount importance.

## Overtraining syndrome or staleness

When the central nervous system cannot cope any more with the total amount of stress, a dysfunction of the neuroendocrine system and changes in behaviour may be encountered (Barron *et al.* 1985). This generalized form of overstress in athletes is generally referred to as overtraining syndrome or staleness (Kuipers & Keizer 1988). The overtraining syndrome is characterized by premature fatigue during exercise, decline in performance, mood swings, emotional instability, and decreased motivation (Stone *et al.* 1991). In addition, overtraining and staleness may be associated with changes in immune function (Fry *et al.* 1992). The proneness for infections has been attributed to changes in glutamine metabolism by Newsholme and associates (1991). They suggested that intensive exercise may cause a decrease in plasma glutamine. Since glutamine is considered to be essential for immune cell functioning, decreased plasma glutamine levels may lead to decreased immune function. Further research is needed to determine whether supplementation of glutamine can decrease the risk of overtraining or can ameliorate the intensity of the symptoms.

Training alone is seldom the primary cause of overtraining syndrome or staleness. It is rather the total amount of stress exceeding the capacity of the organism to cope. Contributing factors for an overtraining syndrome include: too many competitions, too much training, infectious diseases, allergic reactions, mental stress, nutritional deficiencies, and jet lag. Nutritional deficiencies refer specifically to a low carbohydrate intake. Several studies have shown that even elite athletes may consume a suboptimal diet, containing too little carbohydrate and too much fat. Newsholme *et al.* (1991) attributed the overtraining syndrome to an increased uptake of branched-chain amino acids by muscle tissue during exhaustive exercise, leading to changed balance of the ratio of aromatic to branched-chain amino acids. This, in turn, would lead to an increased uptake of tryptophan in the brain and an increased formation of the neurotransmitter 5-hydroxytryptamine. This is supposed to be associated with central fatigue and symptoms of overtraining syndrome. However, recent studies do not provide scientific evidence in support of this hypothesis (Rowbottom *et al.* 1995; Tanaka *et al.* 1997). In a recent study by van Hall *et al.* (1995), in which the ratio between branched-chain amino acids and aromatic amino acids was restored by nutritional intervention, no changes in performance and perception of fatigue were found.

The German literature distinguishes between two forms of overtraining: the sympathetic and the parasympathetic (Israel 1958). The sympathetic, or Basedowian, form is characterized by increased sympathetic tone in the resting state, while in the parasympathetic, or Addisonoid, form the parasympathetic tone dominates in the resting state as well as during exercise. The main characteristics of the sympathetic form of overtraining are:
• increased resting heart rate;
• slow recovery after exercise;
• poor appetite, weight loss;
• mental instability, mood swings and irritability;
• increased blood pressure in the resting state;
• menstrual irregularities, oligomenorrhoea or amenorrhoea in females;
• disturbed sleep: difficulties in falling asleep and early wakening;
• increased resting diastolic and systolic blood pressure.

The main characteristics of the parasympathetic form of overtraining are:
• low or normal resting pulse rate;
• relatively low exercise heart rate;
• fast recovery of heart rate after exercise;
• hypoglycaemia during exercise, good appetite;
• normal sleep, lethargy, depression;
• low resting blood pressure;
• low plasma lactates during submaximal and maximal exercise (lactate paradox).

The sympathetic form of overtraining syndrome is most often observed in team sports and sprint events, while the parasympathetic form is preferentially observed in endurance athletes (Lehmann *et al.* 1993). The characteristics of the parasympathetic form of the overtraining syndrome are misleading to the athletes and the coach, because the symptoms are suggestive of excellent health. Although the pathophysiological mechanism of both forms of overtraining is not clear yet, it is hypothesized that both forms reflect different stages of the overtraining syndrome. The sympathetic form is supposed to be the early stage of the overtraining syndrome, during which the sympathetic system is continuously activated. During advanced overtraining, the activity of the sympathetic system is inhibited, resulting in a dominance of the parasympathetic system. This would also explain the increased proneness for hypoglycaemia during exercise in the parasympathetic form, because glucose counter-regulation is mediated via the sympathetic system.

Because overtraining is difficult to diagnose, it is most important to prevent overtraining. The following rules and advice can be helpful to prevent overtraining.

**1** Develop a well-balanced, flexible and attractive training programme, with individual adjustment when necessary.

**2** Have field or laboratory performance tests at regular intervals—for instance, during the easy week during periodization.

**3** Emphasize proper diet, which supplies sufficient carbohydrate to meet the metabolic requirements (4–8 g·kg⁻¹ body weight during normal training and up to 10 g·kg⁻¹ body weight during heavy training) and also provides sufficient amounts of other nutrients.

**4** Have the athletes keep a training log in which resting heart rate and body weight are registered.

Because behavioural signs seem to be the first consistent signs of overtraining, it can be helpful to use the profile of mood states scale (POMS scale) as described by Morgan and coworkers (1987). The POMS scale yields information about the global measure of mood, tension, depression, anger, vigour, fatigue and confusion. By monitoring the mood state on the POMS scale, overtraining can be detected at an early stage.

In addition, or alternatively, the athletes can fill in a self-designed visual analogue scale questionnaire, containing questions about fatiguability, recovery, motivation, irritability and sleep.

Recent research has shown that a balanced training programme results in an increase in plasma glutamine concentrations, whereas a mismatch between training and recovery is associated with a decline in plasma glutamine concentrations (Rowbottom *et al.* 1996). Therefore, monitoring plasma glutamine concentrations during the training process may be helpful to detect overtraining in its earliest stage. However, more studies are needed to provide clear and practical guidelines about this possibility.

## Treatment of overtraining

When symptoms of increased fatiguability occur, and no other symptoms are observed, overreaching or metabolic overtraining is most likely. In that case, the training should be adjusted, mainly by decreasing the volume.

A decrease in volume is the most important measure to be taken. Most emphasis should be laid on sufficient rest, recovery, and a diet that is rich in carbohydrates and contains sufficient amounts of trace elements, vitamins, and other nutrients (Kuipers & Keizer 1988). Usually metabolic overtraining is reversible within some days.

Systemic overtraining or overtraining syndrome usually requires one to several weeks for recovery. The contributing factors should be identified and sometimes counselling is necessary. There are no specific drugs or treatments known. Although proper nutrition is important, there is no evidence that specific nutritional supplements may be of any help to treat overtraining or to enhance recovery.

## References

Barron, G.L., Noakes, T.D., Levy, W., Smith, C. & Millar, R.P. (1985) Hypothalamic dysfunction in overtrained athletes. *Journal of Clinical Endocrinology and Metabolism* **60**, 803–806.

Fry, R.W., Morton, A.W., Garcia-Webb, P., Crawford, G.P.M. & Keast, D. (1992) Biological responses to overload training in endurance sports. *European Journal of Applied Physiology* **64**, 335–344.

Israel, S. (1958) Die Erscheinungsformen des Ueber-trainings. *Sportmedicine* **9**, 207–209.

Kuipers, H. & Keizer, H.A. (1988) Overtraining in elite athletes: review, and directions for the future. *Sports Medicine* **6**, 79–92.

Lehmann, M., Foster, C. & Keul, J. (1993) Overtraining in endurance athletes: a brief review. *Medicine and Science in Sport and Exercise* **25**, 854–862.

Morgan, W.P., Brown, D.R., Raglin, J.S., O'Connor, P.J. & Ellickson, K.A. (1987) Psychological monitoring of overtraining and staleness. *British Journal of Sports Medicine* **21**, 107–114.

Newsholme, E.A., Parry-Billings, M., McAndrew, N. & Budgett, R. (1991) A biochemical mechanism to explain some characteristics of overtraining. In *Advances in Nutrition and Top Sport* (ed. F. Brouns), pp. 79–93. Karger, Basel.

Rowbottom, D.G., Keast, D., Goodman, C. & Morton, A.R. (1995) The hematological, biochemical and immunological profile of athletes suffering from the overtraining syndrome. *European Journal of Applied Physiology* **70**, 502–509.

Rowbottom, D.G., Keast, D. & Morton, A.R. (1996) The emerging role of glutamine as an indicator of exer-cise stress and overtraining. *Sports Medicine* **22**, 80–96.

Sahlin, K. & Katz, A. (1993) Adenine nucleotide metab-olism. In *Principles of Exercise Biochemistry* (ed. J.R. Poortmans), pp. 137–157. Karger, Basel.

Snyder, A.C. & Foster, C. (1994) Physiology and nutri-tion for skating. In *Perspectives in Exercise Science and Sports Medicine*. Vol. 7. *Physiology and Nutrition for Competitive Sport* (ed. D.R. Lamb, H.G. Knuttgen & R. Murray), pp. 181–219. Cooper Publishing, Carmel, IN.

Stone, M.H., Keith, R.E., Kearny, J.T., Fleck, S.J., Wilson, G.D. & Triplett, N.T. (1991) Overtraining: a review of the signs, symptoms and possible causes. *Journal of Applied Sport Science and Research* **5**, 35–50.

Tanaka, H., West, K.A., Duncan, G.E. & Bassett, D.R. (1997) Changes in plasma tryptophan/branched chain amino acid ratio in responses to training volume variation. *International Journal of Sports Medicine* **18**(4), 270–275.

Van Hall, G., Raaymakers, W.H.M., Saris, J.S.H. & Wagenmakers, A.J.M (1995) Ingestion of branched-chain amino acids and tryptophane during sustained exercise: failure to affect performance. *Journal of Physiology* **486**, 789–794.

# Chapter 38

# Exercise at Climatic Extremes

MARK A. FEBBRAIO

## Introduction

The relationship between nutrition and exercise has been a major scientific interest area for over 150 years. With the popularization of the muscle biopsy technique, arteriovenous (a-v) balance measurements and, more recently, the use of isotope tracers as metabolic probes during exercise, it has become possible to clearly investigate the role of nutrition in exercise physiology and biochemistry. Accordingly, growth in this area has increased exponentially. Much of the research which has examined the interaction between nutrition and exercise has been conducted in comfortable ambient conditions. It is clear, however, that environmental temperature is a major practical issue one must consider when examining nutrition and sport. In extremely low ambient temperatures, when the gradient between the skin and surrounding environment is high, the rate of endogenous heat production, even during exercise, may be insufficient to offset body heat loss. In these circumstances, responses are invoked to reduce heat loss and increase heat production. In contrast, when exercise is conducted in very high ambient temperatures, the gradient for heat dissipation is significantly reduced, which results in changes to thermoregulatory mechanisms designed to promote body heat loss. In both climatic extremes, these physiological adaptations ultimately impact upon hormonal and metabolic responses to exercise which act to alter substrate utilization. Hence, environmental temperature is an important factor to consider when determining optimal nutritional strategies for exercise performance.

## Exercise in a cold environment

### Cold stress or attenuated exercise-induced hyperthermia?

Unlike heat, which can only serve to augment the exercise-induced increase in body temperature, a cold environment may invoke varied physiological responses during exercise. These responses depend on whether the interaction between the environment and the exercising organism promotes excessive heat loss or attenuates the normal rise in body core temperature associated with exercise. Most studies which have observed relative hypothermia during exercise have done so using swimming as the mode of exercise (Holmer & Bergh 1974; Galbo et al. 1979; Doubt & Hsieh 1991), since water is a much greater thermal conductant than air. In contrast, when exercise has been conducted in cold air environments ranging from 3 to 9°C, an attenuated rise, rather than a fall in body core temperature, has been observed (Jacobs et al. 1985; Febbraio et al. 1996a, 1996b). The severity of the 'cold stress' is an important consideration when examining nutritional requirements since a fall in body temperature will result in shivering thermogenesis (Webb 1992) and an enhanced sympathoadrenal response (Galbo et al. 1979), while an attenuated rise in body temperature blunts the exercise-induced increase in adrenaline secretion

497

(Febbraio *et al.* 1996b). Such responses are likely to alter substrate utilization during exercise.

## Substrate utilization during exercise in a cold environment

When the rise in body temperature is attenuated during prolonged exercise in a cold environment, the rate of glycogen utilization in contracting muscle is reduced (Kozlowski *et al.* 1985; Febbraio *et al.* 1996b; Parkin *et al.* 1999) and exercise performance is increased (Hessemer *et al.* 1984; Febbraio *et al.* 1996a; Parkin *et al.* 1999), which is not surprising, since fatigue during prolonged exercise often coincides with glycogen depletion (Coggan & Coyle 1991). In many circumstances, therefore, the cool environment may be viewed as an 'ergogenic aid', since it results in a conservation of finite endogenous carbohydrate stores within contracting muscles. It must be noted, however, that even in some circumstances where measures have been taken to ensure that body heat loss is eliminated, more energy is required to undertake many outdoor activities in a cold than in a temperate environment. Brotherhood (1973, 1985) has demonstrated that walking over ice or snow-covered terrain increases energy demand compared with walking at a similar speed over dry ground. In addition, wearing heavy boots and clothing as a prevention against hypothermia increases metabolic demands and substrate utilization (Campbell 1981, 1982; Romet *et al.* 1986).

There are many athletic events, such as open water swimming and mountaineering, where extreme cold can lead to a fall in body temperature. In these circumstances, thermoregulatory mechanisms are invoked to increase body heat production and consequent substrate utilization. These include shivering and non-shivering thermogenesis. Shivering, an involuntary rhythmic contraction of skeletal muscle, is usually invoked in response to a 3–4°C fall in body temperature (Webb 1992). This increase in muscle contraction results in an approximate 2.5-fold increase in total energy expenditure. More importantly, the carbohydrate oxidation rate increases almost sixfold, while the rise in lipid oxidation is modest (Vallerand & Jacobs 1989). The rise in carbohydrate oxidation is accounted for by increases in plasma glucose turnover, glycolysis and glycogenolysis (Vallerand *et al.* 1995). We have recently observed that when subjects exercised at 3°C, their pulmonary respiratory exchange ratio (RER) was higher than during exercise at 20°C despite contracting muscle glycogenolysis and lactate accumulation being lower (Febbraio *et al.* 1996b). This suggests that involuntary activity associated with shivering in otherwise inactive muscles contributes to an increase in total body carbohydrate oxidation during exercise in a cold environment. Hence, carbohydrate availability is a critical issue during exercise in climatic conditions where a shivering response may be invoked.

Apart from the increase in carbohydrate utilization as a result of shivering, cold exposure may also increase intramuscular carbohydrate utilization via an augmented sympathoadrenal response. Plasma catecholamines are elevated during exercise in response to cold stress (Galbo *et al.* 1979; Young *et al.* 1986) and exogenous increases in adrenaline often results in a concomitant increase in muscle glycogenolysis (Jannson *et al.* 1986; Spriet *et al.* 1988; Febbraio *et al.* 1998) and liver glucose production (Kjær *et al.* 1993). Shivering thermogenesis is not an absolute requirement, therefore, for increases in carbohydrate utilization during exercise in a cold environment.

## Dietary modifications for exercise in a cold environment

In circumstances where exercise in a cold environment attenuates the exercise-induced increase in body temperature, guidelines for nutritional intake require little, if any, modification from that which is recommended for exercise in comfortable ambient conditions. It is generally accepted that a glucose/sucrose beverage of 6–10% carbohydrate is appropriate for ingestion during exercise (Costill & Hargreaves 1992), since this would provide necessary glucose while allowing for optimal gastric emptying and intestinal absorption (Mitchell *et al.* 1989; Rehrer *et al.* 1989; Gisolfi *et al.* 1991). It has been suggested, however, that increasing the carbohydrate content of a fluid beverage may be beneficial during exercise in cooler conditions since the requirement for optimal fluid delivery may be less important, due to the reduction in thermoregulatory stress, while the necessity for sufficient circulating glucose levels is maintained. We have recently tested this hypothesis and found that increasing the carbohydrate content of a fluid beverage which is ingested during exercise in a cool environment is not advantageous (Fig. 38.1). While such a practice does elevate blood glucose levels, it results in increased gastrointestinal discomfort, a less than efficient maintenance of plasma volume and a reduction in exercise performance relative to the ingestion of a 7% carbohydrate beverage (Febbraio *et al.* 1996a). Therefore, when the endogenous heat produced by exercise in cool ambient conditions is sufficient to offset body heat loss, feeding strategies recommended during exercise in comfortable ambient temperatures should be adhered to.

During exercise in extremely cold environments which results in a fall in body core temperature, any dietary modification which results in an increase in whole-body metabolic rate, which would generate warmer body temperatures and improve cold tolerance, would be most beneficial. As a result, recent research has focused on administration of many ergogenic aids designed to increase thermotolerance during cold stress. These ergogenic aids include hormones, pharmacological agents and nutrients. Administration of the pharmacological agent dinitrophenol (Hall *et al.* 1948) and hormones such as thyroxin, catecholamines, cortisol and growth hormone (Sellers 1972; Le Blanc 1975) in cold exposed animals results in a delay in the onset of hypothermia. However, while these studies provide useful information regarding the mechanisms for the induction of thermogenesis, it is impractical to suggest that they be taken by humans as ergogenic aids during exercise and cold stress because of the obvious health risks.

It is possible, that ingestion of β-adrenergic agonists such as caffeine, ephedrine or theophylline may improve cold tolerance, although the literature which has examined such a phenomenon has produced conflicting results. Ingesting the combination of ephedrine and caf-

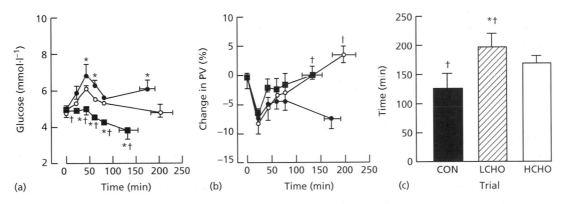

**Fig. 38.1** (a) Plasma glucose, (b) change in plasma volume (PV), and (c) time to exhaustion while consuming a placebo (CON, ■), 7% carbohydrate (LCHO, ○) or 14% carbohydrate (HCHO, ●), beverage during fatiguing exercise at 70% $\dot{V}o_{2max}$ in 5°C conditions. *, difference ($P < 0.05$) compared with CON; †, difference ($P < 0.05$) compared with HCHO. Data expressed as means ±SE ($n = 6$). From Febbraio *et al.* (1996a).

feine (Vallerand *et al.* 1989) or ephedrine, caffeine and theophylline (Vallerand *et al.* 1993) results in a significant increase in heat production in cold-exposed humans, but the ingestion of caffeine alone produces no such effect (Graham *et al.* 1991). Likewise, some researchers (Wang *et al.* 1987) but not others (Vallerand *et al.* 1993) have demonstrated that the ingestion of theophylline during cold exposure attenuates the fall in body temperature. It appears, therefore, that ingestion of β-adrenergic agonists may provide some means of enhancing thermoregulatory thermogenesis, although further work in this area is required to confirm this theory. In addition, since β-adrenergic agonists such as ephedrine and caffeine are substances banned by the International Olympic Committee, they may be impractical as a mechanism for overcoming cold stress during athletic competition.

Since carbohydrate is the major substrate utilized in shivering thermogenesis, it has been suggested that low endogenous glycogen stores may reduce cold tolerance. This is true of very lean individuals (Martineau & Jacobs 1989) but not of moderately lean and fatter individuals (Young *et al.* 1989). Therefore, adequate carbohydrate stores are not only important to fuel muscle contraction during exercise, they possibly allow for a better maintenance of body core temperature, especially in leaner athletes.

In summary, during exercise in a cold environment, effort should be made to ensure that pre-exercise carbohydrate stores are adequate in order to offset the potential increase in carbohydrate oxidation associated with shivering and non-shivering thermogenesis. This is especially important for those individuals who live and repeatedly exercise in a cold environment. The concentration of carbohydrate within a fluid beverage should not be increased to more than 12%, despite the fact that fluid loss via sweating is minimized or abolished, because of potential gastrointestinal distress. Finally, the ingestion of β-adrenergic agonists such as caffeine and theophylline may provide some benefit against acute cold exposure, but further work examining this phenomenon is required.

# Exercise in a hot environment

## Substrate utilization during exercise in the heat

Although there is some conflict in the literature, it is generally accepted that exercise in a hot environment results in a substrate shift towards increased carbohydrate utilization. Muscle glycogenolysis (Fink *et al.* 1975; Febbraio *et al.* 1994a, 1994b), liver glucose production (Hargreaves *et al.* 1996a) and respiratory exchange ratio (Febbraio *et al.* 1994a, 1994b; Hargreaves *et al.* 1996a) are higher during exercise in a hot environment. Furthermore, both muscle (Young *et al.* 1985; Febbraio *et al.* 1994a, 1994b) and plasma (Rowell *et al.* 1968; Fink *et al.* 1975; Powers *et al.* 1985; Young *et al.* 1985; Yaspelkis *et al.* 1993; Febbraio *et al.* 1994a) lactate accumulation are increased in humans during exercise in the heat compared with during similar exercise in a cool environment. The increase in plasma lactate accumulation is likely to reflect an increase in muscle lactate production, since hepatic lactate removal, although decreased during exercise in the heat, does not account for the increase in plasma lactate accumulation (Rowell *et al.* 1968) while muscle lactate efflux is unaffected during exercise and heat stress (Nielsen *et al.* 1990). It must be noted, however, that not all studies have observed an increase in intramuscular glycogen utilization during exercise in the heat (Nielsen *et al.* 1990; Yaspelkis *et al.* 1993; Young *et al.* 1996). It is likely that the discrepancy in the literature is related to methodological differences such as the use of acclimatized subjects (Yaspelkis *et al.* 1993) or differences in pre-exercise glycogen concentrations (Nielsen *et al.* 1990; Young *et al.* 1996) when comparing exercise in the heat with that in a cooler environment. These factors will influence rates of glycogen utilization, since heat acclimation attenuated glycogenolysis during exercise in the heat (King *et al.* 1985) while pre-exercise glycogen concentration is directly related to rates of utilization during submaximal exercise (Chesley *et al.* 1995; Hargreaves *et al.* 1995). In general, the literature suggests that exercise and heat stress results in a shift towards increased carbohydrate catabolism.

The increase in carbohydrate oxidation indicates that lipid utilization is decreased during exercise in the heat. Few studies, however, have examined the effect of exercise and heat stress on lipid catabolism. Plasma free-fatty acid concentration (Fink *et al.* 1975; Nielsen *et al.* 1990) and uptake (Nielsen *et al.* 1990) are similar when comparing exercise in the heat with that in a cooler environment. These findings, however, do not demonstrate unequivocally that lipid utilization is unaffected by heat stress during exercise, since Fink *et al.* (1975) also observed a decreased intramuscular triglyceride utilization. These data, along with the consistent observation of an increased RER during exercise and heat stress, suggest a substrate shift away from lipid.

Recently, Mittleman *et al.* (1998) have demonstrated that branched-chain amino acid (BCAA) supplementation increased endurance performance during exercise in the heat. This finding is in contrast with studies conducted during exercise in cooler environments (van Hall *et al.* 1995; Madsen *et al.* 1996). This discrepancy could arise because protein catabolism may be augmented during exercise in the heat. We have observed an increase in ammonia ($NH_3$) accumulation during exercise and heat stress (Snow *et al.* 1993; Febbraio *et al.* 1994b). Although a major pathway for $NH_3$ production during exercise is via the deamination of adenosine 5'-monophosphate to form $NH_3$ and inosine 5'-monophosphate (IMP), $NH_3$ can also be formed in skeletal muscle via the oxidation of BCAA. Accordingly, BCAA supplementation augments muscle $NH_3$ production during exercise (MacLean *et al.* 1996). During our study (Febbraio *et al.* 1994b), the augmented muscle $NH_3$ accumulation when comparing exercise in the heat with that in a cooler environment was observed in the absence of any difference in IMP accumulation, suggesting that enhanced BCAA oxidation may have accounted for the increase. It should be noted, however, that others (Dolny & Lemon 1988) have estimated protein degradation, as measured by urea excre-

tion, to be reduced during exercise in the heat. Further work examining the effect of exercise and heat stress on protein catabolism is warranted.

## Factors influencing fatigue during exercise in the heat: substrate depletion vs. hyperthermia

During submaximal exercise in comfortable ambient temperatures, the rate of energy utilization is closely matched by rates of energy provision. It is well established that in these circumstances fatigue is often associated with glycogen depletion and/or hypoglycaemia (Coyle *et al.* 1986; Sahlin *et al.* 1990) and endurance can be increased by providing exogenous carbohydrate during exercise (Coyle *et al.* 1986; Coggan & Coyle 1987). At fatigue the muscle is characterized by low glycogen levels and a concomitant elevation in IMP accumulation (Sahlin *et al.* 1990; Spencer *et al.* 1991), since glycogen depletion may impair the tricarboxylic acid cycle and adenosine triphosphate must be generated from alternative pathways such as the adenylate kinase reaction. Since carbohydrate utilization is augmented during exercise in the heat and fatigue often coincides with depletion of this substrate, it is somewhat paradoxical that fatigue during exercise in the heat is often related to factors other than substrate depletion. We (Parkin *et al.* 1999) and others (Nielsen *et al.* 1990) have demonstrated that intramuscular glycogen content is approximately $300 \, mmol \cdot kg^{-1}$ dry weight at fatigue when, during exercise in cooler environments, this figure is usually less than $150 \, mmol \cdot kg^{-1}$ dry weight (Fig. 38.2). This may be because hyperthermia may lead to fatigue prior to carbohydrate stores being compromised. This hypothesis is supported by the observations that, when exercising in the heat to exhaustion, subjects will fatigue at the same body core temperature even if interventions such as acclimatization (Nielsen *et al.* 1993) or fluid/carbohydrate ingestion (Febbraio *et al.* 1996a) alter the duration of exercise. There may be circumstances, however, where carbohydrate may be limiting during exercise in the heat. If the

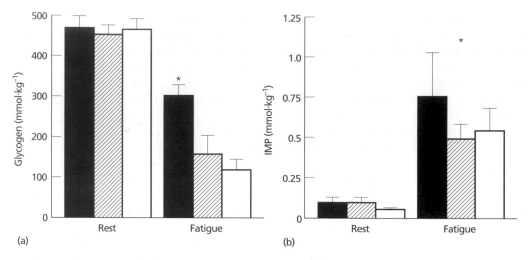

**Fig. 38.2** (a) Glycogen content and (b) inosine 5′-monophosphate (IMP) concentration before (rest) and after (fatigue) submaximal exercise to exhaustion in different ambient temperatures: ■, 40 °C; ▨, 20 °C; □, 3 °C. Data expressed as mean ±SE (*n*=8). From Parkin *et al.* (1999), with permission.

intensity of exercise is moderate, resulting in a relatively low rate of endogenous heat production, or the exercise is intermittent in nature allowing for effective heat dissipation, carbohydrate may be limiting. Accordingly, carbohydrate ingestion may (Murray *et al.* 1987; Davis *et al.* 1988b; Millard-Stafford *et al.* 1992) or may not (Davis *et al.* 1988a; Millard-Stafford *et al.* 1990; Febbraio *et al.* 1996a) increase exercise performance in the heat. The benefit of carbohydrate ingestion during and following exercise in the heat may, however, be related to factors other than exercise performance. Immune function has been demonstrated to be depressed by increases in stress hormones such as catecholamines, corticosteroids and growth hormone (Keast *et al.* 1988). These hormones are elevated when comparing exercise in the heat with that in a cooler environment (Febbraio *et al.* 1994a; Hargreaves *et al.* 1996a). There may be, therefore, a possible relationship between exercise in a hot environment and immune suppression. Indeed, it has been demonstrated that exercise and heat stress results in a decrease in lymphocyte production (Cross *et al.* 1996). Carbohydrate feeding during exercise in comfortable ambient conditions results in a decrease in circulating adrenaline

(McConell *et al.* 1994), cortisol (Mitchell *et al.* 1990) and growth hormone (Smith *et al.* 1996). In addition, plasma elastase, a marker of *in vivo* neutrophil activation, is reduced during exercise with carbohydrate feedings (Smith *et al.* 1996). It is possible, therefore, that carbohydrate ingestion during and following exercise in the heat may attenuate the rise in the counterregulatory hormones which depress immune function, and we are currently undertaking experiments to examine this hypothesis.

As mentioned previously, glycogen content within human skeletal muscle at the point of fatigue during exercise in the heat is often adequate to maintain energy turnover via oxidative phosphorylation. It is somewhat surprising, therefore, that a marked increase in IMP accumulation at fatigue during exercise and heat stress is observed despite glycogen concentration being adequate to maintain the oxidative potential of the contracting skeletal muscle (Fig. 38.2) (Parkin *et al.* 1999).

These data suggest a disruption to mitochondrial function during exercise and heat stress and support recent findings by Mills *et al.* (1996), who observed an increase in plasma concentrations of lipid hydroperoxides, a marker of oxidative stress, in horses exercising in the heat. In addition, when examining the ratio between adenosine diphosphate (ADP) production and mitochondrial oxygen consumption (ADP/O ratio) in isolated rat skeletal muscle mitochondria, Brooks *et al.* (1971) observed a constant ADP/O ratio at temperatures ranging from 25 to 40°C. Above 40°C, however, the ADP/O ratio declined linearly with an increase in temperature, suggesting that for a given oxygen consumption the increase in ADP rephosphorylation was lower than the rate of ATP degradation. Interestingly, in our previous studies in which we observed increased phosphocreatine degradation and IMP formation (Febbraio *et al.* 1994b; Parkin *et al.* 1999), intramuscular temperature was greater than 40°C following exercise in the hot environment but not the control trial. The data indicate, therefore, that the combination of exercise and heat stress may affect mitochondrial function resulting in oxyradical formation. Although speculative, antioxidant supplementation may be of benefit during exercise in the heat and we are currently examining such a phenomenon.

### Benefit of fluid ingestion

Although a more comprehensive review of fluid ingestion is covered in previous chapters of this book (see Chapters 15–17), it is necessary to reiterate the importance of fluid when discussing nutrition for exercise in climatic extremes. In circumstances where the endogenous heat production and high environmental temperature result in fatigue prior to carbohydrate stores being compromised, fluid ingestion, irrespective of whether it contains carbohydrate, is of major importance in delaying the rise in body core temperature. Exercise-induced dehydration is associated with an increase in core temperature (Hamilton *et al.* 1991; Montain & Coyle 1992), reduced cardiovascular function (Hamilton *et al.* 1991; Montain & Coyle 1992) and impaired exercise performance (Walsh *et al.* 1994). These deleterious physiological effects are attenuated, if not prevented, by fluid ingestion (Costill *et al.* 1970;

Candas *et al.* 1986; Hamilton *et al.* 1991; Montain & Coyle 1992), which also improves exercise performance (Maughan *et al.* 1989; Walsh *et al.* 1994; McConell *et al.* 1997). In addition to the physiological alterations caused by dehydration, we have also observed that fluid ingestion reduces muscle glycogen use during prolonged exercise (Fig. 38.3), since it also results in a reduced intramuscular temperature and a blunted sympathoadrenal response (Hargreaves *et al.* 1996b). It is clear from these data that fluid ingestion not only attenuates the rise in body core temperature, thereby preventing hyperthermia, it also reduces the likelihood of carbohydrate depletion. Since sweat rate is exacerbated during exercise in the heat, dehydration progresses more rapidly and therefore the importance of fluid ingestion is increased during exercise in extreme heat. Indeed, Below *et al.* (1995) have demonstrated that fluid ingestion improves exercise performance in a hot environment.

Since the negative effects of dehydration are well documented, it would be desirable to hyperhydrate prior to exercise in a hot environment. Accordingly, glycerol added to a bolus of water

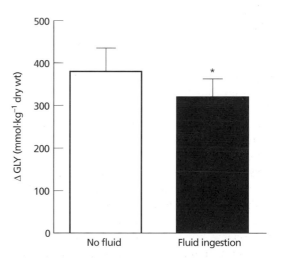

**Fig. 38.3** Net muscle glycogen utilization (GLY; postexercise minus pre-exercise) during 120 min of exercise in the absence or presence of fluid ingestion. *, difference ($P < 0.05$) compared with no fluid. Data expressed as mean ±SE ($n = 5$). From Hargreaves *et al.* (1996b), with permission.

and ingested has been demonstrated by some (Lyons *et al.* 1990; Koenigsberg *et al.* 1991; Freund *et al.* 1995) but not others (Murray *et al.* 1991) to increase fluid retention, reduce sweat rate and consequently result in an enhanced thermoregulatory capacity, especially during exercise in a hot environment (Lyons *et al.* 1990). Although not clearly understood, it appears that the effectiveness of glycerol may be related to an attenuated rate of free water clearance, and/or an increase in the kidney's medullary concentration gradient resulting in increased glomerular reabsorption (Freund *et al.* 1995). On balance, the literature suggests that glycerol hyperhydration may be effective prior to exercise in a hot environment.

As sweat rate increases during exercise in the heat, the potential for electrolyte loss, in particular sodium, is increased. It has been suggested that sodium be included in rehydration beverages to replace sweat sodium losses, prevent hyponatraemia, promote the maintenance of plasma volume and enhance intestinal absorption of glucose and fluid (for detailed review, see Chapter 17). Although the addition of sodium to a fluid beverage will maintain the drive for drinking and minimize urinary fluid loss in recovery from exercise (Nose *et al.* 1988; Maughan & Leiper 1995), we have observed little effect of alterations in beverage sodium content on glucose or fluid bioavailability during exercise (Hargreaves *et al.* 1994).

## Guidelines for dietary intake when exercising in the heat

In examining the literature, it is clear that both carbohydrate and fluid availability are very important when making dietary recommendations for those exercising in the heat. The intake of carbohydrate should be increased with repeated exercise bouts in the heat because even though acclimation reduces glycogenolytic rate (King *et al.* 1985), glycogen use is still higher in an acclimated individual exercising in the heat than in an unacclimated individual exercising in cooler conditions (Febbraio *et al.* 1994a). In addition, those individuals who undergo daily

exercise in hot conditions must pay careful attention to fluid intake, since heat acclimatization increases sweat rate (Armstrong & Maresh 1991) and, hence, body fluid loss. It is important to note that while a high carbohydrate diet may exaggerate the core temperature response in rats (Francesconi & Hubbard 1986), such a diet does not cause any deleterious thermoregulatory responses during exercise in humans (Schwellnus *et al.* 1990).

When exercising, one should ingest a carbohydrate/fluid/electrolyte beverage frequently. Since the relative importance of fluid delivery is increased during exercise in the heat, one may be tempted to ingest water in these circumstances. This practice should be avoided, since the ingestion of a carbohydrate/electrolyte/fluid beverage empties from the gut at the same rate as water (Francis 1979; Owen *et al.* 1986; Ryan *et al.* 1989), while it can spare muscle glycogen (Yaspelkis & Ivy 1991), during exercise in the heat. In addition, the relative importance of electrolyte intake may be increased during exercise in the heat and thus rehydration beverages should include electrolytes. The amount of the carbohydrate within a fluid beverage ingested during exercise in the heat appears to have little effect on fluid availability or exercise performance, provided the carbohydrate is not too concentrated. The change in plasma volume and exercise performance in the heat is not different when ingesting beverages containing 0%, 4.2% and 7% carbohydrate, respectively. Of note, however, when a 14% carbohydrate solution is ingested during exercise in the heat, the maintenance of plasma volume is reduced while the rise in rectal temperature tends to be augmented. Accordingly, exercise performance tends to fall (Fig. 38.4) (Febbraio *et al.* 1996a). It is important, therefore, to keep the concentration of carbohydrate within a fluid beverage to approximately 10% during exercise in the heat, even though carbohydrate utilization is augmented in these circumstances. In terms of volume and frequency, a practical recommendation might be 400 ml every 15 min since the rate of fluid loss during exercise in the heat is approximately $1.6 l \cdot h^{-1}$ (M.

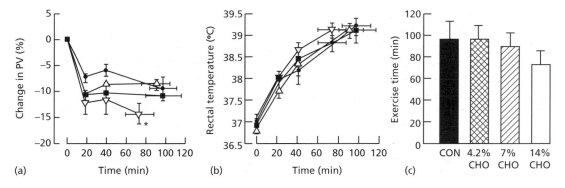

**Fig. 38.4** The change in (a) plasma volume (PV), (b) rectal temperature, and (c) time to exhaustion, while consuming a placebo (CON, ■) or carbohydrate (CHO) beverage of differing concentrations: 4.2% CHO (●), 7% CHO (△) or 14% CHO (▽) during fatiguing exercise at 70% $\dot{V}o_{2max.}$ in 33°C conditions. *, difference ($P<0.05$) from other trials. Data expressed as mean ±SE. Data from Febbraio *et al.* (1996a).

Febbraio, unpublished observations). It is also recommended that the carbohydrate beverage be ingested into recovery to replenish intramuscular glycogen stores and promote rehydration, especially important for those individuals repeatedly exercising in a hot environment.

As previously discussed, there is some evidence to suggest that protein catabolism is increased during exercise in the heat. One may be tempted to recommend that protein intake be increased prior to and during such exercise. However, it must be noted that there is a relative paucity of research examining protein requirements during exercise in the heat and more is required before definitive recommendations can be made. Likewise, there is some evidence to suggest that oxyradical generation may be increased via the combination of exercise and heat stress and it may be of some benefit to supplement those undertaking repeated exercise in a hot environment with antioxidants such as α-tocopherol (vitamin E) and ascorbic acid (vitamin C). This recommendation is speculative, however, since the hypothesis that such supplementation is advantageous during exercise in the heat is yet to be experimentally investigated.

The deleterious effects of dehydration during exercise, especially that which is conducted in a hot environment, have been well documented.

It would be desirable to hyperhydrate before exercise and, as has been demonstrated, glycerol ingestion may provide some benefit in achieving hyperhydration by attenuating urine output. It appears that a regime consisting of 1 g glycerol · kg⁻¹ body weight in approximately 2 l of fluid ingested in the 120 min prior to exercise provides some benefit during subsequent exercise (Lyons *et al.* 1990). Competitive athletes should, however, experiment with this regime during training, since not all individuals may respond favourably to glycerol hyperhydration.

In summary, during exercise in the heat, a balance between preventing hyperthermia and maintaining adequate fuel supply to fuel muscle contraction must be maintained. In order to achieve this, athletes need to closely monitor hydration levels and carbohydrate intake leading up to exercise. Daily monitoring of body weight and ensuring that urine is pallid will provide a guide to hydration status. During competition, a 4–8% carbohydrate/fluid/electrolyte solution should be ingested at approximately 400 ml every 15 min and such ingestion should be maintained during recovery to ensure fluid and energy replacement. Other dietary modifications such as increased protein intake, antioxidant supplementation and glycerol hyperhydration may provide some benefit but further research in these areas is required before definitive recommendations can be made regarding their efficacy.

# References

Armstrong, L.E. & Maresh, C.M. (1991) The induction and decay of heat acclimatisation in trained athletes. *Sports Medicine* **12**, 302–312.

Below, P.R., Mora-Rodriguez, R., Gonzalez-Alonso, J. & Coyle, E.F. (1995) Fluid and carbohydrate ingestion independently improve performance during 1 h of intense exercise. *Medicine and Science in Sports and Exercise* **27**, 200–210.

Brooks, G.A., Hittleman, K.J., Faulkner, J.A. & Beyer, R.E. (1971) Temperature, skeletal muscle mitochondrial functions, and oxygen debt. *American Journal of Physiology* **220**, 1053–1059.

Brotherhood, J.R. (1973) Studies on energy expenditure in the Antarctic. In *Polar Human Biology* (ed. P. Edholm & L. Gunderson), pp. 182–192. Heinemann, London.

Brotherhood, J.R. (1985) Snow, cold and energy expenditure: a basis for fatigue and skiing accidents. *Australian Journal of Science and Medicine in Sports* **17**, 3–7.

Campbell, I.T. (1981) Energy intakes on sledding expedition. *British Journal of Nutrition* **45**, 89–94.

Campbell, I.T. (1982) Nutrition in adverse environments. 2. Energy balance under polar conditions. *Human Nutrition and Applied Nutrition* **36**, 165–178.

Candas, V., Libert, J.P., Brandenberger, G., Sagot, J.C., Amaros, C. & Kahn, J.M. (1986) Hydration during exercise: effects on thermal and cardiovascular adjustments. *European Journal of Applied Physiology* **55**, 113–122.

Chesley, A., Hultman, E. & Spriet, L.L. (1995) Effects of epinephrine infusion on muscle glycogenolysis during intense aerobic exercise. *American Journal of Physiology* **268**, E127–E134.

Coggan, A.R. & Coyle, E.F. (1987) Reversal of fatigue during prolonged exercise by carbohydrate infusion or ingestion. *Journal of Applied Physiology* **63**, 2388–2395.

Coggan, A.R. & Coyle, E.F. (1991) Carbohydrate ingestion during prolonged exercise: effects on metabolism and performance. *Exercise and Sport Science Reviews* **19**, 1–40.

Costill, D.L. & Hargreaves, M. (1992) Carbohydrate nutrition and fatigue. *Sports Medicine* **13**, 86–92.

Costill, D.L., Krammer, W.F. & Fisher, A. (1970) Fluid ingestion during distance running. *Archives of Environmental Health* **21**, 520–525.

Coyle, E.F., Coggan, A.R., Hemmert, M.K. & Ivy, J.L. (1986) Muscle glycogen utilization during prolonged exercise when fed carbohydrate. *Journal of Applied Physiology* **61**, 165–172.

Cross, M.C., Radomski, M.W., Vanhelder, W.P., Rhind, S.G. & Shepherd, R.J. (1996) Endurance exercise with and without a thermal clamp: effects on leukocytes and leukocyte subsets. *Journal of Applied Physiology* **81**, 822–829.

Davis, J.M., Burgess, W.A., Slentz, C.A., Bartoli, W.P. & Pate, R.R. (1988a) Effects of ingesting 6% and 12% glucose/electrolyte beverages during prolonged intermittent cycling in the heat. *European Journal of Applied Physiology* **57**, 563–569.

Davis, J.M., Lamb, D.R., Pate, R.R., Slentz, C.A., Burgess, W.A. & Bartoli, W.P. (1988b) Carbohydrate-electrolyte drinks: effects on endurance cycling in the heat. *American Journal of Clinical Nutrition* **48**, 1023–1030.

Dolny, D.G. & Lemon, P.W.R. (1988) Effect of ambient temperature on protein breakdown during prolonged exercise. *Journal of Applied Physiology* **64**, 550–555.

Doubt, T.J. & Hsieh, S.S. (1991) Additive effects of caffeine and cold water during submaximal leg exercise. *Medicine and Science in Sports and Exercise* **23**, 435–442.

Febbraio, M.A., Snow, R.J., Hargreaves, M., Stathis, C.G., Martin, I.K. & Carey, M.F. (1994a) Muscle metabolism during exercise and heat stress in trained men: effect of acclimation. *Journal of Applied Physiology* **76**, 589–597.

Febbraio, M.A., Snow, R.J., Stathis, C.G., Hargreaves, M. & Carey, M.F. (1994b) Effect of heat stress on muscle energy metabolism during exercise. *Journal of Applied Physiology* **77**, 2827–2831.

Febbraio, M.A., Murton, P., Selig, S.E., Clark, S.A., Lambert, D.L., Angus, D.J. & Carey, M.F. (1996a) Effect of CHO ingestion on exercise metabolism and performance in different ambient temperatures. *Medicine and Science in Sports and Exercise* **28**, 1380–1387.

Febbraio, M.A., Snow, R.J., Stathis, C.G., Hargreaves, M. & Carey, M.F. (1996b) Blunting the rise in body temperature reduces muscle glycogenolysis during exercise in humans. *Experimental Physiology* **81**, 685–693.

Febbraio, M.A., Lambert, D.L., Starkie, R.L., Proietto, J. & Hargreaves, M. (1998) Effect of epinephrine on muscle glycogenolysis during exercise in trained men. *Journal of Applied Physiology* **84**, 465–470.

Fink, W.J., Costill, D.L. & Van Handel, P.J. (1975) Leg muscle metabolism during exercise in the heat and cold. *European Journal of Applied Physiology* **34**, 183–190.

Francesconi, R.P. & Hubbard, R.W. (1986) Dietary manipulation and exercise in the heat: thermoregulatory and metabolic effects in rats. *Aviation, Space and Environmental Medicine* **57**, 31–35.

Francis, K.T. (1979) Effect of water and electrolyte replacement during exercise in the heat on biochemical indices of stress and performance. *Aviation, Space and Environmental Medicine* **50**, 115–119.

Freund, B.J., Montain, S.J., Young, A.J. *et al.* (1995) Glycerol hyperhydration: hormonal, renal and vascular fluid responses. *Journal of Applied Physiology* **79**, 2069–2077.

Galbo, H., Houston, M.E., Christensen, N.J. *et al.* (1979) The effect of water temperature on the hormonal response to prolonged swimming. *Acta Physiologica Scandinavica* **105**, 326–337.

Gisolfi, C.V., Spranger, K.J., Summers, W., Schedl, H.P. & Bleiler, T.L. (1991) Effects of cycle exercise on intestinal absorption in humans. *Journal of Applied Physiology* **71**, 2518–2527.

Graham, T.E., Sathasivam, P. & McNaughton, K.W. (1991) Influence of cold, exercise, and caffeine on catecholamines and metabolism in men. *Journal of Applied Physiology* **70**, 2052–2058.

Hall, V.E., Attardo, F.P. & Perryman, J.H. (1948) Influence of dinitrophenol on body temperature threshold for thermal polypnea. *Proceedings of the Society of Experimental Biology* **69**, 413–415.

Hamilton, M.T., Gonzalez-Alonso, J., Montain, S.J. & Coyle, E.F. (1991) Fluid replacement and glucose infusion during exercise prevent cardiovascular drift. *Journal of Applied Physiology* **71**, 871–877.

Hargreaves, M., Costill, D., Burke, L., McConell, G. & Febbraio, M. (1994) Influence of sodium on glucose bioavailability during exercise. *Medicine and Science in Sports and Exercise* **26**, 365–368.

Hargreaves, M., McConell, G.K. & Proietto, J. (1995) Influence of muscle glycogen on glycogenolysis and glucose uptake during exercise. *Journal of Applied Physiology* **78**, 288–292.

Hargreaves, M., Angus, D., Howlett, K., Marmy Conus, N. & Febbraio, M. (1996a) Effect of heat stress on glucose kinetics during exercise. *Journal of Applied Physiology* **81**, 1594–1597.

Hargreaves, M., Dillo, P., Angus, D. & Febbraio, M. (1996b) Effect of fluid ingestion on muscle metabolism during prolonged exercise. *Journal of Applied Physiology* **80**, 363–366.

Hessemer, V., Langush, D., Brük, K., Bodeker, R. & Breidenbach, T. (1984) Effects of slightly lowered body temperatures on endurance performance in humans. *Journal of Applied Physiology* **57**, 1731–1737.

Holmer, I. & Bergh, U. (1974) Metabolic and thermal responses to swimming in water at varying temperatures. *Journal of Applied Physiology* **37**, 702–705.

Jacobs, I., Romet, T.T. & Kerrigan-Brown, D. (1985) Muscle glycogen depletion during exercise at 9°C

and 21°C. *European Journal of Applied Physiology* **54**, 35–39.

Jansson, E., Hjemdahl, P. & Kaijser, L. (1986) Epinephrine induces changes in muscle carbohydrate metabolism during exercise in male subjects. *Journal of Applied Physiology* **60**, 1466–1470.

Keast, D., Cameron, K. & Morton, A.R. (1988) Exercise and the immune response. *Sports Medicine* **5**, 248–267.

King, D.S., Costill, D.L., Fink, W.J., Hargreaves, M. & Fielding, R.A. (1985) Muscle metabolism during exercise in the heat in unacclimatized and acclimatized humans. *Journal of Applied Physiology* **59**, 1350–1354.

Kjær, M., Engfred, K., Fernandes, A., Secher, N.H. & Galbo, H. (1993) Regulation of hepatic glucose production during exercise in humans: role of sympathoadrenergic activity. *American Journal of Physiology* **265**, E275–E283.

Koeningsberg, P., Lyons, P.T., Nagy, R. & Riedesel, M.L. (1991) 40 hour glycerol-induced hyperhydration *FASEB Journal* **5**, A768 (abstract).

Kozlowski, S., Brzezinska, Z., Kruk, B., Kaciuba-Uscilko, H., Greenleaf, J.E. & Nazar, K. (1985) Exercise hyperthermia as a factor limiting physical performance: temperature effect on muscle metabolism. *Journal of Applied Physiology* **59**, 766–773.

Le Blanc, J. (1975) *Man in the Cold.* Charles C. Thomas, Springfield, IL.

Lyons, T.P., Riedesel, M.L., Meuli, L.E. & Chick, T.W. (1990) Effects of glycerol-induced hyperhydration prior to exercise in the heat on sweating and core temperature. *Medicine and Science in Sports and Exercise* **22**, 477–483.

McConell, G.K., Fabris, S., Proietto, J. & Hargreaves, M. (1994) Effect of carbohydrate ingestion on glucose kinetics during exercise. *Journal of Applied Physiology* **77**, 1537–1541.

McConell, G.K., Burge, C.M., Skinner, S.L. & Hargreaves, M. (1997) Influence of ingested fluid volume on physiological responses during prolonged exercise. *Acta Physiologica Scandinavica* **160**, 149–156.

MacLean, D.A., Graham, T.E. & Saltin, B. (1996) Stimulation of muscle ammonia production during exercise following branched-chain amino acid supplements in human. *Journal of Physiology* **493**, 909–922.

Madsen, K., MacLean, D.A., Kiens, B. & Christensen, D. (1996) Effects of glucose, glucose plus branched chain amino acids, or placebo on bike performance over 100 km. *Journal of Applied Physiology* **81**, 2644–2650.

Martineau, L. & Jacobs, I. (1989) Muscle glycogen availability and temperature regulation in humans. *Journal of Applied Physiology* **66**, 72–78.

Maughan, R.J. & Leiper, J.B. (1995) Sodium intake and post-exercise rehydration in man. *European Journal of Applied Physiology* **71**, 311–319.

Maughan, R.J., Fenn, C.E. & Leiper, J.B. (1989) Effects of fluid, electrolyte and substrate ingestion on endurance capacity. *European Journal of Applied Physiology* **58**, 481–486.

Millard-Stafford, M., Sparling, P.B., Rosskopf, L.B., Hinson, B.T. & Dicarlo, L.J. (1990) Carbohydrate-electrolyte replacement during a simulated triathlon in the heat. *Medicine and Science in Sports and Exercise* **22**, 621–628.

Millard-Stafford, M., Sparling, P.B., Rosskopf, L.B. & Dicarlo, L.J. (1992) Carbohydrate-electrolyte replacement improves distance running performance in the heat. *Medicine and Science in Sports and Exercise* **24**, 934–940.

Mills, P.C., Smith, N.C., Casa, I., Harris, P., Harris, R.C. & Marlin, D.J. (1996) Effects of exercise intensity and environmental stress on indices of oxidative stress and iron homeostasis during exercise in the horse. *European Journal of Applied Physiology* **74**, 60–66.

Mitchell, J.B., Costill, D.L., Houmard, J.A., Fink, W.J., Roberds, R.A. & Davis, J.A. (1989) Gastric emptying: influence of prolonged exercise and carbohydrate concentration. *Medicine and Science in Sports and Exercise* **21**, 269–274.

Mitchell, J.B., Costill, D.L., Houmard, J.A., Flynn, M.G., Fink, W.J. & Belz, J.D. (1990) Influence of carbohydrate ingestion on counterregulatory hormones during prolonged exercise. *International Journal of Sports Medicine* **11**, 33–36.

Mittleman, K., Ricci, M. & Bailey, S.P. (1998) Branched-chain amino acids prolong exercise during heat stress in men and women. *Medicine and Science in Sports and Exercise* **30**, 83–91.

Montain, S.J. & Coyle, E.F. (1992) Influence of graded dehydration on hyperthermia and cardiovascular drift during exercise. *Journal of Applied Physiology* **73**, 1340–1350.

Murray, R., Eddy, D.E., Murray, T.W., Seifert, J.G., Paul, G.L. & Halaby, G.A. (1987) The effect of fluid and carbohydrate feedings during intermittent cycling exercise. *Medicine and Science in Sports and Exercise* **19**, 597–604.

Nielsen, B., Savard, G., Richter, E.A., Hargreaves, M. & Saltin, B. (1990) Muscle blood flow and muscle metabolism during exercise and heat stress. *Journal of Applied Physiology* **69**, 1040–1046.

Nielsen, B., Hales, J.R.S., Strange, S., Juel Christensen, N., Warberg, J. & Saltin, B. (1993) Human circulatory and thermoregulatory adaptations with heat acclimation and exercise in a hot, dry environment. *Journal of Physiology* **460**, 467–485.

Nose, H., Mack, G.W., Shi, X. & Nadel, E.R. (1988) Role of osmolality and plasma volume during rehydration in humans. *Journal of Applied Physiology* **65**, 332–336.

Owen, M.D., Kregel, K.C., Wall, P.T. & Gisolfi, C.V. (1986) Effects of ingesting carbohydrate beverages during exercise in the heat. *Medicine and Science in Sports and Exercise* **18**, 568–575.

Parkin, J.M., Carey, M.F., Zhao, S. & Febbraio, M.A. (1999) Effect of ambient temperature on human skeletal muscle metabolism during fatiguing submaximal exercise. *Journal of Applied Physiology* **86**, 902–908.

Powers, S.K., Howley, E.T. & Cox, R. (1985) A differential catecholamine response during exercise and passive heating. *Medicine and Science in Sports and Exercise* **14**, 435–439.

Rehrer, N.J., Beckers, E.J., Brouns, F., ten Hoor, F. & Saris, W.H.M. (1989) Exercise and training effects on gastric emptying of carbohydrate beverages. *Medicine and Science in Sports and Exercise* **21**, 540–549.

Romet, T.T., Shephard, R.J. & Frim, J. (1986) The metabolic cost of exercising in cold air. *Arctic Medical Research* **44**, 29–36.

Rowell, L.B., Brenglemann, G.L., Blackmon, J.R., Twiss, R.D. & Kusumi, F. (1968) Splanchnic blood flow and metabolism in heat stressed man. *Journal of Applied Physiology* **24**, 475–484.

Ryan, A.J., Bleiler, T.L., Carter, J.E. & Gisolfi, C.V. (1989) Gastric emptying during prolonged cycling exercise in the heat. *Medicine and Science in Sports and Exercise* **21**, 51–58.

Sahlin, K., Katz, A. & Broberg, S. (1990) Tricarboxylic acid cycle intermediates in humans during prolonged exercise. *American Journal of Physiology* **259**, C834–C841.

Schwellnus, M.P., Gordon, M.F., van Zyl, G.G. *et al.* (1990) Effect of a high carbohydrate diet on core temperature during prolonged exercise. *British Journal of Sports Medicine* **24**, 99–102.

Sellers, E.A. (1972) Hormones in the regulation of body temperatures. In *The Pharmacology of Thermoregulation* (ed. E. Schönbaum & P. Lomax), pp. 57–71. Karger, Basel.

Smith, J.A., Gray, B., Pyne, D.B., Baker, M.S., Telford, R.D. & Weidemann, M.J. (1996) Moderate exercise triggers both priming and activation of neutrophil subpopulations. *American Journal of Physiology* **270**, R838–R845.

Snow, R.J., Febbraio, M.A., Carey, M.F. & Hargreaves, M. (1993) Heat stress increases ammonia accumulation during exercise. *Experimental Physiology* **78**, 847–850.

Spencer, M.K., Yan, Z. & Katz, A. (1991) Carbohydrate supplementation attenuates IMP accumulation in human muscle during prolonged exercise. *American Journal of Physiology* **261**, C71–C76.

Spriet, L.L., Ren, J.M. & Hultman, E. (1988) Epinephrine infusion enhances muscle glycogenolysis during prolonged electrical stimulation. *Journal of Applied Physiology* **64**, 1439–1444.

Vallerand, A.L. & Jacobs, I. (1989) Rates of energy substrates utilization during human cold exposure. *European Journal of Applied Physiology* **58**, 873–878.

Vallerand, A.L., Jacobs, I. & Kavanagh, M.F. (1989) Mechanisms of advanced cold tolerance by an ephedrine-caffeine mixture in humans. *Journal of Applied Physiology* **67**, 438–444.

Vallerand, A.L., Tikuisis, P., Ducharme, M.B. & Jacobs, I. (1993) Is energy substrate mobilization a limiting factor for cold thermogenesis? *European Journal of Applied Physiology* **67**, 239–244.

Vallerand, A.L., Zamecnik, J. & Jacobs, I. (1995) Plasma glucose turnover during cold stress in humans. *Journal of Applied Physiology* **78**, 1296–1302.

van Hall, G., Raaymakers, J.S.H., Saris, W.H.M. & Wagenmakers, A.J.M. (1995) Ingestion of branched-chain amino acids and tryptophan during sustained exercise in man: failure to affect performance. *Journal of Physiology* **486**, 789–794.

Walsh, R.M., Noakes, T.D., Hawley, J.A. & Dennis, S.C. (1994) Impaired high-intensity cycling performance time at low levels of dehydration. *International Journal of Sports Medicine* **15**, 392–398.

Wang, L.C.H., Man, S.F.P. & Belcastro, A.N. (1987) Metabolic and hormonal responses in theophylline-increased cold resistance in males. *Journal of Applied Physiology* **63**, 589–596.

Webb, P. (1992) Temperature of skin, subcutaneous tissue, muscle and core in resting men in cold, comfortable and hot conditions. *European Journal of Applied Physiology* **64**, 471–476.

Yaspelkis, B.B. III & Ivy, J.L. (1991) Effect of carbohydrate supplements and water on exercise metabolism in the heat. *Journal of Applied Physiology* **71**, 680–687.

Yaspelkis, B.B. III, Scroop, G.C., Wilmore, K.M. & Ivy, J.L. (1993) Carbohydrate metabolism during exercise in hot and thermoneutral environments. *International Journal of Sports Medicine* **14**, 13–19.

Young, A.J., Sawka, M.N., Levine, L., Cadarette, B.S. & Pandolf, K.B. (1985) Skeletal muscle metabolism during exercise is influenced by heat acclimation. *Journal of Applied Physiology* **59**, 1929–1935.

Young, A.J., Muza, S.R., Sawka, M.N., Gonzalez, R.R. & Pandolf, K.B. (1986) Human thermoregulatory responses to cold air are altered by repeated cold water immersion. *Journal of Applied Physiology* **60**, 1542–1548.

Young, A.J., Sawka, M.N., Neufer, P.D., Muza, S.R., Askew, E.W. & Pandolf, K.B. (1989) Thermoregulation during cold water immersion is unimpaired by low muscle glycogen levels. *Journal of Applied Physiology* **66**, 1809–1816.

# Chapter 39

# Eating Disorders in Athletes

JORUNN SUNDGOT-BORGEN

## Introduction

Athletes seem to be at increased risk of developing eating disorders, and studies indicate that specific risk factors for the development of eating disorders occur in some sport settings.

The diagnosis of an eating disorder in athletes can easily be missed unless specifically searched for. Counselling on wise food choices and eating habits will be helpful for most athletes and the role of the sport nutritionist in working with athletes with eating disorders is crucial. Therefore, nutritionists should have good knowledge of the symptomatology of eating disorders, how to approach the athlete and how to establish trust that can lead to effective treatment.

If untreated, eating disorders can have long-lasting physiological and psychological effects and may even be fatal. For a number of reasons, there is a strong pattern of denial, and a standardized scale or a diagnostic interview specific for athletes must be obtained.

This chapter reviews the characteristics of eating disorders, their prevalence, and risk factors for the development of eating disorders in sport. Practical implications for the identification and treatment of eating-disordered athletes and the need for future research are also discussed.

## Characteristics of eating disorders

As described in the *Diagnostic and Statistical Manual of Mental Disorders* (DSM), eating disorders are characterized by gross disturbances in eating behaviour. They include anorexia nervosa, bulimia nervosa and eating disorder not otherwise specified (American Psychiatric Association 1987).

Anorexia nervosa is characterized in individuals by a refusal to maintain body weight over a minimal level considered normal for age and height, a distorted body image, an intense fear of fatness or weight gain while being underweight, and amenorrhoea (the absence of at least three consecutive menstrual cycles). Individuals with anorexia 'feel fat' while they are underweight (American Psychiatric Association 1987).

Bulimia nervosa is characterized by binge eating (rapid consumption of a large amount of food in a discrete period of time) and purging. This typically involves consumption of calorie-dense food, usually eaten inconspicuously or secretly. By relieving abdominal discomfort through vomiting, the individual can continue to binge (American Psychiatric Association 1987).

The eating disorder not otherwise specified category is for disorders of eating that do not meet the criteria for any specific eating disorder (American Psychiatric Association 1994).

Athletes constitute a unique population and special diagnostic considerations should be applied when working with this group (Szmuckler *et al.* 1985; Sundgot-Borgen 1993; Thompson & Trattner-Sherman 1993). An attempt has been made to identify athletes who show significant symptoms of eating disorders, but who do not meet the DSM criteria for anorexia nervosa or bulimia nervosa. These athletes have been classified as having a subclinical eating disorder termed *anorexia athletica* (Sundgot-Borgen 1994a).

It is assumed that many cases of anorexia nervosa and bulimia nervosa begin as subclinical variants of these disorders. Early identification and treatment may prevent development of the full disorder (Bassoe 1990). Subclinical cases are more prevalent than those meeting the formal diagnostic criteria for anorexia nervosa and bulimia nervosa (Sundgot-Borgen 1994a).

## Prevalence

Data on the prevalence of eating disorders in athletic populations are limited and equivocal. Most studies have looked at symptoms of eating disorders such as preoccupation with food and weight, disturbed body image, or the use of pathogenic weight control methods.

### Female athletes

Estimates of the prevalence of the symptoms of eating disorders and true eating disorders among female athletes range from less than 1% to as high as 75% (Gadpalle *et al.* 1987; Burckes-Miller & Black 1988; Warren *et al.* 1990; Sundgot-Borgen 1994a).

Methodological weaknesses such as small sample size, lack of definition of the competitive level or type of sport(s) and lack of definition of the data collection method used characterize most of the studies attempting to study the prevalence of eating disorders (Sundgot-Borgen 1994b).

Only one study has used clinical evaluation and the DSM criteria applied across athletes and controls (Sundgot-Borgen 1994a). The prevalence of anorexia nervosa (1.3%) seems to be within the same range as that reported in non-athletes (Andersen 1990), whereas bulimia nervosa (8.2%) and subclinical eating disoders (8%) seem to be more prevalent among female athletes than non-athletes (Sundgot-Borgen 1994a). The prevalence of eating disorders was significantly higher among athletes competing in aesthetic and weight-dependent sports than among other sport groups where leanness is considered less important (Fig. 39.1).

### Male athletes

Results from existing studies on male athletes indicate that the frequency of eating disturbances and pathological dieting practices varies from none to 57%, depending on the definition used and the population studied (Dummer *et al.*

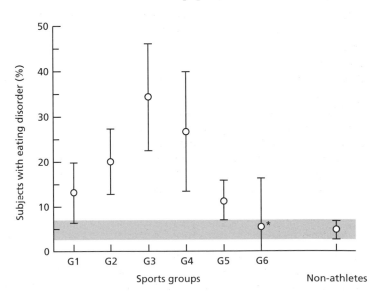

**Fig. 39.1** Prevalence of eating disorders in female elite athletes representing: G1, technical sports (*n*=98); G2, endurance sports (*n*=119); G3, aesthetic sports (*n*=64); G4, weight-dependent sports (*n*=41); G5, ball games (*n*=183); G6, power sports (*n*=17); and non-athletes (*n*=522). The data are shown as mean and 95% confidence intervals. The shaded area is the 95% confidence interval for the control group of non-athletes.

1987; Burckes-Miller & Black 1988; Rosen & Hough 1988; Rucinski 1989).

Only one study on male athletes has used the DSM criteria to diagnose eating disturbances. The prevalence of clinically diagnosed eating disorders in Norwegian male elite athletes is 8% compared to 0.5% in matched controls (Torstveit *et al.* 1998).

In a study by Blouin and Goldfield (1995), bodybuilders reported significantly greater body dissatisfaction, a high drive for bulk, a high drive for thinness, increased bulimic tendencies and more liberal attitudes towards using steroids than runners and martial artists.

Sykora *et al.* (1993) compared eating, weight and dieting disturbances in male and female lightweight and heavyweight rowers. Females displayed more disturbed eating and weight control methods than did males. Male rowers were more affected by weight restriction than were female rowers, probably because they gained more during the off-season. Lightweight males showed greater weight fluctuation during the season and gained more weight during the off season than did lightweight females and heavyweight males and females. Despite the methodological weaknesses, existing studies are consistent in showing that symptoms of eating disorders and pathogenic weight-control methods are more prevalent in athletes than non-athletes, and more prevalent in sports in which leanness or a specific weight are considered important, than among athletes competing in sports where these factors are considered less important (Hamilton *et al.* 1985, 1988; Rosen *et al.* 1986; Dummer *et al.* 1987; Sundgot-Borgen & Corbin 1987; Rosen & Hough 1988; Wilmore 1991; Sundgot-Borgen 1994b; O'Connor *et al.* 1996).

Furthermore, the frequency of eating disorder problems determined by questionnaire only is much higher than the frequency reported when athletes have been clinically evaluated (Rosen & Hough 1988; Rucinski 1989; Sundgot-Borgen 1994b).

### Self reports vs. clinical interview

Elite athletes underreport the use of purging methods such as laxatives, diuretics and vomiting and the presence of an eating disorder, and overreport the use of binge eating when data are obtained in the questionnaire (Sundgot-Borgen 1994a). Therefore, it is the author's opinion that to determine whether an athlete actually suffers from any of the eating disorders described, an interview with a clinician is necessary to assess an athlete's physical and emotional condition, and whether this interferes with everyday functioning.

Firm conclusions about the optimum methods of assessment and the prevalence of disordered eating at different competitive level cannot be drawn without longitudinal studies with a careful classification and description of the competitive level of the athletes investigated.

## Risk factors

Psychological, biological and social factors are implicated in the development of eating disorders (Katz 1985; Garner *et al.* 1987). Athletes appear to be more vulnerable to eating disorders than the general population, because of additional stresses associated with the athletic environment (Hamilton *et al.* 1985; Szmuckler *et al.* 1985). It is assumed that some risk factors (e.g. intense pressure to be lean, increased training volume and perfectionism) are more pronounced in elite athletes.

Hamilton *et al.* (1988) found that less skilled dancers in the United States reported significantly more eating problems than the more skilled dancers. On the other hand, Garner *et al.* (1987) found that dancers at the highest competitive level had a higher prevalence of eating disorders than dancers at lower competitive levels.

A biobehavioural model of activity-based anorexia nervosa was proposed in a series of studies by Epling and Pierce (1988) and Epling *et al.* (1983) and there are some studies indicating that the increased training load may induce an energy deficit in endurance athletes, which in turn may elicit biological and social reinforcements leading to the development of eating disorders (Sundgot-Borgen 1994a). Thus, longitudinal studies with close monitoring of a number of sport-specific factors such as volume, type and intensity of the training in athletes representing different sports are needed before the question regarding the role played by different sports in the development of eating disorders can be answered.

Also, starting sport-specific training at prepubertal age may prevent athletes from choosing the sport most suitable for their adult body type. Athletes with eating disorders have been shown to start sport-specific training at an earlier age than athletes who do not meet the criteria for eating disorders (Sundgot-Borgen 1994a).

In addition to the pressure to reduce weight, athletes are often pressed for time, and they may have to lose weight rapidly to make or stay on the team. As a result, they often experience frequent periods of restrictive dieting or weight cycling (Sundgot-Borgen 1994a). Such periods have been suggested as important risk or trigger factors for the development of eating disorders in athletes (Brownell *et al.* 1987; Sundgot-Borgen 1994a).

Pressure to reduce weight has been the general explanation for the increased prevalence of eating-related problems among athletes. It is not necessarily dieting *per se*, but the situation in which the athlete is told to lose weight, the words used, and whether the athlete receives guidance or not, that are important.

The characteristics of a sport (e.g. emphasis on leanness or individual competition) may interact with the personality traits of the athlete to start or perpetuate an eating disorder (Wilson & Eldredge 1992). Finally, athletes have reported that they developed eating disorders as a result of an injury or illness that left them temporarily unable to continue their normal level of exercise (Katz 1985; Sundgot-Borgen 1994a). An injury can curtail the athlete's exercise and training habits. As a result, the athlete may gain weight due to the reduced energy expenditure, or the athlete may develop an irrational fear of weight

gain. In either case, the athlete may begin to diet as a means of compensating (Thompson & Trattner-Sherman 1993). Thus, the loss of a coach or unexpected illness or injury can probably be regarded as traumatic events similar to those described as trigger mechanisms for eating disorders in non-athletes (Bassoe 1990).

Most researchers agree that coaches do not cause eating disorders in athletes, although inappropriate coaching may trigger the problem or exacerbate it in vulnerable individuals (Wilmore 1991). Therefore, in most cases the role of coaches in the development of eating disorders in athletes should be seen as a part of a complex interplay of factors.

Figure 39.2 illustrates an aetiological model for the development of eating disorders in athletes.

## Medical issues

Whereas most complications of anorexia nervosa occur as a direct or indirect result of starvation, complications of bulimia nervosa occur as a result of binge eating and purging (Thompson & Trattner-Sherman 1993). Hsu (1990), Johnson and Connor (1987) and Michell (1990) provide information on the medical problems encountered in eating-disordered patients.

Studies have reported mortality rates from less than 1% to as high as 18% in patients with anorexia nervosa in the general population (Thompson & Trattner-Sherman 1993).

Death is usually attributable to fluid and electrolyte abnormalities or to suicide (Brownell & Rodin 1992). Mortality in bulimia nervosa is less well studied, but deaths do occur, usually secondary to the complications of the binge–purging cycle or to suicide. Mortality rates from eating disorders among athletes are not known.

For years, athletes have used and abused drugs to control weight. Some athletes use dieting, bingeing, vomiting, sweating and fluid restriction for weight control. It is clear that many of these behaviours exist on a continuum, and may present health hazards for the athlete. Laxatives, diet pills and diuretics are probably the

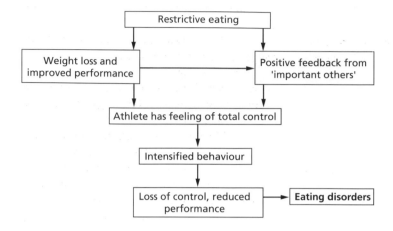

**Fig. 39.2** Aetiological model for the development of eating disorders in athletes.

type of drugs most commonly abused by athletes while eating-disordered dancers also report the use of marijuana, cocaine, tranquillizers and amphetamines (Holderness *et al.* 1994). Eight per cent of the Norwegian elite athletes suffering from eating disorders reported a regular use of diuretics and a significantly higher number reported the use of laxatives, vomiting, and diet pills (Sundgot-Borgen & Larsen 1993b). It should be noted that diet pills often contain drugs in the stimulant class, and that both these and diuretics are banned by the IOC.

## Identifying athletes with eating disorders

### ANOREXIA NERVOSA AND ANOREXIA ATHLETICA

Most individuals with anorexia athletica do not realize that they have a problem, and therefore do not seek treatment on their own. Only if these athletes see that their performance level is levelling off might they consider seeking help. The following physical and psychological characteristics may indicate the presence of anorexia nervosa or anorexia athletica.

The physical symptoms of athletes with anorexia nervosa or anorexia athletica (Thompson & Trattner-Sherman 1993) include:

**1** significant weight loss beyond that necessary for adequate sport performance;

**2** amenorrhoea or menstrual dysfunction;

**3** dehydration;

**4** fatigue beyond that normally expected in training or competition;

**5** gastrointestinal problems (i.e. constipation, diarrhoea, bloating, postprandial distress);

**6** hyperactivity;

**7** hypothermia;

**8** bradycardia;

**9** lanugo;

**10** muscle weakness;

**11** overuse injuries;

**12** reduce bone mineral density;

**13** stress fractures.

The psychological and behavioral characteristics of athletes with anorexia nervosa and anorexia athletica (Thompson & Trattner-Sherman 1993; Sundgot-Borgen 1994b) include:

**1** anxiety, both related and unrelated to sport performance;

**2** avoidance of eating and eating situations;

**3** claims of 'feeling fat' despite being thin;

**4** resistance to weight gain or maintenance recommended by sport support staff;

**5** unusual weighing behavior (i.e. excessive weighing, refusal to weigh, negative reaction to being weighed);

**6** compulsiveness and rigidity, especially regarding eating and exercise;

**7** excessive or obligatory exercise beyond that required for a particular sport;

**8** exercising while injured despite prohibitions by medical and training staff;

9 restlessness—relaxing is difficult or impossible;

10 social withdrawal from teammates and sport support staff, as well as from people outside sports;

11 depression;

12 insomnia.

### BULIMIA NERVOSA

Most athletes suffering from bulimia nervosa are at or near normal weight. Bulimic athletes usually try to hide their disorder until they feel that they are out of control, or when they realize that the disorder negatively affects sport performance. Therefore, the team staff must be able to recognize the following physical symptoms and psychological characteristics.

The physical symptoms of athletes with bulimia nervosa (Thompson & Trattner-Sherman 1993) include:

1 callus or abrasion on back of hand from inducing vomiting;

2 dehydration, especially in the absence of training or competition;

3 dental and gum problems;

4 Oedema, complaints of bloating, or both;

5 electrolyte abnormalities;

6 frequent and often extreme weight fluctuations (i.e. mood worsens as weight goes up);

7 gastrointestinal problems;

8 low weight despite eating large volumes;

9 menstrual irregularity;

10 muscle cramps, weakness, or both;

11 swollen parotid glands.

The psychological and behavioural characteristics of athletes with bulimia nervosa (Thompson & Trattner-Sherman 1993) include:

1 binge eating;

2 agitation when bingeing is interrupted;

3 depression;

4 dieting that is unnecessary for appearance, health or sport performance;

5 evidence of vomiting unrelated to illness;

6 excessive exercise beyond that required for the athlete's sport;

7 excessive use of the restroom;

8 going to the restroom or 'disappearing' after eating;

9 self-critical, especially concerning body, weight and sport performance

10 secretive eating;

11 substance abuse—whether legal, illegal, prescribed, or over-the-counter drugs, medications or other substances;

12 use of laxatives, diuretics (or both) that is unsanctioned by medical or training staff.

Laboratory investigations recommended for all eating-disordered patients, those indicated for particular patients and those of academic interest with expected finding are discussed by Beumont *et al.* (1993).

## Eating pattern and dietary intake in elite eating-disordered athletes

The eating-disordered athlete's attitude to eating and nutrition is often based on myths and misconceptions. Most eating-disordered athletes report that the onset of their eating disorder was preceded by a period of dieting or weight cycling. Apart from the binge eating, most bulimics, as well as the anorexia athletica and anorexia nervosa patients, show restrictive eating pattern.

In a study of female elite athletes, as many as 29% of the anorexia nervosa, 14% of the anorexia athletica and 60% of the bulimia nervosa, and 13% of the healthy athletes reported having two or fewer meals a day (Sundgot-Borgen & Larsen 1993a). Bulimic athletes have fewer meals per day than athletes with anorectic symptoms. For a number of eating-disordered athletes, the duration between meals is 7–11 h. Thus, it is not difficult to understand why such a high number of eating-disordered athletes binge and purge on a regular basis. In the same study, eating-disordered athletes reported that they had irregular eating pattern even before the eating disorder developed. Therefore, this may be an adapted and 'normal' eating pattern for these young female athletes, and as such, a possible risk factor for the development of eating disorders. These results indicate the need for teaching young athletes and their parents about the importance of meal planning and to make it possible to have the meals fitted into their schedule.

Eating-disordered athletes, except for the bulimic athletes, consume a diet that is too low in energy and nutrients. The mean levels of energy and carbohydrate intake for anorexia athletica are lower than recommended for active females, and a significant number of eating-disordered athletes do not reach the protein level recommended for athletes. In addition, low intakes of several micronutrients are reported, most notably calcium, vitamin D and iron (Sundgot-Borgen & Larsen 1993a). The inadequacy reported, combined with the use of different purging methods, are of major concern since a number of eating-disordered athletes are young and still growing individuals. Again, the guidance of qualified nutritionists for the athletic population in general and specifically for the athlete at risk for eating disorder is crucial.

Athletes representing sports emphasizing leanness such as the rhythmic gymnasts are exposed to nutrition and weight-control myths. The author has worked specifically with national level rhythmic gymnasts and these athletes reported a number of nutritional myths that partly explain why such a high number of those athletes are suffering from eating disorders. These include: never eat after 5 p.m.; 3360 kJ·day$^{-1}$ (800 kcal·day$^{-1}$) is enough for rhythmic gymnasts; eat only cold food because you spend more energy digesting cold food; do not eat meat, bread or potatoes; and drinking during training will destroy your practice.

Athletes, coaches, and in some sports also the parents, need to be educated about weight control, sound nutrition, and 'natural' growth and development. The focus on leanness must be de-emphasized and the unwritten rules in some sports changed. Eating disorders are likely to be a special problem within those sports where the competitors are young (still growing) and leanness is considered important for top performance, unless limits are placed on age and percentage fat for participants in sports.

## Effect of eating disorders on sport performance

The nature and the magnitude of the effect of eating disorders on athletic performance are influenced by the severity and chronicity of the eating disorder and the physical and psychological demands of the sport. Loss of endurance due to dehydration impairs exercise performance (Fogelholm 1994). Absolute maximal oxygen uptake (measured as litres per minute) is unchanged or decreased after rapid body weight loss, but maximal oxygen uptake expressed in relation to body weight (millilitres per kilogram body weight per minute) may increase after gradual body weight reduction (Ingjer & Sundgot-Borgen 1991; Fogelholm 1994).

Anaerobic performance and muscle strength are typically decreased after rapid weight reduction even after 1–3 h of rehydration. When tested after 5–24 h of rehydration, performance is maintained at euhydrated levels (Klinzing & Karpowicz 1986; Fogelholm et al. 1993). Loss of coordination due to dehydration is also reported to impair exercise performance (Fogelholm 1994).

Reduced plasma volume, impaired thermoregulation and nutrient exchange, decreased glycogen availability and decreased buffer capacity in the blood are plausible explanations for reduced performance in aerobic, anaerobic and muscle endurance work, especially after rapid weight reduction (Fogelholm 1994).

### Psychological effects

Studies on the psychological effect of dieting and weight cycling are lacking in female athletes, but it is reported that many young wrestlers experience mood alterations (increased fatigue, anger, or anxiety) when attempting to lose body weight rapidly (Fogelholm et al. 1993).

### Long-term health effects

The long-term effects of body-weight cycling and eating disorders in athletes are not clear. Biological maturation and growth have been studied in girl gymnasts before and during puberty: there are sufficient data to conclude that young female gymnasts are smaller and mature later than females in sports which do not require extreme leanness, e.g. swimming (Mansfield & Emans 1993; Theintz *et al.* 1993). It is, however, difficult to separate the effects of physical strain, energy restriction and genetic predisposition to delayed puberty.

Besides increasing the likelihood of stress fractures, early bone loss may prevent normal peak bone mass from being achieved. Thus, female athletes with frequent or longer periods of amenorrhoea may be at high risk of sustaining fractures.

More longitudinal data on fast and gradual body-weight reduction and cycling in relation to health and performance parameters in different groups of athletes are clearly needed.

## Treatment of eating disorders

Eating-disordered athletes usually are involved in outpatient treatment and are likely to be included in several modes of treatment. Typically, these include individual, group and family therapy. Nutritional counselling is usually combined with cognitive therapy. For some athletes, pharmacotherapy may be included as an adjunct. The different types of treatment strategies have been described elsewhere (Thompson & Trattner-Sherman 1993). Nutrition counselling is discussed in this chapter.

Since most athletes with eating disorders are females, the athlete/patient will be referred to as she.

The formal treatment of athletes with eating disorders should be undertaken only by health care professionals. Ideally, these individuals should also be familiar with the sport environment. Treatment of eating-disordered athletes ideally involves a team of a physician, physiologist, nutritionist and, in some cases, a psychologist. The dietitians should be trained and experienced in working with individuals with eating disorders and understand the demands of

the specific sports. The nutritionist must understand how strongly the athlete identifies with the sport as well as what the athlete perceives as demands from coaches and 'important' others.

Once the eating disorder is diagnosed, the goal is to modify the behavioural, cognitive and affective components of the athlete's eating disorder and to develop a rational approach for achieving self-management of healthy diet, optimal weight and integration of these in the training programme (Clark 1993).

### Nutritional counselling

Individuals with eating disorders do not remember what constitutes a balanced meal or 'normal' eating. The major roles for the nutritionist seems to be an evaluator, nutrition educator and counsellor, behaviour manager, and active member of the treatment team. The suggested nutritional counselling programme is the one developed by Hsu (1990). This nutritional programme is based on the assumption that eating disorders are initiated and maintained by semistarvation, and that adequate nutrition knowledge will, in most instances, result in healthy eating behaviour, which in turn will eliminate the semistarvation and the binge–purge cycle. The aims of the nutritional counselling programme are: (i) to enable the patient to understand principles of good nutrition, her nutritional needs, and the relationships between dieting and overeating and (ii) to establish and maintain a pattern of regular eating through meal planning.

### Nutritional status and body-weight history

Nutrition counselling can help the athlete overcome an eating disorder by clarifying misconceptions and focusing on the role of nutrition in promoting health and athletic performance. For athletes who have been suffering for years, readiness to listen should be assessed in conjunction with a mental health professional. Before nutritional counselling can begin, training volume, training intensity, body-weight history and nutritional status should be determined. Bodyweight history of the parents and siblings should be obtained. The eating-disordered athlete's weight and bodybuild expectations may be beyond that which is genetically possible. After gaining the athlete's trust, the dietitian should conduct body-fat measurements. It is crucial to obtain a measure of body fat in order to establish realistic goals, which also depend on the athlete's sport (Eisenman *et al.* 1990).

## Laboratory tests

Blood and urine laboratory tests will provide differential diagnoses for observed symptoms. Such values as haemoglobin, haematocrit, albumin, ferritin, glucose, potassium, sodium, total and high-density lipoprotein cholesterol, and oestrogen (if applicable) should be obtained initially and monitored over time. These can be shared with the athlete during treatment to indicate restoration of health (Beumont *et al.* 1993).

Self-esteem of eating-disordered athletes who have suffered for a longer period tends to be quite low and this may be associated with an experience of decreased performance level and often unrealistic expectations. Therefore, one important issue is to determine the athlete's motivation for continuing competitive sport. The author's experience is that some athletes even try to simulate an eating disorder to legalize the end of their career.

## Treatment goals and expectations

The primary focuses of the nutrition counselling are normalizing eating behaviours, body weight and exercise behaviour. Athletes have the same general concerns as non-athletes about increasing their weight, but they also have concerns from a sport point of view. What they think is an ideal competitive weight, one that they believe helps them be successful in their sport, may be significantly lower than their treatment goal weight. As a result, athletes may have concerns about their ability to perform in their sport following treatment.

## Training and competition

Once an athlete has been found to be in need of treatment, an important question is whether she should be allowed to continue to train and compete while recovering from the disorder.

To continue competition and training, the following list represents what Thompson and Trattner-Sherman (1993) believe are the minimal criteria in this regard.

**1** The athlete must agree to comply with all treatment strategies as best she can.

**2** She must genuinely want to compete.

**3** She must be closely monitored on an ongoing basis by the medical and psychological health care professionals handling her treatment and by the sport-related personnel who are working with her in her sport.

**4** The treatment must always take precedence over sport.

**5** If any question arises at any time regarding whether the athlete is meeting or is able to meet the preceding criteria, competition is not to be considered a viable option while the athlete is in treatment (Clark 1993; Thompson & Trattner-Sherman 1993).

Some athletes should be allowed to compete while in aftercare if not medically or psychologically contraindicated. As mentioned previously, it is extremely important to examine whether the athlete really wants to go back to competitive sport. If so, she should be allowed to do so as soon as she feels ready for it when finishing treatment and if she is in good health.

## Limited training and competition while in treatment

If the criteria mentioned above for competing cannot be met, or if competition rather than physical exertion is a problem, some athletes who are not competing may still be allowed to engage in limited training. The same criteria used to assess the safety of competition (i.e. diagnosis, problem severity, type of sport, competitive level and health maintenance) apply (Thompson & Trattner-Sherman 1993).

If the athlete is ready to get over her disorder, allowing her to continue with her sport with minimal risk when she really wants to continue can enhance the motivation for and the effect of treatment.

It is the author's experience that a total suspension is not a good solution. Therefore, if she wants to compete after treatment and no medical complications are present, she should be allowed to train, but usually at a lower volume and at a decreased intensity.

The athlete's family may be involved in the process of getting the athlete into treatment. One factor affecting this involvement is the athlete's age—the younger the athlete, the more the family's involvement is recommended.

### Health maintenance standards

If the athlete meets the criteria just mentioned, the 'bottom-line standards' regarding health maintenance must be imposed to protect the athlete. The treatment staff determine these and individually tailor them according to the athlete's particular condition. These standards may vary between individual athletes or by sport.

According to Thomson and Trattner-Shermann (1993), athletes should maintain at a minimum a weight of no less than 90% of 'ideal' weight. This is not sport-related, but health-related body weight. The athlete should eat at least three balanced meals a day, consisting of enough energy to sustain the pre-established weight standard the dietitian has proposed. Athletes who have been amenorrhoeic for 6 months or more should undergo a gynaecological examination to consider hormone replacement therapy. In addition, bone-mineral density should be assessed and results should be within the normal range.

## Prevention of eating disorders in athletes

Since the exact causes of eating disorders are unknown, it is difficult to draw up preventive strategies. Coaches should realize that they can strongly influence their athletes. Coaches or others involved with young athletes should not comment on an individual's body size, or require weight loss in young and still-growing athletes. Without offering further guidance, dieting may result in unhealthy eating behaviour or eating disorders in highly motivated and uninformed athletes (Eisenman et al. 1990). Early intervention is also important, since eating disorders are more difficult to treat the longer they progress. However, most important of all is the prevention of circumstances or factors which could lead to an eating disorder. Therefore, professionals working with athletes should be informed about the possible risk factors for the development of eating disorders, the early signs and symptoms, the medical, psychological and social consequences of these disorders, how to approach the problem if it occurs, and what treatment options are available.

### Weight-loss recommendation

A change in body composition and weight loss can be achieved safely if the weight goal is realistic and based on body composition rather than weight-for-height standards.

1 The weight-loss programme should start well before the season begins. Athletes must consume regular meals, sufficient energy and nutrients to avoid menstrual irregularities, loss of bone mass, loss of muscle tissue and the experience of compromised performance.

2 The health care personnel should set realistic goals that address methods of dieting, rate of weight change, and a reasonable target range of weight and body fat.

3 Change in body composition should be monitored on a regular basis to detect any continued or unwarranted losses or weight fluctuations.

4 Measurements of body composition should be done in private to reduce the stress, anxiety, and embarrassment of public assessment.

5 A registered dietitian who knows the demands of the specific sport should be involved to plan individual nutritionally adequate diets.

Throughout this process, the role of overall good nutrition practices in optimizing performance should be emphasized.

6 If the athlete exhibits symptoms of an eating disorder, the athlete should be confronted with the possible problem.

7 Coaches should not try to diagnose or treat eating disorders, but they should be specific about their suspicions and talk with the athlete about the fears or anxieties they may be having about food and performance. Medical evaluation should be encouraged and appropriate support given to the athlete.

8 The coach should assist and support the athlete during treatment.

## Conclusion

1 The prevalence of eating disorders is higher among female athletes than non-athletes, but the relationship to performance or training level is unknown. Athletes competing in sports where leanness or a specific weight are considered important are more prone to eating disorders than athletes competing in sports where these factors are considered less important. The number of male athletes who meet the eating disorder criteria is unknown and such prevalence studies are needed.

2 It is not known whether eating disorders are more common among elite athletes than among less successful athletes. Therefore, it is necessary to examine anorexia nervosa, bulimia nervosa, and subclinical eating disorders and the range of behaviours and attitudes associated with eating disturbances in athletes representing different sport and competitive level to learn how these clinical and subclinical disorders are related.

3 Clinical interviews seem to be superior to self-report methods for determining the prevalence of eating disorders. However, because of methodological weaknesses in the existing studies, including deficient description of the populations investigated and procedures for data collection, the best instruments or interview methods are not known. Therefore, there is a need to validate self-report and interview guides

with athletes and identify the conditions under which self-reporting of eating disturbances is most likely to be accurate.

4 Interesting suggestions about possible sport-specific risk factors for the development of eating disorders in athletes exist, but large-scale longitudinal studies are needed to learn more about risk factors and the aetiology of eating disorders in athletes at different competitive levels and within different sports.

5 Once the eating disorder is diagnosed, the goal is to modify the behavioural, cognitive, and affective components of the athlete's eating disorder. Treatment of athletes ideally involves a team of a physician, physiologist, nutritionist and, in some cases, a psychologist. The dietitians should be trained and experienced in working with individuals with eating disorders and understand the demands of different sports.

6 More knowledge about the short- and long-term effects of weight cycling and eating disorders upon the health and performance of athletes is needed.

## References

American Psychiatric Association (1987) *Diagnostic and Statistical Manual of Mental Disorders*, 3rd edn. American Psychiatric Association, Washington, DC.

American Psychiatric Association (1994) *Diagnostic and Statistical Manual of Mental Disorders*, 4th edn. American Psychiatric Association, Washington, DC.

Andersen, A.E. (1990) Diagnosis and treatment of males with eating disorders. In *Males with Eating Disorders* (ed. A.E. Andersen), pp. 133–162. Brunner/Mazel, New York.

Bassoe, H.H. (1990) Anorexia/Bulimia nervosa: the development of anorexia nervosa and of mental symptoms—treatment and the outcome of the disease. *Acta Psychiatrica Scandinavica* **82**, 7–13.

Beumont, P.J.V., Russell, J.D. & Touyz, S.W. (1993) Treatment of anorexia nervosa. *Lancet* **26**, 1635–1640.

Blouin, A.G. & Goldfield, G.S. (1995) Body image and steroid use in male body builders. *International Journal of Eating Disorders* **2**, 159–165.

Brownell, K.D. & Rodin, J. (1992) Prevalence of eating disorders in athletes. In *Eating, Body Weight and Performance in Athletes: Disorders of Modern Society* (ed. K.D. Brownell, J. Rodin & J.H. Wilmore), pp. 128–143. Lea and Febiger, Philadelphia.

Brownell, K.D., Steen, S.N. & Wilmore, J.H. (1987) Weight regulation practices in athletes: analysis of metabolic and health effects. *Medicine and Science in Sports and Exercise* **6**, 546–560.

Burckes-Miller, M.E. & Black, D.R. (1988) Male and female college athletes: prevalence of anorexia nervosa and bulimia nervosa. *Athletic Training* **2**, 137–140.

Clark, N. (1993) How to help the athlete with bulimia: practical tips and case study. *International Journal of Sport Nutrition* **3**, 450–460.

Dummer, G.M., Rosen, L.W. & Heusner, W.W. (1987) Pathogenic weight-control behaviors of young competitive swimmers. *Physician and Sportsmedicine* **5**, 75–86.

Eisenman, P.A., Johnson, S.C. & Benson, J.E. (1990) *Coaches Guide to Nutrition and Weight Control*, 2nd edn. Leisure Press, Champaign, IL.

Epling, W.F. & Pierce, W.D. (1988) Activity based anorexia nervosa. *International Journal of Eating Disorders* **7**, 475–485.

Epling, W.F., Pierce, W.D. & Stefan, L. (1983) A theory of activity based anorexia. *International Journal of Eating Disorders* **3**, 27–46.

Fogelholm, M. (1994) Effects of bodyweight reduction on sports performance. *Sports Medicine* **4**, 249–267.

Fogelholm, G.M., Koskinen, R. & Laakso, J. (1993) Gradual and rapid weight loss: effects on nutrition and performance in male athletes. *Medicine and Science in Sports and Exercise* **25**, 371–377.

Gadpalle, W.J., Sandborn, C.F. & Wagner, W.W. (1987) Athletic amenorrhea, major affective disorders and eating disorders. *American Journal of Psychiatry* **144**, 939–943.

Garner, M.D., Garfinkel, P.E., Rockert, W. & Olmsted, M.P. (1987) A prospective study of eating disturbances in the ballet. *Psychotherapy and Psychosomatics* **48**, 170–175.

Hamilton, L.H., Brocks-Gunn, J. & Warren, M.P. (1985) Sociocultural influences on eating disorders in professional female ballet dancers. *International Journal of Eating Disorders* **4**, 465–477.

Hamilton, L.H., Brocks-Gunn, J., Warren, M.P. & Hamilton, W.G. (1988) The role of selectivity in the pathogenesis of eating problems in ballet dancers. *Medicine and Science in Sports and Exercise* **20**, 560–565.

Holderness, C.C., Brooks-Gunn, J. & Warren, M.P. (1994) Eating disorders and substance use: a dancing vs. nondancing population. *Medicine and Science in Sports and Exercise* **3**, 297–302.

Hsu, L.K.G. (1990) *Eating Disorders*. Guilford Press, New York.

Ingjer, F. & Sundgot-Borgen, J. (1991) Influence of body weight reduction on maximal oxygen uptake in female elite athletes. *Scandinavian Journal of Medicine and Science in Sports* **1**, 141–146.

Johnson, C. & Connor, S.M. (1987) *The Etiology and Treatment of Bulimia Nervosa*. Basic Books, New York.

Katz, J.L. (1985) Some reflections on the nature of the eating disorders. *International Journal of Eating Disorders* **4**, 617–626.

Klinzing, J.E. & Karpowicz, W. (1986) The effect of rapid weight loss and rehydration on a wrestling performance test. *Journal of Sports Medicine and Physical Fitness* **26**, 149–156.

Mansfield, M.J. & Emans, S.J. (1993) Growth in female gymnasts: should training decrease during puberty? *Pediatrics* **122**, 237–240.

Mitchell, J.E. (1990) *Bulimia Nervosa*. University of Minnesota Press, Minneapolis.

O'Connor, P.J., Lewis, R.D. & Kirchner, E.M. (1996) Eating disorder symptoms in female college gymnasts. *Medicine and Science in Sports Exercise* **4**, 550–555.

Rosen, L.W. & Hough, D.O. (1988) Pathogenic weight-control behaviors of female college gymnasts. *Physician and Sportsmedicine* **9**, 141–144.

Rosen, L.W., McKeag, D.B. & Hough, D.O. (1986) Pathogenic weight-control behaviors in female athletes. *Physician and Sportsmedicine* **14**, 79–86.

Rucinski, A. (1989) Relationship of body image and dietary intake of competitive ice skaters. *Journal of the American Dietetic Association* **89**, 98–100.

Sundgot-Borgen, J. (1993) Prevalence of eating disorders in female elite athletes. *International Journal of Sport Nutrition* **3**, 29–40.

Sundgot-Borgen, J. (1994a) Risk and trigger factors for the development of eating disorders in female elite athletes. *Medicine and Science in Sports and Exercise* **4**, 414–419.

Sundgot-Borgen, J. (1994b) Eating disorders in female athletes. *Sports Medicine* **3**, 176–188.

Sundgot-Borgen, J. & Corbin, C.B. (1987) Eating disorders among female athletes. *Physician and Sportsmedicine* **15**, 89–95.

Sundgot-Borgen, J. & Larsen, S. (1993a) Nutrient intake and eating behavior of female elite athletes suffering from anorexia nervosa, anorexia athletica and bulimia nervosa. *International Journal of Sport Nutrition* **3**, 431–442.

Sundgot-Borgen, J. & Larsen, S. (1993b) Pathogenic weight-control methods and self-reported eating disorders in female elite athletes and controls. *Scandinavian Journal of Medicine and Science in Sports* **3**, 150–155.

Sykora, C., Grilo, C.M., Wilfly, D.E. & Brownell, K.D. (1993) Eating, weight and dieting disturbances in male and female lightweight and heavyweight rowers. *International Journal of Eating Disorders* **2**, 203–211.

Szmuckler, G.I., Eisler, I., Gillies, C. & Hayward, M.E. (1985) The implications of anorexia nervosa in a ballet school. *Journal of Psychiatric Research* **19**, 177–181.

Theintz, M.J., Howald, H. & Weiss, U. (1993) Evidence of a reduction of growth potential in adolescent female gymnasts. *Journal of Pediatrics* **122**, 306–313.

Thompson, R.A. & Trattner-Sherman, R. (1993) *Helping Athletes with Eating Disorders*. Human Kinetics, Champaign, IL.

Torstveit, G., Rolland, C.G. & Sundgot-Borgen, J. (1998) Pathogenic weight control methods and self-reported eating disorders among elite athletes. *Medicine and Science in Sports and Exercise* **5** (Suppl.), 181.

Warren, B.J., Stanton, A.L. & Blessing, D.L. (1990) Disordered eating patterns in competitive female athletes. *International Journal of Eating Disorders* **5**, 565–569.

Wilmore, J.H. (1991) Eating and weight disorders in female athletes. *International Journal of Sport Nutrition* **1**, 104–117.

Wilson, T. & Eldredge, K.L. (1992) Pathology and development of eating disorders: implications for athletes. In *Eating, Body Weight and Performance in Athletes: Disorders of Modern Society* (ed. K.D. Brownell, J. Rodin & J.H. Wilmore), pp. 115–127. Lea and Febiger, Philadelphia.

# Chapter 40

# Sports Nutrition Products

ROBERT MURRAY

## Introduction

In the never-ending quest to improve performance, athletes and coaches are quick to embrace almost any notion that promises quick success. New ideas involving sports equipment, training techniques and nutritional interventions are often greeted enthusiastically, put into practice before ample testing has occurred, and touted anecdotally as the latest and greatest idea to hit the sporting world. While most scientists would advise a more cautious approach to integrating new ideas into an athlete's training regimen, the fact of the matter is that coaches and athletes have always been and will always be the initial arbiters of proposed innovations. More often than not, in the time required for adequate scientific evaluation, the idea has already been superceded by the next 'improvement'. This is particularly so in the area of sports nutrition, where there has historically been a rapid and seemingly endless series of product introductions, some of which make remarkable claims for superior performance.

Confronted with a constantly changing array of sports nutrition products, the claims for which can appear to bear convincing scientific support, it is not surprising that athletes and coaches have difficulty determining which claims are valid. Considering that it often requires sports scientists considerable time in the laboratory to separate fact from fiction when it comes to claims for sports nutrition products, it is entirely understandable that coaches and athletes find it impos-

sible to do the same. This confusion has resulted from the plethora of commercial products targeted at physically active people, from the inability of government agencies to adequately regulate the claims made for such products, from the rapid turnover of sports nutrition products in the marketplace, and from the confusion resulting from the misuse of scientific claims. Although there is little doubt that some sports nutrition products provide demonstrable benefits when properly used, the claims for other products and nutritional interventions are often dubious, ill-founded, unproven, or abysmally deficient of scientific merit.

For the purpose of this chapter, sports nutrition *products* and sports nutrition *supplements* will be considered to be synonymous, as virtually all sports nutrition supplements are available as commercial products. Whereas it is relatively easy to identify a sports nutrition product by virtue of the advertising claims made for it, it is more difficult to gain agreement on what constitutes a sports nutrition supplement.

## What is a sports nutrition supplement?

There is no consensus opinion on the definition of a sports nutrition supplement. In the strictest sense, sport nutritional supplements might be defined as products that include only those macro- or micronutrients included in dietary guidelines such as the US National Research Council's recommended dietary allowances

(National Research Council 1989). In other words, the composition of a sports nutrition supplement would be limited to water, carbohydrate, fat, protein and amino acids, vitamins and minerals. This definition would exclude a wide variety of nutritional supplements already on the market (e.g. creatine, carnitine, vanadyl sulphate, lipoic acid, etc.). In this case, such a strict definition is both unwieldly and unrealistic.

In the broadest sense, sports nutrition supplements could include any food, beverage, tablet, gel, concentrate, powder or potion purported to be of some value to physically active people. Both the value and the limitation of adopting a broad definition of what might constitute a sport nutrition supplement is that the definition is not exclusionary. In this context, everything from aspirin to zinc could be considered a sport nutrition supplement. In addition, one is left to wrestle with ticklish questions such as whether the effect of the ingested substance is nutritional, physiological or pharmacological.

In the United States, the Dietary Supplement Health Education Act of 1994 established a definition for dietary supplements that included the following wording: 'dietary supplement means a product . . . intended to supplement the diet that . . . contains one or more of the following dietary ingredients: a vitamin; a mineral; an herb or other botanical; an amino acid . . . a concentrate, metabolite, constituent, extract'. In the 1994 Act, it is estimated that 4000 such products are currently marketed in the US. Although this description includes many products positioned as sports nutrition supplements, it excludes foods and beverages formulated for use by physically active people.

For the purpose of this chapter, it is necessary to accept a broad definition, complete with its attendant limitations, to allow for discussion of the wide range of products that are marketed for use by physically active people. *A sport nutrition product/supplement is any food, beverage, tablet, gel, concentrate, powder, capsule, gelcap, geltab or liquid droplet purported to affect body structure, function or nutritional status in such a way as to be of value to physically active people.* To narrow the scope of

discussion, it is necessary to exclude alcohol, analgesics, caffeine, amphetamines, anabolic steroids, hormones, β-blockers, diuretics and other *pharmacological* substances that may affect structure and function but are not considered nutrients.

## Objectives of nutritional supplementation

Abiding by the definition above, an *efficacious* sports nutrition product is one that provides a structural, functional and/or nutritional benefit that is documented by scientific research. For example, an iron-deficient female runner who supplements her diet with ferrous sulphate tablets realizes a functional and nutritional benefit that was not achieved by her usual diet. A bodybuilder who is able to gain lean body mass by ingesting a product that provides energy and protein enjoys a structural benefit afforded by that supplement. The cyclist who ingests a high-carbohydrate beverage to help assure adequate carbohydrate intake benefits from both structural (restoration of muscle and liver glycogen stores) and functional (rapid recovery, increased endurance) effects.

From a scientific standpoint, it is possible to experimentally evaluate the ability of a product to affect human structure or function. In fact, the manufacturers of some sports nutrition products require that rigorous scientific and legal standards be met before a product claim can be made. Unfortunately, many manufacturers do not.

## Evaluating product claims

One only has to page through an issue of any health- and fitness-related magazine to find dozens of advertisements and articles on nutritional supplements. For example, the March 1997 US edition of *Muscle and Fitness* (Weider Publications, Inc.), a popular health and fitness magazine with international distribution, contains nine separate articles and nearly 50 advertisements on sports nutrition supplements. Product claims are many and varied, including 'helps your body use oxygen more efficiently', 'help sculpt a leaner, firmer body', 'contains powerful cell volumizing and recovery nutrients', 'the most effective antioxidant nutrients', 'increases muscle protein synthesis while increasing cell hydration', 'promotes protein synthesis and glycogen storage, supports immune function and cell volumizing, and limits catabolism by cortisol for optimal workout recovery', 'increase levels of adenosine triphosphate', 'more lean-gained mass in less time', 'prevents muscle loss during training and dieting', 'improve strength and stamina during workouts', 'increases lean muscle mass and promotes fat loss', and 'increase peak power output, mean body mass, and muscular performance'. Each of these product claims involves a structural or functional benefit that is directly testable through scientific experimentation. Although a few of these advertising claims were accompanied by a scientific reference, the vast majority were not. This observation is similar to that of Grunewald and Bailey (1993), who evaluated the advertising claims for 624 products targeted at bodybuilders. The products were associated with over 800 performance-related claims, the vast majority of which were unsubstantiated by scientific research.

If the stated objective of a sports nutrition supplement is to provide a structural or functional benefit, validation of the claim can be accomplished in two ways. The highest level of scientific validation for the efficacy of a nutrition supplement is generated by research published in peer-reviewed scientific journals. In this context, the strongest such support is developed when numerous laboratories report similar findings of product effectiveness. A case in point is the scientific consensus that has been developed for carbohydrate–electrolyte beverages on the basis of more than 100 scientific studies published in peer-reviewed journals. The other acceptable example of scientific credibility is when the efficacy of a nutrition supplement can be established by face validity—that is, when the claims made for the product are widely recognized as being both truthful and scientifically

valid. For example, if a product containing large amounts of carbohydrate per serving is claimed to provide a supplemental source of dietary carbohydrate that helps in glycogen restoration, the product's efficacy in that regard enjoys the benefit of face validity. The product claim is accepted as true on its face.

Butterfield (1996) and other authors (Burke 1992; Rangachari & Mierson 1995; Sherman & Lamb 1995; Coleman & Nelson Steen 1996) have suggested guidelines for evaluating research results and product claims. Sherman and Lamb (1995) identified 10 essential characteristics that should be present in an acceptable experimental design. These include:

1 use of an appropriate subject population;
2 adequate control of diet and exercise;
3 use of a double-blind design with placebo;
4 random assignment of subjects to treatment groups;
5 repeated measures or cross-over designs to reduce the impact of individual differences;
6 inclusion of appropriate familiarization trials;
7 adequate control of possible mitigating factors such as environmental conditions and hydration status;
8 measurement of variables related to the potential mechanism of effect;
9 an acceptable number of subjects to assure ample statistical power; and
10 proper statistical analyses.

A critical evaluation of research data requires a trained and experienced eye. Even the most sceptical layperson is unprepared to undertake a thorough review of product claims and related literature. As a result, it is the responsibility of the trained sports health professional to be proactive in providing the public with clear and accurate guidance regarding the efficacy of products that claim to provide structural or functional benefits.

The advertisements for some sports nutrition products rely solely upon claims of nutrient content rather than structural or functional claims. The product's label and advertising merely make a statement regarding the product's nutritional content. Examples of such claims include 'contains calcium', 'delivers 2200 low-fat calories per serving', 'contains di- and tripeptides', and 'provides nine important vitamins and minerals'. Provided that these claims conform to the product's actual content, they are nothing more than statements of fact.

## Ethical considerations regarding sports nutrition products

The International Olympic Committee's list of banned drugs provides a relatively clear-cut, but by no means uncontroversial, way of identifying a substance 'which because of its nature, dosage, or application is able to boost the athlete's performance in competition in an artificial and unfair manner' (International Olympic Committee 1995). The IOC regulations also state that 'doping is the administration of or the use by a competing athlete of any substance foreign to the body or of any physiological substance taken in abnormal quantity or by an abnormal route of entry into the body, with the intention of increasing in an artificial and unfair manner his performance in competition'. The wording of this sentence may be instructive in the evaluation of the ethical considerations surrounding the use of some nutritional supplements. However, as with the IOC's restrictions against doping, a clear understanding of the ethical issues regarding nutritional supplementation can be hard to come by. For example, the ingestion of a glucose–electrolyte solution during exercise involves a normal route of administration of a normal quantity of nutrients and consequently presents little in the way of ethical concerns. On the other hand, if a cyclist were to receive the same nutrients intravenously while riding in competition, such administration would surely be considered abnormal and ethically questionable. Yet, it is quite common for athletes to receive intravenous glucose–electrolyte solutions following training and competition under the guise of medical necessity when the actual intent is to hasten recovery.

In discussing the ethical considerations of using nutritional ergogenic aids, Williams (1994) noted that some nutrients given in high doses can exert pharmacological effects, responses that would appear to be at odds with the language of the IOC doping regulations. One such example is niacin (vitamin $B_3$), high doses of which are commonly prescribed to reduce serum cholesterol (DiPalma & Thayer 1991), an effect that is clearly pharmacological. If similarly large doses of a vitamin improved performance, would this be considered a pharmacological or nutritional effect? Similarly, as also noted by Williams (1994), if research confirms the ergogenic effect of creatine loading, what are the attendant ethical considerations? Does the fact that the body normally synthesizes creatine preclude it from being considered a nutrient? Are the effects of creatine feeding pharmacological or physiological, rather than nutritional? Does it matter? These same questions can surely be applied to any nutrient ingested in amounts far exceeding the established values of normal nutritional requirements. Regardless of the murky nature of some issues involving sports nutrition supplements, the reality is that thousands of such products are marketed around the world.

## Categories of sports nutrition products

A variety of authors and organizations have attempted to categorize sports nutrition products to establish a framework by which the efficacy of the products can be more easily evaluated. Three such attempts at categorization are briefly described below. As with all systems of categorization, each has its own merits and limitations.

Burke and Read (1993) suggested a simple two-category approach that classifies sports nutrition supplements as either dietary supplements or nutritional ergogenic aids. According to the authors, dietary supplements provide a convenient and practical means of consuming nutrients to meet the special dietary needs of athletes. In this regard, the supplement itself does not directly improve performance, but simply meets a dietary need. Examples include sports drinks, high-carbohydrate supplements, liquid meal supplements, and vitamin and mineral supplements. For example, ferrous sulphate tablets consumed by an iron-deficient female athlete or a concentrated carbohydrate beverage ingested following training would be considered dietary supplements.

Nutritional ergogenic aids encompass those products whose ingestion is purported to directly and immediately provoke an improvement in performance. Burke (1992) suggests that these supplements are better labelled as 'proposed ergogenic aids' because there is scant scientific support for their effectiveness. Bee pollen, ginseng, vanadium, inosine, molybdenum, carnitine and countless other pills, potions and powders appear to fall neatly into this category. Upon further examination, however, the distinction between dietary supplements and nutritional ergogenic aids can become blurred. When carbohydrate is ingested during exercise, is it meeting a special dietary need or provoking an immediate improvement in performance? Some would argue that it does both.

Butterfield (1996) suggested that sports nutrition products could be categorized into four areas:

**1** Metabolic fuels such as carbohydrate, fat and metabolic intermediates including pyruvate, lactate and components of the Krebs cycle.
**2** Limited cellular components such as creatine, carnitine, vitamins and free amino acids.
**3** Substances with purported anabolic effects such as energy, protein, chromium and vanadium.
**4** Nutrients which enhance recovery, including fluid, carbohydrate and electrolytes.

This categorization system allows for pigeonholing supplements on the basis of functionality, although some nutrients serve multiple functions. For example, carbohydrate could fit equally well in all four categories: as a metabolic fuel, as a limited cellular component (during the latter stages of prolonged exercise), as a nutrient that provokes anabolic effects (via insulin) and as an aid to recovery.

Kanter and Williams (1995) suggested that the purpose of most nutritional ergogenic aids is to enhance energy production during exercise by either (i) providing an additional energy source (as in the case of carbohydrate and fat) or (ii) by benefiting the metabolic processes that produce energy (a catch-all category for protein, amino acids, vitamins, minerals and sundry other substances touted to improve performance). This two-tiered approach to categorizing sports nutrition supplements served the authors well in their review of antioxidants, carnitine and choline (Kanter & Williams 1995), but falls short of providing a niche for supplements with a proposed effect on processes other than energy metabolism (e.g. amino acids, chromium, choline, $\gamma$-oryzanol).

In the not too distant future, it is likely that government agencies will attempt to establish regulatory control over the nutritional supplement industry, including what might be broadly classified as sports foods. In fact, such regulations have either been proposed or enacted in the United States, Australia, Japan and within the European Community. The likely result of each attempt will be the creation of a less than perfect way to define and categorize a group of foods, beverages and supplements that by their very diversity defy a simple manner of categorization.

None the less, faced with the challenge of addressing the role of sports nutrition supplements, the following section provides an admittedly arbitrary attempt at organizing the wide array of sports nutrition supplements into categories that allow for some degree of generalization regarding their proven or purported effects.

## Role of sports nutrition products

The reader wishing a comprehensive review of the science underlying sports nutrition products is referred to the other chapters in this book and to the many review articles and books previously written on this topic.

### Fluid replacement beverages (i.e. sports drinks)

Sports drinks are the most comprehensively

researched of all sports nutrition products. Formulated to rapidly replace fluid lost as sweat during physical activity, sports drinks commonly contain a mixture of mono-, di- and oligosaccharides (as maltodextrins), minerals (most often sodium, potassium and chloride), along with assorted flavourings. The carbohydrate concentration of most commercially available sports drinks ranges from 5% to 8% carbohydrate (i.e. 50–80 g carbohydrate per litre). The physiological effectiveness of sports drink ingestion has been well documented (Lamb & Brodowicz 1986; Murray 1987; Maughan 1991; Maughan *et al.* 1995) and the plethora of related data provided part of the foundation for the position stand on exercise and fluid replacement published by the American College of Sports Medicine (ACSM 1996). Chapters 15–19 of this text provide an excellent review of issues regarding fluid and electrolyte homeostasis and Chapter 8 addresses the topic of carbohydrate feeding during exercise.

### Carbohydrate-rich beverages

The value of ingesting a diet high in carbohydrate content has been well established, as detailed in Chapters 5–8. Any food or beverage high in carbohydrate content could conceivably be termed a carbohydrate-loading supplement, although this designation is usually applied to commercial products, most often beverages. Whether purchased in liquid form or reconstituted from a powder mix, these beverages should contain a carbohydrate concentration in excess of regular soft drinks (10–14% carbohydrate) and common fruit juices (12–16% carbohydrate). It is accepted at face validity that the ingestion of adequate amounts of such products will help athletes meet their goals for dietary carbohydrate intake, the result of which will be effective restoration of glycogen stores in liver and muscle.

### Complete-nutrition/energy beverages

These beverages, usually in the form of milk-shake type drinks, contain varying combinations of carbohydrate, protein, fat, vitamins and minerals. Some of these products contain an array of other nutrients and metabolites. It is accepted at face validity that the ingestion of these supplements will provide the energy and nutrients included in them, the inference being that intake of the nutrients will help athletes meet their daily nutritional needs. Additional claims of product benefits to structure or function (e.g. 'adds lean body mass', 'boosts fat metabolism by 43%') would require direct substantiation by acceptable scientific research.

### Energy bars

This category of supplements includes solid foods in bar form. Most bars provide 140–250 kcal (588–1050 kJ) of energy and contain varying proportions of carbohydrate, protein, fat and micronutrients. Most of these products are associated with statements of nutritional content (e.g. 'contains ginseng'), although a few make structure or function claims (e.g. 'burn more body fat'). In the latter case, the manufacturers must be held accountable for providing acceptable scientific support.

### Carbohydrate gels

These products are often small packets of carbohydrate syrup (20–30 g) positioned for use during prolonged exercise as an alternative means of carbohydrate intake. The claims made for these products are most often statements of nutritional content. Most products advise the user to ingest the gel with ample amounts of fluid to help assure rapid gastric emptying.

### Vitamin supplements

Vitamins are sold as single nutrients (e.g. vitamin C), in combination with other vitamins (e.g. B complex vitamins), or as vitamin–mineral tablets that contain assorted nutrients. Some manufacturers employ a use-specific positioning for their products that imply particular benefits (e.g. 'an antistress formula'). In most cases, however, the claims for vitamin products are limited to statements of nutrient content (e.g. 'provides 100% of the RDA for seven important vitamins').

The benefits of vitamin supplementation in cases of borderline or frank vitamin deficiency are well accepted (Clarkson 1991). Under these circumstances, health status and performance are improved when the deficiency is corrected. Whether ingestion of vitamins in amounts far exceeding the recommended dietary allowances confer benefits to physically active people remains a topic of much discussion and interest (see Chapters 20–22). Future research will undoubtedly determine if vitamin supplementation provides specific benefits to human structure and function, or serves merely as a way for physically active people to assure adequate micronutrient intake. Additional information on vitamin supplementation can be found in Chapters 20–22 of this text and in review articles by Armstrong and Maresh (1996), Clarkson (1991), Haymes (1991), Rosenbloom et al. (1992), Sobal and Marquart (1994) and Williams (1984).

## Mineral supplements

As with vitamins, minerals are also sold singly (e.g. chromium) or in combination (multimineral tablets). Chapters 23–25 provide a detailed review of mineral requirements in physically active people, as do review articles by Armstrong and Maresh (1996), Clarkson (1991) and Haymes (1991). Acute or chronic deficiencies of minerals such as sodium, calcium and iron can occur as a result of physical activity and inadequate dietary intake. Advertising claims for the benefits of minerals such as boron, chromium, molybdenum, selenium and zinc have not been borne out by scientific research (Clarkson 1991; Haymes 1991). Armstrong and Maresh (1996) identified a number of flaws in the experimental designs of supplementation studies that can render the data suspect or useless. Among these are the inability to control for mineral status of the subjects, the absence of placebo groups, and the choice of inappropriate assessment criteria. Some of the

studies that report positive structural or functional effects of mineral supplementation suffer from one or more of the design flaws noted by Armstrong and Maresh (1996).

## Protein and amino-acid supplements

The advertising for protein and amino-acid supplements is often based upon the notion that physically active people, particularly bodybuilders and power lifters, require large amounts of dietary protein. Claims for these products tout benefits such as, 'promotes anticatabolic activity', 'pack on some solid, rock-hard mass', and 'increases lean muscle mass and promotes fat loss'. There is little in the way of scientific evidence to indicate that ingesting protein supplements will fulfil these promises. As indicated in Chapters 9 and 10, although physical activity increases the dietary requirement for protein, the increase is easily met by consuming a normal diet. In brief, protein and amino-acid supplements are expensive substitutes for protein-rich foods that are readily available in the diet (Lemon 1995).

In recent years, attention has been paid to the effects of ingesting individual amino acids such as glycine and glutamine or combinations of amino acids such as the branched-chain amino acids (leucine, isoleucine and valine) for purposes ranging from stimulating growth hormone release to altering serotonin production in the brain. Although future research may generate evidence of benefits associated with the ingestion of amino acids, the current data are not compelling. In addition, the ingestion of amino-acid supplements is not without risk (Butterfield 1991; Beltz & Doering 1993).

## Putative promoters of muscle growth

A number of other substances have been advertised as being able to promote the growth of muscle tissue. Dibencozide, γ-oryzanol, yohimbe, phosphatidylserine and vanadyl sulphate are among the ingredients that can be found in current products promoted as having growth-enhancing properties. Additional substances are reviewed in Chapter 26. Again, there is an absence of scientific research confirming such effects (Rosenbloom *et al.* 1992; Grunewald & Bailey 1993; Coleman & Nelson-Steen 1996).

### Putative enhancers of energy metabolism

In theory, performance should be enhanced if a product ingredient increased the ability of muscle to resynthesize adenosine triphosphate. The most obvious candidates for such a role would be metabolic intermediates such as lactate, pyruvate, citrate and other tricarboxylic acid intermediates, enzyme-system components such as lipoic acid, alternative fuel sources such as medium-chain triglycerides, mediators in fuel oxidation such as carnitine, and components of the high-energy phosphate pool such as inosine and creatine. Of these, creatine ingestion appears to have the most promise as an ergogenic aid (Greenhaff 1995). As indicated in Chapter 27, creatine ingestion is associated with an increase in muscle creatine content, a response that may be associated with increased performance in very high intensity, short-duration activities. However, as promising as creatine appears to be as an ergogenic aid, and notwithstanding the numerous products containing creatine as an ingredient, it may still be premature to draw a definitive conclusion regarding its efficacy. While some laboratories have reported improved sprint performance associated with creatine feeding (e.g. Casey *et al.* 1996), others have failed to find an effect (e.g. Barnett *et al.* 1996). Although the disparate results may merely be an artefact of differences in experimental design, feeding protocols, subject selection, and choice of performance criteria, more research is needed to confirm if this is indeed the case.

## Conclusion

Efficacious sports nutrition products will continue to play an important role in helping athletes achieve and maintain a nutritional status that positively influences body structure and function. The benefits of remaining well hydrated during exercise, the advantages of ingesting a diet high in carbohydrate content, the importance of sodium in stimulating rapid and complete rehydration, and the indispensible nature of consuming adequate energy are examples of well-documented nutritional applications around which many sports nutrition products are based. There are, however, many products that are associated with claims that lack scientific substantiation. Sports health professionals involved in public-education programmes have an obligation to help provide consumers with up-to-date and accurate information regarding the veracity of product claims.

## References

American College of Sports Medicine (1996) position stand on exercise and fluid replacement. *Medicine and Science in Sports and Exercise* **28**, i–vii.

Armstrong, L. & Maresh, C. (1996) Vitamin and mineral supplements as nutritional aids to exercise performance and health. *Nutrition Reviews* **54**, S149–S158.

Barnett, C., Hinds, M. & Jenkins, D. (1996) Effects of oral creatine supplementation on multiple sprint cycle performance. *Australian Journal of Science and Medicine in Sport* **28**, 35–39.

Beltz, S. & Doering, P. (1993) Efficacy of nutritional supplements used by athletes. *Clinical Pharmacology* **12**, 900–908.

Burke, L. (1992) *The Complete Guide to Food for Sports Performance*. Allen and Unwin, Sydney.

Burke, L. & Read, R. (1993) Dietary supplements in sport. *Sports Medicine* **15**, 43–65.

Butterfield, G. (1991) Amino acids and high protein diets. In *Perspectives in Exercise Science and Sports Medicine*. Vol. 4. *Ergogenics: Enhancement of Performance in Exercise and Sport* (ed. D. Lamb & M. Williams), pp. 87–122. Brown and Benchmark, Indianapolis, IN.

Butterfield, G. (1996) Ergogenic aids: evaluating sport nutrition products. *International Journal of Sports Nutrition* **6**, 191–197.

Casey, A., Constantin-Teodosiu, C., Howell, S., Hultman, E. & Greenhaff, P. (1996) Creatine ingestion favorably affects performance and muscle metabolism during maximal exercise in humans. *American Journal of Physiology* **271**, E31–E37.

Clarkson, P. (1991) Vitamins and trace minerals. In *Perspectives in Exercise Science and Sports Medicine*. Vol. 4.

*Ergogenics: Enhancement of Performance in Exercise and Sport* (ed. D. Lamb & M. Williams), pp. 123–182. Brown and Benchmark, Indianapolis, IN.

Coleman, E. & Nelson Steen, S. (1996) *The Ultimate Sports Nutrition Handbook*. Bull Publishing, Palo Alto, CA.

DiPalma, J. & Thayer, S. (1991) Use of niacin as a drug. *Annual Review of Nutrition* **11**, 169–187.

Greenhaff, P. (1995) Creatine and its application as an ergogenic aid. *International Journal of Sports Nutrition* **5** (Suppl.), S100–S110.

Grunewald, K. & Bailey, R. (1993) Commercially marketed supplements for body building athletes. *Sports Medicine* **15**, 90–103.

Haymes, E. (1991) Vitamin and mineral supplementation to athletes. *International Journal of Sports Nutrition* **1**, 146–169.

International Olympic Committee (1995) *Medical Code*. International Olympic Committee, Lausanne.

Kanter, M. & Williams, M. (1995) Antioxidants, carnitine, choline as putative ergogenic aids. *International Journal of Sports Nutrition* **5** (Suppl.), S120–S131.

Lamb, D. & Brodowicz, G. (1986) Optimal use of fluids of varying formulations to minimise exercise-induced disturbances in homeostasis. *Sports Medicine* **3**, 247–274.

Lemon, P. (1995) Do athletes need more dietary protein and amino acids? *International Journal of Sports Nutrition* **5** (Suppl.), S39–S61.

Maughan, R. (1991) Carbohydrate–electrolyte solutions during prolonged exercise. In *Perspectives in Exercise Science and Sports Medicine*. Vol. 4. *Ergogenics: Enhancement of Performance in Exercise and Sport* (ed. D. Lamb & M. Williams), pp. 35–86. Brown and Benchmark, Indianapolis, IN.

Maughan, R., Shirreffs, S., Galloway, D. & Leiper, J. (1995) Dehydration and fluid replacement in sport and exercise. *Sports, Exercise, and Injury* **1**, 148–153.

Murray, R. (1987) The effects of consuming carbohydrate–electrolyte beverages on gastric emptying and fluid absorption during and following exercise. *Sports Medicine* **4**, 322–351.

National Research Council (1989) *Recommended Dietary Allowances*, 10th edn. National Academy Press, Washington, DC.

Rangachari, P. & Mierson, S. (1995) A checklist to help students analyze published articles in basic medical sciences. *American Journal of Physiology* **268**, 13.

Rosenbloom, C., Millard-Stafford, M. & Lathrop, J. (1992) Contemporary ergogenic aids used by strength/power athletes. *Journal of the American Dietetic Association* **92**, 1264–1266.

Sherman, W. & Lamb, D. (1995) Introduction. *International Journal of Sports Nutrition* **5** (Suppl.), Siii–Siv.

Sobal, J. & Marquart, L. (1994) Vitamin/mineral supplement use among athletes: a review of the literature. *International Journal of Sports Nutrition* **4**, 320–334.

Williams, M. (1984) Vitamin and mineral supplements to athletes: do they help? *Clinics in Sports Medicine* **3**, 623–637.

Williams, M. (1994) The use of nutritional ergogenic aids in sports: is it an ethical issue? *International Journal of Sports Nutrition* **4**, 120–131.

# PART 4

## SPORT-SPECIFIC NUTRITION

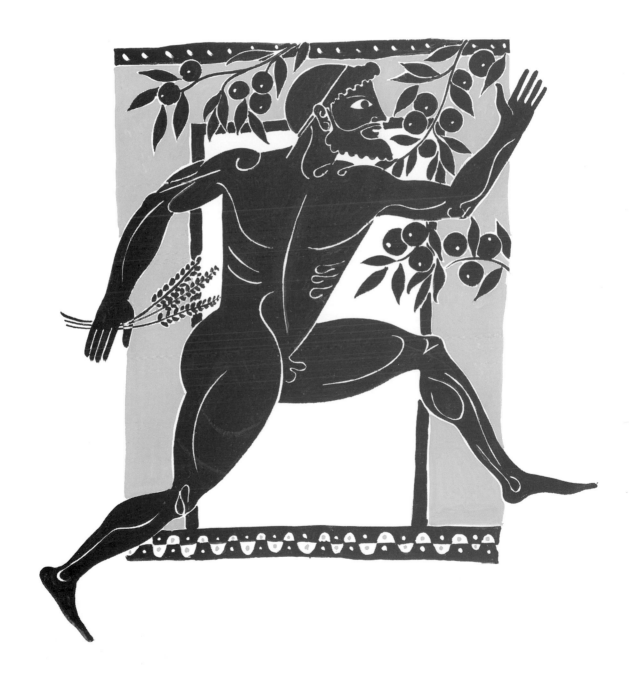

# Chapter 41

# Sprinting

CERI W. NICHOLAS

## Introduction

Of all sports, sprinting is the simplest. All that is required to run the race is a start and finish line, and an accepted method of starting the race. The winner is the first person to cross the finish line. Sprinting over short distances is one of man's earliest athletic pursuits. The pioneering event in the ancient Olympic Games was the 'stade', which was equivalent to the length of the stadium—192m—at Atlis, the theatre of the games (Quercetani 1964). Later, a second race, the *diaulos*, equivalent to two stades (384m), was included as a foot race (Durant 1961).

The earliest records of the Olympic Games credit the winner of the sprint event in the ancient Olympics of 776 BC at Olympia to Coreobus, a cook from the nearby city of Elis. The ancient tradition of honouring the fastest person on the day still holds today in major championships, with the awarding of medals. The introduction of accurate and reliable time-keeping has also led to the establishment of world records. This has allowed athletes to compete against the clock on tracks around the world and far from the record holder (current world sprint records are shown in Table 41.1).

In comparison with the encyclopaedic literature on endurance running, there is little information on sprinting. 'Sprinting' is also a generic term used to describe brief maximum effort during a wide range of activities, including running, cycling, swimming, canoeing, rowing, field hockey, soccer and rugby. Under these circumstances, the duration of the activity is often different from track sprinting. Therefore, for the purpose of this chapter, sprinting is considered as brief maximal exercise, of less than 60s duration. The intensity of exercise is well in excess of that required to elicit maximum oxygen uptake ($\dot{V}o_{2max.}$), and there is no distribution of effort.

Setting aside the influence of natural talent and appropriate training, correct nutrition during training and competition is one of the most important components in the formula for success in sprinting. Athletes are notoriously vulnerable to advertisements for nutritional supplements which make claims about enhancing performance. Before reviewing the pertinent literature on nutrition and sprinting, this chapter will provide a brief overview of physiological and metabolic responses to sprinting, and the onset of fatigue, both on the track and in the laboratory, and adaptations to sprint training.

## Metabolic responses to sprinting

Only a few studies have examined the metabolic responses to 100-m and 400-m track sprinting (Hirvonen *et al.* 1987, 1992; Lacour *et al.* 1990; Hautier *et al.* 1994; Locatelli & Arsac 1995).

Hirvonen *et al.* (1987) measured the muscle adenosine triphosphate (ATP), phosphocreatine (PCr) and lactate concentrations in seven male sprinters before and after running 40, 60, 80 and 100m at maximum speed. The fastest sprinters utilized the greatest amount of PCr in the first 40, 60 and 80m of the run (Fig. 41.2). Most of the PCr

Table 41.1 Current world sprint records (as at January 1999).

| Distance (m) | Men | | | Women | |
| --- | --- | --- | --- | --- | --- |
| | Time (s) | Sprinter | | Time (s) | Sprinter |
| 100 | 9.84 | D. Bailey | | 10.49 | F. Griffith-Joiner |
| 200 | 19.32 | M. Johnson | | 21.34 | F. Griffith-Joiner |
| 400 | 43.29 | H. Reynolds | | 47.6 | M. Koch |

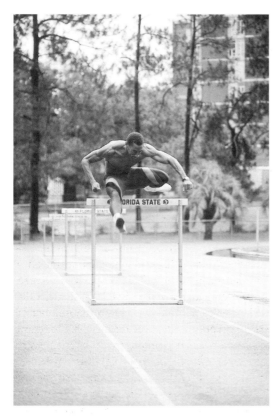

Fig. 41.1 Sprinters and hurdlers in training complete prolonged sessions with many short efforts, even though competitions may involve only a single sprint. Photo courtesy of Ron Maughan.

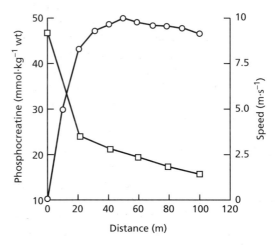

Fig. 41.2 Speed (○) and muscle phosphocreatine concentration (□) during a simulated 100-m track sprint (Hirvonen *et al.* 1987).

was used during the first 5–6 s of the race. The decrease in running speed over the 100 m commenced when the high-energy phosphate stores were markedly reduced and glycolysis was the predominant energy provider. Lactate did not accumulate to a level which could have inhibited glycolysis and is unlikely to have been the principal cause of fatigue. These results show that the rate of PCr utilization is critical to running speed. In agreement with these results, Locatelli and Arsac (1995) showed that anaerobic glycolysis provided approximately 65–70% of the metabolic energy production during a 100-m race in their study of four male and four female national sprinters analysed during the 1994 Italian championships.

The validity of postexercise lactate concentration as an indicator of the rate of anaerobic glycolysis was investigated in 400-m sprinting by Lacour *et al.* (1990), and in 100-m and 200-m sprinting by Hautier *et al.* (1994). In the study by Lacour *et al.* (1990), blood samples were taken from 17 top level athletes within 10 min of completing a 400-m race in a major competition. Postrace blood lactate concentrations were highest in the fastest athletes, as reflected in the strong correlation between running speed and lactate concentration for men ($r=0.85$) and women ($r=0.80$).

A later study by Hirvonen and colleagues (1992) measured the changes in the muscle concentration of ATP, PCr and lactate during a 400-m sprint. A 400-m race was performed (time, 51.9 ±0.7 s) and split times for every 100 m recorded. On subsequent occasions, the six male runners were required to run 100, 200 and 300 m at the same speed as their 400-m split times. Biopsies were taken from the vastus lateralis muscle before and after each sprint and analysed for PCr and lactate concentrations. After the first 100 m, muscle PCr concentration fell from 15.8±1.7–8.3 ±0.3 mmol·kg⁻¹ wet weight (Fig. 41.3), and by the end of the race, PCr concentration had fallen by 89% to 1.7±0.4 mmol·kg⁻¹ wet weight. The average speed over the 400 m decreased after 200 m, even though PCr was not depleted and lactate was not at maximum level at this point in the race (Fig. 41.3). The rate of muscle lactate accumulation for the first 100 m was about half that during

the two subsequent sections of the race (100–200 and 200–300 m), showing an increased contribution of anaerobic glycolysis to energy production up to this point. The rate of ATP yield from glycolysis was maximal between 200 and 300 m, as indicated by the highest rate of lactate accumulation in muscle and blood during this point in the race. Over the last 100 m, the rate of glycolysis declined, resulting in a dramatic decrease in running speed.

## Metabolic responses to sprinting in the laboratory

The development of specific and sensitive laboratory methods to study sprinting provides an opportunity to examine this form of activity in a controlled way (Bar-Or 1978; Lakomy 1986, 1987; Falk et al. 1996).

Sprinting has been studied in the laboratory using a non-motorized treadmill (Lakomy 1987). In the study by Lakomy (1987), performance and metabolic responses during two 30-s sprints were compared. Seven male national level sprinters, whose specialist events ranged from 100 to 400 m, performed one sprint on a non-motorized treadmill, and a second sprint on a running track. Although peak speed and mean speed were slower on the treadmill than on the track, there was no difference in the number of strides taken. In addition, similar physiological and metabolic responses to both runs were observed, demonstrating that the treadmill sprint was a useful tool for the analysis of the physiological demands of sprint running in the laboratory. Postexercise blood lactate concentrations were 16.8 vs. 15.2 mmol·l⁻¹ for treadmill and track runs, respectively. Heart rate averaged 198 beats·min⁻¹ in both 30-s sprints, and postrace blood glucose concentration was 6.4±1.1 mmol·l⁻¹ after the treadmill run, and 6.2±1.0 mmol·l⁻¹ after the track run (H.K.A. Lakomy, unpublished observations).

Cheetham et al. (1986) examined performance during, and the changes in muscle metabolites following, a 30-s sprint on a non-motorized treadmill. Peak power output for eight female

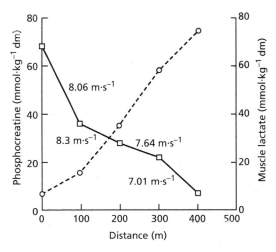

**Fig. 41.3** Muscle phosphocreatine (□) and lactate concentrations (○) at various speeds during a simulated 400-m track sprint (Hirvonen et al. 1992).

subjects was 534±85 W and was 50% of its peak value at the end of the sprint. Biopsy samples were taken from the vastus lateralis muscle before and after the sprint. Muscle glycogen, PCr and ATP declined from resting values by 25%, 64% and 37%, respectively. Three minutes after exercise, muscle and blood lactate increased to 78±26 mmol·l⁻¹ and 13 mmol·l⁻¹, respectively. Similar intramuscular lactate concentrations of 73.9±16.1 mmol·kg⁻¹ dry matter were observed for males by Jacobs *et al.* (1983) after 30 s of maximal cycling using the Wingate anaerobic test (WAnT) protocol. Blood pH decreased by 0.24 units to 7.16±0.07 3 min after the sprint, and heart rate increased over the 30-s sprint, reaching its maximum of approximately 182 beats·min⁻¹ over the last few seconds of the sprint (Cheetham *et al.* 1986). Anaerobic glycogenolysis supplied 64% of the ATP required during the 30-s sprint, calculated from the changes in muscle glycogen, lactate, pyruvate and PCr concentrations. Similar metabolic responses to sprinting were observed in a later study from the same laboratory (Nevill *et al.* 1989).

Costill *et al.* (1983) examined muscle and blood pH along with blood lactate concentration and pH after sprint running. Four male subjects were biopsied from the gastrocnemius muscle before and after a treadmill sprint run at 125% $\dot{V}o_{2max.}$ and a 400-m timed run on a track. After the 400-m sprint, muscle pH in four of the subjects averaged 6.63±0.03 and blood pH and lactate concentration were 7.10±0.03 and 12.3 mmol·l⁻¹, respectively, highlighting the extensive metabolic challenge of this event.

Thirty seconds of treadmill sprinting also provokes a marked increase in endocrine response. Plasma noradrenaline and adrenaline increased from resting values by six- and sevenfold, respectively, and the plasma concentration of β-endorphin doubled following 30 s of treadmill sprinting. (Brooks *et al.* 1988). Plasma growth hormone is elevated to more than eight times its resting value following a 30-s treadmill sprint (Nevill *et al.* 1996). The concentration peaked after 30 min recovery and remained significantly elevated above baseline for the 60 min. A greater endocrine response is observed when maximal

sprints are repeated after a short recovery (Brooks *et al.* 1990). In one study, nine men and nine women performed 10 6-s sprints on a non-motorized treadmill, with 30 s separating each sprint. Peak plasma adrenaline was 9.2±7.3 for the men and 3.7±2.4 nmol·l⁻¹ for the women, and was recorded after only five sprints (Brooks *et al.* 1990).

Most studies reporting the metabolic responses to sprinting have analysed muscle samples which contain a mixture of fibre types. However, studies which have been carried out *in vitro* have suggested that maximal power output and its decline are related to fibre type (Faulkner *et al.* 1986). Energy metabolism in single muscle fibres was measured in a study by Greenhaff and colleagues (1994). Muscle biopsies were taken from the vastus lateralis muscle before and after 30 s of maximal treadmill sprinting and the type I and type II fibres analysed for concentrations of ATP, PCr and glycogen (Fig. 41.4). Prior to the sprint, PCr and glycogen concentrations were highest in the type II fibres and a greater decline was observed in these fibres after the 30-s sprint. Peak power output declined by 65±3% during exercise. Phosphocreatine was almost depleted after the sprint, but those subjects with the higher type II fibre PCr content showed a smaller decline in power output during the sprint ($r=-0.93$; $P<0.01$). The decline in ATP during the sprint was similar in both fibre populations. This illustrates the importance of the contribution of PCr to energy production during maximal exercise.

## Fatigue during sprinting

Elite male sprinters can maintain maximal speed for 20–30 m, whereas females can maintain top speed for only 15–20 m. The explanation, even in elite sprinters, may be due to both mechanical and metabolic factors.

The mechanical limitations to sprinting include failure of neuromuscular coordination (Murase *et al.* 1976), the change in body position relative to the foot striking the ground, and deceleration caused by the grounding foot (Mann & Sprague 1983; Mann 1985). At such

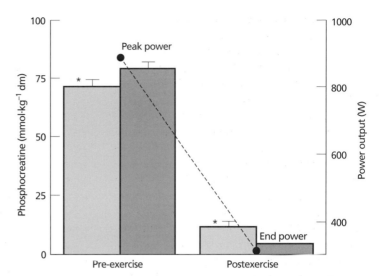

**Fig. 41.4** Muscle phosphocreatine concentrations in type I (☐) and type II (■) fibres before and after a 30-s sprint on a non-motorized treadmill (Greenhaff *et al.* 1994). *, *P* < 0.01, type I vs. type II.

high velocities, it is difficult to maintain such a high limb speed, both in recovery of the driving leg, and in the brief track contact time for force generation (Radford 1990).

Air resistance at high velocities may also be a significant factor in sprinting because it increases with running speed. Davies (1980) calculated that elite 100-m sprinters running 10 m·s⁻¹ would run 0.25–0.5 s faster if they did not have to overcome air resistance. Pugh (1970) estimated that air resistance accounted for 16% of the total energy expended to run 100 m in 10.0 s. Thus, it is advantageous to perform sprints at high altitude. For example, the altitude of Mexico City (2250 m) provides an advantage of approximately 0.07 s (Linthorne 1994).

The metabolic factors contributing to the onset of fatigue are associated with the decrease of PCr or ATP in the muscle (Murase *et al.* 1976; Hirvonen *et al.* 1987, 1992). The consequent decrease in the availability of high-energy phosphates within exercising muscles results in a reduction in the power output. During the middle part of the 100-m sprint, running speed decreases as the contribution of the high-energy phosphate stores is reduced (see Fig. 41.1), and at the end of the 100-m race, anaerobic glycolysis is the main energy source (Hirvonen *et al.* 1987). A decline in running speed or power output towards the end of a 400-m race and a 30-s tread-

mill sprint is also associated with very low PCr values (Hirvonen *et al.* 1992; Greenhaff *et al.* 1994).

The importance of PCr is highlighted because power output declines when PCr utilization decreases, despite adequate stores of ATP and glycogen. For example, during a maximal 30-s treadmill sprint, muscle glycogen was reduced by 27% and 20% in type II and type I fibres, respectively (Greenhaff *et al.* 1994). ATP decreased by a similar amount (20%) in both fibre types. After 30 s of sprint cycling, there was still sufficient glycogen and ATP left in both fibre types in the muscle to sustain energy metabolism (Boobis *et al.* 1987; Vollestad *et al.* 1992). Why, then, do the sprinters fatigue when substrate is still available for energy metabolism? A possible answer is that initial force generation is dependent on the availability of PCr, once intramuscular PCr stores are depleted. Sprinting speed cannot be maintained because the available glycogen cannot be used quickly enough to sustain the high rates of ATP utilization required. In addition, accumulation of inorganic phosphate ($P_i$) may inhibit the cross-bridge recycling between actin and myosin filaments directly (Hultman *et al.* 1987).

The decline in running speed observed towards the end of a 400-m race is due to a reduction in the rate of glycogen hydrolysis, despite

LIVERPOOL
JOHN MOORES UNIVERS
AVRIL ROBARTS LRC
TITHEBARN STREET

ample availability of muscle glycogen. The parallel increase in hydrogen and lactate ions during sprinting may inhibit glycolysis, thus contributing to the development of fatigue (Sahlin 1996). A further explanation for fatigue during the 400-m sprint and repeated shorter sprints during training is that the increase in ammonia observed as a consequence of decreases in PCr and ATP concentrations during sprinting (Schlict et al. 1990; Tullson & Turjung 1990) may be implicated in the fatigue process (Green 1995).

## Influence of sprint training on energy production

The main focus of many studies on the adaptations to sprint training is the changes in energy metabolism underpinning improvements in performance. This approach has led to a greater understanding of the metabolic causes of fatigue during sprinting.

The main and consistent finding in the laboratory and in the field is that sprint training improves performance. This performance is measured as an increase in maximum power output during the initial period of exercise, an increase in the amount of work done during a brief exercise bout, or an increase in exercise duration at high exercise intensities (Brooks et al. 1993).

Nevill et al. (1989), investigated the effect of 8 weeks of high-intensity training on metabolism during a 30-s treadmill sprint. Sixteen matched subjects were assigned to either a training or a control group. After training, peak power increased by 12% during the initial period of exercise, and the total work done during the test was increased by 6%. This improvement in performance was equivalent to a 1.5-s reduction in 200-m running time. Maximum muscle lactate concentration increased by 20% after training, and an equivalent increase in the rate of ATP resynthesis from anaerobic glycolysis was also observed. The excess postexercise oxygen consumption also increased by 18% after training. However, despite the increase in muscle lactate concentration, training did not change muscle pH during maximal treadmill sprinting.

The increased ATP required as a consequence of the improvement in performance after sprint training was provided from anaerobic glycolysis (Nevill et al. 1989). No changes were observed in the contribution from PCr or aerobic metabolism. The increased resynthesis from anaerobic glycolysis was facilitated by an increase in the activity of phosphofructokinase (PFK), the rate-limiting enzyme in anaerobic glycolysis, and by an increased efflux of $H^+$ from the muscle cell after training. This is in agreement with other studies, which have reported that adaptations to sprint training include an increase in the muscle's buffering capacity (Sharp et al. 1986), an increase in the activity of muscle PFK (Fournier et al. 1982; Roberts et al. 1982; Sharp et al. 1986; Jacobs et al. 1987), and an increase in the proportion of type IIa fibres (Jacobs et al. 1987).

However, factors other than increased anaerobic energy production may also contribute to improvement in performance after sprint training. These include an improved regulation of $K^+$ during exercise and changes in the $Na^+$–$K^+$-ATPase concentrations (McKenna et al. 1993), which are important in the excitation–contraction coupling in skeletal muscles. Other factors include the determinants of muscle tension at both the whole muscle and single fibre level. These include action-potential frequency, fibre length and fibre diameter. It is beyond the scope of this review to consider these factors, which are discussed in detail elsewhere (Brooks et al. 1993).

## Nutritional influences on sprinting

### Dietary intake

In contrast to the plethora of information on the dietary intake of endurance athletes, the nutritional habits of sprinters are not well documented. It is a well-established belief in the power- and strength-training community that strength is improved when a diet high in protein is consumed. Quantitatively, the recommended protein intake for these athletes is about 1.4–1.7 g protein·kg$^{-1}$ body mass·day$^{-1}$ (Lemon 1992). A diet containing 12–15% of its energy from protein should be adequate for strength athletes (including sprinters), assuming that the total energy intake is sufficient to cover their high daily energy expenditure (Lemon & Proctor 1991).

Should sprinters consume a particular type of diet? Total energy intake should be increased in order to cover the demands of training and competition. Most of the studies which have reported the energy intakes of runners have focused on endurance athletes. One study of trained university track athletes (Short & Short 1983) reported that the daily energy intake of these sprinters was approximately 16.8 MJ (4000 kcal), similar to the energy intake of university bodybuilders in the same study. Unfortunately, no data on the physical characteristics of these athletes were documented. A well-balanced diet, containing a wide variety of foods, is all that is recommended to ensure that all needs for energy, vitamins and minerals are met. At least 60–70% (7–8 g·kg$^{-1}$) of daily energy intake should come from carbohydrates, about 12% from protein (1.2–1.7 g·kg$^{-1}$), and the remaining energy provided by fat (Devlin & Williams 1991; Lemon 1992). However, only endurance athletes seem to comply with these recommendations (C. Williams 1993). The only nutrient supplementation which may enhance sprinting is creatine (see Chapter 27) and bicarbonate (see Chapter 29). Currently, there is little evidence to suggest that sprinters require any other supplements (including vitamins and minerals) in addition to a normal balanced diet containing a wide range of foods covering the individual's energy requirements. Further research is necessary to establish whether some nutrients and combinations of nutrients have an ergogenic effect during sprinting.

## Carbohydrate loading and sprinting

Muscle glycogen 'supercompensation' improves performance during prolonged exercise (Costill 1988), and is a nutritional strategy used by endurance athletes in preparation for competi-

tion. The importance of the initial glycogen concentration on the performance of maximal or high-intensity exercise remains an issue, although it is clear that very low pre-exercise glycogen concentrations are associated with reductions in performance in high-intensity exercise (Maughan & Poole 1981; Pizza et al. 1995). However, it is unlikely that increased glycogen stores will affect sprinting performance, as glycogen per se is not a limiting factor during sprints over distances of 400 m or less (Hirvonen et al. 1992). Laboratory studies on brief, maximal exercise also support this conclusion. The mean and peak power outputs of athletes performing 30 s of maximal exercise using the WAnT protocol on a cycle ergometer were unchanged after carbohydrate loading (Wootton & Williams 1984).

This lack of ergogenic effect is elucidated when the metabolic responses to sprinting are examined in single fibres of human skeletal muscle (Greenhaff et al. 1994). Biopsies were obtained from six subjects before and after a 30-s sprint on a non-motorized treadmill. Glycogen was reduced by 20% and 27% in the type I and type II fibres, respectively, in agreement with the significant contribution from muscle glycogen during a 30-s sprint reported by Cheetham et al. (1986). However, the 65% decline in power output during the 30-s sprint was probably associated with the large decline in PCr concentration in both type I fibres (83% decrease), and particularly the type II fibres (94% decline).

Varying the carbohydrate intake in the days before exercise has been shown to influence performance during high-intensity (not maximal) exercise when undertaken either continuously (Maughan & Poole 1981; Pizza et al. 1995), or intermittently (Bangsbo et al. 1992; Nicholas et al. 1997). However, a relationship between carbohydrate status and exercise performance during maximum exercise has not been consistently reported (Symons & Jacobs 1989; Vandenberghe et al. 1995). There may, however, be a critical concentration of glycogen below which high-intensity exercise is impaired. Indeed, it has been shown that below a muscle glycogen concentration of 20–30 mmol·kg⁻¹ of wet weight, the rate of energy production is reduced and performance decreased (Costill 1988).

## Carbohydrate loading and repeated sprints

Sprint training involves many sprints during daily training sessions. The metabolic and physiological responses to repeated sprints performed in the laboratory (Gaitanos *et al.* 1993; Trump *et al.* 1996) provide some information on the glycogen demands of a sprint training session, or in sports such as soccer or rugby (Nicholas *et al.* 1994), where maximal sprints are performed briefly between periods of less intense exercise over an 80–90-min period.

Several studies have examined maximal dynamic muscle power output and the associated metabolic changes in muscle during three to four bouts of maximal cycling at 100 r.p.m. (10.5 rad·s⁻¹), separated by 4-min recovery intervals (McCartney *et al.* 1986; Spriet *et al.* 1989; Trump *et al.* 1996). In these studies, power output and work done decreased by 20% in both the second and third exercise periods, but there was no further decrement in performance in the

fourth bout (McCartney *et al.* 1986). Changes in muscle glycogen, lactate and glycolytic intermediates suggested that the rate of glycogenolysis was limited at the PFK level during the first and second exercise periods, and at the phosphorylase level in the third and fourth exercise periods (McCartney *et al.* 1986). In agreement with these findings, Spriet *et al.* (1989) reported that muscle [H⁺] was higher and the glycolytic flux lower after the third exercise bout than after the second, even though ATP and PCr degradation was similar in the two exercise bouts. As a consequence of the reduction in the rate of glycolysis during the third and fourth sprints, there is a greater reliance on aerobic metabolism (Fig. 41.5), and possibly the intramuscular triglyceride stores (McCartney *et al.* 1986).

The laboratory studies on repeated sprints of 30 s duration are relevant to training sessions where sets of 200 or 300 m are performed. However, muscle metabolism during repeated shorter sprints (<6 s) has a wider applicability, not only for sprint training, but also to the multiple sprint sports. Gaitanos *et al.* (1993) examined muscle metabolism during intermittent maximal exercise. The exercise protocol consisted of 10 ×

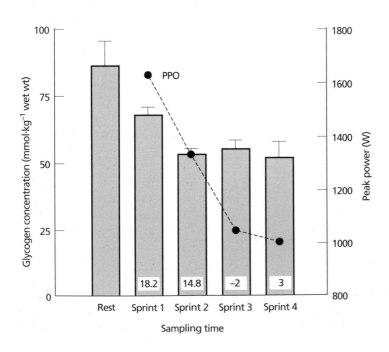

**Fig. 41.5** Post-sprint glycogen concentration and power output during four bouts of 30-s isokinetic cycling (McCartney *et al.* 1986). The amount of glycogen utilized during each bout is also shown (in mmol·kg⁻¹ wet wt). PPO, peak power output.

6-s maximal sprints on a cycle ergometer with 30 s of recovery between each sprint. The applied load for the sprints was calculated as for the WAnT protocol (75 g·kg⁻¹ body mass). Biopsies were taken from the vastus lateralis muscle before and after the first sprint and 10 s before and immediately after the 10th sprint. Mean power output generated over the first 6-s sprint was sustained by an equal contribution from PCr degradation and anaerobic glycolysis. By the end of the first sprint, PCr and glycogen concentration decreased by 57% and 14%, respectively, of resting values, and muscle lactate concentration increased to 28.6 mmol·kg⁻¹ dry matter, an indication of significant glycolytic activity. However, in the 10th sprint, mean power output was reduced to 73% of that generated in the first sprint, despite the fact that there was a dramatic reduction in the energy yield from anaerobic glycolysis. Thus it was suggested that power output during the last sprint was supported by energy that was mainly derived from PCr degradation and an increased aerobic metabolism.

Thus the weight of available evidence shows that it is unlikely that sprinting is limited by muscle glycogen availability, unless the glycogen concentration falls below a critical threshold value of 100 mmol·kg⁻¹ of dry matter. Glycogen availability is also unlikely to limit peak power output during repeated sprints because of the decline in glycogenolysis and lactate production observed under these conditions. However, as reviewed in the next section, evidence shows that an inadequate intake of carbohydrate in the diet is detrimental to sprinting.

### Carbohydrate intake and repeated maximal sprints

An inadequate carbohydrate intake has been shown to decrease performance during a second maximal cycle ergometer interval test performed 2–3 days after the first test (Fulcher & Williams 1992; Jenkins et al. 1993). Fulcher and Williams (1992) studied the effects of 2 days' intake of either a normal carbohydrate (450±225 g) or a low carbohydrate (71±27 g) diet on power

output during maximal intermittent exercise. Two trials were performed, one before, and then one following the 2 days of dietary manipulation. The test protocol comprised five sets of five all-out fixed level sprints with 30 s recovery (65 g·kg⁻¹ applied load) separated by 5 min active recovery. A final, sixth set comprised 10× 6-s sprints, separated by 30 s recovery. Those subjects who ate their normal amount of carbohydrate showed a significant improvement in peak power output during the five sets of sprints in test 2 compared with test 1. No such improvement was shown in test 2 after the low carbohydrate diet. In the study by Jenkins and colleagues (1993), 14 moderately trained individuals completed two intermittent exercise tests, separated by 3 days. Each test comprised five bouts of 60-s cycle performed maximally, with successive exercise periods separated by 5 min of passive recovery. During the 3-day period between trials, each subject was randomly assigned to either a high carbohydrate (83%), moderate carbohydrate (58%) or low carbohydrate (12%) diet. Although performance declined in the low carbohydrate condition in both these studies, the amount of carbohydrate ingested (10% and 12%, respectively, of total energy intake) was significantly lower than the amount normally consumed by athletes. Nevertheless, these studies highlight the importance of an adequate intake of dietary carbohydrate for those individuals performing repeated sprint exercise.

These results emphasize the need for sprinters in training, and sportsmen and women competing in the multiple sprint sports (see Chapter 45 for a more detailed review) to consume adequate amounts of carbohydrate on a daily basis. Much research has been carried out to determine the amount of carbohydrate needed to replenish glycogen stores within 24 h of intense training. A diet which comprised approximately 8–10 g carbohydrate·kg⁻¹ body mass was sufficient to replace muscle glycogen stores after daily 1-h training sessions (Pascoe et al. 1990). High-intensity endurance capacity was also improved following a high carbohydrate recovery diet (Nicholas et al. 1997). However, some studies have shown that when a fixed amount of exercise is performed on a daily basis, performance is not affected when only a moderate amount of carbohydrate is consumed (Simonsen *et al.* 1991; Nevill *et al.* 1993; Sherman *et al.* 1993).

Nevill *et al.* (1993) reported that power output during 1 h of intermittent sprint exercise was unchanged after the carbohydrate intake was manipulated during the 24-h recovery (Fig. 41.6). During the first trial, 18 games players performed 30 maximum 6-s sprints, interspersed with walking and jogging, on a non-motorized treadmill. The subjects were then randomly assigned to three equally matched groups and repeated the test 24 h later, after consuming either a high, low or normal carbohydrate diet (79±3%, 47±8%, 12±1% carbohydrate, respectively). Power output over the 30 sprints was not different between trials; however, the high carbohydrate group did perform better than the low carbohydrate group over the first nine sprints.

However, although no performance decrements were observed in the short term, an increased carbohydrate intake is recommended because it may improve performance after an intensive training period (Simonsen *et al.* 1991). Laboratory studies have shown that one 6-s sprint reduces glycogen by approximately 44 mmol·kg$^{-1}$ dry matter (14%), and after 10 sprints, glycogen is reduced by 36% (Gaitanos *et al.* 1993). A sprinter may train intensively—say, three to five times per week—which may cumulatively reduce glycogen stores, leading to glycogen depletion. Performance during maximal exercise may be reduced by 10–15% when glycogen concentration falls below a critical threshold (Jacobs *et al.* 1982). Although there is no ergogenic benefit of carbohydrate loading in the days prior to a single sprint, an adequate carbohydrate intake is recommended for sprinters in training to support the intense daily training sessions.

## Dietary supplements and sprinting

### Protein and amino acids

Anabolic steroids, used by bodybuilders to increase lean muscle tissue, are illegal in sporting competition, and may pose a number of health risks. A variety of nutrients are believed to provide an effective, safe and legal alternative instead (M.H. Williams 1993). Amino acid supplements have been advertised for strength athletes because they are said to provide a safe anabolic or muscle-building effect. The two most commonly used amino acids are arginine and ornithine because of their stimulatory effects on human growth hormone (HGH) production (Hatfield 1987; Williams 1989). It is well documented that exogenous growth hormone produces anabolic effects in growth hormone-deficient animals and humans, but it is questionable as to whether this same effect exists in normal animals and humans.

However, many athletes believe that supplementation with these amino acids stimulates the release of HGH, which is thought to act by increasing insulin-like growth factors (IGF1 and IGF2). Thus, protein and nucleic acid synthesis is stimulated in skeletal muscle (Lombardo *et al.* 1991). However, many well-controlled studies

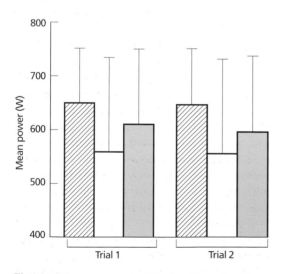

**Fig. 41.6** Mean power output during 30 maximal 6-s sprints during trial 1 and trial 2 for three dietary groups: ▨, high carbohydrate; □, normal carbohydrate; ■, low carbohydrate (Nevill *et al.* 1993).

have failed to observe an increase in the serum concentration of HGH following supplementation with these amino acids. Those studies which have shown some anabolic effect of these amino acid supplements are flawed. Suminski *et al.* (1997) found that the ingestion of 1500 mg of arginine and 1500 mg of lysine immediately before resistance exercise did not alter exercise-induced changes in the concentration of growth hormone in weight-training males. When the same amino acid mixture was ingested under basal conditions, the secretion of growth hormone was increased to levels which were higher than after ingestion of a placebo, 60 min after amino acid ingestion during resting conditions. Additional research is required to evaluate claims for commercial products.

A few studies have examined the effect of arginine and/or ornithine supplementation on body composition, measures of muscular strength or power and reported significant increases in lean body mass. Where increases in lean body mass have been reported (Crist *et al.* 1988; Yarasheski *et al.* 1992), the functional ability of the muscle was not assessed. M.H. Williams (1993) emphasizes the flawed experimental methodology in each study, thus questioning the interpretation of the findings. Although statistical significance was reported in two of the studies, a recalculation, using the appropriate statistical technique, actually revealed no significant differences between the supplement and the placebo. Other studies have reported no significant effect of arginine or a mixture of amino acids on measures of strength, power or HGH in experienced weightlifters (Hawkins *et al.* 1991; Warren *et al.* 1991). The use of both HGH and anabolic steroids is contraindicated for athletes, since they are both proscribed by the IOC and both carry significant health risks (Lombardo *et al.* 1991; M.H. Williams 1993).

The ergogenic effect of supplementing the diet with low-dose oral amino acids has been questioned (Fogelholm *et al.* 1993; Fry *et al.* 1993; Lambert *et al.* 1993). Fogelholm *et al.* (1993) found no difference in the concentrations of serum growth hormone or insulin of competitive weightlifters following 4 days supplementation with L-arginine, L-orthinine and L-lysine. This result was consistent with the findings of Lambert *et al.* (1993), who reported that serum growth hormone concentrations were not elevated in male bodybuilders after the ingestion of commercial amino acid supplements in the quantities specified by the manufacturers. The supplements of amino acids comprised two mixtures: 2.4 g of arginine and lysine, and 1.85 g of ornithine and tyrosine.

Fry and colleagues monitored both hormonal and performance responses to amino acid supplementation in parallel with high-volume training. In this study, 28 elite junior weightlifters were tested for strength before and after 7 days of high-volume training sessions. During this 7 day training period, the subjects' diets were supplemented with capsules containing either amino acids (protein group) or lactose (placebo group). The protein group took 2.4 g of amino acids (containing a mixture of all 20 amino acids) immediately prior to their three daily meals for 7 days, as well as 2.1 g of branched-chain amino acids (L-leucine, L-isoleucine, L-valine, supplemented with L-glutamine and L-carnitine), prior to each training session. It was concluded that hormonal responses, both at rest and following training, were unaltered.

It is important to recognize that brief periods of high-intensity exercise significantly increase the concentration of growth hormone. Growth hormone increased and remained approximately 10 times the basal value in sprint-trained athletes, 1 h after a maximal 30-s sprint on a non-motorized treadmill (Nevill *et al.* 1996). The growth hormone response was greater in sprint-trained than endurance-trained athletes, and no differences were found between males and females. Peak power output and the magnitude of metabolic response to the sprint accounted for 82% of the variation in serum peak growth hormone response. Thus, sprint training *per se* is effective in increasing growth hormone. Whether or not sprinting could promote increases in IGF1 and IGF2 is unknown, but repeated eccentric contractions have been shown to increase the immunoreactivity of IGF1 in muscle 4 days after exercise (Yan *et al.* 1993).

In summary, a high carbohydrate diet is recommended in order to replenish the muscle glycogen depleted during intense training sessions on a daily basis. With the exception of creatine supplementation (reviewed in Chapter 27) and bicarbonate supplementation (reviewed in Chapter 29), there is little evidence to suggest that sprinters need any additional nutrient supplementation (including vitamins and minerals) provided that they eat a normal balanced diet, containing a wide range of foods, which covers the individual's energy requirements (Clarkson 1990; Van Der Beek 1990).

## References

Bangsbo, J., Norregaard, L. & Thorsoe, F. (1992) The effect of carbohydrate diet on intermittent exercise performance. *International Journal of Sports Medicine* **13**, 152–157.

Bar-Or, O. (1978) The Wingate Anaerobic Test: an update on methodology, reliability and validity. *Sports Medicine* **4**, 381–394.

Boobis, L.H., Williams, C., Cheetham, M.E. & Wootton, S.A. (1987) Metabolic aspects of fatigue during sprinting. In *Exercise Benefits, Limits and Adaptations* (ed. D. Macleod, R. Maughan, M. Nimmo, T. Reilly & C. Williams), pp. 116–143. E and FN Spon, London.

Brooks, S., Burrin, J., Cheetham, M.E., Hall, G.M., Yeo, T. & Williams, C. (1988) The responses of the catecholamines and B-endorphin to brief maximal exercise in man. *European Journal of Applied Physiology* **57**, 230–234.

Brooks, S., Nevill, M.E., Meleagros, L., Lakomy, H.K.A., Hall, G.M., Bloom, S.R. & Williams, C. (1990) The hormonal responses to repetitive brief maximal exercise in humans. *European Journal of Applied Physiology* **60**, 144–148.

Brooks, S., Nevill, M.E., Gaitanos, G. & Williams, C. (1993) Metabolic responses to sprint training. In *Intermittent High Intensity Exercise: Preparation, Stresses and Damage Limitation* (ed. D.A.D. Macleod, R.J. Maughan, C. Williams, C.R. Madeley, J.C.M. Sharp & R.W. Nutton), pp. 33–47. E and FN Spon, London.

Cheetham, M.E., Boobis, L.H., Brooks, S. & Williams, C. (1986) Human muscle metabolism during sprint running. *Journal of Applied Physiology* **61**, 54–60.

Clarkson, P.M. (1990) Minerals: exercise performance and supplementation in athletes. *Journal of Sports Sciences* **9**, S91–S116.

Costill, D.L. (1988) Carbohydrates for exercise: dietary demands for optimal performance. *International Journal of Sports Medicine* **9**, 1–18.

Costill, D.L., Barnett, A., Sharp, R., Fink, R.J. & Katz, A. (1983) Leg muscle pH following sprint running. *Medicine and Science in Sports and Exercise* **15**, 325–329.

Crist, D.M., Peake, G. & Egan, P. *et al.* (1988) Body composition response to exogenous GH during training in highly conditioned adults. *Journal of Applied Physiology* **65**, 579–584.

Davies, C.T.M. (1980) The effects of wind assistance and resistance on the forward motion of a runner. *Journal of Applied Physiology* **48**, 702–709.

Devlin, J.T. & Williams, C. (1991) Foods, nutrition and sports performance: a final consensus statement. *Journal of Sports Sciences* **9** (Suppl.), iii.

Durant, J. (1961) *Highlights of the Olympics: From Ancient Times to the Present.* Arco Publications, London.

Falk, B., Weinstein, Y., Dotan, R., Abramson, D.A., Mannsegal, D. & Hoffman, J.R. (1996) A treadmill test of sprint running. *Scandinavian Journal of Medicine and Science in Sports* **6**, 259–264.

Faulkner, J.A., Clafin, D.R. & McCully, K.K. (1986) Power output of fast and slow fibres from human skeletal muscle. In *Human Power Output* (ed. N.L. Jones, N. McCartney & A.J. McComas), pp. 81–89. Human Kinetics Publishers, Champaign, IL.

Fogelholm, G.M., Naveri, H.K., Kiilavuori, K.T.K. & Harkonen, M.H.A. (1993) Low dose amino acid supplementation: no effect on serum growth hormone and insulin in male weightlifters. *International Journal of Sport Nutrition* **3**, 290–297.

Fournier, M., Ricci, J., Taylor, A.W., Ferguson, R.J., Montpetit, R.R. & Chaitman, B.R. (1982) Skeletal muscle adaptation in adolescent boys: sprint and endurance training and detraining. *Medicine and Science in Sports and Exercise* **14**, 453–456.

Fry, A.C., Kraemer, W.J., Stone, M.H. *et al.* (1993) Endocrine and performance responses to high volume training and amino acid supplementation in elite junior weightlifters. *International Journal of Sport Nutrition* **3**, 306–322.

Fulcher, K.Y. & Williams, C. (1992) The effect of diet on high-intensity intermittent exercise performance. *Journal of Sports Sciences* **10**, 550–551A.

Gaitanos, G.C., Williams, C., Boobis, L.H. & Brooks, S. (1993) Human muscle metabolism during intermittent maximal exercise. *Journal of Applied Physiology* **75**, 712–719.

Green, H.J. (1995) Metabolic determinants of activity induced muscular fatigue. In *Exercise Metabolism* (ed. M. Hargreaves), pp. 211–256. Human Kinetics, Champaign, IL.

Greenhaff, P.L., Nevill, M.E., Soderlund, K. *et al.* (1994) The metabolic responses of human type I and II muscle fibres during maximal treadmill sprinting. *Journal of Physiology* **478**, 149–155.

Hatfield, F.C. (1987) *Ultimate Sports Nutrition.* Contemporary Books, Chicago.

Hautier, C.A., Wouassi, D., Arsac, L.M., Bitanga, E., Thiriet, P. & Lacour, J.R. (1994) Relationships between postcompetition blood lactate concentration and average running velocity over 100-m and 200-m races. *European Journal of Applied Physiology* **68**, 508–513.

Hawkins, C.E., Walberg-Rankin, J. & Sebolt, D.R. (1991) Oral arginine does not affect body composition or muscle function in male weight lifters (Abstract). *Medicine and Science in Sports and Exercise* **23**, S15.

Hirvonen, J., Rehunen, S., Rusko, H. & Harkonen, M. (1987) Breakdown of high-energy phosphate compounds and lactate accumulation during short supramaximal exercise. *European Journal of Applied Physiology* **56**, 253–259.

Hirvonen, J., Nummela, H., Rehunen, S. & Harkonen, M. (1992) Fatigue and changes of ATP, creatine phosphate, and lactate during the 400-m sprint. *Canadian Journal of Sport Science* **17**, 141–144.

Hultman, E., Spriet, L.L. & Soderlund, K. (1987) Energy metabolism and fatigue in working muscle. In *Exercise Benefits, Limits and Adaptations* (ed. D. Macleod, R. Maughan, M. Nimmo, T. Reilly & C. Williams), pp. 63–80. E and FN Spon, London.

Jacobs, I., Kaiser, P. & Tesch, P. (1982) The effects of glycogen exhaustion on maximal short-term performance. In *Exercise and Sport Biology* (ed. P.V. Komi), pp. 103–108. Human Kinetics, Champaign, IL.

Jacobs, I., Tesch, P.A., Bar-Or, O., Karlsson, J. & Dotan, R. (1983) Lactate in human skeletal muscle after 10 and 30 s of supramaximal exercise. *Journal of Applied Physiology* **55**, 365–367.

Jacobs, I., Esbjornsson, M., Sylven, C., Holm, I. & Jansson, E. (1987) Sprint training effects on muscle myoglobin, enzymes, fibre types, and blood lactate. *Medicine and Science in Sports and Exercise* **19**, 368–374.

Jenkins, D.G., Palmer, J. & Spillman, D. (1993) The influence of dietary carbohydrate on performance of supramaximal intermittent exercise. *European Journal of Applied Physiology* **67**, 309–314.

Lacour, J.R., Bouvat, E. & Barthelemy, J.C. (1990) Post competition blood lactate concentrations as indicators of anaerobic energy expenditure during 400-m and 800-m races. *European Journal of Applied Physiology* **61**, 172–176.

Lakomy, H.K.A. (1986) Measurement of work and power output using friction-loaded cycle ergometers. *Ergonomics* **29**, 509–517.

Lakomy, H.K.A. (1987) The use of a non-motorized treadmill for analyzing sprint performance. *Ergonomics* **30**, 627–637.

Lambert, M.I., Hefer, J.A., Millar, R.P. & Macfarlane, P.W. (1993) Failure of commercial oral amino acid supplements to increase serum growth hormone concentrations in male body builders. *International Journal of Sport Nutrition* **3**, 298–305.

Lemon, P.W.R. (1992) Effect of exercise on protein requirements. In *Foods, Nutrition and Sports Performance* (ed. C. Williams & J.T. Devlin), pp. 65–86. E. and F.N. Spon, London.

Lemon, P.W.R. & Proctor, D.N. (1991) Protein intake and athletic performance. *Sports Medicine* **12**, 313–325.

Linthorne, N.P. (1994) The effect of wind on 100 m sprint times. *Journal of Applied Biomechanics* **10**, 110–131.

Locatelli, E. & Arsac, L. (1995) The mechanics and energetics of the 100-m sprint. *New Studies in Athletics* **10**, 81–87.

Lombardo, J.A., Hickson, R.C. & Lamb, D.R. (1991) Anabolic/androgenic steroids and growth hormone. In *Perspectives in Exercise Science and Sports Medicine.* Vol. 4. *Ergogenics: Enhancement of Performance in Exercise and Sport* (ed. D.R. Lamb & M.H. Williams), pp. 249–278. Brown and Benchmark, Indianapolis, IN.

McCartney, N., Spriet, L.L., Heigenhauser, G.J.F., Kowalchuk, J.M., Sutton, J.R. & Jones, N.L. (1986) Muscle power and metabolism in maximal intermittent exercise. *Journal of Applied Physiology* **60**, 1164–1169.

McKenna, M.J., Schmidt, T.A., Hargreaves, M., Cameron, L., Skinner, S.L. & Kjeldsen, K. (1993) Sprint training increases human skeletal muscle $Na^+$–$K^+$ ATPase concentration and improves $K^+$ regulation. *Journal of Applied Physiology* **75**, 173–180.

Mann, R. (1985) Biomechanical analysis of the elite sprinter and hurdler. In *The Elite Athlete* (ed. N.K. Butts, T.K. Gushiken & B. Zairns), pp. 43–80. Spectrum Publications, New York.

Mann, R. & Sprague, P. (1983) Kinetics of sprinting. *Track and Field Quarterly Review* **83**, 4–9.

Maughan, R.J. & Poole, D.C. (1981) The effects of a glycogen-loading regimen on the capacity to perform anaerobic exercise. *European Journal of Applied Physiology* **46**, 211–219.

Murase, Y., Hoshikawa, T., Yasuda, N., Ikegami, Y. & Matsui, H. (1976) Analysis of the changes in progressive speed during 100-metre dash. In *Biomechanics V-B* (ed. P.V. Komi), pp. 200–207. University Park Press, Baltimore, MD.

Nevill, M.E., Boobis, L.H., Brooks, S. & Williams, C. (1989) Effect of training on muscle metabolism during treadmill sprinting. *Journal of Applied Physiology* **67**, 2376–2382.

Nevill, M.E., Williams, C., Roper, D., Slater, C. & Nevill, A.M. (1993) Effect of diet on performance during recovery from intermittent sprint exercise. *Journal of Sports Sciences* **11**, 119–126.

Nevill, M.E., Holmyard, D.J., Hall, G.M., Allsop, P., van Oosterhout, A. & Nevill, A.M. (1996) Growth hormone responses to treadmill sprinting in sprint- and endurance-trained athletes. *European Journal of Applied Physiology* **72**, 460–467.

Nicholas, C.W., Williams, C., Boobis, L.H. & Little, N. (1994) Effect of ingesting a carbohydrate–electrolyte beverage on muscle glycogen utilization during high intensity, intermittent shuttle running (Abstract). *Clinical Science* **87**, 26A.

Nicholas, C.W., Green, P.A., Hawkins, R.D. & Williams, C. (1997) Carbohydrate intake and recovery of intermittent running capacity. *International Journal of Sport Nutrition* **7**, 251–260.

Pascoe, D.D., Costill, D.L., Robergs, R.A., Davis, J.A., Fink, W.J. & Pearson, D.R. (1990) Effects of exercise mode on muscle glycogen restorage during repeated days of exercise. *Medicine and Science in Sports and Exercise* **22**, 593–598.

Pizza, F.X., Flynn, M.G., Duscha, B.D., Holden, J. & Kubitz, E.R. (1995) A carbohydrate loading regimen improves high intensity, short duration exercise performance. *International Journal of Sport Nutrition* **5**, 110–116.

Pugh, L.G.C.E. (1970) Oxygen intake in track and treadmill running with observations on the effect of air resistance. *Journal of Physiology* **207**, 823–835.

Quercetani, R.L. (1964) *A World History of Track and Field Athletica*. Oxford University Press, Oxford.

Radford, P.F. (1990) Sprinting. In *Physiology of Sports* (ed. T. Reilly, N. Secher, P. Snell & C. Williams), pp. 71–99. E and FN Spon, London.

Roberts, A.D., Billeter, R. & Howald, H. (1982) Anaerobic muscle enzyme changes after interval training. *International Journal of Sports Medicine* **3**, 18–21.

Sahlin, K. (1996) Acid–base balance during high-intensity exercise. In *Oxford Textbook of Sports Medicine* (ed. M. Harries, C. Williams, W.D. Stanish & L.J. Micheli), pp. 46–52. Oxford University Press, New York.

Schlicht, W., Naretz, W., Witt, D. & Rieckert, H. (1990) Ammonia and lactate: differential information on monitoring training load in sprint events. *International Journal of Sports Medicine* **11** (Suppl. 2), S85–S90.

Sharp, R.L., Costill, D.L., Fink, W.J. & King, D.S. (1986) Effects of eight weeks of bicycle ergometer sprint training on human muscle buffer capacity. *International Journal of Sports Medicine* **7**, 13–17.

Sherman, W.M., Doyle, J.A., Lamb, D.R. & Strauss, R.H. (1993) Dietary carbohydrate, muscle glycogen, and exercise performance during 7 d of training. *American Journal of Clinical Nutrition* **57**, 27–31.

Short, S.H. & Short, W.R. (1983) Four-year study of university athletes' dietary intake. *Journal of the American Dietetic Association* **82**, 632–645.

Simonsen, J.C., Sherman, W.M., Lamb, D.R., Dernbach, A.R., Doyle, J.A. & Strauss, R. (1991) Dietary carbohydrate, muscle glycogen, and power output during rowing training. *Journal of Applied Physiology* **70**, 1500–1505.

Spriet, L.L., Lindinger, M.I., McKelvie, R.S., Heigenhauser, G.J.F. & Jones, N.L. (1989) Muscle glycogenolysis and $H^+$ concentration during maximal intermittent cycling. *Journal of Applied Physiology* **66**, 8–13.

Suminski, R.R., Robertson, R.J., Goss, F.L. *et al.* (1997) Acute effect of amino acid ingestion and resistance exercise on plasma growth hormone concentration in young men. *International Journal of Sport Nutrition* **7**, 48–60.

Symons, J.D. & Jacobs, I. (1989) High-intensity exercise performance is not impaired by low intramuscular glycogen. *Medicine and Science in Sports and Exercise* **21**, 550–557.

Trump, M.E., Heigenhauser, G.J.F., Putman, C.T. & Spriet, L.L. (1996) Importance of muscle phosphocreatine during intermittent maximal cycling. *Journal of Applied Physiology* **80**, 1574–1580.

Tullson, P.C. & Terjung, R.L. (1990) Adenine nucleotide degradation in striated muscle. *International Journal of Sports Medicine* **11** (Suppl. 2), S47–S55.

Van Der Beek, E.J. (1990) Vitamin supplementation and physical exercise performance. *Journal of Sports Sciences* **9**, S77–S89.

Vandenberghe, K., Hespel, P., Vanden Eynde, B., Lysens, R. & Richter, E.A. (1995) No effect of glycogen level on glycogen metabolism during high-intensity exercise. *Medicine and Science in Sports and Exercise* **27**, 1278–1283.

Vollestad, N.K., Tabata, I. & Medbo, J.I. (1992) Glycogen breakdown in different human muscle fibre types during exhaustive exercise of short duration. *Acta Physiologica Scandinavica* **144**, 135–141.

Warren, B.J., Stone, M.H., Kearney, J.T., Fleck, S.J., Kraemer, W.J. & Johnson, R.L. (1991) The effect of amino acid supplementation on physiological responses of elite junior weightlifters (Abstract). *Medicine and Science in Sports and Exercise* **23**, S15.

Williams, C. (1993) Carbohydrate needs of elite athletes. In *Nutrition and Fitness for Athletes* (ed. A.P. Simopoulos & K. Pavlou), pp. 34–60. Karger, New York.

Williams, M.H. (1989) *Beyond Training: How Athletes Enhance Performance Legally and Illegally*. Leisure Press, Champaign, IL.

Williams, M.H. (1993) Dietary supplements, drugs and performance. In *Intermittent High Intensity Exercise: Preparation, Stresses and Damage Limitation* (ed.

D.A.D. Macleod, R.J. Maughan, C. Williams, C.R. Madeley, J.C.M. Sharp & R.W. Nutton), pp. 139–158. E and FN Spon, London.

Wootton, S.A. & Williams, C. (1984) Influence of carbohydrate status on performance during maximal exercise. *International Journal of Sports Medicine* **5**, 126–127.

Yan, Z., Biggs, R.B. & Booth, F.W. (1993) Insulin-like growth factor immunoreactivity increases in muscle after acute eccentric contractions. *Journal of Applied Physiology* **74**, 410–414.

Yarasheski, K.E., Campbell, J.A., Smith, K., Rennie, M.J., Holloszy, J.O. & Bier, D.M. (1992) Effect of growth-hormone and resistance exercise on muscle growth in young men. *American Journal of Physiology* **262**, E261–E267.

# Chapter 42

# Distance Running

JOHN A. HAWLEY, ELSKE-JEANNE SCHABORT AND
TIMOTHY D. NOAKES

## Introduction

Many athletes steadfastly believe that there exists a single nutritional ingredient that will suddenly transform them into world champions. Yet, to the best of our knowledge, the only substances that may confer such advantages to a competitor are already on the International Olympic Committee's list of banned substances. But, ever alert to commercial opportunities, marketers of nutritional supplements for athletes continue to make extravagant claims for the performance-enhancing effects of their products. Sports practitioners need to be aware that there exist few controls to regulate the extent of the claims that such nutritional companies can make for the effectiveness of their products. Unlike the pharmaceutical industry, which requires that all product claims be substantiated by the results of costly, controlled clinical trials, no such control is required in the marketing of nutritional supplements for sport. It is therefore not surprising to find that athletes are often confused about the extent to which nutrition can improve performance.

In this review we analyse the scientific basis for the nutritional practices of athletes, with special reference to distance runners. We believe that although nutrition is important for success, it is only part of a balanced approach. As Olympic gold and silver marathon medallist Frank Shorter has said: 'You don't run 5 minutes a mile for 26 miles on good looks and a secret recipe.'

## What do athletes eat and what should they eat during training?

The major nutritional concern for athletes is the excess energy expended during strenuous training, which, if not matched by an increased energy consumption, will inevitably result in a reduced training capacity and a drop in performance. Top-class athletes undergoing strenuous training can have daily energy expenditures two to three times greater than untrained, weight-matched individuals. This greater energy expenditure may exceed nutritional intake if only normal eating patterns are maintained and could explain the nibbling patterns of eating among athletes.

The macronutrient intakes of well-trained male and female middle- and long-distance runners reported in a review of published studies (Hawley *et al.* 1995a) are summarized in Tables 42.1 and 42.2. A mean weighted carbohydrate (CHO) intake of 48% of total energy consumption was reported by both male and female runners. However, in contrast to male distance runners who usually consume sufficient energy to meet daily training requirements, the energy intake of many of the female athletes was lower than would be expected, given their workload. Among female athletes, iron, zinc, vitamin $B_{12}$ and calcium intakes were also below the recommended daily allowance.

It has long been proposed that the optimum diet for athletes, especially for endurance runners, should contain up to 70% of energy

**Table 42.1** The dietary intakes of well-trained male distance runners. Adapted from Hawley *et al.* (1995a).

| Athletes | *n* | Body mass: kg | Energy: MJ (kcal) | CHO: g (%) [g·kg⁻¹] | Fat: g (%) [g·kg⁻¹] | Protein: g (%) [g·kg⁻¹] |
|---|---|---|---|---|---|---|
| Runners | 10 | — | 17.3 (4121) | 526 (50) | 161 (35) | 144 (15) |
| Endurance runners | 56 | 69 | 13.5 (3226) | 403 (50) [5.84] | 122 (34) [1.76] | 78 (16) [1.40] |
| Distance runners | 35 | — | 12.64 (3020) | 374 (50) | 115 (34) | 119 (16) |
| Distance runners | 10 | — | 12.7 (3034) | 372 (49) | 115 (34) | 129 (17) |
| Marathon runners | 4 | 61 | 13.84 (3309) | 361 (44) [5.92] | 137 (37) [2.24] | 158 (19) [2.59] |
| Marathon runners | 19 | 64 | 14.9 (3570) | 487 (52) [7.6] | 128 (32) [2.0] | 128 (14.5) [2.0] |

**Table 42.2** The dietary intakes of well-trained female distance runners. Adapted from Hawley *et al.* (1995a).

| Athletes | *n* | Body mass: kg | Energy: MJ (kcal) | CHO: g (%) [g·kg⁻¹] | Fat: g (%) [g·kg⁻¹] | Protein: g (%) [g·kg⁻¹] |
|---|---|---|---|---|---|---|
| Endurance runners | 18 | 52 | 9.00 (2151) | 296 (55) [5.69] | 62 (29) [1.19] | 86 (16) [1.65] |
| Distance runners | 17 | — | 8.48 (2026) | 252 (48) | 87 (38) | 74 (14) |
| Distance runners | 18 | 50 | 8.95 (2135) | 224 (47) [4.48] | 89 (39) [1.78] | 74 (14) [1.48] |
| Distance runners | 41 | 55 | 7.84 (1870) | — | — | 70 (15) [1.27] |
| Distance runners | 9 | 53 | 9.21 (2193) | 333 (59) [6.28] | 66 (27) [1.25] | 73 (13) [1.38] |
| Marathon runners | 19 | 53 | 9.62 (2295) | 248 (44) [4.68] | 99 (40) [1.86] | 80 (16) [1.50] |
| US distance runners | 51 | 52 | 14.9 (3570) | 323 (54) [6.2] | 89 (33) [1.7] | 81 (13) [1.5] |

from CHO, with approximately 15% from fat and 15% from protein. However, the *proportional* contribution of CHO, fat and protein to athletes' diets may not be vastly different from that of non-athletes. At first, this paradox may seem confusing. This is because the amount of dietary CHO consumed should not be determined merely as a proportion of total energy intake, but, instead, should rather be based upon the *absolute* amount of CHO consumed relative to the athlete's body mass (BM). Often a 'low' percentage of dietary CHO when calculated from a higher than normal total energy intake results in adequate CHO provision. For example, Costill (1986) reported that a sample of 22 long-distance runners consumed a diet containing only 50% CHO. At first sight, this CHO intake might be considered too low for distance runners, but as their total energy intake was nearly 50% higher than would be expected for individuals of similar size, a more than adequate amount of CHO (375 g·day⁻¹ or 5.7 g·kg⁻¹ body mass·day⁻¹) was being consumed.

The question as to what constitutes an 'adequate' CHO intake has been addressed by several recent studies (Lamb *et al.* 1990; Simonsen *et al.* 1991; Sherman *et al.* 1993). The general consensus is that providing athletes are ingesting 5–6 g CHO·kg⁻¹ body mass·day⁻¹, they are probably not compromising their training capacity. Acute supplementation of the normal diets of trained athletes with additional CHO will, however, elevate muscle glycogen stores and improve performance in competition (for review, see Hawley *et al.* 1997b). Further, when an athlete requires rapid recovery from training, a CHO intake of 8–10 g·kg⁻¹ body mass·day⁻¹ is recommended.

## Muscle glycogen stores and the effect of CHO loading on metabolism

The glycogen content of skeletal muscle of untrained individuals consuming a mixed diet is around 80 mmol·kg⁻¹ wet weight muscle. For individuals involved in regular endurance training and consuming a similar diet, muscle glycogen content is somewhat higher, at approximately 125 mmol·kg⁻¹ wet weight muscle, although this figure will obviously depend on when the measurement was taken in relation to the last training session. After several days of a high (8 g·kg⁻¹ body mass) CHO diet and a reduction in training, the muscle glycogen content may be elevated to values around 175–200 mmol·kg⁻¹ wet weight. There is some evidence that trained athletes who habitually consume a moderate- to high-CHO diet (≈6 g CHO·kg⁻¹ body mass·day⁻¹) do not increase their muscle glycogen contents to the same extent as untrained individuals (Hawley *et al.* 1997a). Indeed, if well-trained athletes consume a moderate- to high-CHO diet, muscle glycogen 'supercompensation' can occur on a day-to-day basis. In this respect, Costill *et al.* (1981) have previously reported that muscle glycogen content was not significantly different when trained runners consumed either 525 or 650 g CHO·day⁻¹, suggesting that the extent of muscle glycogen supercompensation is not further increased by the ingestion of very large (>600 g·day⁻¹) quantities of dietary CHO.

The mechanism(s) explaining the ergogenic effect of CHO loading still needs to be established. One possibility is that the higher muscle glycogen content may delay the onset of fatigue resulting from muscle glycogen depletion during exercise. Alternatively, the increased availability of muscle glycogen could slow the rate of liver glycogen depletion because it would reduce the muscle's demand for blood glucose. Liver glyco-

gen sparing would depend on the rate of hepatic glycogenolysis, which seems to be accelerated by a high liver glycogen content after CHO loading.

## Effect of carbohydrate loading on running performance

The results of studies which have examined the effects of CHO loading and CHO restriction on running performances, are summarized in Tables 42.3 and 42.4. Although there are many laboratory studies which demonstrate a positive relationship between pre-exercise muscle glycogen stores and endurance performance for both cycling and running (for review, see Hawley *et al.* 1997b), to the best of our knowledge only one study has evaluated this effect in the field. Sherman *et al.* (1981) examined the effects of either low-, moderate- or high-CHO diets on muscle glycogen content and utilization during a half-marathon event (20.9 km) in six trained runners. They found that large differences in pre-exercise muscle glycogen contents of the runners had no influence on subsequent performance. In fact, running times were generally a bit slower when athletes started the trials with higher levels of muscle glycogen. Perhaps of physiological interest was that the absolute amount of muscle glycogen left at the end of the three runs was similar regardless of the initial muscle glycogen content.

The results of Sherman *et al.* (1981) were subsequently confirmed in the laboratory by Madsen *et al.* (1990). They reported that 25% higher starting muscle glycogen contents did not improve treadmill run time to exhaustion at 75–80% of maximal oxygen uptake ($\dot{V}o_{2max.}$). In agreement with the data of Sherman *et al.* (1981), the total amount of muscle glycogen utilized during the two treadmill runs was similar. Perhaps the most important finding was that at the point of 'exhaustion', muscle glycogen content was still relatively high in all subjects. These studies strongly suggest that CHO loading has no benefit to performance for athletes who participate in moderate-intensity events lasting up to 90 min.

**Table 42.3** Effects of carbohydrate loading on moderate intensity running lasting 60–90 min. Adapted from Hawley *et al.* (1997b).

| Dietary treatment | Muscle glycogen ($mmol \cdot kg^{-1}$ wet weight) | | Performance measure | Results |
|---|---|---|---|---|
| | Pre-exercise | Postexercise | | |
| A: 3 days LCHO ($1.5\,g \cdot kg^{-1}$ BM, $CHO \cdot day^{-1}$, then 3 days $7.7\,g \cdot kg^{-1}$ BM CHO) | A: $208 \pm 30$ | A: $102 \pm 39$ | 20.9-km run | A: $83 \pm 15$ min ($n = 6$ M) |
| B: 3 days HCHO ($5.0\,g \cdot kg^{-1}$ BM, $CHO \cdot day^{-1}$, then 3 days $7.7\,g \cdot kg^{-1}$ BM CHO) | B: $203 \pm 28$ | B: $96 \pm 17$ | | B: $83 \pm 9$ min |
| C: 6 days NORM ($5.0\,g \cdot kg^{-1}$ BM, $CHO \cdot day^{-1}$) | C: $159 \pm 13$ | C: $96 \pm 28$ | | C: $83 \pm 15$ min |
| A: NORM | A: $135 \pm 28$ | A: $101 \pm 32$ | Run to exhaustion at 75–80% $\dot{V}o_{2max.}$ | A: $70 \pm 20$ min ($n = 3$ M, 3 F) |
| B: 3 days 50% CHO 3 days 70% HCHO | B: $168 \pm 19$ | B: $129 \pm 40$ | | B: $77 \pm 30$ min |

BM, body mass; F, female; HCHO, high carbohydrate intake; LCHO, low carbohydrate intake; M, male; NORM, normal diet; $1\,mmol \cdot kg^{-1}$ wet weight = $4.3\,mmol \cdot kg^{-1}$ dry weight.
All values are mean $\pm$ SD.

In contrast, there is some evidence to indicate that elevating pre-exercise muscle glycogen contents extend endurance time in events lasting longer than 90 min (Table 42.4). Evidence for the important role of muscle glycogen in continuous endurance exercise also comes from studies of the effects of high-CHO diets on running times to fatigue at 70–75% of $\dot{V}o_{2max.}$. The largest increases in running endurance were found in an investigation by Galbo *et al.* (1967). In that study, the subjects ingested extreme diets with either a low (10%) or a high (77%) CHO content. Compared with the low-CHO diet, the high-CHO diet increased muscle glycogen content by about 150% and subsequently extended running times to exhaustion by approximately 66%.

In addition to increasing running times to fatigue, CHO loading may also improve running performance during prolonged exercise in which a set distance must be covered as quickly as possible (i.e. in a race situation). Karlsson and Saltin (1971) reported that the consumption of a diet high in CHO for several days before exercise resulted in improvements of about 6% in race

times during a 30-km event. Interestingly, the twofold higher starting muscle glycogen contents did not increase the initial running speed but, instead, allowed the athletes to maintain a fast race pace for longer. Williams *et al.* (1992) have also reported a similar finding. They observed that a high-CHO diet before exercise increased the speed over the last 5 km of a 30-km treadmill running time-trial and improved overall performance by approximately 2%.

## Fluid and energy replacement during distance running

The pioneering studies showing that CHO ingested during prolonged exercise could enhance endurance performance were conducted on runners competing in the 1924 and 1925 Boston Marathon. The results of these investigations clearly highlighted the importance of CHO loading *before* and CHO ingestion *during* prolonged, steady-state running. Unfortunately for the athletic community, these findings were completely ignored. So too, it seems, were the

**Table 42.4** Effects of carbohydrate loading on prolonged running lasting longer than 90 min. Adapted from Hawley *et al.* (1997b).

| Dietary treatment | Muscle glycogen (mmol·kg⁻¹ wet weight) | | Performance measure | Results |
|---|---|---|---|---|
| | Pre-exercise | Postexercise | | |
| A: 4 days LCHO (10.5% CHO, 76% fat, 13.5% protein) | A: 45±19 | A: 35±21 | Run to exhaustion at 70% $\dot{V}o_{2max}$ | A: 64±16 min (*n*=7 M) |
| B: 4 days HCHO (77% CHO, 13.5% protein, 9.5% fat) | B: 112±61 | B: 75±19 | | B: 106±13 min |
| A: NORM<br>   Trial 1: 4.6±1.3 g·kg⁻¹ BM CHO·day⁻¹<br>   Trial 2: 5.1±1.4 | — | — | Run to exhaustion at 70% $\dot{V}o_{2max}$ | A  Trial 1: 119±19 min<br>   (*n*=15 M, 15 F)<br>   Trial 2: 122±22 min |
| B: COMPLEX CHO<br>   Trial 1: 4.6±1.3 g·kg⁻¹ BM CHO·day⁻¹<br>   Trial 2: 7.7±1.8 | | | | B  Trial 1: 106±24 min<br>   Trial 2: 133±46 min* |
| C: SIMPLE CHO<br>   Trial 1: 4.0±0.7 g·kg⁻¹ BM CHO·day⁻¹<br>   Trial 2: 7.0±1.2 | | | | C  Trial 1: 114±16 min<br>   Trial 2: 141±27 min* |
| A: 3.5 days 6.1 g·kg⁻¹ BM CHO·day⁻¹ (pasta) | A: 103±49 | — | Run to exhaustion at 75% $\dot{V}o_{2max}$ | A: 153±49 min (*n*=14 M) |
| B: 3 days 2.4 g·kg⁻¹ BM CHO·day⁻¹ and depletion exercise, then 3.5 days 11.2 g·kg⁻¹ BM CHO·day⁻¹ (pasta) | B: 130±47 | | | B: 169±30 min |
| C: 3.5 days 6.3 g·kg⁻¹ BM CHO·day⁻¹ (beverage) | C: 107±32 | | | C: 139±26 min |
| D: 3 days 2.5 g·kg⁻¹ BM CHO·day⁻¹ and depletion exercise, then 3.5 days 11.6 g·kg⁻¹ BM CHO·day⁻¹ (beverage) | D: 150±44 | | | D: 168±27 min† |
| A: NORM | A: 100±39 | A: 29±33 | 30-km running race | A: 143±20 min (*n*=10 M) |
| B: HCHO—3 days no CHO, then 3 days 9 g·kg⁻¹ BM CHO·day⁻¹ | B: 194±66 | B: 105±72 | | B: 135.3±18 min |
| A: NORM<br>   Trial 1: 5±1 g·kg⁻¹ BM CHO·day⁻¹<br>   Trial 2: 7 days 5.4±0.8 | — | — | 30-km treadmill run | A: Trial 1: 135.3±14.1 min<br>   (*n*=12 M, 6 F)<br>   Trial 2: 135.3±14.1 min |
| B: HCHO<br>   Trial 1: 5.1±0.8 g·kg⁻¹ BM CHO·day⁻¹<br>   Trial 2: 3 days 8.6±1.3<br>   4 days 6.9±1.2 | | | | B: Trial 1: 137.5±16.5 min<br>   Trial 2: 134.9±16.5 min‡ |

BM, body mass; F, female; HCHO, high carbohydrate intake; LCHO, low carbohydrate intake; M, male; NORM, normal diet; 1 mmol·kg⁻¹ wet weight=4.3 mmol·kg⁻¹ dry weight.
All values are mean±SD.
* $B_2 > B_1$, $C_2 > C_1$ ($P < 0.01$).
† $D > C$ ($P < 0.05$).
‡ 1.9% improvement; increase in speed over last 5 km during Trial 2 ($P < 0.001$).

early investigations showing the importance of adequate fluid replacement during prolonged exercise in the heat. In fact, the earliest reference to fluid replacement during long-distance running is found in the 1953 International Amateur Athletic Federation (IAAF) Handbook controlling marathon events. The handbook stated that 'refreshments shall only be provided by the organizers of a race after 15 km', and that 'no refreshments could be carried or taken by a competitor other than that provided by the organizers'. As water was the only drink available to runners, it was clear that the IAAF had also ignored the pioneering studies conducted in the 1920s showing the benefits of CHO ingestion during long-distance running.

In the 1960s, the IAAF modified their rules slightly, so that by 1967 refreshments were available after only 11 km of a race. Although competitors could now make up their own drink, only water was provided by the race organizers. Between 1960 and 1970, the notion that water was more important than CHO replacement during exercise gained popularity. This was because studies showed that runners who were the most dehydrated after distance races had the highest postrace rectal temperatures. Indeed, the belief that fluid replacement alone was of primary importance for optimizing performance during prolonged exercise was promoted to such an extent that CHO ingestion was actively discouraged. As a result of the perceived importance of fluid replacement, the IAAF again altered their rules in 1977 to allow runners to ingest water earlier and more frequently during competition.

The question of whether water or CHO replacement should be practised during endurance exercise was not really resolved until the late 1970s and early 1980s, when commercial interests in the US revived research into the value of CHO ingestion during exercise. These laboratory controlled studies *conducted on cyclists* confirmed the findings reported some 50 years earlier, which demonstrated that the ingestion of CHO-containing solutions enhanced performance and endurance during prolonged exercise (for review, see Coggan & Coyle 1991). Today, the consumption of CHO–electrolyte beverages is advocated by the IAAF in all races of 10 km and longer. But, the exact amounts that should be consumed to provide sufficient fluid, CHO and electrolytes to replace sweat and energy losses during exercise remain to be established.

### Fluid loss and replacement

Fluid loss during exercise is determined principally by the athlete's sweat rate, which is proportional to their metabolic rate and the prevailing ambient temperature. Estimated sweat rates for endurance runners, along with their rates of fluid intake and measured weight losses, are shown in Table 42.5. One study conducted in the 1960s reported very low rates of fluid intake during a 32-m race ($150\,\text{ml}\cdot\text{h}^{-1}$), with resultant weight losses of more than 2.4 kg and significantly elevated postrace rectal temperatures (Wyndham & Strydom 1969). Largely on the basis of this single finding, it was recommended that runners

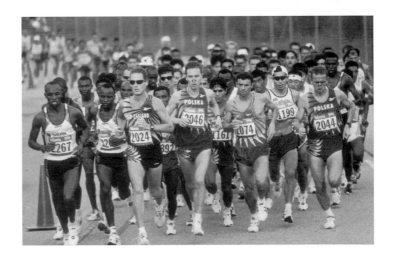

**Fig. 42.1** Endurance events provide an opportunity for intake of fluids and substrate—usually carbohydrate—during the event itself. Photo © Allsport / G. Prior.

**Table 42.5** The rate of fluid loss and fluid ingestion during various long-distance running races. Adapted from Noakes *et al.* (1995).

| Race distance (km) | Fluid intake ($l \cdot h^{-1}$) | Estimated sweat rate ($l \cdot h^{-1}$) | Weight loss (kg) |
|---|---|---|---|
| 32 | 0.15 | 1.35 | 2.4 |
| 42* | 0.4±0.2 | 1.1±1.1 | 2.4±0.3 |
| 56 | 0.5 | 0.9 | 2.0 |
| 67 | 0.4 | 0.8 | 2.4 |
| 90 | 0.5 | 0.85 | 3.5 |

The total fluid intake of runners was determined as the sum of their individual intakes, as reported at various recording points during the race. Sweat rate was estimated from the rate of water loss, minus estimated respiratory losses. Total weight loss was determined as the sweat loss, plus metabolic fuel loss plus fluid intake minus urine output.
*42-km values are means±SD of the average values from seven studies on male subjects. Female sweat rates were lower than those for males over distances of 42 km ($0.6 l \cdot h^{-1}$ vs. $1.1 l \cdot h^{-1}$) and 67 km ($0.5 l \cdot h^{-1}$ vs. $0.8 l \cdot h^{-1}$).

needed to drink 'at least 900 ml of fluid per hour during competition in order not to collapse from heat stroke' (Wyndham & Strydom 1969). Modern studies show that runners do not voluntary consume much more than $500 ml \cdot h^{-1}$ during distance races. In contrast to these moderate rates of fluid intake, sweat rates are invariably around $1.0–1.2 l \cdot h^{-1}$ during events lasting 2 h or more (for review, see Noakes 1993).

One explanation for the failure of runners to match their fluid intake to their fluid losses during exercise is that they develop symptoms of 'fullness' when they attempt to drink fluid at high rates. Feelings of abdominal fullness may, in part, be due to limited rates of fluid absorption, as duodenal and jejunal perfusion studies show the maximum rate of water absorption occurs from isotonic solutions containing glucose, and is limited to about $0.8 l \cdot h^{-1}$ (Davies *et al.* 1980). Similarly, in studies in which sufficient fluid was ingested to match fluid losses during exercise,

not all of the ingested fluid appeared in the extracellular or intracellular fluid pools. Thus, the maximum rate of fluid absorption by the small bowel during exercise may be less than the high rates of fluid loss incurred by some athletes during more intensive exercise, leading to progressive or 'involuntary' dehydration (Noakes 1993).

An alternative hypothesis is that man, unlike other mammals, may develop progressive dehydration during exercise because of the sodium chloride (NaCl) losses in sweat. Large sodium losses attenuate the rise in serum osmolality during exercise-induced dehydration in humans, and since thirst is regulated by changes in both serum osmolality and plasma volume, dipsogenic drive in dehydrated humans ceases before either fluid or sodium losses are fully replaced. Ingestion of NaCl solutions also terminates drinking prematurely by restoring plasma and extracellular volumes before intracellular fluid losses have been replaced. The practical significance of this observation is that whether dehydrated humans drink plain water or NaCl solutions, they tend to stop drinking before they are fully rehydrated. These complex interactions may explain why some humans are unable to prevent the development of 'involuntary' dehydration during prolonged exercise. Additionally, the rapid alleviation of the symptoms that indicate drinking, such as dryness of the mouth, may also cause premature cessation of drinking before full rehydration has occurred.

## Carbohydrate ingestion and oxidation during exercise

Runners are often confused as to the optimum fluid replacement regimen to enhance their performance. Although the addition of high (>15 g per 100 ml) concentrations of CHO to fluid replacement beverages may impair intestinal fluid absorption, inadequate CHO ingestion impairs performance by limiting the rates of CHO oxidation late in exercise. Accordingly, recent attention has focused on strategies to optimize the rate of CHO ingestion and its subsequent oxidation by the working muscles during prolonged exercise. In this regard, gastric volume along with solute energy content and osmolality are critical determinants of the rate of gastric emptying during exercise. With regard to gastric volume, the maximum rate at which CHO and water can be delivered to the intestine from an ingested solution is strongly influenced by the average volume of fluid in the stomach. This, in turn, is governed by the drinking pattern of the athlete. The principal findings of studies that have simultaneously measured rates of gastric emptying and the oxidation of CHO solutions that have been ingested in repeated doses during exercise are, firstly, that the amount of a solution emptied from the stomach is at least double the amount that is ultimately oxidized by the active muscles and, second, provided sufficient is consumed, the peak rates of ingested CHO oxidation

rise to approximately $1\,g\cdot min^{-1}$ after 70–90 min of exercise (for review, see Hawley *et al.* 1992).

An interesting observation from those studies which have fed runners CHO during exercise is that when there is a performance improvement, it coincides with a faster running pace over the *latter* stages of a race or trial. This effect is similar to that seen when subjects CHO-load. That is, the additional CHO does not allow athletes to run faster, but merely resist fatigue and maintain a given pace for longer (for review, see Maughan 1994). Unlike submaximal cycling, CHO ingestion during steady-state running has been shown to result in muscle glycogen sparing (Table 42.6). Although this effect seems limited to the type I fibres, it could potentially have a profound influence on performance during long-distance races. More research specifically related to running needs to be conducted to confirm the results of these preliminary studies.

**Table 42.6** The effects of carbohydrate ingestion on distance running performance.

| Dietary treatment | Drinking regimen | Performance measure | Results/comments | Reference |
|---|---|---|---|---|
| A: Placebo 4 h prior, CHO solution at start and during<br>B: CHO meal 4 h prior, water at start and during | Placebo 10 ml·kg⁻¹ BM fluid CHO meal: 2 g CHO· kg BM At start (8 ml·kg⁻¹ BM) and every 5 km (2 ml·kg⁻¹ BM): water or 6.9% CHO solution | 30-km treadmill time-trial | A: 121.7±13.0 min*<br><br>B: 121.8±11.4 min* | Chryssanthopoulos *et al.* (1994) |
| A: Water<br>B: 5% CHO | 250 ml fluid immediately prior, 150 ml fluid every 5 km | 30-km road race | A: 131.2±18.7 min<br>B: 128.3±19.9 min† | Tsintzas *et al.* (1993) |
| A: Water<br>B. Glucose solution (50 g CHO+20 g glucose)<br>C: Fructose solution (50 g CHO+20 g fructose) | 250 ml fluid before warm-up, 5 min prior to trial, then: 150 ml at 5-km intervals | 30-km treadmill time-trial | A: 129.3±17.7 min‡<br>B: 124.8±14.9 min‡<br><br>C: 125.9±17.9 min‡ | Williams *et al.* (1990) |

*Continued*

**Table 42.6** *Continued.*

| Dietary treatment | Drinking regimen | Performance measure | Results/comments | Reference |
|---|---|---|---|---|
| A: Water<br>B: 7% CHO solution: glucose polymer/fructose solution | 200 ml fluid at time 0, 30, 60 and 90 min | 2-hour treadmill run at 60–65% $\dot{V}o_{2max}$. | CHO solution abolished rise in plasma cortisol and decreased exercise-induced rise in FFA | Deuster *et al.* (1992) |
| A: Water<br>B: 5.5% CHO–electrolyte solution | 5 min prior to exercise: 8 ml · kg$^{-1}$ BM, then: 2 ml · kg$^{-1}$ BM after 20, 40 min | 60-min treadmill run at 70% $\dot{V}o_{2max}$. | CHO ingestion resulted in muscle glycogen sparing in type I muscle fibres | Tsintzas *et al.* (1995) |
| A: Water<br>B: 5.5% CHO solution<br>C: 6.9% CHO solution | 8 ml·kg$^{-1}$ BM CHO solution ingested prior to exercise, then: 2 ml · kg$^{-1}$ BM ingested at 20-min intervals during first hour; thereafter, water until exhaustion | Run until exhaustion at 70% $\dot{V}o_{2max}$. | A: 109.6±31.8 min<br>B: 124.5±26.6 min§<br><br>C: 121.4±29.7 min | Tsintzas *et al.* (1996) |
| A: Placebo<br>B: 7% CHO solution (glucose polymer/sucrose) | 250 ml prior to exercise and 125 ml at 15-min intervals during exercise | Run until exhaustion at 80% $\dot{V}o_{2max}$. | A: 92±27 min<br>B: 115±25 min§ | Wilber and Moffatt (1992) |
| A: Placebo<br>B: Sucrose (81±18 g)<br>C: Caffeine (384±13 mg)<br>D: Sucrose (72±22 g) and caffeine (396±29 mg) | 200 ml 60 min before, 250 ml prior to the start, 250 ml after 45 min | Run until exhaustion at 80% $\dot{V}o_{2max}$. | A: 39.45±11.19 min<br>B: 58.29±15.25 min ‖<br>C: 53.02±9.16 min ‖<br><br>D: 56:58±11:10 min ‖ | Sasaki *et al.* (1987) |
| A: No fluid<br>B: Water<br>C: 5% CHO solution (glucose polymer and fructose) | 240 ml at 15, 30, 45, 60 and 75 min | Run until exhaustion at 85% $\dot{V}o_{2max}$. | A: 56.0±4.39 min<br>B: 78.25±4.93 min¶<br>C: 102.3±7.28 min¶ | Macaraeg (1983) |
| A: Placebo<br>B: 7% CHO–electrolyte drink | 400 ml 30 min prior to exercise and 250 ml at 5-km intervals during the run | 40-km run in the heat: 35 km training pace + 5 km race pace | A: 24.4±4.2 min<br>B: 21.9±2.8 min** | Millard-Stafford *et al.* (1992) |

*Not significant.<br>
†B<A ($P<0.01$).<br>
‡Not significant overall; however, significant decrease in running speed ($P<0.05$) over last 10 km of trial A from 4.14±0.55 to 3.75±0.86 m · s$^{-1}$.<br>
§B>A ($P<0.05$).<br>
‖ B, C, D>A ($P<0.05$).<br>
¶ B, C>A ($P<0.01$).<br>
**B<A ($P<0.03$).

## Conclusions and recommendations for optimal fluid replacement during distance running

The principal aims of fluid ingestion during distance running are to improve performance by:
- limiting any dehydration-induced decreases in plasma volume and skin blood flow;
- limiting any rise in serum sodium osmolality or serum osmolality;
- diminishing progressive rises in rectal temperature;
- decreasing the subjective perception of effort; and
- supplementing endogenous CHO stores.

Although it has been assumed that the optimum rate of fluid ingestion is the rate that closely tracks the rate of fluid loss, the exact composition of the solution that will optimize electrolyte and fluid replacement of the extracellular space has not been established. Furthermore, the rates of fluid ingestion needed to replace the high ($>1 l \cdot h^{-1}$) sweat rates typically induced during prolonged exercise probably exceed the maximal intestinal absorptive capacity for water. Most runners will not be able to achieve such fluid intakes without great difficulty. However, fluid consumption can be maximized during distance running by paying careful attention to the temperature and palatability of the drink and the addition of electrolytes, particularly sodium, to the beverage.

CHO ingestion during distance running is recommended whenever the exercise is of sufficient duration or intensity to deplete endogenous CHO stores. If CHOs are ingested frequently enough and in appropriate volumes, it appears that, with the exception of fructose:
- the type of CHO consumed does not greatly influence the rate of gastric emptying of isoenergetic solutions;
- there are no physiologically important differences in the rates of CHO oxidation resulting from repeated ingestion of a variety of mono-, di- and oligosaccharides during exercise; and
- all ingested CHOs are oxidized at a maximum

rate of approximately $1 g \cdot min^{-1}$ after the first 70–90 min of exercise.

The reason for similar peak rates of ingested CHO oxidation from different CHOs is because, in all likelihood, it is the prevailing concentrations of glucose and insulin normally present during prolonged, moderate-intensity exercise that set the upper limit for the rate of glucose uptake and oxidation by skeletal muscle (Hawley *et al.* 1995b).

The following practical guidelines are suggested for runners participating in prolonged, moderate-intensity exercise of up to 6 h duration:
- Immediately before exercise or during the warm-up, the athlete should ingest up to $5 ml \cdot kg^{-1}$ of body mass of cool, flavoured water.
- For the first 60–75 min of exercise, the athlete should ingest 100–150 ml of a cool, dilute (3.0–5.0 g per 100 ml) glucose polymer solution at regular intervals (10–15 min). It seems unwarranted to consume CHO in amounts much greater than 30 g during this period, as only 20 g of ingested CHO are oxidized in the first hour of moderate-intensity exercise, irrespective of the type of CHO consumed or the drinking regimen.
- After about 90 min of exercise, the concentration of the ingested solution should be increased to 7–10 g per 100 ml, to which 20 mEq $\cdot l^{-1}$ of sodium should be added. Higher sodium concentrations may not be palatable to most athletes, although they may be beneficial. Potassium, which may facilitate rehydration of the intracellular fluid compartment, could also be included in the replacement beverage in small amounts (2–4 mEq $\cdot l^{-1}$). For the remainder of the race, the athlete should consume 100–150 ml of this solution at regular (10–15 min) intervals. Such a drinking regimen will ensure optimal rates of both *fluid* and *energy* delivery, thereby limiting any dehydration-induced decreases in plasma volume, and maintaining the rate of ingested CHO oxidation at approximately $1 g \cdot min^{-1}$ late in exercise.

## References

Chryssanthopoulos, C., Williams, C., Wilson, W.,

Asher, L. & Hearne, L. (1994) Comparison between carbohydrate feedings before and during exercise on running performance during a 30-km treadmill time trial. *International Journal of Sport Nutrition* **4**, 374–386.

Coggan, A.R. & Coyle, E.F. (1991) Carbohydrate ingestion during prolonged exercise: effects on metabolism and performance. In *Exercise and Sports Science Reviews*, Vol. 19 (ed. J.O. Holloszy), pp. 1–40. Williams and Wilkins, Baltimore.

Costill, D.L. (1986) *Inside Running: Basics of Sports Physiology*. Benchmark Press, Indianapolis, IN.

Costill, D.L., Sherman, W.M. & Fink, W.J. (1981) The role of dietary carbohydrates in muscle glycogen resynthesis after strenuous running. *Americal Journal of Clinical Nutrition* **34**, 1831–1836.

Davies, G.R., Santa Ana, C.A., Morawski, S.G. & Fordtran, J.S. (1980) Development of a solution associated with minimal water and electrolyte absorption or secretion. *Gastroenterology* **78**, 991–995.

Deuster, P.A., Singh, A., Hofmann, A., Moses, F.M. & Chrousos, G.C. (1992) Hormonal responses to ingesting water or a carbohydrate beverage during a 2 h run. *Medicine and Science in Sports and Exercise* **24**, 72–79.

Galbo, H., Holst, J. & Christensen, N.J. (1967) The effect of different diets and of insulin on the hormonal response to prolonged exercise. *Acta Physiologica Scandinavica* **107**, 19–32.

Hawley, J.A., Dennis, S.C. & Noakes, T.D. (1992) Oxidation of exogenous carbohydrate ingested during prolonged exercise. *Sports Medicine* **14**, 27–42.

Hawley, J.A., Dennis, S.C., Lindsay, F.H. & Noakes, T.D. (1995a) Nutritional practices of athletes: are they sub-optimal? *Journal of Sports Sciences* **13**, S63-S74.

Hawley, J.A., Dennis, S.C. & Noakes, T.D. (1995b) Carbohydrate, fluid, and electrolyte requirements during prolonged exercise. In *Sports Nutrition: Minerals and Electrolytes* (ed. C.V. Kies & J.A. Driskell), pp. 235–265. CRC Press, Boca Raton, FL.

Hawley, J.A., Palmer, G. & Noakes, T.D. (1997a) Effect of carbohydrate supplementation on muscle glycogen content and utilisation during one hour cycling performance. *European Journal of Applied Physiology and Occupational Physiology* **75**, 407–412.

Hawley, J.A., Schabort, E.J., Noakes, T.D. & Dennis, S.C. (1997b) Carbohydrate loading and exercise performance: an update. *Sports Medicine* **24**, 73–81.

Karlsson, J. & Saltin, B. (1971) Diet, muscle glycogen, and endurance performance. *Journal of Applied Physiology* **31**, 203–206.

Lamb, D.R., Rinehardt, K.F., Bartels, R.L., Sherman, W.M. & Snook, J.T. (1990) Dietary carbohydrate and intensity of interval swim training. *American Journal of Clinical Nutrition* **52**, 1058–1063.

Macaraeg, P.V.J. (1983) Influence of carbohydrate electrolyte ingestion on running endurance. In *Nutrient Utilization During Exercise* (ed. E.L. Fox), pp. 91–96. Ross Laboratories, Columbus, OH.

Madsen, K., Pedersen, P.K. & Rose, P. (1990) Carbohydrate supercompensation and muscle glycogen utilization during exhaustive running in highly trained athletes. *European Journal of Applied Physiology* **61**, 467–472.

Maughan, R. (1994) Physiology and nutrition for middle distance and long distance running. In *Perspectives in Exercise Science and Sports Medicine*. Vol. 7. *Physiology and Nutrition for Competitive Sport* (ed. D.R. Lamb, H.G. Knuttgen & R. Murray), pp. 329–364. Cooper Publishing, Carmel, IN.

Millard-Stafford, M.L., Sparling, P.B., Rosskopf, L.B. & Dicarlo, L.J. (1992) Carbohydrate–electrolyte replacement improves distance running performance in the heat. *Medicine and Science in Sport and Exercise* **24**, 934–940.

Noakes, T.D. (1993) Fluid replacement during exercise. In *Exercise and Sports Science Reviews*, Vol. 21 (ed. J.O. Holloszy), pp. 297–330. Williams and Wilkins, Baltimore.

Noakes, T.D., Hawley, J.A. & Dennis, S.C. (1995) Fluid and energy replacement during prolonged exercise. In *Current Issues in Sports Medicine*, 3rd edn (ed. R.J. Shephard & J.S. Torg), pp. 571–520. Mosby, Philadelphia.

Sasaki, H., Maeda, J., Usui, S. & Ishiko, T. (1987) Effect of sucrose and caffeine ingestion on performance of prolonged strenuous running. *International Journal of Sports Medicine* **8**, 261–265.

Sherman, W.M., Costill, D.L. & Fink, W.J. (1981) The effect of exercise and diet manipulation on muscle glycogen and its subsequent use during performance. *International Journal of Sports Medicine* **2**, 114–118.

Sherman, W.M., Doyle, J.A., Lamb, D.R. & Strauss, R.H. (1993) Dietary carbohydrate, muscle glycogen and exercise performance during 7 d of training. *American Journal of Clinical Nutrition* **57**, 27–31.

Simonsen, J.C., Sherman, W.M., Lamb, D.R., Dernbach, A.R., Doyle, J.A. & Strauss, R. (1991) Dietary carbohydrate, muscle glycogen, and power output during rowing training. *Journal of Applied Physiology* **70**, 1500–1505.

Tsintzas, K., Liu, R., Williams, C., Campbell, I. & Gaitanos, G. (1993) The effect of carbohydrate ingestion on a performance during a 30-km race. *International Journal of Sport Nutrition* **3**, 127–139.

Tsintzas, K., Liu, R., Williams, C., Boobis, L. & Greenhaff, P. (1995) Carbohydrate ingestion and glycogen utilization in different fibre types in man. *Journal of Physiology* **489**, 243–250.

Tsintzas, K., Williams, C., Wilson, W. & Burrin, J. (1996)

Influence of carbohydrate supplementation early in exercise on endurance running capacity. *Medicine and Science in Sports and Exercise* **28**, 1373–1379.

Wilber, R.L. & Moffatt, R.J. (1992) Influence of carbohydrate ingestion on blood glucose and performance in runners. *International Journal of Sport Nutrition* **2**, 317–327.

Williams, C., Nute, M.G., Broadbank, L. & Vinall, S. (1990) Influence of fluid intake on endurance running performance. *European Journal of Applied Physiology* **60**, 112–119.

Williams, C., Brewer, J. & Walker, M. (1992) The effect of a high carbohydrate diet on running performance during a 30-km treadmill time trial. *European Journal of Applied Physiology* **65**, 18–24.

Wyndham, C.H. & Strydom, N.B. (1969) The danger of inadequate water intake during marathon running. *South African Medical Journal* **43**, 893–896.

# Chapter 43

# Cycling

ASKER E. JEUKENDRUP

## Introduction

Without doubt, cycling is the sport most intensively studied by exercise physiologists and sport nutritionists. Christensen and Hansen (1939) were among the first to report the effect of different diets on cycling performance. These early reports already demonstrated the importance of carbohydrates (CHO) for improving or maintaining exercise performance. Since then, many studies have investigated the effect of CHO feedings during cycling, and the role of CHO after exercise to replenish glycogen stores and improve recovery (see Chapters 5–8). This chapter will review some of the nutritional habits of cyclists and will define some recommendations for nutrition during bicycling races or intensive training. Although cycling obviously has many disciplines (including road racing, time trialing, track cycling, mountain biking, BMX), this chapter will focus on road racing and time trialling.

## Energy cost of cycling

Cycling, triathlon and cross-country skiing are among the sports with the highest reported energy turnovers. The levels of energy expenditure in these endurance sports have been measured in the field by using doubly labelled water, an accurate technique which allows measurements over longer periods (days) in the field (Westerterp et al. 1986). Of particular interest are the data obtained during the most demanding

cycling race in the world: the Tour de France (Saris et al. 1989). This race has 20 stages and lasts about 3 weeks in which the riders cover almost 4000 km. During these 3 weeks, energy expenditures of up to 35 MJ·day$^{-1}$ (8300 kcal·day$^{-1}$) have been reported during the long (300 km) stages (Saris et al. 1989). Recently, we performed measurements of power output during the stages of the Tour de France using a power-measuring system (SRM Training System, Germany) which is claimed to be accurate to ±1%, and to record and store power data at 1-s intervals (G. Leinders & A.E. Jeukendrup, unpublished findings). These data show that average power output during a 6-h stage may be over 240 W, which indicates a very high energy turnover. With an estimated average efficiency of 22%, this represents an energy expenditure of about 24 MJ (5700 kcal) during the race itself. In order to maintain energy balance, a similar amount of energy has to be consumed on a daily basis.

Most of the energy intake is derived from CHO (Saris et al. 1989), which is less energy-dense than lipid, and many CHO-rich foods are bulky and rich in fibre. A high-CHO/high-energy diet entails a large food volume and considerable eating time. Since cyclists in the Tour de France are usually on the bike for 4–6 h·day$^{-1}$ and they avoid eating 1–3 h before the start, there is barely time left to eat the large meals. Besides this, appetite is usually depressed after strenuous exercise. These factors make it very hard to maintain energy balance on a daily basis.

Studies on energy balance have usually

employed indirect calorimetry or doubly labelled water as techniques to measure energy expenditure, while energy intake is usually estimated by the reported food intakes of athletes. The reported energy intakes, however, display large variation and are susceptible to a number of methodological errors. Besides that, there are only a few studies available in the literature which systematically looked at the food intake of cyclists. Nevertheless, the few available studies report mean energy intakes which are similar to those of other groups of endurance athletes and which range from 15 to 25 MJ·day$^{-1}$ (3500–6000 kcal·day$^{-1}$) for male athletes (Erp van-Baart et al. 1989), cyclists in the Tour de France and

Tour de l'Avenir having the highest energy intakes (Table 43.1).

During the Tour de France, mean food intake was 24.3 MJ·day$^{-1}$ (5800 kcal·day$^{-1}$) while the highest recorded values reached 32.4 MJ (7600 kcal) on the days of the long (300 km) stages (Saris et al. 1989). This indicates that the athletes in the Tour de France match their energy expenditures quite well with their food intake (Fig. 43.1), and they remain weight stable (i.e. maintain energy balance) during the entire race. Only during the long stages with extremely high energy expenditures could food intake not completely compensate for the energy expended. In general, riders in the Tour de France remain

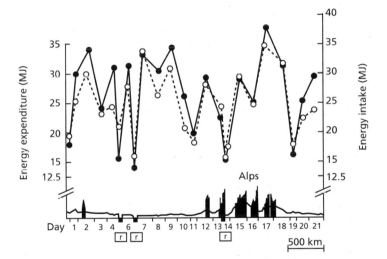

**Fig. 43.1** Daily energy expenditure (●) and energy intake (○) as measured in a cyclist during the Tour de France. The profile of the race as well as the length of the stages are indicated at the bottom of this figure. r, days of rest. From Saris et al. (1989).

**Table 43.1** Daily energy expenditures (EE) and energy intakes (EI) in cyclists.

| Race/category | EE | EI (MJ) | Reference |
|---|---|---|---|
| 24-h race | NR | 43.4 | Lindeman et al. 1991 |
| Race across America | NR | 35.4 | Lindeman et al. 1991 |
| Tour de France (peak) | 32.7 MJ | 32.4 | Saris et al. 1989 |
| Tour de France (mean) | 25.4 MJ | 24.7 | Saris et al. 1989 |
| Tour de France | NR | 24.3 | Van Erp-Baart et al. 1989 |
| Tour de l'Avenir | NR | 23.3 | Van Erp-Baart et al. 1989 |
| Amateur cyclists | NR | 18.3 | Van Erp-Baart et al. 1989 |

NR, not recorded.

remarkably weight stable (Saris *et al.* 1989; A.E. Jeukendrup & G. Leinders, unpublished findings). Anecdotal evidence suggests that racers who lose weight may not be able to finish the race.

Brouns and colleagues (Brouns *et al.* 1989b–d) performed a simulation study in the laboratory in which the effect of diet manipulation was studied in athletes expending 26 MJ·day$^{-1}$ (6200 kcal·day$^{-1}$) by exercising for 5 h in a respiration chamber. Subjects received *ad libitum* a conventional solid diet with a high carbohydrate content (62.5% CHO diet) supplemented with water or the same diet supplemented with a 20% CHO solution (80% CHO diet). Although food intake was allowed *ad libitum* in both trials, the CHO supplement enabled the subjects to maintain their daily energy balance, which they could not when supplemented with water. As a consequence, exercise performance was improved. These data show that during stage races or multiple days of intensive training, energy expenditure is very high and CHO-containing drinks may be required to maintain energy balance in cyclists involved in such rigorous programmes, since digestion and absorption of solid meals will be impaired and hunger feelings are suppressed during intensive physical exercise (Brouns 1986).

Other reports in the literature regarding energy intake of cyclists include those of the Race Across America, a race from the West coast to the East coast of the United States (Lindeman 1991). Energy intake in one individual taking part in this race was 35.4 MJ (8429 kcal) daily of which 78% was derived from CHO. During the preparation, this individual rode a 24-h race where his energy intake was as much as 43.4 MJ·day$^{-1}$ (10 343 kcal·day$^{-1}$) with 75% of the energy from CHO.

## Eating behaviour of cyclists

An important observation from several of the investigations which have reported very high energy intakes in athletes is that a significant amount of the day's nutrient intake may be consumed while the individual is exercising. For example, CHO-rich foods and drinks consumed while riding provided nearly 50% of the total energy, and 60% of the daily CHO intake of cyclists competing in the Tour de France stages (Saris *et al.* 1989). Only by adopting such a nutritional regimen do these cyclists maintain energy balance over the 20 days of the Tour de France. Suitable food choices to attain such goals include concentrated sports drinks and portable CHO-rich foods such as fruit, confectionery, bread, cakes and sports bars. It has also been reported that a large part of the carbohydrates is from snacks. These snacks usually contain simple carbohydrates, a fair amount of fat and little or no micronutrients, and therefore it has often been recommended that riders should replace these snacks by fruit and snacks that contain less fat and more micronutrients (Brouns 1986).

## Preparing for a race

Athletes involved in prolonged moderate- to high (>70% of maximal oxygen uptake) intensity exercise not only have unusually high energy requirements but they also have greatly increased CHO needs. The extra CHO is necessary to optimize fuel availability during training sessions used, and to promote postexercise muscle glycogen resynthesis. A well-known method to restore glycogen levels to the preexercise level or even above that is known as glycogen loading or glycogen supercompensation.

### Glycogen loading

Muscle glycogen depletion and low blood glucose levels have been shown to be major factors in the development of fatigue during endurance exercise. It is therefore important to ensure optimal glycogen storage prior to exercise and optimal delivery of CHO during exercise. These aspects have been discussed in detail in Chapter 7. Supercompensation protocols as described by Bergström and Hultman (Bergström *et al.* 1967) and later adapted by

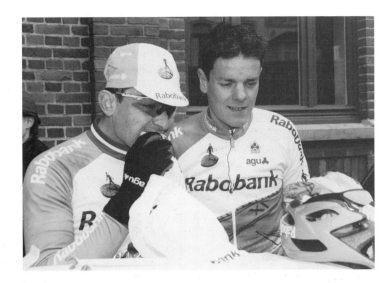

**Fig. 43.2** Pre-exercise feedings will top up liver glycogen. Photo © Cor Vos.

Sherman *et al.* (1981) do not usually apply to cycling at the highest level. Professional cyclists and top-level amateurs have too many races in a short time period and a week of nutritional preparation is usually not possible. For this group of cyclists, it is often recommended that they eat high-CHO diets which are often expressed in percentages of CHO in daily energy intake. However, the absolute amounts may be more important. In a 70-kg subject, the body CHO stores are believed to amount to about 600–700 g (about 10 g · kg$^{-1}$ body weight). It is believed that ingesting more than 600–700 g (10 g · kg$^{-1}$ body weight) of CHO to replenish these stores will not further improve glycogen storage (Rauch *et al.* 1995). This is especially important for sports with repeated days of exercise with very high energy expenditures, such as in the Tour de France (Saris *et al.* 1989). If these athletes would consume a 70% CHO diet (as often recommended), they would consume more than a kilo of CHO, assuming an energy intake of 25 MJ (6000 kcal).

Recently, however, we observed increased glycogen storage after ingestion of 12–13 g · kg$^{-1}$ body weight · day$^{-1}$ compared to 9 g · kg$^{-1}$ · day$^{-1}$ when athletes trained on a daily basis (A.E. Jeukendrup *et al.*, unpublished observations).

### Prerace feedings

It is often recommended that CHO ingestion should be avoided in the hours preceding the race in order to prevent rebound hypoglycaemia. CHO ingestion 30–120 min prior to exercise raises plasma glucose and insulin levels, which stimulates glucose uptake and inhibits fat mobilization and oxidation during exercise. Early studies showed that CHO ingestion in the fasted state, about 45–60 min prior to an acute bout of exercise, may result in a drop in the blood glucose concentration as soon as exercise begins (Foster *et al.* 1979; Koivisto *et al.* 1981). During intense exercise, this was shown in one study to result in hypoglycaemia and decreased performance (Foster *et al.* 1979). However, more recent studies, in the fasted state (Gleeson *et al.* 1986) as well as in the non-fasted state, as is usual in athletes going into competition, have not shown these detrimental effects (Brouns *et al.* 1991). Due to strong individual differences in response, however, it is always possible that an individual is prone to an exercise-induced insulin rebound response after a CHO-rich solid or liquid meal. In addition, pre-exercise CHO feedings 2–4 h before the race may inhibit lipolysis, decrease the availability of plasma fatty acids and thereby deprive the muscle of substrate. This, in turn, may accelerate glycogenolysis and increase whole-body CHO oxidation. Large pre-exercise CHO feedings may compensate for the excess oxidized CHO by providing sufficient glucose through the blood, whereas small CHO feedings may not provide sufficient substrate and result in premature glycogen depletion and fatigue. So, pre-exercise CHO feedings should be large enough (>200 g) to provide substrate to the muscle to compensate for the accelerated glycogen breakdown and increased CHO oxidation.

## Recommendations for precompetition nutrition

**1** Ensure a CHO intake of 10 g·kg$^{-1}$ body weight·day$^{-1}$ during the 3 days before the race. This amount of CHO should maximize glycogen storage.
**2** Drink plenty of fluids during the days before the race, to ensure euhydration at the start. If large sweat losses are to be expected, add a little sodium (a pinch of salt) to the drinks.
**3** Avoid food with a high dietary fibre content during the days before the competition to prevent gastrointestinal problems.
**4** Eat a CHO-rich meal 2–4 h before the race to replenish the liver glycogen stores: before short races, light digestible CHO foods or energy drinks; before long races, semisolid or solid food such as energy bars and bread. Too much protein and fat should be avoided since this may slow gastric emptying and may cause gastrointestinal discomfort. This meal should contain a fair amount of CHO (>200 g) to compensate for the increased glycogen breakdown and CHO oxidation.
**5** Although in general the intake of CHO in the hours before a race does not have adverse effects on performance, some individuals may develop rebound hypoglycaemia when ingesting a high-CHO meal or drinks before the race. These individuals should delay eating CHO until the warming up or 5 min before the race. An oral glucose tolerance test can be used to determine which individuals are prone to develop rebound hypoglycaemia.

## Nutrition during exercise

### Nutrition during exercise longer than 90 min

CHO ingestion during exercise has been shown to improve exercise performance in events of 90 min duration and longer by maintaining high plasma glucose levels and high levels of CHO oxidation. The increased availability of plasma glucose enables the athlete to postpone fatigue or to develop a higher power output in a final sprint following endurance exercise (Hargreaves et al. 1984; Coggan & Coyle 1987, 1988, 1989; Mitchell et al. 1988; Goodpaster et al. 1996). From numerous studies, we know that most of the soluble CHO (glucose, maltose, sucrose, glucose polymers, soluble starch) are oxidized at similar rates, as reviewed by Hawley et al. (1992), and similar improvements in cycling performance have been observed when ingesting glucose, maltodextrins or soluble starch (Goodpaster et al. 1996). Exceptions are fructose, galactose and insoluble starch, which are oxidized at slightly lower rates (Saris et al. 1993; Leijssen et al. 1995) and do not seem to have the same positive effect on performance (Goodpaster et al. 1996). Therefore, glucose, maltose, sucrose, glucose polymers and soluble starch are all good CHO types to ingest during exercise. Ingested CHO may be oxidized at rates up to 1 g·min$^{-1}$, which appears to be the maximal exogenous CHO oxidation rate (for review, see Hawley et al. 1992). Recently, we reported that the oxidation rate of ingested CHO was similar in well-trained cyclists and untrained individuals when they are exercising at the same relative intensity and same rates of total CHO oxidation (Jeukendrup et al. 1997b). The oxidation of exogenous CHO seems related to the amount ingested (up to a certain limit) and the exercise intensity and active muscle mass rather than any other variables. Its maximal oxidation rate may be determined by the absorption rate or by liver metabolism (Jeukendrup 1997; Jeukendrup et al. 1999). However, additional research is required to study the factors limiting exogenous CHO oxidation. In order to maximize the contribution of oral CHO to total energy expenditure, it may be advised that 1–1.2 g CHO·min$^{-1}$ (60–70 g·h$^{-1}$)

should be ingested during exercise while slightly higher rates of ingestion during the first hour may speed up the achievement of these high levels of oxidation. However, ingesting more than $1.5 \, g \cdot min^{-1}$ during exercise may not result in increased exogenous CHO oxidation (Wagenmakers *et al.* 1993) and increases the risk of gastrointestinal problems.

Most studies of cyclists have shown that CHO ingestion does not alter the rate of muscle glycogen breakdown during exercise, although during intermittent exercise glycogen may be resynthesized during the low-intensity cycles (Hargreaves *et al.* 1984; Kuipers *et al.* 1986). So the mechanism by which CHO ingestion during cycling improves performance in road races may not only be maintaining the plasma glucose concentration, but also the resynthesis of muscle glycogen during periods of low intensity.

### Nutrition during high-intensity exercise of about 1h

Although previous studies suggested that CHO feedings can improve exercise performance during exercise of longer than 90 min duration, recent evidence shows that CHO feedings can also be effective during high-intensity exercise of shorter duration (60 min) (Anantaraman *et al.* 1995; Below *et al.* 1995; Jeukendrup *et al.* 1997a).

We recently found improved time-trial performance (comparable to a 40-km time trial) in well-trained cyclists when they ingested a carbohydrate–electrolyte solution during exercise (75 g of CHO) compared with placebo (Fig. 43.3) (Jeukendrup *et al.* 1997a). Seventeen out of 19 subjects showed improved time-trial performance, while two athletes displayed a decreased performance with the carbohydrate–electrolyte solution. The average power output during the time trial when the carbohydrate–electrolyte solution was ingested was $298 \pm 10 \, W$ vs. $291 \pm 10 \, W$ with placebo. Although the beneficial effect of the CHO ingestion during high intensity exercise of about 1 h duration has now been confirmed by several studies, the mechanism behind this performance effect remains unclear and central effects of glucose on the brain cannot be excluded at this point (Jeukendrup *et al.* 1997a). Optimally, athletes should ingest a carbohydrate–electrolyte solution throughout exercise in order to maintain a certain volume of fluid in the stomach which will enhance gastric emptying (Rehrer *et al.* 1990). It has recently been shown that ingestion of CHO throughout exercise improves performance more than ingestion of an identical amount of CHO late in exercise (McConell *et al.* 1996). Again, these results suggest that CHO ingestion improves performance through mechanisms other than, or in

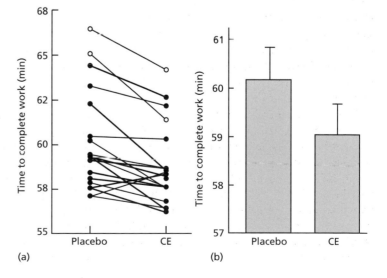

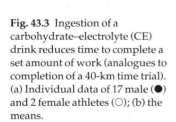

**Fig. 43.3** Ingestion of a carbohydrate–electrolyte (CE) drink reduces time to complete a set amount of work (analogues to completion of a 40-km time trial). (a) Individual data of 17 male (●) and 2 female athletes (○); (b) the means.

addition to, an increased CHO availability to the contracting muscles.

## Medium-chain triacylglycerol ingestion during exercise

Recently it has been suggested that medium-chain triacylglycerol (MCT) ingestion during cycling exercise may provide an additional fuel, thereby possibly sparing endogenous CHO stores and improving exercise capacity. MCT is derived from coconut oil and contains medium-chain fatty acids which are rapidly absorbed and oxidized (Massicotte *et al.* 1992; Jeukendrup *et al.* 1995, 1996a). However, despite its rapid metabolism, several studies show that ingestion of small amounts of MCT (25–45 g of MCT over the course of 1–3 h) may not be sufficient to alter fat oxidation, glycogen breakdown or cycling performance (Ivy *et al.* 1980; Jeukendrup *et al.* 1995, 1996a, 1996b, 1998). Larger amounts generally cause gastrointestinal problems and can therefore not be recommended.

## Fluid intake during exercise

Besides CHO, cyclists need to maintain their water balance. Exercise-induced dehydration may augment hyperthermia and multiple studies show that prevention of dehydration by fluid ingestion improves performance (see Chapter 16). Dependent on the weather conditions, fluid losses may vary from 0.5 to up to almost $3 \cdot h^{-1}$. Individual fluid loss can be estimated from weight loss although this also includes a small amount of weight loss due to glycogen and fat oxidation. During 90 min of exercise, 100–300 g of glycogen and fat may be oxidized. By regularly monitoring body weight before and after training sessions and competitions, it is possible to predict the fluid loss in a certain race. However, since the main limitation seems to be the amount of beverage that can be tolerated in the gastrointestinal tract, in most conditions it is advisable to drink as much as possible. Completely compensating for sweat loss by fluid consumption may not always be pos-

sible because sweat losses may exceed $2 \cdot h^{-1}$ and ingestion of such amounts cannot be tolerated by the gastrointestinal tract. Observations in professional cyclists during the Mediterranean Tour in France and the Ruta del Sol in Spain show that riders lose about 2.1–4.5 kg during a 4–5-h stage, indicating that even cyclists who are well aware of the importance of drinking cannot drink sufficiently during a race (G. Leinders & A.E. Jeukendrup, unpublished findings). Therefore, fluid and CHO consumption is usually limited by the practical situation and by the amount of drink that can be tolerated after ingestion. This highlights the importance of making 'drinking during exercise' a part of the regular training programme.

Also during high-intensity exercise of about 1 h duration, water seems to be beneficial to performance. Below *et al.* (1995) showed that water ingestion, independently of CHO, improved time-trial performance (time trial of about 10 min duration after 50 min at 80% $\dot{V}o_{2max.}$), while the CHO and water had an additive effect on performance.

Palatability of drinks and food is a very important aspect because it will stimulate consumption and with it increase the intake of fluid and CHO. In addition, taste and flavour perception may also influence the rate of gastric emptying. Disliked flavour or aroma may slow gastric emptying and may even cause nausea.

## Nutrition during exercise: some observations in professional cyclists

In general, professional cyclists tend to eat solid food during the first hours of their stages, usually consisting of chunks of banana, apple, white bread with jamor rice cakes. The pace during the first hours is usually slow and there is plenty of time to digest the solid food. As soon as the speed increases, the cyclists switch to fluid ingestion and solid food will only be eaten when the speed drastically drops or their stomachs feel empty. Since they have only two bottles on their bike, usually containing 0.5l each, they have to get new bottles regularly during the race. Profes-

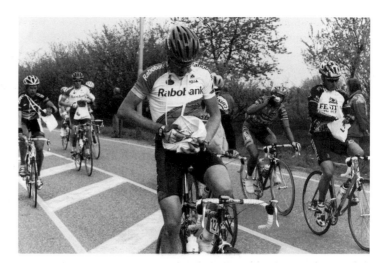

**Fig. 43.4** Feeding zone where bags with solid and liquid food are given to the riders. Photo © Cor Vos.

sional cyclists often receive their new bottles from the team director in the car behind the pack. One or two riders of the team will go to the car and bring bottles for the whole team. Also they usually have the opportunity to get additional bottles at the feeding zone (2–4 h into the race). At these feeding zones the athletes will receive a little bag containing one or two bottles of fluid and some solid food in case they get hungry or get an empty feeling in their stomach (Fig. 43.4). Often riders will take the bottles and throw away the solid food.

### Recommendations for nutrition during exercise

**1** During intense exercise lasting 45 min or more, a CHO solution should be ingested. This may improve performance by reducing/delaying fatigue.

**2** Consume 60–70 g CHO·h–1 of exercise. This can be optimally combined with fluid in quantities related to needs determined by environmental conditions, individual sweat rate and gastrointestinal tolerance.

**3** During exercise of up to 30–45 min duration, there appears to be little need to consume CHO.

**4** The type of soluble CHO (glucose, sucrose, glucose polymer, etc.) does not make much difference when ingested in low to moderate quantities. Fructose and galactose are less effective.

**5** Athletes should consume CHO beverages throughout exercise, rather than only water early in exercise followed by a CHO beverage late in exercise.

**6** Avoid drinks extremely high in CHO and/or osmolality (>15–20% CHO) because fluid delivery will be hampered and gastrointestinal problems may occur.

**7** Try to predict the fluid loss during endurance events of more than 90 min. The amount of fluid to be ingested should in principle equal the predicted fluid loss. In warm weather conditions with low humidity, athletes have to drink more and the drinks can be more dilute. In cold weather conditions, athletes will drink only small amounts and drinks have to be more concentrated.

**8** Large drink volumes stimulate gastric emptying more than small volumes. Therefore, it is recommended to ingest a fluid volume of 6–8 ml·kg–1 body weight 3–5 min prior to the start to 'prime' the stomach, followed by smaller volumes (2–3 ml·kg–1 body weight) every 15–20 min.

**9** The volume of fluid that athletes can ingest is usually limited. Athletes should 'learn' to drink during exercise. This aspect can be trained.

**10** After drinking a lot, the stomach may feel empty and uncomfortable. In this case it may be wise to eat some light digestible solid food (CHO). During long, low-intensity races, solid food can be eaten also in the first phase of the race.

**11** Factors such as fibre content, protein content, high osmolality and high CHO concentrations have been associated with the development of gastrointestinal symptoms during exercise, and thus should be avoided during exercise.

## Nutrition after exercise

Quick recovery is an extremely important aspect of training and frequent competitions. Especially during repeated days of training or in stage races, it is important to recover as quickly as possible. Dietary measures have been shown to influence recovery significantly. The restoration of muscle glycogen stores and fluid balance after heavy training or competition is probably the most important factor determining the time needed to recover. The rate at which glycogen can be formed (synthesized) is dependent on several factors:

**1** The quantitative CHO ingestion.
**2** The type of CHO.
**3** The timing of CHO ingestion after exercise.
**4** Coingestion of other nutrients.

### Amount of CHO ingestion

The quantity of CHO is by far the most important factor determining the rate of glycogen resynthesis. In studies, it appeared that the muscle glycogen resynthesis rate of 50 g CHO ingested every 2 h was double that of 25 g CHO ingested every 2 h (Blom *et al.* 1987; Ivy *et al.* 1988b). When more than 50 g was ingested (100–225 g), muscle glycogen storage did not further increase (Blom *et al.* 1987; Ivy *et al.* 1988b). Thus, 50 g in 2 h (or 25 g · h$^{-1}$) appears to result in a maximum rate of postexercise muscle glycogen resynthesis. Frequent small meals do not appear to have an advantage over a few large meals.

### Type of CHO

To optimally restore glycogen levels after exercise, a source of CHO which is easily digested and absorbed is needed. The rate of absorption of a certain CHO is reflected by the glycaemic index. Foods with a moderate to high glycaemic

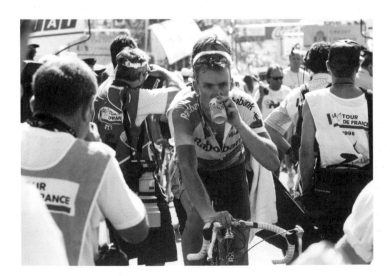

**Fig. 43.5** Rehydration and carbohydrate loading start immediately after the race. Photo © Cor Vos.

index enter the bloodstream relatively rapidly, resulting in a high rate of glycogen storage. Foods with a low glycaemic index enter the bloodstream slowly and result in a lower rate of glycogen resynthesis. Therefore it is recommended that low glycaemic index foods should not comprise the bulk of CHO after exercise when a quick recovery is required.

### Timing of CHO intake

During the first hours following exercise, glycogen resynthesis proceeds at a somewhat higher rate than later on (Ivy *et al.* 1988a). Therefore, in cases of short recovery times, CHO intake should take place immediately after exercise. Although this can maximize the rate of glycogen resynthesis in the early phase, the full process of glycogen storage still takes considerable time. Depending on the degree of glycogen depletion and the type of meals consumed, it may take 10–36h to refill the glycogen stores to pre-exercise values. Therefore, it is impossible to perform two or more workouts per day without affecting the initial glycogen stores. Even when CHO intake between training bouts or competitions is very high, the muscle glycogen levels will be suboptimal when the next activity is started within 8–16h.

The rate at which fluid balance can be restored depends on (i) the quantity of fluid consumed and (ii) the composition of the fluid, especially the sodium content. Recent studies show that the postexercise fluid retention approximates 50% when the fluid that is consumed is low in sodium. This is the case with most tap and mineral waters as well as fruit juices. After the consumption of carbohydrate–electrolyte solutions containing 25–100mmol·l⁻¹ sodium, the water retention may be as high as 70–80% (Maughan & Leiper 1995; Shirreffs *et al.* 1996). From these findings, it can also be concluded that, in order to restore fluid balance, the postexercise fluid consumption must be considerably higher (150–200%) than the amount of fluid lost as sweat.

### Practical considerations

Usually, appetite is suppressed after exercise and there is a preference for drinking fluids rather than eating a meal. Therefore, beverages which contain high-glycaemic-index CHO sources in sufficient quantity (6g·100ml⁻¹ or more) should be made available.

If preferred, the athlete may also ingest easily digestible solid CHO-rich food such as ripe banana, rice cake and sweets. When the desire for normal meals returns, approximately 10g CHO·kg⁻¹ body weight of moderate- to high-glycaemic-index CHO sources should be eaten within 24h. This can easily be realized by consuming foods that are low in fat. For practical reasons, a certain amount of low-glycaemic CHO cannot be excluded from the diet.

Sleeping hours interrupt the feeding possibilities. Therefore, it is recommended to ingest an amount of CHO prior to sleeping which is sufficient to supply the required 25g·h⁻¹ (e.g. 250g for a 10-h period).

### Guidelines for postexercise nutrition

1 To maximize glycogen storage, it is recommended to ingest 100g CHO during the first 2h after exercise in the form of liquids or easily digestible solid or semisolid meals. In total, about 10g CHO·kg⁻¹ body weight should be eaten within 24h, with two thirds of this preferably as high glycaemic index foods.
2 It is recommended to consume CHO sources with moderate to high glycaemic index to hasten recovery.
3 Addition of 25–100mmol·l⁻¹ sodium to postexercise rehydration beverages improves fluid retention and the recovery of fluid balance.

## Acknowledgements

The author would like to thank Dr G. Leinders and the Rabobank professional cycling team for their friendly co-operation.

# References

Anantaraman, R., Carmines, A.A., Gaesser, G.A. & Weltman, A. (1995) Effects of carbohydrate supplementation on performance during 1 h of high intensity exercise. *International Journal of Sports Medicine* **16**, 461–465.

Below, P.R., Mora-Rodríguez, R., Gonzáles Alonso, J. & Coyle, E.F. (1995) Fluid and carbohydrate ingestion independently improve performance during 1 h of intense exercise. *Medicine and Science in Sports and Exercise* **27**, 200–210.

Bergström, J., Hermansen, L., Hultman, E. & Saltin, B. (1967) Diet, muscle glycogen and physical performance. *Acta Physiologica Scandinavica* **71**, 140–150.

Blom, P.C.S., Høstmark, A.T., Vaage, O., Kardel, K.R. & Maehlum, S. (1987) Effect of different post-exercise sugar diets on the rate of muscle glycogen resynthesis. *Medicine and Science in Sports and Exercise* **19**, 491–496.

Brouns, F. (1986) Dietary problems in the case of strenuous exertion. *Journal of Sports Medicine and Physical Fitness* **26**, 306–319.

Brouns, F., Rehrer, N.J., Saris, W.H.M., Beckers, E., Menheere, P. & ten Hoor, F. (1989a) Effect of carbohydrate intake during warming up on the regulation of blood glucose during exercise. *International Journal of Sports Medicine* **10**, S68–S75.

Brouns, F., Saris, W.H.M., Beckers, E. *et al.* (1989b) Metabolic changes induced by sustained exhaustive cycling and diet manipulation. *International Journal of Sports Medicine* **10**, S49–S62.

Brouns, F., Saris, W.H.M., Stroecken, J. *et al.* (1989c) Eating, drinking, and cycling: a controlled Tour de France simulation study. Part I. *International Journal of Sports Medicine* **10**, S32–S40.

Brouns, F., Saris, W.H.M., Stroecken, J. *et al.* (1989d) Eating, drinking, and cycling: a controlled Tour de France simulation study. Part II. Effect of diet manipulation. *International Journal of Sports Medicine* **10**, S41–S48.

Brouns, F., Rehrer, N.J., Beckers, E., Saris, W.H.M., Menheere, P. & ten Hoor, F. (1991) Reaktive hypoglykamie. *Deutsche Zeitschrift fuer Sportmedizin* **42**, 188–200.

Christensen, E.H. & Hansen, O. (1939) Arbeitsfahigkeit und ernahrung. *Scandinavian Archives of Physiology* **81**, 160–171.

Coggan, A.R. & Coyle, E.F. (1987) Reversal of fatigue during prolonged exercise by carbohydrate infusion or ingestion. *Journal of Applied Physiology* **63**, 2388–2395.

Coggan, A.R. & Coyle, E.F. (1988) Effect of carbohydrate feedings during high-intensity exercise. *Journal of Applied Physiology* **65**, 1703–1709.

Coggan, A.R. & Coyle, E.F. (1989) Metabolism and performance following carbohydrate ingestion late in exercise. *Medicine and Science in Sports and Exercise* **21**, 59–65.

Coyle, E.F. & Coggan, A.R. (1984) Effectiveness of carbohydrate feeding in delaying fatigue during prolonged exercise. *Sports Medicine* **1**, 446–458.

Erp van-Baart, A.M.J., Saris, W.H.M., Binkhorst, R.A., Vos, J.A. & Elvers, J.W.H. (1989) Nationwide survey on nutritional habits in elite athletes. Part I. Energy carbohydrate, protein. *International Journal of Sports Medicine* **10**, S3–S10.

Foster, C., Costill, D.L. & Fink, W.J. (1979) Effects of preexercise feedings on endurance performance. *Medicine and Science in Sports and Exercise* **11**, 1–5.

Gleeson, M., Maughan, R.J. & Greenhaff, P.L. (1986) Comparison of the effects of pre-exercise feeding of glucose, glycerol and placebo on endurance and fuel homeostasis in man. *European Journal of Applied Physiology* **55**, 645–653.

Goodpaster, B.H., Costill, D.L., Fink, W.J. *et al.* (1996) The effects of pre-exercise starch ingestion on endurance performance. *International Journal of Sports Medicine* **17**, 366–372.

Hargreaves, M., Costill, D.L., Coggan, A., Fink, W.J. & Nishibata, I. (1984) Effect of carbohydrate feedings on muscle glycogen utilisation and exercise performance. *Medicine and Science in Sports and Exercise* **16**, 219–222.

Hawley, J.A., Dennis, S.C. & Noakes, T.D. (1992) Oxidation of carbohydrate ingested during prolonged endurance exercise. *Sports Medicine* **14**, 27–42.

Ivy, J.L., Costill, D.L., Fink, W.J. & Maglischo, E. (1980) Contribution of medium and long chain triglyceride intake to energy metabolism during prolonged exercise. *International Journal of Sports Medicine* **1**, 15–20.

Ivy, J.L., Katz, A.L., Cutler, C.L., Sherman, W.M. & Coyle, E.F. (1988a) Muscle glycogen synthesis after exercise: effect of time of carbohydrate ingestion. *Journal of Applied Physiology* **64**, 1480–1485.

Ivy, J.L., Lee, M.C., Brozinick, J.T. & Reed, M.J. (1988b) Muscle glycogen storage after different amounts of carbohydrate ingestion. *Journal of Applied Physiology* **65**, 2018–2023.

Jeukendrup, A. (1997) *Aspects of Carbohydrate and Fat Metabolism during Exercise.* De Vrieseborch, Haarlem.

Jeukendrup, A.E., Saris, W.H.M., Schrauwen, P., Brouns, F. & Wagenmakers, A.J.M. (1995) Metabolic availability of medium chain triglycerides co-ingested with carbohydrates during prolonged exercise. *Journal of Applied Physiology* **79**, 756–762.

Jeukendrup, A.E., Saris, W.H.M., Van Diesen, R., Brouns, F. & Wagenmakers, A.J.M. (1996a) Effect of endogenous carbohydrate availability on oral medium-chain triglyceride oxidation during prolonged exercise. *Journal of Applied Physiology* **80**, 949–954.

Jeukendrup, A.E., Wagenmakers, A.J.M., Brouns, F., Halliday, D. & Saris, W.H.M. (1996b) Effects of carbohydrate (CHO) and fat supplementation on CHO metabolism during prolonged exercise. *Metabolism* **45**, 915–921.

Jeukendrup, A.E., Brouns, F., Wagenmakers, A.J.M. & Saris, W.H.M. (1997a) Carbohydrate feedings improve 1 H time trial cycling performance. *International Journal of Sports Medicine* **18**, 125–129.

Jeukendrup, A.E., Mensink, M., Saris, W.H.M. & Wagenmakers, A.J.M. (1997b) Exogenous glucose oxidation during exercise in trained and untrained subjects. *Journal of Applied Physiology* **82**, 835–840.

Jeukendrup, A.E., Thielen, J.J.H.C., Wagenmakers, A.J.M., Brouns, F. & Saris, W.H.M. (1998) Effect of MCT and carbohydrate ingestion on substrate utilization and cycling performance. *American Journal of Clinical Nutrition* **67**, 397–404.

Jeukendrup, A.E., Raben, A., Gijsen, A. *et al.* (1999) Glucose kinetics during prolonged exercise following glucose ingestion: a comparison of tracers. *Journal of Physiology* **515**, 579–589.

Koivisto, V.A., Karonen, S.-L. & Nikkila, E.A. (1981) Carbohydrate ingestion before exercise: comparison of glucose, fructose and placebo. *Journal of Applied Physiology* **51**, 783–787.

Kuipers, H., Costill, D.L., Porter, D.A., Fink, W.J. & Morse, W.M. (1986) Glucose feeding and exercise in trained rats: mechanisms for glycogen sparing. *Journal of Applied Physiology* **61**, 859–863.

Leijssen, D.P.C., Saris, W.H.M., Jeukendrup, A.E. & Wagenmakers, A.J.M. (1995) Oxidation of orally ingested [13C]-glucose and [13C]-galactose during exercise. *Journal of Applied Physiology* **79**, 720–725.

Lindeman, A.K. (1991) Nutrient intake in an ultraendurance cyclist. *International Journal of Sport Nutrition* **1**, 79–85.

McConell, G., Kloot, K. & Hargreaves, M. (1996) Effect of timing of carbohydrate ingestion on endurance exercise performance. *Medicine and Science in Sports and Exercise* **28**, 1300–1304.

Massicotte, D., Peronnet, F., Brisson, G.R. & Hillaire-Marcel, C. (1992) Oxidation of exogenous medium-chain free fatty acids during prolonged exercise:

comparison with glucose. *Journal of Applied Physiology* **73**, 1334–1339.

Maughan, R.J. & Leiper, J.B. (1995) Sodium intake and post-exercise rehydration in man. *European Journal of Applied Physiology and Occupational Physiology* **71**, 311–319.

Mitchell, J.B., Costill, D.L., Houmard, J.A., Flynn, M.G., Fink, W.J. & Beltz, J.D. (1988) Effects of carbohydrate ingestion on gastric emptying and exercise performance. *Medicine and Science in Sports and Exercise* **20**, 110–115.

Rauch, L.H.G., Rodger, I., Wilson, G.R. *et al.* (1995) The effect of carbohydrate loading on muscle glycogen content and cycling performance. *International Journal of Sport Nutrition* **5**, 25–36.

Rehrer, N.J., Brouns, F., Beckers, E.J., ten Hoor, F. & Saris, W.H.M. (1990) Gastric emptying with repeated drinking during running and bicycling. *International Journal of Sports Medicine* **11**, 238–243.

Saris, W.H.M., van Erp-Baart, M.A., Brouns, F., Westerterp, K.R. & ten Hoor, F. (1989) Study on food intake and energy expenditure during extreme sustained exercise: the Tour de France. *International Journal of Sports Medicine* **10**, S26–S31.

Saris, W.H.M., Goodpaster, B.H., Jeukendrup, A.E., Brouns, F., Halliday, D. & Wagenmakers, A.J.M. (1993) Exogenous carbohydrate oxidation from different carbohydrate sources during exercise. *Journal of Applied Physiology* **75**, 2168–2172.

Sherman, W.M., Costill, D.L., Fink, W.J. & Miller, J.M. (1981) The effect of exercise and diet manipulation on muscle glycogen and its subsequent utilization during performance. *International Journal of Sports Medicine* **2**, 114–118.

Shirreffs, S.M., Taylor, A.J., Leiper, J.B. & Maughan, R.J. (1996) Post-exercise rehydration in man: effects of volume consumed and drink sodium content. *Medicine and Science in Sports and Exercise* **28**, 1260–1271.

Wagenmakers, A.J.M., Brouns, F., Saris, W.H.M. & Halliday, D. (1993) Oxidation rates of orally ingested carbohydrates during prolonged exercise in man. *Journal of Applied Physiology* **75**, 2774–2780.

Westerterp, K.R., Saris, W.H.M., van Es, M. & ten Hoor, F. (1986) Use of doubly labeled water technique in man during heavy sustained exercise. *Journal of Applied Physiology* **61**, 2162–2167.

# Chapter 44

# Team Sports

JENS BANGSBO

## Introduction

In determining proper nutritional recommendations in a sport discipline, it is important to assess the requirements of the sport and determine whether substrate availability may limit performance. In team sports such as basketball, rugby, soccer, hockey, ice-hockey, volleyball and team handball, the players perform many different types of exercise. The intensity can alter at any time and range from standing still to sprinting (Fig. 44.1). This is in contrast to sports disciplines such as a 100-m sprint and a marathon run, in which during the entire event continuous exercise is performed at a very high or at a moderate intensity, respectively. Due to the intermittent nature of team sports, performance may not only be impaired toward the end of a match, but also after periods of intense exercise. Both types of fatigue might be related to the metabolic processes that occur during match-play. Therefore, before discussing the diet of athletes in team sports, energy provision and substrate utilization during intermittent exercise and in team sports will be considered.

## Energy production and substrate utilization in team sports

In most team sports, the exercise performed is intermittent. It is therefore important to know how metabolism and performance during an exercise bout are influenced by previous exercise. Through the years, this has been investigated

systematically by changing one of the variables at a time. Such studies form the basis for understanding the physiology of intermittent exercise. It has to be recognized, however, that in most laboratory studies the variations in exercise intensity and duration are regular, whereas in many intermittent sports the changes in exercise intensity are irregular and can be almost random.

### Anaerobic energy production

In one study, subjects performed intermittent cycle exercise for 1 h, alternating 15 s rest and 15 s of exercise at a work rate that for continuous cycling demanded maximum oxygen uptake (Essen *et al.* 1977). Considerable fluctuations in muscle levels of adenosine triphosphate (ATP) and phosphocreatine (PCr) occurred. The PCr concentration after an exercise period was 40% of the resting level, and it increased to about 70% of the initial level in the subsequent 15-s recovery period, whereas the increase in muscle lactate was low.

Also during competition in team sports, the PCr concentration probably alternates continuously as a result of the intermittent nature of the game. Figure 44.2 shows an example of the fluctuations of PCr determined by nuclear magnetic resonance (NMR) during three 2-min intermittent exercise periods that each included short maximal contractions, low-intensity contractions and rest. A pronounced decrease of PCr was observed during the maximal contractions, but it almost reached pre-exercise value at the end of

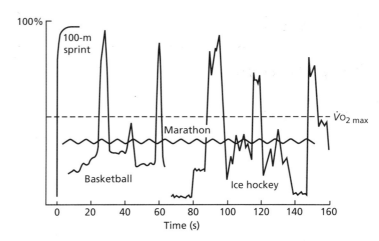

**Fig. 44.1** Examples of pattern of exercise intensities in various sports.

each 2-min intermittent contraction period (Fig. 44.2). Thus, although the net utilization of PCr is quantitatively small during competition in team sports, PCr has a very important function as an energy buffer, providing phosphate for the resynthesis of ATP reaction during rapid elevations in the exercise intensity, and the availability of PCr may determine performance during some intense periods of a game.

Lactate in the blood taken during match-play may reflect, but underestimate, the lactate production in a short period prior to the sampling. Thus, the concentration of lactate in the blood is often used as an indicator of the anaerobic lactacid energy production in sports. In several team sports like basketball and soccer, high lactate concentrations are often found, suggesting that lactate production during a match can be very high.

### Aerobic energy production

Heart rate determinations during match-play can give an indication of the extent to which the aerobic energy system is taxed. In many team sports, such as basketball, team handball and soccer, the aerobic energy production is high. For example, it has been estimated that the mean relative work rate in soccer is around 70% of maximum oxygen uptake, although the players are standing or walking for more than one third of the game (Bangsbo 1994a). One explanation of

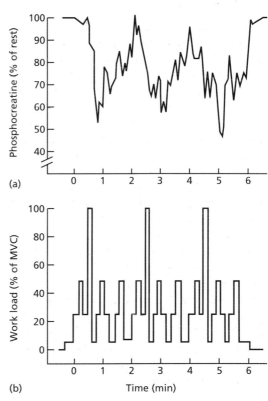

**Fig. 44.2** (a) Phosphocreatine concentration in the gastrocnemius muscle determined by NMR during isometric contractions with the calf muscles at alternating work loads (b). The exercise consisted of three identical 2-min contraction periods, each including a maximal contraction. MVC, maximum voluntary force of contraction. Adapted from Bangsbo (1994a), with permission from *Acta Physiologica Scandinavica*.

the high aerobic energy utilization is that oxygen uptake in the recovery periods after intense exercise is high (Bangsbo 1994a).

## Substrate utilization

The large aerobic energy production and the pronounced anaerobic energy turnover during periods of a match in many team sports are associated with a large consumption of substrates. The dominant substrates are carbohydrate and fat, either stored within the exercising muscle or delivered via the blood to the muscles.

The carbohydrate used during a match is mainly the glycogen stored within the exercising muscles, but glucose extracted from the blood may also be utilized by the muscles. Information about the use of muscle glycogen during a match can be obtained from determinations of glycogen in muscle samples taken before and after the match. The difference in glycogen content represents the net utilization of muscle glycogen, but it does not show the total glycogen turnover, since some resynthesis of glycogen probably occurs during the rest and low-intensity exercise periods during a match (Nordheim & Vøllestad 1990; Bangsbo 1994a). Muscle glycogen utilization may be high in team sports. As an example,

in a study of Swedish soccer players the average thigh muscle glycogen concentrations of five players were 96, 32 and 9 mmol · kg$^{-1}$ wet weight before, at half-time and after a non-competitive match, respectively (Saltin 1973). An important aspect to consider in intermittent sport is that even though the muscle glycogen stores are not completely depleted, the level of muscle glycogen may be limiting for performance (see below).

Fat oxidation is probably high during most team sports. Studies focusing on recovery from intense exercise and intermittent exercise suggest that fat is oxidized to a large extent after intense exercise (Essen 1978; Bangsbo *et al.* 1991). The primary source of the fat oxidized in the rest periods in between the more intense exercise may be muscle triacylglycerol (Bangsbo *et al.* 1991).

The role of protein in metabolism in team sports is unclear, but studies with continuous exercise at a mean work rate and duration similar to team sports such as soccer and basketball have shown that oxidation of proteins may contribute less than 10% of the total energy production (Wagenmakers *et al.* 1990).

As an example, an estimation of substrate utilization and energy production during a soccer game is shown in Fig. 44.3. It is clear that muscle

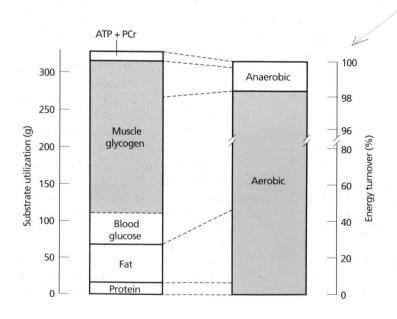

**Fig. 44.3** Estimated relative aerobic and anaerobic energy turnover (right) and corresponding substrate utilization (left) during a soccer match. Adapted from Bangsbo (1994a), with permission from *Acta Physiologica Scandinavica.*

glycogen is the most important substrate in soccer and likely also in other team sports.

It should be noted that in team sports large interindividual differences exist in the energy production during a match due to the variety of factors influencing the exercise intensity, e.g. motivation, physical capacity and tactical limitations. Therefore, there may be major individual variations in the demand of players in the same team.

## Diet in team sports

In this section the importance of nutrition in team sports is discussed and dietary recommendations to accommodate nutritional requirements for training and matches are provided. It should be emphasized that maintaining an adequate diet will improve the potential to reach a maximum level of performance, but does not ensure good performance during a match. There are many other factors that influence performance, including technical abilities and tactical understanding.

### Diet and performance in intermittent exercise

It is well established that performance during long-term continuous exercise is improved by intake of a carbohydrate-rich diet in the days before the exercise. In order to evaluate whether a diet high in carbohydrate also affects performance during prolonged intermittent exercise, a study of eight top-class Danish players was performed.

A soccer-specific intermittent exercise test was used to evaluate performance (Fig. 44.4). The players ran intermittently until they were exhausted and the test result was the total distance covered. The average exercise intensity during the tests was 70–80% of maximum oxygen uptake, which resembles the average intensity during several team sports such as team handball, soccer and basketball. The players performed the test on two occasions separated by 14 days. On one of the occasions, the test was carried out with the players having ingested a diet containing 39% carbohydrate (control diet; C-diet) during the days before the test, and on the other occasion the players performed the test having consumed a high (65%) carbohydrate diet (CHO-diet) prior to the test. Both tests were carried out 3 days after a competitive soccer match, with the diets maintained during the 2 days following the match. The order of the tests was assigned randomly. The total running distance of 17.1 km after the CHO-diet was significantly longer (0.9 km) than after the C-diet. Thus, increasing the carbohydrate content in the diet from 39% or 355 g to 65% or 602 g·day$^{-1}$ (4.6 and 7.9 g·kg$^{-1}$ body mass) improved intermittent endurance performance. Similarly, it has been observed that performance during long-term intermittent exercise consisting of 6-s work periods separated by 30-s rest periods was related to the initial muscle glycogen concentration (Balsom 1995).

The findings in the above mentioned studies suggest that elevated muscle glycogen levels prior to competition can increase the mean work rate during a team sport match. In agreement with this suggestion are findings in a study of soccer players. It was observed that the use of glycogen was more pronounced in the first than in the second half of a game (Saltin 1973). Furthermore, the players with initially low glycogen covered a shorter distance and sprinted significantly less, particularly in the second half, than the players with normal muscle glycogen levels prior to a match (Saltin 1973). It can be assumed that the players would have been better prepared for the second half if the muscle glycogen stores had been higher prior to the match.

In may not only be towards the end of a match that the level of muscle glycogen affects performance. In a study using 15 repeated 6-s sprints separated by 30-s rest periods, it was found that performance was significantly increased when the subjects had elevated the muscle glycogen stores prior to the exercise (Fig. 44.5). In agreement with this finding, it has been observed that high muscle glycogen levels did not affect performance in single intense exercise periods, but when exercise was repeated 1 h later, fatigue

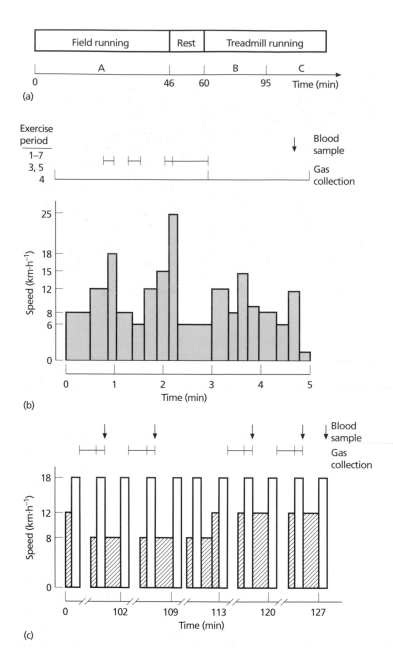

**Fig. 44.4** Protocol of an intermittent endurance test. (a) The test consisted of 46 min of intermittent field running followed by 14 min of rest and then by two parts of intermittent treadmill running to exhaustion. (b) The first part of the treadmill running consisted of seven identical 5-min intermittent exercise periods. (c) The second part of the treadmill running shows where the treadmill speed was alternated between 8 and 18 km · h⁻¹ for 10 s (□) and 15 s (▨), respectively. After 17 min, the lower speed was elevated to 12 km · h⁻¹, and the running was continued until exhaustion. Adapted from Bangsbo *et al.* (1992b), with permission from the *International Journal of Sport Medicine*.

occurred at a later stage when the subjects started with superior muscle glycogen concentrations (Bangsbo *et al.* 1992a). It is worthwhile to note that in both studies the muscle glycogen level was still high at the point of fatigue where fatigue was defined as an inability to maintain the required power output. During intense intermittent exercise, both slow-twitch (ST) and fast-twitch (FT) fibres are involved (Essen 1978) and a partial depletion of glycogen in some fibres, particular the FT fibres, may result in a reduction in performance. These studies demonstrate that if

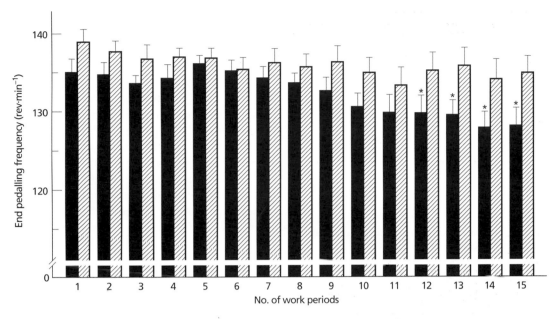

**Fig. 44.5** Pedalling frequency during the last 2 s of 15 × 6-s periods of intense cycling separated by 30-s rest periods with a diet low (■) and high (▨) in carbohydrates in the days before the test. The subjects were supposed to maintain a pedalling frequency of 140 rev · min⁻¹. Note that after the high-carbohydrate diet the subjects were better able to keep a high pedalling frequency. *, significant difference between high- and low-carbohydrate diet. Adapted from Balsom (1995), with permission.

the muscle glycogen levels are not high prior to a game, performance of repeated intense exercise during the game may be impaired.

## Diets of athletes in team sports

The above mentioned studies clearly show that high glycogen levels are essential to optimize performance during intense intermittent exercise. However, athletes in team sports may not actually consume sufficient amounts of carbohydrate, as illustrated in a study of Swedish elite soccer players. After a competitive match played on a Sunday, the players were monitored until the following Wednesday, when they played a European Cup match. One light training session was performed on the Tuesday. Immediately after the match on Sunday, and on the following 2 days, muscle samples were taken from a quadriceps muscle for determination of glycogen content (Fig. 44.6). After the match, the

muscle glycogen content was found to be reduced to approximately 25% of the level before the match. Twenty-four hours (Monday) and 48 h (Tuesday) later, the glycogen stores had only increased to 37% and 39% of the prematch level, respectively. Muscle samples were not taken on the Wednesday because of the European Cup match, but it can be assumed that the glycogen stores were less than 50% of the prematch levels. Thus, the players started the match with only about half of their normal muscle glycogen stores, which most likely reduced their physical performance potential.

The food intake of each player was analysed during the same period (Sunday to Wednesday). The average energy intake per day was 20.7 MJ (4900 kcal), with a variation between players from 10.5 to 26.8 MJ (2500–6400 kcal). By use of the activity profile and body weight of each player, it was calculated that most of the players should have had an intake of at least 20 MJ

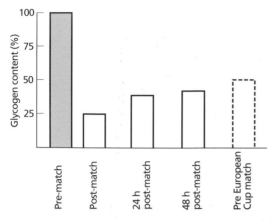

**Fig. 44.6** The muscle glycogen content of a quadriceps muscle for players in a Swedish top-class soccer team, before and just after a league match (Sunday). The figure also gives muscle glycogen values 24 and 48 h after the match, and an estimate of the level before a European Cup match on the following Wednesday (dashed bar). The values are expressed in relation to the level before the league match (100%). Note that muscle glycogen was only restored to about 50% of the 'normal level' before the European Cup match. Adapted from Bangsbo (1994b), with permission from HO + Storm.

(4800 kcal). Therefore, for some of the players the total energy consumption was much lower than required.

The quality of the diet must also be considered, e.g. the proportion of protein, fat and carbohydrate. The players' diet contained, on average, 14% protein of total energy intake (which lies within the recommended range), 47% carbohydrate and 39% fat. If these percentages are compared with those recommended of at least 60% carbohydrate and no more than 25% fat, it is evident that the carbohydrate intake by the players was too low on the days before the European Cup match. This factor, together with the relatively low total energy consumption of some players after the Sunday match, can explain the low muscle glycogen stores found on the days prior to the European Cup match. Thus, the diet of the players was inadequate for optimal physical performance.

It is evident that many athletes in team sports are not aware of the importance of consuming large amounts of carbohydrates in the diet. It may be possible to achieve major changes in dietary habits just by giving the players appropriate information and advice.

In the study concerning the effect of a carbohydrate-rich diet on intermittent exercise performance, 60% of the soccer players' diet was controlled and within given guidelines they could select the remaining 40% themselves. Using this procedure, the average carbohydrate intake was increased from about 45% in the normal diet to 65% in the high-carbohydrate diet. The foods that were consumed in the carbohydrate-rich diet are found in most households. This means it is not necessary to drastically change dietary habits in order to obtain a more appropriate diet.

**Everyday diet**

### CARBOHYDRATES

It is clear that eating a carbohydrate-rich diet on the days before a match is of importance for performance. To consume a significant amount of carbohydrate in the everyday diet is also beneficial to meet the demands of training. Figure 44.7 illustrates how the muscle glycogen stores may vary during a week of training for a player that consumed either a high-carbohydrate diet or a 'normal' diet. During training, some of the glycogen is used, and between training sessions the stores are slowly replenished. If the diet contains large amounts of carbohydrate, it is possible to restore glycogen throughout the week. This may not be achieved if the diet is low in carbohydrates.

An increase in glycogen storage is followed by an enhanced binding of water (2.7 g water·$g^{-1}$ glycogen). Thus, a high-carbohydrate diet is likely to result in an increase in body weight, which might adversely affect performance in the early stage of the match. However, this effect is probably small and the benefit of high muscle-glycogen concentrations before a match will probably outweigh the disadvantages of any

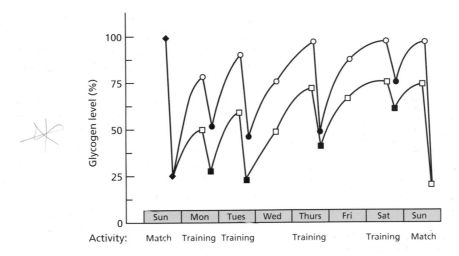

**Fig. 44.7** A hypothetical example of how muscle glycogen stores can vary during a week for a soccer player with a high-carbohydrate (circles) and a 'normal' (squares) diet. There is a match on Sunday, a light training session on Monday, an intensive training session on Tuesday and Thursday, and a light training session on Saturday. The filled symbols indicate the values after the match and training. Note that the glycogen stores are replenished at a faster rate with the high-carbohydrate diet, thus allowing for proper preparation for training and the subsequent match. In contrast, consuming a 'normal' diet may result in reduced training efficiency and the glycogen stores may be lowered before the match. Adapted from Bangsbo (1994b), with permission from HO + Storm.

increase in body weight. The maximal additional muscle-glycogen synthesis when consuming a high-carbohydrate diet as compared with a normal diet should be 150 g, which corresponds to a weight gain of less than 0.5 kg. Furthermore, a more pronounced breakdown of glycogen will enhance the release of water, which will reduce the net loss of water.

PROTEIN

Protein is used primarily for maintaining and building up tissues, such as muscles. The amount of protein required in the diet is a topic frequently discussed, particularly with respect to those sports where muscle strength is important or where muscle injuries often occur. Most team sports can be included in both of these categories. However, in most cases the athletes take in sufficient amount of proteins (see Chapter 10). For example, the daily intake of protein by Swedish and Danish soccer players was 2–3 g · kg⁻¹ body weight, which is above the recommended daily intake for athletes of 1–2 g · kg⁻¹ (Jacobs *et al.* 1982; Bangsbo *et al.* 1992b). In general, supplementing protein intake by tablets or protein powders is unnecessary for athletes in team sports, even during an intensive strength-training period.

FAT

Fat exists in two forms—saturated fat and unsaturated fat. The saturated fats are solid at room temperature (butter, margarine and fat in meat) while unsaturated fats are liquid or soft at room temperature (vegetable oil, vegetable margarine and fat in fish). An adequate intake of unsaturated fats is essential for the body, and, in contrast to saturated fats, unsaturated fats may aid in lowering the amount of cholesterol in the blood, thereby reducing the risk of heart disease. Therefore, it is important that saturated fats are replaced with unsaturated fats where possible. The total content of fat in the average diet for an athlete is often too high and a general lowering of fat intake is advisable.

## MINERALS AND VITAMINS

Food and drink supplies the body with fluids, energy-producing substrates, and other important components, such as salt, minerals, and vitamins. In a well-balanced diet, most nutrients are supplied in sufficient amounts. However, there can be some exceptions.

Iron is an important element in haemoglobin, which binds to the red blood cells and aids in the transport of oxygen throughout the body. Therefore, an adequate iron intake is essential for athletes and especially for female athletes, who lose blood and, thus, haemoglobin during menstruation (see Chapter 24). The recommended daily intake of iron for a player is approximately 20 mg, which should be ingested via solid foods rather than in tablet form, as iron found in solid foods is more effectively absorbed from the intestine to the blood. Animal organs (liver, heart and kidneys), dried fruits, bread, nuts, strawberries and legumes are foods with a high content of iron. It is advisable to increase iron intake in periods when players are expected to increase their red blood cell production, e.g. during the preseason or when training at a high altitude.

A question commonly asked is whether or not players should supplement their diet with vitamins. In general, vitamin supplementation is not necessary, but there are conditions where it might be beneficial. For example, it is advisable to enhance vitamin E intake when training at high altitudes, and to use vitamin C and multiple B-vitamin supplements in hot climates (see Chapters 20 and 26).

## CREATINE

In team sports, the rate of muscle PCr utilization is high during periods of match play and in the following recovery periods PCr is resynthesized (see above). This leads to the question whether an athlete in team sports can benefit from ingestion of creatine in a period before a match, as it has been shown that intake of creatine increases the PCr and particularly creatine levels in muscles (Harris *et al.* 1992). For example, it was found that five subjects increased their total muscle creatine level (PCr and creatine) by 25% after a creatine intake of 20 g·day$^{-1}$ for 5 days (Greenhaff *et al.* 1994). The effect of intake of creatine is discussed in detail in Chapter 27 and the discussion here will focus on issues relevant to the team games players.

An elevated level of creatine and PCr may affect PCr resynthesis after exercise (Greenhaff *et al.* 1994), which may have an impact on the ability to perform intermittent exercise. In one study, subjects performed 10 6-s high-intensity exercise bouts on a cycle-ergometer separated by 24 s of rest, after they had ingested either creatine (20 g·day$^{-1}$) or placebo for a week (Balsom *et al.* 1993a). The group which ingested creatine had a lower reduction in performance as the test progressed than the placebo group. On the other hand, as one would expect, creatine ingestion appears to have no effect on prolonged (>10 min) continuous exercise performance (Balsom *et al.* 1993b).

Although creatine ingestion increases muscle PCr and creatine concentration, it is doubtful that athletes in team sports, except probably for vegetarians, will benefit from creatine supplementation, since creatine ingestion also causes an increase in body mass. It is still unclear what causes this increase, but it is most likely due to an increased accumulation of water. Nevertheless, a gain in body weight has a negative influence in sports in which the athletes have to move their body mass against gravity. For example, no difference in performance during intense intermittent running (Yo-Yo intermittent recovery test) was observed when a group of subjects performed the test after 7 days of creatine intake (20 g·day$^{-1}$) compared with a test under control conditions. Furthermore, it is unclear how ingesting creatine for a period influences the body's own production of creatine and the enzymes that are related to creatine/PCr synthesis and breakdown. It may be that an athlete, through regular intake of creatine, reduces his ability to produce PCr and creatine, which may result in a reduction in the PCr and creatine levels when the athlete no longer is ingesting creatine. In addition, very little is known about any possible side-effect of a frequent intake of creatine. Regular high concentrations of creatine in the blood may, on a long-term basis, have negative effects on the kidney, which is the organ that has to eliminate the excess creatine. One should also consider that ingestion of creatine can be considered as doping, even though it is not on the IOC doping list. It may be argued that creatine is a natural compound and that it is contained in the food. However, it is almost impossible to get doses of creatine corresponding to those used in the experiments which showed enhanced performance, as the content of creatine in 1 kg of raw meat is around 5 g.

### Pretraining and precompetition meal

On the day of a match, the intake of fat and protein (especially derived from meat) should be restricted. The pretraining or prematch meal should be ingested 3–4 h prior to competition or training. If too much food is ingested after this time, there still may be undigested food in the stomach and intestine when the training or match begins. The meal should mainly consist of a sufficient amount of carbohydrate. It has been demonstrated that ingestion of 312 g of carbohydrate 4 h prior to strenuous continuous exercise resulted in a 15% improvement in exercise performance, but no improvement was observed when either 45 or 156 g of carbohydrate was ingested (Sherman *et al.* 1989). A snack high in carbohydrate, e.g. bread with jam, may be eaten about 1.5 h before the match. However, these time references are only guidelines. There are great individual differences in the ability to digest food. It is a good idea for players to experiment with a variety of different foods at different times before training sessions.

An improvement in exercise performance has been observed if carbohydrate was ingested immediately before exercise (Neufer *et al.* 1987). On the other hand, glucose ingestion 30–60 min prior to severe exercise has been shown to produce a rapid fall in blood glucose with the onset of exercise, an increase in muscle glycogen utilization and a reduction in exercise time to exhaustion (Costill *et al.* 1977). However, not all studies have shown a detrimental effect of ingesting carbohydrate before exercise, and some studies have shown improved performance after carbohydrate ingestion in the last hour prior to strenuous exercise (Gleeson *et al.* 1986). The differences seem to be closely related to the glucose and insulin responses. When exercising with a high insulin concentration, there is an abnormally large loss of glucose from the blood, resulting in a low blood glucose concentration. Consequently, the muscles and the brain gradually become starved of glucose, which eventually leads to fatigue.

### Food intake after exercise

Physical activity is a powerful stimulus to glycogen resynthesis, as was elegantly shown in a study where a glycogen-depleted leg attained muscle glycogen levels twice as high as the resting control leg during a 3-day period (Bergström & Hultman 1966). In addition, it seems that the muscles are particularly sensitive to glucose uptake and glycogen resynthesis in the period immediately after exercise (Ploug *et al.* 1987). It was found that the rate of glycogen resynthesis during the first 2 h after carbohydrate intake was faster if carbohydrate was ingested immediately following an exercise bout, rather than delaying the intake by 2 h (Ivy *et al.* 1988). Thus, to secure a rapid resynthesis of glycogen, an athlete should take in carbohydrates immediately after training and a match. For specific recommendations about amount and type of carbohydrate, see Chapter 7.

An inverse relationship between the rate of glycogen rebuilding and the muscle-glycogen concentration after prolonged continuous exercise or soccer match-play has been demonstrated (Piehl *et al.* 1974; Jacobs *et al.* 1982). Therefore, in team sports the players should be able to replenish the muscle glycogen stores within 24 h after a match, irrespective of the magnitude of the decrease of carbohydrates during the game. However, other factors have been shown to influence the rate of glycogen synthesis. Glycogen restoration is impaired after eccentric exercise and after exercise causing muscle damage (Blom *et al.* 1987; Widrick *et al.* 1992). In most team sports the players are often performing some eccentric exercise and muscle damage can occur due to physical contact. It has been demonstrated that an increased ingestion of carbohydrate can partially overcome the effect of the muscle damage on glycogen resynthesis (Bak & Peterson 1990). Thus, also in this respect the players can benefit from a high carbohydrate intake following match-play and training.

## Fluid intake in team sports

In many team sports, the loss of body water, mainly due to the secretion of sweat, can be large during competition. For example, under normal weather conditions the decrease in body fluid during a soccer match is approximately 2 l, and under extreme conditions the reduction in body water can be higher, e.g. in a World Cup soccer match in Mexico, one Danish player lost about 4.5 l of fluid. Such changes in body fluid can influence performance negatively during match-play (Saltin 1964). Thus, it is important for the players to take in fluid during a game and also during a training session to maintain the efficiency of the training. The question is what and how much to drink before, during and after a training session or a game.

### Before a training session or match

It is important that the players are not dehydrated before a match. The players should begin the process of 'topping-up' with fluid on the day before a match. For example, an additional litre of juice can be drunk on the evening before a match, which will also provide an extra supply of sugar.

On the match day, the players should have plenty to drink and be encouraged to drink even when they are not feeling thirsty. The content of sugar should be less than 10%. During the last hour before the match, the players should not have more than 300 ml (a large cup) of a liquid with a sugar concentration less than 5% every 15 min.

The intake of coffee should be limited, as coffee contains caffeine, which has a diuretic effect and causes the body to lose a larger amount of water than is absorbed from the coffee.

### During a training session or match

Besides reducing the net loss of body water, the intake of fluid can supply the body with carbohydrates. As low muscle glycogen concentrations in some team sports might limit performance at the end of a match, intake of carbohydrate solutions during a match is useful.

Questions remain concerning the optimum composition of the drink, particularly with respect to its concentration, form of carbohydrates, electrolyte content, osmolality, pH, volume and temperature. These considerations depend, among other things, on the temperature and humidity of the environment, which should determine the ratio between the need for fluid and need for carbohydrates. In a cold environment, there is little need for water, and a drink with a sugar concentration up to 10% can be used, whereas in a hot environment the carbohydrate content should be much less. Before using drinks with high sugar concentrations in a match, however, the players should have tried these drinks during training to ensure that stomach upset does not occur. There are large individual differences in the ability to tolerate drinks and to empty fluid from the stomach. While some players are unaffected by large amounts of fluid in the stomach, others find it difficult to tolerate even small quantities of fluid. The players will benefit by experimenting with different drinks and drinking habits during training. For further discussion of the compositions of the fluid, see Chapters 17 and 39.

During a match, small amounts of fluid should be drunk frequently. It is optimal to drink between 100 and 300 ml with a 2–5% sugar concentration every 10–15 min. In a soccer match, this will give a total fluid intake of between 1 and 2 l, plus 30–50 g of sugar during the match. This is sufficient to replace a significant amount of the water lost through sweat, and to cover some of the demand for sugar. Although fluid intake during a match is important, it should not interfere with the game. The players should only drink when there is a natural pause in the game as the drinking may disturb the playing rhythm. In some team sports, such as basketball and ice-hockey, the players can drink during time-outs or when they are on the bench, whereas in other sports, such as soccer, it is more difficult. In the latter case, it is convenient to place small bottles of fluid at different positions around the field in order to avoid long runs to the team bench.

### After a training session or match

The players should drink plenty of fluid after a match and training. Several studies have demonstrated that restoration of fluid balance is a slow process and that it is not sufficient merely to increase fluid intake immediately after a match (see Chapter 19). It is not unusual for players to be partially dehydrated on the day after a match. The body can only partially regulate water balance through the sensation of thirst, as thirst is quenched before a sufficient amount of fluid has been drunk. Thus, in order to maintain fluid balance, more fluid has to be drunk than just satisfies the sensation of thirst.

The colour of urine is a good indicator of the fluid balance and the need for water. If the body is dehydrated, the amount of water in the urine is reduced and the colour becomes a stronger yellow.

### Recommendations

The following recommendations regarding fluid intake may be helpful for an athlete in team sports:
• Drink plenty of fluid the day before a match

and on the day of the match—more than just to quench thirst.
• Drink frequently just before and during a match as well as at half-time, but only small amounts at a time—not more than 300 ml of fluid every 15 min.
• Drinks consumed just before and during a match should have a sugar concentration lower than 5% and a temperature between 5 and 10 °C.
• Drink a lot after a match—even several hours afterwards.
• Use the colour of the urine as an indication of the need for fluid—the yellower the urine, the greater the need for fluid intake.
• Experiment with drinking habits during training so that any difficulties in absorbing fluid during exercise can be overcome.

## Conclusion

In most team sports, the players perform high-intensity intermittent exercise, at times for a long duration. The intense exercise periods require a high rate of energy turnover and the total energy cost of a game can be high. Muscle glycogen appears to the most important substrate in team sports, and performance may be limited due to a partial depletion of the muscle glycogen stores.

Athletes that are taking part in team sports should have a balanced diet that contains large amounts of carbohydrate to allow for a high training efficiency and for optimal preparation for matches. Therefore, it is important for the players to be conscious of the nutritive value of the food that they consume. The highest potential for storing glycogen in the muscles is immediately after exercise. It is therefore advisable to consume carbohydrate, either in solid or liquid form, shortly after a match or training session. This is particularly important if the players are training twice on the same day. On the day of competition, the last meal should be ingested 3–4 h before the start, and it should mainly consist of carbohydrates that can be rapidly absorbed. During the last hour before a match, solid food or liquid with a high carbohydrate content may be avoided.

To limit the extent of dehydration and to provide the body with carbohydrate during match-play, the players should take in fluid with a low carbohydrate content both before and during a match. Also, fluid ingestion should be high after a match.

# References

Bak, J.F. & Peterson, O. (1990) Exercise enhanced activation of glycogen synthase in human skeletal muscle. *American Journal of Physiology* **258**, E957–E963.

Balsom, P.D. (1995) *High intensity intermittent exercise: performance and metabolic responses with very high intensity short duration work periods.* Doctoral thesis, Karolinska Institutet, Sweden.

Balsom, P.D., Ekblom, B., Söderlund, K., Sjödin., B. & Hultman, E. (1993a) Creatine supplementation and dynamic high-intensity intermittent exercise. *Scandinavian Journal of Medicine and Science in Sports* **3**, 143–149.

Balsom, P.D., Harridge, S.D.R., Söderlund, K., Sjödin, B. & Ekblom, B. (1993b) Creatine supplementation per se does not enhance endurance exercise performance. *Acta Physiologica Scandinavica* **149**, 521–523.

Bangsbo, J (1994a) The physiology of soccer: with special reference to intense intermittent exercise. *Acta Physiologica Scandinavica* **151** (Suppl. 610), 1–156.

Bangsbo, J (1994b) *Fitness Training for Football: A Scientific Approach.* HO + Storm, Bagsværd, Copenhagen, Denmark.

Bangsbo, J., Gollnick, P.D., Graham, T.E. & Saltin, B. (1991) Substrates for muscle glycogen synthesis in recovery from intense exercise in humans. *Journal of Physiology* **434**, 423–440.

Bangsbo, J., Graham, T.E., Kiens, B. & Saltin, B. (1992a) Elevated muscle glycogen and anaerobic energy production during exhaustive exercise in man. *Journal of Physiology* **451**, 205–222.

Bangsbo, J., Nørregaard, L. & Thorsøe, F. (1992b) The effect of carbohydrate diet on intermittent exercise performance. *International Journal of Sports Medicine* **13**, 152–157.

Bergström, J & Hultman, E. (1966) Muscle glycogen synthesis after exercise: an enhancing factor localized to the muscle cells in man. *Nature* **210**, 309–310.

Blom, P.C.S., Costill, D.L. & Völlestad, N.K. (1987) Exhaustive running: inappropriate as a stimulus of muscle glycogen supercompensation. *Medicine and Science in Sports and Exercise* **19**, 398–403.

Costill, D.L., Coyle, E.F., Dalsky, G., Evans, W., Fink, E. & Hoppes, D. (1977) Effects of elevated plasma FFA and insulin on muscle glycogen usage during exercise. *Journal of Applied Physiology* **43**, 695–699.

Essén, H. (1978) Studies on the regulation of metabolism in human skeletal muscle using intermittent exercise as an experimental model. *Acta Physiologica Scandinavica* (Suppl.) **454**, 1–32.

Gleeson, M., Maughan, R.J & Greenhaff, P.L. (1986) Comparison of the effects of pre-exercise feeding of glucose, glycerol and placebo on endurance and fuel homeostasis in man. *European Journal of Applied Physiology* **55**, 645–653.

Greenhaff, P.L., Bodin, K., Söderlund, I. & Hultman, E. (1994) The effect of oral creatine supplementation on skeletal muscle phosphocreatine resynthesis. *American Journal of Physiology* **266**, E725–E730.

Harris, R.C., Söderlund, K. & Hultman, E. (1992) Elevation of creatine in resting and exercise muscles of normal subjects by creatine supplementation. *Clinical Science* **83**, 367–374.

Ivy, J.L., Katz, A.L., Cutler, C.L., Sherman, W.M. & Coyle, E.F. (1988) Muscle glycogen synthesis after exercise: effect of time of carbohydrate ingestion. *Journal of Applied Physiology* **64**, 1480–1495.

Jacobs, I., Westlin, N., Karlsson, J., Rasmusson, M. & Houghton, B. (1982) Muscle glycogen and diet in elite soccer players. *European Journal of Applied Physiology* **48**, 297–302.

Neufer, P.D., Costill, D.L., Glynn, M.G., Kirwan, J.P., Mitchell, J.B. & Houmard, J (1987) Improvements in exercise performance: effects of carbohydrate feedings and diet. *Journal of Applied Physiology* **62**, 983–988.

Nordheim, K. & Vøllestad, N.K. (1990) Glycogen and lactate metabolism during low-intensity exercise in man. *Acta Physiologica Scandinavica* **139**, 475–484.

Piehl, K., Adolfsen, S. & Nazar, K. (1974) Glycogen storage and glycogen synthetase activity in trained and untrained muscle of man. *Acta Physiologica Scandinavica* **90**, 779–788.

Ploug, T., Galbo, H., Vinten, J., Jørgensen, M. & Richter, E.A. (1987) Kinetics of glucose transport in rat muscle: effects of insulin and contractions. *American Journal of Physiology* **253**, E12–E20.

Saltin, B. (1964) Aerobic work capacity and circulation at exercise in man: with special reference to the effect of prolonged exercise and/or heat exposure. *Acta Physiologica Scandinavica* **62** (Suppl.), 1–52.

Saltin, B. (1973) Metabolic fundamentals in exercise. *Medicine and Science in Sports and Exercise* **5**, 137–146.

Sherman, W.M., Brodowicz, G., Wright, D.A., Allen, W.K., Simonsen, J. & Dernback., A. (1989) Effects of

4 h pre-exercise carbohydrate feedings on cycling performance. *Medicine and Science in Sports and Exercise* **21**, 598–604.

Wagenmakers, A.J.M., Coakley, J.H. & Edwards, R.H.T. (1990) Metabolism of branched-chain amino acids and ammonia during exercise: clues from McArdle's disease. *International Journal of Sports Medicine* **11**, 101–113.

Widrick, J., Costill, D.L., McConell, G.K., Anderson, D.E., Pearson, D.R. & Zachwieja, J.J (1992) Time course of glycogen accumulation after eccentric exercise. *Journal of Applied Physiology* **75**, 1999–2004.

# Chapter 45

# Gymnastics

DAN BENARDOT

## Introduction

Enrolment in gymnastics programmes continues to flourish for a variety of reasons. There is an increasing availability of good gymnastics schools and coaches in more locations, and a high level of media attention has been afforded gymnastics during recent Olympic Games (gymnastics coverage for the 1996 Summer Olympic Games in Atlanta represented the most coverage given to any sport). The ever-increasing number of young gymnastics competitors requires that those in sports medicine pay careful attention to their health and well-being, especially as these athletes are assessed for growth, weight, bone-health, eating behaviour, and other developmentally important factors. For the seasoned competitors, every effort must be made to ensure an evolution of nutritional habits that will optimize performance while guaranteeing the opportunity for good health.

The concern for improving the nutritional health of gymnasts is real. The traditional paradigm in gymnastics is to develop gymnasts who are small, and gymnasts themselves commonly view this small body image as the ideal for their sport. The issue of *weight* is a prevailing theme, regardless of the gymnastics discipline. Even in men's gymnastics, it is ordinarily suggested that controlling energy intake to achieve lower weight is an appropriate and desired act if a gymnast is to achieve success (Maddux 1970). It is also a common practice to regularly weigh gymnasts as a normal part of training, but the results of these weigh-ins are not often used constructively. Since there is a normal expectation for growth in children, there should be a concomitant expectation for increasing weight. Failure to accept this fact may place abnormal pressures on young gymnasts to achieve an arbitrarily low weight through unhealthy means. Adolescent females, as a group, are the most vulnerable to disordered eating patterns, and this group constitutes the majority of competitive women in gymnastics. This makes it imperative that those working with gymnasts become sensitive to the possibility that some of these athletes may have a predisposition to eating behaviours that could put them at health risk. Thus, while a lowering of excess body fat will reduce body mass and, perhaps, lower the risk of traumatic injuries to joints, excessive attention to weight carries with it its own set of health and injury risks (Houtkooper & Going 1994).

There has been a consistent drop in the age at which gymnasts compete at the elite level. In 1960, the United States Olympic gymnasts had an average height of about 157.5 cm and an average weight of 50 kg. In 1992, the United States Olympic gymnasts had an average height of 146 cm and an average weight of 37.5 kg. During this same time, the average age of these competitors dropped from 18.5 to 16 years (Nattiv & Mendelbaum 1993). The Fédération Internationale de Gymnastique (FIG) has addressed this issue by making 16 the minimum age for competing at the Olympic Games, beginning in the year 2000. However, the pace at which gymnasts must learn increasingly difficult skills continues to accelerate, placing a higher value on curtailing adolescent body changes that could inhibit the gymnastics learning curve. To make matters more difficult, the means commonly used by gymnasts to attain a desired body composition is counterproductive in several ways. Restrained eating, besides being associated with inadequate energy intake, is also associated with a lowering of metabolic rate and a lowering of nutrient intake. A lower metabolic rate makes it more difficult for the gymnast to eat normally without increasing fat storage, and consumption of less energy is associated with inadequate nutrient intake, just at a time (adolescence) when nutrient demands are high. For instance, there is ample survey evidence that gymnasts tend to consume an inadequate level of calcium, a nutrient critical for proper bone development. This malnutrition may predispose gymnasts to stress fractures, and may also increase the risk for early development of osteoporosis. Inadequate energy and nutrient intake may also reduce the benefits gymnasts derive from training, because the conditioning benefit from intense activity is likely to be minimized when working muscles have insufficient fuel and metabolites to work at an optimal level. Since the same primary fuel responsible for muscular work (glucose) is also the primary fuel for brain and nervous system function, there is also good reason to suspect that injury rates may be higher when there is a failure to provide sufficient energy to support the activity.

## Background

Elite level gymnastics has four separate disciplines, including men's gymnastics, women's artistic gymnastics, women's rhythmic gymnastics, and women's rhythmic group gymnastics.
• Women's artistic gymnastics: Competitions include four different events, including the floor exercise, vault, uneven bars and balance beam.
• Men's artistic gymnastics: Competitions include six different events, including the floor exercise, side horse, horse vault, parallel bars and horizontal bar.
• Rhythmic sportive gymnastics (women): Competitions include four different routines, each performed as a floor exercise, with four of the five rhythmic apparatus (rope, ball, hoop, clubs and ribbon). The four apparatus to be used are determined by FIG every 2 years following the World Championships.
• Rhythmic group gymnastics (women): Competitions include two different routines performed by teams of six gymnasts. Each routine is performed with a combination of rhythmic apparatus. For instance, at the 1996 Olympic Games, the rhythmic group teams performed one routine with two ribbons and three balls, and another routine with hoops. The apparatus combinations to be used is determined every 2 years by FIG following the World Championships.

Gymnastics training at the elite level takes place 5 or 6 days per week, for 3–5 h each day. In some cases, gymnasts have two practices each day, a morning practice that lasts for 1 or 2 h, and an afternoon practice that lasts for 2–3 h. Although the total time spent in gymnastics practice is high for elite gymnasts (up to 30 h of practice each week), the actual time spent in conditioning and skills training is considerably less. Gymnasts begin practice with a series of stretches, and then initiate a series of basic skills on the floor mat as part of the warm-up routine. Following warm-up, each gymnast takes a turn practicing one of the events. The time performing a skill in practice never exceeds that of the competition maximum, and is usually a small fraction of it. Because practice involves repeated bouts of highly intense, short-duration activity, gymnasts rest between each practice bout to regenerate strength. With the exception of the group competition in rhythmic gymnastics, none of the competition events within each of these disciplines has a duration longer than 90 s. This duration categorizes gymnastics as a high-intensity, anaerobic sport (Table 45.1).

As anaerobes, gymnasts rely heavily on type IIb (pure fast twitch) and type IIa (intermediate fast twitch) muscle fibres (Bortz *et al.* 1993). These

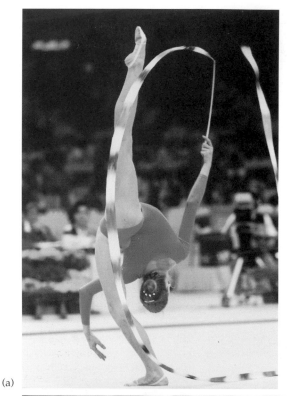

(a)

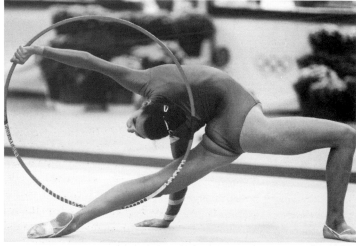

(b)

**Fig. 45.1** Many studies show that estimates of the energy intake of elite gymnasts are less than the estimated energy requirements. Photos © IOC / Olympic Museum Collections.

fibres, while capable of producing a great deal of power, are generally regarded as incapable of functioning at high intensity for longer than 90 s. Type II fibres have a low oxidative capacity, a factor that limits fat usage as an energy substrate during gymnastic activity, and a poor capillary supply, which deprives these fibres of nutrient, oxygen, and carbon dioxide exchange during intensive work. Because of these factors, gymnastics activity is heavily dependent on creatine phosphate and carbohydrate (both glucose and glycogen) as fuels for activity.

**Table 45.1** Gymnastics disciplines and duration (in seconds) of each competitive event.

| Activity | Rhythmic (individual) | Rhythmic (group) | Women's artistic | Men's artistic |
|---|---|---|---|---|
| Floor exercise | 75–90 | 135–150 | 60–90 | 50–70 |
| Balance beam | — | — | 70–90 | — |
| Horizontal bar | — | — | — | 15–30 |
| Parallel bars | — | — | — | 20–30 |
| Uneven parallel bars | — | — | 20–30 | — |
| Pommel horse | — | — | — | 20–30 |
| Vault | — | — | 6–8 | 6–8 |
| Rings | — | — | — | 20–30 |

**Table 45.2** Comparison of energy intakes vs. requirements of different artistic gymnastic populations.

| Subject age (years) | Population evaluated* (n) | Intake (kJ) | Intake (kcal) | RDA† (%) | Predicted requirement (%) | Reference |
|---|---|---|---|---|---|---|
| 9.4±0.8 | US junior elite (29) | 6934±1525 | 1651±363 | — | 76 | Benardot et al. (1989) |
| 11.4±0.9 | US junior elite (22) | 7165±1768 | 1706±471 | — | 76 | Benardot et al. (1989) |
| 11.5±0.5 | Turkish club (20) | 6586 | 1568 | 59 | — | Ersoy (1991) |
| 12.3±1.7 | Italian club (26) | 6518±2138 | 1552±509 | 78 | — | Reggiani et al. (1989) |
| 14.8 | US Level I, II (20) | 7325 | 1744 | 99 | — | Calabrese (1985) |
| 14.8±1.2 | Swedish elite (22) | 8106±1911 | 1930±455 | — | 73 | Lindholm et al. (1995) |
| 15.2±4.1 | US high school (13) | 8077±2831 | 1923±674 | 96 | 84 | Moffatt (1984) |
| 15.8±0.9 | US national team (14) | 6283±1743 | 1496±415 | 71 | 66 | Benardot (1996) |
| 19.7±0.2 | US college team (26) | 5800±458 | 1381±109 | 63 | 47 | Kirchner et al. (1995) |
| — | US college team (male) (10) | 8736 | 2080 | 72 | — | Short and Short (1983) |
| 36.3±1.0 | Former competitive (18) | 11 004±1100 | 2620±262 | 119 | 119 | Kirchner et al. (1996) |

* All data are for female gymnasts, except for data from Short and Short (1983).
† RDAs are country specific.

Gymnastics competition typically involves those who have not yet reached the age of 25, with those who are between 16 and 19 years old constituting the majority of the elite ranks (Nattiv & Mendelbaum 1993). However, there are increasing numbers of junior gymnasts who are already seasoned competitors at age 12 (Benardot et al. 1989, 1993).

### Energy and nutrient intake

A number of studies have evaluated the nutrient intake of elite gymnasts. In general, these studies demonstrate an inadequacy in the intake of total energy, iron and calcium. Heavy gymnastic training and inadequate nutrient intake are implicated as causative factors in the primary amenorrhoea experienced by many young gymnasts, and may also contribute to the secondary amenorrhoea experienced by older gymnasts. Inadequate calcium intake is associated with poor bone development and increased risk of stress fracture (see Chapter 23). Inadequate iron intake is associated with anaemia, which is a risk factor in the development of amenorrhoea (Loosli 1993) (see Chapter 24).

ENERGY INTAKE

Table 45.2 presents a summary of selected published energy intake data obtained from several gymnastics populations. Included in this summary are young, beginning gymnasts averaging age 9, club gymnasts, college male and female gymnasts, competitive gymnasts, national team gymnasts, and former competitive gymnasts. Of these groups, only the former competitive gymnasts had average energy intakes that exceeded the recommended level. College team gymnasts from the United States were the oldest of the competitive gymnasts evaluated (mean age, 19.7 years) and had the lowest daily energy intakes of all the groups evaluated. The second lowest daily energy intake was seen in the USA national team members. It appears from this summary that gymnasts involved in the highest levels of competition are most likely to have the greatest differential between energy intake and energy requirement.

The youngest gymnasts to be evaluated for energy intake were junior elite gymnasts ranging in age from 7 to 10 years (mean age, 9.4 years; Benardot et al. 1989). These gymnasts were serious about gymnastics, spending approximately 3–4 h in the gym each day. Despite this heavy practice schedule, they had an average energy intake of 69.1 MJ (1650 kcal), which was predicted to be 76% of their energy requirement. The findings for an older group (11–14 years) of junior elite gymnasts were similar, with gymnasts consuming an average of 7.1 MJ (1700 kcal) (Benardot et al. 1989).

An even greater energy deficit was found in a group of 20 Turkish gymnasts, averaging 11.5 years of age, who trained between 5 and 6 h daily (Ersoy 1991). These gymnasts had an energy intake of 6.6 MJ (1570 kcal), a level of intake that was predicted to be only 59% of the recommended level. A majority of these gymnasts (75%) had reported feeling dizzy, weak, and short of breath during gymnastics practices (Ersoy 1991).

A survey of Italian club gymnasts (involved in competitions but not at the 'elite' level) who averaged 12.3 years of age revealed a similar trend in underconsumption of total energy (Reggiani et al. 1989). These gymnasts had an average energy intake of 6.5 MJ·day$^{-1}$ (1550 kcal·day$^{-1}$), which was 78% of the recommended level. The

authors point out that this level of intake is consistent for the standard of intake when adjusted by body weight (180 kJ·kg$^{-1}$, 43 kcal·kg$^{-1}$). However, it appears that this level of energy intake does not meet the additional energy demands of growth, which should be an expectation for 12-year-olds. According to the World Health Organization, the daily energy requirement of 10–14-year-old children with average activity levels is between 189 and 227 kJ·kg$^{-1}$ (45.2–54.2 kcal·kg$^{-1}$) (Lemons 1989).

In a study of recreational club gymnasts (mean age, 14.8 years), it was found that energy intake was 7.3 MJ·day$^{-1}$ (1744 kcal·day$^{-1}$), or 99% of the standard requirement (Calabrese 1985). A similar finding was observed in a group of 13 female high-school gymnasts, who consumed 8 MJ·day$^{-1}$ (1923 kcal·day$^{-1}$), or 96% of the recommended intake and 84% of the predicted requirement (Moffatt 1984). It is important to note that these two groups were performing at the lowest competitive level of the groups evaluated, and came the closest to meeting energy requirements.

In a study of 22 elite adolescent female Swedish gymnasts (mean age, 14.8 years) evaluated for energy intake, it was determined that they consumed approximately 3035±2436 kJ (725±582 kcal) of energy less than their predicted requirement (11.1±1.36 MJ, 2653±325 kcal) (Lindholm et al. 1995). This value takes into account the gymnasts' current height, weight, gender, age (growth requirement), and daily activity (including an average daily gymnastics practice of approximately 3 h). This value can be compared to that of a reference group of equivalently aged non-gymnast females who experienced an average predicted energy deficit of 1879 ±1528 kJ (449±365 kcal) compared to their need (8883±1005 kJ, 2122±240 kcal) (Lindholm et al. 1995). Compared to established standards, over 50% of these gymnasts were below the standard, while the majority of the non-gymnasts fell within the standard of intake (Lindholm et al. 1995).

Members of the United States National Team (average age, 15.8) were evaluated in 1994, and were found to consume either 5119 or 6258 kJ·

day⁻¹ (1223 or 1495 kcal·day⁻¹), depending on the technique used to obtain food intake data (Benardot 1996). These values represent approximately 60–70% of the recommended intake and 66% of the gymnasts' predicted energy requirement. In this study there was a statistically significant relationship between energy intake and body-fat percentage. Gymnasts with the lowest energy intake had the highest body fat levels, and gymnasts with the greatest number of within-day energy deficits greater than 1255 kJ (300 kcal) also had the highest body-fat percentages. These data were sufficiently powerful that body fat could be predicted from the largest energy deficit (Benardot 1996):

$$\text{Body fat \%}_{DEXA}{}^* = \text{Largest energy deficit} \\ (0.00385893) + 7.92609$$

Standard error of estimation = 2.438

Multiple $R^2$ = 0.582

$P$ = 0.0035

These data suggest that the gymnasts' adaptive mechanism to energy inadequacy is to increase energy storage (fat), probably through a decrease in the metabolic rate and a heightened insulin response to food. These data also support the idea that regular energy restriction is counterproductive in the attainment of low body fat, and may create an increasingly difficult cycle of continually greater food restrictions to maintain the desired body composition.

A group of older United States college gymnasts, averaging 19.7 (±0.2) years of age, reported an energy intake of 5780 kJ·day⁻¹ (1380 kcal·day⁻¹), representing 63% of the RDA and 47% of the predicted energy expenditure of 12.2 MJ (2911 kcal) (Kirchner et al. 1995). The difference between reported energy intake and predicted energy requirement represents an energy intake that provided only 47% of the predicted requirement for this group. This was the oldest group of competitive gymnasts studied, and a group

with the greatest average height and weight. Nevertheless, this group had the greatest differential between predicted energy expenditure and energy intake. They also consumed significantly less daily energy than age-, height- and weight-matched non-gymnast controls (5780 vs. 7304 kJ, 1381 vs. 1745 kcal) (Kirchner et al. 1995).

The only reviewed published survey of energy and nutrient intake in male gymnasts determined that these athletes had the lowest energy intake (approximately 8707 kJ·day⁻¹ or 2080 kcal·day⁻¹) of college athletes involved in various college sports (Short & Short 1983). The other sports evaluated in this survey included wrestling, basketball, football (American), crew, track, track and field, lacrosse, football (soccer), mountain climbing and body building.

A study of 18 former competitive gymnasts (female), with a mean age of 36.3 years at the time of the study, were found to consume 10.9 MJ·day⁻¹ (2620 kcal·day⁻¹) (Kirchner et al. 1996). This level of intake is 119% of the RDA and 12% higher than a group of age-, height- and weight-matched controls (Kirchner et al. 1996). This is a dramatic departure from the energy intake of gymnasts who are actively competing, and may indicate a degree of liberalized eating behaviour that follows years of restrained eating.

### Energy substrate distribution

The intake of energy substrates in gymnastics should be based on usage rate and the association of different energy substrates with other needed nutrients. Because gymnastics activity in both competition and practice is primarily anaerobic, there is a heavy reliance on glycogen and creatine phosphate as fuels. Glycogen storage is best accomplished on diets that are high in starchy carbohydrates. Creatine storage, which can be synthesized from the amino acids glycine, arginine and methionine, is best obtained in the diet through consumption of skeletal muscle (meat protein) (Crim et al. 1976; Coggan & Coyle 1988). (For information related to creatine metabolism and creatine monohydrate supplementation, see Chapter 27.)

---

*Body fat percentage derived by dual energy X-ray absorptiometry (DEXA).

The anaerobic nature of gymnastics should place limitations on the total quantity of fat consumed, since there would be difficulty in metabolizing fat as an energy substrate during training. Therefore, it appears that a conservative distribution of energy substrates for gymnasts should be as follows: 20–25% of total calories from fat, 15% of total calories from protein, and 60–65% of total calories from carbohydrate. This represents an energy distribution that is only slightly lower in fat and slightly higher in carbohydrate than that recommended for the general population (30% from fat, 15% from protein, and 55% from carbohydrate) (Table 45.3) (Whitney et al. 1994).

Some studies suggest that intense exercise for 1 h can significantly lower liver glycogen, and 2 h of intense exercise may deplete both liver glycogen and the glycogen in specific muscles involved in the activity, particularly when carbohydrate intake is inadequate (Bergstrom et al. 1967; Costill et al. 1971; Coggan & Coyle 1988). Studies have also established the importance of glycaemic index and timing of carbohydrate ingestion as important factors in glycogen repletion. (For issues related to glycogen storage, see Chapter 7.) Results of these studies suggest that the most rapid rise in postexercise muscle glycogen occurs with high glycaemic index foods, and that consumption of foods immediately following exercise results in a better glycogen storage than if food ingestion is delayed (Ivy et al. 1988; Burke et al. 1993).

While the requirement for carbohydrate is high in gymnastic activities, it is unclear whether gymnasts would benefit by pursuing a glycogen-loading technique to enhance total glycogen storage (Maughan & Poole 1981; Wooton & Williams 1984). There is a particular concern that a supersaturation of the tissues with glycogen may cause excessive stiffness and a feeling of heaviness because of the increased water retention associated with stored glycogen (2.7 g $H_2O$ for each g of glycogen stored) (McArdle et al. 1986). This would be unacceptable in a sport where flexibility is needed for achieving the required skills. A reasonable approach therefore would be one that encourages a high level of carbohydrate intake as a regular part of the diet rather than the initiation of a protocol that would lead to a supercompensation of carbohydrate in the tissues.

Total energy intake in gymnasts is inadequate and, of the energy consumed, too great a proportion is derived from fats and too little from carbohydrates (see Table 45.3). Of the 11 studies reviewed, only one had a carbohydrate intake greater than 60% from total kilocalories, and seven of the studies had fat intakes greater than 30% of total kilocalories. The highest carbohy-

**Table 45.3** Energy substrate distribution in different gymnastic populations, organized by age of subjects.

| Subject age (years) | Total energy (kJ) | Total energy (kcal) | Energy from carbohydrate (%) | Energy from protein (%) | Energy from fat (%) | Reference |
|---|---|---|---|---|---|---|
| 9.4±0.8 | 6934±1525 | 1651±363 | 52.3 | 15.9 | 32.1 | Benardot et al. (1989) |
| 11.4±0.9 | 7165±1768 | 1706±421 | 52.7 | 15.0 | 32.5 | Benardot et al. (1989) |
| 11.5±0.5 | 6586 | 1568 | 57.1 | 15.2 | 27.4 | Ersoy (1991) |
| 12.3±1.7 | 6518±2138 | 1552±509 | 47.7 | 15.3 | 36.0 | Reggiani et al. (1989) |
| 14.8 | 7325 | 1744 | 50.0 | 12.8 | 38.7 | Calabrese (1985) |
| 14.8±1.2 | 8106±1911 | 1930±455 | 52.0 | 15.0 | 32.0 | Lindholm et al. (1995) |
| 15.2±4.1 | 8077±2831 | 1923±674 | 46.1 | 15.4 | 28.3 | Moffatt (1984) |
| 15.8±0.9 | 6283±1743 | 1496±415 | 64.9 | 18.6 | 16.4 | Benardot (1996) |
| 19.7±0.2 | 5800±458 | 1381±109 | 52.1 | 15.5 | 31.1 | Kirchner et al. (1995) |
| — | 8736 | 2080 | 44.0 | 15.0 | 39.0 | Short and Short (1983) |
| 36.3±1.0 | 11 004±1100 | 2620±262 | 48.1 | 13.9 | 26.2 | Kirchner et al. (1996) |

drate and lowest fat intake is seen in national team gymnasts, and the lowest carbohydrate and highest fat is seen in college male gymnasts. An increase in fat and protein intake has been proposed recently as a means of increasing athletic performance (Sears 1995), but there is little evidence that such a diet would actually improve athletic performance (Coleman 1996). There is good evidence that increasing dietary fat intake may not influence energy metabolism to the degree that increasing carbohydrate intake does (Schutz et al. 1989). Therefore, increasing fat intake may make it easier for a gymnast to increase body fat than would increasing carbohydrate intake. This relationship between dietary fat intake and body-fat percentage is well elaborated. In a review of five studies that evaluated this relationship in both males and females, all have shown a positive relationship between fat intake and body fat storage (Dattilo 1992). Assuming that the gymnastics surveys represent a true reflection of the energy distribution of gymnasts, it appears that most gymnasts would benefit by lowering fat intake and increasing the intake of carbohydrates. However, since carbohydrates provide energy in a lower density package than fats, it is conceivable that gymnasts could consume a greater volume of food and still obtain less total energy. Therefore, care must be taken that this shift in the intake of energy substrates does not further reduce the already inadequate energy intake of gymnasts.

To further discourage gymnasts from consuming a low-carbohydrate diet, there is evidence that low-carbohydrate diets, consumed in conjunction with exercise and training, adversely affect the mood state of the athlete (Keith et al. 1991). While there are limited data on male gymnasts, two surveys indicated that protein intake in male gymnasts is $2.0 \, \text{g} \cdot \text{kg}^{-1} \cdot \text{day}^{-1}$, or more than 20% of total energy from protein (Short & Short 1983; Brotherhood 1984). By most measures, this level of protein intake is excessive and is not likely to be optimal for gymnasts (Tarnopolsky et al. 1988; Kaufman 1990; Butterfield et al. 1992). (For information on protein requirements in athletes, see Chapter 10.)

The issue of creatine intake (either as preformed creatine from dietary meat, or as a creatine monohydrate supplement) is an important one to consider, since several studies have reported that athletes involved in high-intensity anaerobic sports may benefit from a higher level of creatine intake (Harris et al. 1992; Greenhaff et al. 1993; Balsom et al. 1995; Maughan 1995). In a recently completed study on elite female gymnasts, it was found that those consuming creatine monohydrate during an intensive 3-day training camp were better able to maintain anaerobic power and anaerobic endurance than those consuming an energy-equivalent placebo (Kozak et al. 1996). Since these gymnasts consumed less than their predicted requirement for energy, it is not possible to know if the same result would have been seen with adequate energy consumption. (Creatine metabolism, phosphocreatine and creatine monohydrate supplementation are subjects covered in Chapter 27.)

Given the substantial scientific evidence that diets high in carbohydrates, moderate in protein, and low in fat provide the best mix of fuels for both aerobic and anaerobic activities, there is little reason to support another type of a dietary regimen. A starting point for gymnasts would be to increase complex carbohydrate intake and decrease fat intake, all with an eye toward supplying sufficient nutrient and energy to meet physiological needs.

## Nutrient intake

What follows is a review of surveys that have evaluated nutrient intake in gymnasts. In general, these surveys indicate that gymnasts typically have intakes that are below established recommended levels in one or more nutrients, likely because total energy intake is also below desired levels. It is difficult to predict the true requirement for nutrients in this population because, although growing, they are small in stature with a higher proportion of metabolic mass than the average for people their age.

Most nutrient requirements for highly active anaerobic (power) athletes have not been well

Table 45.4 Summary of selected nutrient intakes in surveys of artistic gymnasts. Values are average intakes.

| Subject group (n) | Vit. A ($\mu g^{RE}$) | Vit. C (mg) | Vit. $B_1$ (mg) | Vit. $B_2$ (mg) | Niacin ($mg^{NE}$) | Calcium (mg) | Iron (mg) | Reference |
|---|---|---|---|---|---|---|---|---|
| College elite male (10) | 1100 | 97.0 | 1.10 | 1.20 | 16.00 | 1059 | 12.0 | Short and Short (1983) |
| High-school female (13) | 883 | 83.6 | 1.04 | 1.39 | 13.36 | 706 | 11.3 | Moffatt (1984) |
| 7–10-year-old competitive female (29) | 1031 | 129.0 | 1.40 | 1.80 | 17.50 | 840 | 11.0 | Benardot et al. (1989) |
| 11–14-year-old competitive female (22) | 1127 | 145.0 | 1.50 | 1.80 | 18.20 | 867 | 11.0 | Benardot et al. (1989) |
| 12–13-year-old competitive female (26) | 771 | 56.1 | 0.60 | 0.70 | 8.70 | 539 | 6.2 | Reggiani et al. (1989) |
| 10–12 year-old competitive female (20) | 834 | 64.0 | 0.74 | 1.45 | 8.50 | 397 | 8.4 | Ersoy (1991) |
| Elite adolescent female (22) | 1200 | 79.0 | — | — | — | 1215 | 14.0 | Lindholm et al. (1995) |
| College elite female (26) | — | — | — | — | — | 683 | 11.8 | Kirchner et al. (1995) |

studied. Therefore, it is unclear whether small stature would translate into a generally lower requirement for a nutrient, or the higher lean mass would translate into a generally higher requirement for a nutrient. In addition, there is no clear way to predict how anaerobic activities might influence nutrient usage (and requirement) in this population (Table 45.4).

### Vitamin A (retinol)

In three studies evaluating vitamin A intake in gymnasts, subjects consumed less than the recommended level of 1000 $\mu g^{RE}$ (Moffatt 1984; Reggiani et al. 1989; Ersoy 1991). In four other surveys, gymnasts were found to consume adequate levels of vitamin A (Short & Short 1983; Benardot et al. 1989; Lindholm et al. 1995). There is no apparent pattern of vitamin A intake among younger, older, elite and non-elite gymnasts. When a value of 75% of the RDA is applied to the intake of vitamin A, all surveys indicate that the consumption of vitamin A in gymnasts is adequate. (See Chapters 20 and 21 for information on vitamins.)

### Vitamin C (ascorbic acid)

Only one study, which evaluated vitamin C

consumption in 12–13-year-old competitive gymnasts in Italy, noted an intake that was marginally below the recommended intake (56.1 vs. 60.0 mg; Reggiani et al. 1989). The intake of vitamin C in four other studies was only marginally better than the recommended intake of 60 mg·day$^{-1}$ (Short & Short 1983; Moffatt 1984; Ersoy 1991; Lindholm et al. 1995). In one survey of 7–10-year-old and 11–14-year-old gymnasts, the intake of vitamin C was approximately double the recommended level (adjusted for age and gender; Benardot et al. 1989). (See Chapters 20 and 21 for information on vitamins.)

### Vitamin $B_1$ (thiamin)

The intake of vitamin $B_1$ was below the recommended level of 1.3–1.5 mg·day$^{-1}$ in three surveys of gymnasts (Short & Short 1983; Moffatt 1984; Reggiani et al. 1989; Ersoy 1991). A marginally adequate intake of vitamin $B_1$ was found in 7–10-year-old and 11–14-year-old competitive female gymnasts (Benardot et al. 1989). The gymnastic survey data are troubling because of the strong and well-established association between thiamin intake and athletic performance. It is likely that athletes consuming an adequate level of energy would obtain a sufficient level of vitamin $B_1$ if a wide variety of foods, emphasizing complex carbohydrates, are consumed. Since most of the gymnastic surveys indicate an under-consumption of energy, an appropriate strategy for improving vitamin $B_1$ intake in gymnasts is an improvement in total energy consumption. (See Chapters 20 and 21 for information on vitamins.)

### Vitamin $B_2$ (riboflavin)

With the exception of a single survey (Benardot et al. 1989), all other nutrient intake studies indicate that riboflavin intake is below the RDA of 1.5–1.8 mg·day$^{-1}$. However, when evaluated as 0.6 mg per 4.2 MJ (1000 kcal) consumed (the basis of the RDA, assuming normal energy consumption), the vitamin $B_2$ intake of gymnasts meets or exceeds the required level in all of the surveys. There are some reports, however, that athletes may have higher rates of vitamin $B_2$ utilization, and may have a predisposition to mild symptoms of riboflavin deficiency (particularly cheilosis), especially when involved in aerobic work (Belko et al. 1983). It is unclear whether gymnasts, who consume less energy than their predicted requirements and who have less total vitamin $B_2$ intake than the RDA, would be at similar risk, especially since the majority of their training is anaerobic. (See Chapters 20 and 21 for information on vitamins.)

### Niacin

Using the niacin RDA for young and adolescent females of 15 mg$^{NE}$, three groups of surveyed gymnasts had niacin intakes below the recommended level (Moffatt 1984; Reggiani et al. 1989; Ersoy 1991). These groups, including gymnasts in high school, elite gymnasts and very young competitive gymnasts, had intakes of niacin that ranged between 89% and 57% of the recommended levels. There is no discernible pattern in the intake of niacin in the published surveys, so it is not clear whether a recommendation should be made for an additional intake on niacin in gymnasts. It is clear, however, that with a balanced intake of food high in complex carbohydrates,

moderate in protein, and moderately low in fat, gymnasts would have little difficulty in obtaining the needed niacin from consumed foods. (See Chapters 20 and 21 for information on vitamins.)

### Calcium

The results of several surveys on gymnasts indicate a level of calcium intake that is significantly lower than the recommended level of intake (see Table 45.4). With the exception of the survey conducted by Lindholm et al. (1995) on elite adolescent females, which found an average calcium intake at the recommended level of 1200 mg, all other surveys indicate a calcium intake ranging between 397 mg (10–12-year-old females) and 1059 mg (college-age males). Given the frequency with which gymnasts suffer from musculoskeletal injury, and the degree to which calcium intake is associated with a reduction of skeletal injury risk, it is alarming that the calcium intake of gymnasts appears to be so inadequate across all groups evaluated (Dixon & Fricker 1993; Nattiv & Mandelbaum 1993; Sands et al. 1993).

Even with inadequate calcium intakes, there is evidence that gymnasts have higher bone mineral densities than those of age-matched controls (Nichols et al. 1994; Kirchner et al. 1995). It is likely that the physical stresses placed on the skeleton from gymnastics activity stimulates calcium deposition in the bone (Slemenda et al. 1991; Carbon 1992; Fehily et al. 1992; VandenBergh et al. 1995). It is confounding, however, that gymnasts have high bone densities despite having multiple risk factors related to poor bone development and bone loss, including primary and secondary amenorrhoea (Sundgot-Borgen 1994), high cortisol levels (Licata 1992), low calcium intake (VandenBergh et al. 1995), low weights (Miller et al. 1991), and low heights (Miller et al. 1991). Given the high level of lean body (muscle) mass found in gymnasts (in the 75th percentile for their height and age (Benardot & Czerwinski 1991), it may be that bone density, while high, remains insufficient to support this level of muscular force. This latter possibility is supported by the disproportionately high level of skeletal injuries suffered in gymnastics (Dyment 1991). It is prudent therefore to encourage gymnasts to consume at least 1200 mg calcium·day⁻¹. There is some evidence that a higher level of calcium (up to 1500 mg calcium·day⁻¹) may be even more beneficial in supporting bone development and reducing skeletal injury risk, especially for young athletic females (Carbon 1992). (See Chapter 23 for information on calcium.)

### Iron

The iron intake of gymnasts was found to be below the recommended level (15 mg·day⁻¹ in females between 11 and 24 years) in all of the surveys reviewed (see Table 45.4). This has numerous implications for the gymnasts' resistance to disease, but also has implications for growth, strength, and the ability to concentrate (Loosli 1993). The current recommendation of 15 mg iron·day⁻¹ for adolescents is based on the 10-mg adult male and postmenopausal female requirement, plus an allowance for menstrual losses and growth (National Research Council 1989). In fact, linear growth velocity and enlargement of blood volume during adolescence is the reason the male recommended intake is only slightly lower (12 mg·day⁻¹) than that for females (National Research Council 1989). Since gymnasts have delayed menarche and a slower growth velocity than non-gymnasts, it is possible to conclude that the requirement for iron intake in gymnasts is lower than that for the general population. With only limited published data on the actual haemoglobin, haematocrit, and ferritin status of gymnasts, it is impossible to fully understand if current iron intakes match actual need. There are some data indicating, however, that a significant number of gymnasts do have low low serum iron and a high rate of anaemia (Lindholm *et al.* 1995).

The typical diet in industrialized nations provides approximately 6 mg of iron per 4.2 MJ (1000 kcal) of energy (Whitney *et al.* 1994). Given the energy intakes seen in past surveys of gymnasts, it is doubtful that gymnasts would consume more than 12 mg iron·day⁻¹. With the exception of the subjects in the Lindholm *et al.* study (1995), where gymnasts consumed close to the recommended intake of 14 mg iron·day⁻¹, and where a number of gymnasts were found to have low serum iron, all other nutrient intake surveys indicate that gymnasts consume between 6.2 and 12.0 mg iron·day⁻¹. Therefore, even assuming no growth or menstrual losses of iron, the intake of iron in gymnasts must be considered inadequate.

A commonly used strategy for reducing anaemia risk or improving a known low blood iron level is to supplement gymnasts with a daily dose of oral iron (Loosli 1993). However, this strategy may not be the most effective technique for assuring normal iron status. Recent data suggest that administration of oral iron every 3–7 days is as good as daily dosing in children, and produces fewer side-effects (Viteri *et al.* 1992; Gross *et al.* 1994; Stephenson 1995). It also appears that daily oral iron supplementation may reduce weight gain and growth velocity by interfering with normal absorptive mechanisms (Idjradinata *et al.* 1994). Therefore, it seems reasonable to suggest that gymnasts consider taking a weekly or bi-weekly supplement of iron and consume more iron-rich foods to reduce the risk of developing iron-deficiency anaemia. (See Chapter 24 for information on iron.)

## Nutritionally related problems studied in gymnasts

### Female athlete triad

This triad of disorders represents eating disorders (anorexia nervosa, anorexia athletica, bulimia, and other restrictive eating behaviours), amenorrhoea (both primary and secondary), and early development of osteoporosis (Smith 1996). The degree to which the *female athlete triad* occurs in gymnastics remains unclear because a symptom of eating disorders is denial of the disease, and surveys typically rely on the respondent to provide clear and accurate information (Benardot *et al.* 1994). There are additional weaknesses in the reliability of the Eating Disorder

Inventory (Garner *et al.* 1983) and the Eating Attitude Test (Garner & Garfinkel 1979) when applied to athlete populations (Sundgot-Borgen 1994). Despite these problems in determining incidence data, there is no question that the female athlete triad exists, and represents a serious and potentially life-threatening reality in gymnastics (Rosen & Hough 1988; Sundgot-Borgen 1994). Therefore, it is important for everyone associated with gymnastics, including team and personal physicians, nutritionists, judges, coaches, parents, and the athletes themselves, to become sensitized to the warning signs of the triad to ensure that its frequency and seriousness is controlled.

Weight preoccupation appears to be associated with gymnastics training, but disordered eating patterns are reduced following retirement from gymnastics (O'Connor *et al.* 1996b). It also appears that, in initiating disordered eating behaviours, gymnasts are trying to achieve an ideal body (i.e. small, muscular, strong appearance) rather than trying to achieve an ideal body fat (O'Connor *et al.* 1996b).

Eating disorders have also been shown to have a negative impact on athletic performance, although this area has not been well studied. Athletes who lower water intake or increase water loss to lower weight have been shown to lose endurance and have reduced exercise performance (Webster *et al.* 1990). Fasting, which would encourage a faster depletion of muscle glycogen (a critical factor in high-intensity activity such as gymnastics), has also been shown to reduce performance (Sundgot-Borgen 1994).

There is a relationship between dietary restraint and menstrual cycle difficulties (shortened luteal phase length), both of which may be associated with lower bone density of predominantly trabecular bone (Prior *et al.* 1990; Barr *et al.* 1994). Trabecular bone, which has a higher turnover rate than cortical bone, is more sensitive to low circulating oestrogen, while cortical bone may be stabilized or even increase in density with physical activity, even in the presence of inadequate oestrogen (Slemenda *et al.* 1991; Carbon 1992). This has been clearly demon-strated in one study evaluating elite college gymnasts, which showed an increase in bone mineral density despite the presence of amenorrhoea or oligomenorrhoea (Nichols *et al.* 1994). (See Chapter 40 for information on eating disorders in athletes, Chapter 32 for information on the young athlete, and Chapter 31 for information on the female athlete.)

## Gymnastics injuries

Although gymnastics is commonly mentioned as a hazardous sport, a review of all the injuries reported between 1982 and 1991 in 42 male and 74 Australian female elite artistic gymnasts found a low number of severe injuries and no catastrophic injuries (Dixon & Fricker 1993). In a study analysing posture, spinal sagittal mobility, and subjective back problems in former female elite gymnasts, it was determined that the gymnasts had fewer problems than an age-matched control group (27% vs. 38%, respectively; Tsai & Wredmark 1993).

Despite these data, it is clear that gymnastics injuries do occur, and often it is an injury that takes talented gymnasts out of the sport. In the study by Dixon and Fricker (1993), stress fractures of the lumbosacral spine accounted for 45% of all bony injuries in female gymnasts. The feet accounted for 32% of stress fractures and 28% of all bony injuries. In male gymnasts, stress fractures of the lumbosacral spine accounted for 33% of all stress fractures and 16% of all bony injuries. In the male gymnasts, there were approximately the same number of stress fractures and fractures (Dixon & Fricker 1993). A 5-year prospective study by Sands *et al.* (1993) determined that a new injury was expected to occur nine out of every 100 training exposures, with the most frequent injuries related to repetitive stress syndrome. There was a higher injury incidence associated with competitions and performance of full routines than training (Sands *et al.* 1993).

The nutritional relationship to injury is difficult to prove, but several studies have demonstrated a relationship between injury frequency and nutritional factors. Muscle-glycogen depletion is associated with fatigue, muscle fibre damage, and joint weakness that could predispose an athlete to skeletal injury (Schlabach 1994). An adequate calcium intake of 1500 mg·day⁻¹ may impart some degree of safety in helping to reduce fracture risk (Heaney 1991), and if it is not possible to obtain sufficient calcium through food consumption, calcium supplementation has been found to be effective in increasing bone mineral density in children (Johnston *et al.* 1992).

## Attainment of ideal body composition

The literature is filled with data showing that competitive gymnasts, regardless of age, have body fat levels that are lower than those of age-matched control groups (O'Connor *et al.* 1996a). The best male gymnasts, who attain their top athletic performances in late adolescence, tend to have low body fat levels (3–4% has been reported in the literature), and an average lean body weight of 63.5 kg (Bale & Goodway 1990). When female gymnasts reach the elite ranks in mid- to late adolescence, they tend to have weights of about 50 kg, with body fat levels of between 10% and 16% (Bale & Goodway 1990).

Gymnasts appear to be particularly susceptible to methods of achieving desirable weight and body composition that are commonly described

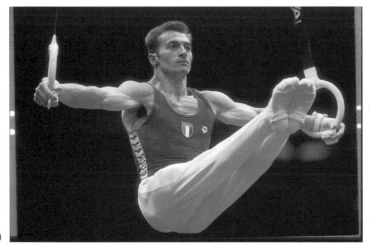

(a)

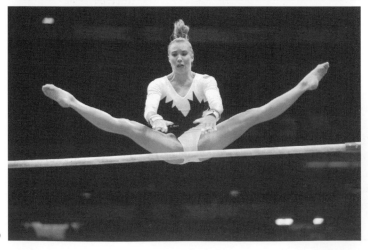

(b)

**Fig. 45.2** In both men's and women's gymnastics, a high power to mass ratio is essential. Elite competitors are characterized by good muscle development and low body fat content. (a) Photo © Allsport / M. Powell. (b) Photo © Allsport / D. Pensinger.

as 'pathogenic' (Rosen *et al.* 1986). In fact, gymnasts are often seen as having a body composition that is most similar to that seen in anorexics and female long-distance runners. The only major difference observed between these groups is a slightly higher body-fat percentage and lower lean body mass in the anorexics (Bale *et al.* 1996). The physical development of the upper body may exacerbate the development of eating problems. It has been shown that gymnasts have a well-developed upper-body musculature that may limit movement of the thorax to reduce its resting end-expiratory size. This limitation may reduce a gymnast's ventilation efficiency, lowering oxygen flow to the working muscles (Barlett

*et al.* 1984). This reduction in oxygen exchange may exacerbate the difficulties many gymnasts experience in maintaining ideal body weight by reducing fat metabolism capability, and may help to explain why so many gymnasts are driven to pathogenic weight control methods to achieve the desired body composition.

Data from several surveys (Tables 45.5, 45.6) generally indicate a steady rise in height and weight by age. Using the statistical technique of meta-analysis, it was determined that age is significantly correlated to body-fat percentage ($r=0.712$; $P=0.004$), height ($r=0.720$; $P=0.002$) and weight ($r=0.829$; $P=0.000$). However, body-fat percentage is not significantly correlated to

**Table 45.5** Heights, weights and body-fat percentages of gymnasts.

| Population, age in years ($n$) | Height (cm) | Weight (kg) | Body fat (%) | Method | Reference |
|---|---|---|---|---|---|
| Junior elite, age 9.1 (100) | 131.1±6.6 | 27.3±4.1 | 8.6±2.0 | Skinfolds | Benardot and Czerwinski (1991) |
| Junior elite, age 9.4 (51) | 134.9 | 30.6 | 9.3 | Skinfolds | Benardot *et al.* (1989) |
| Junior elite, age 11.3 (46) | 141.0±6.9 | 32.8±4.9 | 9.2±1.9 | Skinfolds | Benardot and Czerwinski (1991) |
| Junior elite, age 11.5 (19) | 142.0+2.8 | 31.6±1.5 | 21.5 | Skinfolds | Ersoy (1991) |
| Junior club, age 12.3 (26) | 145.8±8.5 | 37.9±6.9 | 15.0±3.5 | Bioelectrical impedence | Reggiani *et al.* (1989) |
| Junior elite, age 12.3 (22) | 142.0±1.3 | 33.2±1.0 | 14.9±0.7 | Skinfolds | Theintz *et al.* (1993) |
| Junior elite, age 13.3 (20) | 148.0±9.6 | 39.9±7.9 | 10.9±3.2 | Hydrostatic weighing | Bale *et al.* (1996) |
| Club level, age 14.8 (20) | 152.0 | 43.5 | — | — | Calabrese (1985) |
| Junior elite, age 14.8 (22) | 158.0 | 46.8 | 13.2 | Skinfolds | Lindholm *et al.* (1995) |
| High school, age 15.2 (13) | 161.1±3.8 | 50.4±6.5 | 13.1±5.1 | Hydrostatic weighing | Moffatt (1984) |
| National team, age 15.8 (22) | 153.3±5.9 | 46.9±6.1 | 11.3±3.7 | DEXA | Benardot (1996) |
| College, age 19.5 (21) | 159.4±4.3 | 55.0±6.5 | 15.6±2.9 | DEXA | Robinson *et al.* (1995) |
| College, age 19.7 (10) | 158.7±4.8 | 53.0±6.1 | 16.8±3.2 | Hydrostatic weighing | Barlett *et al.* (1984) |
| College, age 19.7 (26) | 158.0±1.1 | 54.1±1.2 | 17.0±0.5 | DEXA | Kirchner *et al.* (1995) |
| Former elite, age 36.3 (18) | 161.6±1.5 | 59.7±1.8 | 23.9±1.0 | DEXA | Kirchner *et al.* (1996) |

**Table 45.6** Meta-analysis: Pearson correlation coefficients of means.

|  | Age (years) | Body fat (%) | Height (cm) | Weight (kg) |
|---|---|---|---|---|
| Age (years) | 1.000 | 0.712* | 0.720* | 0.829* |
| Body fat (%) | 0.712* | 1.000 | 0.505 | 0.520 |
| Height (cm) | 0.720* | 0.505 | 1.000 | 0.961* |
| Weight (kg) | 0.829* | 0.520 | 0.961* | 1.000 |

*Correlation is significant at the 0.01 level (2-tailed).

height and weight in these populations. This is due to the notable exceptions in body-fat trends seen in the more competitive groups analysed. These more competitive gymnasts have higher weights, but lower body fat, indicating that the more elite gymnasts have more muscle mass per unit weight. The least competitive of the groups analysed are the tallest, weigh the most, and have the highest body fats for their age groups. This finding is in agreement with a study of young highly elite gymnasts, who were in the 25th percentile for height/age and weight/age, but in the 75th percentile for arm-muscle circumference and arm-muscle area (Benardot & Czerwinski 1991).

It was pointed out in a study by Grediagin *et al.* (1995) that exercise of different intensities is not related to differential changes in body fat if the total energy burned is equivalent. In this study, it was determined that change in body fat was equivalent in high- and low-intensity activity, but low-intensity exercise (aerobic) caused a greater change in weight because the high-intensity activity was better able to maintain (or increase) lean body mass. Therefore, seeing low body fat levels and high lean body mass in highly active gymnasts involved in high-intensity anaerobic activity is not unexpected.

A standard technique used by gymnasts to attain (or retain) what they perceive to be an ideal body for gymnastics is restrained eating. There are several questions about whether restrained eating is, ultimately, a good strategy for achieving this end since we have adaptive mechanisms that tend to stabilize tissue composition, even in the presence of altered energy intake (Flatt 1987;

Saltzman & Roberts 1995). A study by Benardot (1996) demonstrated this point. In evaluating energy balance by monitoring within-day energy imbalances on national team gymnasts, he found that the size of the largest energy deficit within a day was significantly correlated ($r=0.583$; $P=0.004$) to body-fat percentage, and the number of energy deficits within a day that were greater than 300 kcal explained a sufficient amount of variance in body-fat percentage that it could be predicted (see section on energy intake, above). In addition, total energy intake had a significant negative correlation with body-fat percentage ($r=0.418$; $P=0.038$). That is, the lower the energy intake, the higher the body-fat percentage. This adaptive response of lower energy expenditure and higher body-fat storage with inadequate energy intake may drive gymnasts to continually eat less to achieve the desired body profile. Sadly, this restrained eating pattern may also be the stimulus to the eventual development of disordered eating and related problems that are so often seen in gymnasts.

### Growth retardation

Gymnasts are significantly smaller than non-gymnasts of the same age and they appear to be missing the distinct growth spurt typically seen in adolescence (Lindholm *et al.* 1994). However, it remains unclear whether this shorter stature is due to a self-selection in the sport, which may attract and retain small individuals, or if there is a real stunting of growth that occurs as a result of participation in gymnastics. It has been reported that gymnasts who train more than 18 h·week[-1] before and during puberty do, if fact, have marked stunting of growth (Theintz *et al.* 1993). Theintz *et al.* (1993) also pointed out that, if this intensive exercise schedule occurred before puberty, the gymnasts would permanently alter the growth rate and keep them from ever reaching full adult height. It was particularly noted in this study that leg length was significantly stunted in gymnasts, resulting in a marked difference in sitting height/leg-length ratio when compared to age-equivalent swimmers. This stunting of leg length was associated with a related reduction in predicted height. However, these data do not agree with those of Claessens *et al.* (1992), who found that artistic gymnasts do not differ from non-athletes in leg length, but do have broader shoulders relative to hips. The data of Claessens *et al.* (1992) and Theintz *et al.* (1993) do agree in the area of height and weight. These data demonstrate that gymnasts between the ages of 13 and 20 are considerably shorter and lighter with narrower hips than age-matched non-gymnasts.

It is unclear whether the reduced growth in gymnasts is due to a diet-related inhibition of the hypothalamic–pituitary–gonadal axis from inadequate energy and nutrient intake, or from the combination of inadequate energy and nutrients coupled with a heavy training regimen (Lindholm *et al.* 1994). It is possible that iron status plays a role in this reduced growth. Anaemia, which is seen in about one-third of the gymnasts evaluated, is associated with poor growth velocity in children (Lifshitz *et al.* 1987; Benardot *et al.* 1989; Lindholm *et al.* 1995). Gymnasts have significantly delayed age of menarche when compared to non-gymnasts, and are also shorter and lighter.

It has been suggested that, because gymnasts fail to achieve normal growth velocity during what should be the adolescent growth spurt, gymnastic training should be decreased (Mansfield & Emans 1993). It is hypothesized that decreased training would reduce the incidence of athletic amenorrhoea and the associated hypooestrogenaemia that is associated with decreased bone density and delayed puberty.

## Summary recommendations

### General guidelines

Exercise causes two fundamental physiological events: the body burns energy at a faster rate, and the increase in energy usage causes body temperature to rise, causing a greater rate of water loss through sweat. Therefore, gymnasts should consume sufficient energy to meet the needs of activity *plus* the needs of growth, and should consume sufficient fluids to ensure adequate hydration. Both the provision of sufficient energy and fluids will improve athletic performance by assuring sufficient glycogen and normal muscle function (muscles are approximately 70% water when optimally hydrated) (Hargreaves 1996).

The majority of food consumed should be from complex carbohydrates, but the consumption of fibrous vegetables should be avoided for several hours before training or competition because they are gas causing and may make the gymnast feel uncomfortable from distention. It is not necessary to avoid fat consumption, but a slight lowering of fat intake coupled with an increase in carbohydrate intake may be a desirable dietary change for many gymnasts. This can most easily be achieved through limited consumption of fried foods, visible fats (butter, margarine, meat fat, etc.), and fatty dairy products. There should be a reliance on food rather than vitamin and mineral supplements for obtaining needed nutrients, but the intake of certain mineral supplements (calcium and iron in particular) may be advisable under some circumstances. Periodic consumption of lean red meat is advisable, in that it is an excellent source of iron and zinc, and may improve the availability of creatine or its precursors (amino acids).

Restrained eating behaviours are counterproductive and may initiate more serious pathologic disordered eating patterns. Therefore, gymnasts should try to maintain a frequent eating and snacking pattern to maintain metabolic rate and blood glucose, and improve total energy and nutrient intake. Small but frequent meals and snacks are better than larger less frequent meals, even when the total energy and nutrient content of the meals is similar.

Fluid consumption should be constant to maintain optimal hydration status. Both water and sports beverages are appropriate for gymnasts. Avoidance of thirst is important, since the thirst sensation does not occur until there has been a significant lowering of total body water (Harkins *et al.* 1993). Returning the body to normal hydration after this occurs is time consuming, and may interfere with a normal training schedule.

### Precompetition/pretraining eating

The two main goals for the precompetition/pretraining eating (PCPTE) include the provision of energy to see the athlete through a significant portion of the PCPTE, and sufficient fluid to assure optimally hydrated muscles. The PCPTE is not a time to experiment with untried eating regimens or new foods. In general, the PCPTE should focus on providing starch-based carbohydrates (bread, pasta, rice, etc.) and fluids. Provision of a nutritionally balanced meal should not be a major concern at this time, especially if nutritious foods are commonly consumed during other times.

There should be adequate opportunity for gastric emptying before the initiation of exercise. Because fats cause a delay in gastric emptying, fat intake for the PCPTE should be kept as low as possible. If the meal consumed is large, it should be completed 3.5–4.0 h prior to the initiation of the PCPTE. Small meals can be completed 2.0–3.0 h before exercise. Light carbohydrate snack (crackers, etc.) may be consumed within 1 h of exercise, but solid foods should always be consumed with fluids (Harkins *et al.* 1993).

Athletes with nervous stomachs may not tolerate solid food well before competition, yet they still require energy to fuel the activity. One possible solution for this group is to consume large amounts of carbohydrate the day before the competition, and consume only small periodic snacks with fluids on the day of competition.

Fluid consumption should be sufficient before the PCPTE to produce clear urine. The usual recommendation is the consumption of 235–470 ml of fluid 2 h before the PCPTE, followed by 115–235 ml of fluid immediately before the PCPTE (Burke 1996; O'Connor 1996).

### Eating during competition/practice

Gymnasts require some source of energy during training and competition. Two main strategies may be tried during training. One strategy is to consume a sports beverage that contains carbohydrate energy throughout the practice. Consumption of approximately 115–235 ml of beverage every 15–20 min is the generally accepted recommendation (American College of Sports Medicine 1996), but the amount should be adjusted by the size of the gymnast and environmental heat and humidity. It is important to avoid drinking a great deal all at one time, since that may cause difficulties with training. Instead, the gymnast must become accustomed to sipping on the beverage periodically. Another strategy is to consume water (115–235 ml of water every 15–20 min), and take a brief (10 min) snack break 2.5–3.0 h after the initiation of practice. A snack may include several crackers and some sports beverage, or several bites of a bagel with some sports beverage. The goal is to assure that blood glucose is maintained.

During gymnastics competition, it is not reasonable to assume that the gymnast will be able to take a snack break. Therefore, gymnasts should periodically sip small amounts of sports beverage between events throughout the competition (115–235 ml every 15–20 min when possible; O'Connor 1996). Since this is the only logical technique to be following during competition, gymnasts should consider this the best technique to follow during practice, so as to become well practiced in this consumption pattern.

### Postcompetition/postpractice eating

Muscles are very receptive to replacing glycogen within the first hour following strenuous activity.

Therefore, gymnasts should have carbohydrate snacks available to consume immediately following training or competition. Ideally, the gymnast should consume 840–1670 kJ (200–400 kcal) (one medium-sized bagel is 695 kJ or 165 kcal; 1 cup pasta is 900 kJ or 215 kcal) immediately following the activity, and then consume an additional 840–1260 kJ (200–300 kcal) of carbohydrate within the next several hours (Harkins *et al.* 1993). As always, fluids should be consumed when solid foods are consumed. Every effort should be made by the gymnast to return hydration to a precompetition state (Burke 1996).

## References

American College of Sports Medicine (1996) Exercise and fluid replacement (position stand). *Medicine and Science in Sports and Exercise* **28**, i–vii.

Bale, P. & Goodway, J. (1990) Performance variables associated with the competitive gymnast. *Sports Medicine* **10**, 139–145.

Bale, P., Doust, J. & Dawson, D. (1996) Gymnasts, distance runners, anorexics body composition and menstrual status. *Journal of Sports Medicine and Physical Fitness* **36**, 49–53.

Balsom, P.D., Soderlund, K., Sjodin, B. & Ekblom, B. (1995) Skeletal muscle metabolism during short duration high intensity exercise: influence of creatine supplementation. *Acta Physiologica Scandinavica* **154**, 303–310.

Barlett, H.L., Mance, M.J. & Buskirk, E.R. (1984) Body composition and expiratory reserve volume in female gymnasts and runners. *Medicine and Science in Sports and Exercise* **16**, 311–315.

Barr, S.I., Prior, J.C. & Vigna, Y.M. (1994) Restrained eating and ovulatory disturbances: possible implications for bone health. *American Journal of Clinical Nutrition* **59**, 92–97.

Belko, A.Z., Obarzanke, E., Kalkwarf, H.J. *et al.* (1983) Effects of exercise on riboflavin requirements of young women. *American Journal of Clinical Nutrition* **37**, 509–517.

Benardot, D. (1996) Working with young athletes: views of a nutritionist on the sports medicine team. *International Journal of Sport Nutrition* **6**, 110–120.

Benardot, D. & Czerwinski, C. (1991) Selected body composition and growth measures of junior elite gymnasts. *Journal of the American Dietetic Association* **91** (1), 29–33.

Benardot, D., Schwarz, M. & Heller, D.W. (1989) Nutrient intake in young, highly competitive gymnasts. *Journal of the American Dietetic Association* **89**, 401–403.

Benardot, D., Joye, A. & Shah, B. (1993) Talent opportunity program (TOPS) gymnasts: nutrient intake and body composition assessment results. *Technique* **13**, 17–20.

Benardot, D., Engelbert-Fenton, K., Freeman, K., Hartsough, C. & Steen, S.N. (1994) *Eating Disorders in Athletes: the Dietician's Perspective.* Sports Science Exchange Roundtable, Gatorade Sports Science Institute, Series No. 5.

Bergstrom, J., Hermansen, L., Hultman, E. & Saltin, B. (1967) Diet, muscle glycogen, and physical performance. *Acta Physiologica Scandinavica* **71**, 140–150.

Bortz, S., Schoonen, J.C., Kanter, M., Kosharek, S. & Benardot, D. (1993) Physiology of anaerobic and aerobic exercise. In *Sports Nutrition: A Guide for the Professional Working with Active People* (ed. D. Benardot), pp. 2–10. The American Dietetic Association, Chicago, IL.

Burke, L.M. (1996) Rehydration strategies before and after exercise. *Australian Journal of Nutrition and Diet* **53** (Suppl. 4), S22–S26.

Burke, L.M., Collier, G.R. & Hargreaves, M. (1993) Muscle glycogen storage after prolonged exercise: effect of the glycemic index of carbohydrate feedings. *Journal of Applied Physiology* **75**, 1019–1023.

Butterfield, G., Cady, C. & Moynihan, S. (1992) Effect of increasing protein intake on nitrogen balance in recreational weight lifters. *Medicine and Science in Sports and Exercise* **24**, S71.

Brotherhood, J.R. (1984) Nutrition and sports performance. *Sports Medicine* **1**, 350–389.

Calabrese, L.H. (1985) Nutritional and medical aspects of gymnastics. *Clinics in Sports Medicine* **4**, 23–30.

Carbon, R.J. (1992) Exercise, amenorrhoea and the skeleton. *British Medical Bulletin* **48**, 546–560.

Claessens, A.L., Malina, R.M., Lefevre, J. *et al.* (1992) Growth and menarcheal status of elite female gymnasts. *Medicine and Science in Sports and Exercise* **24**, 755–763.

Coggan, A.R. & Coyle, E.F. (1988) Effect of carbohydrate feedings during high-intensity exercise. *Journal of Applied Physiology* **65**, 1703–1705.

Coleman, E.J. (1996) The BioZone Nutrition System: A dietary panacea? *International Journal of Sport Nutrition* **6**, 69–71.

Costill, D.L., Bowers, R., Branam, G. & Sparks, K. (1971) Muscle glycogen utilization during prolonged exercise on successive days. *Journal of Applied Physiology* **31**, 834–838.

Crim, M.C., Calloway, D.H. & Margen, S. (1976) Creatine metabolism in men: creatine pool size and turnover in relation to creatine intake. *Journal of Nutrition* **106**, 371–381.

Dattilo, A.M. (1992) Dietary fat and its relationship to body weight. *Nutrition Today* **27**, 13–19.

Dixon, M. & Fricker, P. (1993) Injuries to elite gymnasts

over 10 years. *Medicine and Science in Sports and Exercise* **25**, 1322–1329.

Dyment, P.G. (ed.) (1991) *Sports Medicine: Health Care for Young Athletes*, 2nd edn. American Academy of Pediatrics, Elk Grove Village, IL.

Ersoy, G. (1991) Dietary status and anthropometric assessment of child gymnasts. *Journal of Sports Medicine and Physical Fitness* **31**, 577–580.

Fehily, A.M., Coles, R.J., Evans, W.D. & Elwood, P.C. (1992) Factors affecting bone density in young adults. *American Journal of Clinical Nutrition* **56**, 579–586.

Flatt, J.P. (1987) Dietary fat, carbohydrate balance, and weight maintenance: effects of exercise. *American Journal of Clinical Nutrition* **45**, 296–306.

Garner, D.M. & Garfinkel, P.E. (1979) An index of symptoms of anorexia nervosa. *Psychological Medicine* **9**, 273–279.

Garner, D.M., Olmsted, M.P. & Polivy, J. (1983) Development and validation of a multidimensional eating disorder inventory for anorexia nervosa and bulimia. *International Journal of Eating Disorders* **2**, 15–34.

Grediagin, A., Cody, M., Rupp, J., Benardot, D. & Shern, R. (1995) Exercise intensity does not effect body composition change in untrained, moderately overfat women. *Journal of the American Dietetic Association* **95**, 661–665.

Greenhaff, P.C., Casey, A., Short, A.H., Harris, R., Soderlund, K. & Hultman, E. (1993) Influence of oral creatine supplementation of muscle torque during repeated bouts of maximal voluntary exercise in man. *Clinical Science* **84**, 565–571.

Gross, R., Schultink, W. & Juliawati (1994) Treatment of anemia with weekly iron supplementation. *Lancet* **344**, 821.

Hargreaves, M. (1996) Physiological benefits of fluid and energy replacement during exercise. *Australian Journal of Nutrition and Dietetics* **53** (Suppl. 4), S3–S7.

Harkins, C., Carey, R., Clark, N. & Benardot, D. (1993) Protocols for developing dietary prescriptions. In *Sports Nutrition: A Guide for the Professional Working with Active People* (ed. D. Benardot), pp. 170–185. American Dietetic Association, Chicago, IL.

Harris, R.C., Soderlund, K. & Hultman, E. (1992) Elevation of creatine in resting and exercised muscle of normal subjects by creatine supplementation. *Clinical Science* **83**, 367–374.

Heaney, R.P. (1991) Effect of calcium on skeletal development, bone loss, and risk of fractures. *American Journal of Medicine* **91** (Suppl. 5B), 23–28.

Houtkooper, L.B. & Going, S.B. (1994) Body composition: how should it be measured? Does it affect sport performance? *Gatorade Sports Science Exchange* **7** (5s), SSE#52.

Idjradinata, P., Watkins, W.E. & Pollitt, E. (1994) Adverse effect of iron supplementation on weight gain of iron-replete young children. *Lancet* **343**, 1252–1254.

Ivy, J.L., Katz, A.L., Cutler, C.L., Sherman, W.M. & Coyle, E.F. (1988) Muscle glycogen synthesis after exercise: effect of time of carbohydrate ingestion. *Journal of Applied Physiology* **64**, 1480–1485.

Johnston, C.C., Miller, J.Z., Slemenda, C.W., Reister, T.K., Hui, S., Christian, J.C. & Peacock, M. (1992) Calcium supplementation and increases in bone mineral density in children. *New England Journal of Medicine* **327**, 82–87.

Kaufman, D.A. (1990) Protein as an energy substrate during intense exercise. *Annals of Sports Medicine* **5**, 142.

Keith, R.E., O'Keeffe, K.A., Blessing, D.L. & Wilson, G.D. (1991) Alterations in dietary carbohydrate, protein, and fat intake and mood state in trained female cyclists. *Medicine and Science in Sports and Exercise* **23**, 212–216.

Kirchner, E.M., Lewis, R.D. & O'Connor, P.J. (1995) Bone mineral density and dietary intake of female college gymnasts. *Medicine and Science in Sports and Exercise* **27**, 543–549.

Kirchner, E.M., Lewis, R.D. & O'Connor, P.J. (1996) Effect of past gymnastics participation on adult bone mass. *Journal of Applied Physiology* **80**, 226–232.

Kozak, C.J. (1996) *The effect of creatine monohydrate supplementation on anaerobic power and anaerobic endurance in elite female gymnasts*. Master's Thesis, Georgia State University.

Lemons, P.W.R. (1989) Nutrition for muscular development of young athletes. In *Perspectives in Exercise Science and Sports Medicine*. Vol. 2. *Youth, Exercise, and Sport* (ed. C.V. Gisolfi & D.R. Lamb), pp. 370–371. Benchmark Press, Indianapolis, IN.

Licata, A.A. (1992) Stress fractures in young athletic women: case reports of unsuspected cortisol-induced osteoporosis. *Medicine and Science in Sports and Exercise* **24**, 955–957.

Lifshitz, S., Moses, N., Cervantes, C. & Ginsberg, L. (1987) Nutritional dwarfing in adolescents. *Seminars in Adolescent Medicine* **3**, 255–266.

Lindholm, C., Hagenfeldt, K. & Ringertz, B.-M. (1994) Pubertal development in elite juvenile gymnasts: effects of physical training. *Acta Obstetrica et Gynaecologica Scandinavica* **73**, 269–273.

Lindholm, C., Hagenfeldt, K. & Hagman, U. (1995) A nutrition study in juvenile elite gymnasts. *Acta Paediatrica* **84**, 273–277.

Loosli, A.R. (1993) Reversing sports-related iron and zinc deficiencies. *Physician and Sportsmedicine* **21**, 70–78.

McArdle, W.D., Katch, F.I. & Katch, V.L. (1986) *Exercise*

*Physiology: Energy, Nutrition, and Human Performance*, 2nd edn. Lea & Febiger, Philadelphia, PA.

Maddux, G.T. (1970) *Men's Gymnastics*. Good year Publishing, Pacific Palisades, CA.

Mansfield, M.J. & Emans, S.J. (1993) Growth in female gymnasts: should training decrease during puberty? *Journal of Pediatrics* **122**, 237–240.

Maughan, R.J. (1995) Creatine supplementation and exercise performance. *International Journal of Sport Nutrition* **5**, 94–101.

Maughan, R. & Poole, D. (1981) The effects of a glycogen-loading regimen on the capacity to perform anaerobic exercise. *European Journal of Applied Physiology* **46**, 211–214.

Miller, J.Z., Slemenda, C.W., Meaney, F.J., Reister, T.K., Hui, S. & Johnston, C.C. (1991) The relationship of bone mineral density and anthropometric variables in healthy male and female children. *Bone and Mineral* **14**, 137–152.

Moffatt, R.J. (1984) Dietary status of elite female high school gymnasts: inadequacy of vitamin and mineral intake. *Journal of the American Dietetic Association* **84**, 1361–1363.

National Research Council Committee on Dietary Allowances (1989) *Recommended Dietary Allowances*. National Academy of Sciences, Washington, DC.

Nattiv, A. & Mandelbaum, B.R. (1993) Injuries and special concerns in female gymnasts: detecting, treating, and preventing common problems. *Physician and Sportsmedicine* **21**, 66–81.

Nichols, D.L., Sanborn, C.F., Bonnick, S.L., Ben-ezra, V., Gench, B. & DiMarco, N.M. (1994) The effects of gymnastics training on bone mineral density. *Medicine and Science in Sports and Exercise* **26**, 1220–1225.

O'Connor, H. (1996) Practical aspects of fluid replacement. *Australian Journal of Nutrition and Dietetics* **53** (Suppl. 4), S27–S34.

O'Connor, P.J., Lewis, R.D. & Boyd, A. (1996a) Health concerns of artistic women gymnasts. *Sports Medicine* **21**, 321–325.

O'Connor, P.J., Lewis, R.D., Kirchner, E.M. & Cook, D.B. (1996b) Eating disorder symptoms in former female college gymnasts: relations with body composition. *American Journal of Clinical Nutrition* **64**, 840–3.

Prior, J.C., Vigna, Y.M., Schechter, M.T. & Burgess, A.E. (1990) Spinal bone loss and ovulatory disturbances. *New England Journal of Medicine* **323**, 1221–1227.

Reggiani, E., Arras, G.B., Trabacca, S., Senarega, D. & Chiodini, G. (1989) Nutritional status and body composition of adolescent female gymnasts. *Journal of Sports Medicine* **29**, 285–288.

Robinson, T.L., Snow-Harter, C., Taaffe, D.R., Gillis, D., Shaw, J. & Marcus, R. (1995) Gymnasts exhibit higher bone mass than runners despite similar prevalence

of amenorrhea and oligomenorrhea. *Journal of Bone and Mineral Research* **10**, 26–35.

Rosen, L.W. & Hough, D.O. (1988) Pathogenic weight-control behaviors of female college gymnasts. *Physician and Sportsmedicine* **16**, 141–146.

Rosen, L.W., McKeag, D.B., Hough, D.O. & Curley, V. (1986) Pathogenic weight control behavior in female athletes. *Physician and Sportsmedicine* **14**, 79.

Saltzman, E. & Roberts, S. (1995) The role of energy expenditure in energy regulation: findings from a decade of research. *Nutrition Reviews* **53**, 209–220.

Sands, W.A., Shultz, B.B. & Newman, A.P. (1993) Women's gymnastics injuries: a 5-year study. *American Journal of Sports Medicine* **21**, 271–276.

Schlabach, G. (1994) Carbohydrate strategies for injury prevention. *Journal Athletic Training* **29**, 245–254.

Schutz Y., Flatt, J.P. & Jequier, E. (1989) Failure of dietary fat intake to promote fat oxidation: a factor favoring the development of obesity. *American Journal of Clinical Nutrition* **50**, 307–314.

Sears, B. (1995) *The Zone*. ReganBooks, New York.

Short, S.H. & Short, W.R. (1983) Four-year study of university athletes' dietary intake. *Journal of the American Dietetic Association* **82**, 632–645.

Slemenda, C.W., Miller, J.Z., Hui, S.L., Reister, T.K. & Johnston, C.C. (1991) Role of physical activity in the development of skeletal mass in children. *Journal of Bone and Mineral Research* **6**, 1227–1233.

Smith, A.D. (1996) The female athlete triad: causes, diagnosis, and treatment. *Physician and Sportsmedicine* **24**, 67–76.

Stephenson, L.S. (1995) Possible new developments in community control of iron-deficiency anemia. *Nutrition Reviews* **53**, 23–30.

Sundgot-Borgen, J. (1994) Eating disorders in female athletes. *Sports Medicine* **17**, 176–188.

Tarnopolsky, M.A., MacDougall, J.D. & Atkinson, S.A. (1988) Influence of protein intake and training status on nitrogen balance and lean body mass. *Journal of Applied Physiology* **64**, 187–193.

Theintz, G.E., Howald, H., Weiss, U. & Sizonenko, C. (1993) Evidence for a reduction of growth potential in adolescent female gymnasts. *Journal of Pediatrics* **122**, 306–313.

Tsai, L. & Wredmark, T. (1993) Spinal posture, sagittal mobility, and subjective rating of back problems in former female elite gymnasts. *Spine* **18**, 872–875.

VandenBergh, M.F.Q., DeMan, S.A., Witteman, J.C.M., Hofman, A., Trouerbach, W. & Grobbee, D.E. (1995) Physical activity, calcium intake, and bone mineral content in children in the Netherlands. *Journal Epidemiology and Community Health* **49**, 299–304.

Viteri, F.E., Liu, X.-N. & Morris, M. (1992) Iron (Fe) retention and utilization in daily vs. every 3 days Fe supplemented rats. *FASEB Journal* **6**, A1091.

Webster, S., Rutt, R. & Weltman, A. (1990) Physiological effects of weight loss regimen practiced by college wrestlers. *Medicine and Science in Sports and Exercise* **22**, 229–233.

Whitney, E.N., Cataldo, C.B. & Rolfes, S.R. (1994) *Understanding Normal and Clinical Nutrition*, 4th edn. West Publishing, Minneapolis/St Paul, MO.

Wooton, S.A. & Williams, C. (1984) Influence of carbohydrate status on performance during maximal exercise. *International Journal of Sports Medicine* **5**, S126.

# Chapter 46

# Swimming

RICK L. SHARP

## Introduction

Competitive swimming is a sport practised worldwide and includes swimming events of varied distances (50–1500 m, 22 s to 16 min) and stroke styles (freestyle or crawl stroke, backstroke, breaststroke and butterfly). Competitive swimming meets are held year-round and the age range of the swimmers is between 6 and 80 years. In the United States alone there are between 1.0 and 1.5 million competitive swimmers affiliated with community club teams, high school teams, college teams, and masters swimming teams (M.L. Unger, personal communication).

Each swimming practice session can last up to about 3 h and may include a total swimming volume of 10000 metres or yards. During this time, swimmers are engaged in various types of training that include long-distance endurance training, interval training, sprint training, and stroke instruction. The specific stroke styles swum during training depend on the athlete's specialty, but most swimmers swim at least 75% of their total training volume in freestyle. This training is frequently done twice per day and 6 days per week. In addition to this, many swimmers also participate in dry land training such as strength training or supplemental endurance running or cycling. Thus, the nutritional demands of training in this sport can be quite extraordinary.

## Energy demands of swimming training

The large volume of intensive training of these athletes imposes a tremendous demand on energy supply. Sherman and Maglischo (1992) have estimated the energy requirement of swimming training at approximately 16.8–22.6 MJ · day$^{-1}$ (4000–5400 kcal · day$^{-1}$) for males working 4 h · day$^{-1}$ and between 14.2 and 16.8 MJ · day$^{-1}$ (3400–4000 kcal · day$^{-1}$) for females working 4 h · day$^{-1}$. Certainly, these values will vary considerably according to such factors as the intensity of the exercises used, the swimmer's body mass, and mechanical efficiency. Nevertheless, these high energy needs can be difficult for swimmers to meet.

Several studies have examined the daily diets of competitive swimmers to determine if energy needs are being met. Van Handel et al. (1984) used diet records to examine the energy intakes of 14 female and 13 male competitive swimmers who had competed in the US National Championships and were preparing for the Olympic Trials. Their findings indicate that the energy intake of the men averaged 18.2 MJ · day$^{-1}$ (4350 kcal · day$^{-1}$), with a range between 12.6 and 28.6 MJ · day$^{-1}$ (3010–6830 kcal · day$^{-1}$). Expressed relative to body weight, these men were consuming an average of 0.22 MJ · kg$^{-1}$ (50 kcal · kg$^{-1}$). The women had energy intakes averaging 9.6 MJ · day$^{-1}$ (2300 kcal · day$^{-1}$), with a range between 6.3 and 13.8 MJ · day$^{-1}$ (1500–3300 kcal · day$^{-1}$). Relative to body weight, these women consumed an average of 0.15 MJ·kg⁻¹ (36 kcal·kg⁻¹). Distribution of energy for these athletes was 49% of energy from carbohydrate and 34% of energy from fat for the men, while the women reported 53% of energy from carbohydrate and 30% of energy from fat.

Berning *et al.* (1991) reported energy intakes of adolescent developmental level swimmers attending a training camp. Males consumed an average of 21.9 MJ·day⁻¹ (5230 kcal·day⁻¹) while females reported 15.0 MJ·day⁻¹ (3580 kcal·day⁻¹). Distribution of energy among the energy macronutrients was not different from the general population, prompting the authors to conclude that these swimmers consumed too much fat and inadequate carbohydrate.

In an attempt to determine the influence of training volume on the energy intake of competitive swimmers, Barr and Costill (1992) examined diet records of 24 males during a period of 'low volume' training (22 km·week⁻¹) and during 'high volume' training (44 km·week⁻¹). Energy intake averaged 15.3 MJ·day⁻¹ (3650 kcal·day⁻¹) during the lower volume training and increased significantly to 17.7 MJ·day⁻¹ (4230 kcal·day⁻¹) during the 6 weeks of high-volume training. It was noted that this increase in energy intake did not fully compensate for the higher energy demand of the longer training, since the swimmers maintained their body weight while they lost subcutaneous fat.

Costill *et al.* (1988a) examined male collegiate swimmers before, during and after 10 days of increasing training. Their training distance was increased from 4266 to 8970 m·day⁻¹ while average intensity was maintained at 94% of their maximum oxygen uptake. This resulted in an average energy cost during training of 9.6 MJ·day⁻¹ (2300 kcal·day⁻¹). It was noted that four of the 12 swimmers could not tolerate the higher training volume and were forced to swim their training bouts at slower speeds. In addition, these swimmers had reduced muscle glycogen concentration as a consequence of the combined effect of the intensified training and their low carbohydrate intakes. These findings led the authors to conclude that some swimmers have

difficulty in meeting the energy demands of high-volume training and experience chronic muscle fatigue as a result of their failure to ingest sufficient carbohydrate to match the energy demands.

The studies reviewed above suggest that male competitive swimmers in the age range of 16–23 years typically ingest approximately 18.0 MJ·day⁻¹ (4300 kcal·day⁻¹), while females consume only about 10.9 MJ·day⁻¹ (2600 kcal·day⁻¹) despite the fact that female and male swimmers perform similar training volume and intensity. When these data are compared with the estimated energy requirements of swimming training proposed by Sherman and Maglischo (1992), males tend to remain in energy balance (18.0 MJ·day⁻¹ average intake vs. 16.8–22.6 MJ·day⁻¹ (4300 vs. 5400 kcal·day⁻¹) estimated requirement) while female swimmers tend to maintain a negative energy balance (10.9 MJ·day⁻¹ average intake vs. 14.2–16.8 MJ·day⁻¹ (2600 vs. 3400–4000 kcal·day⁻¹) estimated requirement). These data illustrate the nutritional dilemma facing competitive swimmers, especially females, and their coaches. The tremendous training demands imposed on these athletes require careful consideration of the swimmer's diet to make sure that adequate amounts of food are eaten to provide the energy, macronutrients and micronutrients necessary to support the enormous training loads.

## Body composition

With such high energy demands of daily training in competitive swimming, one might wonder why body fat percentages of swimmers are not lower than they are. Typically, male competitive swimmers have body fat percentages in the range of 8–15% and females at 15–22%. Indeed, studies have confirmed that body composition of competitive swimmers is usually about 4–6% greater than age- and ability-matched endurance runners (Novak *et al.* 1977; Thorland *et al.* 1983).

There are a number of possible explanations for the tendency of swimmers to carry more fat than runners despite similar training loads. One explanation is that although running tends to have a somewhat anorexic effect, especially in the few hours after exercise, swimming may have an opposite effect by stimulating appetite (Harri & Kuusela 1986). This would imply that swimmers tend to increase their energy consumption in parallel with their training where runners may not. To this author's knowledge, there have been no published studies comparing the effects of running and swimming on the postexercise appetite. Under this assumption of increased appetite in swimmers, swimmers would not be expected to lose a great deal of body fat during their training. A study by Johnson *et al.* (1989) with female university swimmers supports this argument since no changes in body composition were observed over a 25-week season of training. In contrast, however, Barr *et al.* (1991) reported decreased body fat, increased lean body mass, and no change in body weight in male college swimmers training $22\,000\,m \cdot week^{-1}$ during a 25-week season. In agreement with this study showing changing body composition in males during swim training is a study by Meleski and Malina (1985) showing decreased body weight, decreased absolute and relative fat mass, and increased lean body mass in a group of female college swimmers during the first 2 months of a training season.

Another explanation that has been proposed for the higher body fat percentages in competitive swimmers is a possible difference in fuel utilization both during and following the exercise that promotes fat storage in swimmers. As support for this argument, some have pointed to studies of cold exposure which is known to stimulate fat storage both in animal models and in humans. To determine if swimming training alters fuel utilization and the hormonal milieu differently from running, Flynn *et al.* (1990) monitored energy expenditure and fuel utilization of eight male swimmers and runners while exercising at 75% of maximum oxygen uptake and during 2 h of recovery. Although the energy cost of recovery was similar between the two exercise modes, the respiratory exchange ratio results suggested increased fat oxidation after swimming compared with running. In contrast, serum glycerol concentration was elevated to a greater extent after running than after swimming, suggesting enhanced mobilization of triglycerides with running. Whether this different response can account for the differences in body composition between runners and swimmers remains to be studied.

## Carbohydrate needs in training

The high volume and intensity of swimming

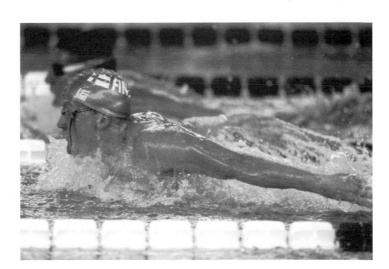

**Fig. 46.1** Swimmers favour high training volumes. This means that a high energy intake is essential, but opportunities for eating may be limited when long training sessions must be combined with work or study. Photo © Allsport.

training places a great demand not only on dietary energy, but also on the carbohydrate needs of these athletes. Maglischo (1993) has estimated that dietary carbohydrate needs of swimmers range between 500 and 800 g·day⁻¹. Thus, a swimmer who consumes a diet providing 16.8 MJ·day⁻¹ (4300 kcal·day⁻¹) with 50% of the energy from carbohydrate will be consuming approximately 500 g·day⁻¹ of carbohydrate and therefore may not meet the carbohydrate demand of the daily training. Clearly, these athletes should make carbohydrate intake a priority in their daily diet.

To determine the amount of muscle glycogen depletion that can occur during typical swim training bouts, Costill *et al.* (1988b) examined muscle glycogen levels of male collegiate swimmers before and after swimming either 2743 or 5486 m. Each swimmer performed the 5486 m of training twice; once by doing 60×91.4 m swims and once by performing 12×457.2 m swims. Biopsies were taken from the anterior deltoid before, at the half-way point of the training session (2743 m), and at the end of each training session and analysed for glycogen concentration. Additional biopsies were taken after 8 h of recovery and ingestion of 112 g carbohydrate to assess the amount of glycogen repletion that might occur in this amount of time. When the training sessions were performed with repeated 91.4-m swims, muscle glycogen concentration declined by 68% at 2743 m, and by 87% at 5486 m (Fig. 46.2). Using repeated 457.2-m swims, muscle glycogen declined by 54% at 2743 m, and by 63% at 5486 m. The greater amount of glycogen depletion with 91.4-m repeats than with 457.2-m repeats was accounted for by a significantly faster swimming speed during the 91.4-m repeats (≈7% faster than during the 457.2-m repeats). In recovery, glycogen repletion was 52% complete after 8 h and ingestion of 112 g of carbohydrate.

These findings show the large loss of muscle glycogen that can occur during a single training session among competitive swimmers. When one considers that many swimmers perform this kind of training on a daily basis, and in many

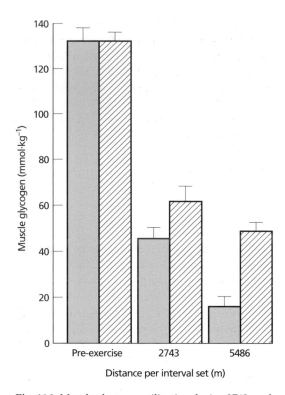

**Fig. 46.2** Muscle glycogen utilization during 2743- and 5486-m interval swim training using repeated 91.4-m (■) or 457-m (▨) swims. Adapted from Costill *et al.* (1988b).

instances twice per day, the probability of chronic glycogen depletion is great, especially considering the incomplete glycogen repletion in the 8 h of recovery. Chronic glycogen depletion may then result in poor performances in subsequent training sessions and in competitions that may follow a period of such training. An obvious solution to this problem is to train only once per day and consume a diet containing at least 500 g·day⁻¹ of carbohydrate. Less frequent training would likely not deplete glycogen from working muscles as much as twice per day training, and the higher intake of dietary carbohydrate would tend to accelerate glycogen repletion in the 24 h between training sessions, especially if a large quantity of carbohydrate is ingested during the first 2 h after the training is finished (MacDougall *et al.* 1977; Ivy *et al.* 1988).

Lamb *et al.* (1990) tested whether a diet in which 80% of calories came from carbohydrate was superior to a 43% carbohydrate diet in supporting the daily training of collegiate swimmers. Both diets provided $19.6 MJ \cdot day^{-1}$ (4680 $kcal \cdot day^{-1}$) and were maintained for 9 days. During the last 5 days of each diet, swimmers performed intervals of various distances ranging from 50 m up to 3000 m and mean swim velocities were recorded. These authors found no significant differences between the two diets in performance of the interval sets. However, they did note that the swimmers who regularly consumed a high carbohydrate diet tended to perform better than those who generally consumed a low carbohydrate diet. A possible reason for the lack of difference in performance between the high and moderate carbohydrate diets could be that even in the moderate carbohydrate diet, enough carbohydrate was supplied to support the demands of their training. At $19.6 MJ \cdot day^{-1}$ (4680 $kcal \cdot day^{-1}$) and 43% carbohydrate, these subjects were consuming an average of 503 g carbohydrate $\cdot day^{-1}$. Costill and Miller (1980) reported that muscle glycogen repletion is proportional to the mass of carbohydrate consumed until carbohydrate intake reaches approximately 600 g $\cdot$ $day^{-1}$. Therefore, it is possible that the 935 g of carbohydrate that were provided in the 80% carbohydrate diet did not stimulate any greater rate of glycogen repletion than the 503 g of carbohydrate provided in the 43% carbohydrate diet.

In light of the observations of Costill *et al.* (1988a), wherein four of the 12 swimmers studied failed to eat enough carbohydrate to prevent chronic muscle glycogen depletion during $8970 m \cdot day^{-1}$ training, it would seem prudent to recommend that swimmers consume a diet that (i) meets the energy requirements of training and (ii) provides at least 600 g carbohydrate $\cdot day^{-1}$.

## Carbohydrate ingestion during training sessions

A number of studies have shown improved endurance performance when carbohydrate is ingested at frequent intervals during the exercise (Coyle *et al.* 1983, 1986; Coggan & Coyle 1987; Davis *et al.* 1988; Tsintzas *et al.* 1993). Typically, the exercise modes studied in these investigations have been either cycling or running. The hypothesized benefit of carbohydrate ingestion is improved maintenance of blood glucose throughout the duration of the activity and/or muscle glycogen sparing leading to increased carbohydrate availability at a time when the low endogenous carbohydrate supplies generally limit muscular performance.

To determine if carbohydrate ingestion during exercise would have similar beneficial effects on the performance of swimming training bouts, O'Sullivan *et al.* (1994) measured swimming performances during a standardized training session once while ingesting a placebo and once while ingesting a liquid carbohydrate supplement. In each of these trials, the nine male collegiate swimmers performed a 5944-m training session composed of a mixture of low- and high-intensity interval training bouts. The final 914 m of the training session was $10 \times 91.4 m$ swims with 20 s rest between each as a performance trial. Performance was measured as each swimmer's average velocity during the first 5, second 5, and for the whole set of $10 \times 91.4 m$. During the carbohydrate supplementation trial, the swimmers were given $1 g \cdot kg^{-1}$ of glucose polymers in 50% solution 10 min into the training session, and $0.6 g \cdot kg^{-1}$ of glucose polymers in 20% solution every 20 min thereafter according to the feeding schedule of Coggan and Coyle (1988). The placebo trial was the same as the carbohydrate trial, but an artificially sweetened placebo drink was substituted for the carbohydrate drink. The trials were conducted 7 days apart in a randomized, double-blind manner. Blood samples were taken before the training session, immediately before each feeding, and at the conclusion of the $10 \times 91.4 m$ performance trial. During the placebo trial, blood glucose concentration remained fairly stable throughout the first 100 min of the training but rose significantly during the $10 \times 91.4 m$ performance test to a final level of $6.3 mmol \cdot l^{-1}$ (Fig. 46.3). In the carbohydrate feeding trial, blood glucose concentration was slightly elevated over the placebo trial at all time points, but no significant differences were observed. Performance times for the 10×91.4 m training set at the end of training averaged 59.1 s in the placebo trial and 59.9 s during the carbohydrate trial. The authors concluded that carbohydrate supplementation was not effective in improving performance late in a swimming practice because blood glucose remains stable even without supplemental carbohydrate. However, individual differences in their responses were presented. Two of the subjects did

experience a substantial decline in blood glucose concentration during the training in the placebo trial. During his placebo trial, one swimmer's blood glucose concentration dropped from 4.3 mmol·l⁻¹ before the training to a low of 2.6 mmol·l⁻¹ immediately before the 10×91.4 m performance trial (Table 46.1). The ingestion of carbohydrate completely prevented this decline and his performance time improved by 1.3 s from 64.3 s in the placebo trial to 63.0 s in the carbohydrate trial. Another subject experienced a drop in blood glucose concentration from 5.6 mmol·l⁻¹ pre-exercise to 3.7 mmol·l⁻¹ immediately before the performance trial. Again, the carbohydrate supplementation prevented this decline and performance improved by 1.1 s from 58.4 to 57.3 s. Thus, it seems that the carbohydrate supplementation protocol used in this study is effective in improving late-practice performance but only for those individuals who normally experience declining blood glucose concentration during the training.

Because it would be impossible for swimmers to know if they normally experience declining blood glucose concentration during training without taking blood samples, coaches may want to recommend carbohydrate supplementation for the entire team. In those individuals who are able to maintain their blood glucose concentrations without supplemental carbohydrate, there is little, if any, risk in consuming the carbohydrate. Therefore, supplementing the entire team would be one way of assuring that those swimmers who need the extra carbohydrate would get it. Alternatively, coaches could watch their swimmers for signs of excessive muscle

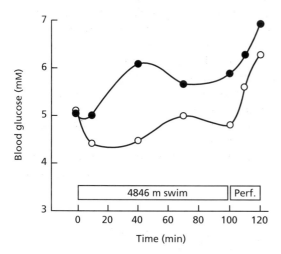

**Fig. 46.3** Blood glucose concentration throughout a 5486-m swim training session when fed placebo (○) or carbohydrate (●) every 20 min. Perf., performance trial of 10 × 91.4-m swims. Adapted from O'Sullivan *et al.* (1994).

**Table 46.1** Responses of two subjects who had declining blood glucose concentration during placebo and carbohydrate trials. Adapted from O'Sullivan *et al.* (1994).

| | Trial | Pre-exercise (mmol·l⁻¹) | Preperformance (mmol·l⁻¹) | Time/91.4 m (s) |
|---|---|---|---|---|
| Subject 1 | Placebo | 4.3 | 2.6 | 64.3 |
| | Carbohydrate | 4.5 | 4.3 | 63.0 |
| Subject 2 | Placebo | 5.6 | 3.7 | 58.4 |
| | Carbohydrate | 5.7 | 7.2 | 57.3 |

fatigue during the latter part of training sessions and prescribe a carbohydrate supplement only to those who consistently seem to have difficulty maintaining their work output.

There is a more fundamental question than whether or not carbohydrate supplementation is effective in improving training performance. By preventing the decline in blood glucose concentration during training, we effectively eliminate one of the physiological/metabolic stresses imposed by the training. Since training is a careful dosage of physical stress to create long-term adaptations that will ultimately improve competitive performance potential, elimination of these stresses may lessen the degree of adaptation experienced by the athlete. Whether or not one adapts in a performance-enhancing way to low carbohydrate availability is not currently known, but this may be part of the stimulus that improves glycogen storage in endurance athletes (Gollnick *et al.* 1973; Piehl *et al.* 1974; Costill *et al.* 1985a).

## Carbohydrate ingestion after training

Studies have shown that muscle glycogen resynthesis is accelerated when carbohydrate is ingested within 1–2 h after the exercise is stopped (Ivy *et al.* 1988). In this immediate postexercise period, evidence suggests that high glycaemic index sugars may be the preferred carbohydrate source since insulin is known to be a potent activator of muscle glycogen synthase. A recent study also suggests including some protein in the postexercise meal because the protein will augment the insulin response to the carbohydrate and thereby stimulate an even greater rate of muscle glycogen storage (Zawadzki *et al.* 1992). Since competitive swimmers likely experience large decrements in muscle glycogen concentration during single training sessions, it seems wise to provide a carbohydrate source soon after the training session ends. This strategy may be helpful in preventing the chronic muscle glycogen depletion that undoubtedly occurs in many swimmers, especially those training twice per day.

## Chronic muscle glycogen depletion and overtraining

With all the training competitive swimmers do, it is not surprising that overtraining has become almost an epidemic in swimming. The frequent, high-volume, and high-intensity training these athletes perform often results in a chronic muscle fatigue that, if unchecked, may lead to the development of an overtraining state. Chronic muscle fatigue has been linked to failure to adequately replace the muscle glycogen stores between training sessions due to the combination of heavy training and inadequate dietary carbohydrate intake. Since a competitive swimming season may last as long as 25 weeks before a break from training is taken, swimmers can suffer from chronic depletion for up to 6 months. At the end of most swimming seasons, swimmers gradually reduce both the volume and intensity of training in preparation for their season-ending competition. This 'taper period' has not been studied extensively, but the few studies that have been done indicate that improved strength or power and increased muscle glycogen stores may be partly responsible for the enhanced performance that typically occurs with the taper.

## Protein requirements during swimming training

The prior discussion concerning carbohydrate needs of competitive swimmers suggests that many swimmers may experience chronic muscle glycogen depletion during their daily training. Lemon and Mullin (1980) have shown that protein catabolism is accelerated when exercising while glycogen depleted. Therefore, competitive swimming training may often result in increased protein catabolism that needs to be compensated for with extra dietary protein intake. Furthermore, the relatively low energy intake that has been reported for some swimmers may also trigger an increase in protein catabolism.

Lean body mass has been shown to significantly correlate with swimmers' performance in a 91.4-m freestyle (Stager *et al.* 1984). In addition, numerous studies have shown the importance of muscle strength and power in performance of competitive swimming (Sharp *et al.* 1982; Costill *et al.* 1985b, 1986; Sharp 1986; Cavanaugh & Musch 1989). Thus, development and maintenance of lean mass to preserve muscle strength and power should be a priority for competitive swimmers. Unfortunately, this seems to be a difficult task during the heavy training phase of their season as studies have shown decrements in muscle power despite continued resistance training during midseason (Sharp 1986; Cavanaugh & Musch 1989) followed by increased power during the taper phase of training (Costill *et al.* 1985b). Whether these changes in muscle power are related to a chronic increase in muscle protein catabolism followed by an attenuation of muscle wasting during the taper phase has not been studied.

There are other studies which provide indirect evidence of an enhanced protein need during swimming training. Kirwan *et al.* (1988) and Morgan *et al.* (1988) showed evidence of muscle damage with a twofold increase in serum creatine kinase activity and increased muscle soreness in male college swimmers when training volume was increased from $4266\,\text{m}\cdot\text{day}^{-1}$ to $8970\,\text{m}\cdot\text{day}^{-1}$. In another study on the effects of swimming training on protein catabolism, Lemon *et al.* (1989) observed an increase in serum urea concentration and urinary urea excretion after a 4572-m training session in competitive swimmers. Conversely, Mussini *et al.* (1985) found no evidence of increased muscle proteolysis using postexercise urinary 3-methyl-histidine excretion in a group of 16–20-year-old males performing a 2000-m competitive swimming training session. It should be noted, however, that the training volume used in this study was considerably less than that used in the previous studies and less than that typically used by most competitive swimmers.

Although the United States recommended daily allowance (RDA) for protein is set at $0.8\,\text{g}\cdot\text{kg}^{-1}$ for adults, Friedman and Lemon (1989)

suggest that a protein intake of approximately $1.5\,\text{g}\cdot\text{kg}^{-1}$ may be more appropriate to support endurance exercise training. In addition, Marable *et al.* (1979) recommend a protein intake up to $2\text{–}3\,\text{g}\cdot\text{kg}^{-1}$ to support the muscle building requirements of resistance training. Since competitive swimming training employs considerable involvement in both endurance and resistance training, their protein needs may lie somewhere within this range of about $1.5\text{–}2\,\text{g}\cdot\text{kg}^{-1}\cdot\text{day}^{-1}$. The typical young-adult female competitive swimmer in the Netherlands consumes approximately $50\text{–}60\,\text{g}$ protein $\cdot$ day$^{-1}$, translating to about a protein intake of $0.9\text{–}1.2\,\text{g}\cdot\text{kg}^{-1}\cdot\text{day}^{-1}$ (van Erp-Baart *et al.* 1989). These authors also report the typical protein intake of male swimmers in the range of $80\text{–}100\,\text{g}\cdot\text{day}^{-1}$, or a protein intake of about $1.1\text{–}1.3\,\text{g}\cdot\text{kg}^{-1}\cdot\text{day}^{-1}$.

Perhaps if swimmers maintained a higher protein intake and a higher carbohydrate intake, and consumed enough calories to match the energy demands of their training, responses such as loss of muscle power in the middle of the season, chronic muscle fatigue, overtraining, and recovery of power and performance ability during taper would be lessened. Elimination of these responses might be expected to result in improved performance of these athletes throughout their competitive season, instead of only at the end of a taper period. However, many coaches worry that the large performance improvement usually observed with the season-ending taper would no longer occur if the swimmers were not pushed to the edge of overtraining throughout the early and midseason phases. In addition, they often fear that physiological capacities such as aerobic endurance and anaerobic power will not be fully developed in their athletes if training volume is reduced. Consequently, training for competitive swimming will likely continue to place extraordinary demands on the young athletes who choose this as their sport.

## Micronutrient requirements in competitive swimming

The only vitamin or mineral that has received much attention in the literature on dietary habits of competitive swimmers is iron. Perhaps the reason for this is that swimmers tend to consume a large amount of food and typically exceed the RDA for most of the nutrients. However, there is evidence of iron deficiency, particularly among female swimmers, even when RDA is met.

Brigham *et al.* (1993) determined iron status in 25 female college swimmers on a biweekly basis throughout a 25-week competitive season. In addition, they examined the effectiveness of iron supplementation during this season. Before breaking the swimmers into an experimental (iron supplement) and placebo group, these authors observed that 17 of the swimmers had depleted iron stores (defined as serum ferritin concentration $< 12 \mu g \cdot l^{-1}$) while five of the swimmers were defined as anaemic (haemoglobin $< 12 g \cdot dl^{-1}$). During the 5 weeks in which the experimental group received 39 mg elemental iron as an iron supplement per day, haemoglobin concentration increased in 24% of the subjects and plasma ferritin concentration increased in 68% of the subjects. In the control group who did not ingest an iron supplement, haemoglobin concentration decreased despite consuming a diet containing 16.3 mg iron·day$^{-1}$. These authors concluded that moderate iron supplementation is effective in preventing a decline in iron status during swimming training but a higher dose may be needed to reverse a pre-existing iron deficiency.

Ganzit *et al.* (1993; cited in Burke 1993) tested the effectiveness of 80 mg iron supplementation per day in male and female swimmers. Swimmers in the experimental group maintained their plasma ferritin levels while those swimmers in the placebo group experienced a decrease in plasma ferritin concentration. These authors also noted an improvement in anaerobic capacity and reduced lactic acid response to submaximal exercise that was more marked in the experimental group than in the placebo group. In the

females, these improvements were confined only to the group that received the dietary iron supplement. Since haemoglobin concentrations did not change in either of the groups, these authors concluded that performance gains were made at the level of iron-associated muscle enzymes.

Walsh and McNaughton (1989) studied the effects of 150 mg iron supplementation per day on the haematology and $\dot{V}o_{2max.}$ of competitive female swimmers training at least 2 h·day$^{-1}$ and 7 days a week. During this period, the experimental group had an increase in haemoglobin concentration from 12.5 g·dl$^{-1}$ before supplementation to 13.6 g·dl$^{-1}$ after supplementation with no change in the placebo group. Plasma ferritin concentration dropped in the placebo group from 28 to 16 μg·l$^{-1}$ while no signficant change was observed in the experimental group (26 to 21 μg·l$^{-1}$). By the end of the study, 40% of the subjects in the placebo group were classified as iron deficient (serum ferritin $\leq 12 \mu g \cdot l^{-1}$, haemoglobin $\geq 12 g \cdot dl^{-1}$) and 10% of the subjects were classified as anaemic (serum ferritin $\leq 12 \mu g \cdot l^{-1}$, haemoglobin $\leq 12 g \cdot dl^{-1}$). These data are shown in Fig. 46.4. None of the swimmers who received the iron supplement was classified as either iron deficient or anaemic. These authors concluded that young female swimmers should be routinely tested for iron status and that iron supplementation undertaken when deemed necessary.

## Conclusion

The nutritional problems that have been summarized in this chapter may all be linked to the volume, frequency and intensity of training these athletes perform. Thus, the difficulties in trying to meet the energy demands, supply adequate carbohydrate to fuel the exercise and aid recovery, minimize muscle proteolysis, and prevent iron depletion and the associated negative effects on haematology could be avoided most simply by reducing training. At the very least, swimming coaches should design training programmes that lessen the risk of developing the

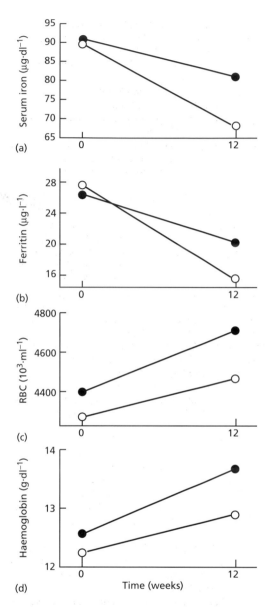

**Fig. 46.4** Iron status and haematology of female competitive swimmers taking either placebo (○) or 150 mg iron supplement (●) daily during 12 weeks of swim training. Adapted from Walsh and McNaughton (1989).

educating swimmers and their parents about general nutritional principles and specific nutritional problems of their sport are all ways swimming coaches can help assure that nutrition supports the efforts of these dedicated athletes instead of limiting their performance.

## References

Barr, S.I. & Costill, D.L. (1992) Effect of increased training volume on nutrient intake of male collegiate swimmers. *International Journal of Sports Medicine* **13**, 47–51.

Barr, S.I., Costill, D.L., Fink, W.J. & Thomas, R. (1991) Effect of increased training volume on blood lipids and lipoproteins in male collegiate swimmers. *Medicine and Science in Sports and Exercise* **23**, 795–800.

Berning, J.R., Troup, J.P., Van Handel, P.J., Daniels, J. & Daniels, N. (1991) The nutritional habits of young adolescent swimmers. *International Journal of Sport Nutrition* **1**, 240–248.

Brigham, D.E., Beard, J.L., Krimmel, R.S. & Kenney, W.L. (1993) Changes in iron status during competitive season in female collegiate swimmers. *Nutrition* **9**, 418–422.

Burke, L.M. & Read, R.S.D. (1993) Dietary supplements in sport. *Sports Medicine* **15**, 43–65.

Cavanaugh, D.J. & Musch, K.I. (1989) Arm and leg power of elite swimmers increase after taper as measured by Biokinetic variable resistance machines. *Journal of Swimming Research* **5**, 7–10.

Coggan, A.R. & Coyle, E.F. (1987) Reversal of fatigue during prolonged exercise by carbohydrate infusion or ingestion. *Journal of Applied Physiology* **63**, 2388–2395.

Coggan, A.R. & Coyle, E.F. (1988) Effect of carbohydrate feedings during high-intensity exercise. *Journal of Applied Physiology* **65**, 1703–1709.

Costill, D.L. & Miller, J.M. (1980) Nutrition for endurance sport: carbohydrate and fluid balance. *International Journal of Sports Medicine* **1**, 2–14.

Costill, D.L., Fink, W.J., Hargreaves, M., King, D.S. & Thomas, R. (1985a) Metabolic characteristics of skeletal muscle during detraining from competitive swimming. *Medicine and Science in Sports and Exercise* **17**, 339–343.

Costill, D.L., King, D.S., Thomas, R. & Hargreaves, M. (1985b) Effects of reduced training on muscular power in swimmers. *Physician and Sportsmedicine* **13**, 94–101.

Costill, D.L., Rayfield, R., Kirwan, J. & Thomas, R. (1986) A computer based system for the measurement of force and power during front crawl swimming. *Journal of Swimming Research* **2**, 16–19.

nutritional problems outlined in this chapter. Alternating between high and lower volume training days, allowing adequate time between intense practices for muscle glycogen recovery,

Costill, D.L., Flynn, M.G., Kirwan, J.P. *et al.* (1988a) Effects of repeated days of intensified training on muscle glycogen and swimming performance. *Medicine and Science in Sports and Exercise* **20**, 249–254.

Costill, D.L., Hinrichs, D., Fink, W.J. & Hoopes, D. (1988b) Muscle glycogen depletion during swimming interval training. *Journal of Swimming Research* **4**, 15–18.

Coyle, E.F., Hagberg, J.M., Hurley, B.F., Martin, W.H., Ehsani, A.A. & Hollszy, J.O. (1983) Carbohydrate feeding during prolonged strenuous exercise can delay fatigue. *Journal of Applied Physiology* **55**, 230–235.

Coyle, E.F., Coggan, A.R., Hemmert, M.K. & Ivy, J.L. (1986) Muscle glycogen utilization during prolonged exercise when fed carbohydrate. *Journal of Applied Physiology* **61**, 165–172.

Davis, J.M., Lamb, D.R., Pate, R.R., Slentz, C.A., Burgess, W.A. & Bartoli, W.P. (1988) Carbohydrate–electrolyte drinks: effects on endurance cycling in the heat. *American Journal of Clinical Nutrition* **48**, 1023–1030.

Flynn, M.G., Costill, D.L., Kirwan, J.P. *et al.* (1990) Fat storage in athletes: metabolic and hormonal responses to swimming and running. *International Journal of Sports Medicine* **11**, 433–440.

Friedman, J.E. & Lemon, P.W. (1989) Effect of chronic endurance exercise on retention of dietary protein. *International Journal of Sports Medicine* **10**, 118–123.

Ganzit, G.P., Giribaudo, C.G. & Biancotti, P.P. (1989) Effetti della somministrazione di supplemento di ferro ferritinico sull' adaltamento funzionale aerobico e anaerobico all' alienamento, in nuotatori maschi e femmine. *Medicina dello Sport* **42**, 7–15.

Gollnick, P.D., Armstrong, R.B., Saltin, B., Saubert, C.W., Sembrowich, W.L. & Shepherd, R.J. (1973) Effects of training on enzyme activity and fiber composition of human skeletal muscle. *Journal of Applied Physiology* **34**, 107–111.

Harri, M. & Kuusela, P. (1986) Is swimming exercise or cold exposure for rats? *Acta Physiologica Scandinavica* **126**, 189–197.

Ivy, J.L., Katz, A., Cutler, C.L., Sherman, W.M. & Coyle, E.F. (1988) Muscle glycogen synthesis after exercise: effect of time of carbohydrate ingestion. *Journal of Applied Physiology* **64**, 1480–1485.

Johnson, G.O., Nebelsick-Gullett, L.J., Thorland, W.G. & Housh, T.J. (1989) The effect of a competitive season on the body composition of university female athletes. *Journal of Sports Medicine and Physical Fitness* **29**, 314–320.

Kirwan, J.P., Costill, D.L., Flynn, M.G. *et al.* (1988) Physiological responses to successive days of intense training in competitive swimmers. *Medicine and Science in Sports and Exercise* **3**, 255–259.

Lamb, D.R., Rinehardt, K.F., Bartels, R.L., Sherman,

W.M. & Snook, J.T. (1990) Dietary carbohydrate and intensity of interval swim training. *American Journal of Clinical Nutrition* **52**, 1058–1063.

Lemon, P.W. & Mullin, J.P. (1980) Effect of initial muscle glycogen levels on protein catabolism during exercise. *Journal of Applied Physiology* **48**, 624–629.

Lemon, P.W., Deutsch, D.T. & Payne, W.R. (1989) Urea production during prolonged swimming. *Journal of Sports Science* **7**, 241–246.

MacDougall, J.D., Ward, G.R., Sale, D.G. & Sutton, J.R. (1977) Muscle glycogen repletion after high-intensity intermittent exercise. *Journal of Applied Physiology* **42**, 129–132.

Maglischo, E.W. (1993) *Swimming Even Faster.* Mayfield Publishing, Mountain View, CA.

Marable, N.L., Hickson, J.F., Korslund, M.K., Herbert, W.G., Desjardins, R.F. & Thye, F.W. (1979) Urinary nitrogen excretion as influenced by a muscle-building exercise program and protein intake variation. *Nutrition Reports International* **19**, 795–805.

Meleski, B.W. & Malina, R.M. (1985) Changes in body composition and physique of elite university-level female swimmers during a competitive season. *Journal of Sports Science* **3**, 33–40.

Morgan, W.P., Costill, D.L., Flynn, M.G., Raglin, J.S. & O'Connor, P.J. (1988) Mood disturbance following increased training in swimmers. *Medicine and Science in Sports and Exercise* **4**, 408–414.

Mussini, E., Colombo, L., De Ponte, G., Calzi, M. & Marcucci, F. (1985) Effect of swimming on protein degradation: 3-methylhistidine and creatinine excretion. *Biochemical Medicine* **34**, 373–375.

Novak, L.P., Woodward, W.A., Bestit, C. & Mellerowicz, H. (1977) Working capacity, body composition and anthropometry of olympic female athletes. *Journal of Sports Medicine* **17**, 275–283.

O'Sullivan, S., Sharp, R.L. & King, D.S. (1994) Carbohydrate ingestion during competitive swim training. *Journal of Swimming Research* **10**, 35–40.

Piehl, K., Adolfsson, S. & Nazar, K. (1974) Glycogen storage and glycogen synthase activity in trained and untrained muscle of man. *Acta Physiologica Scandinavica* **90**, 779–788.

Sharp, R.L. (1986) Muscle strength and power as related to competitive swimming. *Journal of Swimming Research* **2**, 5–10.

Sharp, R.L., Troup, J.P. & Costill, D.L. (1982) Relationship between power and sprint freestyle swimming. *Medicine and Science in Sports and Exercise* **14**, 53–56.

Sherman, W.M. & Maglischo, E.W. (1992) Minimizing athletic fatigue among swimmers: special emphasis on nutrition. In *Sports Science Exchange*, Gatorade Sports Science Institute. **4**, 35.

Stager, J.M., Cordain, L. & Becker, T.J. (1984) Relationship of body composition to swimming performance in female swimmers. *Journal of Swimming Research* 1, 21–26.

Thorland, W.G., Johnson, G.O., Housh, T.J. & Refsell, M.J. (1983) Anthropometric characteristics of elite adolescent competitive swimmers. *Human Biology* 55, 735–748.

Tsintzas, K., Liu, R., Williams, C., Campbell, I. & Gaitanos, G. (1993) The effect of carbohydrate ingestion on performance during a 30 km race. *International Journal of Sport Nutrition* 3, 127–129.

Van Erp-Baart, A.M.J., Saris, W.H.M., Binkhorst, R.A., Vos, J.A. & Elvers, J.W.H. (1989) Nationwide survey on nutritional habits in elite athletes. Part I. Energy, carbohydrate, protein, and fat intake. *International Journal of Sports Medicine* 10 (Suppl. 1), 3–10.

Van Handel, P.J., Cells, K.A., Bradley, P.W. & Troup, J.P. (1984) Nutritional status of elite swimmers. *Journal of Swimming Research* 1, 27–31.

Walsh, R. & McNaughton, L. (1989) Effects of iron supplementation on iron status of young female swimmers during the pre-season phase of competition. *Journal of Swimming Research* 5, 13–18.

Zawadzki, K.M., Yaspelkis, B.B. & Ivy, J.L. (1992) Carbohydrate–protein complex increases the rate of muscle glycogen storage after exercise. *Journal of Applied Physiology* 72, 1854–1859.

# Chapter 47

# Weightlifting and Power Events

VICTOR A. ROGOZKIN

## Introduction

The success of athletes in many competitive sports is determined by the extent to which they have developed their strength–velocity characteristics: these include strength, speed and power of muscle function. Peak expression of the functional capability of the athlete requires the maximum voluntary effort that can be achieved, and thus depends not only on the characteristics of the muscle, but also on the initiation of impulses in the motor centres of the central nervous system, on the maintenance of high firing rates in the motor nerves, and on the coordination of the activation of synergistic and antagonistic muscles. Important muscle characteristics include, in addition to muscle size itself, the orientation of the muscle fibres, the proportions of the different fibre types present, and the amount and structure of the connective tissue.

The basics of muscle structure and function have been reviewed in Chapter 2, and will be discussed only briefly here. The following characteristics of muscle are important for the development of force and power:

**1** The maximum muscular effort that can be achieved is directly proportional to the length of the individual sarcomeres (Faulkner & White 1990). This cannot be changed with training, but will be influenced by joint angle, which will in turn change the length of the muscle. In a whole muscle, maximum force-generating capacity in an isometric contraction is largely determined by cross-sectional area (Maughan *et al.* 1983).

Adding more sarcomeres in parallel will increase the maximum force that can be achieved, but adding more sarcomeres in series will have no effect on maximum force other than by shifting the position on the length–tension relationship at any given joint angle.

**2** The maximum velocity of shortening of a muscle is dependent on the load applied. For single muscle fibres, the maximum velocity of shortening, and therefore the maximum speed of movement, is a function of the myosin adenosine triphosphatase (ATPase) activity: this determines the rate at which ATP can be used to power the interactions between actin and myosin. In fast-contracting (type IIb) muscle fibres, the maximum velocity of shortening is four times higher than in slow-contracting (type I) fibres (Burke & Edgerton 1975).

**3** The power that can be developed by a muscle is a linear function of the maximum ATPase activity, and thus is closely related to the proportions of the different fibre types present. Muscles with a high proportion of type II fibres will be able to achieve higher power outputs than those where type I fibres predominate. Muscles of elite sprinters typically contain more than 60% type I fibres, whereas type I fibres predominate in the muscles of endurance athletes (Costill *et al.* 1976).

**4** The characteristic relationship between force, or strength, and velocity referred to above was described by Hill (1938). Force is greatest during an isometric activation of the muscle, where the applied load exceeds the force generating capacity of the muscle and the velocity of shortening is zero: the maximum velocity, in an isolated muscle or an individual fibre, occurs during unloaded shortening. This situation cannot be achieved with the muscle *in situ* because of the mass of the limb segments that must be moved and other biomechanical factors, and maximum velocity is achieved when the load applied is less than 20% of the maximum isometric force that can be generated. The maximum values of isometric force that can be achieved by human muscle are approximately $15-30 \times 10^4 \, N \cdot m^2$ (Saltin & Gollnick 1982). The maximum force per unit cross-sectional area of the muscle is not significantly different between the different fibre types (Faulkner & White 1990).

The known relationships between strength and velocity of muscle contraction allow identification of the main components of a programme designed for developing the strength and power characteristics of an athlete. For development of the maximum isometric strength, training should be carried out at forces between 70% and 100% of the maximum voluntary isometric strength. To improve performance where high speeds of movement are required, the force should not exceed 70% of maximum isometric strength. Where high rates of power generation are to be developed, the force applied during training should be in the range of 40–70% of maximum isometric force.

## Speed–strength sports

The 1996 Olympic Games included a number of very different types of sport where strength and speed are primary requirements for the participants (Table 47.1). These include:
• Boxing: open to men only, including 12 weight categories ranging from 48 kg to over 91 kg.
• Judo: open to men (weight categories from 60 kg to over 80 kg) and women (from 48 to over 72 kg).

**Table 47.1** Profile of major championship sports with a high strength component and in which competition is by weight category.

| Parameters | Boxing | Judo | | Weightlifting | | Wrestling |
| | Male | Male | Female | Male | Female | Greco-Roman and freestyle |
|---|---|---|---|---|---|---|
| Weight classes (kg) | 48 | 60 | 48 | 54 | 46 | 48 |
| | 51 | 65 | 51 | 59 | 50 | 52 |
| | 54 | 71 | 56 | 64 | 54 | 57 |
| | 57 | 78 | 61 | 70 | 59 | 62 |
| | 60 | 86 | 66 | 76 | 64 | 68 |
| | 63.5 | 90 | 72 | 83 | 70 | 74 |
| | 67 | Over 90 | Over 72 | 91 | 76 | 82 |
| | 71 | | | 99 | 83 | 90 |
| | 75 | | | 108 | Over 83 | 100 |
| | 81 | | | Over 108 | | 130 |
| | 91 | | | | | |
| | Over 91 | | | | | |
| Match rules | Three 2-min rounds | One 5-min bout | | Three lifts | | One 5-min period |
| Matches per day | No more than one | No more than three recommended in 2 days | | No more than one | | No more than three are recommended |
| Weigh-in rules | 3 h before competition | 2 h before competition each day | | 2 h before competition | | Night before competition |

• Weightlifting: open to men only, with 10 weight classes from 54 to over 108 kg.

• Wrestling: Greco-Roman and freestyle competition, open to men only, with 10 weight classes from 48 kg to over 130 kg, giving a total of 20 competitions.

In addition, strength and speed are vital components of the sprint events on the track and of all field events, including long jump, high jump, triple jump, pole vault, shot, discus, javelin, hammer throw. In cycling, there are sprint events on the track for men and women. In the Winter Olympic competition, speed skating and bobsleigh (two-man and four-man) also require similar characteristics: indeed many speed skaters are also top class cyclists, and bobsleigh competitors often compete at 100 m on the track in the summer. It is clear that sports in this grouping account for the majority of medals awarded at the Olympic Games.

Non-Olympic sports involving similar characteristics and demands include a variety of martial arts (karate, Tae Kwondo). Bodybuilding training follows broadly similar principles, although the training loads and numbers of repetitions performed may be somewhat different and the demands of competition are also different.

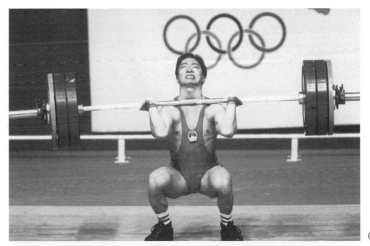

(a)

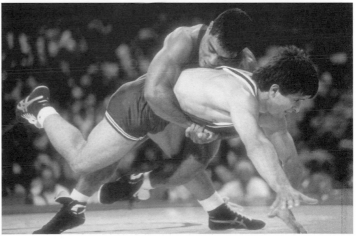

(b)

**Fig. 47.1** In all weight category sports, a high power to mass ratio is essential. Increasing body mass moves the competitor up into a higher weight category. (a) Photo © Allsport; (b) photo © Allsport / J. Jacobsohn.

The two main characteristics of this group of sports, therefore, are that, at least in most of them, competition is open to men and women, and that, in many, athletes compete in specific weight categories. This latter fact places particular demands on the athlete, with special consideration required for training and diet in preparation for competition.

## General nutritional principles for athletes

The requirements of the athlete for energy and for individual nutrients are different in different sports, and will be influenced very much by the total training load that is carried out (Rogozkin 1978). Body mass is also a major factor, as is immediately obvious when looking at the requirements of a light-flyweight boxer (48 kg weight class), a track athlete, or a wrestler in the super-heavyweight class (over 130 kg). Even for athletes with similar body size, however, the nutritional requirements will vary greatly depending on the training load: this is set in part by the demands of the sports but will also vary within any given event depending on the programme selected by the athlete and coach. Recommended energy intakes for male and female athletes in different sports are clearly influenced by many factors, but are likely to be about 14.6–23.0 MJ (3500–5500 kcal) daily for male athletes and 12.5–18.8 MJ (3000–4500 kcal) for female athletes during periods of hard training (Rogozkin 1978).

The protein requirement of athletes in different sports is described in detail in Chapter 10. It is clear that the requirement for protein will depend to some extent on the specific nature of the sport, but will also be very much influenced by the amount and intensity of the training load, which will vary at different times of the season. In Russia, it is generally recommended that the daily protein intake for athletes in hard training should be about $1.4–2.0\,g\cdot kg^{-1}$ body mass (Rogozkin 1978). The requirement for carbohydrate will be closely related to the power output required in training and competition, and a daily

carbohydrate intake of $8–10\,g\cdot kg^{-1}$ would be considered normal. Depending on the type of sport, fat intake should be about $1.7–2.4\,g\cdot kg^{-1}\cdot day^{-1}$. These recommendations are made in absolute amounts related to body weight rather than as a fraction of total energy intake, but if the guidelines are followed, this will give a diet with the following composition: 15–16% of total energy intake from protein, 25–26% from fat and 58–60% from carbohydrate.

The fundamental principles of nutritional support which have been developed in the Russian Federation for athletes competing in strength and power events have been described in detail by Rogozkin (1993). These are summarized in the following recommendations.

**1** The body must be provided with sufficient energy to meet its needs. For athletes, the energy requirement will be largely determined by the total training load. If the energy demand is not met, it will not be possible to continue with the same intensity and duration of training.

**2** An appropriate nutritional balance among the various essential nutrients must be maintained. The proportions of the different macronutrients and micronutrients necessary to achieve this balance will depend on the total energy intake and on the period of preparation relative to competition. Protein intake must provide an appropriate balance of all the essential amino acids, and the dietary fat must supply all of the essential fatty acids. In addition, the intake of vitamins, minerals and fibre must be adequate for the athlete's needs.

**3** The choice of foods and nutritional products that will meet the nutrient requirements will be different during periods of intensive training, during the period of preparation for competition, during competition itself, and during the recovery phase after competition.

**4** Several nutrients, mostly vitamins and minerals, play a key role in the activation and regulation of intracellular metabolic processes, and a deficiency of any of these in the diet will impair performance during training and competition.

**5** Biosynthetic processes involved in tissue repair and recovery after exercise will be influenced by the hormonal environment: important factors include the catecholamines, insulin, corticosteroids, growth hormone, cyclic nucleotides and others. Dietary influences on the metabolic environment in the recovery phase will influence the extent of recovery from training and competition.

**6** A varied diet is essential to provide all the nutrients needed by that athlete in adequate amounts, but other factors, including especially those associated with the storage and preparation of foods, will affect the availability of these nutrients from the diet.

**7** The diet must be chosen to include foodstuffs that will provide all of the essential nutrients, but care must be taken to ensure that, during periods when the athlete is training two or three times per day, the meals are readily digested and absorbed and do not result in gastrointestinal disturbances.

**8** Where there is a need to increase body mass, usually in the form of lean tissue, and specifically in the form of muscle, the diet must contain sufficient protein and other nutrients to ensure that the increased requirement is met. For athletes competing in weight category sports, and for others where a low body mass or a low body fat content are important, there must be special attention to the composition of the diet to ensure that all nutritional requirements are met from the restricted total energy intake.

**9** The diet must be chosen to take account of the individual physiological, metabolic and anthropometric characteristics of the individual athlete, and should consider the condition of the athlete's digestive system. It must also take personal tastes and preferences into account.

Only if the diet is selected in the light of these considerations is it possible to meet all of the requirements imposed by training and competition and to optimize the athlete's performance.

## Strength training

Muscle, fat and bone are the three major structural components that determine the body shape and size of the individual. Body build is to a large degree genetically determined, as is the ability to achieve success in sport. Specific types of physical training can modify the expression of the individual's genetic endowment, resulting in changes in body composition. Weight training is effective when the aim is to increase muscle mass, whereas endurance training can alter energy balance and reduce fat mass. An appropriate weight-training regimen, however, will also be effective in reducing body fat content if combined with a suitable diet.

There are several categories of strength exercise that can be included in a weight training programme: these include isometric (static) contractions, which are not truly contractions, as the muscle is not allowed to shorten during activation and the angle of the limb is fixed. Because of stretching of the elastic components, however, there will be some shortening of individual sarcomeres. Isokinetic exercise involves shortening of the muscle at a fixed velocity, and requires special apparatus to keep the velocity of shortening constant while measuring the applied force. Isotonic exercise, in which a constant load is applied to the muscle is the type of training most familiar to and popular with coaches and athletes (Fahey 1986). The applied load may be in the form of free weights or a resistance machine. Isotonic strength-training techniques may include constant or variable load, and may involve lengthening of the muscle (eccentric activation) as well as the more normal shortening (concentric activation) when the load is applied. Plyometric and speed loading techniques may also be included in a strength programme.

It has been shown that greater increases in strength can be achieved following a programme of maximum-force concentric and eccentric activation than when concentric activation alone is used (Fahey 1986). The available evidence suggests that eccentric activity results in some degree of damage to the muscle, involving disruption of the muscle membrane and possibly also some disruption of the contractile components, and the subsequent repair process seems to be important for the increase in the size of muscle fibres that results from a strength training programme (Faulkner & White 1990). Strength training with high loads leads to an increase in the cross-sectional area of the muscle without any appreciable change in muscle length, and changes in cross-sectional area of the muscle can be used as an index of the gain in muscle mass. Both type I and type II fibres increase in size in response to this type of training stimulus, and increases in cross-sectional area of 39% for type I fibres and 31% for type II fibres have been reported after a programme of heavy resistance exercise (MacDougall *et al.* 1980). Increases in force-generating capacity after strength training may be large (30–40%) in the early stages of a training programme, and are invariably greater than the increase in cross-sectional area (Maughan 1984). Some of the increase in muscle strength is therefore likely to be the result of changes in the muscle recruitment pattern and in neural drive. In pennate muscles, where the individual fibres lie at an angle to the long axis of the muscle, increases in the size of the individual fibres will result in an increase in the angle of pennation, which will have the effect of decreasing the force relative to the anatomical cross-sectional area (Maughan 1984).

Release of a variety of hormones is stimulated during and after high resistance training: these include growth hormone, testosterone, catecholamines and cortisol (Sutton *et al.* 1990). The release of these hormones will be influenced by the intensity of training, the length of rest periods allowed, and the level of training of the athlete. The response to training is specific to the muscle, so there must be a change in the sensitivity of the active muscle to the circulating hormones and growth factors so that changes in the systemic concentration results in specific changes in protein synthesis. This may involve a change in receptor number or sensitivity and/or release of local growth factors (including insulin-like growth factor) in the working muscle in response to hormonal stimulation.

Increases in muscle strength and muscle hypertrophy have been shown to be greater after prolonged fatiguing contractions than after short, intermittent contractions (Schott *et al.* 1995). The authors speculated that the enhanced response after fatiguing contractions indicated an involvement of changes in intracellular metabolite levels and pH in determining the response of the muscle.

In addition to the changes in muscle size and strength, weight training will have a significant effect on bone mass. Peak bone mass, which is normally reached in the third decade of life, can be increased by any form of weight-bearing exercise, and will help to protect the skeleton against the stresses imposed on it. These processes are described in detail in Chapter 23.

As the muscle becomes stronger with training and the load that can be applied increases, so the stimulus for new bone formation should also be increased to a degree consistent with the imposed load or relative intensity of the exercise. The imposed load is more important for determining the response of bone than the number of loading cycles completed. Progressive resistance training should therefore allow the bone mass to increase until it reaches the genetically determined peak bone mass. Given the greater length of time required for new bone formation relative to the adaptation of skeletal muscle, which is apparent within a few days of training beginning, changes in bone mass require long-term adherence to a training programme that will effectively load the skeleton.

## Training diet

The adaptive changes that occur in the various organs and tissues of the athlete in response to the training load occur in a phasic manner. The acute responses to a single bout of exercise are translated into a permanent (at least as long as the training persists) condition by a series of events that may be described as fatigue, restoration and supercompensation. The adaptations which occur in response to training result in an increased capacity for force generation, power output or endurance, depending on the type of training. This will be manifested during the effort itself, but there must be, during the post-exercise period, an altered gene expression to cause an enhanced synthesis of specific proteins.

To achieve these aims during the training period, athletes normally follow a training programme containing microcycles lasting 3–5 days. Each training microcycle is constructed to allow adaptation of all of the different functions which respond to the specific training undertaken. Complete adaptation in response to this type of training usually appears after three to five repetitions of the cycle (Lamb 1984).

The diet consumed by the athlete during this training phase should be designed to supply the necessary energy and nutrients in order to maximize the efficiency of the training process. Preparation of the diet requires a knowledge of the total energy demand, but also some understanding of the specific character of the training programme at any given time. Energy expenditure of strength and power athletes during periods of heavy training is typically about 14.6–18.8 MJ (3500–4500 kcal), depending on body weight, and the preparation of a balanced diet is not difficult to achieve. However, it appears that at some times in the training cycle of these athletes, there is a need for an increase in the dietary protein intake if muscular development is to occur. To meet the protein requirement of weightlifters, sprinters and throwers, for example, it is recommended that the daily protein intake should be 1.4–2.0 g · kg$^{-1}$ body mass (Rogozkin 1993). This is slightly higher than the intake of 1.4–1.7 g · kg$^{-1}$ recommended by Lemon (1991). It is not only the total protein intake that is important, but also the content and balance of the essential amino acids, and the proteins in meat, fish and dairy produce have a higher biological value than those in other foods. Dairy products have a high content of the sulphur-containing amino acid methionine, which is indispensable for the synthesis of muscle protein (Williams 1976).

The fat intake for athletes from these sports should be approximately 2 g · kg$^{-1}$ · day$^{-1}$, and a significant part of this will be provided by the protein-rich foods in the diet, especially meat and dairy produce. Vegetable oils, however, including sunflower seed, corn and nut oils, are valuable sources of the essential polyunsaturated fats, which may comprise as much as 50–60% of their total fat content. Dietary fat is also important in ensuring an adequate supply and uptake of the fat-soluble vitamins A, D and E. A carbohydrate intake of 8–10 g · kg$^{-1}$ · day$^{-1}$ should be sufficient to meet the needs of the organism even during the heaviest training.

The requirements of the strength athlete for vitamins and minerals have been identified, and the recommended intakes are shown in Table 47.2 (Rogozkin 1993).

The following general and specific recommendations are made.

**1** The energy requirement for the athlete in training should be completely satisfied from non-protein sources (carbohydrate and fat).

**2** The diet should contain an increased amount (15–20%) of energy from protein, consisting of biologically valuable and easily assimilated proteins from various sources, including meat, fish, milk and eggs.

**3** Meals with a high protein content should be eaten no less than five times per day.

**4** There must be optimal conditions for the assimilation of the protein components of foods. After training, meat should be taken together with vegetables, and during the intervals

Table 47.2 Recommended daily intakes of vitamins and minerals for athletes during periods of intensive strength training.

| Vitamins | | Minerals | |
| --- | --- | --- | --- |
| C | 175–200 mg | Phosphorus | 2.5–3.0 g |
| B$_1$ | 2.5–4.0 mg | Calcium | 2.0–2.4 g |
| B$_2$ | 4.0–5.5 mg | Potassium | 5.0–6.0 g |
| B$_3$ | 20 mg | Magnesium | 0.5–0.7 g |
| B$_6$ | 7–10 mg | Iron | 25–35 mg |
| B$_9$ | 0.5–0.6 mg | Zinc | 25–35 mg |
| B$_{12}$ | 4–9 µg | Iodine | 150–200 mg |
| PP | 25–45 mg | Chromium | 10–15 mg |
| A | 2.8–3.8 mg | | |
| E | 20–30 mg | | |

between training sessions, special protein supplements should be taken.

5 It is necessary to ensure an adequate intake of vitamins ($B_1$, $B_2$, $B_6$, C and PP) which promote protein synthesis and the accumulation of muscle mass.

Careful attention to diet is necessary during periods of intensive weight training in order to create the appropriate metabolic environment to allow increases in muscle mass to occur.

## Diet and weight control

Restriction of energy intake sufficient to result in a negative energy balance is an essential part of any successful weight-control programme (Williams 1976). Most fad diets that promise rapid loss of body weight stress weight loss rather than fat loss, and may seriously affect the athlete's performance because loss of lean tissue is likely to account for much of the loss in weight. These diets are often unpalatable and unhealthy, and do not represent an eating pattern that would be possible to sustain on a long-term basis. A rebound gain of the lost weight is almost inevitable. The goal of the dietary programme when weight loss is required should be a loss of body fat followed by maintenance of that loss.

Many popular diets promote a low carbohydrate intake, and these diets may be successful in causing large weight losses, perhaps as much as 5–10 kg in a few weeks. However, a diet that is low in carbohydrate will result in depletion of the liver and muscle glycogen stores and in a loss of water from tissues. Although the weight loss seems impressive, there may be little loss of body fat. Additionally, glycogen depletion greatly diminishes exercise capacity, leading to a decreased exercise level, which in turn means a decreased level of energy expenditure. Periods of low exercise levels in combination with restricted energy intake result in a loss of muscle tissue.

A successful weight-loss programme requires a negative energy balance. Given that the energy content of 0.45 kg of fat is about 14.7 MJ (3500 kcal), which is as much as most athletes expend

in day, it is clearly impossible to lose more than a few pounds of fat in a week. Empirical evidence suggests that, if weight is lost at a faster rate, the loss must come increasingly from loss of muscle mass. Diets that promise large decreases in fat in a short time are misleading: they are potentially dangerous and will impair performance.

## Weight loss and making weight

The aim of all weight-loss programmes should be to restrict food intake so that the body's fat reserve is gradually reduced while the normal functions of the body are maintained. The only successful approach is to reduce energy intake while ensuring that the nutrient density, and in particular the carbohydrate content, is kept high. The reducing diet will therefore be achieved by restricting fat, rather than carbohydrate, intake. Foods should be chosen to provide not only carbohydrate, which should be present mostly in the form of complex carbohydrates, but also vitamins, minerals and trace elements in adequate amounts, rather than simply being high in fibre. All visible fat should be removed from meat, and low-fat foods should be substituted for high-fat alternatives where these are available. If the diet is already very low in fat, the only available option is to reduce the overall amount of food being eaten.

Making weight is a different situation from a gradual weight-loss programme. This situation arises when athletes have to prepare to compete in a particular weight category. Most athletes participating in sports with specific weight categories, including boxing, judo, wrestling and weightlifting, compete in a class that is 5–10% below their usual weight. Typical weight reduction techniques used to induce large weight losses in a short time include dietary restriction, fluid restriction, dehydration through exercise in the heat or in a rubber suit, or sitting or exercising in a sauna or steam room. Less commonly used techniques include the use of diuretics and laxatives, vomiting and spitting.

Athletes will commonly lose weight rapidly in the last few days before competition (3–4 kg in the space of 3–4 days) by a combination of sweating and severe restriction of food and fluid intake. This practice of making weight may be repeated very often in a competitive season, as the lost weight is quickly regained. A more gradual weight loss (3–4 kg over 3–4 weeks) achieved by a more modest restriction of energy intake and increased energy expenditure would probably allow a better hydration state to be maintained. Prolonged dietary restriction, however, would inevitably involve restriction of protein and carbohydrate intake, and might lead to some loss of body proteins and glycogen stores. Although dehydration has a much smaller impact on high-intensity exercise than on endurance activities, and does not seem to compromise muscle strength or performance in events lasting less than 30 s, some reduction in function may occur (Sawka & Pandolf 1990). Dehydration is better tolerated by trained athletes than by sedentary individuals, with less impact on thermoregulation and exercise performance (Sawka & Pandolf 1990). The trained person has an increased body water reserve, and may be able to tolerate a fluid deficit of up to 5% of body mass without a significant detrimental effect on some aspects of physiological function (Rehrer 1991).

Athletes should be encouraged to maintain a relatively stable body weight and to lose unwanted fat gradually. The practical experience of athletes and coaches, however, indicates that the most successful performers often undergo severe weight-loss regimens in the few days before competition. The use of diuretics, and competition after their use, is to be discouraged. Not only does this impair performance, but also poses a health risk.

## Gaining weight

A high body mass is an advantage in many sports, including the throwing events in athletics, and the top weight categories in weightlifting, wrestling and judo. If too much of this weight is made up of fat, however, performance will suffer. The principles of weight gain are the same as those for weight loss: a positive energy balance will result in weight gain, and a negative energy balance will result in weight loss. Athletes who are seeking to gain weight should strive to ensure that as much as possible of the gain is in the form of lean tissue. This can be achieved most effectively through a vigorous weight-training programme that stresses the large muscle groups in the legs, hips, shoulders, arms and chest. Increases in muscle mass occur only slowly, and may take many years to be fully realized, but this is preferable to the increase in body fat that is quickly added by the use of high-energy weight-gain supplements.

Eating a high-protein diet will not in itself result in an increase in muscle mass (Lemon 1991). Any protein consumed in excess of the body's requirement will simply be used as a fuel for oxidative metabolism, and the excess nitrogen will be excreted. The common practice of eating large amounts of meat, dairy produce and eggs is expensive, and is potentially detrimental to the athlete's health and performance. Abnormal eating habits established during the years of training are not easily altered in later life, and consumption of a relatively high fat diet, which almost invariably accompanies a high intake of these foods, may lead to an increased risk of cardiovascular disease. In addition, if the intake of protein and fat is too high, there will be little room left in the diet for high-carbohydrate foods. Without an adequate dietary carbohydrate intake, the athlete is unlikely to be able to train to full potential and will be unable to maximize the benefits that accrue from consistent intensive training.

Many weightlifters and bodybuilders use specific amino acid supplements in an attempt to stimulate output of growth hormone and insulin, as both of these hormones are involved in the stimulation of protein synthesis and thus in the processes of muscle growth and repair. In a carefully controlled trial, however, supplementation with the amino acids that are purported to be effective at a dosage equal to that commonly used by power athletes (1 g arginine, 1 g ornithine and 1 g lysine, twice daily), had no effect on serum growth hormone or insulin concentrations (Fogelholm *et al.* 1993). There seems to be no substantial evidence to support the use of these supplements.

The addition of medium-chain triglycerides, which include fatty acids with a carbon chain 6–12 atoms long, to the diet of athletes is a new phenomenon (Manore *et al.* 1993). Medium-chain triglycerides are metabolized differently from longer chain fatty acids. They are absorbed rapidly in the gut and transported via the portal vein to the liver, rather than through the lymphatic system in the form of chylomicrons. As with longer chain fatty acids, oxidation occurs in the mitochondria, but carnitine is not required for transport across the mitochondrial membrane. They are rapidly oxidized after ingestion. The use of medium-chain triglycerides is becoming popular with athletes, especially bodybuilders, because they are energy dense ($35.3\,kJ\cdot g^{-1}$, $8.4\,kcal\cdot g^{-1}$), providing twice the energy of carbohydrate on a weight basis. A single dose of 25–30 g of medium-chain triglycerides does not cause any gastrointestinal problems, but some symptoms may occur with higher doses (Berning 1996). They are, however, relatively expensive. Also, ingestion of large amounts will stimulate ketone body formation if not consumed with an adequate amount of carbohydrate, and have a strong thermogenic effect.

Creatine supplementation in an appropriate dose can provide improved performance for athletes in explosive events: these include all events lasting from a few seconds to a few minutes. The effects and use of creatine are described fully in Chapter 27. One commonly reported side-effect is a gain in weight of 1–2 kg within a week of beginning supplementation. Most of this extra weight is accounted for by water, but this may have implications for athletes in weight category sports.

# References

Berning, J.R. (1996) The role of medium-chain triglycerides in exercise. *International Journal of Sport Nutrition* **6**, 121–133.

Burke, R.E. & Edgerton, V.R. (1975) Motor unit properties and selective involvement in movement. In *Exercise and Sport Science Reviews*, Vol. 3, pp. 33–81 (ed. J.H. Wilwore & J.F. Keogh). Academic Press, New York.

Costill, D.L., Fink, W.J. & Pollock, M.L. (1976) Muscle fiber composition and enzyme activities of elite distance runners. *Medicine and Science in Sports* **8**, 96–100.

Fahey, T. (ed.) (1986) *Athletic Training: Principles and Practice*. Mayfield, Mountain View, CA.

Faulkner, J.A. & White, T.P. (1990) Adaptations of skeletal muscle to physical activity. In *Exercise, Fitness and Health* (ed. C. Bouchard, R.J. Shephard, T. Stephans, J.R. Sutton & B.D. McPherson), pp. 265–279. Human Kinetics, Champaign, IL.

Fogelholm, G.M., Naveri, H.K., Kiilavouri, K.T. & Härkönen, M.H. (1993) Low-dose amino acid supplementation: no effect on serum human growth hormone and insulin in male weight lifters. *International Journal of Sport Nutrition* **3**, 290–297.

Hill, A.A. (1938) The heat of shortening and the dynamic constants of muscle. *Nutrition* **126**, 136–195.

Lamb, D.R. (1984) *Physiology of Exercise: Responses and Adaptations*. Macmillan, New York.

Lemon, P.W. (1991) Effect of exercise on protein requirements. *Journal of Sports Science* **9**, 53–70.

MacDougall, J.D., Elder, G.C., Sale, D.G., Moroz, J.R. & Sutton, J.R. (1980) Effects of strength training and immobilisation on human muscle fibres. *European Journal of Applied Physiology* **43**, 25–34.

Manore, M., Thompson, J. & Russo, M. (1993) Diet and exercise strategies of a world-class bodybuilder. *International Journal of Sport Nutrition* **3**, 76–86.

Maughan, R.J. (1984) The relationship between muscle strength and muscle cross-sectional area and the implications for training. *Sports Medicine* **1**, 263–269.

Maughan, R.J., Watson, J.S. & Weir, J. (1983) Strength and cross-section area of human skeletal muscle. *Journal of Physiology* **338**, 37–49.

Rehrer, N.J. (1991) Aspects of dehydration and rehydration during exercise. In *Advances in Nutrition and Top Sport Medicine and Sport Science* (ed. F. Brouns), pp. 128–146. Karger, Basel.

Rogozkin, V. (1978) Some aspects of athletes' nutrition. In *Nutrition, Physical Fitness and Health. International Series on Sport Science* (ed. J. Parizkova & V. Rogozkin), pp. 119–123. University Park Press, Baltimore, MD.

Rogozkin, V.A. (1993) Principles of athletes' nutrition in the Russian federation. *World Review of Nutrition and Diet* **71**, 154–182.

Saltin, B. & Gollnick, P.D. (1982) Skeletal muscle adaptability: significance for metabolism and performance. In *Handbook of Physiology* (ed. L.D. Peachey,

R.H. Adrian & S.R. Geiger), pp. 555–631. Williams & Wilkins, Baltimore, MD.

Sawka, M.N. & Pandolf, K.B. (1990) Effects of body water loss on physiological function and exercise performance. In *Perspectives in Exercise Science and Sports Medicine*. Vol. 3. *Fluid Homeostasis during Exercise* (ed. C.V. Gisolfi & D.R. Lamb), pp. 1–38. Benchmark Press, Carmel, IN.

Schott, J., McCully, K. & Rutherford, O.M. (1995) The role of metabolites in strength training: short vs. long isometric contractions. *European Journal of Applied Physiology* **71**, 337–341.

Sutton, J.R., Farrel, P.A. & Harber, V.J. (1990) Hormonal adaptation to physical activity. In *Exercise, Fitness and Health* (ed. C. Bouchard, R.J. Shepard, T. Stephans, J.R. Sutton & B.D. McPherson), pp. 217–257. Human Kinetics, Champaign, IL.

Williams, M.H. (1976) *Nutritional Aspects of Human Physical and Athletic Performance*. Charles C. Thomas, Springfield, IL.

# Chapter 48

# Racquet Sports

MARK HARGREAVES

## Introduction

Racquet sports are played in all parts of the world and, in addition to being a popular form of recreational activity, have well-developed professional circuits and are represented at the Olympic Games. These games are played either on a divided court area across a net (e.g. tennis, badminton) or on a common court against a wall (e.g. squash, racquetball). Table tennis provides a slight variation on these general themes. The nutritional requirements for racquet sports will vary greatly between the sports and between individuals and are likely to be determined by a number of factors. Of most importance is the level of energy expenditure which, in turn, is influenced by the game duration, level of participation and quantity of training/competition, type of match (singles vs. doubles), ability of opponent and the extent to which they dictate playing patterns and, in the case of tennis, court surface. Environmental conditions will have an additional impact and are a major determinant of fluid needs. For the purposes of this chapter, discussion will be limited to tennis, squash and badminton; however, the general principles should apply to all racquet sports. Given the complexity of these sports and the interactions between cognitive and physical performance, the racquet sports have been less studied by scientists with an interest in sports performance.

## Physiological and metabolic demands of racquet sports

The physiological and metabolic demands of racquet sports have been well summarized by Reilly (1990). In general, they can be characterized as intermittent exercise, with relatively short bursts of activity, involving both the upper and lower limb muscles, followed by periods of rest. The average duration of a rally is in the range of 4–12 s (Docherty 1982; Dawson *et al.* 1985; Christmass *et al.* 1995; Faccini & Dal Monte 1996), but competitive matches may last from just under an hour up to several hours depending upon the number of games/sets played. For example, some years ago a tennis match in the Davis Cup team competition, when advantage rather than tiebreak sets were played, lasted for over 6 h! Of the racquet sports, tennis has the greatest range of court surfaces, the consequence of which is variation in the duration of rallies and matches. Matches on grass courts tend to be characterized by shorter rallies and dominated by the serve and volley. In contrast, matches on hard and clay courts usually involve longer rallies from the baseline. In general, rallies in squash tend to be longer than those in badminton and tennis (Docherty 1982), which may be a function of the walled court allowing potential 'out balls' to remain in play.

Measurements of heart rate and $\dot{V}o_{2max.}$ during racquet sports support the contention that these sports can be classified as moderate- to high-intensity aerobic activities, with values in the

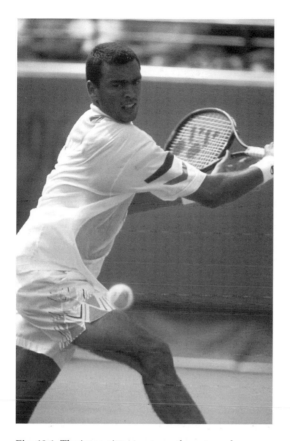

**Fig. 48.1** The intermittent nature of sports such as tennis combines the demands of an endurance event with those of repeated sprints. Photo © Allsport / G.M. Prior.

range of 60–90% of maximal heart rate and 50–80% $\dot{V}o_{2max.}$ (Docherty 1982; Elliott *et al.* 1985; Garden *et al.* 1986; Reilly 1990; Bergeron *et al.* 1991; Therminarias *et al.* 1991; Christmass *et al.* 1995; Faccini & Dal Monte 1996). The heart rate and blood pressure responses tend to be higher in squash and this has led to some discussion about the risk of cardiovascular events in susceptible individuals who play squash vigorously.

The metabolic changes during racquet sports are consistent with the cardiorespiratory responses. Blood glucose usually increases or remains at pre-exercise levels during relatively short periods (45–90 min) of play (Noakes *et al.* 1982; Garden *et al.* 1986; Bergeron *et al.* 1991;

Therminarias *et al.* 1991; Christmass *et al.* 1995). It is possible that, in the absence of carbohydrate supplementation, blood glucose may fall during an extended duration match (Burke & Ekblom 1982). Blood lactate levels are generally within the 1–4 mmol·l⁻¹ range (Noakes *et al.* 1982; Garden *et al.* 1986; Bergeron *et al.* 1991; Therminarias *et al.* 1991), although values as high as 5–6 mmol·l⁻¹ have been observed (Reilly 1990; Christmass *et al.* 1995). While this may reflect a period of intense activity just prior to sampling, it nevertheless suggests the potential for significant lactate production during racquet sports. Although no data on muscle metabolites during racquet sports exist, there is likely to be a large reliance on muscle glycogen, particularly during longer matches. The observed increases in plasma glycerol and free fatty acids (Noakes *et al.* 1982; Garden *et al.* 1986; Christmass *et al.* 1995), which correlate with match duration, suggest an increase in lipolysis. Increases in the plasma levels of catecholamines, adrenocorticotrophic hormone, growth hormone, renin and vasopressin, and decreases in insulin, have been observed during racquet sports (Noakes *et al.* 1982; Garden *et al.* 1986; Therminarias *et al.* 1991).

The intermittent nature of racquet sports results in a thermal load which is less than that encountered during continuous exercise of similar intensity. Environmental heat and humidity will potentially have a greater impact on thermoregulation and fluid balance during racquet sports. For example, it is not uncommon for the on-court temperature to be as high as 45–50°C on some days of the Australian Open tennis tournament (held during the summer month of January) and this creates a major challenge to the thermal and fluid balance of elite players. Medical treatment for heat illness (i.v. fluids and postmatch monitoring) was required for two players in the 1997 tournament. In addition, factors such as air-conditioning, ventilation, humidity, and heat generation from lighting will influence the environmental conditions when squash, badminton and tennis are played indoors. Increases in rectal temperature of 0.8–1.5°C have been observed following tennis

(Elliot *et al.* 1985; Therminarias *et al.* 1991) and squash (Blanksby *et al.* 1980; Noakes *et al.* 1982) in moderate conditions and greater increases are reported during exercise in the heat (Dawson *et al.* 1985). Losses of body mass have been reported in the range of 0.9–2 kg (Therminarias *et al.* 1991; Bergeron *et al.* 1995), a relatively large fluid loss which is determined by the balance between sweat fluid losses and fluid replacement. The opportunities for fluid replacement tend to be greater in tennis, where there is a change of ends every two games and a 90-s rest period. In contrast, during squash and badminton, fluid intake is usually limited to the end of a game. Another concern for the tournament tennis player is the need to sometimes play more than one match per day and to play a number of matches on successive days. During the course of several days of tournament play, it is possible that the fluid and electrolyte status of players is challenged (Bergeron *et al.* 1995).

## Nutrition for racquet sports

In general, the nutritional strategies adopted by racquet sport competitors should adhere to the guidelines suggested for most athletes. Total energy intake should be sufficient to cover the energy requirements of competition and training, which in the case of players at the elite level can be large. For the recreational racquet sports participant, where total energy expenditure is less and the need to maintain an optimal body weight by energy restriction may be greater, there should be a greater emphasis on carbohydrate intake. Particular attention should be paid to carbohydrate and fluid requirements for the reasons that have been well described in previous chapters. Tournament play will create certain difficulties in achieving nutritional goals. The need for international travel will cause disruption to normal cycles and eating patterns and provide food choices that differ from those usually consumed. Adequate preparation prior to an international trip is essential and this may be as simple as becoming familiar with food

choices available at a tournament venue or as involved as taking certain foods and/or supplements as part of the luggage. Most international tournaments have excellent catering services; however, delays due to bad weather, prolonged matches and/or alterations in playing schedules can interfere with eating plans. Under such circumstances, it is advisable to have a range of light, easily digested, high carbohydrate-containing meals available. Liquid meals/supplements are often appropriate. The other nutritional challenge for the tournament player is the need for rapid recovery, since matches are scheduled on a daily basis and if a successful competitor is also involved in doubles, there can be many matches over a relatively short period. Towards the end of a tournament, it is not uncommon for successful competitors to play multiple games on successive days. To facilitate rapid recovery and optimize liver and muscle glycogen reserves and whole body hydration, carbohydrate and fluid replacement should be emphasized early in the recovery period. The principles underlying this practice have been well described in Chapters 7 and 19, respectively.

Another aspect of nutritional practice related to the racquet sports is the need for carbohydrate and fluid replacement during activity. The beneficial effects of carbohydrate and fluid supplementation on performance during exercise, and the underlying mechanisms, have been well described in the literature (see Chapters 8, 16 and 17). It could be argued that any nutritional intervention that minimizes the risk of fatigue during prolonged, strenuous racquet sport activity would contribute to at least maintained, if not improved, performance. Furthermore, given the heavy reliance on perceptual and motor skills in the racquet sports, attenuation of the effects of carbohydrate depletion and dehydration on central nervous system function is likely to enhance performance. Relatively few studies have directly tested such hypotheses. Mitchell *et al.* (1992) observed no benefit of carbohydrate supplementation on indices of tennis performance (serve velocity/accuracy, error rates) during 3h of tennis play. Because a decline in blood glucose was not observed during exercise in the control trial, the authors speculated that glucose availability was not limiting during the tennis match and accordingly, carbohydrate supplementation would have little effect. In contrast, Burke and Ekblom (1982) observed that the addition of carbohydrate to a rehydration beverage enhanced indices of tennis performance to a greater extent than water alone or no fluids. Furthermore, Vergauwen *et al.* (1998) recently observed that carbohydrate ingestion during 2h of strenuous tennis training increased performance during a shuttle running test and a specific tennis performance test that assessed error rates, ball velocity and precision of ball placement when compared with ingestion of a sweet placebo. Based on previous work demonstrating the benefits of energy and fluid replacement during continuous and intermittent exercise, it is recommended that such practices be adopted during racquet sports. There is little argument that fluids should be ingested. The need for carbohydrate supplementation will depend upon the intensity and duration of the match and is likely to be of most benefit the longer the match progresses. Athletes should experiment with energy replacement beverages during training and competition of varying duration to identify a practice that best suits their needs.

In summary, the physiological and metabolic demands of racquet sport training and competition are such that total energy, carbohydrate and fluid intakes should be increased. The training diet should contain sufficient amounts of these nutrients, together with vitamins and minerals. During periods of intense training and tournament competition, carbohydrate and fluid intake may need to be increased to facilitate rapid recovery on a daily basis. Ingestion of fluid during matches will minimize the risk of dehydration and carbohydrate supplementation should also be considered, especially when duration is extended. Given the large number of factors that will influence the nutritional needs of racquet sport competitors, nutritional guidelines should be formulated on an individual basis.

# References

Bergeron, M.F., Maresh, C.M., Kraemer, W.J., Abraham, A., Conroy, B. & Gabaree, C. (1991) Tennis: a physiological profile during match play. *International Journal of Sports Medicine* **12**, 474–479.

Bergeron, M.F., Maresh, C.M., Armstrong, L.E. *et al.* (1995) Fluid–electrolyte balance associated with tennis match play in a hot environment. *International Journal of Sport Nutrition* **5**, 180–193.

Blanksby, B.A., Elliott, B., Davis, K.H. & Mercer, M.D. (1980) Blood pressure and rectal temperature responses of middle-aged sedentary, middle-aged active and 'A' grade competitive male squash players. *British Journal of Sports Medicine* **14**, 133–138.

Burke, E.R. & Ekblom, B. (1982) Influence of fluid ingestion and dehydration on precision and endurance performance in tennis. *Athletic Training* **17**, 275–277.

Christmass, M.A., Richmond, S.E., Cable, N.T. & Hartmann, P.E. (1995) A metabolic characterisation of single tennis. In *Science and Racket Sports* (ed. T. Reilly, M. Hughes & A. Lees), pp. 3–9. E & FN Spon, London.

Dawson, B., Elliott, B., Pyke, F. & Rogers, R. (1985) Physiological and performance responses to playing tennis in a cool environment and similar intervalized treadmill running in a hot climate. *Journal of Human Movement Studies* **11**, 21–24.

Docherty, D. (1982) A comparison of heart rate responses in racquet games. *British Journal of Sports Medicine* **16**, 96–100.

Elliott, B., Dawson, B. & Pyke, F. (1985) The energetics of singles tennis. *Journal of Human Movement Studies* **11**, 11–20.

Faccini, P. & Dal Monte, A. (1996) Physiologic demands of badminton match play. *American Journal of Sports Medicine* **24**, S64–S66.

Garden, G., Hale, P.J., Horrocks, P.M., Crase, J., Hammond, J. & Nattrass, M. (1986) Metabolic and hormonal responses during squash. *European Journal of Applied Physiology* **55**, 445–449.

Mitchell, J.B., Cole, K.J., Grandjean, P.W. & Sobczak, R.J. (1992) The effect of a carbohydrate beverage on tennis performance and fluid balance during prolonged tennis play. *Journal of Applied Sport Science Research* **6**, 96–102.

Noakes, T.D., Cowling, J.R., Gevers, W. & Van Niekark, J.P. de V. (1982) The metabolic response to squash including the influence of pre-exercise carbohydrate ingestion. *South African Medical Journal* **62**, 721–723.

Reilly, T. (1990) The racquet sports. In *Physiology of Sports* (ed. T. Reilly, N. Secher, P. Snell & C. Williams), pp. 337–369. E & FN Spon, London.

Therminarias, A., Dansou, P., Chirpaz-Oddou, M.-F., Gharib, C. & Quirion, A. (1991) Hormonal and metabolic changes during a strenuous tennis match: effect of ageing. *International Journal of Sports Medicine* **12**, 10–16.

Vergauwen, L., Brouns, F. & Hespel, P. (1998) Carbohydrate supplementation improves stroke performance in tennis. *Medicine and Science in Sports and Exercise* **30**, 1289–1295.

# Chapter 49

# Weight Category Sports

JACK H. WILMORE

## Introduction

Most athletes are concerned with either attaining or maintaining an optimal body weight and composition for their sport, or event within their sport. For some athletes, increased body size can be an advantage (e.g. basketball, rugby and American football), providing that the increase in size is the result of an increase in the athlete's fat-free mass. For other athletes, body size is not nearly as important, but it is critical to maintain a low relative body fat (% fat mass) and a high relative fat-free mass (% fat-free mass) to optimize performance (e.g. distance running, soccer and swimming). For still other athletes, their body weight is dictated by a specific weight category (range of weights) within which the athlete must fall in order to be eligible to compete (i.e. weight category sports).

Weight category sports include all sports in which the athlete must compete within a given weight category. Examples of weight category sports are provided in Table 49.1. There are also sports, or events within a sport, which are weight controlled. In these sports or events, competition is not organized by weight categories, yet the tradition of the sport or event dictates a slim figure, and thus a low body weight. For example, in diving and figure skating, athletes are rated by judges as to how well they perform a certain dive or skating routine. While the emphasis in judging is to be placed on the athlete's performance, appearance does play a significant role, and a leaner body is associated

with success. Examples of weight-controlled sports are provided in Table 49.1. Weight-controlled sports are included with weight category sports in this chapter as they share a number of common nutritional concerns. Weight-controlled sports are also addressed in Chapter 39.

Weight category and weight-controlled sports and events present a unique challenge from the nutritional perspective (Wilmore 1992). Many of these athletes are consciously trying to either reduce weight or maintain a weight well below what would be considered normal or optimal for them. This leads to a variety of unhealthy nutritional practices, including skipping meals, avoiding specific foods or food groups which are necessary for meeting the minimum daily requirement for certain vitamins, minerals or macronutrients, and the binge–purge syndrome, including the use of diuretics and laxatives, among others. This chapter will focus on nutritional issues unique to weight category and weight-controlled sports. It will address techniques used to achieve weight loss and weight maintenance for these sports, the health, physiological and performance consequences of weight loss and maintenance through these techniques, and practical considerations as to how to best achieve and maintain an optimal body weight for these sports.

## Weight loss and weight maintenance techniques

For both weight category sports and weight-controlled sports, the rate of weight loss can be rapid (i.e. within 24–72 h), moderate (from 72 h to several weeks), or gradual (from several weeks to months). In some sports, moderate and rapid weight loss will occur many times over a single season. Tipton has stated that in wrestling, this process can be repeated between five and 30 times per season (Tipton 1981). Thus, the consequences of not only an acute period of moderate or rapid weight loss must be considered, but also the cumulative effects over the course of a season where there are multiple bouts of weight loss and

weight regain, or what has been termed weight cycling. The magnitude of the weight loss per cycle can also be substantial. Steen and Brownell (1990), in their survey of 63 college wrestlers and 368 high school wrestlers, reported that 41% of the college wrestlers reported weight losses of 5.0–9.1 kg each week of the season while 23% of the high school wrestlers lost 2.7–4.5 kg weekly.

For sports like wrestling, where both rapid and moderate rates of weight loss are used, the techniques for achieving a given weight loss are quite varied. Horswill (1994) has listed a number of common methods of weight loss used by wrestlers which are presented in Table 49.2. The technique of negative energy balance is common across rapid, moderate and gradual rates of weight loss. Dehydration, purging and the other techniques listed in Table 49.2 are most common for rapid weight loss, but can extend across the moderate rate of weight loss category as well.

Establishing a negative energy balance is the preferred technique for weight loss. However, this technique has limited efficacy when the athlete must lose weight in a short period of time. Ideally, the athlete will establish a goal weight well in advance of his or her need to achieve that weight. A negative energy balance of 2100–4200 kJ (500–1000 kcal) daily is ideal, and this should be achieved through a balance of

**Table 49.1** Examples of weight category and weight-controlled sports and events.

| Weight category sports | Weight-controlled sports |
| --- | --- |
| Body building | Dance (ballet) |
| Boxing | Distance running |
| Horse racing (jockeys) | Diving |
| Martial arts (e.g. judo, karate) | Figure skating |
| Rowing | Gymnastics |
| Weight lifting | Synchronized swimming |
| Wrestling | |

**Table 49.2** Methods of weight loss used by wrestlers. Adapted from Horswill (1994).

| Method | Example | Weight loss compartment |
| --- | --- | --- |
| Negative energy balance | | Body cell mass |
|    Increase energy output | Aerobic training | |
|    Decrease energy intake | Diet, fasting | |
| Intentional dehydration | | Body water |
|    Metabolic | Exercise | |
|    Thermal | Sauna, sweat suit, rubber suit | |
|    Diuresis | Diuretics, high-protein diet | |
|    Bloodletting | | |
| Purging | Laxatives, vomiting | Gastrointestinal tract |
| Other | Haircut | Body cell mass |
| | Inversion* | |

*Inversion involves the wrestler standing on his head to redistribute his blood and body fluids, which some wrestlers believe affects the scale reading.

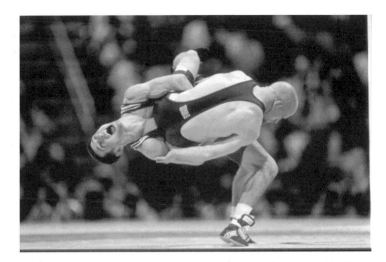

**Fig. 49.1** Rapid weight loss to make weight for competition can pose health risks and can impair performance. However, as long as competitors perceive an advantage, the practice will persist. Photo © Allsport / D. Leah.

increased energy expenditure and decreased energy intake. The objective is to reach the desired goal weight over a reasonable period of time, minimizing the potential loss of fat-free mass (Wilmore 1992).

It has been clearly established that for both rapid and moderate rates of weight loss, a substantial percentage of the weight loss, i.e. 50% or more of the weight, can be derived from the fat-free mass, predominantly from the total body water and protein stores. In fact, with very low energy diets (i.e. 1680–3360 kJ·day$^{-1}$, 400–800 kcal·day$^{-1}$) or low energy diets extended over longer periods of time, water and protein can still constitute a substantial percentage of the weight lost. Keys *et al.* (1950), in their classic series of studies on human starvation, fed non-obese adult men a test diet of 6570 kJ·day$^{-1}$ (1570 kcal·day$^{-1}$) for 24 weeks. The subjects' diet which maintained stable weight prior to going on the low energy diet was 14.5 MJ·day$^{-1}$ (3468 kcal·day$^{-1}$). Over the first 11 weeks, approximately 40% of the weight lost was from fat, 12% from protein, and 48% from water, with an average rate of weight loss of 0.15 kg per day. In a study of obese subjects, Yang and Van Itallie (1976) reported an average rate of weight loss of 0.45 kg per day in obese subjects on a 5020 kJ·day$^{-1}$ (1200 kcal·day$^{-1}$) mixed diet over the first 5 days on the diet. Water comprised 66% of the total weight loss. The relatively high contribution of water to initial weight losses is at least partially the result of obligatory water loss accompanying the metabolism of glycogen and protein. Both glycogen and protein have hydration ratios of approximately 3–4 g water·g$^{-1}$ of substrate, both for storage and degradation (Van Itallie & Yang 1977). Thus, athletes must be very careful when dieting to maximize weight loss while minimizing loss of fat-free tissue. Again, it is important to combine exercise with diet to achieve a given energy deficit per day. Including exercise as a component of the energy deficit attenuates the loss of fat-free mass when compared to diet alone (Ballor & Poehlman 1994; Saris 1995).

Dehydration is the most widely used technique for rapid weight loss. Intentional dehydration is probably a better phrase to use since the intent of the technique is specific to producing body water loss, where unintentional dehydration is an unexpected consequence of negative energy balance resulting from the obligatory water loss associated with glycogen and protein degradation. With intentional dehydration, both metabolic and thermal techniques are intended to induce water loss through sweating, although an added bonus from exercise is the obligatory water loss from depletion of the body's glycogen stores as discussed previously. Sweat losses, which are composed mostly of water, can be as high as $2–3 l \cdot h^{-1}$ in men acclimatized to heat over the short term, and up to $10–15 l \cdot day^{-1}$ (Wenger 1988). Sauna and sudation or water vapour-barrier garments have been widely used to promote sweating, and the subsequent loss of water can be considerable. These techniques are not without risk or negative consequences (Vuori & Wilmore 1994), but dehydration remains a powerful tool for major losses of weight in short periods of time.

Dehydration can potentially be induced by the use of a high-protein diet, as water loss has been associated with a high-protein diet. However, the contribution of a high-protein diet to water loss is most likely associated with the fact that carbohydrate intake is reduced. This forces the body to rely more on fats, with the resulting production of ketone bodies. It has been clearly established that an excessive formation of ketone bodies, or ketosis, leads to diuresis. Also, as the intake of carbohydrate is limited, muscle and liver glycogen stores are gradually depleted, resulting in further water loss, i.e. the obligatory water loss associated with glycogen degradation. Prescription diuretics are also used to induce dehydration, although these are on the banned list of substances for use by athletes (Wadler & Hainline 1989). Certain foods, particularly alcohol and those foods containing caffeine, have substantial diuretic properties. However, caffeine is a banned substance when ingested in excessive quantities, e.g. 6–8 cups of coffee in one sitting (Wadler & Hainline 1989). Refer to Chapter 28 for further details.

Bloodletting has been stated as a method used for weight loss by wrestlers (Horswill 1994); however, it is unclear if this is widely practised. This was not mentioned as a technique for weight loss in the comprehensive review of Fogelholm (1994), and was not included as a technique for weight loss in a large survey of high school wrestlers (Weissinger et al. 1991). Most likely, bloodletting is not widely used for weight loss in athletes, as most athletes do not like invasive techniques and recognize the obvious physiological and performance disadvantages of blood loss.

Purging behaviours are discussed in detail in Chapter 39, and will not be addressed in detail in this chapter. Self-induced vomiting and the use of laxatives are the primary purging behaviours. These behaviours can lead to transient weight losses, but have substantial clinical risk, are potentially addictive, and can negatively impact athletic performance. While haircuts and inversion might be used in hopes of reducing the athlete's weight, there is no evidence to support the efficacy of these techniques.

## Health consequences of weight loss

Athletes generally lose weight for one of three purposes: to qualify for a specific weight category, to achieve a more aesthetic appearance, and to improve performance potential. There are a number of questions raised concerning the potential for detrimental health consequences of weight loss. While most critical attention has been focused on rapid and moderate rates of weight loss, there is also concern over gradual, long-term weight loss. Each of these will be addressed.

The primary concern with rapid and moderate rates of weight loss is the consequences of severe dehydration. Wrestlers have reduced body weight by 4–5% in 12–24h, and losses of up to 12% of body weight have been reported (Brownell et al. 1987; Fogelholm 1994). The greatest percentage of the weight lost is from the total body water stores. Water accounts for approximately 60% of the total weight of an adult man. Thus, for a 70-kg man, total body water would represent about 42 kg, or 42 l, assuming a water density of 1.000. The intracellular fluid accounts for about 67% of the total body water, or 28 l, and the extracellular fluid accounts for the remaining 14 l. Of the 14 l of extracellular fluid, plasma volume would account for 3 l and the interstitial fluid would account for the remaining 11 l (Guyton & Hall 1996). With rapid weight loss, water is lost from each of the fluid compartments. It has been estimated that the intracellular compartment can contribute 30–60% of the total; the interstitial fluid, 30–60% of the total; and the plasma volume, 8–12% of the total (Mack & Nadel 1996).

In a study by Costill *et al.* (1976), eight healthy men cycled at 70% of $\dot{V}o_{2max.}$ in an environmental chamber ($T_{amb}$ =39°C) until they were progressively dehydrated by 2%, 4% and 6% of their initial body weight during a single, prolonged exercise bout. After achieving each level of dehydration, the subjects rested for 30 min in a supine position while a blood sample and muscle biopsy were obtained. Plasma and muscle water contents were reduced by 2.4% and 1.2%, respectively, for each percentage decrease in body weight. Figure 49.2 illustrates the changes in the plasma, interstitial and intracellular fluid compartments at each level of dehydration.

What are the health implications of such major changes in total body water? Of obvious concern is the potential for disturbances in thermoregulation. Sawka (1992) concludes from his review of the literature that hypohydration, consequent to dehydration, causes greater heat storage (i.e. increased core temperature) and reduces tolerance to heat strain. This is the result of reductions in the rate of sweating and skin blood flow. Even with decreased skin blood flow, there is still considerable displacement of blood to the skin for cooling, making it difficult to maintain central venous pressure and an adequate cardiac output.

Excessive sweat or urine loss could also result in large losses of electrolytes, which could possibly have serious health consequences, such as cardiac dysrhythmias. However, Costill (1977) has concluded that even those electrolyte losses can be large, they are largely derived from the extracellular compartment, and that losses of ions in sweat and urine have little effect on the K+ content of plasma or muscle.

Further, concern has been expressed as to the effects of chronic dehydration on renal function. Zambraski (1990), in a review of renal function, fluid homeostasis and exercise, concluded that exercise, particularly in conjunction with hypo-

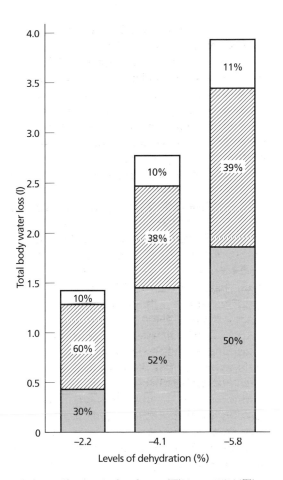

**Fig. 49.2** Changes in the plasma (□), interstitial (▨) and intracellular water (■) compartments with exercise and thermal dehydration of 2%, 4% and 6% of body weight. Adapted from Costill *et al.* (1976), with permission.

hydration, sodium deprivation, and/or heat stress, presents a major stress to the kidneys. Renal vasoconstriction and antinatriuretic responses are increased in magnitude when dehydration and/or heat stress are combined with exercise. Exercise proteinuria and haematuria have been reported, indicating dramatic changes in renal function. However, the incidence of acute renal failure is relatively small. The long-term consequences of repeated episodes of acute renal stress are unknown.

Repeated bouts of weight cycling have also

been postulated to have negative health consequences (Brownell *et al.* 1987). These would include an increased energy efficiency, thus an increased risk of weight gain, increased deposition of fat in the upper body (i.e. visceral fat), lipid and lipoprotein disorders, reproductive disorders such as delayed menarche and secondary amenorrhoea, and bone mineral disturbances consequent to secondary amenorrhoea. Fortunately, most of these concerns have now been clearly established to be unrelated to weight cycling (van der Kooy *et al.* 1993; Anonymous 1994; Jeffery 1996).

Athletes attempting to maintain a body weight which is lower than that which is normal and healthy for them is also a cause for concern. These athletes are often in a state of chronic energy deficit (i.e. energy expenditure>energy intake for many days, weeks or months). In female athletes, Loucks and Heath (1994a, 1994b) have demonstrated that once the energy deficit exceeds a certain critical level, reproductive and thyroid function are suppressed, which might serve as a trigger for athletic amenorrhoea (secondary amenorrhoea in the athletic population). Amenorrhoea in athletes is associated with low concentrations of 17β-oestradiol and progesterone, which are, in turn, associated with low bone mineral density in the spine (Snead *et al.* 1992). The combination of disordered eating (including energy deficit), amenorrhoea and bone mineral disorders has been termed the 'female athlete triad,' with the assumption that disordered eating can lead to menstrual dysfunction, which, in turn, can lead to bone mineral disorders (Wilmore 1991). The female athlete triad has become a topic of great concern and is the focus of a recent position statement by the American College of Sports Medicine (Otis *et al.* 1997).

## Physiological and performance consequences of weight loss

With rapid and moderate rates of weight loss, there will be reductions in total body water, muscle and liver glycogen stores, as well as in other components of the fat-free mass (Oppliger *et al.* 1996). For the most part, these athletes are already very lean prior to weight loss, and so very little of the weight lost will be derived from the fat stores. In fact, Friedl *et al.* (1994) have reported that there is likely a lower limit to the loss of body fat with weight loss in lean individuals. In a group of 55 soldiers participating in an 8-week Ranger Training Course, those who achieved a minimum relative body fat of 4–6% by 6 weeks demonstrated only small additional total and subcutaneous fat losses in the final 2 weeks and lost increasingly larger proportions of fat-free mass. Therefore, as the athlete reaches a low total fat mass, there is a reduced likelihood of further losses of body fat with weight loss. Consequently, the percentage of the actual weight loss from the fat-free mass during rapid and moderate rates of weight loss is likely to be high. Generally, decrements in performance are associated with losses in the body's fat-free mass (Wilmore 1992).

Several recent papers have reviewed the research literature on the effects of rapid and moderate rates of weight loss on physiological function and performance (Fogelholm 1994; Horswill 1994; Oppliger *et al.* 1996). The results of these reviews are summarized in Table 49.3. Since there is typically an interval of time between weigh-in and actual competition for most sports, ranging from a few minutes up to 20 h or more, it is extremely important to understand how physiological function and performance respond following a variable period of rehydration and replenishment of nutrients. Unfortunately, while a great deal is known about the effects of acute dehydration on physiological function and performance, far less is known about the regain in function and performance with rehydration and intake of nutrients.

From this table, it is very clear that rapid or moderate rates of weight loss can have major effects on both physiological function and performance. What is less certain are the potential changes that occur with rehydration and food intake during the interval of time between weigh-in and competition. It appears that some

**Table 49.3** Alterations in physiological function and performance consequent to rapid and moderate rates of dehydration. Data from reviews of Fogelholm (1994), Horswill (1994), Keller *et al.* (1994) and Oppliger *et al.* (1996).

| Variables | Dehydration | Rehydration |
|---|---|---|
| *Physiological function* | | |
| Cardiovascular | | |
| Blood volume/plasma volume | $\downarrow$ | $\downarrow$* |
| Cardiac output | $\downarrow$ | ? |
| Stroke volume | $\downarrow$ | ? |
| Heart rate | $\uparrow$ | ? |
| Metabolic | | |
| Aerobic capacity ($\dot{V}O_{2max.}$) | $\leftrightarrow, \downarrow$ | $\leftrightarrow$* |
| Anaerobic power (Wingate test) | $\leftrightarrow, \downarrow$ | $\leftrightarrow, \downarrow$ |
| Anaerobic capacity (Wingate test) | $\leftrightarrow, \downarrow$ | $\leftrightarrow, \downarrow$ |
| Blood lactate (peak value) | $\downarrow$ | $\downarrow$* |
| Buffer capacity of the blood | $\downarrow$ | ? |
| Lactate threshold (velocity) | $\downarrow$ | ? |
| Muscle and liver glycogen | $\downarrow$ | $\downarrow$ |
| Blood glucose during exercise | Possible $\downarrow$ | ? |
| Protein degradation with exercise | Possible $\uparrow$ | ? |
| Thermoregulation and fluid balance | | |
| Electrolytes (muscle and blood) | $\downarrow$ | $\leftrightarrow$ |
| Exercise core temperature | $\uparrow$ | ? |
| Sweat rate | $\downarrow$, delayed onset | ? |
| Skin blood flow | $\downarrow$ | ? |
| *Performance* | | |
| Muscular strength | $\leftrightarrow, \downarrow$ | $\leftrightarrow, \downarrow$ |
| Muscular endurance | $\leftrightarrow, \downarrow$ | $\leftrightarrow, \downarrow$ |
| Muscular power | ? | $\downarrow$† |
| Speed of movement | ? | ? |
| Run time to exhaustion | $\downarrow$ | ? |
| Total work performed | $\downarrow$ | $\downarrow$* |
| Wrestling simulation tests† | $\downarrow$ | $\leftrightarrow \downarrow$† |

$\downarrow$, decrease; $\uparrow$, increase; $\leftrightarrow$, no known change, or return to normal values; ?, unknown.
*From Burge *et al.* (1993).
†From Oopik *et al.* (1996).

of the function and performance that was lost during an acute episode of a rapid or a moderate rate of weight loss can be regained within 5–20 h providing ample food and beverage are available and the athlete is willing to eat. There are still many questions to be answered regarding the total efficacy of eating and drinking during this period between weigh-in and competition with respect to regaining normal physiological function and performance. The issue of replacing carbohydrate postexercise is covered in Chapter 7, and rehydration after exercise-induced sweat loss is covered in Chapter 19.

## Practical considerations for weight loss

As stated in a previous section of this paper, the ideal way to lose weight for competition is to establish a goal weight several months in advance of the start of the competitive season, and achieve this goal weight by gradual reductions in body fat of not more than 0.45–0.9 kg· week⁻¹ while maintaining or increasing the fat-free mass. Koutedakis *et al.* (1994) have shown that weight reduction of the same magnitude (6–7% of body weight) over 2 months vs. 4

months in the same athletes 1 year later adversely altered fitness-related performance parameters in international lightweight oarswomen. Unfortunately, for many athletes a prolonged weight loss protocol is not possible. Since most of them are already very lean (low fat mass), they are able to achieve their competitive weight only by losing large amounts of fat-free weight with minimal losses of fat mass. This is accomplished primarily through decreases in the total body water stores, and the muscle and liver glycogen stores, both of which are critical to successful performance. Therefore, the length of time between the weigh-in and competition is extremely important, as is the fluid and nutrient replenishment protocol. While a solid data base is not yet available, it would seem logical that the longer the period of repletion of fluid and energy stores, and the more fluid and energy the athlete can ingest during this period, the better will be the subsequent performance.

What might be an optimal rehydration/ refeeding protocol? Of primary concern would be the need to replenish both fluid and glycogen stores. Of secondary concern would be the replacement of electrolytes lost during the process of dehydration. However, electrolyte replacement is essential for the restoration of fluid balance (Maughan & Leiper 1995; Shirreffs *et al.* 1996). Thus, it would seem logical to use both a sports drink (5–10% carbohydrate and electrolytes) plus a high-carbohydrate food source such as sports bars (providing there is at least 2–3 h before competition). The combination of the sports drink and sports bar should provide optimal replenishment for the time available. Since there is not a good data base on this issue, athletes should be encouraged to experiment with different combinations to see what works best for them, keeping in mind that they need to replenish both fluids and glycogen.

Effective strategies to make weight would include each of the following.

• Compete in an attainable weight category — do not drop down to an unrealistic category.

• Lose most of the weight preseason, and lose it gradually to maximize fat loss.

• Ideally, if you need to lose 10% of body weight, lose the first 6% gradually during the preseason, and the last 4% through dehydration 24–48 h prior to competition.

• Eat a high-carbohydrate diet during training and during periods of weight loss to maintain as best as possible muscle and liver glycogen stores.

• Supplement vitamins and minerals if restricting food to lose weight.

• Maintain normal hydration during training, except for the 24–48-h period before weigh-in if it becomes necessary to dehydrate to make weight.

• Maximize the period of time between weigh-in and competition to replenish both water and energy stores.

## References

Anonymous (1994) Weight cycling: National Task Force on the Prevention and Treatment of Obesity. *Journal of the American Medical Association* **272**, 1196–1202.

Ballor, D.L. & Poehlman, E.T. (1994) Exercise-training enhances fat-free mass preservation during diet-induced weight loss: a meta-analytical finding. *International Journal of Obesity* **18**, 35–40.

Brownell, K.D., Steen, S.N. & Wilmore, J.H. (1987) Weight regulation practices in athletes: analysis of metabolic and health effects. *Medicine and Science in Sports and Exercise* **19**, 546–556.

Burge, C.M., Carey, M.F. & Payne, W.R. (1993) Rowing performance, fluid balance, and metabolic function following dehydration and rehydration. *Medicine and Science in Sports and Exercise* **25**, 1358–1364.

Costill, D.L. (1977) Sweating: its composition and effects on body fluids. *Annals of the New York Academy of Sciences* **301**, 160–174.

Costill, D.L., Cote, R. & Fink, W. (1976) Muscle water and electrolytes following varied levels of dehydration in man. *Journal of Applied Physiology* **40**, 6–11.

Fogelholm, M. (1994) Effects of bodyweight reduction on sports performance. *Sports Medicine* **18**, 249–267.

Friedl, K.E., Moore, R.J., Martinez-Lopez, L.E. *et al.* (1994) Lower limit of body fat in healthy active men. *Journal of Applied Physiology* **77**, 933–940.

Guyton, A.C. & Hall, J.E. (1996) *Textbook of Medical Physiology*, 9th edn, pp. 298–299. Saunders, Philadelphia, PA.

Horswill, C.A. (1994) Physiology and nutrition for wrestling. In *Physiology and Nutrition for Competitive Sport* (D.R. Lamb, H.G. Knuttgen & R. Murray), Vol. 7, pp. 131–174. Cooper, Carmel, IN.

Jeffery, R.W. (1996) Does weight cycling present a health risk? *American Journal of Clinical Nutrition* **63** (Suppl.), 452S–455S.

Keller, H.L., Tolly, S.E. & Freedson, P.S. (1994) Weight loss in adolescent wrestlers. *Pediatric Exercise Science* **6**, 211–224.

Keys, A., Brozek, J., Henschel, A., Mickelsen, O. & Taylor, H.L. (1950) *The Biology of Human Starvation.* University of Minnesota Press, Minneapolis, MN.

Koutedakis, Y., Pacy, P.J., Quevedo, R.M. *et al.* (1994) The effects of two different periods of weight-reduction on selected performance parameters in elite lightweight oarswomen. *International Journal of Sports Medicine* **15**, 472–477.

Loucks, A.B. & Heath, E.M. (1994a) Dietary restriction reduces luteinizing hormone (LH) pulse frequency during waking hours and increases LH pulse amplitude during sleep in young menstruating women. *Journal of Clinical Endocrinology and Metabolism* **78**, 910–915.

Loucks, A.B. & Heath, E.M. (1994b) Induction of low-$T_3$ syndrome in exercising women occurs at a threshold of energy availability. *American Journal of Physiology* **266**, R817–R823.

Mack, G.W. & Nadel, E.R. (eds) (1996) *Body Fluid Balance during Heat Stress in Humans.* Oxford University Press, New York.

Maughan, R.J. & Leiper, J.B. (1995) Sodium intake and post-exercise rehydration in man. *European Journal of Applied Physiology* **71**, 311–319.

Oopik, V., Paasuke, M., Sikku, T. *et al.* (1996) Effect of rapid weight loss on metabolism and isokinetic performance capacity: a case study of two well trained wrestlers. *Journal of Sports Medicine and Physical Fitness* **36**, 127–131.

Oppliger, R.A., Case, H.S., Horswill, C.A., Landry, G.L. & Shelter, A.C. (1996) Weight loss in wrestlers: an American College of Sports Medicine position stand. *Medicine and Science in Sports and Exercise* **28**, ix–xii.

Otis, C.L., Drinkwater, B., Johnson, M., Loucks, A. & Wilmore, J. (1997) The Female Athlete Triad. *Medicine and Science in Sports and Exercise* **29**, i–ix.

Saris, W.H.M. (1995) Exercise with or without dietary restriction and obesity treatment. *International Journal of Obesity* **19** (Suppl. 4), S113–S118.

Sawka, M.N. (1992) Physiological consequences of hypohydration: exercise performance and thermoregulation. *Medicine and Science in Sports and Exercise* **24**, 657–670.

Shirreffs, S.M., Taylor, A.J., Leiper, J.B. & Maughan, R.J. (1996) Post-exercise dehydration in man: effects of volume consumed and drink sodium content. *Medicine and Science in Sports and Exercise* **28**, 1260–1271.

Snead, D.B., Weltman, A., Weltman, J.Y. *et al.* (1992) Reproductive hormones and bone mineral density in women runners. *Journal of Applied Physiology* **72**, 2149–2156.

Steen, S.N. & Brownell, K.D. (1990) Patterns of weight loss and regain in wrestlers: has the tradition changed? *Medicine and Science in Sports and Exercise* **22**, 762–768.

Tipton, C.M. (1981) Consequences of rapid weight loss. In *Nutrition and Athletic Performance* (ed. W.L. Haskell, J. Scala & J.H. Whittam), pp. 176–197. Bull, Palo Alto, CA.

van der Kooy, K., Leenen, R., Seidell, J.C., Deurenberg, P. & Hautvast, J.G.A.J. (1993) Effect of a weight cycle on visceral fat accumulation. *American Journal of Clinical Nutrition* **58**, 853–857.

Van Itallie, T.B. & Yang, M.-U. (1977) Current concepts in nutrition: diet and weight loss. *New England Journal of Medicine* **297**, 1158–1161.

Vuori, I. & Wilmore, J.H. (1994) Adjuvants to physical activity: do they help in any way? In *Physical Activity, Fitness, and Health* (ed. C. Bouchard, R.J. Shephard & T. Stephens), pp. 270–284. Human Kinetics, Champaign, IL.

Wadler, G.I. & Hainline, B. (1989) *Drugs and the Athlete.* F.A. Davis, Philadelphia, PA.

Weissinger, E., Housh, T.J., Johnson, G.O. & Evans, S.A. (1991) Weight loss behavior in high school wrestling: wrestler and parent perceptions. *Pediatric Exercise Science* **3**, 64–73.

Wenger, C.B. (1988) Human heat acclimatization. In *Human Performance Physiology and Environmental Medicine at Terrestrial Extremes* (ed. K.B. Pandolf, M.N. Sawka & R.R. Gonzalez), pp. 153–197. Benchmark Press, Indianapolis, IN.

Wilmore, J.H. (1991) Eating and weight disorders in the female athlete. *International Journal of Sports Nutrition* **1**, 104–117.

Wilmore, J.H. (1992) Body weight standards and athletic performance. In *Eating, Body Weight and Performance in Athletes: Disorders of Modern Society* (ed. K.D. Brownell, J. Rodin & J.H. Wilmore), pp. 315–329. Lea & Febiger, Philadelphia, PA.

Yang, M.-U. & Van Itallie, T.B. (1976) Composition of weight lost during short-term weight reduction: metabolic responses of obese subjects to starvation and low-calorie ketogenic and nonketogenic diets. *Journal of Clinical Investigation* **58**, 722–730.

Zambraski, E.J. (1990) Renal regulation of fluid homeostasis during exercise. In *Perspectives in Exercise Science and Sports Medicine. Vol. 3. Fluid Homeostasis during Exercise* (ed. C.V. Gisolfi & D.R. Lamb), pp. 247–276. Benchmark Press, Carmel, IN.

# Chapter 50

# Skating

ANN C. SNYDER AND CARL FOSTER

## Introduction

Speed skating, ice hockey and figure skating, while quite different activities, all make up the sport of skating. The different types of skating vary from each other and also within discipline. Speed skating is rhythmical, continuous and fast, and includes long and short track, pack style, in-line, and marathon skating. Ice hockey has numerous starts, stops and direction changes and thus is non-rhythmical, and is played by forwards, defensemen and goalies. Finally, figure skating is more rhythmical than hockey skating, and is also slower and graceful, with the various jumps being of particular importance in competition in singles, pairs and ice dancing. While the different activities vary in nature, the basic skating motion involves contraction of the hip and knee extensors during the stroke. The three types of skating will be discussed independently in this chapter.

## Speed skating

Skating has been performed in cold weather locations since the 1200s as a means of travel wherever there was sufficient ice. Initially, skating was performed with wooden runners attached to shoes, with iron runners first used in the late 1500s.

An Olympic sport for men since 1924, and for women since 1960, long-track speed skating is performed on a 400-m oval ice rink. Five events are performed by both men (500–10000 m) and

women (500–5000 m) lasting approximately 0.59–13.50 and 0.63–7.05 min, respectively (Table 50.1). In long-track events, two skaters race at one time, thus a time trial is performed, with the fastest skater of all pairs the event winner. World championships are contested annually in both sprint (500 and 1000 m) and all-around (500, 1500, 3000/5000 and 5000/10000 m) events, with two events usually held per day.

Short-track skating is generally performed on a hockey rink converted to an 111-m oval. Short-track skating was a demonstration sport in the 1988 Olympic Games and has been a medal sport ever since. Both men and women perform the 500-and 1000-m events, as well as a 3000-m relay for women and a 5000-m relay for men at the Olympics. At world championship events, men and women also perform the 1500- and 3000-m events. With short-track skating, multiple skaters (at least four) are on the ice during each race, with multiple heats per event and many events per day.

Finally, marathon skating generally entails more than 1 h of skating (on a course of at least 40 km), and includes such races as the 11 cities speed skating race/tour (De Elfstedentocht). This 200-km event is held whenever the channels of the northern Netherlands are frozen (the event in 1997 was the 15th) with a limit of 20000 participants. Skating times for the event range from 6.75 to 18 h.

Thus, speed-skating events last from 0.6 min to 18 h. As very little has been written concerning the non-Olympic speed-skating events and the

**Table 50.1** Current fastest recorded times for long-track speed-skating events.

| Event (m) | Women | Men |
|---|---|---|
| 500 | 0:37.55 | 0:34.76 |
| 1 000 | 1:14.61 | 1:08.55 |
| 1 500 | 1:56.95 | 1:46.43 |
| 3 000 | 4:01.67 | 3:53.06 |
| 5 000 | 6:58.63 | 6:21.49 |
| 10 000 | | 13:08.71 |

athletes who participate in them, long-track skating will be discussed in greater detail throughout this chapter as it occurs more widely in the literature.

Propulsion in the speed-skating stroke is obtained from a sideward push-off caused by extension of the hip and knee joint muscles. Generally, 60–80 skating strokes are performed per minute (de Boer & Nilsen 1989). The propulsion or push-off phase of the stroke lasts 0.15–0.20 s and is in the middle of the glide (0.50–0.75 s) and recovery (0.05–0.20 s) phases (de Boer & Nilsen 1989). The muscle contraction time/total stroke time (duty cycle) of the hip and leg muscles is approximately 55% of the activity (de Boer 1986).

## Characteristics of speed skaters

The average body composition (men, 10% body fat; women, 21% body fat), height (men, 177 cm) and weight (men, 74 kg; women, 63 kg) of speed skaters for the most part are similar to that of the average man and woman (Snyder & Foster 1994). Muscular strength and endurance (i.e. anaerobic ability) are up to 20–35% greater in speed skaters relative to body weight than the sedentary individual (Foster & Thompson 1990). Maximal aerobic power in speed skaters is approximately $65 \, \text{ml} \cdot \text{kg}^{-1} \cdot \text{min}^{-1}$ for men and $58 \, \text{ml} \cdot \text{kg}^{-1} \cdot \text{min}^{-1}$ for women. Skaters reach only 85–90% of their running or cycling aerobic power during a skating event, more than likely due to the reduced blood flow caused by the isometric muscle contractions of the hip and knee extensors (Foster & Thompson 1990).

## Training practices

Due to a lack of year-round venue availability, speed skaters, like most winter sports athletes, face unique training problems. Even though there are now eight indoor 400-m ice ovals in the world, very few venues have ice the whole year round, with most venues open only from September to March. Thus, many dry land training techniques are needed. The general training year for speed skaters can be broken down into preparation, competition and transition phases (Crowe 1990; van Ingen Schenau et al. 1992). Overall conditioning is the primary goal of the preparation phase, with general activities progressing to specific skating activities (June to October). Skating technique is emphasized and conditioning maintained during the competition phase (November to March). Finally, recovery is emphasized during the transition period (April to June) with activities other than skating performed.

Generally, elite skaters spend about 30–35 h in 14 different exercise sessions per week during the preparation phase (Pollock et al. 1982; van Ingen Schenau et al. 1992). As the energy source of the different speed-skating races varies depending on the distance (Fig. 50.1), training activities include: (i) aerobic (distance running and cycling) activities (40%), (ii) high-intensity interval/anaerobic activities (20%), (iii) strength and endurance resistance training (15%), and (iv) skating-related training (25%) (Pollock et al. 1982). During the preparation phase, 3 weeks of intensive training are followed by 1 week of easier training (Knapp et al. 1986; van Ingen Schenau et al. 1992). The aerobic activities of skaters are quite similar to those of distance athletes and are intended to build an aerobic base. The muscular strength and endurance activities involve primarily high-intensity (or high weight), low repetition and tempo work of the hip and knee extensor muscles (Figs 50.2, 50.3).

Due to the general lack of ice availability, specific dry land skating activities have been developed and used with varying degrees of success. Dry skating (Fig. 50.4) and low walking are two

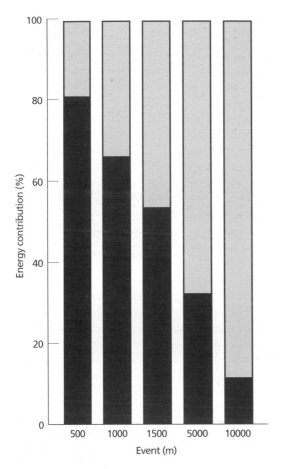

Fig. 50.1 The aerobic (□) and anaerobic (■) energy contributions in long-track speed-skating events energy contributions. Adapted from van Ingen Schenau *et al.* (1990).

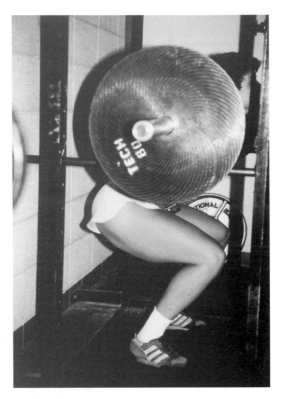

Fig. 50.2 Long-track speed skater performing heavy weight resistance training. From Foster and Thompson (1990), with permission.

activities which can be performed anywhere, but low walking is usually performed going up a hill (Fig. 50.5). Physiologically and biomechanically, a skater responds differently to low walking and dry skating, therefore activities more similar to speed skating such as slide board exercise (Fig. 50.6) or in-line skating should also be performed (de Boer *et al.* 1987a, 1987b, 1987c; de Groot *et al.* 1987; Kandou *et al.* 1987). Because maximal speed between speed skating and in-line skating is different, heart rate may be a better indicator of exercise intensity than speed (de Boer *et al.* 1987c). However, since trained individuals may

require high speeds to obtain cardiovascular benefits from in-line skating, skating up hill may be required (Hoffman *et al.* 1992; Snyder *et al.* 1993).

Technique and skating endurance become the goals once the skater gets on the ice. To facilitate the skating endurance, goal measurement of lactate ice-profiles may be important. From the lactate ice-profiles we have observed that when skaters use correct skating posture, with low pre-extension angles of the knee and hip joints, no matter how slow the skater is skating, blood lactate concentrations of at least 5–7 mM occur (Foster & Thompson 1990). We have also observed a right shifting of the lactate ice-profile (i.e. a lower blood lactate concentration at any given skating speed) when an athlete is training and/or muscle glycogen depleted (Foster *et al.* 1988).

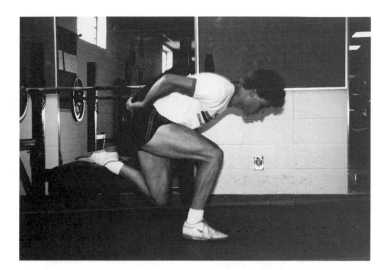

**Fig. 50.3** Long-track speed skater performing light resistance/ endurance resistance training. From Snyder and Foster (1994), with permission.

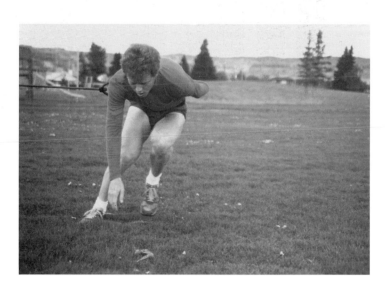

**Fig. 50.4** Long-track speed skater performing dry skating.

### Nutrition practices

Historically, skaters have spent no more than 4–8 weeks at one location, and often not even that long; thus, proper and balanced nutrient intake was not always easily obtainable. Also, as skaters spend a lot of time in training (as described above) and sharpening skates, not much time is generally spent on food preparation. Thus, food choices end up not always being what they could or should be. Also, as a great deal of exercise is performed every day by speed skaters, glycogen depletion can be a significant problem. In 1983, skaters' diets consisted primarily of fat (50%) with rather low levels of carbohydrate (30%) (Snyder & Foster 1994). Through much effort devoted to education and the addition of carbohydrate supplements, by 1989 the diet of comparable groups of skaters consisted of 63% carbohydrates for the women and 56% carbohydrates for the men (Snyder *et al.* 1989). Thus, in general, speed skaters do not consume sufficient carbohydrate to meet the recommendation (Costill & Miller 1980), although this can

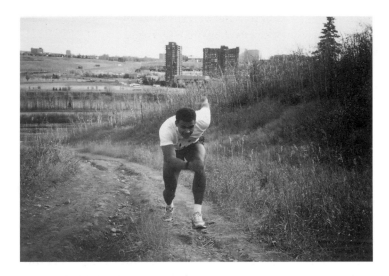

**Fig. 50.5** Long-track speed skater performing low walking up a hill. From Snyder and Foster (1994), with permission.

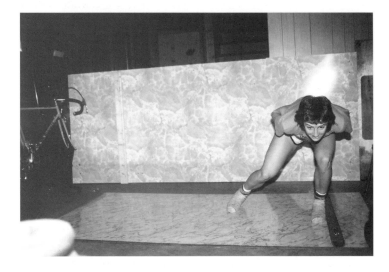

**Fig. 50.6** Long-track speed skater performing slide board exercise. From Foster and Thompson (1990), with permission.

be achieved with the use of carbohydrate supplements.

As proper nutrition has been shown to be important to exercise performance, skaters could benefit from paying special attention throughout the preparation and competitive phases to ensure that:

1 carbohydrates make up a large percentage (minimally 60%) of their daily energy intake (Costill & Miller 1980);

2 enhancement of muscle glycogen replenishment occurs through consumption of 100 g of carbohydrates within 2 h after the completion of an exercise bout; this carbohydrate can be either in liquid or solid form (Ivy *et al.* 1988a, 1988b); and

3 body protein and thus muscle strength is maintained, if not enhanced, by consumption of 1.6 g protein·kg⁻¹ body weight daily (Snyder & Naik 1998).

On the day of skating competitions, a prerace high-carbohydrate meal should be consumed approximately 4 h prior to competition, with a light carbohydrate snack consumed between events if time permits. A high-carbohydrate meal should be consumed following the completion of the events, in addition to the 100 g of carbohydrates within the first 2 h after competition discussed above, so that muscle glycogen levels are replenished for the next day of competition.

Fluid should be readily available at all exercise and competition sites, and should be consumed according to a predetermined schedule but also as needed, as the thirst mechanism does not always indicate when the body is in the early stages of dehydration. Monitoring body weight before and after exercise sessions can be used to detect dehydration via weight loss. Through the use of these guidelines and constant education of the athletes regarding food intake and supplementation, especially that of carbohydrates, the speed skater's diet should be appropriate for their exercise and training needs.

# Ice hockey

Canadians began playing ice hockey in the early 1800s and it became an Olympic sport for men in 1920 and for women in 1998. An ice hockey oval is approximately $61 \times 30.5$ m and is usually indoors. The ice hockey game consists of three 20-min periods, with a 12-min intermission between periods. Six players are on the ice at one time for each team: three forwards, two defencemen and one goalie. A team generally has 9–12 (3–4 lines or shifts) forwards and 4–6 (2–3 lines) defencemen. The most recent time–motion analysis has shown that the average skating time per shift is about 40 s, with a large number of shifts in the playing rotation (Montgomery 1988). As there are fewer defencemen on a team, defencemen generally play for more minutes, at a slower velocity (62% of forwards' velocity) than forwards.

Even though the ice hockey skate (shorter blade, stiffer/taller boot) is different from the speed skate, the ice hockey skating stroke, like that of the speed skater, involves three components: (i) glide with single support, (ii) propulsion with single support, and (iii) propulsion with double support (Marino & Weese 1979).

Propulsion during the stroke therefore occurs using both one and two legs.

## Characteristics of ice hockey players

As ice hockey is a relatively new sport for women, very little information is available concerning women ice hockey players; therefore, the characteristics referred to will be those of men. Ice hockey players tend to weigh approximately 80 kg, are 180 cm tall and have about 10% body fat (Green & Houston 1975; Houston & Green 1976; Orvanova 1987; Agre et al. 1988). Ice hockey players, even more so than speed skaters, tend to have relatively ordinary aerobic abilities ($55 \text{ ml} \cdot \text{kg}^{-1} \cdot \text{min}^{-1}$). Finally, as was observed with the speed skaters, the maximal aerobic ability of ice hockey players was slightly less while skating than while running.

## Training practices

A typical ice hockey season can last from 5 to 8 months and may involve upwards of 100 games. Two to three games can be played in a week during the season, with practices usually held on non-game days. During the season, practice sessions generally involve developing skill and getting ready for the next game, as games occur frequently. During a typical practice, a short warm-up period will occur along with repeat bouts of high-intensity skating, instruction, special plays and controlled scrimmages, all within 1.5–2 h (Daub et al. 1982). As with a number of athletes, during the season aerobic ability and muscular strength and endurance are generally not enhanced in ice hockey players, and can actually be lower at the end of the season than after preseason training (Green & Houston 1975; Cotton et al. 1979; Green et al. 1979; Quinney et al. 1982; Daub et al. 1983; Johansson et al. 1989; Posch et al. 1989).

In an attempt to increase the aerobic and/or muscular ability of ice hockey players during the hockey season, additional on-ice or non-ice training was incorporated into the training programme for a short period (6–7 weeks), with improvements in aerobic ability and skating speed and acceleration observed (Hollering & Simpson 1977; Hutchinson *et al.* 1979; Greer *et al.* 1992). However, addition of a low-intensity ($\approx 74\%$ $\dot{V}_{O_{2max}}$) cycling exercise to a hockey training programme did not cause any changes in aerobic ability (Daub *et al.* 1983).

### Nutrition practices

Very little literature is available concerning the nutrition practices of ice hockey players. One 7-day diet survey of seven players reported that they consumed per day: 2.8 servings of meat or equivalent, 2.3 servings of milk or equivalent, 1.6 servings of vegetables, 1.2 servings of fruit, 4.6 servings of grain, 2.1 servings of soft drinks and sweets, and 3.0 servings of alcohol (Houston 1979). Breads, pasta and crackers made up the primary grain consumed, while french fries comprised about half of the vegetable servings. Approximately 2.4 meals per day were consumed by the ice hockey players, with almost half (45%) of the meals consumed away from home. Finally, breakfast was skipped 67% of the time by the players.

Two potential limitations to ice hockey performance are those imposed by energy metabolism and disturbances in temperature regulation. Due to the nature of the game, very high intensity exercise is performed for a short period of time and repeated many times during a game. The result for the ice hockey player is great utilization of muscle glycogen, elevated levels of blood lactate concentration, and slow recovery from the metabolic acidosis due to the sedentary nature of the brief recovery period. In an attempt to enhance performance by enhancing muscle glycogen levels, ice hockey players consumed 360 g of supplemental carbohydrate for 3 days prior to a championship series and obtained muscle glycogen levels twice as high as those of players who did not consume the supplement (Rehunen & Liitsola 1978). As suggested with the speed skaters, regular consumption of a high-carbohydrate supplement may be necessary to

ensure normal muscle glycogen levels in ice hockey players.

Due to the high-intensity exercise performed and the protective clothing worn by ice hockey players, they can lose 2–3 kg of body weight during a game despite *ad libitum* fluid intake (Green *et al.* 1978; MacDougall 1979). Some things can be done to reduce the protective clothing, such as removing the helmet and gloves when not playing, but greater consumption of fluids is probably also necessary to ensure proper hydration of the ice hockey players.

As the ice hockey season is long and the games and practice sessions relatively strenuous, proper nutrient intake is important. Similar to the recommendations for speed skaters, ice hockey players need to consume large amounts of carbohydrate ($\approx 60\%$ of total energy intake) and protein ($\approx 1.6$ g $\cdot$ kg$^{-1}$ body weight) to ensure replenishment of muscle and liver glycogen stores and strength maintenance/development. Likewise, fluid intake before, during and after a game should be encouraged to reduce the loss of body fluids.

## Figure skating

The sport of figure skating has four very different events which are performed by different groups of athletes: men's singles (Olympic sport since 1908), women's singles (Olympic sport since 1920), pairs (Olympic sport since 1920) and ice dancing (Olympic sport since 1976). The figure skating rink is maximally 60×30 m, and is usually indoors. The figure skate blade is wider than that of a speed skate, but narrower than that of an ice hockey skate, with the boot being of leather (similar to the speed skate) and extending above the ankle joint (similar to the ice hockey skate). Figure skaters perform a short programme (maximum time, 2.5 min) and a long programme (maximum time, 4.0 min) during their event.

### Characteristics of figure skaters

Figure skaters tend to be shorter (men, 170 cm; women, 160 cm), lighter (men, 63 kg; women, 50 kg) and leaner (men, 7% body fat; women, 11% body fat) than speed skaters and ice hockey players (Brock & Striowski 1986; Niinimaa 1982). Compared to the sedentary individual, the elite figure skater is also generally leaner and lighter. Maximal aerobic ability of figure skaters tends to be comparable (men, 66 ml·kg$^{-1}$·min$^{-1}$, women, 57 ml·kg$^{-1}$·min$^{-1}$) to that of speed skaters and slightly higher than that of ice hockey players (Kjaer & Larsson 1992).

### Training practices

At elite level, figure skaters typically spend most of their training time skating, with total training time being approximately 5 h·day$^{-1}$ (Niinimaa 1982; Brock & Striowski 1986; Smith & Ludington 1989). Of this time, approximately: (i) 0.1 h·day$^{-1}$ are spent in preskating warm-up, (ii) 0.9 h·day$^{-1}$ are spent performing strength and aerobic activities, and (iii) 4 h·day$^{-1}$ are spent with on-ice activities (Brock & Striowski 1986). Others (Smith & Micheli 1982) have also reported that less than 5 min off-ice and on-ice warm-up activities were performed by elite figure skaters before each training session.

Heart rate during figure skating is dependent upon the skill being performed, but averages approximately 92% of the maximal value (Woch *et al.* 1979; Kjaer & Larsson 1992). Similarly, oxygen uptake averages approximately 80% of maximal for men, and 75% of maximal for women during a figure-skating programme (Niinimaa 1982).

A major component of a figure-skating performance is the jumps, with a high jump usually producing a greater score for technical merit (Podolsky *et al.* 1990). Muscular strength would therefore seem to be important to the figure skater. Historically, however, figure skaters have performed very little resistance training off the ice, with almost all of their muscular develop-

ment occurring through repetitions of jumps on the ice (Podolsky *et al.* 1990).

### Nutrition practices

The nutrition practices of 17 men and 23 women figure skaters using the Eating Attitude Test (EAT) and a 3-day diet record were examined by Rucinski (1989). Daily energy intake was 4.9±1.9 MJ (1170±450 kcal) for the women and 12.1±4.5 MJ (2890±1075 kcal) for the men. Because of their low energy intake, the women consumed less than 60% of the US recommended daily allowance for vitamin B$_6$, vitamin B$_{12}$, vitamin D, folacin, pantothenic acid, iron, and calcium, whereas the men consumed less than 60% of the RDA for only folacin. Additionally, 48% of the women were within the anorexic range.

Figure skaters, similar to the speed skaters and ice hockey players, perform demanding exercise sessions throughout a very long season. The figure skaters, however, unlike the other skaters, have had to be conscious of their body weight and physique, and disordered eating is thus more than likely very prevalent, especially among the women. However, the demands of the sport still require adequate nutrient intake, with high amounts of complex carbohydrates (≈60%) and appropriate levels of protein (≈1.6 g·kg$^{-1}$ body weight). Athletes consuming less than these recommendations will not only be impairing their exercise performance, but could also be impairing their health both currently and/or in the future.

## Conclusion

The sport of skating involves many different types of activities, most of which are anaerobic in nature. Although preparing to perform their events on ice, skaters quite often must perform a portion of their training with dry land activities. The dry land activities need to be as skill-specific as possible and also must stress the anaerobic and aerobic energy systems. Due to the long hours of training performed by all types of skaters, as well as the multiple bouts of high-intensity exercise, proper food and fluid intake are a requirement for good performance. Finally, proper warm-up and cool-down activities, flexibility exercises, and strength development are important in the overall programme of a skater.

## Acknowledgements

The United States Olympic Committee (USOC) and United States Speedskating (formerly USISA) have funded most of our work with the speed skaters. We also need to acknowledge the assistance and co-operation of the coaches (Dave Besteman, Mike Crowe, Dianne Holum, Gerard Kempers, Stan Klotkowski, Jeroun Otter, Susan Schobe, Guy Thiboult and Nick Thometz) and athletes who allowed us to test them over the years, and also allowed us to learn from them. Finally, we would like to acknowledge Ken Rundell, Nancy Thompson, Matt Schrager and Ralph Welsh, who assisted us in the testing of the athletes.

## References

Agre, J.C., Casal, D.C., Leon, A.S., McNally, C., Baxter, T.L. & Serfass, R.C (1988) Professional ice hockey players: physiologic, anthropometric, and musculoskeletal characteristics. *Archives in Physical and Medical Rehabilitation* **69**, 188–192.

Brock, R.M. & Striowski, C.C. (1986) Injuries in elite figure skaters. *Physician and Sportsmedicine* **14**, 111–115.

Costill, D.L. & Miller, J.M. (1980) Nutrition for endurance sport: carbohydrate and fluid balance. *International Journal of Sports Medicine* **1**, 2–14.

Cotton, C.E., Reed, A., Hansen, H. & Gauthier, R. (1979) Pre and post seasonal muscular strength tests of professional hockey players. *Canadian Journal of Applied Sport Science* **4**, 245–251.

Crowe, M. (1990) Year-round preparation of the winter sports athlete. In *Winter Sports Medicine* (ed. M.J. Casey, C. Foster & E.G. Hixson), pp. 7–13. F.A. Davis, Philadelphia, PA.

Daub, W.B., Green, H.J., Houston, M.E., Thompson, J.A., Fraser, I.G. & Ranney, D.A. (1982) Cross-adaptive responses to different forms of leg training: skeletal muscle biochemistry and histochemistry. *Canadian Journal of Physiology and Pharmacology* **60**, 628–633.

Daub, W.B., Green, H.J., Houston, M.E., Thompson, J.A., Fraser, I.G. & Ranney, D.A. (1983) Specificity of physiological adaptations resulting from ice-hockey training. *Medicine and Science in Sports and Exercise* **15**, 290–294.

de Boer, R.W. (1986) *Training and Technique in Speed Skating*. Free University Press, Amsterdam.

de Boer, R.W. & Nilsen, K.L. (1989) The gliding and push-off technique of male and female Olympic speed skaters. *International Journal of Sport Biomechanics* **5**, 119–134.

de Boer, R.W., de Groot, G. & van Ingen Schenau, G.J. (1987a) Specificity of training in speed skating. In *Biomechanics X-B*. (ed. B. Jonsson), pp. 685–689. Human Kinetics, Champaign, IL.

de Boer, R.W., Ettema, G.J.C., Faessen, B.G.M. *et al.* (1987b) Specific characteristics of speed skating: implications for summer training. *Medicine and Science in Sports and Exercise* **19**, 504–510.

de Boer, R.W., Vos, E., Hutter, W., de Groot, G. & van Ingen Schenau, G.J. (1987c) Physiological and biomechanical comparison of roller skating and speed skating on ice. *European Journal of Applied Physiology* **56**, 562–569.

de Groot, G., Hollander, A.P., Sargeant, A.J., van Ingen Schenau, G.J. & de Boer, R.W. (1987) Applied physiology of speed skating. *Journal of Sport Science* **5**, 249–259.

Foster, C. & Thompson, N. (1990) The physiology of speed skating. In *Winter Sports Medicine* (ed. M.J. Casey, C. Foster, and E.G. Hixson), pp. 221–240. F.A. Davis, Philadelphia, PA.

Foster, C., Snyder, A.C., Thompson, N.N. & Kuettel, K. (1988) Normalization of the blood lactate profile in athletes. *International Journal of Sports Medicine* **9**, 198–200.

Green, H.J. & Houston, M.E. (1975) Effect of a season of ice hockey on energy capacities and associated functions. *Medicine and Science in Sports* **7**, 299–303.

Green, H.J., Houston, M.E. & Thompson, J.A. (1978) Inter- and intragame alterations in selected blood parameters during ice hockey performance. In *Ice Hockey* (ed. F. Landry & W.A.R. Orban), pp. 37–46. Symposia Specialists, Miami, FL.

Green, H.J., Thompson, J.A., Daub, W.D., Houston, M.E. & Ranney, D.A. (1979) Fiber composition, fiber size and enzyme activities in vastus lateralis of elite athletes involved in high intensity exercise. *European Journal of Applied Physiology* **41**, 109–117.

Greer, N., Serfass, R., Picconatto, W. & Blatherwick, J. (1992) The effects of a hockey-specific training program on performance of bantam players. *Canadian Journal of Sport Science* **17**, 65–69.

Hoffman, M.D., Jones, G.M., Bota, B., Mandli, M. & Clifford, P.S. (1992) In-line skating: physiological responses and comparison with roller skiing. *International Journal of Sports Medicine* **13**, 137–144.

Hollering, B.L. & Simpson, D. (1977) The effects of three types of training programs upon skating speed of college ice hockey players. *Journal of Sports Medicine* **17**, 335–340.

Houston, M.E. (1979) Nutrition and ice hockey performance. *Canadian Journal of Applied Sport Science* **4**, 98–99.

Houston, M.E. & Green, H.J. (1976) Physiological and anthropometric characteristics of elite Canadian ice hockey players. *Journal of Sports Medicine and Physical Fitness* **16**, 123–128.

Hutchinson, W.W., Maas, G.M. & Murdoch, A.J. (1979) Effect of dry land training on aerobic capacity of college hockey players. *Journal of Sports Medicine* **19**, 271–276.

Ivy, J.J., Katz, A.L., Cutler, C.L., Sherman, W.M. & Coyle, E.F. (1988a) Muscle glycogen synthesis after exercise: effect of time on carbohydrate ingestion. *Journal of Applied Physiology* **64**, 1480–1485.

Ivy, J.J., Lee, M.C., Brozinick, J.T. & Reed, M.J. (1988b) Muscle glycogen storage after different amounts of carbohydrate ingestion. *Journal of Applied Physiology* **65**, 2018–2023.

Johansson, C., Lorentzon, R. & Fugl-Meyer, A.R. (1989) Isokinetic muscular performance of the quadriceps in elite ice hockey players. *American Journal of Sports Medicine* **17**, 30–34.

Kandou, T.W.A., Houtman, I.L.D., Bol, E.V.D., de Boer, R.W., de Groot, G. & van Ingen Schenau, G.J. (1987) Comparison of physiology and biomechanics of speed skating with cycling and with skateboard exercise. *Canadian Journal of Sport Science* **12**, 31–36.

Kjaer, M. & Larsson, B. (1992) Physiological profile and incidence of injuries among elite figure skaters. *Journal of Sports Science* **10**, 29–36.

Knapp, D.N., Gutmann, M.C., Rogowski, B.L., Foster, C. & Pollock, M.L. (1986) Perceived vulnerability to illness and injury among olympic speedskating candidates: effects on emotional response to training. In *Sport and the Elite Performer* (ed. D. Landers), pp. 103–112. Human Kinetics, Champaign, IL.

MacDougall, J.D. (1979) Thermoregulatory problems encountered in ice hockey. *Canadian Journal of Applied Sport Science* **4**, 35–38.

Marino, G.W. & Weese, R.G. (1979) A kinematic analysis of the ice skating stride. In *Science in Skiing, Skating and Hockey* (ed. J. Terauds & H.J. Gros), pp. 65–74. Academic Publishers, Del Mar, CA.

Montgomery, D.L. (1988) Physiology of ice hockey. *Sports Medicine* **5**, 99–126.

Niinimaa, V. (1982) Figure skating: what do we know about it? *Physician and Sportsmedicine* **10**, 51–56.

Orvanova, E. (1987) Physical structure of winter sports athletes. *Journal of Sports Science* **5**, 197–248.

Podolsky, A., Kaufman, K.R., Cahalan, T.D., Aleshinskky, S.Y. & Chao, E.Y.S. (1990) The relationship of strength and jump height in figure skaters. *American Journal of Sports Medicine* **18**, 400–405.

Pollock, M.L., Foster, C., Anholm, J. *et al.* (1982) Body composition of Olympic speed skating candidates. *Research Quarterly* **53**, 150–155.

Posch, E., Haglund, Y. & Eriksson, E. (1989) Prospective study of concentric and eccentric leg muscle torques, flexibility, physical conditioning, and variation of injury rates during one season of amateur ice hockey. *International Journal of Sports Medicine* **2**, 113–117.

Quinney, H.A., Belcastro, A. & Steadward, R.D. (1982) Seasonal fitness variations and pre-playoff blood analysis in NHL players. *Canadian Journal of Applied Sport Science* **7**, 237 (Abstract).

Rehunen, S. & Liitsola, S. (1978) Modification of the muscle-glycogen level of ice-hockey players through a drink with high carbohydrate content. *Deutsche Zeitschrift fuer Sportmedizin* **26**, 15–25.

Rucinski, A. (1989) Relationship of body image and dietary intake of competitive ice skaters. *Journal of American Dietetic Association* **89**, 98–100.

Smith, A.D. & Ludington, R. (1989) Injuries in elite pair skaters and ice dancers. *American Journal of Sports Medicine* **17**, 482–488.

Smith, A.D. & Micheli, L.J. (1982) Injuries in competitive skaters. *Physician and Sportsmedicine* **82**, 36–47.

Snyder, A.C. & Foster, C. (1994) Physiology and nutrition for skating. In *Perspectives in Exercise Science and Sports Medicine*. Vol. 7. *Physiology and Nutrition for Competitive Sport* (ed. D.R. Lamb, H.G. Knuttgen & R. Murray), pp. 181–219. Cooper Publishing Group, Carmel, IN.

Snyder, A.C. & Naik, J. (1998) Protein requirements of athletes. In *Sports Nutrtion for the 90s: The Health Professional's Handbook* (ed. J. Berning & S. Nelson Steen), Vol. 2, pp. 45–58. Aspen Publishers, Gaithersburg, MD.

Snyder, A.C., Schulz, L.O. & Foster, C. (1989) Voluntary consumption of a carbohydrate supplement by elite speed skaters. *Journal of the American Dietetic Association* **89**, 1125–1127.

Snyder, A.C., O'Hagan, K.P., Clifford, P.S., Hoffman, M.D. & Foster, C. (1993) Exercise responses to in-line skating: comparisons to running and cycling. *International Journal of Sports Medicine* **14**, 38–42.

van Ingen Schenau, G.J., Bakker, F.C., de Groot, G. & de Koning, J.J. (1992) Supramaximal cycle tests do not detect seasonal progression in performance in groups of elite speed skaters. *European Journal of Applied Physiology* **64**, 292–297.

Woch, Z.T., Niinimaa, V. & Shephard, R.J. (1979) Heart rate responses during free figure skating manoeuvres. *Canadian Journal of Sport Science* **4**, 274–276.

# Chapter 51

# Cross-country Skiing

BJORN EKBLOM AND ULF BERGH

## Introduction

Recreational touring and racing skiing are common activities in many countries today but cross-country skiing has been practised for several thousand years in northern countries. Ski-racing equipment has changed considerably, and the dimensions of the ski have changed from being 3 m long, 10 cm wide, and weighing 2–3 kg at the beginning of this century to 2 m, 4 cm and about 0.5 kg in the modern era. There are specialized skis for classic and free-style ski racing. The courses on which competition takes place have changed as well. Now grooming machines are used at least for the more advanced levels of competition, which makes the tracks very hard and durable, thus making the conditions more equal for all competitors. It must be emphasized that racing conditions vary due to changes in snow and weather conditions.

Skiing competitions are classified into two different styles: classic skiing and free style. Three main techniques are used in classic skiing: double pole, kick double pole, and diagonal. In free-style events, skating techniques dominate: these are characterized by leg movements similar to those in ice-skating combined with various forms of double poling.

Elite skiing competitions are performed over distances ranging from 5 to 90 km. In the Olympic Games and the world championships, the distances range from 5 to 30 km in female events and from 10 to 50 km for males. Relay races are 4×5 km and 4×10 km for women and men, respectively. At present, individual races last 12–90 min for women and 22–140 min for men.

Modern rules stipulate that the courses for international races must in length be equally divided into uphill, downhill, and level skiing. Since the racing speed differs greatly among these three parts of the course, the time spent in uphill skiing is more than half of the total racing time, while downhill skiing time correspondingly occupies less than 10%. Even so, downhill skiing ability is important. A fall in a downhill part causes loss of speed and rhythm in skiing. Compared to the winner, the time 'lost' is greatest in uphill and level skiing. The exact relation between time spent in the different parts is, of course, dependent on many factors such as level of competition and type of terrain.

## Characteristics of elite skiers

International elite competitors are often relatively old—average ages are reported to be 27 and 29 years for females and males, respectively, indicating that it takes years of training to achieve that level of performance. These elite athletes do not differ very much in body size, body weight and appearance from other non-obese persons, having relatively little body fat but not to the extreme degree observed in some endurance sports.

The leg muscles of elite cross-country skiers have been found to consist of predominantly slow-twitch fibres but the variability is considerable. A similar pattern has been found in the deltoid muscle, where there is an even greater variation. Young elite skiers have been found to have a lower percentage of slow-twitch fibres than older skiers (Rusko 1976), which can be an effect either of training or further selection. The predominance of slow-twitch fibres is logical, since the metabolism in cross-country skiing is predominantly aerobic and slow-twitch fibres have a high oxidative capacity. Furthermore, the number of capillaries is greater around a slow-twitch than a fast-twitch fibre. This enhances the transportation of gases and nutrients between blood and muscle cells, allowing for an effective aerobic metabolism. All these findings are consistent with the hypothesis that physical training for many years increases local aerobic metabolic capacity (Saltin & Gollnick 1983).

However, the physiological variable that most evidently distinguishes elite cross-country skiers from the average person as well as less successful cross-country skiers is the maximum oxygen uptake, expressed as litres per minute as well as in relation to body size ($ml \cdot min^{-1} \cdot kg^{-1}$ body mass). Over the decades, reports have confirmed that elite cross-country skiers have, without exceptions, very high values (Table 51.1). World-class skiers have displayed a higher maximum oxygen uptake than less successful skiers (Bergh 1987; Ingjer 1991). Skiers of junior age display lower values than adults (Rusko 1976; Bergh & Forsberg 1992). These differences are also reflected in differences in racing speed and, thus, racing success.

The power facilitated by the metabolism is necessary for moving the body mass, and more power increases speed. On the other hand, a higher body mass demands more power at a given speed. Thus, there is a need to compensate for differences in body mass, otherwise it is not possible to compare the values obtained in different skiers. Traditionally, such compensations have been made by means of dividing maximum oxygen uptake by body mass. However, it has been demonstrated that the power needed to ski at a given speed on level terrain increases less than proportional to body mass. Thus, it is not logical to divide oxygen uptake by body mass in order to equate heavy and light skiers. Therefore, dimensional analysis and empirical findings suggest that a division by body mass raised to the second or third power may be more valid for cross-country skiing (Bergh 1987). This is supported by a study of Ingjer (1991), which demonstrated that world-class skiers differed significantly from medium-class and less successful skiers if the maximum oxygen uptake was divided by body mass raised to the second or third power, whereas a division by body mass did not reveal any significant difference. Thus, it seems logical to relate maximum oxygen uptake body mass raised to the second or third power if the purpose is to predict the capacity for cross-county skiing.

**Table 51.1** Different measurements of maximum oxygen uptake in elite cross-country male skiers.

| $O_{2max.}$ uptake ($l \cdot min^{-1}$) | | $O_{2max.}$ uptake ($ml \cdot kg^{-1} \cdot min^{-1}$) | | |
|---|---|---|---|---|
| Mean | SD | Mean | SD | Reference |
| 5.5 | 0.2 | 80.1 | 1.4 | Åstrand (1955) |
| 5.6 | 0.3 | 82.5 | 1.5 | Saltin & Åstrand (1967) |
| 5.5 | 0.2 | 75 | 2.7 | Hanson (1973) |
| 6.5 | 0.5 | 83.8 | 6.4 | Bergh (1987) |
| 6.7 | 0.6 | 87.0 | 6.9 | Bergh & Forsberg (1992) |

Although all groups can be characterized as elite skiers, there were differences in the performance level both within and between groups.

The high values of maximum oxygen uptake in elite cross-country skiers are the result of a high maximum cardiac output elicited by a large stroke volume. Maximum cardiac output over $40 \, l \cdot min^{-1}$ and stroke volumes over $200 \, ml$ have been measured in skiers with maximum oxygen uptake values over $6 \, l \cdot min^{-1}$ (Ekblom & Hermansen 1968). The maximum heart rates and the arteriovenous differences were close to values obtained in less successful athletes and non-athletes and cannot account for the observed differences between the different groups of individuals. Blood volume is also high in these athletes, while haemoglobin concentrations are within the normal ranges of non-athletes and less successful athletes (Ekblom & Hermansen 1968).

The information on muscular strength of the elite competitor is not very extensive. Available data indicate that the maximum strength of the legs is only slightly greater than that of the average person. However, in endurance tests—such as 50 consecutive knee joint extensions—skiers show superior endurance values to those of most other endurance athletes. The arm muscle strength for poling and, thus, skiing performance, is also of the utmost importance.

## Ski racing

### Energy expenditure

The skier has to expend power in order to move forward. This power is used for:
1 overcoming friction between ski and snow;
2 elevating the body mass in uphill skiing and for each stride during level skiing;
3 accelerating the different body segments and the centre of mass; and
4 overcoming air resistance.

The relative importance of these factors for energy expenditure during skiing is dependent on several factors, including body composition, type of skiing technique, level of coordination and technique, type of terrain, snow conditions, and racing speed. Hence, quantitative information will only be valid under specific conditions.

It is, however, safe to state that on uphill terrain the cost of elevating the centre of mass accounts for the major part of the energy expenditure. In downhill sections, the main resistances are the friction between the ski and the snow and the air resistance. The power to sustain this power expenditure comes from the metabolism except in downhill terrain. Hence, skiing speed will depend on the power producing capacity of the metabolism.

As stated above, the capacity and effectiveness of the aerobic energy system is the most important factor for physical performance during ski racing, indicating that the central circulation and the regulation of its distribution are of primary importance for skiing capacity. Maximal uphill skiing produces higher oxygen uptake than maximal running (Stromme et al. 1977). There is no difference in maximum oxygen uptake between maximal uphill skiing using the classic or free-style technique (Bergh & Forsberg 1991). Thus, the muscle mass used during maximal skiing has a metabolic potential which exceeds the transport capacity of oxygen of the central circulation. Any variation in the amount of oxygen from the heart to the peripheral muscles will undoubtedly influence skiing performance. During uphill skiing, the heart rate is close to or even exceeds peak heart rate obtained during conventional all-out maximal running on a treadmill. During the downhill parts, the heart rate is some 20 beats $\cdot min^{-1}$ below maximum, mainly because the strain on the circulation is still high. During level skiing, the heart rate is on the average 10–15 beats $\cdot min^{-1}$ below maximum and, during longer races, such as the 50 km, the heart rate is on the average somewhat lower than in the shorter races on the same parts of the track due to the lower average speed in the longer race.

## Training

Important characteristics of cross-country skiing are as follows.
1 Metabolism is mainly aerobic.
2 Oxygen uptake can be taxed maximally.
3 Certain techniques cannot elicit maximum

oxygen uptake and, in these cases, the attainable level can vary considerably between individuals.

**4** The technique has to be learned.

**5** The duration of races may be such that the glycogen stores become emptied.

**6** The training necessary to obtain the performance level of elite competitors is such that only an extremely well-trained individual can endure this.

As a consequence of these characteristics, the training should contain practices that: (i) challenge the cardiovascular system considerably, (ii) activate all of the muscles used during competetive skiing, (iii) improve the technical skill, and (iv) last for periods of up to several hours.

Moreover, the amount of training should be increased gradually during the course of each year and from one year to the next. Otherwise, there is a considerable risk of overtraining and overuse injuries.

Running and roller-skiing can elicit approximately the same oxygen uptake as that achieved in all-out skiing (Bergh 1982). Ski-walking (walking up a steep hill using poles to imitate skiing) and cross-country skiing have been found to produce slightly higher levels of oxygen uptake than running in individuals trained for cross-country skiing (Hermansen 1973; Stromme *et al.* 1977). Roller-skiing has an advantage over running in regard to training of the upper body: the activity patterns of the muscles are similar in skiing on snow and roller-skiing. This is advantageous for the development of the local aerobic power. This is important because the muscles involved in poling must have endurance since this activity contributes significantly to performance in skiing. Moreover, it has been demonstrated that individuals who can attain a relatively high oxygen uptake during upper-body exercise benefit in regard to the maximum oxygen uptake that can be attained during combined arm and leg exercise (Bergh *et al.* 1976).

Elite skiers rarely use barbells or other resistance devices in order to improve maximum muscle strength. However, repeated double-poling on roller-skis at maximal speed for 10–30 s is used as strength training. This exercise is a minor part of the training (3–5% of the time during summer and early fall).

Skiing technique should be learned by skiing, because other exercises, e.g. roller-skiing and ski-walking, do not display the same muscular activity patterns as in skiing, judging from electromyographic recordings. In general, it is preferable to concentrate on technique with youngsters because they learn more easily than adults. In total, elite male and female skiers train about 650–750 and 500–700 h·year$^{-1}$, respectively. In addition, they normally compete in about 35–45 ski races·year$^{-1}$.

**Metabolic energy yield**

In order to evaluate the average metabolic energy yield during a ski race, heart-rate recordings during the race and blood lactate and core temperature measurements after the race have been used. Using these measures, it can be estimated that the average energy expenditure during ski racing between 5 and 30 km is in the range of 90–95% of maximum oxygen uptake. During the longer ski races, it is some 5–10% lower. There are no reasons to believe that genders differ in this respect.

Combining this information on fractional utilization of oxygen with data on maximum oxygen uptake of elite skiers, racing metabolic cost can be estimated. Such calculations indicate that the metabolic rate of an average male elite skier is about 1.5–2 kW during the shorter races. During longer races (50 km and longer), the metabolic rate is about 10% lower. The total energy yield for a normal 15-km race is about 4–5 MJ (950–1200 kcal) and for a 50-km race about 13–15 MJ (3100–3600 kcal). Corresponding calculations for females indicate that they use about 30% less energy than males for a given distance, which is due to the lower maximum aerobic power and body mass in the females.

**Heat balance**

Since cross-country skiing is often performed in cold climates, problems related to cold injuries, breathing problems, and hypothermia might be expected. For the body as a whole, the metabolic heat production during ski racing is usually greater than the heat loss due to convection, conduction and radiation. Therefore, the skier must sweat to maintain heat balance. During ski racing, the weight loss, mainly due to water loss, might be some 2–3% of body mass during 15- to 30-km races. This will undoubtedly impair performance. Therefore, fluid replacement during races longer than 15–20 km is needed.

Although heat production is high, cold injuries to peripheral parts of the body, such as fingers, toes, nosetip and ears, are not uncommon during cold weather, since the wind velocity is high, especially during long downhill segments of a course. Furthermore, pulmonary ventilation may be at least $100–150 l \cdot min^{-1}$ and, in many cases or parts of a track, over $200 l \cdot min^{-1}$. This puts large demands on the airways, since cold air is very dry and must be heated and saturated with water before it reaches the alveolae. Many skiers experience coughing problems during races and after exercise. Therefore, many top elite skiers use antiasthmatic medications. To avoid local cold injuries and breathing problems, competitions and hard training sessions should be avoided at temperatures below –20°C.

### Total energy yield

The energy cost of cross-country skiing is high, as mentioned earlier. During the preparation or main training part of the year, which often includes two training sessions per day, the estimated total energy turnover is some 20–$25 MJ \cdot day^{-1}$ (4800–6000 kcal $\cdot day^{-1}$). During training camps, it can be 4–8 MJ (950–1900 kcal) higher. The total energy turnover for a 15- and 50-km race is about 4–5 MJ (950–1200 kcal) and 13–15 MJ (3100–3600 kcal), respectively.

One of the main nutritional problems is to cover this high energy demand. In many cases, this problem is solved by having three main meals — breakfast, lunch and dinner — and, added to that, small meals after each training session. A carbohydrate-rich meal just before bedtime facilitates restoring the muscle glycogen.

### Quality of the meal

The glycogen concentration in activated arm and leg muscles is low or almost empty in many muscle cells at the end of a race or a long training session. Thus, a meal rich in carbohydrates is an essential part of an elite cross-country skier's diet. The post-training meal is especially important, since the rate of glycogen resynthesis and accumulation in the muscles seems to be faster when a high-carbohydrate meal is consumed just after the exercise. It is a general experience that most skiers are not hungry immediately after a race, but failure to eat at this time may delay recovery and limit the training load. Of interest for the hard training cross-country skier, therefore, is the observation that postexercise muscle glycogen concentration can be enhanced above normal with a carbohydrate–protein supplement as a result of the interaction of carbohydrate and protein on insulin secretion.

During the racing season, there may be specific nutritional problems at hand. Racing and prolonged hard training sessions may damage the muscle cells as indicated by a leakage of protein and other molecules from slow-twitch fibres. If this occurs, the rate of glycogen resynthesis may be reduced after exhaustive exercise. Therefore, it might not always be possible to fully replenish glycogen stores within 24–48 h after hard races and training sessions.

### Rehydration during skiing

During races, skiers may sweat a lot even in a cold climate. The body mass loss for a 15- and 50-km race may be in the range of 2–4% of initial value of body mass. It is a well-known fact that this can impair physical performance. Rehydration is therefore of great importance for counteracting the negative influence of the dehydration. However, not only rehydration is of importance. During prolonged exercise, as in cross-country skiing, a carbohydrate intake during prolonged exercise will also enhance performance. The mechanism is not clear but it is most likely that the glucose uptake from the bloodstream may contribute considerably to the aerobic metabolism.

Therefore, most skiers consume some 100–200 ml of a 5–10% carbohydrate drink about each 10–15 min in races with a duration longer than 1 h. The intake is of the same order of magnitude as the minimum of $40–60 g \cdot h^{-1}$ suggested by Coyle (1991). However, some skiers also take in a solution with up to 25–30% of carbohydrates. The reason for this is that the net uptake of glucose is higher in such a solution than with a traditional 5–8% concentration, although the water uptake is, of course, less.

During training camps at altitude, the water turnover is increased because of the increased urine output and the high respiratory water losses. Some elite skiers drink up to $8–10 l \cdot day^{-1}$ in order to compensate for the increased rate of dehydration during altitude training.

**Vitamins and minerals**

Vitamins and minerals are essential nutrients for optimal performance. It is well known that deficiencies impair general health and human functions but, in present-day society, obvious vitamin deficiencies are rare. Cross-country skiers have a high energy intake. Since the amount of nutrient intake mainly follows energy intake when the athlete consumes 'normal' food (Blixt 1965), there is a general agreement that the risk of an inadequate nutrient intake is low in athletes with high total energy intakes.

# Conclusion

Cross-country skiing is dynamic exercise involving a large muscle mass. There are many different skiing techniques. The energy yield is mainly aerobic and the cardiovascular system can be taxed maximally during skiing. Therefore, cross-country skiing is effective in regard to endurance training. The elite skier is characterized by an extremely high maximum oxygen uptake and the skeletal muscles contain predominantly slow-twitch fibres. Body size is not very different from the average person of corresponding gender and age. Training is mainly performed by skiing, roller-skiing and running. The energy demand is very high, and in longer races, the glycogen stores may be emptied. Proper rehydration procedures during races are of greatest importance.

# References

Åstrand, P.O. (1955) New records in human power. *Nature* **176**, 922–923.

Bergh, U. (1982) *Physiology of Cross-Country Ski Racing*. Human Kinetics, Champaign, IL.

Bergh, U. (1987) The influence of body mass in cross-country skiing. *Medicine and Science in Sports and Exercise* **19**, 324–331.

Bergh, U. & Forsberg, A. (1991) Cross-country ski racing. In *Endurance in Sports* (ed. R. Shephard & P.O. Åstrand), pp. 570–581. Blackwell Science, Oxford.

Bergh, U. & Forsberg, A. (1992) Influence of body mass on cross-country ski racing performance. *Medicine and Science in Sports and Exercise* **24**, 1033–1039.

Bergh, U., Kanstrup-Jensen, I.-L. & Ekblom, B. (1976) Maximal oxygen uptake during exercise with various combinations of arm and leg work. *Journal of Applied Physiology* **41**, 191–196.

Blixt, G. (1965) A study on the relation between total calories and single nutrients in Swedish food. *Acta Sociologica et Medica Upsallieusis* **70**, 117–125.

Coyle, E.F. (1991) Carbohydrate feedings: effects on metabolism, performance and recovery. In *Advances in Nutrition and Top Sport* (ed. F. Brouns), pp. 1–4. Medicine and Sports Science No. 32. Karger, Basels.

Ekblom, B. & Hermansen, L. (1968) Cardiac output in athletes. *Journal of Applied Physiology* **25**, 619–625.

Hanson, J. (1973) Maximal exercise performance in members of the US nordic ski team. *Journal of Applied Physiology* **35**, 592–595.

Hermansen, L. (1973) Oxygen transport during exercise in human subjects. *Acta Physiologica Scandinavica* Suppl. 339, 1–104.

Ingjer, F. (1991) Maximal oxygen uptake as a predictor of performance in women and men elite cross-country skiers. *Scandinavian Journal of Medicine and Science in Sports* **1**, 25–30.

Rusko, H. (1976) *Physical performance characteristics in Finnish athletes*. Studies in Sports, Physical Education and Health Vol. 8. University of Jyvèskylè, Jyvèskylè, Finland.

Saltin, B. & Åstrand, P.O. (1967) Maximal oxygen uptake in athletes. *Journal of Applied Physiology* **23**, 353–358.

Saltin, B. & Gollnick, P.D. (1983) Skeletal muscle adaptability: significance for metabolism and performance. In *Handbook of Physiology* (ed. L.D. Peachy, R.H. Adrian & S.R. Geiger), pp. 555–631. Williams and Wilkins, Baltimore, MD.

Stromme, S.B., Ingjer, F. & Meen, H.D. (1977) Assessment of maximal aerobic power in specifically trained athletes. *Journal of Applied Physiology* **42**, 833–837.

# Index

Page numbers in **bold** refer to tables; page numbers in *italic* refer to figures.

LIVERPOOL
JOHN MOORES UNIVERSITY
AVRIL ROBARTS LRC
TITHEBARN STREET
LIVERPOOL L2 2ER
TEL. 0151 231 40?